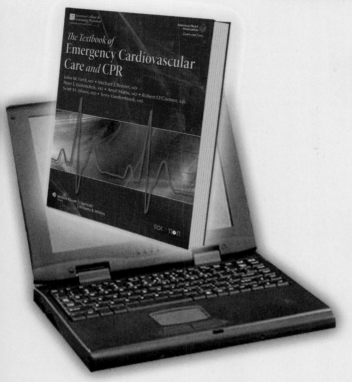
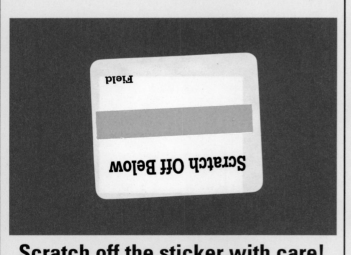
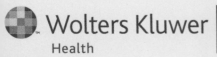
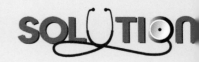

The Textbook of
Emergency Cardiovascular Care *and* CPR

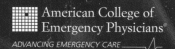

American College of
Emergency Physicians®
ADVANCING EMERGENCY CARE

American Heart
Association®
Learn and Live℠

The Textbook of
Emergency Cardiovascular
Care *and* CPR

EDITOR-IN-CHIEF

John M. Field, MD, FAHA, FACEP, FACC

American Heart Association ECC Senior Science Editor
Professor of Medicine and Surgery
Pennsylvania State University College of Medicine
Heart and Vascular Institute
Hershey, Pennsylvania

Wolters Kluwer | Lippincott Williams & Wilkins
Health

Philadelphia · Baltimore · New York · London
Buenos Aires · Hong Kong · Sydney · Tokyo

Acquisitions Editor: Frances R. DeStefano
Managing Editors: Chris Potash and Julia Seto
Project Manager: Rosanne Hallowell
Manufacturing Manager: Kathleen Brown
Marketing Manager: Kimberly Schonberger
Creative Director: Doug Smock
Cover Designer: Joseph DePinho
Production Services: Aptara, Inc.

Printed in China

Library of Congress Cataloging-in-Publication Data

The textbook of emergency cardiovascular care and CPR / editor-in-chief, John M. Field ; ACEP associate editors, Michael J. Bresler, Amal Mattu, Scott M. Silvers ; AHA associate editors, Peter J. Kudenchuk, Robert O'Connor, Terry VandenHoek.
    p. ; cm.
  Includes bibliographical references and index.
  ISBN-13: 978-0-7817-8899-1 (alk. paper)
  ISBN-10: 0-7817-8899-4 (alk. paper)
  1. Cardiovascular emergencies. 2. CPR (First aid) I. Field, John M.
  [DNLM: 1. Cardiovascular Diseases—therapy. 2. Cardiopulmonary Resuscitation—methods. 3. Emergency Medical Services—methods. WG 166 T3545 2009]
  RC675.T49 2009
  616.1′025—dc22

2008028088

Care has been taken to confirm the accuracy of the information presented and to describe generally accepted practices. However, the authors, editors, and publisher are not responsible for errors or omissions or for any consequences from application of the information in this book and make no warranty, expressed or implied, with respect to the currency, completeness, or accuracy of the contents of the publication. Application of this information in a particular situation remains the professional responsibility of the practitioner.

The authors, editors, and publisher have exerted every effort to ensure that drug selection and dosage set forth in this text are in accordance with current recommendations and practice at the time of publication. However, in view of ongoing research, changes in government regulations, and the constant flow of information relating to drug therapy and drug reactions, the reader is urged to check the package insert for each drug for any change in indications and dosage and for added warnings and precautions. This is particularly important when the recommended agent is a new or infrequently employed drug.

Some drugs and medical devices presented in this publication have Food and Drug Administration (FDA) clearance for limited use in restricted research settings. It is the responsibility of health care providers to ascertain the FDA status of each drug or device planned for use in their clinical practice.

The publishers have made every effort to trace copyright holders for borrowed material. If they have inadvertently overlooked any, they will be pleased to make the necessary arrangements at the first opportunity.

To purchase additional copies of this book, call our customer service department at (800) 638-3030 or fax orders to (301) 223-2320. International customers should call (301) 223-2300.

Visit Lippincott Williams & Wilkins on the Internet: at LWW.com. Lippincott Williams & Wilkins customer service representatives are available from 8:30 am to 6 pm, EST.

10 9 8 7 6 5 4 3 2 1

To LaDora and Julie

Contents

Contributors

Benjamin S. Abella, MD, MPhil
Assistant Professor
Department of Emergency Medicine
Clinical Research Director
Center for Resuscitation Science
University of Pennsylvania
Philadelphia, Pennsylvania

Christopher J. Andrews, BE, MBBS, MEngSc, PhD, DipCSc, EDIC, FACLM
General Practitioner and Consultant in Electrical and
    Lightning Injuries
Indooroopilly Medical Center
Queensland, Australia

Jill M. Baren, MD, FACEP, FAAP, MBE
Associate Professor of Emergency Medicine
    and Pediatrics
University of Pennsylvania School of Medicine
Attending Physician
Emergency Medicine
Hospital of the University of Pennsylvania
Philadelphia, Pennsylvania

Lance B. Becker, MD, FAHA
Professor of Emergency Medicine
University of Pennsylvania School of Medicine
Center for Resuscitation Science and Department of
    Emergency Medicine
Translational Research Laboratory
University of Pennsylvania
Philadelphia, Pennsylvania

Joost Bierens, MD, PhD
Professor of Emergency Medicine
Director, Department of Anesthesiology
VU University Medical Center
Amsterdam, The Netherlands

Michael J. Bresler, MD, FACEP
Clinical Professor
Division of Emergency Medicine
Stanford University School of Medicine
Palo Alto, California

Anthony J. Busti, PharmD, BCPS
Associate Professor
Department of Internal Medicine
Diplomate, Accreditation Council for Clinical
    Lipidology
Texas Tech University Health Sciences Center
School of Pharmacy Dallas/Ft. Worth Regional
    Campus
Dallas, Texas

Diana M. Cave, RN, MSN
Emergency Services
Legacy Health System
Legacy Emanuel Hospital & Health
    Center
Portland, Oregon

Mary Ann Cooper, MD
Professor
Departments of Bioengineering and Emergency
    Medicine
University of Illinois at Chicago
University of Illinois Hospital
Chicago, Illinois

Beatrice M. Correa, MD
Department of Internal Medicine
Rosalind Franklin University of Medicine and Science/
    The Chicago Medical School
North Chicago, Illinois

Todd J. Crocco, MD
Associate Professor and Chair
Department of Emergency Medicine
West Virginia University Hospital
Morgantown, West Virginia

Anthony J. Dean, MD
Assistant Professor of Emergency Medicine
University of Pennsylvania School of Medicine
Director of Emergency Ultrasound
Department of Emergency Medicine
University of Pennsylvania Medical Center
Philadelphia, Pennsylvania

Martin Dünser, MD
Department of Anesthesiology and Critical Medicine
Innsbruck Medical University
Innsbruck, Austria

Timothy B. Erickson, MD, FACEP, FACMT, FAACT
Professor
Department of Emergency Medicine
Division of Clinical Toxicology
University of Illinois at Chicago College
    of Medicine
Chicago, Illinois

John M. Field MD, FAHA, FACEP, FACC
Professor of Medicine and Surgery
Penn State University College of Medicine
Penn State Heart and Vascular Institute
Hershey, Pennsylvania

Raúl J. Gazmuri, MD, FCCM, PhD
Professor of Medicine and Associate Professor
    of Physiology
Rosalind Franklin University of Medicine
    and Science
Section Chief, Critical Care Medicine
North Chicago VA Medical Center
Chicago, Illinois

Edward P. Grimes, MD
Assistant Professor of Anesthesiology
University of Connecticut School of Medicine
Hartford Anesthesiology Associates
Farmington, Connecticut

Anthony J. Handley, MD, FRCP
Chief Medical Adviser
Royal Life Saving Society
Chairman
BLS/AED Subcommittee, Resuscitation
    Council
United Kingdom

Kane High, MD, MS
Associate Professor
Department of Anesthesiology
Penn State University
Milton S. Hershey Medical Center
Hershey, Pennsylvania

Judd E. Hollander, MD
Professor of Emergency Medicine
University of Pennsylvania School of Medicine
Clinical Research Director
Department of Emergency Medicine
Hospital of the University of Pennsylvania
Philadelphia, Pennsylvania

Ronald L. Holle, MS
Meteorologist
Holle Meteorology & Photography
Oro Valley, Arizona

Kenneth V. Iserson, MD, FACEP, FAAEM, MBA
Professor Emeritus
Department of Emergency Medicine
The University of Arizona
Tucson, Arizona

Edward C. Jauach, MD, MS, FAHA, FACEP
Associate Professor
Division of Emergency Medicine
Department of Neurosciences
Medical University of South Carolina
Charleston, South Carolina

Richard E. Kerber, MD
Professor of Medicine
Department of Internal Medicine
University of Iowa School of Medicine
Director, Echocardiography Lab
Department of Internal Medicine
University of Iowa Hospitals and Clinics
Iowa City, Iowa

Karl B. Kern, MD, FACC
Professor of Medicine
Section of Cardiology
University of Arizona Health Sciences Center
Director, Cardiac Catheterization Laboratories and the
    Interventional Cardiology Fellowship Program
Sarver Heart Center
Tucson, Arizona

Peter J. Kudenchuk, MD, FAHA, FACC, FACP, FHRS
Professor of Medicine
University of Washington School of Medicine
Division of Cardiology, Arrhythmia Services
University of Washington Medical Center
Seattle, Washington

Amal Mattu, MD, FACEP, FAAEM
Associate Professor
Department of Emergency Medicine
University of Maryland School of Medicine
Program Director
Emergency Medicine Residency
University of Maryland Medical System
Baltimore, Maryland

Steven H. Mitchell, MD, FACEP
Acting Instructor of Medicine
Division of Emergency Medicine
University of Washington School of Medicine
Attending Physician
Emergency Services
Harborview Medical Center
Seattle, Washington

Vincent N. Mosesso Jr, MD, FACEP
Associate Professor of Emergency Medicine
University of Pittsburgh School of Medicine
Medical Director, Prehospital Care
University of Pittsburgh Medical Center
Medical Director, Sudden Cardiac Arrest Association
Pittsburgh, Pennsylvania

Allan R. Mottram, MD
Department of Emergency Medicine
Section of Toxicology
John Stroger-Cook County Hospital
Chicago, Illinois

Robert W. Neumar, MD, FACEP, PhD
Associate Professor
Department of Emergency Medicine
University of Pennsylvania School of Medicine
Philadelphia, Pennsylvania

Graham Nichol, MD MPH
Associate Professor of Medicine & Medic One
    Foundation Chair
University of Washington
Seattle, Washington

Jerry P. Nolan, MD, FRCA, FCEM
Consultant in Anesthesia and Intensive Care Medicine
Royal United Hospital
Bath, United Kingdom

Robert O'Connor, MD, FACEP
Professor and Chair
Department of Emergency Medcine
University of Virginia Health System
Charlottesville, Virginia

Joseph P. Ornato, MD, FACP, FACC, FACEP, FAHA
Professor and Chairman
Department of Emergency Medicine
Virginia Commonwealth University
Richmond, Virginia

W. Frank Peacock, MD, FACEP
Professor of Emergency Medicine
Department of Emergency Medicine
Cleveland Clinic
Cleveland, Ohio

Charles V. Pollack Jr, MD, FAHA, FACEP, MA
Professor
Department of Emergency Medicine
University of Pennsylvania
Chairman
Department of Emergency Medicine
Pennsylvania Hospital
Philadelphia, Pennsylvania

Linda Quan, MD
Professor
Division of Pediatric Emergency Medicine
Department of Pediatrics
University of Washington School of Medicine
Attending Physician, Emergency Services
Children's Hospital Regional Medical Center
Seattle, Washington

Helmut Raab, MD
Department of Anesthesiology and Critical Medicine
Innsbruck Medical University
Innsbruck, Austria

Cheryl Rickens, RN, BSN
AED Program Coordinator
University of Pittsburgh Medical Center
Pittsburgh, Pennsylvania

Michael R. Sayre, MD
Associate Professor
Department of Emergency Medicine
The Ohio State University
Columbus, Ohio

Michael Shuster, MD, FRCPC
Emergency Physician
Department of Emergency Medicine
Mineral Springs Hospital
Banff, Canada

Mark E. Silverman, MD, FACC, MACP, FRCP
Professor of Medicine
Emory University
Chief of Cardiology
Piedmont Hospital
Atlanta, Georgia

Scott M. Silvers, MD, FACEP
Assistant Professor and Vice Chair
Department of Emergency Medicine
Mayo Clinic
Jacksonville, Florida

Elizabeth H. Sinz, MD
Associate Professor of Anesthesiology, Critical Care
    Medicine, and Neurosurgery
Pennsylvania State University College of Medicine
Director, Simulation Development and Cognitive Science
    Laboratory
Penn State University Hershey Medical Center
Hershey, Pennsylvania

Sarah A. Stahmer, MD, FACEP
Professor of Emergency Medicine
University of Medicine and Dentistry of New Jersey/Robert
    Wood Johnson Medical School
Residency Program Director
Department of Emergency Medicine
Cooper University Hospital
Camden, New Jersey

Richard L. Summers, MD, FACEP
Professor of Emergency Medicine
University of Mississippi Medical Center
Emergency Physician
Emergency Department
University of Mississippi Hospitals and Clinics
Jackson, Mississippi

David Szpilman, MD
Founder, Ex-President, and Medical Director
Brazilian Life Saving Society (SOBRASA)
Director, Drowning Resuscitation Center, Barra da Tijuca
Director, Adult Intensive Care Unit
Hospital Municipal Miguel Couto
Rio de Janeiro, Brazil

Terry L. Vanden Hoek, MD, FACEP
Associate Professor
Section of Emergency Medicine
University of Chicago Hospital
Chicago, Illinois

Rafáel Vasconcellos
Medical Rescue Team
Rio de Janeiro, Brazil

Eric A. Weiss, MD, FACEP
Associate Professor of Emergency Medicine
Stanford University School of Medicine
Medical Director, Office of Disaster Planning
Stanford University Hospital and Lucille Packard's
    Children's Hospital
Medical Director, Stanford Wilderness
    Medicine Fellowship
Medical Director, San Mateo County EMS Agency
Palo Alto, California

Volker Wenzel, MD, MSc
Department of Anesthesiology and Critical Medicine
Innsbruck Medical University
Innsbruck, Austria

Roger D. White, MD, FACC
Professor
Department of Anesthesiology
Mayo Clinic College of Medicine
Consultant
Department of Anesthesiology and Internal Medicine
Mayo Clinic
Rochester, Minnesota

Michael E. Winters, MD, FACEP, FAAEM
Assistant Professor
Departments of Emergency Medicine & Medicine
University of Maryland School of Medicine
University of Maryland Medical Center
Baltimore, Maryland

Carolyn M. Zelop, MD
Professor
Department of Obstetrics and Gynecology
University of Connecticut School of Medicine
Director
Maternal Fetal Medicine Associate Department
    Chair of OB/GYN
Saint Francis Hospital and Medical Center
Hartford, Connecticut

Foreword

In the 1950s and 1960s anesthesiologists, engineers, and cardiologists ushered in the modern era of resuscitation, combining mouth-to-mouth ventilation, closed-chest compressions, and electrical defibrillation of the heart. Early pioneers summarized their science and treatment recommendations in the *First Conference on CPR* sponsored by the National Academy of Science in 1966. Over the following half century, emergency cardiovascular care and resuscitation science have continued to provide a bench-to-bedside approach for improving timely emergency care to patients suffering from an acute cardiovascular event, such as sudden cardiac death.

As recognized by those early pioneers, improving patient outcomes requires dedicated effort from many: multiple specialties and sub-specialties, national and international scientists and clinicians, and millions of individuals trained and ready to act. Collaboration, cooperation, and participation of these many dedicated groups and individuals are required for the successful translation of science into clinical practice, including the effective transmission of both information and skills to prepare individuals who are not only skilled, but also willing and able to take appropriate action.

The American Heart Association and the American College of Emergency Physicians have assumed leadership roles in emergency cardiovascular care, recognizing that successful patient outcomes depend on not only effective action in the first minutes to hours of the acute event, but also the decisions made over the next days to weeks. The placement of a stent for an acute ST-segment elevation myocardial infarction (STEMI) or an automated implantable cardioverter/defibrilla-tor (AICD) for survivors of sudden cardiac death begins within the community and is facilitated by knowledgeable healthcare providers, EMS systems, and skilled emergency physicians.

This textbook represents the recognition and sponsorship of these principles and educational efforts. The textbook is the first major cooperative collaboration in this area. Experts in clinical emergency cardiovascular care summarize state-of-the art strategies to promote interdisciplinary excellence in resuscitation and emergency medicine, and scientists and educators provide insight into implementation strategies and careers. Key AHA and ACEP guidelines and clinical policies are immediately available and referenced and provide science and consensus recommendations in critical areas.

Continuing collaboration will have one objective: to provide the best care and the most favorable outcomes for victims of sudden cardiac arrest and other cardiovascular emergencies by optimizing what is done in the first minutes and hours and days, when critical interventions often make the difference between survival and death, between functional recovery and disability.

Timothy J. Gardner, MD, FAHA, President
AMERICAN HEART ASSOCIATION

Linda L. Lawrence, MD, FACEP, President
AMERICAN COLLEGE OF EMERGENCY PHYSICIANS

Preface

This first edition of *The Textbook of Emergency Cardiovascular Care and CPR* is a humble effort by the editors to bring together the work of many others in the field of emergency cardiovascular care. Special emphasis is placed on the practicing physician and other healthcare providers who strive to intervene on behalf of patients with an acute cardiovascular emergency within the first several hours after onset—often the most critical moments that determine short-term survival and long-term prognosis.

The core content of the book has been written and edited by experts in the field of resuscitation and emergency cardiovascular care, but more broadly, it brings together the collective efforts of many others who have committed their time and effort to this field. As such, the components of this book and its electronic version are intended to provide expeditious and efficient access to evidence-based materials, clinical guidelines, and scientific treatises in the relevant topics.

Each core chapter is an up-to-date summary of current research and clinical practice. Within each chapter, links to AHA ECC Guidelines, ACEP Clinical Policies, International Liaison Committee on Resuscitation (ILCOR) and AHA Scientific Statements and worksheets, and ACC AHA Guidelines are available so the reader can reference and review the evidence in context. Where applicable, audiovisual aids are also included to integrate the material. Readers can access AVI clips online that demonstrate performance of a technique or diagnostic procedure.

This format recognizes that the *individual practitioner* and *healthcare providers* must ultimately apply group data and consensus recommendations to each patient in an emergent situation in a timely and comprehensive manner. In this regard, the editors dedicate this text to healthcare providers who strive on a daily basis to treat cardiovascular emergencies, preventing or reversing cardiac arrest when possible, optimizing recovery and functional disability, and supporting the patient and family humanely when death is imminent.

Acknowledgments

The original framework for this textbook was developed by the AHA ACLS Subcommittees over many years and expertly edited by Richard Cummins, MD, MPH, MSc, in its most recent version. This core was expanded by the editors and focused on evidence-based medicine. In this context, it now summarizes and includes the work of many too numerous to include here: the writing groups, task forces, contributors and editors of the contained guidelines, clinical policies, and statements referenced in the links or reproduced by the authors and editors. Their expertise, original work, and material are recognized and were invaluable to this work.

The leadership and foresight of the American Heart Association and the American College of Emergency Physicians are summarized in the Foreword. In particular the editors would like to recognize three individuals. Mary Ann McNeely, PhD, AHA Director of ECC Product Development during inception, had the insight and provided the foundation for the text, and Mr. Stephen Prudhomme, AHA Vice President, Healthcare Quality, directed and facilitated its execution and publication. Ms. Marta Foster, Director and Senior Editor, ACEP Educational and Professional Publications, was invaluable in coordinating the ACEP leadership and selection of the dedicated ACEP editors.

Special Contributors

Owing to the extensive evidence-based nature of the text, the complexity of the material, and the coordination of media involved, many additional people were instrumental in executing the final version of this text. We would like to especially recognize Kara Robinson, ECC Publications Editor, for her writing, editing, and coordination of graphics; Julie A. Linick, ELS, for her writing and editing; and Erik Soderberg, Senior Product Manager, AHA ACLS Products, for his coordination and editing of audiovisual material.

Note on Drugs and Medication Dosing

Emergency cardiovascular care is a dynamic and fluid topic. At the time of this publication, work is in progress for the evidence evaluation leading to the publication of updated guidelines in many areas discussed in this text. Every effort has been made to ensure the correct and most accurate dosing of ECC medications. In this effort, we would like to recognize the detailed review and contribution of Anthony Busti, PharmD, BCPS. However, readers are advised to check carefully for changes in drugs, dosing and indications.

One

Acute Coronary Syndromes

Chapter 1
Pathophysiology and Initial
Triage of Acute Coronary
Syndromes

John M. Field

In patients with symptoms of possible ACS, some of the traditional risk factors for CAD (e.g., hypertension, hypercholesterolemia, cigarette smoking, family history) are only weakly predictive of acute ischemia. Therefore, the presence or absence of these traditional risk factors ordinarily should not be used to determine whether an individual should be admitted or treated for ACS. Patients who present with ischemic symptoms should undergo early risk stratification using a risk-stratification model.[1,2]

- A Disrupted Plaque as the Proximate Cause of ACS
- Usually a Nonocclusive Plaque in the Infarct-Related Artery
- Triage Priorities for ACS—Not Only the Traditional Risk Factors
- A Systematic Approach—Key to Selecting a Strategy

Introduction to Acute Coronary Syndromes

An acute coronary syndrome (ACS) due to a disrupted plaque is present in the majority of patients with adult cardiac arrest.[3,4] Alarmingly, the first prolonged episode of ischemic discomfort has a 34% fatality rate. More than half the patients with sudden cardiac death (SCD) have no prior symptoms; in 17%, SCD is the first, last, and only symptom.[5–7] Additionally, the consequences of coronary atherosclerosis and ACS are responsible for the epidemiologic pool of patients at risk for SCD and those with significant cardiovascular morbidity. A conservative estimate for the number of discharges from patients with ACS from hospitals from 2005 is 772,000.[7]

It is, therefore, appropriate for a textbook on emergency cardiovascular care to begin with a section on acute coronary syndromes. The following chapters by Drs. Nichol and

Mitchell, Hollander, Ornato, Pollock and Summers, Peacock, Dean, and Stahmer set the stage for the broad spectrum of patients who present with cardiovascular emergencies. Currently, there are approximately 15.8 million individuals in the United States with coronary artery disease (CAD). There will be at least 1.4 million new, recurrent, or silent episodes of ACS. About 325,000 of these patients will experience out-of-hospital or emergency department SCD.[7]

This introductory chapter provides a broad general overview of ACS, focusing on an understanding of the pathophysiology necessary to apply triage and risk-stratification principles. In the following chapters, the authors mentioned above review these principles in current detail for health care providers who are charged with managing patients with ACS during the first several hours after presentation.

Overview of the Acute Coronary Syndrome

Definition and Spectrum of Acute Coronary Syndromes

The formation and accumulation of lipid and oxidative byproducts in an arterial wall is called atherosclerosis. When this deposit involves the coronary arteries, it is called coronary atherosclerosis. This process is gradual (Fig. 1-1) and gives rise to no symptoms for the many years of pathologic progression.[8]

Almost all regional ACS are caused by disruption of an atherosclerotic plaque, either plaque rupture or plaque erosion. Many of these disruptions are subclinical events; but when symptoms occur, a spectrum of clinical syndromes can result in which the disrupted plaque is a common and proximate feature. These syndromes are unstable angina pectoris, non–ST-segment-elevation myocardial infarction (NSTEMI), and ST-segment-elevation MI (STEMI). SCD can occur with any of these syndromes (Fig. 1-2).

Stable and Unstable Plaques

Coronary atherosclerosis is a diffuse process with segmental lesions called *coronary plaques;* these gradually enlarge and extend, causing variable degrees of coronary artery luminal occlusion. Intravascular ultrasound of the coronary arteries has shown that the majority of the atheroma burden is subluminal and not visible by coronary angiography. Coronary arteries are usually closed about 70% (by angiography; 90% closed when viewed by a pathologist) before they cause symptoms and are considered for percutaneous coronary intervention or surgery[9] (Fig. 1-3, top).

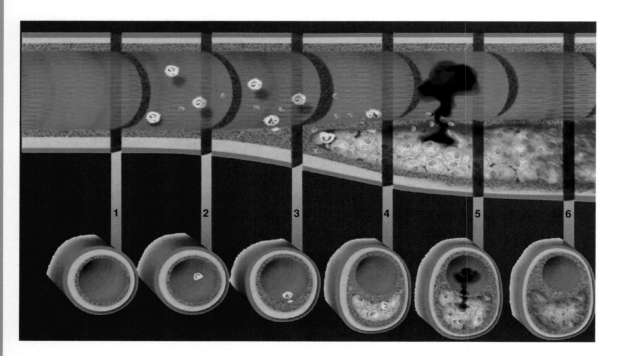

FIGURE 1-1 • Acute coronary syndromes (ACS). This figure illustrates the chronology of the progression of plaque formation and the onset and complications of STEMI, along with relevant management considerations at each stage. The longitudinal section of an artery depicts the "timeline" of atherogenesis from a normal artery (1) to (2) lesion initiation and accumulation of extracellular lipid in the intima, to (3) the evolution to the fibrofatty stage, to (4) lesion progression with procoagulant expression and weakening of the fibrous cap. An ACS develops when the vulnerable or high-risk plaque undergoes disruption of the fibrous cap (5); disruption of the plaque is the stimulus for thrombogenesis. Thrombus resorption may be followed by collagen accumulation and the growth of smooth muscle cells (6). (Modified from Libby P. Current concepts of the pathogenesis of the acute coronary syndromes. *Circulation* 2001;104[3]:365–372, with permission.)

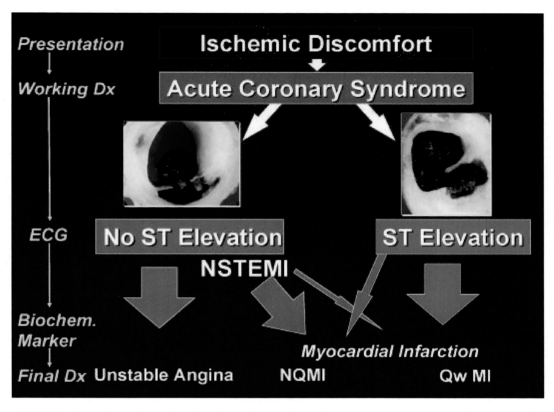

FIGURE 1-2 • Following disruption of a vulnerable or high-risk plaque, patients experience ischemic discomfort resulting from a reduction of flow through the affected epicardial coronary artery. This flow reduction may be caused by a completely occlusive thrombus (bottom half, right side) or subtotally occlusive thrombus (bottom half, left side). Patients with ischemic discomfort may present with or without ST-segment elevation on the ECG. Of patients with ST-segment elevation, most (large red arrow in bottom panel) ultimately develop a Q-wave MI (QwMI), while a few (small red arrow) develop a non–Q-wave MI (NQMI). Patients who present without ST-segment elevation are suffering from either unstable angina (UA) or a non–ST-segment elevation MI (NSTEMI) (large open arrows), a distinction that is ultimately made on the presence or absence of a serum cardiac marker such as CK-MB or a cardiac troponin detected in the blood. Most patients presenting with NSTEMI ultimately develop a NQMI on the ECG; a few may develop a QwMI. The spectrum of clinical presentations ranging from UA through NSTEMI and STEMI are referred to as the ACSs. (Modified from Libby P. Current concepts of the pathogenesis of the acute coronary syndromes. *Circulation* 2001;104[3]:365–372; Hamm CW, Bertrand M, Braunwald E. Acute coronary syndrome without ST elevation: implementation of new guidelines. *Lancet* 2001;358: 1533–1538; and Davies MJ. The pathophysiology of acute coronary syndromes. *Heart* 2000;83:361–366.)

Most plaques do not cause symptoms and are nonocclusive. But nonocclusive plaques are the ones most prone to cause ACS (Fig. 1-3, bottom). They have little if any hemodynamic effect before rupture, and stress testing and angiography cannot predict which ones will rupture and cause an ACS. Plaques can be classified as *stable* or *vulnerable* on the basis of their lipid content, the thickness of the cap that covers and separates them from the arterial lumen, and the degree of inflammation in the plaque itself.

1. A **"stable"** intracoronary plaque (Fig. 1-4A) has a lipid core that is separated from the arterial lumen by a thick fibrous cap. Stable plaques have less lipid, and the thick cap makes them resistant to fissuring and the formation of thrombi. Over time, the lumen of the vessel becomes progressively narrower, leading to flow limitations, supply-demand imbalance, and exertional angina. Stable plaques may progress to complete occlusion but do not usually cause STEMI because of the development over time of collateral supply to the myocardium at risk, thus preventing or limiting MI.

2. A **"vulnerable"** intracoronary plaque (Fig. 1-4B) has a lipid-rich core combined with an active inflammatory process that makes the plaque soft and prone to rupture. These plaques rarely restrict blood flow enough to cause clinical angina, and functional studies (e.g., stress tests) often yield negative results. Imaging techniques such as cardiac CT and MRI are being investigated as tools to identify unstable and inflamed plaques and may prove to be helpful in the future.

3. Inflammation is often found in the plaque. Inflammatory processes are concentrated in the leading edge affected by coronary blood flow. It is here that most plaque ruptures occur. A plaque that is inflamed and prone to rupture is called **unstable** (Fig. 1-4C).

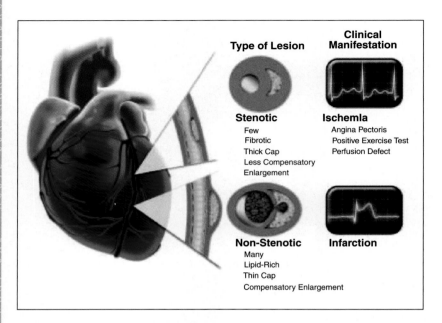

FIGURE 1-3 • Clinical manifestations of CAD in relation to degree of stenosis. Stenotic lesions tend to have smaller lipid cores, more fibrosis, and calcification as well as thick fibrous caps and less compensatory enlargement (positive remodeling). They typically produce exertional ischemia when, with exercise or emotion, demand for coronary blood flow exceeds supply. Nonstenotic lesions generally outnumber stenotic plaques and tend to have large lipid cores and thin fibrous caps susceptible to rupture and thrombosis. They often undergo substantial compensatory enlargement leading to underestimation of lesion size by angiography. Nonstenotic plaques may cause no symptoms for many years; when disrupted, however, they can provoke an episode of unstable angina or MI. (From Libby P, Theroux P. Pathophysiology of coronary artery disease. *Circulation* 2005;111[25]:3481–3488, with permission.)

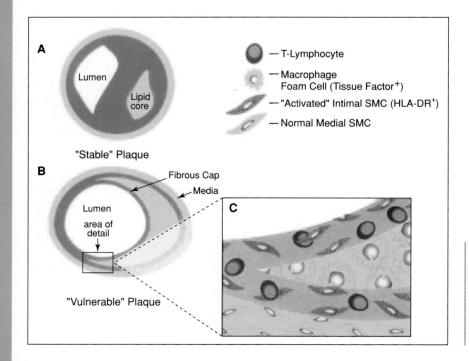

FIGURE 1-4 • Stable and vulnerable plaques. A. Stable plaque. B. Vulnerable plaque. C. Area of detail of vulnerable plaque showing infiltration of inflammatory cells. SMC, smooth muscle cell. (From Libby P. Molecular bases of the acute coronary syndromes. *Circulation* 1995;91:2844–2850, with permission. ©1995 American Heart Association.)

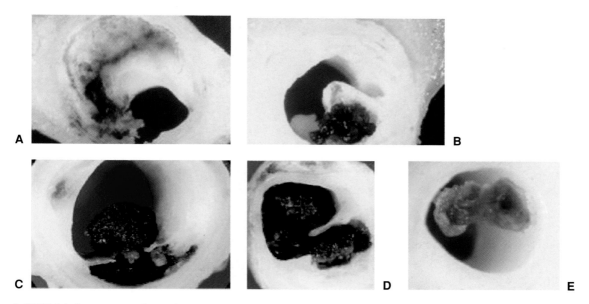

FIGURE 1-5 • Coronary plaque disruption can result in several clinical outcomes. A. Superficial erosion of a plaque has occurred but the coronary artery is patent. B. Rupture of a coronary plaque, which may progress to incomplete (C) or complete (D) coronary occlusion. In the ACSs, emboli (E) from a disrupted plaque may lodge distal in the coronary tree and cause microvascular dysfunction in the absence of complete epicardial occlusion or after restoration of coronary patency.

Progression to Acute Coronary Syndrome

Triggers of Acute Coronary Syndrome/Myocardial Infarction Most episodes of ACS occur at rest or with modest daily activity. Heavy physical exertion or mental stress is present in a minority of patients, perhaps 10% to 15%.[11,12] Regular exercise appears to be protective and reduces the incidence of coronary events and SCD precipitated by exertion.[12–14] Conversely, individuals who engage in little physical activity are at increased risk.[15]

There has been a documented circadian variation in the occurrence and presentation of acute coronary syndromes.[16] A diurnal pattern has been observed for acute MI (AMI), ischemic episodes, SCD, and stroke.[11,17–19] A peak incidence from 6 A.M. to noon has been noted, usually in the first 2 to 3 hours after arising.[20–22] Most likely the variation involves an interaction between the internal and external triggers of plaque instability, thrombosis, and ischemia.[23] There is an early-morning increase in sympathetic activity accentuated by assumption of the erect posture. Coronary artery disease and abnormal endothelial responses appear to be a prerequisite for these factors to precipitate ACS.[24]

Plaque Rupture When spontaneous or triggered plaque disruption occurs, a spectrum of pathologic changes and intraluminal events occur that act in concert with platelet factors and the coagulation cascade to determine the clinical presentation. For example, if superficial erosion occurs in the setting of extracardiac stress, microemboli may result in elevation of cardiac troponin levels without manifest clinical symptoms (Fig. 1-5E). Rupture or erosion of a coronary plaque (Fig. 1-5A and B) can be asymptomatic; but if the resulting thrombus partially and intermittently occludes the epicardial coronary artery, unstable angina or NSTEMI occurs (Fig. 1-5C). If the thrombus completely and persistently occludes the coronary artery, STEMI occurs, and infarct size is determined by the amount of myocardium at risk, the degree and duration of occlusion, and the presence and extent of coronary collateral supply (Fig. 1-5D).

Triage of the Patient with Possible Acute Coronary Syndrome

The 12-lead electrocardiogram is central to the triage of patients with chest discomfort. A 12-lead ECG should be performed and shown to an experienced emergency physician within 10 minutes of ED arrival on all patients with chest discomfort.

The 12-lead electrocardiogram is central to the triage of patients with chest discomfort. A 12-lead ECG should be performed and shown to an experienced emergency physician within 10 minutes of ED arrival on all patients with chest discomfort. The 12-lead ECG is imprecise but can be used to initially classify patients into groups that trigger further diagnostic testing and therapeutic strategies. Three groups can initially be defined: ST-segment elevation, ST-segment depression and/or dynamic T-wave inversion, and nonspecific or normal ECG (Fig. 1-7). In the Gusto IIB Trial electrocardiographic substudy, presenting ST-segment elevation predicted AMI on presentation in 89% of patients.[25] In addition, ST-segment deviation was

| TABLE 1-1 • Subsequent Confirmation of Acute MI on Presentation, and the Occurence of Death and Reinfarction Based on ST-Segment and T-Wave Abnormalities[25]

	ST-Segment Elevation and Depression	ST-Segment Elevation Only	ST-Segment Depression Only	Isolated T-Wave Inversion
Patients	15%	28%	35%	22%
AMI (within 16 hours)	89%	81%	48%	32%
Death (30 days)	6.6%	5.1%	5.1%	1.7%
Reinfarction (30 days)	7.1%	5.0%	7.0%	4.2%

prognostic for AMI on presentation, SCD, and reinfarction in hospital (Table 1-1).

ST-Segment Elevation Myocardial Infarction

Patients with STEMI are candidates for immediate reperfusion, and the outcome is time-sensitive. Mortality increases with the location of infarct and the degree and extent of ST-segment elevation.[26] This fact can be used in association with time of onset to assess risk and benefit for reperfusion therapy. Findings consistent with STEMI trigger an assessment for rapid reperfusion therapy, either fibrinolytic therapy or percutaneous coronary intervention (PCI).

Unstable Angina/Non–ST-Segment-Elevation MI

Patients with possible ischemic chest discomfort are a heterogeneous group with variable risk for the occurrence of major cardiac events ("MACE"- SCD, MI, and need for urgent revascularization). Historical features and objective findings are helpful in a minority of patients. In the majority of patients, a definitive diagnosis is not obvious on presentation and an estimation of the likelihood that symptoms are due to obstructive CAD must be made. Traditional risk factors for the development of CHD have been developed

| TABLE 1-2 • Likelihood That Signs and Symptoms Represent an ACS Secondary to CAD

Feature	High Likelihood Any of the following:	Intermediate Likelihood Absence of high-likelihood features and presence of any of the following:	Low Likelihood Absence of high- or intermediate-likelihood features but may have:
History	Chest or left arm pain or discomfort as chief symptom reproducing prior documented angina Known history of CAD, including MI	Chest or left arm pain or discomfort as chief symptom Age >70 years Male sex Diabetes mellitus	Probable ischemic symptoms in absence of any of the intermediate likelihood characteristics Recent cocaine use
Examination	Transient MR murmur, hypotension, diaphoresis, pulmonary edema, or rales	Extracardiac vascular disease	Chest discomfort reproduced by palpation
ECG	New or presumably new transient ST-segment deviation (≥1 mm) or T-wave inversion in multiple precordial leads	Fixed Q waves ST-segment depression 0.5–1 mm or T-wave inversion ≥1 mm	T-wave flattening or inversion <1 mm in leads with dominant R waves Normal ECG
Cardiac markers	Elevated cardiac TnI, TnT, or CK-MB	Normal	Normal

ACS, acute coronary syndrome; CAD, coronary artery disease; CK-MB, MB fraction of creatine kinase; ECG, electrocardiogram; MI, myocardial infarction; MR, mitral regurgitation; TnI, troponin I; TnT, troponin T.
Source: Modified with permission from Braunwald E, Mark DB, Jones RH, et al. Unstable angina: diagnosis and management. AHCPR publication no. 94-0602 (124). Rockville, MD: Agency for Health Care Policy and Research and the National Heart, Lung, and Blood Institute, U.S. Public Health Service, U.S. Department of Health and Human Service, 1994.

from long-term epidemiologic studies.[27] However, traditional risk factors are weak predictors of an ACS, and prognostic scores have been developed from clinical trials to help physicians assess the risk of adverse cardiovascular events in patients likely to have symptoms due to CAD.[28–30] Although typical chest discomfort increases the probability of CAD, atypical features do not exclude ACS. In the Multicenter Chest Pain Study focusing on the subgroup of patients with chest discomfort presenting to an emergency department (ED), 15% of patients with pleuritic chest pain and 22% of those with stabbing pain were "ruled in" for AMI.[29]

Assessment of the Risk of CAD Using Initial History, Physical Examination, Electrocardiogram, and Cardiac Markers

In this context, two key questions are asked when patients are evaluated for possible ischemic discomfort:

- **What is the likelihood that symptoms are due to obstructive coronary artery disease (Table 1-2)?**
- **If the answer to this question is yes (intermediate or high likelihood), what is the risk of an adverse major cardiac event (Table 1-3)?**

| TABLE 1-3 • Short-Term Risk of Death or Nonfatal MI in Patients With UA/NSTEMI[a]

Feature	High Risk At least 1 of the following features must be present:	Intermediate Risk No high-risk feature, but must have 1 of the following:	Low Risk No high- or intermediate-risk feature but may have any of the following features:
History	Accelerating tempo of ischemic symptoms in preceding 48 h	Prior MI, peripheral or cerebrovascular disease, or CABG; prior aspirin use	
Character of pain	Prolonged ongoing (>20 min) rest pain	Prolonged (>20 min) rest angina, now resolved, with moderate or high likelihood of CAD Rest angina (>20 min) or relieved with rest or sublingual NTG Nocturnal angina New-onset or progressive CCS class III or IV angina in the preceding 2 weeks without prolonged (>20 min) rest pain but with intermediate or high likelihood of CAD	Increased angina frequency, severity, or duration Angina provoked at a lower threshold New onset angina with onset 2 weeks to 2 months prior to presentation
Clinical findings	Pulmonary edema, most likely due to ischemia New or worsening MR murmur S3 or new/worsening rales Hypotension, bradycardia, tachycardia Age >75 years	Age >70 years	
ECG	Angina at rest with transient ST-segment changes >0.5 mm Bundle-branch block, new or presumed new Sustained ventricular tachycardia	T-wave changes Pathologic Q waves or resting ST-segment depression <1 mm in multiple lead groups (anterior, inferior, lateral)	Normal or unchanged ECG
Cardiac markers	Elevated cardiac TnT, TnI, or CK-MB (e.g., TnT or TnI >0.1 ng/mL)	Slightly elevated cardiac TnT, TnI, or CK-MB (e.g., TnT >0.01 but <0.1 ng/mL)	Normal

CABG, coronary artery bypass grafting; CAD, coronary artery disease; CCS, Canadian Cardiovascular Society; CK-MB, creatine kinase, MB fraction; ECG, electrocardiogram; MI, myocardial infarction; MR, mitral regurgitation; NTG, nitroglycerin; TnI, troponin I; TnT, troponin T; UA/NSTEMI, unstable angina/non–ST-elevation myocardial infarction.
[a]Estimation of the short-term risks of death and nonfatal cardiac ischemic events in UA (or NSTEMI) is a complex multivariable problem that cannot be fully specified in a table such as this; therefore, this table is meant to offer general guidance and illustration rather than rigid algorithms. Adapted from the Agency for Health Care Practice and Research (AHCPR) Clinical Practice Guidelines No. 10, Unstable Angina: Diagnosis and Management, May 1994 (124).

Braunwald Risk Stratification

Braunwald had initially proposed risk stratification based on the history, physical examination, and ECG.[31] Patients were classified as having a low (0.01–0.14), intermediate (0.15–0.84), or high (0.85–0.99) likelihood of coronary events. The American College of Cardiology/American Heart Association (ACC/AHA) Guidelines Committee later refined and incorporated cardiac markers into this classification and updated it.[32] This clinical risk stratification has continued as a basis for determining the initial clinical risk of patients with unstable angina and NSTEMI and has been prospectively validated.[33–35] Table 1-2 is derived from the most recent update of the ACC/AHA Guidelines for the Management of Patients with Unstable Angina Non-ST Elevation MI[2] addressing the first key question of risk stratification: What is the likelihood that symptoms are due to CAD?

Based upon this initial assessment, patients who are at intermediate to high risk for symptoms due to CAD are then evaluated for their short-term risk of SCD or nonfatal MI. Again, they are classified as being at high, intermediate, or low risk (Table 1-3).

TIMI Risk Score

The TIMI investigators developed a risk-stratification scheme to quantify risk in a broad, heterogeneous group of patients with unstable angina and NSTEMI. Seven risk variables were identified in the TIMI 11B and ESSENCE trials from a cohort of patients with clinical ACS and ST-segment deviation. The risk score was then validated in three separate cohorts of patients in those trials. Seven variables of equal risk magnitude were identified: age 65 years or older, at least three traditional cardiac risk factors, prior coronary stenosis of 50% or more, ST-segment deviation on ECG at presentation, at least two anginal events in the preceding 24 hours, use of aspirin in the prior 7 days, and elevated serum cardiac markers. One point was assigned to each of these factors and a gradient of risk identified in patients presenting and felt to have unstable angina or myocardial infarction without ST-segment elevation (Fig. 1-6). Application of the TIMI risk score has been useful in assessing risk and the benefit of interventions such as an invasive or conservative strategy,[30,36] use of low-molecular-weight heparins, and glycoprotein IIb/IIIa inhibitor therapy.[37]

Conclusions

Patients presenting with chest discomfort and possible ACS represent a heterogeneous group with a spectrum of pathophysiology and graded risks for major adverse cardiac events. The challenge to the clinician is significant and the body of evidence-based medicine enormous. To date, over 1

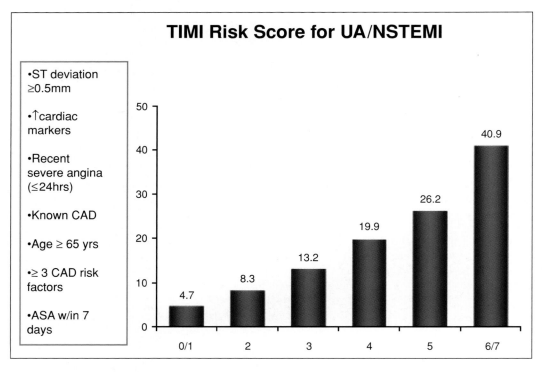

FIGURE 1-6 • TIMI Risk Score for unstable angina/non–ST-segment-elevation myocardial infarction (UA/NSTEMI). Each of seven variables is assigned 1 point: age ≥65 years, at least three traditional cardiac risk factors, prior coronary stenosis ≥50%, ST-segment deviation on ECG at presentation, at least two anginal events in the preceding 24 hours, use of aspirin in the prior 7 days, and elevated serum cardiac markers. The total score reveals a gradient of risk for all-cause mortality, nonfatal MI, and urgent target-vessel revascularization. Patients with a score of 0 to 2 are considered at low risk; 3 to 4, intermediate risk; and 5 to 7, high risk.

million patients have been randomized to clinical trials comprising ACS patients. An organized and systematic approach to diagnosis is helpful in gauging prognosis and risk stratification is mandatory. STEMI patients should be immediately identified and assigned to an institutional protocol for rapid reperfusion. The remaining patients require a careful,

logical, and thoughtful approach matching each individual's risk to an appropriate strategy and treatment using initial clinical and prognostic parameters. In general, three prognostic groups can be designated and assigned to immediate reperfusion, intensive antiplatelet and anticoagulant therapy, aspirin and further diagnostic and functional assessment (Fig. 1-7).

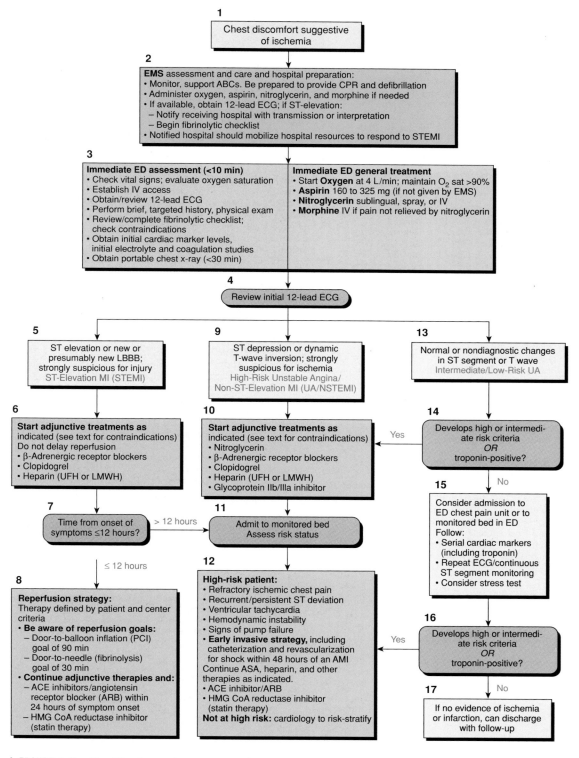

| FIGURE 1-7 • Algorithm for acute coronary syndromes.

References

1. Antman EM, Anbe DT, Armstrong PW, et al. ACC/AHA guidelines for the management of patients with ST-elevation myocardial infarction—executive summary. A report of the American College of Cardiology/American Heart Association Task Force on Practice Guidelines (Writing Committee to Revise the 1999 Guidelines for the Management of Patients With Acute Myocardial Infarction). *J Am Coll Cardiol* 2004;44(3):671–719.
2. Anderson JL, Adams CD, Antman EM, et al. ACC/AHA 2007 guidelines for the management of patients with unstable angina/non–ST-elevation myocardial infarction: a report of the American College of Cardiology/American Heart Association Task Force on Practice Guidelines (Writing Committee to Revise the 2002 Guidelines for the Management of Patients With Unstable Angina/Non–ST-Elevation Myocardial Infarction): developed in collaboration with the American College of Emergency Physicians, the Society for Cardiovascular Angiography and Interventions, and the Society of Thoracic Surgeons: endorsed by the American Association of Cardiovascular and Pulmonary Rehabilitation and the Society for Academic Emergency Medicine. *Circulation* 2007;116(7):e148–304.
3. Davies MJ. Anatomic features in victims of sudden coronary death: coronary artery pathology. *Circulation* 1992;85(Suppl)(1):I19–I24.
4. Davies MJ, Thomas AC. Plaque fissuring: the cause of acute myocardial infarction, sudden ischaemic death, and crescendo angina. *Br Heart J* 1985;53(4):363–373.
5. Kannel WB, McGee DL. Epidemiology of sudden death: insights from the Framingham Study. *Cardiovasc Clin* 1985;15(3):93–105.
6. Kannel WB, Schatzkin A. Sudden death: lessons from subsets in population studies. *J Am Coll Cardiol* 1985;5(6 Suppl):141B–149B.
7. Rosamond W, Flegal K, Furie K, et al. Heart Disease and Stroke Statistics – 2008 Update. A report from the American Heart Association Statistics Committee and Stroke Statistics Subcommittee.*Circulation*. 2008 Jan 29;117(4):e25-146. Epub 2007 Dec 17.
8. Libby P. Current concepts of the pathogenesis of the acute coronary syndromes. *Circulation* 2001;104(3):365–372.
9. Libby P, Theroux P. Pathophysiology of coronary artery disease. *Circulation* 2005;111(25):3481–3488.
10. Libby P. Molecular bases of the acute coronary syndromes. *Circulation* 1995;91(11):2844–2850.
11. Behar S, Halabi M, Reicher-Reiss H, et al. Circadian variation and possible external triggers of onset of myocardial infarction. SPRINT Study Group. *Am J Med* 1993;94(4):395–400.
12. Smith M, Little WC. Potential precipitating factors of the onset of myocardial infarction. *Am J Med Sci* 1992;303(3):141–144.
13. Siscovick DS, Weiss NS, Fletcher RH, et al. The incidence of primary cardiac arrest during vigorous exercise. *N Engl J Med* 1984;311(14):874–877.
14. Siscovick DS, Weiss NS, Hallstrom AP, et al. Physical activity and primary cardiac arrest. *JAMA* 1982;248(23):3113–3117.
15. D'Avanzo B, Santoro L, La Vecchia C, et al. Physical activity and the risk of acute myocardial infarction. GISSI–EFRIM Investigators. Gruppo Italiano per lo Studio della Sopravvivenza nell'Infarto–Epidemiologia dei Fattori di Rischio dell'Infarto Miocardico. *Ann Epidemiol* 1993;3(6):645–651.
16. Cannon CP, McCabe CH, Stone PH, et al. Circadian variation in the onset of unstable angina and non–Q-wave acute myocardial infarction (the TIMI III Registry and TIMI IIIB). *Am J Cardiol* 1997;79(3):253–258.
17. Figueras J, Lidon RM. Early morning reduction in ischemic threshold in patients with unstable angina and significant coronary disease. *Circulation* 1995;92(7):1737–1742.
18. Muller JE, Stone PH, Turi ZG, et al. Circadian variation in the frequency of onset of acute myocardial infarction. *N Engl J Med* 1985;313(21):1315–1322.
19. Willich SN, Levy D, Rocco MB. Circadian variation in the incidence of sudden cardiac death in the Framingham Heart Study population. *Am J Cardiol* 1987;60(10):801–806.
20. Peters RW. Circadian patterns and triggers of sudden cardiac death. *Cardiol Clin* 1996;14(2):185–194.
21. Peters RW, Mitchell LB, Brooks MM, et al. Circadian pattern of arrhythmic death in patients receiving encainide, flecainide or moricizine in the Cardiac Arrhythmia Suppression Trial (CAST). *J Am Coll Cardiol* 1994;23(2):283–289.
22. Tofler GH, Gebara OC, Mittleman MA, et al. Morning peak in ventricular tachyarrhythmias detected by time of implantable cardioverter/defibrillator therapy. The CPI Investigators. *Circulation* 1995;92(5):1203–1208.
23. Krantz DS, Kop WJ, Santiago HT, et al. Mental stress as a trigger of myocardial ischemia and infarction. *Cardiol Clin* 1996;14(2):271–287.
24. el-Tamimi H, Mansour M, Pepine CJ, et al. Circadian variation in coronary tone in patients with stable angina. Protective role of the endothelium. *Circulation* 1995;92(11):3201–3205.
25. Savonitto S, Ardissino D, Granger CB, et al. Prognostic value of the admission electrocardiogram in acute coronary syndromes. *JAMA* 1999;281(8):707–713.
26. Mauri F, Gasparini M, Barbonaglia L, et al. Prognostic significance of the extent of myocardial injury in acute myocardial infarction treated by streptokinase (the GISSI trial). *Am J Cardiol* 1989;63(18):1291–1295.
27. Lloyd-Jones DM, Wilson PW, Larson MG, et al. Framingham risk score and prediction of lifetime risk for coronary heart disease. *Am J Cardiol* 2004;94(1):20–24.
28. Jayes RL Jr, Beshansky JR, D'Agostino RB, et al. Do patients' coronary risk factor reports predict acute cardiac ischemia in the emergency department? A multicenter study. *J Clin Epidemiol* 1992;45(6):621–626.
29. Lee TH, Cook EF, Weisberg M, et al. Acute chest pain in the emergency room: identification and examination of low-risk patients. *Arch Intern Med* 1985;145(1):65–69.
30. Antman EM, Cohen M, Bernink PJ, et al. The TIMI risk score for unstable angina/non–ST elevation MI: A method for prognostication and therapeutic decision making. *JAMA* 2000;284(7):835–842.
31. AHCPR Unstable Angina Panel. Agency for Health Care Policy and Research Unstable Angina Panel: Diagnosing and managing unstable angina. *Clin Pract Guidel Quick Ref Guide Clin* 1994(10):1–25.
32. Braunwald E, Antman EM, Beasley JW, et al. ACC/AHA guidelines for the management of patients with unstable angina and non–ST-segment elevation myocardial infarction: executive summary and recommendations. A report of the American College of Cardiology/American Heart Association Task Force on Practice Guidelines (Committee on the Management of Patients With Unstable Angina). *Circulation* 2000;102(10): 1193–1209.
33. van Miltenburg–van Zijl AJ, Simoons ML, Veerhoek RJ, et al. Incidence and follow-up of Braunwald subgroups in unstable angina pectoris. *J Am Coll Cardiol* 1995;25(6):1286–1292.
34. Calvin JE, Klein LW, VandenBerg BJ, et al. Risk stratification in unstable angina. Prospective validation of the Braunwald classification. *JAMA* 1995;273(2):136–141.
35. Brotons C, Permanyer-Miralda G, Calvo F, et al. Validation of the Agency for Health Care Policy and Research (AHCPR) classification for managing unstable angina. *J Clin Epidemiol* 1999;52(10): 959–965.
36. Cannon CP, Weintraub WS, Demopoulos LA, et al. Comparison of early invasive and conservative strategies in patients with unstable coronary syndromes treated with the glycoprotein IIb/IIIa inhibitor tirofiban. *N Engl J Med* 2001;344(25): 1879–1887.
37. Morrow DA, Antman EM, Snapinn SM, et al. An integrated clinical approach to predicting the benefit of tirofiban in non–ST elevation acute coronary syndromes. Application of the TIMI Risk Score for UA/NSTEMI in PRISM–PLUS. *Eur Heart J* 2002;23(3):223–229.

Chapter 2
Sudden Cardiac Death: Epidemiology, Pathophysiology, and Future Directions

Steven H. Mitchell and Graham Nichol

Cardiac arrest is the cessation of cardiac mechanical activity as confirmed by the absence of signs of circulation.[1] SCD describes the unexpected natural death from a cardiac cause within a short time period, generally 1 hour from the onset of symptoms, in a person without any prior condition that would appear fatal.[2]

- The incidence of ventricular fibrillation/ventricular tachycardia (VF/VT) cardiac arrest is decreasing, but there is little improvement in survival from cardiac arrest over time.
- The median reported survival to discharge from cardiac arrest is only 6.4%.
- Most community-based cardiac arrests occur in a low-risk subset of the population.
- Only broad implementation and ongoing maintenance of adequately funded emergency medical services (EMS)—staffed by highly trained, experienced providers—can have a meaningful impact on death due to out-of-hospital cardiac arrest.

Definition of Cardiac Arrest

The terms "cardiac arrest" and "sudden cardiac death" (SCD) are used interchangeably to refer to similar clinical conditions. SCD describes the unexpected natural death from a cardiac cause within a short time period, generally 1 hour from the onset of symptoms, in a person without any prior condition that would appear fatal.[2] An international consensus workshop classified cardiac arrest as the "cessation of cardiac mechanical activity, as confirmed by the absence of signs of circulation."[1]

See Web site for AHA/ILCOR Statement on Definition of Cardiac Arrest and Cardiopulmonary Resuscitation

This definition emphasizes that cardiac arrest is a clinical syndrome that involves the sudden (usually <1 hour from onset of first symptoms until death) loss of detectable pulse or cessation of spontaneous breathing. If an EMS provider or physician did not witness the event, whether a primary cardiac arrest has occurred may be uncertain, especially if spontaneous circulation has returned. The World Health Organization proposed an alternate definition acknowledging that many cardiac arrests are not witnessed: for those patients without an identifiable noncardiac etiology, cardiac arrest includes death within 1 hour of symptom onset for witnessed events or within 24 hours of having been observed alive and symptom-free for unwitnessed events.[3]

Such definitions have several limitations despite their widespread use. First, "presumed cardiac etiology" is frequently used as an inclusion criterion, but it can accurately be determined only by conducting a postmortem examination. Since it is impractical to perform an autopsy on every fatal arrest, classification must rely on the limited information that is available to emergency providers in the out-of-hospital setting or physicians in the emergency department (ED).[4] It is frequently difficult for emergency providers—when they are trying to provide acute resuscitation in the field—to ascertain whether and how long the patient had symptoms beforehand. In the absence of precise definitions, use of the etiology of arrest as an inclusion criterion can create bias. Therefore, episodes should be included in epidemiologic studies regardless of their etiology.

Since the likelihood of underlying disease is uncertain, many studies presume that an arrest is of cardiac origin unless there is another obvious cause. Specifically, unless the episode is known or likely to have been caused by trauma, submersion, drug overdose, asphyxia, exsanguinations, or any other noncardiac cause as determined by the rescuers, SCD is assumed to have occurred.[1]

Second, many epidemiologic studies of cardiac arrest use EMS as the sampling frame; therefore, unwitnessed deaths that did not result in a call for aid are difficult to ascertain and not included. The exclusion of such patients from a study would underestimate episode incidence and overestimate survival compared to a study that included them.

Third, there is geographic variation in the frequency of "do not attempt resuscitation" declarations by individuals and family members and whether EMS providers can choose to not initiate or cease efforts in the field. The inclusion or exclusion of such patients in different epidemiologic studies makes it difficult to compare the incidence and outcome of cardiac arrest in different jurisdictions.

Reasonable alternative definitions that address these limitations are cardiac arrest without any reference to duration of symptoms and EMS-treated cardiac arrest. The latter would apply to any person evaluated by organized EMS personnel who (1) receives attempts at external defibrillation (from lay responders or emergency personnel) or receives chest compressions by organized EMS personnel or (2) is pulseless but does not receive attempts to defibrillate or provide cardiopulmonary resuscitation (CPR) from EMS personnel. This would include those with "do not attempt resuscitation" directives, a history of terminal illness or intractable disease, or a request from the patient's family to not treat.

Cardiac arrest generally occurs in persons with known or previously unrecognized ischemic heart disease.[5,6] Other causes of cardiac arrest include nonischemic heart disease (especially arrhythmic, including ventricular fibrillation, Wolff–Parkinson–White syndrome, long-QT syndrome, Brugada's syndrome, short-coupled torsade de pointes, and catecholamine-induced polymorphic ventricular tachyarrhythmia), pulmonary diseases including embolus, cerebral nervous system disease, vascular catastrophes including ruptured aneurysms, as well as drugs and poisons. Patients without identifiable abnormalities are categorized as idiopathic. Traumatic sudden death is usually considered separately from unexpected cardiac death because the treatment and prognosis of traumatic and nontraumatic arrest differ so much from each other.

See Web site for ACC/AHA/ESC Guidelines for Management of Patients with Ventricular Arrhythmias and the Prevention of Sudden Cardiac Death

Epidemiology of Cardiac Arrest

Much of what we understand today about the basic pathophysiology of cardiac arrest has been gained through observational rather than randomized studies of patients at risk for or in a state of cardiac arrest. This is only natural, since cardiac arrest is a relatively unpredictable event that usually

RISK FACTORS FOR SUDDEN CARDIAC DEATH

- Clinical (CAD)
- Cellular–genetic (long-QT syndrome)
- Environmental (stress)
- Behavioral (smoking)
- Educational and social

occurs out of hospital and is initially treated by EMS providers; the patient is then transported to hospital for further triage and treatment in the ED. The epidemiologic study of cardiac arrest not only provides information about risk factors for the onset of arrest and the current status of treatment of the condition but also suggests how to improve treatment and directs physicians toward future studies of resuscitation.

In broad terms, epidemiologic data are used to identify risk factors for cardiac arrest. These include cellular factors (e.g., gene mutations that predispose to arrhythmias); environmental, social, educational, behavioral factors (e.g., activity level, smoking); clinical factors (e.g., atherosclerosis, reduced ventricular function, diabetes); and health-system risk factors that predispose individuals to cardiac arrest or particular outcomes after the onset of arrest. By identifying risk factors that are amenable to modification, such as diet or smoking, physicians have attempted to improve survival through prevention, including use of pharmaceutical agents (e.g., beta-blockers) which can reduce an individual's risk of cardiac arrest (Fig. 2-1).

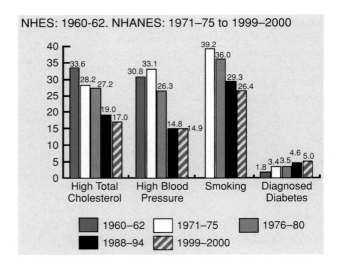

FIGURE 2-1 • Trends in cardiovascular risk factors in the U.S. population, ages 20–74. In this study group, high total cholesterol was defined as ≥240 mg/dL; high blood pressure was defined as ≥140/90 mm Hg. Smoking data not available for 1960–1962. (From Gregg EW et al. Secular trends in cardiovascular disease risk factors according to body mass index in U.S. adults. *JAMA* 2005;293:1868–1874, with permission.)

By identifying favorable interventional factors for survival, such as early CPR, physicians have improved the acute treatment of sudden death. The ability to identify individuals who have survived cardiac arrest enables physicians to use implantable cardioverter-defibrillators to reduce the risk of further cardiac arrest.[8] Implantation of these devices shortly after an acute cardiovascular event is deleterious,[9] but noninvasive alternatives exist for high-risk individuals.[10]

During the early twentieth century, the incidence of coronary artery disease (CAD) in the United States and other high-income countries increased dramatically. In the 1940s, cardiovascular disease (CVD) became the leading cause of death, overtaking deaths caused by infectious agents. In the early twenty-first century, CVD has become a ubiquitous cause of morbidity in most countries.[11] This epidemiologic transition reflects increased longevity in low- and middle-income countries and thereby increased exposure to cardiovascular risk factors. It also reflects adverse lifestyle changes, including increased inactivity, obesity, tobacco use, and consumption of saturated fats.

There has been a steady decline in morbidity and mortality from most CVD in high-income countries over the last 30 years.[12–14] Much of this reduction has been attributed to risk-factor modification.[15] Globally, CVD contributes 30.9% of global mortality and 10.3% of the global burden of disease.[16–18] It is responsible for more deaths than any other disease in industrialized countries and three-quarters of mortality due to noncommunicable diseases in developing countries. Eighty percent of deaths due to CVD occur in low- and middle-income countries.

In the United States, CVD is the leading cause of death among individuals aged above 65 years of age; it is the second leading cause of death among individuals 0 to 14 years and 25 to 64 years of age and the fourth leading cause of death among individuals 15 to 24 years of age (http://www.americanheart.org/presenter.jhtml?identifier=3000963, accessed April 24, 2008). CVD is estimated to have cost $448.5 billion in the United States in 2008 (http://www.nhlbi.nih.gov/about/factbook/chapter4.htm#4_7, accessed April 24, 2008).

Incidence

Incidence is the occurrence rate per year for a disease within a population at risk. It is usually calculated by taking a ratio of the number of persons developing a disease each year divided by the population at risk. This "simple" measurement becomes quite complicated when applied to cardiac arrest because of the effect of age on the incidence. Many cardiac arrest studies reported incidence as the number of cardiac arrests per year divided by the population within the region. If we use Seattle—with a census population of 460,000 aged 20 years or older—as an example, there were 372 cardiac arrests within the metropolitan area during the year 2000, which is an incidence of 372/460,000/yr or 0.81 cardiac arrests/1,000/yr. Focusing on the adult population

like this is convenient, yet underestimates the total number of arrests slightly, but not the incidence, since cardiac arrest is uncommon in the pediatric population.

A separate but related issue is that incidence rates are usually based on the census population of the catchment area of the EMS agency, even though the number of individuals fluctuates by time of day and day of week. A city that has a large population ingress during the working week may appear, falsely, to have an elevated rate of unexpected cardiac death.

If large, unaccountable differences in incidence are present, there are important public health questions that require investigation and may prove critical for efforts to improve survival. Likewise, this information may be useful for comparing survival statistics from different communities. Therefore, incidence should be routinely reported in cardiac arrest studies.

The true incidence of out-of-hospital cardiac arrest is unknown. About half of coronary heart deaths are sudden.[19] Since there were 7.2 million coronary heart deaths worldwide in 2002 (http://www3.who.int/whosis/), this implies that there were 3.6 million unexpected cardiac deaths. About two-thirds of these occur without prior recognition of cardiac disease. About 60% are treated by EMS.[20] Although the proportion of those treated by EMS is likely less in those countries that have limited access to emergency services, this implies that as many as 2.2 million cardiac arrests are treated by EMS worldwide annually.

The reported incidence of out-of-hospital cardiac arrest in the United States is 1.9/1,000 person-years among those aged 50 to 79 years. Since the U.S. population aged 50 to 79 is estimated to be 78 million (http://www.census.gov/), this implies 148,000 out-of-hospital cardiac arrests. The reported incidence of EMS-treated cardiac arrest is 36/100,000 to 81/100,000 total population (Fig. 2-2).[20,21] Since the total U.S. population is 301 million (http://www.census.gov/), this implies 107,000 to 240,000 treated arrests occur in the United States annually. Of these, 20% to 38% have ventricular fibrillation/ventricular tachycardia (VF/VT) as the first recorded rhythm (Fig. 2-3).[21,22] This implies 21,000 to 91,000 treated VF arrests annually. Although the incidence of VF and cardiac arrest with any first initial rhythm is decreasing over time,[21] there has been little improvement in survival from cardiac arrest.[23,24]

The reported incidence of unexpected cardiac arrest in Europe is 1/1000 population.[25] Since the European Union's population is 492,646,492 (http://www.populationdata.net/, accessed April 24, 2008), this implies that 490,000 out-of-hospital arrests occur annually in European Union countries.

See Web site for AHA Heart Disease and Stroke Statistics

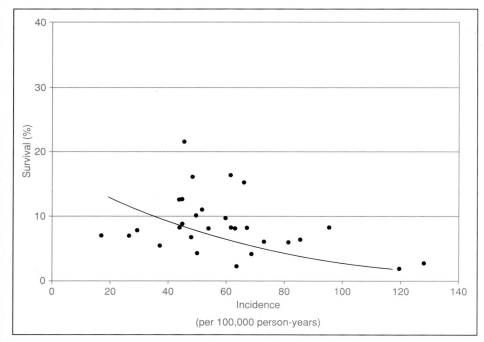

FIGURE 2-2 • Incidence of
EMS-treated cardiac arrest.
(From Rea TD, Pearce RM,
Raghunathan TE, et al.
Incidence of out-of-hospital
cardiac arrest. *Am J Cardiol*
2004;93[12]:1455–1460,
with permission.)

Cardiac Arrest in Children

Cardiac arrest in children merits special consideration in the field of acute resuscitation because its characteristics differ from those of out-of-hospital adult episodes. SCD accounts for 19% of sudden deaths in children aged 1 to 13 and 30% in those aged between 14 and 21 years.[26] The reported incidence of out-of-hospital pediatric cardiac arrest is 2.6 to 19.7 annual cases per 100,000.[27] These are usually due to trauma, sudden infant death syndrome, respiratory causes, or submersion,[28] but VF is still commonly

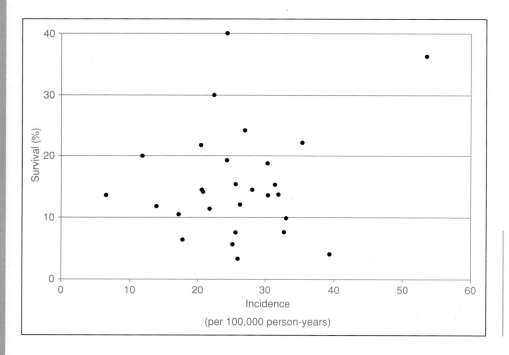

FIGURE 2-3 • Incidence of
ventricular fibrillation.
(From Rea TD, Pearce RM,
Raghunathan TE, et al.
Incidence of out-of-hospital
cardiac arrest. *Am J Cardiol*
2004;93[12]:1455–1460, with
permission.)

observed.[29] The reported average survival to discharge is 6.7%. Children with submersion or traumatic injury have a poorer prognosis.

Cardiac Arrest in Hospital

Cardiac arrest in hospital also merits special consideration because of its unique characteristics. A large multicenter cohort study of in-hospital cardiopulmonary arrest events excluded events that occurred out of hospital so as to avoid double counting.[30] For adults, the reported incidence of unexpected cardiac death in hospital was 0.17 ± 0.09 per bed per year. The commonest causes of these events were arrhythmia, respiratory distress, hypotension, or myocardial infarction (MI). The average survival to discharge was 17%.

Epidemiology of High-Risk Subgroups

The patients at highest risk for cardiac arrest account for only a small portion of arrests in the community.[31] The largest number of cardiac arrests in the community occur in the low-risk general public simply because there are so many more of these individuals in that group than in the high-risk subgroups.

Coronary Artery Disease and Acute Coronary Syndromes

Nonetheless certain populations are at increased risk for cardiac arrest. The rates of cardiac arrest parallel the prevalence of risk factors for CAD (Fig. 2-4). Known CAD or a previous episode of sudden death remains the greatest risk factor for sudden death.

Patients with acute coronary syndromes (ACS) that include MI are at high risk of mortality (i.e., >5%) within 30 days of presentation, regardless of whether ST-segment elevation is present or absent.[32] The risk of death remains elevated for at least 6 months in patients with ACS[33] and for

at least a year in patients with MI.[34] Patients with ventricular dysfunction are at higher risk than those without.[35] At least one-half of these deaths are suspected to have an arrhythmic mechanism.[36]

Several noninvasive diagnostic tests can identify patients who are at high risk of cardiac arrest, but they have low sensitivity and specificity[37] and are generally available only in tertiary care centers. An estimated 1,413,000 people will be discharged with a diagnosis of ACS this year. Of these, 838,000 will be for MI and 670,000 will be for unstable angina.[26] Since >16% of patients with MI have a left ventricular ejection fraction (LVEF) <40%,[38] thousands of individuals are annually at increased risk of cardiac arrest.

Ischemia and reperfusion, which occur commonly during the early phases of MI, are clearly associated with arrhythmias. Because only 20% of cardiac arrests involve an acute infarction, it has been assumed that transient ischemia rather than infarction has a major role in triggering sudden death. Transient systemic factors, such as hypoxia, hypotension, acidosis, or electrolyte abnormalities, can affect electrophysiologic stability and susceptibility to arrhythmias. However, a vigilant search should be made for an underlying cause of arrhythmia even in the setting of electrolyte abnormalities such as hypokalemia, which may be a cause or consequence of cardiac arrest.[39]

Congenital or acquired arrhythmias are a known risk factor for cardiac arrest. Unfortunately, the severity of risk is not well defined because of the many associated factors that may confound evaluation of a particular patient. Deaths in athletes have drawn considerable public interest to this problem. Although known arrhythmias increase the chance of cardiac arrest, the degree to which various arrhythmias do so is difficult to predict precisely. Screening of athletes for risk of arrhythmia lacks sensitivity and specificity.[40]

 See Web site for AHA Scientific Statement for Prescreening Athletes for Competitive Sports

Age, Race, and Traditional Risk Factors

The rate of cardiac arrest increases exponentially with increasing age. The rates for cardiac arrest are substantially higher at any given age for men than for women. Since there are more women in the population than older men, the overall incidences by gender are similar. However women are at less risk at any particular age.

Race is an important risk factor for many CVDs. Blacks have a higher rate of hypertension, LV hypertrophy, renal disease, and diabetes than do whites. As a consequence of these differences in the distribution of risk factors, the incidence of cardiac arrest is significantly higher among blacks than among whites.[41]

Hypertension predisposes patients to develop CAD, cardiac hypertrophy, congestive heart failure, stroke, renal disease, and sudden death. The risk is continuous, without

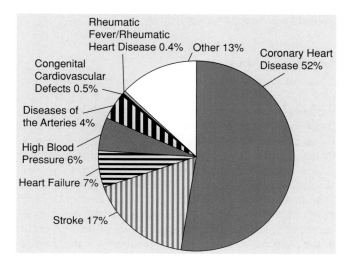

FIGURE 2-4 • Percentage breakdown of deaths from cardiovascular diseases, United States, 2004. (From *CDC/NCHS.*)

evidence of a threshold, down to blood pressures as low as 115/75 mm Hg.[42] Twofold to threefold increases in CAD are seen in patients with systolic blood pressures above 160 mm Hg or diastolic blood pressures above 95 mm Hg.[43] Hypertension affects about 65 million persons in the United States[44] and affects >90% of individuals at some time during their lives.[45] As many as two-thirds of affected Americans are untreated or undertreated.[46] This care gap has important public health implications, since randomized trials have definitively shown that treatment of hypertension reduces the risk of cardiovascular events and mortality.[47]

Elevations of serum cholesterol and triglycerides are known risk factors for cardiac death. The risk of CAD increases as total cholesterol increases, with low-density-lipoprotein cholesterol (LDL-C) associated with elevated risk and high-density-lipoprotein cholesterol (HDL-C) associated with decreased risk.[48] Elevated triglycerides are of special concern for women.[49] The levels of lipids are thought to be mediated through an unclear combination of hereditary predisposition and diet. Strict control of diet (<10 g of fat per day) may cause regression of preexisting CAD.[50] Reduction of dietary saturated fat and partial replacement by unsaturates for at least 2 years reduces cardiovascular events as well as cardiovascular and all-cause mortality.[51]

Obesity is an independent risk factor for cardiac disease. The prevalence of obesity among adults aged 20 to 74 years has risen from 13% to 31% during the past 25 years[52-54] despite a decrease in the prevalence of all other risk factors except diabetes that has decreased over time across all body mass index groups in the United States.[55] Similar increases in obesity have been observed in other high-income countries.

Diabetes is associated with increased CAD. The prevalence of diabetes is increasing over time in the United States.[56] About 10% of the population have diagnosed or undiagnosed diabetes. Diet, exercise, and tighter control of glucose levels may moderate the risk of CAD associated with diabetes. Since diabetics have an elevated incidence of hypertension, control of blood pressure will also reduce the risk of CAD and renal failure. The latter is associated with an increased incidence of cardiac arrest.[57]

Male patients presenting with impotence related to vascular disease are at high risk for sudden death.[58] More than two-thirds of males admitted with acute MI were found to have had significant complaints of sexual dysfunction before infarction.[59] Therefore, physicians evaluating patients with noncardiac vascular disease should ensure that these patients are evaluated for cardiac risk as well.

Triggers of Cardiac Arrest

Despite considerable study, the underlying and proximate causes of cardiac arrest remain poorly defined. This problem of predicting how a complex system with multiple interrelated elements responds to a variation in an individual component is a general one in systems biology. Atherosclerosis is likely a factor in the majority of cases; structural and congenital abnormalities, fibrosis, and conditions such as myocarditis contribute to most of the rest.[20] Many risk factors for cardiac

arrest, such as hypertension and hypercholesterolemia, are present for long periods of time and are likely to be identified when an individual is evaluated. Others are evanescent, difficult to document and less understood. Here risk factors are classified as cellular, phenotypic, environmental, social, behavioral, clinical, or health-system risk factors. A combination of these factors is usually present. In each group, risk factors can be divided into those that are fixed ("fate" factors) and those that can be modified to some extent. The latter may evolve over time or be transient. Evolving factors that may modify the risk of lethal arrhythmia include cell-membrane levels of polyunsaturated fatty acids,[60] ion-channel function,[61] and local or systemic inflammation.[62] Transient factors that may suddenly trigger a lethal arrhythmia include transient ischemia and reperfusion, transient systemic factors, transient autonomic and neurohumoral factors, and toxic/proarrhythmic effects.[19] The interplay of these factors is complex, as socioeconomic gradients exist in some circulating factors that are not fully explained by health-related behaviors or risk factors for CAD.[63] Efforts should be made to modify risk whenever feasible.

Cellular Factors

Animal experimental, cell biology, genetic, nutritional, and epidemiologic studies demonstrate that cellular constituents such as cell-membrane and free fatty acid levels of n-3 polyunsaturated fatty acids (PUFAs) alter cardiac ion-channel function, modify cardiac action potentials, and reduce myocardial vulnerability to VF.[64] These findings have important clinical and public health implications, because n-3 PUFA levels can be altered by inexpensive changes in dietary intake. Specifically, ingestion of one fatty fish meal a week is associated with a marked reduction in cardiac arrest.

Elevations in plasma nonesterified fatty acid (NEFA) levels[65] and high-sensitivity C-reactive protein (CRP) levels[62] or decreased long-chain n-3 fatty acid levels are independently associated with an elevated risk of unexpected cardiac death. It remains unclear whether elevation of CRP indicates an underlying pathologic inflammatory process or whether it is directly proarrhythmic.

Genetic Factors

Genetically based risk factors for cardiac arrest include factors that facilitate the onset of ischemia and infarction, including activators of plaque rupture and thrombogenesis; alterations in neuroendocrine signaling, including differences in transmitter pathways that contribute to sympathetic–parasympathetic imbalance; and potential triggers or attenuators of cardiomyocyte membrane excitability and transcellular conduction.[66,67] Molecular genetic analysis has identified an inherited disease and likely cause of death in 40% of families with at least one member who experienced unexplained cardiac death at age 40 years or less.[68] A caveat to the potential role of genetic screening to identify mutations that predispose to arrhythmia is that familial clustering of cardiac death could reflect either shared environmental or genetically transmissible abnormalities. Regardless of which of these is correct, familial risks for sudden death are separable from familial risks for MI.[65,69]

Identification of cellular and genetics risk factors for cardiac arrest could have therapeutic implications. For example, individuals with KvLTQ1 gene mutations are predisposed to arrhythmias that may be more responsive to beta-blockers;[70] carriers of SCN5A gene mutations are predisposed to arrhythmias that appear to be more responsive to electrical defibrillation.[71] The marked reduction in the incidence of ventricular fibrillation over time suggests that genetics have a relatively small contribution to population attributable risk.

Environmental and Circadian-Rhythm Factors

The incidence and outcome of cardiac arrest varies by time of day, day of week, and also season of the year.[72–77] Data from the Framingham study show that the highest risk for MI is on awakening and that it decreases progressively during the day. Various physiologic processes have been considered to explain this phenomenon, such as increased clotting or increased parasympathetic instability. Some researchers have suggested that part of the morning peak in cardiac arrest may be due to a reporting artifact (i.e., when patients really die during the night but are not discovered until early morning). Potential interventions to reduce periodic variation in unexpected cardiac death include resource allocation of EMS and hospital resources to match anticipated need.

Social Factors

Disparities in the incidence of cardiac arrest are observed across socioeconomic gradients as well as geographic region.[41,78–83] CVD is the leading cause of income-related differences in premature mortality in the United States[84] and Canada.[85] Non-Hispanic blacks bear a disproportionate burden of morbidity and mortality due to CVD.[86] These disparities may be caused by differences in genetic risk, health behaviors, educational attainment, socioeconomic disadvantage, access to preventive care, or other yet to be identified variables. As our understanding of the magnitude and causes of these disparities increases, potential interventions include culturally appropriate public health initiatives, community support, and equitable access to quality care.

Behavioral Factors

Cigarette smoking is thought to be the single most important cause of preventable death in the United States. An estimated 438,000 persons in the United States die prematurely each year owing to exposure to tobacco smoke.[87] The deleterious effects of smoking may be mediated through increased plasma catecholamines, heart rate, and arterial blood pressure, resulting in coronary spasm and increases in myocardial work and oxygen demand with a concomitant reduction in oxygen supply.[88] Collectively these effects lower VF thresholds. In patients who successfully quit smoking, rates of sudden death return to near normal over time. Of great concern is the effect of "passive smoking," which has been associated with an increase in smoking-related disease, primarily heart disease.[89]

Exercise can be both good and bad. Persons who exercise regularly have a decreased incidence of CAD compared to those who are sedentary[90] and decreased mortality in those with CAD who exercise compared with those who do not.[91] Nevertheless, heavy exertion with exercise is associated with an increase in acute events, such as MI. A period of strenuous activity has been associated with a temporary increase in the risk of having an MI for about 1 hour after the exertion.[92] Heavy exertion in persons who do not exercise regularly was associated with the highest risk.

Use of **street drugs** is associated with cardiac arrest. Cocaine use is associated with severe and catastrophic heart disease in many individuals. It increases adrenergic stimulation by blocking the presynaptic reuptake of norepinephrine and dopamine, thus causing an increased sensitivity to catecholamines. The combined effects of cocaine and cigarette smoke are worse than either one alone.[93] Opioids are also associated with cardiac arrest.[94] Both cocaine and methadone prolong QT intervals, predisposing to ventricular arrhythmias.[95]

Moderate alcohol intake is associated with reduced cardiovascular mortality compared with no alcohol intake, although the mechanisms by which alcohol is protective remain unclear. This effect is thought to be mediated through increased levels of HDL-C.[96] However, heavy consumption is associated with increased mortality—an effect sometimes referred to as "holiday heart," because it is often associated with binge drinking in otherwise healthy people during weekends.[97] In the Physicians' Health Study, after controlling for multiple confounders, men who consumed two to six drinks per week had a 60% to 80% reduced risk of unexpected cardiac death compared with those who rarely or never consumed alcohol.[98] In the British Regional Heart Study, the relative risk of unexpected cardiac death in those who drank more than six drinks per day was twice as high as that among occasional or light drinkers.[99]

Emotional factors influence the occurrence of cardiac disease. However, characteristics such as anger, chronic stress, aggressiveness, anxiety, and hostility are difficult to measure objectively, and there are many confounding issues. Educational attainment moderates the risk of acute infarction due to anger.[100] However, studies have yet to confirm a definite relationship between emotional factors and cardiac arrest.

Pharmacologic Agents

A variety of prescription and nonprescription pharmaceutical agents increase or decrease the risk of arrhythmia or cardiac arrest (Table 2-1). Drugs that have the most significant impact on mortality due to cardiac arrest lack direct electrophysiologic effects on myocardial excitability.[101] This implies that these agents act on proximate events that can predispose to lethal arrhythmias (e.g., ischemia, fibrosis). Other agents decrease cardiovascular or all-cause mortality but have not been demonstrated to decrease cardiac arrest. The latter likely reflects lack of statistical power to detect a difference in an event that is infrequent compared with events or mortality. However lack of demonstrated benefit specific to cardiac

PART ONE • ACUTE CORONARY SYNDROMES

| TABLE 2-1 • Effect of Drugs on Long-Term Risk of Cardiovascular Death and Cardiac Arrest[d]

Drug	Effect of Cardiovascular Mortality	Effect of Cardiac Arrest Mortality
ACE Inhibitors	−	−
Aldosterone antagonists	−	−
Amiodarone	−	−
Angiotensin receptor blockers	±	±
Aspirin	−	±
Beta-blockers	−	−
Clopidogrel	−	±
Cyclooxygenase inhibitors (COX-2)	+	+
Digoxin	±	±
Drugs that prolong QT interval[a]	±	+
HMG-CoA reductase inhibitors	−	−
Iib/Iia receptor antagonists	±	±
Inotropes	±	+
Low-molecular-weight heparin	±	±
Thrombolytic therapy	−	−
Vaughan-Williams class IC[b]	+	+
Vaughan-Williams class III[c]	+	+
Warfarin	−	±

[a] Includes but not limited to selected antiarrhythmic agents, fluoquinolone antibiotics, cocaine, methadone.
[b] Flecainide, encainide.
[c] D-sotalol, dofetilide.
[d] − indicates decrease; + indicates increase.

arrest should not be interpreted as lack of need to prescribe agents that are otherwise effective in persons with CVD.

Survival

There is a wide variation in reported survival after the onset of cardiac arrest. The median reported survival to discharge after any first recorded rhythm is 6.4%.[102] Published rates of survival after treatment of any initial rhythm range from 0% to >20% (Fig. 2-5). As well, survival from admission after resuscitation from cardiac arrest to discharge from hospital varies widely between hospitals (Fig. 2-6).[103] These survival disparities reemphasize that effective emergency cardiovascular care can decrease death and disability due to acute cardiovascular events in the out-of-hospital setting.

The wide variation in survival is attributable in part to regional differences in the availability of out-of-hospital and hospital-based emergency cardiovascular care.[104] Interventions

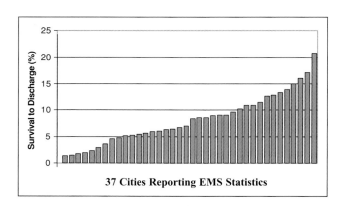

FIGURE 2-5 • Survival after EMS-treated cardiac arrest. Statistics from 37 cities. (Adapted from Nichol G, Stiell IG, Laupacis A, et al. A cumulative metaanalysis of the effectiveness of defibrillator-capable emergency medical services for victims of out-of-hospital cardiac arrest. (From *Ann Emerg Med* 1999;34[4]:517–525, with permission.)

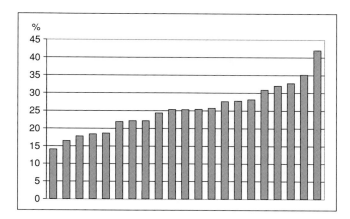

FIGURE 2-6 • Survival among those admitted to hospital after cardiac arrest. Survival to 1 month in 21 corresponding hospitals among all patients who were alive on hospital admission after out-of-hospital cardiac arrest (crew-witnessed cases not included). (From Herlitz J, Engdahl J, Svensson L, et al. Major differences in 1-month survival between hospitals in Sweden among initial survivors of out-of-hospital cardiac arrest. *Resuscitation* 2006;70[3]:404–409, with permission.)

for cardiac arrest include bystander CPR, lay responder defibrillation programs,[105] experienced EMS providers,[106] and specific interventions provided by EMS providers[107,108] or at receiving hospitals.[109,110] Bystander CPR is simple, inexpensive, and known to be lifesaving, in numerous studies conferring a two- to threefold increase in survival rate[111–113] but performed in a minority of cases of out-of-hospital cardiac arrest.[102] However, only lay responder defibrillation[105] and therapeutic hypothermia[110] have been shown in randomized trials to significantly improve outcomes to hospital discharge after cardiac arrest.

There is substantial regional variation in EMS structures and processes (e.g., EMS service level provided, number of EMS providers responding, use of procedures or drugs in the field, training, quality assurance/feedback, and response-time intervals). Some of these factors have been associated with differences in survival or quality of life after resuscitation,[102,115–118] although no analysis has had adequate power to detect the independent effect of each.

Some recent studies have been interpreted as suggesting that prehospital emergency care interventions do not improve outcomes after cardiac arrest.[119–121] However, these studies did not account for the prior experience of EMS providers, which is an important predictor of outcome after cardiac arrest.[106] Highly qualified EMS providers, such as those who work in the Seattle Medic One program, can be trained to achieve central vascular access in the field,[122] and others administer thrombolytic therapy in the field to patients with acute MI.[123–125] Thus broad implementation and ongoing maintenance of adequately funded EMS systems staffed by highly trained, experienced providers may be necessary to have a meaningful impact on death due to out-of-hospital cardiac arrest.

Witnessed VF is commonly used to assess the efficacy of an EMS agency because it provides a homogeneous population for analysis that is readily responsive to timely intervention.[126] It is hoped that survival figures become more closely comparable between communities by use of such a definition; but this could be untrue, because VF is correlated with response time.[127] A potential limitation to this approach is that as the subgroup becomes smaller, the results become less applicable to the larger population. Also, focusing on a subgroup of patients with a particular initial rhythm rather than all treated cardiac arrests could give an optimistic sense of outcomes. By considering only patients with VF, one underestimates the burden of illness and improvements in treatment, since the incidence of VF has decreased and rates of survival to hospital admission or discharge have been static over time for VF but not for pulseless electrical activity or asystole.[21] The updated Utstein template and recommendations offer some logical guidelines for investigators reporting on subgroups.[1]

OUT-OF-HOSPITAL CARDIAC ARREST

- According to the National Center for Health Statistics, 325,000 CHD deaths occur outside of hospitals or in hospital emergency departments annually (ICD-10 codes I20–I25). (Vital Statistics of the U.S., Data Warehouse, NCHS 2003. http://www.cdc.gov/nchs/datawh.htm.)
- About 60% of unexpected cardiac deaths are treated by EMS personnel. (*J Am Coll Cardiol* 2004;44:1268–1275.)
- On average, 27.4% of out-of-hospital cardiac arrests receive bystander cardiopulmonary resuscitation (CPR). (*Ann Emerg Med* 1999;34:517–525.)
- The incidence of lay responder defibrillation is low—2.05% in 2002—but increasing over time. (*Circulation* 2004;109:1859–1863.)
- Unexpected death in the pediatric patient is usually due to trauma, sudden infant death syndrome, respiratory causes, or submersion. (*Pediatrics* 2004;114:157–164.)
- The incidence of in-hospital cardiac arrest is unknown.

Dynamic Cellular Changes at the Time of Cardiac Arrest

Cardiac arrest involves sudden, global ischemia. Reperfusion occurs during CPR and restoration of circulation and is associated with marked release of cytokines/chemokines (e.g., the interleukins: IL-1ra, IL-6, IL-8, and IL-10), activated complement, and polymorphonuclear leukocytes as well as endothelial cell adhesion molecules.[128–131] These fluxes are associated with endothelial dysfunction, thrombosis, and impairment of fibrinolysis.[128,132–134] After cardiac arrest, nonsurvivors demonstrate plasma IL-6 concentrations 20-fold greater than those of survivors,[128] which is approximately 50-fold greater than normal human baseline values.[135] These inflammatory and coagulation changes contribute to poor capillary perfusion, tissue ischemia, multiorgan dysfunction, and death.[136–139] The extent of such reperfusion injury is associated with the duration of ischemia and adequacy of resuscitation.

However, early hemodynamic failure is not predictive of a poor neurologic outcome, and many patients with early hemodynamic dysfunction have a good neurologic outcome.[128,140] Therefore, treatments that decrease early mortality related to intractable shock could increase the number of survivors with good neurologic outcomes.

Recent and Ongoing Approaches to Resuscitation Research

The U.S. Institute of Medicine has described the future of emergency care, including acute, unscheduled health care delivered outside the hospital by a system that responds to calls for medical aid (http://www.annemergmed.com/content/iomsummary, accessed June 26, 2006). A common reason for such a response is treatment of out-of-hospital cardiac arrest. A challenge to defining the needs of such care is the relative paucity of evidence of the effectiveness of resuscitation interventions, since most prior experimental studies of interventions for those in cardiac arrest have been conducted in a small number of sites without sufficient power to detect the minimum clinically important difference. However, the absence of evidence does not indicate evidence of absence. This absence of evidence has been addressed in part by increased investment in fundamental, translational, and clinical resuscitation research in North America by the National Institutes of Health and other agencies.

Resuscitation Outcomes Consortium

The Resuscitation Outcomes Consortium (ROC) is a prehospital emergency care research network that has the necessary infrastructure to conduct multiple randomized trials to aid rapid translation of promising scientific and clinical advances aimed at improving resuscitation outcomes. Such large, simple trials have been highly successful at rapidly and definitively evaluating interventions in order to accelerate the pace of evidence-based change to improve outcomes in patients with acute MI.[32,141-151] ROC consists of 11 clinical sites located throughout North America as well as a central coordinating center. As of June 7, 2007, ROC has implemented cohort studies of consecutive cases of patients who experience out-of-hospital cardiac arrest or life-threatening traumatic injury. These disorders are being studied together by ROC because they have in common the factors of epidemiology, physiology, and initial care providers. ROC has initiated enrollment in a partial factorial trial of an active versus sham impedance threshold device and early analysis (about 30 seconds of CPR before rhythm analysis) versus late analysis (about 3 minutes of CPR before rhythm analysis). ROC has also initiated enrollment in randomized trials of normal saline versus hypertonic saline versus hypertonic saline with dextran in patients with traumatic brain injury or shock after trauma.

Future Directions

In the future, significant changes in resuscitation are likely to occur. Observational studies will continue to improve the field of resuscitation. New epidemiologic data are needed to answer the following questions:

- What is the current incidence and survival rate of out-of-hospital cardiac arrest? Why has the survival rate after cardiac arrest remained static?
- Can the proportion of cases that receive bystander CPR be increased?
- Can outcomes be improved by broad implementation of quality assurance of EMS care?
- Is training and equipping family members of those at risk of cardiac arrest an effective method of reducing time to defibrillation and increasing survival?
- Can differences in incidence and survival according to race and socioeconomic status be reduced?

To find answers to these questions and to test future therapies, more accurate and larger quantities of data are needed than are currently available. It is plausible that implementing mandatory reporting of out-of-hospital cardiac arrest incidence and outcome would increase the availability of such data. National or international databases offer the best opportunities to do so. Data accuracy must be improved so that real verifiable time intervals can be measured. A critical step towards improving outcomes is for every community to monitor and improve its rate of survival after out-of-hospital cardiac arrest. Finally, new therapies must be developed to improve treatment.

References

1. Jacobs I, Nadkarni V, Bahr J, et al. Cardiac arrest and cardiopulmonary resuscitation outcome reports: update and simplification of the Utstein templates for resuscitation registries: a statement for healthcare professionals from a task force of the International Liaison Committee on Resuscitation (American Heart Association, European Resuscitation Council, Australian Resuscitation Council, New Zealand Resuscitation Council, Heart and Stroke Foundation of Canada, InterAmerican Heart Foundation, Resuscitation Councils of Southern Africa). *Circulation* 2004;110(21):3385–3397.
2. Zipes DP, Wellens HJ. Sudden cardiac death. *Circulation* 1998; 98(21):2334–2351.
3. Working Group on Ischemic Heart Disease Registers. Report of a Working Group. Parts I and II. Copenhagen, Denmark: Regional Office for Europe, World Health Organization, 1969.
4. Kurkciyan I, Meron G, Behringer W, et al. Accuracy and impact of presumed cause in patients with cardiac arrest. *Circulation* 1998;98(8):766–771.
5. Uretsky BF, Thygesen K, Armstrong PW, et al. Acute coronary findings at autopsy in heart failure patients with sudden death: results from the assessment of treatment with lisinopril and survival (ATLAS) trial. *Circulation* 2000;102(6):611–616.
6. Soo LH, Gray D, Hampton JR. Pathological features of witnessed out-of-hospital cardiac arrest presenting with ventricular fibrillation. *Resuscitation* 2001;51(3):257–264.
7. Zipes DP, Camm AJ, Borggrefe M, et al. ACC/AHA/ESC 2006 guidelines for management of patients with ventricular arrhythmias and the prevention of sudden cardiac death: a report of the American College of Cardiology/American Heart Association Task Force and the European Society of Cardiology Committee for Practice Guidelines (Writing Committee to Develop

Guidelines for Management of Patients With Ventricular Arrhythmias and the Prevention of Sudden Cardiac Death). *J Am Coll Cardiol* 2006;48(5):e247–e346.

8. Connolly SJ, Hallstrom AP, Cappato R, et al. Meta-analysis of the implantable cardioverter defibrillator secondary prevention trials. *Eur Heart J* 2000;21(24):2071–2078.

9. Hohnloser SH, Kuck KH, Dorian P, et al. Prophylactic use of an implantable cardioverter-defibrillator after acute myocardial infarction. *N Engl J Med* 2004;351(24):2481–2488.

10. Feldman AM, Klein H, Tchou P, et al. Use of a wearable defibrillator in terminating tachyarrhythmias in patients at high risk for sudden death: results of the WEARIT/BIROAD. *Pacing Clin Electrophysiol* 2004;27(1):4–9.

11. Reddy KS, Yusuf S. Emerging epidemic of cardiovascular disease in developing countries. *Circulation* 1998;97(6):596–601.

12. Gillum RF. Sudden coronary death in the United States: 1980–1985. *Circulation* 1989;79:756–765.

13. Higgins MW, Luepker RV. *Trends in Coronary Heart Disease Mortality: The Influence of Medical Care.* New York: Oxford University Press, 1988.

14. Rosamond WD, Chambless LE, Folsom AR, et al. Trends in the incidence of myocardial infarction and in mortality due to coronary heart disease, 1987 to 1994. *N Engl J Med* 1998;339: 861–867.

15. Tillinghast SJ, Doliszny KM, Gomez-Marin O, et al. Change in survival from out-of-hospital cardiac arrest and its effect on coronary heart disease mortality—Minneapolis–St. Paul: the Minnesota Heart Survey. *Am J Epidemiol* 1991;134(8):851–861.

16. Yusuf S, Reddy S, Ounpuu S, et al. Global burden of cardiovascular diseases: part I: general considerations, the epidemiologic transition, risk factors, and impact of urbanization. *Circulation* 2001;104(22):2746–2753.

17. World Health Report 2002: *Reducing Risks and Promoting Healthy Life.* Geneva: World Health Organization; 2002.

18. Mathers CD, Stein C, Fat Ma D, et al. *Global Burden of Disease 2000.* Version 2: *Methods and Results.* Geneva: World Health Organization; 2002.

19. Myerburg RJ, Kessler KM, Castellanos A. Sudden cardiac death: epidemiology, transient risk, and intervention assessment. *Ann Intern Med* 1993;119(12):1187–1197.

20. Chugh SS, Jui J, Gunson K, et al. Current burden of sudden cardiac death: multiple source surveillance versus retrospective death certificate-based review in a large U.S. community. *J Am Coll Cardiol* 2004;44(6):1268–1275.

21. Cobb LA, Fahrenbruch CE, Olsufka M, et al. Changing incidence of out-of-hospital ventricular fibrillation, 1980–2000. *JAMA* 2002;288(23):3008–3013.

22. Rea TD, Pearce RM, Raghunathan TE, et al. Incidence of out-of-hospital cardiac arrest. *Am J Cardiol* 2004;93(12):1455–1460.

23. Rea TD, Eisenberg MS, Becker LJ, et al. Temporal trends in sudden cardiac arrest: a 25-year emergency medical services perspective. *Circulation* 2003;107(22):2780–2785.

24. Herlitz J, Bang A, Gunnarsson J, et al. Factors associated with survival to hospital discharge among patients hospitalised alive after out of hospital cardiac arrest: change in outcome over 20 years in the community of Goteborg, Sweden. *Heart* 2003; 89(1):25–30.

25. de Vreede-Swagemakers JJ, Gorgels AP, Dubois-Arbouw WI, et al. Out-of-hospital cardiac arrest in the 1990s: a population-based study in the Maastricht area on incidence, characteristics and survival. *J Am Coll Cardiol* 1997;30(6):1500–1505.

26. Rosamond W, Flegal K, Furie K, et al. Heart disease and stroke statistics—2008 update. A Report From the American Heart Association Statistics Committee and Stroke Statistics Subcommittee. *Circulation* 2008.

27. Donoghue A, Nadkarni V, Berg RA, et al. Out-of-hospital pediatric cardiac arrest: an epidemiologic review and assessment of current knowledge. *Ann Emerg Med* 2005;46:512–522.

28. Young KD, Gausche-Hill M, McClung CD, et al. A prospective, population-based study of the epidemiology and outcome of out-of-hospital pediatric cardiopulmonary arrest. *Pediatrics* 2004;114(1): 157–164.

29. Mogayzel C, Quan L, Graves L, et al. Out-of-hospital ventricular fibrillation in children and adolescents: causes and outcomes. *Ann Emerg Med* 1995;25:484–491.

30. Peberdy MA, Kaye W, Ornato JP, et al. Cardiopulmonary resuscitation of adults in the hospital: A report of 14, 720 cardiac arrest from the National Registry of Cardiopulmonary Resuscitation. *Resuscitation* 2003;58:297–308.

31. Huikuri HV, Castellanos A, Myerburg RJ. Sudden death due to cardiac arrhythmias. *N Engl J Med* 2001;345(20):1473–1482.

32. A comparison of recombinant hirudin with heparin for the treatment of acute coronary syndromes. The Global Use of Strategies to Open Occluded Coronary Arteries (GUSTO) IIb investigators. *N Engl J Med* 1996;335(11):775–782.

33. Alexander JH, Sparapani RA, Mahaffey KW, et al. Association between minor elevations of creatine kinase-MB level and mortality in patients with acute coronary syndromes without ST-segment elevation. PURSUIT steering committee. Platelet glycoprotein IIb/IIIa in unstable angina: receptor suppression using integrilin therapy. *JAMA* 2000;283(3):347–353.

34. Califf RM, Pieper KS, Lee KL, et al. Prediction of 1-year survival after thrombolysis for acute myocardial infarction in the global utilization of streptokinase and TPA for occluded coronary arteries trial. *Circulation* 2000;101(19):2231–2238.

35. Pinski SL, Yao Q, Epstein AE, et al. Determinants of outcome in patients with sustained ventricular tachyarrhythmias: the antiarrhythmics versus implantable defibrillators (AVID) study registry. *Am Heart J* 2000;139(5):804–813.

36. Moss AJ, DeCamilla J, Davis H. Cardiac death in the first 6 months after myocardial infarction: potential for mortality reduction in the early posthospital period. *Am J Cardiol* 1977;39(6):816–820.

37. Bailey JJ, Berson AS, Handelsman H, et al. Utility of current risk stratification tests for predicting major arrhythmic events after myocardial infarction. *J Am Coll Cardiol* 2001;38(7):1902–1911.

38. La Rovere MT, Bigger JT Jr, Marcus FI, et al for the ATRAMI investigators. Baroflex sensitivity and heart-rate variability in prediction of total cardiac mortality after myocardial infarction. *Lancet* 1998;351:478–484.

39. Thompson RG, Cobb LA. Hypokalemia after resuscitation from out-of-hospital ventricular fibrillation. *JAMA* 1982;248(21): 2860–2863.

40. Estes NA III, Link MS, Cannom D, et al. Report of the NASPE policy conference on arrhythmias and the athlete. *J Cardiovasc Electrophysiol* 2001;12(10):1208–1219.

41. Becker LB, Han BH, Meyer PM, et al. Racial differences in the incidence of cardiac arrest and subsequent survival. The CPR Chicago Project. *N Engl J Med* 1993;329(9):600–606.

42. Lewington S, Clarke R, Qizilbash N, et al. Age-specific relevance of usual blood pressure to vascular mortality: a meta-analysis of individual data for one million adults in 61 prospective studies. *Lancet* 2002;360(9349):1903–1913.

43. Castelli WP. Epidemiology of coronary heart disease: the Framingham study. *Am J Med* 1984;76(2A):4–12.

44. Fields LE, Burt VL, Cutler JA, et al. The burden of adult hypertension in the United States 1999 to 2000: a rising tide. *Hypertension* 2004;44(4):398–404.

45. Vasan RS, Beiser A, Seshadri S, et al. Residual lifetime risk for developing hypertension in middle-aged women and men: The Framingham Heart Study. *JAMA* 2002;287(8):1003–1010.

46. Hajjar I, Kotchen TA. Trends in prevalence, awareness, treatment, and control of hypertension in the United States, 1988–2000. *JAMA* 2003;290(2):199–206.

47. Psaty BM, Lumley T, Furberg CD, et al. Health outcomes associated with various antihypertensive therapies used as first-line agents: a network meta-analysis. *JAMA* 2003;289(19):2534–2544.

48. Stamler J, Wentworth D, Neaton JD. Is relationship between serum cholesterol and risk of premature death from coronary heart disease continuous and graded? Findings in 356,222 primary screenees of the Multiple Risk Factor Intervention Trial (MRFIT). *JAMA* 1986;256(20):2823–2828.

49. Castelli WP. The triglyceride issue: a view from Framingham. *Am Heart J* 1986;112(2):432–437.

50. Gould KL, Ornish D, Kirkeeide R, et al. Improved stenosis geometry by quantitative coronary arteriography after vigorous risk factor modification. *Am J Cardiol* 1992;69(9):845–853.

51. Hooper L, Summerbell CD, Higgins JPT, et al. Reduced or modified dietary fat for preventing cardiovascular disease. *Cochrane Database Syst Rev* 2005(3).

52. Flegal KM, Carroll MD, Kuczmarski RJ, et al. Overweight and obesity in the United States: prevalence and trends, 1960–1994. *Int J Obes Relat Metab Disord* 1998;22(1):39–47.

53. Flegal KM, Carroll MD, Ogden CL, et al. Prevalence and trends in obesity among US adults, 1999–2000. *JAMA* 2002;288(14):1723–1727.

54. Mokdad AH, Serdula MK, Dietz WH, et al. The spread of the obesity epidemic in the United States, 1991–1998. *JAMA* 1999;282(16):1519–1522.

55. Gregg EW, Cheng YJ, Cadwell BL, et al. Secular trends in cardiovascular disease risk factors according to body mass index in US adults. *JAMA* 2005;293(15):1868–1874.

56. Mokdad AH, Bowman BA, Ford ES, et al. The continuing epidemics of obesity and diabetes in the United States. *JAMA* 2001;286(10):1195–1200.

57. Karnik JA, Young BS, Lew NL, et al. Cardiac arrest and sudden death in dialysis units. *Kidney Int* 2001;60(1):350–357.

58. Michal V. Arterial disease as a cause of impotence. *Clin Endocrinol Metab* 1982;11(3):725–748.

59. Wabrek AJ, Burchell RC. Male sexual dysfunction associated with coronary heart disease. *Arch Sex Behav* 1980;9(1):69–75.

60. Leaf A, Kang JX, Xiao YF, et al. Clinical prevention of sudden cardiac death by n-3 polyunsaturated fatty acids and mechanism of prevention of arrhythmias by n–3 fish oils. *Circulation* 2003;107(21):2646–2652.

61. Roden DM, Yang T. Protecting the heart against arrhythmias: potassium current physiology and repolarization reserve. *Circulation* 2005;112(10):1376–1378.

62. Albert CM, Ma J, Rifai N, et al. Prospective study of C-reactive protein, homocysteine, and plasma lipid levels as predictors of sudden cardiac death. *Circulation* 2002;105(22):2595–2599.

63. Kumari M, Marmot M, Brunner E. Social determinants of von Willebrand factor: the Whitehall II study. *Arterioscler Thromb Vasc Biol* 2000;20(7):1842–1847.

64. Siscovick DS, Lemaitre RN, Mozaffarian D. The fish story: a diet-heart hypothesis with clinical implications: n-3 polyunsaturated fatty acids, myocardial vulnerability, and sudden death. *Circulation* 2003;107(21):2632–2634.

65. Jouven X, Desnos M, Guerot C, et al. Predicting sudden death in the population: the Paris Prospective Study I. *Circulation* 1999;99(15):1978–1983.

66. Spooner PM, Albert C, Benjamin EJ, et al. Sudden cardiac death, genes, and arrhythmogenesis: consideration of new population and mechanistic approaches from a National Heart, Lung, and Blood Institute workshop. Part II. *Circulation* 2001;103(20):2447–2452.

67. Spooner PM, Albert C, Benjamin EJ, et al. Sudden cardiac death, genes, and arrhythmogenesis: consideration of new population and mechanistic approaches from a national heart, lung, and blood institute workshop. Part I. *Circulation* 2001;103(19):2361–2364.

68. Tan HL, Hofman N, van Langen IM, et al. Sudden unexplained death: heritability and diagnostic yield of cardiological and genetic examination in surviving relatives. *Circulation* 2005;112(2):207–213.

69. Friedlander Y, Siscovick DS, Weinmann S, et al. Family history as a risk factor for primary cardiac arrest. *Circulation* 1998;97(2):155–160.

70. Priori SG, Barhanin J, Hauer RN, et al. Genetic and molecular basis of cardiac arrhythmias: impact on clinical management parts I and II. *Circulation* 1999;99(4):518–528.

71. Schwartz PJ, Priori SG, Spazzolini C, et al. Genotype-phenotype correlation in the long-QT syndrome: gene-specific triggers for life-threatening arrhythmias. *Circulation* 2001;103(1):89–95.

72. Page RL, Zipes DP, Powell JL, et al. Seasonal variation of mortality in the Antiarrhythmics Versus Implantable Defibrillators (AVID) study registry. *Heart Rhythm* 2004;1(4):435–440.

73. Fall-related injuries during the holiday season—United States, 2000–2003. *MMWR* 2004;53(48):1127–1129.

74. Crawford JR, Parker MJ. Seasonal variation of proximal femoral fractures in the United Kingdom. *Injury* 2003;34(3):223–225.

75. Allegra JR, Cochrane DG, Allegra EM, et al. Calendar patterns in the occurrence of cardiac arrest. *Am J Emerg Med* 2002;20(6):513–517.

76. Herlitz J, Eek M, Holmberg M, et al. Diurnal, weekly and seasonal rhythm of out of hospital cardiac arrest in Sweden. *Resuscitation* 2002;54(2):133–138.

77. Gruska M, Gaul GB, Winkler M, et al. Increased occurrence of out-of-hospital cardiac arrest on Mondays in a community-based study. *Chronobiol Int* 2005;22(1):107–120.

78. Iwashyna TJ, Christakis NA, Becker LB. Neighborhoods matter: a population-based study of provision of cardiopulmonary resuscitation. *Ann Emerg Med* 1999;34(4 Pt 1):459–468.

79. Sampson RJ, Raudenbush SW, Earls F. Neighborhoods and violent crime: a multilevel study of collective efficacy. *Science* 1997;277(5328):918–924.

80. Sampson RJ, Morenoff JD, Raudenbush S. Social anatomy of racial and ethnic disparities in violence. *Am J Public Health* 2005;95(2):224–232.

81. Dunn L, Henry J, Beard D. Social deprivation and head injury: a national study. *J Neurol Neurosurg Psychiatry* 2003;74(8):1060–1064.

82. Cubbin C, LeClere FB, Smith GS. Socioeconomic status and the occurrence of fatal and nonfatal injury in the United States. *Am J Public Health* 2000;90(1):70–77.

83. Cubbin C, LeClere FB, Smith GS. Socioeconomic status and injury mortality: individual and neighbourhood determinants. *J Epidemiol Commun Health* 2000;54(7):517–524.

84. Singh GK, Siahpush M. Increasing inequalities in all-cause and cardiovascular mortality among U.S. adults aged 25–64 years by area socioeconomic status, 1969–1998. *Int J Epidemiol* 2002;31(3):600–613.

85. Wilkins R, Berthelot J-M, Ng E. Trends in mortality by neighbourhood income in urban Canada from 1971 to 1996. *Health Reports* 2002(Dec. 11).

86. Health disparities experienced by black or African Americans – United States. *MMWR* 2005;54(1):1–3.

87. Annual smoking-attributable mortality, years of potential life lost, and productivity losses – United States, 1997–2001. *MMWR* 2005;54(25):625–628.

88. Mehta MC, Jain AC, Mehta A, et al. Cardiac Arrhythmias following intravenous nicotine: experimental study in dogs. *J Cardiovasc Pharmacol Ther* 1997;2(4):291–298.

89. Jamrozik K. Estimate of deaths attributable to passive smoking among UK adults: database analysis. *BMJ* 2005;330(7495):812.

90. Berlin JA, Colditz GA. A meta-analysis of physical activity in the prevention of coronary heart disease. *Am J Epidemiol* 1990;132(4):612–628.

91. Taylor RS, Brown A, Ebrahim S, et al. Exercise-based rehabilitation for patients with coronary heart disease: systematic review and meta-analysis of randomized controlled trials. *Am J Med* 2004;116(10):682–692.

92. Mittleman MA, Maclure M, Tofler GH, et al. Triggering of acute myocardial infarction by heavy physical exertion. Protection against triggering by regular exertion. Determinants of Myocardial Infarction Onset Study Investigators. *N Engl J Med* 1993;329(23):1677–1683.

93. Moliterno DJ, Willard JE, Lange RA, et al. Coronary-artery vasoconstriction induced by cocaine, cigarette smoking, or both. *N Engl J Med* 1994;330(7):454–459.

94. Paredes VL, Rea TD, Eisenberg MS, et al. Out-of-hospital care of critical drug overdoses involving cardiac arrest. *Acad Emerg Med* 2004;11(1):71–74.

95. Krantz MJ, Rowan SB, Mehler PS. Cocaine-related torsade de pointes in a methadone maintenance patient. *J Addict Dis* 2005;24(1):53–60.

96. Gaziano JM, Buring JE, Breslow JL, et al. Moderate alcohol intake, increased levels of high-density lipoprotein and its subfractions, and decreased risk of myocardial infarction. *N Engl J Med* 1993;329(25):1829–1834.

97. Kupari M, Koskinen P. Alcohol, cardiac arrhythmias and sudden death. *Novartis Found Symp* 1998;216:68–79.

98. Albert CM, Manson JE, Cook NR, et al. Moderate alcohol consumption and the risk of sudden cardiac death among U.S. male physicians. *Circulation* 1999;100(9):944–950.

99. Wannamethee G, Shaper AG. Alcohol and sudden cardiac death. *Br Heart J* 1992;68(5):443–8.

100. Mittleman MA, Maclure M, Nachnani M, et al. Educational attainment, anger, and the risk of triggering myocardial infarction onset. The Determinants of Myocardial Infarction Onset Study Investigators. *Arch Intern Med* 1997;157(7):769–775.

101. Alberte C, Zipes DP. Use of nonantiarrhythmic drugs for prevention of sudden cardiac death. *J Cardiovasc Electrophysiol* 2003;14(9 Suppl):S87–S95.

102. Nichol G, Stiell IG, Laupacis A, et al. A cumulative metaanalysis of the effectiveness of defibrillator-capable emergency medical services for victims of out-of-hospital cardiac arrest. *Ann Emerg Med* 1999;34(4):517–525.

103. Herlitz J, Engdahl J, Svensson L, et al. Major differences in 1-month survival between hospitals in Sweden among initial survivors of out-of-hospital cardiac arrest. *Resuscitation* 2006;70(3): 404–409.

104. Eisenberg MS, Horwood BT, Cummins RO, et al. Cardiac arrest and resuscitation: a tale of 29 cities. *Ann Emerg Med* 1990;19: 179–186.

105. Public-access defibrillation and survival after out-of-hospital cardiac arrest. *N Engl J Med* 2004;351(7):637–646.

106. Soo LH, Gray D, Young T, et al. Influence of ambulance crew's length of experience on the outcome of out-of-hospital cardiac arrest. *Eur Heart J* 1999;20(7):535–540.

107. Kudenchuk PJ, Cobb LA, Copass MK, et al. Amiodarone for resuscitation after out-of-hospital cardiac arrest due to ventricular fibrillation. *N Engl J Med* 1999;341(12):871–878.

108. Dorian P, Cass D, Schwartz B, et al. Amiodarone as compared with lidocaine for shock-resistant ventricular fibrillation. *N Engl J Med* 2002;346(12):884–890.

109. Bernard SA, Gray TW, Buist MD, et al. Treatment of comatose survivors of out-of-hospital cardiac arrest with induced hypothermia [see comment]. *N Engl J Med* 2002;346(8):557–563.

110. Mild therapeutic hypothermia to improve the neurologic outcome after cardiac arrest. The Hypothermia after Cardiac Arrest Study Group.[erratum appears in N Engl J Med 2002;346(22): 1756]. *N Engl J Med* 2002;346(8):549–556.

111. Weaver WD, Cobb LA, Hallstrom AP, et al. Considerations for improving survival from out-of-hospital cardiac arrest. *Ann Emerg Med* 1986;15:1181–1186.

112. Thompson RG, Hallstrom AP, Cobb LA. Bystander-initiated cardiopulmonary resuscitation in the management of ventricular fibrillation. *Ann Intern Med* 1979;90(5):737–740.

113. Herlitz J, Ekstrom L, Wennerblom B, et al. Effect of bystander initiated cardiopulmonary resuscitation on ventricular fibrillation and survival after witnessed cardiac arrest outside hospital. *Br Heart J* 1994;72:408–412.

114. Fato R, Di Bernardo S, Estornell E, et al. Saturation kinetics of coenzyme Q in NADH oxidation: rate enhancement by incorporation of excess quinone. *Mol Aspects Med* 1997;18(S):269–273.

115. van der Hoeven J, de Koning J, van der Weyden P, et al. Improved outcome for patients with a cardiac arrest by supervision of the emergency medical services system. *Netherlands J Med* 1995;46: 123–130.

116. Bergner L, Bergner M, Hallstrom AP, et al. Service factors and health status of survivors of out-of-hospital cardiac arrest. *Am J Emerg Med* 1983;1(3):259–263.

117. Frandsen F, Nielsen JR, Gram L, et al. Evaluation of intensified prehospital treatment in out-of-hospital cardiac arrest: survival and cerebral prognosis. The Odense Ambulance Study. *Cardiology* 1991;79:256–264.

118. Stiell IG, Wells GA, Field BJ, et al. Improved out-of-hospital cardiac arrest survival through the inexpensive optimization of an existing defibrillation program: OPALS study phase II. Ontario Prehospital Advanced Life Support. *JAMA* 1999;281(13): 1175–1181.

119. Stiell IG, Wells GA, Field B, et al. Advanced cardiac life support in out-of-hospital cardiac arrest. *N Engl J Med* 2004;351(7): 647–656.

120. Gausche M, Lewis RJ, Stratton SJ, et al. Effect of out-of-hospital pediatric endotracheal intubation on survival and neurological outcome: a controlled clinical trial. *JAMA* 2000;283(6):783–790.

121. Gausche M, Tadeo RE, Zane MC, et al. Out-of-hospital intravenous access: unnecessary procedures and excessive cost. *Acad Emerg Med* 1998;5(9):878–882.

122. Waugh R. *University of Washington School of Medicine Paramedic Training Program Handbook*, 2006.

123. Morrison LJ, Verbeek PR, McDonald AC, et al. Mortality and prehospital thrombolysis for acute myocardial infarction: A meta-analysis. *JAMA* 2000;283(20):2686–2692.

124. Morrow DA, Antman EM, Sayah A, et al. Evaluation of the time saved by prehospital initiation of reteplase for ST-elevation myocardial infarction: results of the Early Retavase-Thrombolysis in Myocardial Infarctoin (ER-TIMI) 19 trial. *J Am Coll Cardiol* 2002;40(1):71–77.

125. Bonnefoy E, Lapostolle F, Leizorovicz A, et al. Primary angioplasty versus prehospital fibrinolysis in acute myocardial infarction: a randomised study. *Lancet* 2002;360(9336):825–829.

126. Eisenberg MS, Cummins RO, Damon S, et al. Survival rates from out-of-hospital cardiac arrest: recommendations for uniform definitions and data to report. *Ann Emerg Med* 1990;19:1249–1259.

127. Holmberg M, Holmberg S, Herlitz J. An alternate estimate of the disappearance rate of ventricular fibrillation in out-of-hospital cardiac arrest in Sweden. *Resuscitation* 2001;49:219–220.

128. Adrie C, Adib-Conquy M, Laurent I, et al. Successful cardiopulmonary resuscitation after cardiac arrest as a "sepsis-like" syndrome. *Circulation* 2002;106(5):562–568.

129. Shyu KG, Chang H, Lin CC, et al. Concentrations of serum interleukin-8 after successful cardiopulmonary resuscitation in patients with cardiopulmonary arrest. *Am Heart J* 1997;134(3): 551–556.

130. Gando S, Nanzaki S, Morimoto Y, et al. Alterations of soluble L- and P-selectins during cardiac arrest and CPR. *Intens Care Med* 1999;25(6):588–593.

131. Bottiger BW, Motsch J, Braun V, et al. Marked activation of complement and leukocytes and an increase in the concentrations of soluble endothelial adhesion molecules during cardiopulmonary resuscitation and early reperfusion after cardiac arrest in humans. *Crit Care Med* 2002;30(11):2473–2480.

132. Bottiger BW, Motsch J, Bohrer H, et al. Activation of blood coagulation after cardiac arrest is not balanced adequately by activation of endogenous fibrinolysis. *Circulation* 1995;92(9): 2572–2578.

133. Gando S, Kameue T, Nanzaki S, et al. Massive fibrin formation with consecutive impairment of fibrinolysis in patients with out-of-hospital cardiac arrest. *Thromb Haemost* 1997;77(2):278–282.

134. Laurent I, Adrie C, Vinsonneau C, et al. High-volume hemofiltration after out-of-hospital cardiac arrest: a randomized study. *J Am Coll Cardiol* 2005;46(3):432–437.

135. Vgontas AN, Bixler EO, Lin H-M, et al. I-6 and its circadian secretion in humans. *Neuroimmunomodulation* 2005;12(3):131–140.

136. Lefer DJ, Granger DN. Oxidative stress and cardiac disease. *Am J Med* 2000;109(4):315–323.

137. Anderson T, Vanden Hoek TL. Preconditioning and the oxidants of sudden death. *Curr Opin Crit Care* 2003;9(3):194–198.

138. Chen Q, Vazquez EJ, Moghaddas S, et al. Production of reactive oxygen species by mitochondria: central role of complex III. *J Biol Chem* 2003;278(38):36027–36031.

139. Nolan JP, Morley PT, Vanden Hoek TL, et al. Therapeutic hypothermia after cardiac arrest: an advisory statement by the advanced life support task force of the International Liaison Committee on Resuscitation. *Circulation* 2003;108(1): 118–121.

140. Laurent I, Monchi M, Chiche JD, et al. Reversible myocardial dysfunction in survivors of out-of-hospital cardiac arrest. *J Am Coll Cardiol* 2002;40(12):2110–2116.

141. Assessment of the Safety and Efficacy of a New Thrombolytic (ASSENT-2) Investigators. Single-bolus tenecteplase compared with front-loaded alteplase in acute myocardial infarction: the ASSENT-2 double-blind randomized trial. *Lancet* 1999;354(9180): 716–722.

142. Van de Werf F, Cannon CP, Luyten A, et al. Safety assessment of single-bolus administration of TNK tissue-plasminogen activator in acute myocardial infarction: the ASSENT-1 trial. The ASSENT-1 Investigators. *Am Heart J* 1999;137(5): 786–791.

143. The GUSTO Investigators. An international randomized trial comparing four thrombolytic strategies for acute myocardial infarction,. *N Engl J Med* 1993;329:673–682.

144. Randomized trial of intravenous heparin versus recombinant hirudin for acute coronary syndromes. The Global Use of Strategies to Open Occluded Coronary Arteries (GUSTO) IIa Investigators. *Circulation* 1994;90(4):1631–1637.

145. Randomised trial of intravenous atenolol among 16,027 cases of suspected acute myocardial infarction: ISIS-1. First International

PART ONE • ACUTE CORONARY SYNDROMES

Study of Infarct Survival Collaborative Group. *Lancet* 1986;2(8498):57–66.

146. Effectiveness of intravenous thrombolytic treatment in acute myocardial infarction. Gruppo Italiano per lo Studio della Streptochinasi nell'Infarto Miocardico (GISSI). *Lancet* 1986;1(8478):397–402.

147. GISSI-2: a factorial randomised trial of alteplase versus streptokinase and heparin versus no heparin among 12,490 patients with acute myocardial infarction. Gruppo Italiano per lo Studio della Sopravvivenza nell'Infarto Miocardico [see comments]. *Lancet* 1990;336(8707):65–71.

148. In-hospital mortality and clinical course of 20,891 patients with suspected acute myocardial infarction randomised between alteplase and streptokinase with or without heparin. The International Study Group [ee comments]. *Lancet* 1990;336(8707):71–75.

149. GISSI-3: effects of lisinopril and transdermal glyceryl trinitrate singly and together on 6-week mortality and ventricular function after acute myocardial infarction. Gruppo Italiano per lo Studio della Sopravvivenza nell'infarto Miocardico [see comments]. *Lancet* 1994;343(8906):1115–1122.

150. Randomised trial of intravenous streptokinase, oral aspirin, both, or neither among 17,187 cases of suspected acute myocardial infarction: ISIS-2. ISIS-2 (Second International Study of Infarct Survival) Collaborative Group [see comments]. *Lancet* 1988; 2(8607):349–360.

151. ISIS-3: a randomised comparison of streptokinase vs tissue plasminogen activator vs anistreplase and of aspirin plus heparin vs aspirin alone among 41,299 cases of suspected acute myocardial infarction. ISIS-3 (Third International Study of Infarct Survival) Collaborative Group [see comments]. *Lancet* 1992;339(8796):753–770.

Chapter 3
Evaluation, Differential Diagnosis, and Approach to the Patient with Possible Acute Coronary Syndrome

Judd E. Hollander

The standard 12-lead electrocardiogram is the single best test to identify patients with acute myocardial infarction and ST-segment Elevation MI (STEMI) immediately upon ED presentation,[1] despite the fact that it has relatively low sensitivity for detection of acute coronary syndromes.

- Significance of history and physical findings in possible ACS patients
- The 12-lead electrocardiogram (ECG) as central to evaluation
- Utility of cardiac markers in decision making and risk stratification
- Imaging modalities in ED patients with chest pain
- Disposition from the ED—home, hospital, decision unit

Introduction

Chest pain is the most common potential life-threatening complaint for patients presenting to the emergency department (ED), occurring in approximately 8 million patients annually in the United States.[2]

Chest pain, shortness of breath, and other symptoms of potential acute coronary syndrome (ACS) present an initial diagnostic challenge. Demographics, traditional risk factors, chest pain characteristics, and physical examination can assist disposition decisions but are insufficient by themselves to identify patients safe for ED release.[3–9] Patients with acute myocardial infarction (AMI) can present with a wide variety of symptoms, making diagnosis difficult.[10–12] Some patients may have objective evidence of a clear-cut diagnosis; however, the majority do not.[13]

Physicians maintain a low threshold for admitting patients to exclude an ACS. As a result, the percentage of patients admitted to coronary care units who actually suffer cardiac ischemia has been reported to be as low as 15% to 30% historically, and up to $8 billion to $10 billion a year is spent on hospital stays to rule out AMI and ACS.[7,12–16] Despite this high rate of admission, up to 2% to 5% of patients with AMI are still inappropriately discharged from the ED, with concomitant increased morbidity and mortality.[10,12,15–16] Missed AMI ranks as the highest single diagnosis in terms of dollars paid and third highest in terms of frequency of claims in malpractice against emergency physicians.[17]

History

A carefully conducted history and physical examination comprise the initial assessment of patients presenting with potential ACS. The precision of clinical features for the evaluation of chest pain is quite variable.[18–21] Hickan et al. found that features associated with a lower probability of AMI, such as pleuritic, positional, and sharp chest pain, showed poor to fair interphysician reliability (kappa values of 0.27–0.44). High-risk features (radiation to left arm, substernal location, and history of AMI) were more reliable (kappa 0.74–0.89).[18] Thus, history is most reliable in "ruling in" high-risk patients but is less reliable when being used to "rule out" ACS. Likelihood ratios for several clinical features are shown in Table 3-1.

Cardiac Risk Factors

In the presence of symptoms, cardiac risk factors are poor predictors of risk for MI or ACS.[9,22] Traditional cardiac risk factors, such as hypertension, diabetes mellitus, tobacco use, family history of coronary artery disease (CAD) at an early age, and hypercholesterolemia, are not predictive of the cardiac risk in ED patients with chest pain. Traditional cardiac risk factors were derived from population-based longitudinal cohort studies of asymptomatic patients. In contrast, ED patients with chest pain have already been identified as being at increased risk by the very fact that they have symptoms.

| TABLE 3-1 • Likelihood Ratios for Clinical Features That Increase or Decrease Risk of AMI in Patients Presenting With Chest Pain

Clinical Feature	Likelihood Ratio (95% CI)
Increased Likelihood of AMI	
Described as pressure	1.3 (1.2–1.5)
Pain in chest or left arm	2.7[a]
Chest pain radiation	
• To right arm or shoulder	4.7 (1.9–12)
• To left arm	2.3 (1.7–3.1)
• To both left and right arms	7.1 (3.6–14.2)
• To both arms or shoulders	4.1 (2.5–6.5)
Chest pain most important symptom	2.0[a]
Chest pain associated with exertion	2.4 (1.5–3.8)
Worse than previous angina or similar to prior AMI	1.8 (1.6–2.0)
History of MI	1.5–3.0[b]
Nausea or vomiting	1.9 (1.7–2.3)
Diaphoresis	2.0 (1.9–2.2)
Third heart sound	3.2 (1.6–6.5)
Hypotension (systolic BP <80 mm Hg)	3.1 (1.8–5.2)
Pulmonary crackles	2.1 (1.4–3.1)
Decreased Likelihood of AMI	
Pleuritic chest pain	0.2 (0.1–0.3)
Described as sharp	0.3 (0.2–0.5)
Positional chest pain	0.3 (0.2–0.5)
Reproduced by palpation	0.3 (0.2–0.4)
Inframammary location	0.8 (0.7–0.9)
Not associated with exertion	0.8 (0.6–0.9)

[a]Data not available to calculate confidence intervals.
[b]In heterogeneous studies the likelihood ratios are reported as ranges.
Sources: Adapted from Panju AA, Hemmelgarm BR, Guyatt GH, et al. Is this patient having a myocardial infarction? *JAMA* 1998;280:1256–1263, and Swap CJ, Nagurney JT. Value and limitations of chest pain history in the evaluation of patients with suspected acute coronary syndromes. *JAMA* 2005;294:2623–2629.

The presence of symptoms outweighs the predictive abilities of cardiac risk factors. A lack of cardiac risk factors does not sufficiently decrease cardiac risk in ED patients such that they can be expeditiously released from the ED unless they are <40 years old and have normal ECGs.[22–25]

A lack of cardiac risk factors does not sufficiently decrease cardiac risk in ED patients such that they can be expeditiously released from the ED, unless the patient is less than 40 years old and has a normal electrocardiogram.

Physical Examination

Likewise, the use of the physical examination to distinguish patients with ACS from patients with noncardiac chest pain is suboptimal. Patients with ACS may appear deceptively well without any clinical signs of distress or may be uncomfortable, pale, cyanotic, and in respiratory distress. Heavy reliance on individual physical examination findings is not wise. The first and second heart sounds may be diminished due to poor myocardial contractility, even in the absence of myocardial ischemia. An S3 is present in only 15% to 20% of patients with AMI, but it is also common in those with heart failure. An S4 is common in patients with long-standing hypertension or myocardial dysfunction with or without acute ischemia. The presence of a murmur can be an ominous sign (flail leaflet of the mitral valve or a ventricular septal defect), or it can reflect long-standing valvular heart disease. Signs and symptoms of congestive heart failure have poor interrater reliability (S3 gallop, kappa = 0.14–0.37; rales, 0.12–0.31; neck vein distention, 0.31–0.51; hepatomegaly, 0.00–0.16; and dependent edema, 0.27–0.64).[19] Thus the use of these individual signs and symptoms as strong guides to management can be misleading in the ED setting.

Atypical Presentations

Atypical presentations and silent myocardial ischemia are common. Some 22% to 40% of patients with Q-wave MI are clinically unrecognized.[26] Women and the elderly are more likely to have atypical presentations. The prognosis for patients who have atypical symptoms at the time of their infarction is worse than that of patients who had more typical symptoms.

The response to initial therapy is not useful in "ruling in" or "ruling out" an ACS. Relief of symptoms with either nitroglycerin or a "GI cocktail" occurs in pain related and unrelated to myocardial ischemia.[27–30]

Differential Diagnosis

The differential diagnosis of chest pain and shortness of breath is extensive, with ACS being the most common potentially life-threatening condition. Other life-threatening conditions include aortic dissection, pulmonary embolism, tension pneumothorax, pericardial tamponade, and mediastinitis.

Approximately 15% to 30% of patients who present to the ED with nontraumatic chest pain have ACS.[7,12–16,31–32] The 28-day case mortality rate for an ACS among patients in developed nations is approximately 10% but varies with the severity of disease and the treatment provided.

Aortic Dissection

The incidence of aortic dissection is estimated at 3 per 100,000 patients per year.[33] Aortic dissection most commonly affects patients with systemic hypertension in their seventh decade of life. The probability of aortic dissection increases when pain is of abrupt onset with a sharp, tearing, and/or ripping character; there is a variation in pulse (absence of a proximal extremity or carotid pulse) and/or blood pressure (difference of >20 mm Hg between the right and left arms), and the chest radiography shows mediastinal or aortic widening.[34,35]

Pulmonary Embolism

The incidence of pulmonary embolism (PE) is estimated at over 1 in 1,000 patients, but the diagnosis is often missed and the incidence may be higher.[36] Risk stratification depends on the pretest probability for PE. Several scoring systems exist to characterize patient risk for PE, including the Canadian (Wells) score, the Charlotte rule, the Geneva score, and others.[37–40] Patients with symptoms suggestive of PE and right ventricular dysfunction or hemodynamic instability are at high risk for PE and major comorbidity and death.

Pneumothorax

Pneumothorax can occur spontaneously or following trauma or pulmonary procedures. Patients with primary spontaneous pneumothorax tend to be younger males who are tall and thin. Secondary spontaneous pneumothorax occurs with greatest frequency in patients with chronic obstructive pulmonary disease, cystic fibrosis, or asthma.[41] Tension pneumothorax is diagnosed clinically by the presence of unilateral decreased breath sounds, hypotension, and shifting of the trachea in the opposite direction.

Mediastinitis

Mediastinitis is less frequent and occurs following odontogenic infections, esophageal perforation, and iatrogenic complications of cardiac surgery or upper gastrointestinal and airway procedures. "Hamman's crunch," heard over the anterior chest, is strongly suggestive. Mortality for patients with mediastinitis remains high (14%–42%), even when it is treated with operative debridement and antibiotics.[42–45]

Pericardial Tamponade

Pericardial tamponade results in a direct compromise in cardiac filling, producing a picture resembling cardiogenic shock that requires emergent reduction in pericardial pressure by pericardiocentesis. Tamponade may occur with aortic dissection, after thoracic trauma, or as a consequence of acute pericarditis from infection, malignancy, uremia, or other causes.

Other Conditions

Other conditions are more common but less serious. Gastroesophageal reflux disease, esophageal spasm, hiatal hernias, as well as upper abdominal processes can cause chest pain. Gastrointestinal causes account for the symptoms of a sizable number of patients who complain of chest pain and do not have an ACS. Respiratory infections such as pneumonia and bronchitis are frequently accompanied by chest discomfort but can usually be identified on the basis of cough and fever. Chest tightness is a common complaint in patients with acute exacerbations of asthma, which can often be distinguished by wheezing on examination.

Acute decompensated heart failure can result in chest discomfort that may or may not represent an ACS because heart failure is the result of chronic CAD and other cardiovascular conditions in some patients.[46,47] Valvular heart disease, such as aortic stenosis, can result in chest pain that often signifies severe disease, while mitral valve prolapse is associated with chest pain that may have few if any long-term consequences. Infectious or inflammatory causes of chest discomfort include pericarditis, myocarditis, and endocarditis.

Chest heaviness or discomfort may be noted with pleural effusions. Pulmonary malignancy can cause chest pain if there is pleural involvement. Musculoskeletal causes of chest pain include muscle strains and costochondritis as well as overuse syndromes. Herpes zoster can usually be identified as the cause of chest pain, but in rare instances the pain may be evident prior to the exanthem.

Electrocardiogram

The standard 12-lead electrocardiogram (ECG) is the single best test to identify patients with STEMI immediately upon ED presentation,[7] despite the fact that it has relatively low sensitivity for the detection of ACS. The sensitivity of ST-segment deviation for the detection of AMI is 35% to 50%, leaving more than half of all AMI patients unidentified.[7,48]

However, even among patients with ST-segment-elevation MI (STEMI), ECG variables can further risk-stratify the likelihood of 30-day mortality (Table 3-2).[49] ECG criteria that increase the risk of AMI in ED patients with chest pain are shown in Tables 3-2 and 3-3.[20] Patients with normal or nonspecific ECGs have a 1%–5% incidence of AMI and a 4% to 23% incidence of unstable angina.[7,48,50,51] Patients with nondiagnostic ECGs or with ischemia that is not known to be old have a 4% to 7% incidence of AMI and a 21% to 48% incidence of unstable angina. Demonstration of new ischemia increases the risk of AMI to 25% to 73%, and the unstable angina risk to 14% to 43%.[7] A normal diagnostic 12-lead ECG cannot conclusively exclude ACS.[7,52] The ECG should be used in conjunction with clinical history and cardiac markers to determine admission location and treatment for patients with ACS.

Continuous ECG Monitoring

Because of the relatively poor sensitivity of the standard 12-lead ECG to detect patients with ACS, additional electrocardiographic strategies have been proposed. A continuous 12-lead ECG monitors and records new ECGs every

| TABLE 3-2 • Multivariate Significance of the Electrocardiogram in Patients With STEMI Enrolled in GUSTO-1

Electrocardiographic Feature	Odds Ratio (95% CI)
Sum of ST-segment deviation (19 vs. 8 mm)	1.53 (1.38–1.69)
Sum of ST-segment decrease (–1 vs. –7 mm)	0.77 (0.72–0.83)
Heart rate (84 vs. 60 bpm)	1.49 (1.41–1.59)
Sum ST-segment increase in II, III, and aVF (6 vs. 0 mm)	0.79 (0.71–0.89)
QRS duration 100 vs. 80 msec	
• Anterior infarct	1.55 (1.43–1.68)
• Other location	1.08 (1.03–1.13)
Anterior infarction	
• QRS duration 100 msec	1.08 (1.03–1.13)
• QRS duration 50 msec	0.61 (0.43–0.86)
Inferior infarction	
• No prior AMI	0.67 (0.50–0.90)
• Prior AMI	1.41 (0.98–2.02)
Prior infarction	
• Inferior infarction	2.47 (2.02–3.00)
• Other location	1.17 (0.98–1.41)

Source: Hathaway WR, Peterson ED, Wagner GS, et al. Prognostic significance of the initial electrocardiogram in patients with acute myocardial infarction. *JAMA* 1998;279:387–391.

| TABLE 3-3 • Electrocardiographic Features Predictive of AMI in Patients With Acute Chest Pain

Electrocardiographic Feature	Likelihood Ratio (95% CI)
New ST-segment elevation ≥1 mm	5.7–53.9[a]
New Q wave	5.3–24.8[a]
Any ST-segment elevation	11.2 (7.1–17.8)
New conduction defect	6.3 (2.5–15.7)
New ST-segment depression	3.0–5.2[a]
Any Q wave	3.9 (2.7–5.7)
Any ST-segment depression	3.2 (2.5–4.1)
T wave peaking and/or inversion ≥1 mm	3.1[b]
New T-wave inversion	2.4–2.8[a]
Any conduction defect	2.7 (1.4–5.4)

[a]In heterogeneous studies the likelihood ratios are reported as ranges.
[b]Data not available to calculate confidence intervals.
Source: Panju AA, Hemmelgarm BR, Guyatt GH, et al. Is this patient having a myocardial infarction? *JAMA* 1998;280:1256–1263, with permission.

20 seconds. When the ST-segment baseline is altered, it sets off an alarm and prints a copy of the new ECG. This technology is most often employed in chest pain–observation units, where it might be useful for monitoring patients who present with non-AMI ACS for ECG evidence of injury.[48] Because of costs, concerns regarding labile ST-segment and T-wave changes from hyperventilation or patient movement, and a lack of ED-based prospective studies demonstrating clinically relevant differences in outcome, continuous 12-lead ECGs have not been recommended for routine use.[48]

Additional ECG Leads

Other ECGs with 15, 18, and 22 leads have been studied.[48,53] In one study, addition of V4R, V8, and V9 increased the sensitivity to detect ST-segment elevation to 59% without a loss of specificity.[53] The addition of V4R to V6R and V7 to V9 as posterior leads led to an 8% increase in sensitivity for AMI relative to a standard 12-lead ECG but at the cost of a 7% decrease in specificity.[54] Twenty-two–lead and body-surface-mapping ECGs have not been sufficiently studied to recommend their use. Right-sided leads (rV4) should be used in the setting of inferior wall infarction to assess possible RV involvement.[48]

ECG Confounders

There are several clinical conditions where ECG interpretation of ACS is difficult, particularly paced rhythms and

left-bundle-branch block (LBBB) (Table 3-4). In the setting of a LBBB, the presence of ST-segment elevation ≥1 mm and concordance with the QRS complex or ST-segment depression ≥1 mm in leads V1, V2, or V3 suggest AMI.[55] ST-segment elevation ≥5 mm that is discordant with the QRS complex increases the likelihood of AMI but has poor specificity.

Uncomplicated right ventricular pacing causes secondary repolarization changes of opposing polarity to that of the predominant QRS complex. Most leads have predominant negative QRS complexes followed by ST-segment elevation and positive T waves. ST-segment elevation ≥5 mm is most indicative of AMI in leads with predominantly negative QRS complexes. Any ST-segment elevation concordant with the QRS complex in a predominantly positive QRS complex is highly specific for AMI. The QRS complex is predominantly negative in leads V1 to V3. ST-segment depression in these leads had 80% specificity for AMI.[56]

Risk-Stratification Algorithms

Although clinical and computer algorithms can successfully risk-stratify patients, they are not able to reliably identify a group of patients at such low risk of an ACS that they could be safely and immediately released from the Emergency Department.

Several risk-stratification algorithms have been studied and validated.

TABLE 3-4 • Some Clinical Conditions Where the Electrocardiogram Interpretation Can Be Difficult

May have ST Segment Elevation in the Absence of AMI
Early repolarization
Left ventricular hypertrophy
Pericarditis
Myocarditis
Left ventricular aneurysms
Idiopathic hypertrophic subaortic stenosis (IHSS)
Hypothermia
Paced rhythms
Left bundle-branch block

May have ST-segment Depressions in the Absence of Ischemia
Hypokalemia
Digoxin effect
Cor pulmonale and right heart strain
Early repolarization
Left ventricular hypertrophy
Paced rhythms
Left bundle-branch block

May have T-wave Inversions in the Absence of Ischemia
Persistent juvenile pattern
Stokes–Adams syncope or seizures
Posttachycardia T-wave inversion
Postpacemaker T-wave inversion
Intracranial pathology (CNS bleeds)
Mitral valve prolapse
Pericarditis
Primary or secondary myocardial diseases
Pulmonary embolism or cor pulmonale from other causes
Spontaneous pneumothorax
Myocardial contusion
Left ventricular hypertrophy
Paced rhythms
Left bundle-branch block

Source: Hollander JE. Acute coronary syndromes: unstable angina, myocardial ischemia and infarction. In Tintanelli JE, Kelen GD, Stapczynski JS, eds. *Emergency Medicine: A Comprehensive Study Guide*, 6th ed. New York: McGraw-Hill, 2003:343–352.

Goldman Risk Score

The Goldman risk score was derived through analysis of clinical data on a large cohort of patients presenting to the ED with chest pain. It has been prospectively validated and is useful as an initial risk stratification tool.[4] The final algorithm is heavily based on ECG findings and chest pain characteristics (Fig. 3-1). It does not incorporate cardiac marker results. The Goldman algorithm stratifies patients into groups with risks of AMI that vary from 1% to 77%. The sensitivity of the Goldman chest pain protocol for predicting AMI is 88% to 91% with a specificity of 78% to 92%.[57] It does not identify any group with <1% risk who might be safe for ED release. Even in the group of patients deemed to be low risk, the addition of initially negative cardiac troponin I was still associated with a 5% rate of 30-day adverse outcomes.[58] The Goldman algorithm can be used to predict the need for intensive care unit (ICU) admission, development of cardiovascular complications, and outcome in a clinical decision or short-stay observation unit.[14]

The Goldman criteria protocol does not identify any group with <1% risk who might be safe for ED release. Even in the group of patients deemed to be low risk, the addition of initially negative cardiac troponin I was still associated with a 5% rate of 30-day adverse outcomes.

ST-segment elevation or Q waves on the ECG, other ECG findings indicating myocardial ischemia, low systolic blood pressure, pulmonary rales above the bases, or an exacerbation of known ischemic heart disease all predicted complications. This algorithm has been independently validated and strict adherence to the protocol would reduce ICU admissions by 16%, resulting in potentially large cost savings.[59]

ACI-TIPI

The ACI-TIPI is a computer-generated method to determine the likelihood of ACS at the time of initial clinical evaluation. The ACI-TIPI ECG incorporates age, sex, presence of chest or left arm pain, a chief symptom of chest or left arm pain, pathologic Q waves, and the presence and degree of ST-segment elevation or depression and T-wave elevation or inversion. It reports the percent likelihood of "acute cardiac ischemia" on the electrocardiographic record. Four studies including 5,496 patients have found that when combined with physician impression, the ACI-TIPI has a sensitivity of 86% to 95% and a specificity of 78% to 92% for predicting ACS.[57] When house staff without prior emergency medicine training use the ACI-TIPI, it can speed the time to a disposition decision.[60] In a study of over 10,000 patients with potential ACS, in the subset of patients ultimately not felt to have cardiac ischemia, use of ACI-TIPI was associated with a non–statistically significant reduction in coronary care unit (CCU) admissions from 15% to 12% and a slight increase in ED discharges to home from 49% to 52%.[61] The ACI-TIPI has not been widely incorporated into clinical practice in EDs. The ACI-TIPI has not been shown to make a clinically relevant difference in diagnostic accuracy compared with contemporary emergency physician judgment.

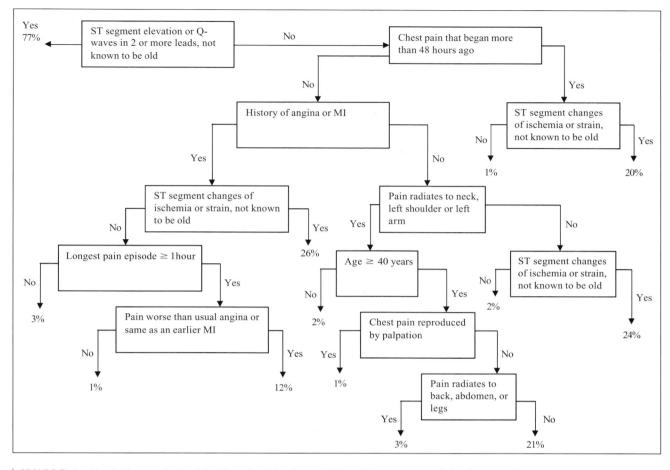

FIGURE 3-1 • The Goldman risk-stratification algorithm for prediction of acute myocardial infarction. (From Lee TH, Juarez G, Cook EF, et al. Ruling out myocardial infarction: a prospective multicenter validation of a 12-hour strategy for patients at low risk. *N Engl J Med* 1991;324:1239–1246.)

The ACI-TIPI has not been shown to make a clinically relevant difference in diagnostic accuracy compared with contemporary emergency physician judgment.

Artificial Neural Networks

The artificial neural network is a nonlinear statistical paradigm shown to be a powerful modality for the recognition of complex patterns; it can maintain accuracy even when some input data are missing. It is thought that the network's ability to allow variable weighting to input information, as opposed to the fixed weighting of other statistical approaches, allows it to perform more accurately than these other approaches.

The artificial neural network can accurately identify the presence of myocardial infarction in patients with anterior chest pain.[62–64] When initial cardiac troponin I and CK-MB determinations are added to the variables used by the network, the network had a sensitivity of 95% and a specificity of 96% despite the fact that an average of 5% of the input data

required by the network were missing on all patients.[63] For prediction of AMI, the neural network has better sensitivity and specificity than the Goldman risk score and ACI-TIPI score. In the same data set, a Goldman risk of ≥7% had a sensitivity of 74% and specificity of 68%. An ACI-TIPI score ≥25% had a sensitivity of 62% and specificity of 73%.[64] The artificial neural network achieved these predictive properties using only data available at the time of ED arrival. It incorporates more clinical information than either the Goldman score or ACI-TIPI (Table 3-5). Despite the improved performance, clinicians seem unwilling to incorporate this "black box" feedback into clinical decision making.[65]

TIMI Risk Score

The TIMI risk score is a seven-item score (Table 3-6) that helps the emergency physician to risk-stratify patients with ACS. It was derived in a high-risk unstable angina/non–ST-segment-elevation MI (UA/NSTEMI) patient population where 14-day event rates increased significantly as the TIMI risk score increased: 4.7% for a score of 0/1; 8.3% for 2; 13.2% for 3; 19.9% for 4; 26.2% for 5; and 40.9% for 6 or

| TABLE 3-5 • Clinical Criteria Included in Several ED Risk Stratification Schemes

	Goldman Score	ACI–TIPI	Baxt Neural Network
Demographics	Age ≥40 years	Age	Age
		Gender	Gender
			Race
Presentation characteristics	Chest pain duration ≥48 hours	Presence of chest or left arm pain	Left anterior chest pain Left arm pain
	Longest pain episode >1 hour	Chief symptom of chest or left arm pain	
	History of angina or MI		History of prior coronary disease, AMI, angina, or CHF
	Pain worse than usual angina or same as prior MI		Pain pressing in nature Pain crushing in nature
	Pain radiates to neck, left shoulder, or left arm		Pain radiating to neck Pain radiating to left arm
	Pain radiates to back, abdomen, or legs		
	Chest pain reproduced by palpation		
	Chest pain is stabbing		
			Shortness of breath Diaphoresis Nausea and vomiting
History			Hypertension Diabetes mellitus Elevated cholesterol Family history of coronary artery disease
Electrocardiographic criteria	ST-segment elevation or Q waves in two or more leads, not known to be old	Pathologic Q waves	Q waves old Q waves not known to be old
	ST-segment changes of ischemia or strain, not known to be old	Presence and degree of ST-segment elevation or depression	ST-segment elevation old ST-segment elevation not known to be old
		T-wave elevation or inversion	T-wave inversion old T-wave inversion not known to be old
			ST-segment depression old ST-segment depression not known to be old
			Left bundle-branch block old Left bundle-branch block not known to be old
			Hyperacute T waves old Hyperacute T waves not known to be old
Cardiac marker determination			Including presentation CK, CK-MB, and troponin I

| TABLE 3-6 • Elements of the TIMI Score for Unstable Angina

Age ≥65 years

Three or more traditional risk factors for coronary artery disease

Prior coronary stenosis of 50% or more

ST-segment deviation on presenting electrocardiogram

Two or more anginal events in prior 24 hours

Aspirin use within the 7 days prior to presentation

Elevated cardiac markers

The presence of each of the above is assigned 1 point. The maximum possible score is 7.

7.[66] When it was applied to a broad-based patient population with chest pain in two studies,[67,68] it performed similarly and was able to risk-stratify the patients with respect to 30-day death, AMI, and revascularization. Moreover, it performed well with regard to both males and females.[69]

Presence of Alternative Diagnoses

One theoretical reason why clinical and computer algorithms cannot identify patients that do *not* have ACS is that they have focused on symptoms consistent *with* a diagnosis of either an AMI[2,3,66] or an ACS.[64,66,67] No risk-stratification algorithm for patients with potential ACS has incorporated information about noncardiac conditions.[13] Three studies have evaluated whether a strong clinical impression of an alternative noncardiac diagnosis might reduce the likelihood of death or cardiovascular events to a low enough level to allow safe and immediate release from the ED.

Miller et al. studied whether a physician impression of noncardiac chest pain was adequate to exclude an ACS.[70] In a large multicenter study of 17,737 patients, they found that 6.8% of patients felt to have noncardiac disease at the conclusion of the ED evaluation had had possible and 2.8% definite 30-day adverse cardiovascular events.

Disla et al. examined patients given a diagnosis of costochondritis.[71] Despite a diagnosis of costochondritis in the ED that was confirmed by a rheumatologist, 6% sustained an AMI. This AMI rate was similar to that observed in many studies of a broad population of ED patients with chest pain.[32,63,64]

Hollander et al., in a study of 1,995 ED patients with potential ACS, found that the presence of a definite alternative noncardiac diagnosis was associated with a reduced risk of an in-hospital triple composite endpoint (death/MI/ revascularization) with a risk ratio of 0.32 (95% CI, 0.19– 0.55), and 30-day triple composite endpoint with a risk ratio of 0.45 (95% CI, 0.29–0.69).[13] However, patients with a definite alternative

noncardiac diagnosis still had a 4% event rate at 30 days (95% confidence interval, 2.4%–5.6%).[13] Thus, use of this criterion alone for safe and immediate release of ED patients that present with potential ACS is not possible.

Markers of Myocardial Injury

The utility of individual cardiac markers depends upon their ability to detect and risk stratify patients with potential ACS. Ideally, a marker with a high sensitivity and high negative predictive value is useful to allow expeditious evaluation and discharge from the ED. Markers with high specificity and positive predictive values are ideal to tailor aggressive care for patients at high risk of cardiovascular complications.

Creatine Kinase MB Fraction

Levels of creatine kinase MB fraction (CK-MB) rise to twice the normal limit within 6 hours and peak within 12 to 24 hours of AMI. Serial CK-MB mass measurements have nearly a 90% sensitivity 3 hours after ED presentation (approximately 6 hours after symptom onset) but are only 36% to 48% sensitive when utilized at or shortly after presentation.[57,72] Single CK-MB measurements cannot be safely used to assist in the admission/discharge decision since they result in an unacceptably high miss rate for AMI and cardiovascular complications. Serial CK-MB measurements over 6 to 9 hours have been widely employed in chest pain observation units and, if negative, are considered sufficient, to safely exclude AMI or allow further diagnostic testing or ED release, depending upon the clinical scenario.[73] An alternative strategy is to examine the change in CK-MB values within 2 hours of ED presentation (Δ CK-MB). A rise in CK-MB ≥1.6 ng/mL over the 2-hour period following presentation achieves a sensitivity for detection of AMI of 94%, which is better than using the 2-hour CK-MB value alone (75%).[74]

Patients with skeletal muscle disease, acute muscle exertion, chronic renal failure, and cocaine use can have elevations in levels of CK-MB in the absence of infarction.[75–78] To distinguish "true positive" elevations (secondary to myocardial injury) from the "false positive" elevations (due to skeletal muscle injury), the measurement of CK-MB as a percentage of total CK has been used (relative index).[79–80] The use of relative index rather than absolute CK-MB at the time of ED presentation to detect AMI improves specificity (96% vs. 93%) and positive predictive value (46% vs. 36%) but decreases sensitivity (52% vs. 47%) without significantly affecting negative predictive value (96% vs. 96%).[80]

Cardiac Troponins

Cardiac troponin I is the most specific marker for myocardial injury. Following AMI, cardiac troponin I becomes elevated at the same rate as CK-MB—it peaks at 12 to 24 hours but remains elevated for 7 to 10 days. Troponin I has a higher specificity for myocardial necrosis than CK-MB in selected subsets of patients with ACS, such as patients with recent surgery, cocaine use, chronic renal failure, and skeletal muscle disease.[69–72] In patients without these confounding conditions, cardiac troponin I has similar sensitivity and specificity for detection of AMI.[76,81,82] In both ED patients with unselected chest pain syndromes and those with definite ACS, elevations in cardiac troponin I predict cardiovascular complications independent of CK-MB and the ECG.[8,81–89]

Cardiac troponin T is released from the cell within 3 to 6 hours following symptom onset. Like troponin I, it remains elevated for 7 to 10 days after injury. Cardiac troponin T is also an independent marker of cardiovascular risk in patients with ACS.[81,83,84]

Combined analysis of four studies assessing the predictive properties of single cardiac troponin-I values (cTnI) at the time of presentation for AMI found a sensitivity of 39% and specificity of 93% (Table 3-7).[57] Analysis of six cardiac troponin-T (cTnT) studies found similar results.[57] Serial sampling increases sensitivities to 90% to 100% with specificities

of 83% to 96% for cTnI and 76% to 91% for cTnT.[57] Elevated values of the cardiac troponins at presentation in patients with NSTEMI increase the short-term risk of death 3.1-fold (1.6% vs. 5.2%).[84] Although the cardiac troponins are useful for both diagnosis and risk stratification of patients with chest pain,[85] and AMI, cardiac-marker testing in the ED will not identify most ED patients who subsequently develop adverse events.[86,87] Thus, patients with negative markers still require evaluation and testing as dictated by their clinical presentations. Elevation in cTnT (and less so cTnI) have been noted in patients with chronic renal failure.[90] Although these have been considered to be falsely positive, they do predict a worse outcome.

Myoglobin

Myoglobin has a lower molecular weight and is released more rapidly than CK-MB and the cardiac troponins during AMI. Serum myoglobin levels rise faster than CK-MB, reaching twice the normal values within 2 hours and peaking within 4 hours of AMI symptom onset. Myoglobin achieves its maximal diagnostic sensitivity within 5 hours of symptom onset.[89–91] The sensitivity of myoglobin at the time of ED presentation is 49%, exceeding that of CK-MB or troponins, but the specificity is lower (only 87%).[57] Serial quantitative testing over 1 hour, evaluating both absolute values

| TABLE 3-7 • Summary of Predictive Properties of Cardiac Markers of Diagnosis of AMI

Marker	No. Studies	No. Subjects	Sensitivity (95% CI)	Specificity (95% CI)	Diagnostic Odds Ratio (95% CI)
At Time of Presentation					
Creatine kinase	12	3,195	37 (31–44)	87 (80–91)	3.9 (2.7–5.7)
CK-MB	19	6,425	42 (36–48)	97 (95–98)	25 (18–36)
Myoglobin	18	4,172	49 (53–55)	91 (87–94)	11 (8–15)
Troponin I	4	1,149	39 (10–78)	93 (88–97)	11 (3.4–34)
Troponin T	6	1,348	39 (26–53)	93 (90–96)	9.5 (5.7–16)
CK-MB and myoglobin	3	2,283	83 (51–96)	82 (68–90)	17 (7.6–40)
Serial Markers					
Creatine kinase	2	786	69–99	68–84	12–220
CK-MB	14	11,625	79 (71–86)	96 (95–97)	140 (65–310)
Myoglobin	10	1,277	89 (80–94)	87 (80–92)	84 (44–160)
Troponin I	2	1,393	90–100	83–96	230–460
Troponin T	3	904	93 (85–97)	85 (76–91)	83 (33–210)
CK-MB and myoglobin	2	291	100	75–91	4.3–14

Source: Lau J, Ioannidis JPA, Balk EM, et al. Diagnosing acute cardiac ischemia in the emergency department: A systematic review of the accuracy and clinical effect of current technologies. Ann Emerg Med 2001;37:453–460.

and a change of 40 ng/mL, has 91% sensitivity and up to a 99% negative predictive value for AMI within 1 hour of ED presentation (approximately 3–4 hours after symptom onset).[92] An elevated myoglobin predicted a 3.4-fold risk of adverse cardiovascular events and identified some high-risk patients not otherwise identified by clinical characteristics, CK-MB, or cTnT.[88] The main advantage of myoglobin is early detection of patients with AMI. The disadvantage is that it has poor specificity for AMI in patients with concurrent trauma or renal failure. When myoglobin is used in appropriately selected patients, these issues are not a significant clinical problem.

Discordant Cardiac Markers

An elevation in CK-MB in the setting of a normal total CK is still predictive of ACS.[93] Most commonly, both CK-MB and troponin are either both elevated or both negative, thus facilitating the diagnosis of AMI. When the CK-MB is elevated in the absence of a cTnI elevation, it is most often a "false positive" CK-MB, but this situation is still associated with a 2.2-fold likelihood of ACS.[93] When one of the cardiac troponins is elevated in the absence of a CK-MB elevation, it is associated with a 4.8-fold increase in ACS diagnosis[93] and usually represents a delayed presentation reflecting the longer time period of troponin elevations than of CK-MB. Patients presenting very early (<2–3 hours after symptom onset) may have elevations in myoglobin in the absence of CK-MB or troponin elevations. Serial testing will clarify if this is the case.

Markers of Inflammation and Platelet Activation

Some markers of inflammation and platelet activation are related to long-term prognosis in selected groups of patients; however, they do not have any proven utility in the acute setting. Markers of platelet activation, such as P-selectin and other integrins, are theoretically attractive because they can detect platelet activation prior to myocardial injury; however, when P-selectin was evaluated in the ED setting, it did not identify patients with AMI and ACS relative to patients with nonischemic chest pain syndromes any better than CK-MB (initial sensitivity, 46%; specificity, 76%).[94] The favorable predictive properties observed with inflammatory markers in longitudinal cohort studies of patients with potential CAD may not generalize to the ED, where most patients with potential ACS have confounding medical conditions that are likely to increase the prevalence of inflammatory markers.

Marker Combinations

When used individually at the time of ED presentation, markers of myocardial injury do not attain sufficient negative predictive value to safely allow immediate ED discharge. However, multimarker panels increase the early predictive value of these types of strategies. Although both troponins and CK-MB have approximately the same rate of rise, they have independent predictive value.[81–89] At the time of ED presentation, the use of both markers rather than either alone increases diagnostic sensitivity more than 25%.[88] Myoglobin and CK-MB, when used in combination, have a sensitivity of 85% at the time of presentation; in one study, they attained 100% sensitivity, specificity, and negative predictive value within 4 hours of ED presentation.[95] When patients with diagnostic ECGs were excluded, the sensitivity of this combination strategy was 80%, with a specificity of 84% at the time of presentation. Both sensitivity and specificity were 100% within 4 hours of ED arrival.[95] A combination of myoglobin and troponin I can achieve a diagnostic sensitivity of 97%, with a 99% negative predictive value, within 90 minutes of ED presentation.[96] The addition of CK-MB does not improve diagnostic accuracy within this time frame, but the CK-MB and myoglobin combination did have a 92% sensitivity and 99% negative predictive value within this same period.

The addition of B-type natriuretic peptide (BNP)—a neurohormone secreted from the cardiac ventricles in response to pressure or volume overload of the ventricle—to markers of cell death (CK-MB, troponin, and myoglobin) increases detection of patients with adverse cardiovascular outcomes early in the hospital course[97,98] and at the time of ED arrival.[99] The sensitivity of the initial markers for detection of a 30-day adverse outcome was 63% (95% CI, 53%–73%), specificity was 65% (95% CI, 61%–70%); negative predictive value, 93% (95% CI, 90%–96%) and positive predictive value, 20% (95% CI, 14%–26%).[99]

Imaging Modalities

Resting Sestamibi Imaging

Resting sestamibi imaging is useful for the early risk stratification of patients with potential ACS. Technetium sestamibi is taken up by the myocardium in proportion to myocardial blood flow and has prolonged retention in the myocardium with minimal redistribution after injection. This allows injection during symptomatic episodes, with subsequent imaging after patient stabilization. Confirming early small studies,[100,101] Tatum et al. reported that none of 338 patients with normal scans sustained AMI or cardiac death within 12 months.[102] An abnormal sestamibi scan was associated with a 50-fold increased risk of AMI and a 14.5-fold increased risk of revascularization over the next 30 days. There was a 30-fold increased risk of death over the ensuing 12 months.[102] Early perfusion imaging was as sensitive as serial cTnI measurements and considerably more sensitive than initial cTnI determinations.[103] The use of early resting sestamibi imaging can reduce unnecessary hospitalizations among patients without ACS without reducing appropriate admissions for patients with ACS.[104]

There are, however, significant practical issues that have prevented widespread implementation.[105] Radioisotope preparation in "batches" makes use in a single patient costly. Decreased accuracy occurs if injection does not occur during or shortly after pain, making timely injection essential. Timely injection by certified nuclear technologists is difficult to attain at most sites.

CT Coronary Angiography

Electron-beam CT (EBCT) alone has been demonstrated to have high sensitivity (92%) and specificity (94%) for the detection of high-grade stenosis and occlusion[106] and has high negative predictive value for cardiac events at both 30 days and 1 year[107–109]. Raggi, in a Bayesian analysis, found that EBCT provided a cost savings of 45% to 65% over a pathway including treadmill testing.[110]

EBCT detects coronary calcium but does not detect plaque without calcification or coronary stenosis, making it difficult to detect disease in young patients who might have plaque without significant calcifications. Studies in ED patients have demonstrated the safety of using the absence of coronary calcifications as criteria for risk stratification;[106–109] however, the addition of CT coronary angiography to calcium scoring further enhances this diagnostic test by detecting both coronary calcification and coronary atherosclerosis. Compared to coronary angiography by cardiac catheterization, CT coronary angiography has a mean difference in percent stenosis of 1.3% $\pm$ 14.2%;[111] it has a sensitivity of 86% to 96% and specificity of 91% to 95% for significant stenosis.[112,113]

Clinical studies assessing the utility of CT coronary angiography have focused on testing following "rule out" protocols in observation units as well as "immediate" testing, meaning in the early hours of the ED evaluation.

Gallagher et al.[114] compared the accuracy of CT coronary angiography with stress myocardial perfusion imaging for the detection of an ACS or 30-day major adverse cardiac events in low-risk chest pain patients following a "rule out" in an observation unit. All patients had both rest and stress myocardial perfusion imaging and CT coronary angiography. Patients with abnormal myocardial perfusion imaging (reversible perfusion defects) or CT coronary angiography results (stenosis >50% or calcium score >400) were considered for cardiac catheterization, and those with discordant results had a 30-day reevaluation. Of 85 study patients, 7 (8%) were found to have significant coronary stenosis and none had myocardial infarction or an adverse cardiovascular event during 30-day follow-up. The sensitivity of myocardial perfusion imaging was 71% (95% CI, 36%–92%); for CT coronary angiography, it was 86% (95% CI, 49%–97%). The specificity was 90% (81%–95%) and 92% (84%–96%), respectively. The negative predictive value of myocardial perfusion imaging and CT coronary angiography was 97% (90%–99%) and 99% (93%–100%), respectively, and the positive predictive value was 38% (18%–64%) and 50% (25%–75%), respectively. In this study, the performance of CT coronary angiography was at least as good as myocardial perfusion imaging in low-risk chest pain patients.

Goldstein et al.[115] studied 197 patients admitted to an observation unit who were randomized to either standard evaluation or CT coronary angiography. CT coronary angiography patients with minimal disease were discharged home. CT coronary angiography excluded or identified a cardiac etiology of chest pain in 75% of cases. As a result, 67 patients with normal coronary arteries were discharged home and 8 with severe disease were referred for immediate invasive evaluation. The CT coronary angiography findings necessitated referral for stress testing in 24% of patients, including 13 with intermediate stenoses. Compared with the standard evaluation, the use of CT coronary angiography resulted in reduced diagnostic time (3.4 vs. 15.0 hours, P <0.0001) and lowered costs ($1,586 vs. $1,872, P <0.0001). No patient in either group died or had an AMI.

Hollander et al.[116] reported results with the use of "immediate" CTA. Their clinical algorithm evaluated low-risk (defined as TIMI score $\leq$2) patients in the ED with CT coronary angiography after obtaining a serum creatinine level and a single set of cardiac markers. Patients with a negative CT coronary angiogram (no stenosis or a stenosis <50% and calcium score <100) were immediately discharged home without a complete rule-out or other provocative testing. Of the 54 patients enrolled, 46 (85%) were discharged from the ED after having negative CT coronary angiograms. None of the patients in the study had an adverse event during index hospitalization or at 30-day follow up (0%; 95% CI, 0%–6.6%). They used a 64-slice CT scanner for the majority of the patients. Some studies suggest that older model CT scanners (for example, 16-slice) do not appear to have the same diagnostic accuracy.[117–119]

Preliminary data from other groups also suggests that CT coronary angiography is useful for the risk stratification of patients with potential ACS.[119–121]

Immediate Provocative Testing

Stress testing is common in chest pain observation units despite a paucity of evidence to show that they are cost-effective tools for risk stratification of ED patients with chest pain. There are no large studies demonstrating the sensitivity and specificity for detection of CAD in this patient population, and some studies in this patient population have more "false positive" than "true positive" tests.[122] Exercise treadmill or pharmacologic testing with or without nuclear imaging as well as stress echocardiography are safe and can assist cardiovascular risk stratification in the ED.[123–125] Patients with an uneventful observation period, negative cardiac markers, and a normal stress test can be safely discharged with a referral for follow-up. There is some evidence supporting the use of immediate exercise testing in low-risk ED patients with chest pain without known ventricular dysfunction and with normal or nonspecific ECGs, even without serial cardiac-marker determination.[126,127]

Utility of Previous Diagnostic Testing for Coronary Artery Disease

The most common diagnostic imaging modality used to evaluate patients with potential ACS is an exercise or pharmacologic stress test. Relative to patients with an abnormal stress test, patients with normal tests are at lower risk for subsequent AMI.[128] However, patients that present to the ED with chest pain syndromes have often been previously evaluated.

Nerenberg et al. found that knowledge of a prior negative stress test did not affect the emergency physician's disposition decision when patients returned to the ED.[128,129] They also found that patients with a prior normal stress test are at the same risk of adverse cardiovascular events as those who have not previously undergone stress testing. Thus, knowledge of a previously normal stress did not and should not affect clinical decision making in the ED. Exercise-induced angina is caused by a fixed obstruction to flow; however, unstable angina, NSTEMI, and STEMI are caused by plaque rupture and thrombus formation in a lesion that may or may not have been significant enough to result in angina (or a positive stress test) prior to the acute process. Stress testing assesses whether or not a fixed obstruction to flow is present and cannot predict subsequent plaque rupture resulting in ischemia.

Patients with a prior normal stress test are at the same risk of adverse cardiovascular events as those who have not previously undergone stress testing. Thus, knowledge of a previously normal stress did not and should not affect clinical decision making in the ED.

Prior cardiac catheterization results are useful for risk stratification. Patients who have previously been documented to have minimal (<25%) stenosis or normal coronary arteriograms have an excellent long-term prognosis, with >98% free from myocardial infarction 10 years later.[130] Repeat cardiac catheterizations an average of 9 years later found that approximately 90% of patients did not develop even single-vessel CAD.[131] Thus, a recent cardiac catheterization with normal or minimally diseased vessels almost eliminates the possibility of an ACS, unlike a recent negative stress test, which is still associated with a 5% event rate at 30 days.[128]

ED Disposition

Once other life-threatening conditions have been excluded, patients without definite ACS on the ECG should be risk-stratified based upon the likelihood that they may have an ACS. The single best tool for the initial risk stratification of chest pain patients is the ECG,[7] despite the fact that it will not identify almost half of the patients with AMI. Validated tools (such as the TIMI score) should be used rather than simply clinical impression.[73]

Patients with a <1% risk of 30-day adverse events could be released home from the ED without further diagnostic testing or observation.

Patients with stable anginal patterns do not require inpatient evaluation.[73] Patients <40 years of age without any cardiac risk factors and without a prior cardiac history have a <1% risk of ACS and <1% risk of 30-day death, AMI, or revascularization. Likewise, patients <40 years old with a normal ECG and no prior cardiac history also have a <1% risk of ACS or adverse 30-day cardiovascular events.[23,24] These groups would be considered at very low risk for ACS; it would be reasonable to discharge them without further evaluation. Sestamibi imaging during acute chest pain or CT coronary angiography can sufficiently exclude ACS such that many patients with negative studies can be safely discharged from the ED without further observation or cardiac marker testing.[104,116]

Most patients at low risk should be treated in an ED observation unit or inpatient setting. Chest pain observation units allow brief periods of observation while obviating the need for more costly hospital admission in a large cohort of patients with nonspecific chest pain syndromes.[4,132–134] A variety of different protocols exist, but most observation protocols incorporate frequent testing of serial markers (at intervals of 1–4 hours) for at least 6 hours, telemetry monitoring, and some form of objective testing for patients that "rule out" for MI and presume that there are no cardiovascular complications during the observation period.[4,132–134] Patients without recurrent symptoms or cardiovascular complications and with negative cardiac marker determinations are safe for release from the ED.[4,132–134] If they are released without objective testing, low-risk patients should have follow-up testing arranged.[73] Delayed testing of this patient population does not appear to increase short-term risk.[135] Aggressive multiple marker strategies—including serial CK-MB, myoglobin, and cardiac troponin I values over 90 minutes—for low-risk chest pain patients may also allow for the safe, rapid release of some of these patients.[96]

Intermediate-risk patients should receive serial cardiac markers and objective testing. Elevated cardiac markers on initial determination may warrant "upgrading" of some patients originally triaged to non-ICU settings, since this increases the risk of adverse events. Patients with abnormal but nondiagnostic ECGs may benefit from more intensive observation and monitoring when initial cardiac markers are elevated.[49–51,82–84,86–87] Patients with normal or nonspecific ECGs are at low risk for complications and, therefore, do not automatically warrant more than a non-ICU telemetry setting unless dictated by other clinical parameters (ECG changes, continued chest pain, or cardiovascular complications).[136] Initial determinations of cardiac markers should not be used to make admission/discharge decisions. Even when an undetectable troponin I on presentation is combined with a Goldman AMI risk of <4%, there is a 5% rate of adverse events at 30 days (1% death, 2% AMI, and 2% revascularization).[58]

Inpatient Telemetry for Low-Risk Patients

Patients with ACS who spend extended time in the ED are less likely to receive guideline-appropriate care and are more likely to have adverse outcomes.

Ideally, patients should not wait in the ED for more 2 to 3 hours for telemetry beds. Patients with ACS who spend extended time in the ED are less likely to receive guideline-appropriate care and are more likely to have adverse outcomes.[137,138] Since telemetry has not been shown to be useful in low-risk patients, the risks of extending the ED stay solely for inpatient telemetry monitoring does not appear to exceed the benefit of early transfer to an inpatient setting.[138,139]

CCUs were created to identify and immediately treat serious dysrhythmias in patients with AMI. Due to high costs of CCUs and the low "rule in" rate for AMI, non-ICU monitored beds (telemetry beds) were established for monitoring low-risk patients. Recently several studies have questioned the utility of this strategy, consistently finding that <1% of these patients are ever upgraded to higher levels of care and even fewer have a demonstrable intervention as a result of the telemetry,[140,141] especially in the absence of known or suspected CAD, heart failure, or documented dysrrhythmias.[136,142]

Schull et al., in a retrospective study of 8,932 patients admitted to telemetry, found that only 20 patients (0.2%) suffered a cardiac arrest.[143] The onset of cardiac arrest was not detected by the telemetry monitors in half of these patients. Only 3 cardiac arrest patients survived to hospital discharge and only 1 was detected by the monitor.

Hollander et al. identified a cohort of 1,029 low-risk patients with chest pain (Goldman risk <8 and negative initial set of markers) admitted from the ED to monitored non-ICU beds and followed them prospectively throughout hospitalization.[144] None of these patients developed sustained ventricular dysrhythmias identified through routine monitoring. No patients died from preventable cardiovascular causes. Two retrospective reports document the Australian experience with predominantly intermediate-risk patients actually admitted to nonmonitored beds.[45,146] No patients in these studies were felt to have had an adverse outcome that could have been averted.[145,146]

Similarly, studies examining the utility of telemetry monitoring during transport have not found any benefit.[147,148] In a study of 315 patients admitted to telemetry beds or to the ICU, there were no life-threatening ventricular dysrhythmias during transport.[147] No interventions by the transporting nurse were performed. No patients developed new chest pain or dyspnea. Similar results were found in another cohort of patients from Australia.[148]

Summary

The clinical evaluation of chest pain patients is difficult. No single historical feature, clinical symptom or diagnostic test can reliably exclude an acute coronary syndrome. An experienced clinician using the initial 12-lead ECG can further risk stratify patients into diagnostic groups for further testing and indicated treatment. Most patients with chest pain without an obvious noncardiac cause will require some diagnostic and functional testing. Only those found to be at very low risk of coronary artery disease can be safely discharged home from the ED after initial assessment.

References

1. Lee TH, Cook EF, Weisberg M, et al. Acute chest pain in the emergency room: identification and examination of low-risk patients. *Arch Intern Med* 1985;145:65–69.
2. McCaig LF, Nawar EW. National Hospital Ambulatory Medical Care Survey: 2004 emergency department summary. *Adv Data* 2006;372:1–29.
3. Goldman, L, Weinberg M, Weisberg M, et al. A computer-derived protocol to aid in the diagnosis of emergency room patients with acute chest pain. *N Engl J Med* 1982;307:588–596.
4. Goldman L, Cook EF, Brand DA, et al. A computer protocol to predict myocardial infarction in emergency department patients with chest pain. *N Engl J Med* 1988;318:797–803.
5. Lee TH, Juarez G, Cook EF, et al. Ruling out myocardial infarction: a prospective multicenter validation of a 12-hour strategy for patients at low risk. *N Engl J Med* 1991;324:1239–1246.
6. Hutter AM Jr, Amsterdam EA, Jaffe AS. 31st Bethesda Conference. Emergency Cardiac Care. Task Force 2: Acute coronary syndromes: Section 2B – chest discomfort evaluation in the hospital. *J Am Coll Cardiol* 2000;35(4):853–862.
7. Lloyd-Jones DM, Camargo CA, Lapuerta P, et al. Electrocardiographic and clinical predictors of acute myocardial infarction in patients with unstable angina pectoris. *Am J Cardiol* 1998;81(10):1182–1186.
8. Zucker Dr, Griffith JL, Beshansky JR, et al. Presentations of acute myocardial infarction in men and women. *J Gen Intern Med* 1997;12(2):79–87.
9. Jayes RL, Beshansky JR, D'Agostino RB, et al. Do patients' coronary risk factor reports predict acute cardiac ischemia in the emergency department? A multicenter study. *J Clin Epidemiol* 1992;45(6):621–626.
10. Lee TH, Rouan GW, Weisberg MC, et al. Clinical characteristics and natural history of patients with acute myocardial infarction sent home from the emergency room. *Am J Cardiol* 1987;60:219–224.
11. Rouan GW, Lee TH, Cook EF, et al. Clinical characteristics and outcome of acute myocardial infarction in patients with initially normal or nonspecific electrocardiograms. *Am J Cardiol* 1989;64:1087–1092.
12. Pope JH, Aufderheide TP, Ruthazer R, et al. Missed diagnosis of acute cardiac ischemia in the emergency department. *N Engl J Med* 2000;342:1163–1170.
13. Hollander JE, Robey JL, Chase M, et al. Relationship between a clear-cut alternative noncardiac diagnosis and 30 day outcome in emergency department patients with chest pain. *Acad Emerg Med* 2007;14:210–215.

14. Goldman L, Cook EF, Johnson PA, et al. Prediction of the need for intensive care in patients who come to emergency departments with acute chest pain. *N Engl J Med* 1996;334:1498–1504.

15. Kontos MC, Jesse RL. Evaluation of the emergency department chest pain patient. *Am J Cardiol* 2000;85:32B–39B.

16. Tatum JL, Jesse RL, Kontos MC, et al. Comprehensive strategy for the evaluation and triage of the chest pain patient. *Ann Emerg Med* 1997;29:116–125.

17. Freeman L, Antill T. Ten things emergency physicians should not do unless they want to become defendants. *Foresight* 2000;49:1–10.

18. Hickan DH, Sox HC, Sox CH. Systematic bias in recording history in patients with chest pain. *J Chronic Dis* 1985;38:91–100.

19. Gadsboll N, Hoiland-Carlsen PF, Nielsen GG, et al. Symptoms and signs of heart failure in patients with myocardial infarction: reproducibility and relationship to chest x-ray, radionuclide ventriculography and right heart catheterization. *Eur Heart J* 1989;10:1017–1028.

20. Panju AA, Hemmelgarn BR, Guyatt GH, et al. Is this patient having a myocardial infarction? *JAMA* 1998;280:1256–1263.

21. Swap CJ, Nagurney JT. Value and limitations of chest pain history in the evaluation of patients with suspected acute coronary syndromes. *JAMA* 2005;294:2623–2629.

22. Han JH, Lindsell CJ, Storrow AB, et al. Cardiac risk factor burden and its association with acute coronary syndrome. *Ann Emerg Med* 2007;49:145–152.

23. Walker NJ, Sites FD, Shofer FS, et al. Characteristics and outcomes of young adults who present to the emergency department with chest pain. *Acad Emerg Med* 2001;8(7):703–708.

24. Marsan RJ Jr, Shaver KJ, Sease KL, et al. Evaluation of a clinical decision rule for young adult patients with chest pain. *Acad Emerg Med* 2005;12(1):26–31.

25. Christenson J, Innes G, McKnight D, et al. A clinical prediction rule for early discharge of patients with chest pain. *Ann Emerg Med* 2006;47:1–10.

26. Sheifer SE, Manolio TA, Gersh BJ. Unrecognized myocardial infarction. *Ann Intern Med* 2001;135:801–811.

27. Diercks DB, Boghos E, Guzman H, et al. Changes in the numeric descriptive scale for pain after sublingual nitroglycerin do not predict cardiac etiology of chest pain. *Ann Emerg Med* 2005;45:581–585.

28. Henrikson CA, Howell EE, Bush DE, et al. Chest pain relief by nitroglycerin does not predict active coronary artery disease. *Ann Intern Med* 2003;139:979–986.

29. Wrenn K, Slovis CM, Gongaware J. Using the "GI cocktail": a descriptive study. *Ann Emerg Med* 1995;26:687–690.

30. Servi RJ, Skiendzielewski JJ. Relief of myocardial ischemia pain with a gastrointestinal cocktail. *Am J Emerg Med* 1985;3:208–209.

31. Launbjerg J, Fruergaard P, Hesse B, et al. Long-term risk of death, cardiac events and recurrent chest pain in patients with acute chest pain of different origin. *Cardiology* 1996;87:60.

32. Lindsell CJ, Anantharaman V, Diercks D, et al. The internet tracking registry of acute coronary syndromes (i*trACS): a multicenter registry of patients with suspicion of acute coronary syndromes reported using the standardized reporting guidelines for emergency department chest pain studies. *Ann Emerg Med* 2006;48:666–677.

33. Meszaros I, Morocz J, Szlavi J, et al. Epidemiology and clinicopathology of aortic dissection. *Chest* 2000;117:1271–1278.

34. von Kodolitsch Y, Schwartz A, Nienaber C. Clinical prediction of acute aortic dissection. *Arch Intern Med* 2000;160:2977–2982.

35. Hagan PG, Nienaber CA. Isselbacher EM, et al. The International Registry of Acute Aortic Dissection (IRAD): new insights into an old disease. *JAMA* 2000;283:897–903.

36. Goldhaber SZ, Visani L, De Rosa M. Acute pulmonary embolism: clinical outcomes in the International Cooperative Pulmonary Embolism Registry (ICOPER). *Lancet* 1999;353:1386–1389.

37. Kline JA, Wells PS. Methodology for a rapid protocol to rule out pulmonary embolism in the emergency department. *Ann Emerg Med* 2003;42:266–275.

38. Wicki J, Perneger TV, Junod AF, et al. Assessing clinical probability of pulmonary embolism in the emergency ward: a simple score. *Arch Intern Med* 2001;161:92–97.

39. Le Gal G, Righini M, Roy PM, et al. Prediction of pulmonary embolism in the emergency department: the revised Geneva score. *Ann Intern Med* 2006;144:165–171.

40. Wells PS, Ginsberg JS, Anderson DR, et al. Use of a clinical model for safe management of patients with suspected pulmonary embolism. *Ann Intern Med* 1998;129:997–1005.

41. Sahn SA, Heffner JE. Spontaneous pneumothorax. *N Engl J Med* 2000; 342:86–74.

42. Estrera AS, Landay MJ, Grisham JM, et al. Descending necrotizing mediastinitis. *Surg Gynecol Obstet* 1983; 157:545–552.

43. Burnett CM, Rosemurgy AS, Pfeiffer EA. Life-threatening acute posterior mediastinitis due to esophageal perforation. *Ann Thorac Surg* 1990; 9:979–983.

44. Sancho LM, Minamoto H, Fernandez A, et al. Descending necrotizing mediastinitis: a retrospective surgical experience. *Eur J Cardiothorac Surg* 1999;16:200–205.

45. Makeieff M, Gresillon N, Berthet JP, et al. Management of descending necrotizing mediastinitis. *Laryngoscope* 2004; 114:772–775.

46. Glauser J, Erickson J, Bhatt D, et al. Elevated serum cardiac markers predict coronary artery disease in patients with a history of heart failure who present with chest pain: insights from the itracs registry. *Cong Heart Failure* 2007;13:142–148.

47. Lettman NA, Sites FD, Shofer FS, et al. Congestive heart failure patients with chest pain: incidence and predictors of acute coronary syndrome. *Acad Emerg Med* 2002;9(10):903–909.

48. Selker HP, Zalenski RJ, Antman EM, et al. An evaluation of technologies for identification of acute cardiac ischemia in the emergency department: a report form a National Heart Attack Alert Program Working Group. *Ann Emerg Med* 1997;29:13–81.

49. Hathaway WR, Peterson ED, Wagner GS, et al. Prognostic significance of the initial electrocardiogram in patients with acute myocardial infarction. *JAMA* 1998;279:387–391.

50. Slater DK, Hlatky MA, Mark DB, et al. Outcome in suspected acute myocardial infarction with normal or minimally abnormal admission electrocardiographic findings. *Am J Cardiol* 1987;60:766–770.

51. Brush JE, Brand DA, Acampora D, et al. Use of the initial electrocardiogram to predict in-hospital complications of acute myocardial infarction. *N Engl J Med* 1985;312:1137–1141.

52. Chase M, Brown AM, Robey JL, et al. Prognostic value of symptoms during a normal or nonspecific electrocardiogram in emergency department patients with potential acute coronary syndrome. *Acad Emerg Med* 2006;13(10):1037–1039.

53. Zalenski RJ, Cooke D, Rydman R, et al. Assessing the diagnostic value of an ECG containing leads V4R, V8 and V9: The 15 lead ECG. *Ann Emerg Med* 1993;22:786–793.

54. Zalenski RJ, Rydman RJ, Sloan EP, et al. Value of posterior and right ventricular leads in comparison to standard 12 lead electrocardiogram in evaluation of ST segment elevation in suspected acute myocardial infarction. *Am J Cardiol* 1997;79:1579–1585.

55. Sgarbossa EB, Pinski SL, Barbagelata A, et al. Electrocardiographic diagnosis of evolving acute myocardial infarction in the presence of left bundle branch block. *N Engl J Med* 1996;334:481–487.

56. Sgarbossa EB, Pinski SL, Gates KB, et al. Early electrocardiographic diagnosis of acute myocardial infarction in the presence of ventricular paced rhythm. *Am J Cardiol* 1996;77:423–424.

57. Lau J, Ioannidis JPA, Balk EM, et al. Diagnosing acute cardiac ischemia in the emergency department: a systematic review of the accuracy and clinical effect of current technologies. *Ann Emerg Med* 2001;37:453–460.

58. Limkakeng A Jr, Gibler WB, Pollack C, et al. Combination of Goldman risk and initial cardiac troponin I for emergency department chest pain patient risk stratification. *Acad Emerg Med* 2001;8:696–702.

59. Qamar A, McPherson C, Babb J, et al. The Goldman algorithm revisited: prospective evaluation of a computer-derived algorithm versus unaided physician judgment in suspected acute myocardial infarction. *Am Heart J* 1999;138:705–709.

60. Sarasin FP, Reymond JM, Griffith JL, et al. Impact of the acute cardiac ischemia time insensitive predictive instrument (ACI-TIPI) on the speed of triage decision making for emergency

department patients presenting with chest pain: a controlled clinical trial. *J Gen Intern Med* 1994;9:187–194.

61. Selker HP, Beshanski JR, Griffith JL, et al. Use of the acute cardiac ischemia time-insensitive predictive instrument (ACI-TIPI) to assist with triage of patients with chest pain or other symptoms suggestive of acute cardiac ischemia: a multicenter, controlled clinical trial. *Ann Intern Med* 1998;129:845–855.

62. Kennedy RL, Harrison RF, Burton AM, et al. An artificial neural network system for diagnosis of acute myocardial infarction (AMI) in the accident and emergency department: evaluation and comparison with serum myoglobin measurements. *Comput Methods Progr Biomed* 1997;52(2):93–103.

63. Baxt WG, Shofer FS, Sites FD, et al. A neural computational aid to the diagnosis of acute myocardial infarction. *Ann Emerg Med* 2002;39(4):366–373.

64. Baxt WG, Shofer FS, Sites FD, et al. A neural network for the prediction of cardiac ischemia in patients presenting to the Emergency Department with chest pain. *Ann Emerg Med* 2002;40(6):575–583.

65. Hollander JE, Sease KL, Sparano DM, et al. Effects of neural network feedback to physicians on admit/discharge decision for emergency department patients with chest pain. *Ann Emerg Med* 2004;44:199–205.

66. Antman EM, Cohen M, Bernink PJ, et al. The TIMI risk score for unstable angina/non-ST elevation MI: a method for prognostication and therapeutic decision making. *JAMA* 2000:284:835–834.

67. Pollack CV Jr, Sites FD, Shofer FS, et al. Application of the TIMI risk score for unstable angina and non-ST elevation acute coronary syndrome to an unselected emergency department chest pain population. *Acad Emerg Med* 2006;13:13–18.

68. Chase M, Robey JL, Zogby KE, et al. Prospective validation of the TIMI risk score in the emergency department chest pain patient population. *Ann Emerg Med* 2006;48:252–259.

69. Karounos M, Chang AM, Robey JL, et al. TIMI risk score: does it work equally well in both males and females. *Emerg Med J* 2007;24:471–474.

70. Miller CD, Lindsell CJ, Khandelwal S, et al. Is the initial diagnostic impression of "noncardiac chest pain" adequate to exclude cardiac disease? *Ann Emerg Med* 2004;44:565–574.

71. Disla E, Rhim HR, Reddy A, et al. Costochondritis: a prospective analysis in an emergency department setting. *Arch Intern Med* 1994;154:2466–2469.

72. Gibler WB, Lewis LM, Erb RE, et al. Early detection of acute myocardial infarction in patients presenting with chest pain and nondiagnostic ECGs: serial CK-MB sampling in the emergency department. *Ann Emerg Med* 1990;19:1359–1366.

73. Braunwald E, Antman EM, Beasley JW, et al. American College of Cardiology/American Heart Association Task Force on Practice Guidelines (Committee on the Management of Patients With Unstable Angina). ACC/AHA guideline update for the management of patients with unstable angina and non-ST-segment elevation myocardial infarction—2002: summary article: A report of the American College of Cardiology/American Heart Association Task Force on Practice Guidelines (Committee on the Management of Patients With Unstable Angina). *Circulation* 2002;106:1893.

74. Fesmire FM, Percy RF, Bardoner JB, et al. Serial creatinine kinase MB testing during emergency department evaluation of chest pain. Utility of a 2 hour delta CK-MB of + 1.6 ng.ml. *Am Heart J* 1998;136:237–244.

75. Adams JE III, Bodor GS, Davila-Roman VG, et al. Cardiac troponin I: a marker with high specificity for cardiac injury. *Circulation* 1993;88:101–196.

76. Brogan GX Jr, Hollander JE, McCuskey CF, et al. Evaluation of a new assay for cardiac troponin I vs creatine kinase-MB for the diagnosis of acute myocardial infarction. *Acad Emerg Med* 1997;4:6–12.

77. Hollander JE, Levitt MA, Young GP, et al. Effect of recent cocaine use on the specificity of cardiac markers for diagnosis of acute myocardial infarction. *Am Heart J* 1998;135:245–252.

78. Morrow DA, Cannon CP, Jesse RL, et al. National Academy of Clinical Biochemistry Laboratory Medicine practice guidelines: clinical characteristics and utilization of biochemical markers in acute coronary syndromes. *Circulation* 2007;115:356–375.

79. Tunstall-Pedoe H, Kuulasmaa K, Annouyel P, et al. The WHO MONICA project. Myocardial infarction and coronary deaths in the World Health Organization MONICA project. *Circulation* 1994;90:588–612.

80. Capellan O, Hollander JE, Pollack C, et al. Prospective evaluation of emergency department patients with potential acute coronary syndromes using initial absolute CK-MB vs. CK-MB relative index. *J Emerg Med* 2003;24:361–367.

81. Green GB, Li DJ, Bessman ES, et al. The prognostic significance of troponin I and troponin T. *Acad Emerg Med* 1998;5:758–767.

82. Antman EM, Tanasijevic MJ, Thompson B, et al. Cardiac specific troponin I levels predict the risk of mortality in patients with acute coronary syndromes. *N Engl J Med* 1996;335:1342–1349.

83. Ohman EM, Armstrong PW, Christenson RH, et al. Cardiac troponin-T levels for risk stratification in acute myocardial ischemia. *N Engl J Med* 1996;335:1333–1341.

84. Heidenreich PA, Alloggiamento T, Melsop K, et al. The prognostic value of troponin in patients with non-ST elevation acute coronary syndromes: a meta-analysis. *J Am Coll Cardiol* 2001;38:478–485.

85. Hamm CW, Goldmann BU, Heeschen C, et al. Emergency room triage of patients with acute chest pain by means of rapid testing for cardiac troponin T or troponin I. *N Engl J Med* 1997;337:1648–1653.

86. McErlean ES, Deluca SA, van Lente F, et al. Comparison of troponin T versus creatine kinase MB in suspected acute coronary syndromes. *Am J Cardiol* 2000;85:421–426.

87. Kontos MC, Anderson FP, Alimard R, et al. Ability of troponin I to predict cardiac events in patients admitted from the Emergency Department. *J Am Coll Cardiol* 2000;36:1818–1823.

88. Green GB, Beaudreau RW, Chan DW, et al. Use of troponin T and creatine kinase MB subunit levels for risk stratification of emergency department patients with possible myocardial ischemia. *Ann Emerg Med* 1998;31:19–29.

89. Newby LK, Storrow AB, Gibler WB, et al. Bedside multi-marker testing for risk stratification in chest pain units: the chest pain evaluation by creatine kinase-MB, myoglobin, and troponin I (CHECKMATE) study. *Circulation* 2001;103:1832–1837.

90. Wayand D, Baum M, Schatzle G, et al. Cardiac troponin T and I in end stage renal failure. *Clin Chem* 2000;46:1345–1350.

91. DeWinter RJ, Lijmer JG, Koster RW, et al. Diagnostic accuracy of myoglobin concentration for the early diagnosis of acute myocardial infarction. *Ann Emerg Med* 2000;35:113–120.

92. Brogan GX Jr, Friedman S, McCuskey C, et al. Evaluation of a new rapid quantitative immunoassay for serum myoglobin versus CK-MB for ruling out acute myocardial infarction in the emergency department. *Ann Emerg Med* 1994;24:665–671.

93. Storrow AB, Lindsell CJ, Han JH, et al. Discordant cardiac biomarkers: frequency and outcomes in emergency department patients with chest pain. *Ann Emerg Med* 2006;48:660–665.

94. Hollander JE, Muttreja MR, Dalesandro MR, et al. Risk stratification of ED patients with acute coronary syndromes using P-selectin. *J Am Coll Cardiol* 1999;34:95–105.

95. Kontos MC, Anderson FP, Hanbury CM, et al. Use of the combination of myoglobin and CKMB mass for the rapid diagnosis of acute myocardial infarction. *Am J Emerg Med* 1997;15:14–19.

96. McCord J, Nowak RM, McCullough PA, et al. Ninety-minute exclusion of acute myocardial infarction by use of quantitative point-of-care testing of myoglobin and troponin I. *Circulation* 2001;104(13):1483–1488.

97. Morrow DA, de Lemos JA, Sabatine MS, et al. Evaluation of B-type natriuretic peptide for risk assessment in unstable angina/Non-ST-elevation myocardial infarction. B-type natriuretic peptide and prognosis in TACTICS-TIMI 18. *J Am Coll Cardiol* 2003;41:1264–1272.

98. de Lemos JA, Morrow DA, Bentley JH, et al. The prognostic value of B-type natriuretic peptide in patients with acute coronary syndromes. *N Engl J Med* 2001;345:1014–1021.

99. Brown AM, Sease KL, Robey JL, et al. The impact of BNP in addition to troponin I, CK-MB, and myoglobin on the risk stratification

of ED chest pain patients with potential ACS. *Ann Emerg Med* 2007;49:153–163.

100. Varetto T, Cantalupi D, Altieri A, et al. Emergency room technetium-99m sestamibi imaging to rule out acute myocardial ischemia events in patients with nondiagnostic electrocardiograms. *J Am Coll Cardiol* 1993;22:1804–1808.

101. Hilton TC, Thompson RC, Williams HJ, et al. Technetium-99m sestamibi myocardial perfusion imaging in the emergency room evaluation of chest pain. *J Am Coll Cardiol* 1994;23:1016–1022.

102. Tatum JL, Jesse RL, Kontos MC, et al. Comprehensive strategy for the evaluation and triage of the chest pain patient. *Ann Emerg Med* 1997;29:116–125.

103. Kontos MC, Jesse RL, Anderson FA, et al. Comparison of myocardial perfusion imaging and cardiac troponin I in patients admitted to the emergency department with chest pain. *Circulation* 1999;99:2073–2078.

104. Udelson JE, Beshansky JR, Ballin DS, et al. Myocardial perfusion imaging for evaluation and triage of patients with suspected acute cardiac ischemia. A randomized controlled trial. *JAMA* 2002;288:2693–2700.

105. Hollander JE. The continuing search to identify the very low risk chest pain patient (editorial). *Acad Emer Med* 1999;6:979–981.

106. Achenbach S, Moshage W, Ropers D, et al. Value of electron beam computed tomography for the noninvasive detection of high grade coronary artery stenosis and occlusions. *N Engl J Med* 1998;339:1964–1971.

107. McLaughlin VV, Balogh T, Rich S. Utility of electron beam computed tomography to stratify patients presenting to the emergency room with chest pain. *Am J Cardiol* 1999;84:327–328.

108. Laudon DA, Vukov LF, Breen JF, et al. Use of electron beam computed tomography in the evaluation of chest pain patients in the emergency department. *Ann Emerg Med* 1999;33:15–21.

109. Georgiou D, Budoff MJ, Kaufer E, et al. Screening patients with chest pain in the emergency department using electron beam tomography: a follow-up study. *J Am Coll Cardiol* 2001;38:105–110.

110. Raggi P, Callister TQ, Cooil B, et al. Evaluation of chest pain in patients with low to intermediate pretest probability of coronary artery disease by electron beam computed tomography. *Am J Cardiol* 2000;85:283–288.

111. Raff GL, Gallagher MJ, O'Neill WW, et al. Diagnostic accuracy of noninvasive coronary angiography using 64-slice spiral computed tomography. *J Am Coll Cardiol* 2005;46:552–557.

112. Leber AW, Knez A, von Ziegler F, et al. Quantification of obstructive and nonobstructive coronary lesions by 64-slice computed tomography. *J Am Coll Cardiol* 2005;46:147–154.

113. Ropers D, Rixe J, Anders K, et al. Usefulness of multidetector row spiral computed tomography with 64 x 0.6-mm collimation and 330-ms rotation for the noninvasive detection of significant coronary artery stenosis. *Am J Cardiol* 2006;97:343–348.

114. Gallagher MJ, Ross MA, Raff GL, et al. The diagnostic accuracy of 64-slice CT coronary angiography compared with stress nuclear imaging in emergency department low risk chest pain patients. *Ann Emerg Med* 2007;49:125–136.

115. Goldstein JA, Gallagher MJ, O'Neill WW, et al. A randomized controlled trial of multislice coronary computed tomography for evaluation of acute chest pain. *J Am Coll Cardiol* 2007;49:863–871.

116. Hollander JE, Litt HI, Chase M, et al. Computed tomography coronary angiography for rapid disposition of low risk emergency department patients with chest pain syndromes. *Acad Emerg Med* 2007;14:112–116.

117. White CS, Kuo D, Kelemen M, et al. Chest pain evaluation in the emergency department: can MDCT provide a comprehensive evaluation? *Am J Roentgenol* 2005;185:533–540.

118. Ghersin E, Litmanovich D, Dragu R, et al. 16-MDCT coronary angiography versus invasive coronary angiography in acute chest pain syndrome: a blinded prospective study. *Am J Roentgenol* 2006;186(1):177–184.

119. Moloo J, Pena AJ, Nichols JH, et al. Multidetector computed tomography coronary angiography vs myocardial perfusion imaging for early triage of patients with suspected acute coronary syndromes (abstract). *Acad Emerg Med* 2006;13:S104.

120. Nagurney JT, Moselewski F, Pena AJ, et al. Multidetector computerized tomography of the coronary arteries improves path probabilities in emergency department patients being admitted with chest pain. *Acad Emerg Med* 2006;13(5 Suppl):S104–S105.

121. Khare RK. Cost effective decision analysis model comparing 64 slice computed tomography with other means of evaluating chest pain. *Acad Emerg Med* 2006;13:S105.

122. Lindsay J Jr, Bonnet YD, Pinnow EE. Routine stress testing for triage of patients with chest pain. Is it worth the candle? *Ann Emerg Med* 1998;32:600–603.

123. Diercks DB, Gibler WB, Liu T, et al. Identification of patients at risk by graded exercise testing in an emergency department chest pain center. *Am J Cardiol* 2000;86:289–292.

124. Trippi JA, Lee KS, Kopp G, et al. Dobutamine stress tele-echocardiography for evaluation of emergency department patients with chest pain. *J Am Coll Cardiol* 1997;30:627–632.

125. Colon PJ III, Guarisco JS, Murgo J, et al. Utility of stress echocardiography in the triage of patients with atypical chest pain from the emergency department. *Am J Cardiol* 1998;82:1282–1284.

126. Kirk JD, Turnipseed S, Lewis WR, et al. Evaluation of chest pain in low risk patients presenting to the emergency department: the role of immediate exercise testing. *Ann Emerg Med* 1998;32:1–7.

127. Amsterdam EA, Kirk JD, Diercks DB, et al. Immediate exercise testing to evaluate low-risk patients presenting to the emergency department with chest pain. *J Am Coll Cardiol* 2002;40:251–256.

128. Nerenberg RH, Shofer FS, Robey JL, et al. Impact of a negative prior stress test on emergency physician disposition decision in ED patients with chest pain syndromes. *Am J Emerg Med* 2007;25:39–44.

129. Shaver KJ, Marsan RJ, Sease KL, et al. Impact of a negative evaluation for underlying coronary artery disease on 1 year resource utilization for patients admitted with potential acute coronary syndromes. *Acad Emerg Med* 2005;11:1272–1277.

130. Pitts WR, Lange RA, Cigarroa JE, et al. Repeat coronary angiography in patients with chest pain and previously normal coronary angiogram. *Am J Cardiol* 1997;80:1086–1087.

131. Papanicolaou MN, Califf RM, Hlatky MA, et al. Prognostic implications of angiographically normal and insignificantly narrowed coronary arteries. *Am J Cardiol* 1986;58:1181–1187.

132. Farkouh ME, Smars PA, Reeder GS, et al. for the Chest Pain Evaluation in the Emergency Room (CHEER) Investigators. A clinical trial of a chest pain observation unit for patients with unstable angina. *N Engl J Med* 1998;339:1882–1888.

133. Zalenski RJ, Rydman RJ, McCarren M, et al. Feasibility of a rapid diagnostic protocol for an emergency department chest pain unit. *Ann Emerg Med* 1997;29(1):88–108.

134. Gibler WB, Runyon JP, Levy RC, et al. A rapid diagnostic and treatment center for patients with chest pain in the emergency department. *Ann Emerg Med* 1995; 25:1–8.

135. Chan GW, Sites FD, Shofer FS, et al. Impact of stress testing on 30-day cardiovascular outcomes for low risk chest pain patients admitted to non-intensive care telemetry beds. *Am J Emerg Med* 2003;21(4):282–287.

136. Hollander JE, Valentine SM, McCuskey C, et al. Are monitored telemetry beds necessary for patients with nontraumatic chest pain and normal or nonspecific electrocardiograms? *Am J Cardiol* 1997;79:1110–1111.

137. Diercks DB, Roe MT, Chen AY, et al. Prolonged emergency department stays of non-ST-segment elevation myocardial infarction patients are associated with worse adherence to the ACC/AHA guidelines for management and increased adverse events. *Ann Emerg Med* 2007;50:489–496.

138. Pines JM, Hollander JE. The impact of emergency department crowding on cardiac outcomes in ED patients with acute chest pain. *Ann Emerg Med* 2007;50(3 Suppl):S3.

139. Hollander JE, Pines JM. The ED crowding paradox: the longer you stay, the less care you get. *Ann Emerg Med* 2007;50:497–499.

140. Estrada CA, Prasad NK, Rosman HS, et al. Outcomes of patients hospitalized to a telemetry unit. *Am J Cardiol* 1994;74:357–362.

141. Estrada CA, Rosman HS, Prasad NK, et al. Role of telemetry monitoring in the non-intensive care unit. *Am J Cardiol* 1995;76:960–965.

142. Lipskis DJ, Dannehl KN, Silverman ME. Value of radiotelemetry in a community hospital. *Am J Cardiol* 1984;53:1284–1287.

143. Schull MJ, Redelmeier DA. Continuous electrocardiographic monitoring and cardiac arrest outcomes in 8,932 telemetry ward patients. *Acad Emerg Med* 2000;7:647–652.

144. Hollander JE, Sites FD, Pollack CV Jr, et al. Lack of utility of telemetry monitoring for identification of cardiac death and life threatening ventricular dysrhythmias in low risk patients with chest pain. *Ann Emerg Med* 2004;43(1):71–76.

145. Kelly AM, Kerr D. It is safe to manage selected patients with acute coronary syndromes in unmonitored beds. *J Emerg Med* 2001;21:227–233.

146. Sultana RV, Kerr D, Kelly AM, et al. Validation of a tool to safely triage selected patients with chest pain to nonmonitored beds. *Emerg Med* 2002;14:393–399.

147. Pines JM, Rich VL, Schwartz AR, et al. Lack of utility of telemetry monitoring during transport to inpatient beds for identification of dysrhythmias for emergency department patients with potential and known acute coronary syndromes. *Crit Path Cardiol* 2005;4:117–120.

148. Lin A, Kerr D, Kelly AM. Is cardiac monitoring during transport of low risk chest pain patients from the emergency department necessary? *Emerg Med Australasia* 2007;19:229–233.

Chapter 4
Community and Prehospital Strategies for Managing Patients with Acute Coronary Syndromes

Joseph P. Ornato

Just as in cardiac arrest, a STEMI 'chain of survival' metaphor can be used to emphasize the need for rapid (1) symptom recognition and a call for help, (2) emergency medical services (EMS) evaluation and treatment, (3) emergency department (ED) evaluation and treatment, and (4) reperfusion therapy.[1]

- ■ Early symptom recognition activates a STEMI Chain of Survival providing access to optimized time-sensitive care for patients with chest discomfort and possible ACS.
- ■ Prehospital electrocardiograms identify patients with STEMI for rapid reperfusion and appropriate destination hospital selection.
- ■ STEMI systems of care, provide rapid reperfusion for STEMI patients and optimize resource utilization for possible ACS patients.

Introduction

The 2005 American Heart Association (AHA) Guidelines for Cardiopulmonary Resuscitation (CPR) and Emergency Cardiovascular Care (ECC) state that half of all patients who die from acute myocardial infarction (AMI) will do so before reaching the hospital, with most deaths due to ventricular tachycardia (VT) or fibrillation (VF) in the first 3 to 4 hours after onset of symptoms.[2] The guidelines encourage communities to "develop programs to respond to out-of-hospital cardiac arrest that include prompt recognition of symptoms of acute coronary syndromes (ACS), early activation of the emergency medical services (EMS) system, and, if needed, early CPR and early access to an automated external defibrillator (AED) through community AED programs."[2]

Effective interventions exist for the majority of ACS patients, but these interventions are extremely time-sensitive, particularly for those with acute ST-segment-elevation myocardial infarction (STEMI). Just as in cardiac arrest, a STEMI "chain of survival" metaphor (Fig. 4-1) can be used to emphasize the need for rapid (1) symptom recognition and a call for help; (2) EMS evaluation and treatment; (3) emergency department (ED) evaluation and treatment; and (4) reperfusion therapy.[1] This chapter focuses on

See Web site for Dr. Ornato's editorial "The STEMI Chain of Survival," originally published in *Circulation*.

community and prehospital evidence-based guideline management strategies that can be used to reduce ACS morbidity and mortality.[3–6]

Symptom Recognition

Many laypersons do not know or recognize the symptoms of cardiac ischemia or infarction (i.e., a "heart attack"), which often delays seeking medical evaluation and care. The longest interval from STEMI symptom onset to definitive treatment is usually due to delay in patient symptom recognition and arrival at the point of care.[7] Failure to recognize symptoms as being caused by a heart attack can be due to inadequate knowledge of AMI symptoms, maladaptive coping strategies, or misattribution of the symptoms to another, noncardiac cause.[8–10] Common reasons why STEMI patients delay seeking emergency medical attention are listed in Table 4-1.[5]

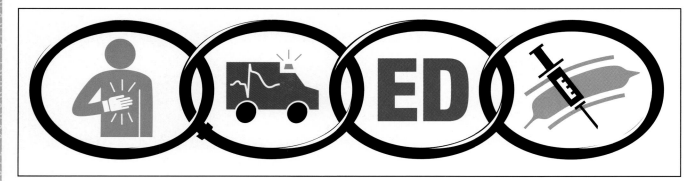

FIGURE 4-1 • The STEMI "Chain of Survival": (1) symptom recognition and a call for help; (2) EMS evaluation and treatment; (3) emergency department (ED) evaluation and treatment; and (4) rapid reperfusion therapy.[1]

The longest interval from STEMI symptom onset to definitive treatment is usually due to delay in patient symptom recognition and health-seeking behavior.

Goff et al.[11] conducted random-digit-dialed telephone surveys of the 1,294 adults in 20 U.S. cities involved in the National Institutes of Health (NIH)–sponsored Rapid Early Action for Coronary Treatment (REACT) trial to determine how frequently laypersons could identify common symptoms of a heart attack (chest discomfort, arm or shoulder pain or discomfort, jaw or neck pain, back pain, shortness of breath, nausea or vomiting, sweating, lightheadedness, and weakness). Chest discomfort was reported as a symptom by 89.7% of respondents and was thought to be the most important symptom by 56.6%. Knowledge of arm pain or numbness (67.3%), shortness of breath (50.8%), sweating (21.3%), and other heart attack symptoms was less common. In a multivariable-adjusted model,

| TABLE 4-1 • Reasons Why STEMI Patients Delay in Seeking Emergency Medical Attention

- Expected a dramatic presentation
- Thought symptoms were not serious/would go away
- Took a "wait and see" approach to the initial symptoms that included self-evaluation, self-treatment, and reassessment until "certain"
- Tended to attribute symptoms to other chronic conditions (e.g., arthritis, muscle strain) or common illnesses (e.g., influenza)
- Lacked awareness of the benefits of rapid action, reperfusion treatment, or of the importance of calling EMS/911 for AMI symptoms
- Expressed fear of embarrassment if symptoms turned out to be a false alarm; reluctant to "bother" physicians or EMS unless "really sick"; needed "permission" from others such as health care providers, spouses, family to take rapid action
- Few ever discussed symptoms, responses, or actions for a heart attack in advance with family or providers
- Stereotypes of who is at risk for a heart attack
- Not perceived at risk if:
  - Young and healthy
  - A woman
  - Under a doctor's care or making lifestyle changes (especially men with risk factors)

From Antman EM, Anbe DT, Armstrong PW, et al. ACC/AHA guidelines for the management of patients with ST-elevation myocardial infarction—executive summary: a report of the American College of Cardiology/American Heart Association Task Force on Practice Guidelines (Writing Committee to Revise the 1999 Guidelines for the Management of Patients With Acute Myocardial Infarction). *Circulation* 2004;110(5):588–636, with permission.

significantly higher mean numbers of correct symptoms were reported by non-Hispanic whites than by other racial or ethnic groups, by middle-aged persons than by older and younger persons, by persons with higher socioeconomic status than by those with lower, and by persons with versus those without previous heart attack experience. The authors concluded that, although the public's knowledge of chest discomfort as an important heart attack symptom is relatively high, knowledge of the complex constellation of heart attack symptoms is deficient in the U.S. population, especially in low-socioeconomic and racial or ethnic minority groups.

Atypical Symptoms

Atypical symptom presentations for ACS, including STEMI, are more commonly seen in elderly, female, and diabetic patients.[12–17] A surprisingly large percentage of patients presenting to the hospital proven subsequently to have AMI do not have chest discomfort. Canto et al.[18] found that 142,445 of 434,877 patients (33%) with confirmed AMI in the National Registry of Myocardial Infarction-2 did not have chest discomfort on presentation to the hospital. This group of AMI patients was, on average, 7 years older than those with chest discomfort (74.2 vs. 66.9 years) and included a higher proportion of women (49.0% vs. 38.0%) and patients with diabetes mellitus (32.6% vs. 25.4%), or prior heart failure (26.4% vs. 12.3%). AMI patients without chest discomfort had a longer delay before hospital presentation (mean, 7.9 vs. 5.3 hours), were less likely to be diagnosed as having confirmed AMI at the time of admission (22.2% vs. 50.3%) and were less likely to receive fibrinolysis or a primary percutaneous intervention (PCI) (25.3% vs. 74.0%), aspirin (ASA; 60.4% vs. 84.5%), beta-blockers (28.0% vs. 48.0%), or heparin (53.4% vs. 83.2%) compared with those with chest discomfort. AMI patients without chest discomfort had a 23.3% in-hospital mortality rate, compared with 9.3% among patients with chest pain (adjusted odds ratio for mortality, 2.21 [95% CI, 2.17–2.26]). The authors concluded that patients without chest pain on hospital presentation represent a large segment of the AMI population and are at increased risk for delays in seeking medical attention, less aggressive treatments, and in-hospital mortality.

Atypical symptom presentations for ACS, including STEMI, are more commonly seen in elderly, female, and diabetic patients. A surprisingly large percentage of patients presenting to the hospital proven subsequently to have AMI do not have chest discomfort.

Prodromal unstable angina symptoms are present in roughly half of AMI patients and are associated with a more favorable prognosis, probably by ischemic preconditioning of the myocardium.[19–22] Prodromal unstable angina was a strong predictor of a smaller infarct size as judged by creatine kinase release ($P = 0.017$) and was associated with an increased odds ratio (3.83; 95% CI, 1.27–11.47) for 5-year survival in the Global Utilization of Streptokinase and Tissue Plasminogen Activator for Occluded Coronary Arteries (GUSTO-I) study.[21]

Women

Women are particularly likely to have prodromal symptoms prior to AMI. In a recent study, 489 of 515 (95%) of women diagnosed with AMI treated at five different hospitals reported prodromal symptoms in the weeks prior to their infarction.[23] The most frequent prodromal symptoms experienced >1 month before AMI were unusual fatigue (70.7%), sleep disturbance (47.8%), and shortness of breath (42.1%). Only 29.7% reported chest discomfort. The most frequent acute symptoms in women were chest discomfort (57%), shortness of breath (57.9%), weakness (54.8%), and fatigue (42.9%).

Media Campaigns and Public Education to Improve Symptom Recognition

Intense public education can increase patient knowledge of heart attack symptoms and the need to call 911/seek medical attention quickly, but it has not been consistently successful in shortening patient delay in executing these actions.[24,25] Ho et al.[25] were the first U.S. investigators to prospectively evaluate the effect of a 7-month public education campaign on AMI patient health-seeking delay and EMS use in King County, WA. The goal of the educational intervention was to increase the public's knowledge of AMI symptoms and encourage anyone with such symptoms to "Call 911, Call Fast." The investigators showed that the public's knowledge of AMI symptoms and the need to call 911 quickly increased significantly in the postmessage period (premessage, 53%; postmessage, 74%; $P < 0.0001$). However, the campaign failed to shorten significantly AMI patient delay in seeking medical care (median delay premessage, 2.6 hours; postmessage, 2.3 hours) or alter the distribution of patients in the time intervals of <2 hours, 2 to 4 hours, and >4 hours. The rate of EMS use did not change significantly (premessage, 42%; postmessage, 44%), prompting the authors to conclude that the short-duration public educational campaign increased knowledge of AMI symptoms and appropriate health-seeking actions but did not alter AMI patient behavior.

Soon after this publication, Herlitz et al.[26] reported the results of a media campaign aimed at reducing delay times in suspected AMI on the volume of emergency department (ED) chest pain patients in Goteborg, Sweden. During the first week of the campaign, the mean number of patients with chest pain increased from 10.5 to 25.4 per day. However, the number declined rapidly over the next several months. The average ED volume increased by 9% during the entire media campaign, while the number of confirmed AMI patients increased by only 6%. The greatest increase was observed in patients with chest discomfort in whom AMI was not suspected after physician evaluation.

Intense public education can increase patient knowledge of heart attack symptoms and the need to call 911/seek medical attention quickly, but it has not been consistently successful in shortening patient delay in executing these actions. Despite these somewhat "mixed" results, prudence would dictate that public education is necessary, albeit perhaps insufficient, to improve ACS patient health-seeking behavior.

In 1996, Blohm et al.[27] analyzed results of all seven preceding educational campaigns that attempted to reduce the delay between onset of AMI symptoms and treatment. The impact on delay time ranged from no reduction to a 35% decrease in patient decision time. One study reported a sustained reduction that cut the delay time in half during the 3 years after the campaign. The overall use of ambulances for transport to the ED did not increase. There was a temporary increase in the numbers of patients presenting to the ED with noncardiac chest discomfort in the initial phase of educational campaigns.

The NIH-sponsored REACT trial was conducted in 20 paired U.S. cities in 10 states to further explore the effect of public education on AMI patient health-seeking behavior.[24] One city in each pair was assigned randomly to an 18-month intervention targeting mass media, community organizations, and professional, public, and patient education to increase appropriate patient actions for AMI symptoms. The other city in each pair served as the control population. Patient delay from symptom onset to hospital arrival at baseline (median, 140 minutes) was identical in the intervention and control communities. Delay time decreased in intervention communities by −4.7% per year (95% CI; −8.6% to −0.6%), but the change did not differ significantly from that observed in reference communities (−6.8% per year; 95% CI, −14.5% to 1.6%; $P = 0.54$). Total numbers of ED presentations for chest discomfort and patients with chest discomfort discharged from the ED, as well as EMS use among patients with chest discomfort released from the ED, did not change significantly. The one promising finding was that EMS use increased significantly (20%; 95% CI, 7%–34%; $P < 0.005$) in intervention compared with control communities.

Despite these somewhat "mixed" results, no one would argue that public education is necessary, albeit perhaps insufficient, to improve ACS patient health-seeking behavior. In September 2001, the NIH National Heart Attack Alert Program (NHAAP) and the AHA launched a national educational campaign urging patients and providers to "Act in Time to Heart Attack Signs."[28] The campaign urges those who feel heart attack symptoms or observe the signs in others to wait no more than a few minutes, 5 minutes at most, before calling 911 (Fig. 4-2). Patients are encouraged to talk with their doctor about heart attack symptoms, how to reduce their risk of having a heart attack, and how to develop a "plan for survival" in the event of a suspected heart attack.

The ACC/AHA STEMI Guidelines encourage health care providers to specifically target educational efforts on patients at increased risk for STEMI, *focusing on those with known CHD, peripheral vascular disease, or cerebral vascular disease, those with diabetes, and patients with 10-year Framingham risk of CHD of >20%*.[5] The health care provider should stress that the chest discomfort is rarely dramatic, as is commonly misrepresented on television or in the movies as a "Hollywood heart attack."[29] Health care providers should review anginal equivalents and the commonly associated symptoms of STEMI (e.g., shortness of breath, a cold sweat, nausea, or light-headedness) in both men and women and point out the increased frequency of atypical symptoms in women, elderly, and diabetic patients. The STEMI Guidelines advise family members of STEMI (or, for that matter, ACS) patients to take CPR training and familiarize themselves with the use of an AED.

The ACC/AHA STEMI Guidelines encourage health care providers to review instructions for taking nitroglycerin in response to chest discomfort when coronary artery disease (CAD) patients are given a prescription for nitroglycerin (Fig. 4-3).[5] Specifically, the patient should be advised to take one nitroglycerin dose sublingually promptly for chest discomfort. If symptoms are unimproved or worsening 5 minutes later, he or she should call 911 immediately. Further doses of nitroglycerin should be discouraged until after EMS activation to avoid additional time delays to reperfusion therapy if the patient is found to have STEMI. Self-treatment with prescription medication, including nitrates and with nonprescription medication (e.g., antacids) should also be discouraged since they are a frequent cause of STEMI patient delay.[30] Family members, close friends, or advocates should be included in these discussions and enlisted to ensure rapid action (such as a prompt call to 911).[31,32] Physicians should consider a selected, more tailored message that takes into account the frequency and character of the patient's angina and their typical time course of response to nitroglycerin for patients with frequent chronic angina.

Taking an ASA in response to acute symptoms by patients is also associated with delay in calling EMS.[33] Patients and family members should be instructed to focus on calling 911 to activate the EMS system promptly rather than self-medication. Patients with suspected STEMI symptoms should be transported to the hospital by ambulance rather than by friends or relatives because approximately 1 in every 300 patients with chest pain transported to the ED by private vehicle goes into cardiac arrest while en route[34] and time to repefusion is reduced.

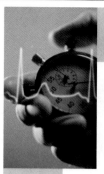

Act in Time to
Heart Attack Signs

Use the T.I.M.E. Method To Help Your Patients Make a Heart Attack Survival Plan

Why Your Patients Need To Act in Time to Heart Attack Signs

Coronary heart disease is the leading killer of both men and women in the United States. Each year, about 1.1 million Americans suffer a heart attack. About 460,000 of those heart attacks are fatal. Disability and death from heart attack can be reduced with prompt thrombolytic and other artery-opening therapies–ideally given within the first hour after symptom onset. Patient delay is the largest barrier to receiving therapy quickly.

Heart Attack Warning Signs
- **Chest discomfort** (pressure, squeezing, fullness, or pain in the center of the chest)
- **Discomfort in one or both arms, back, neck, jaw, or stomach**
- **Shortness of breath** (often comes with or before chest discomfort)
- **Breaking out in a cold sweat, nausea, or light-headedness**

Uncertainty Is Normal

Most people think a heart attack is sudden and intense, like a "movie heart attack." The fact is that many heart attacks start slowly as mild pain or discomfort. People who feel such symptoms may not be sure what is wrong.

Delay Can Be Deadly

 Most heart attack victims wait 2 or more hours after symptoms begin before they seek medical help. People often take a wait-and-see approach or deny that their symptoms are serious. Every minute that passes without treatment means that more heart muscle dies.

Calling 9-1-1 Saves Lives

Minutes matter. Anyone with heart attack symptoms should not wait more than a few minutes– 5 minutes at most–to call 9-1-1.

Use the T.I.M.E. Method:

Talk with your patients about—
- Risk of a heart attack.
- Recognition of symptoms.
- Right action steps to take/rationale for rapid action.
- Rx–give instructions for when symptoms occur (based on patient history).
- Remembering to call 9-1-1 quickly– within 5 minutes.

Investigate—
- Feelings about heart attack.
- Barriers to symptom evaluation and response.
- Personal and family experience with AMI and emergency medical treatment.

Make a plan—
- Help patients and their family members to make a plan for exactly what to do in case of heart attack symptoms.
- Encourage patients and their family members to rehearse the plan.

Evaluate—
- The patient's understanding of risk in delaying.
- The patient's understanding of your recommendations.
- The family's understanding of risk and their plan for action.

Additional Resources

Find information and educational materials at the National Heart, Lung, and Blood Institute Web site: www.nhlbi.nih.gov and the American Heart Association Web site: www.americanheart.org

NATIONAL INSTITUTES OF HEALTH
NATIONAL HEART, LUNG, AND BLOOD INSTITUTE

FIGURE 4-2 • The NIH National Heart Attack Alert Program "Act in Time to Heart Attack Signs." (From: Act in Time to Heart Attack Signs. Action Plan. U.S. Department of Health and Human Services. Public Health Service. National Institutes of Health. National Heart, Lung, and Blood Institute. NIH Publication No. 01-3313, September 2001, http://nhlbi.nih.gov/health/prof/heart/mi/provider/pdf.)

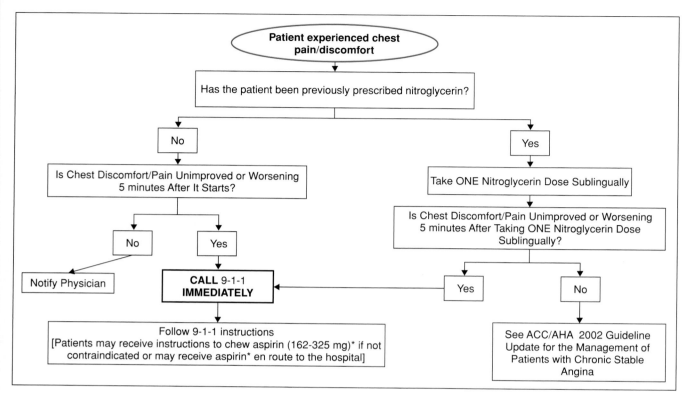

FIGURE 4-3 • Current ACC/AHA Guidelines recommendations for patient use of nitroglycerin. The decision scheme is based upon whether patient's have been previously prescribed nitroglycerin and whether chest discomfort is improving after one sublingual or spray administration.

EMS System Roles in ACS Evaluation and Management

EMS systems have three major components: emergency medical dispatch, public safety (fire and law enforcement) first response, and EMS ambulance response.

Emergency Medical Dispatch

Early access to EMS is promoted by a 911 system currently available to >95% of the U.S. population. Enhanced 911 systems provide the caller's location to the dispatcher, which permits rapid dispatch of prehospital personnel to locations even if the caller is not capable of verbalizing or the dispatcher cannot understand the location and telephone number of the emergency. Although cellular phones have been problematic because they do not stay in a fixed location, new technology exists that allow triangulation of a cellular phone caller's location. This technology is being phased in throughout the country at a rapid pace.

In most communities, law enforcement or public safety officials are responsible for operating 911 centers. Dispatchers who staff 911 centers may have minimal med-

ical training or be emergency medical technicians (EMTs) or paramedics trained and certified as emergency medical dispatchers (EMDs). Dispatchers usually operate under standardized, written (often computerized) protocols. At least one of these protocol systems has been shown to increase the sensitivity of detection of critical cardiac emergencies (e.g., cardiac arrest) based on information provided by layperson callers.[35,36] An increasing number of communities use protocols developed nationally. The ACC/AHA STEMI Guidelines recommend use of medically trained dispatchers staffing 911 center calls, nationally developed and maintained protocols, and quality improvement to ensure compliance with protocols.[5] The document also encourages 911 medical dispatchers to advise suspected ACS patients to chew an ASA tablet (162–325 mg) if there is no history of allergy to it while awaiting arrival of prehospital EMS providers.

Public Safety First Responders

To minimize time to lifesaving treatment, most communities have volunteer and/or paid firefighters and/or law enforcement officers capable of administering first aid, oxygen, CPR, and, increasingly, early defibrillation using AEDs until the ambulance team arrives.[37–41] The goal is to have a sufficient number of personnel to have a trained, equipped first responder at the victim's side in ≤5 minutes of the call. Most EMS systems will dispatch a first responder unit along with an ambulance on suspected STEMI calls, such as those involving chest pain or equivalent complaints, as well as other potentially life-threatening calls (e.g., cardiac arrest, difficulty breathing).

In some areas, law enforcement personnel who are trained and equipped to use AEDs have improved survival from out-of-hospital cardiac arrest compared to that achieved by conventional EMS services.[42-44] The strategy has been successful in some areas,[44-46] but not others.[47,48] To shed light on possible reasons for the differing results from law enforcement AED programs, Groh et al.[49] conducted a prospective survey questionnaire of law enforcement officers in Marion County, IN, in which 66.4% of officers were certified in CPR and 11.3% had received AED training. Only 40.1% believed that AED usage by local law enforcement was needed, and 35.6% stated that they would feel comfortable using an AED if trained. A 100-point attitude score (mean ± SD: 32.1 ± 21.0) was higher in officers who had CPR certification (38.2, 95% CI, 35.6–40.8), who had performed CPR while on duty (40.6, 95% CI, 37.7–43.5), and who were AED-trained (39.5, 95% CI, 35.6–43.4). The authors concluded that law enforcement officers often have limited knowledge and negative attitudes about treating cardiac arrest and the use of AEDs, all of which can have a negative impact on law enforcement AED programs. In 2002, the National Center for Early Defibrillation hosted a blue-ribbon consensus panel to review national and international experiences with law enforcement AED programs.[50] The panel identified 10 key attributes of successful law enforcement AED programs, as listed in Table 4-2.

The ACC/AHA STEMI Guidelines recommend training and equipping all EMS first responders that respond to patients with chest pain and/or suspected cardiac arrest to provide early defibrillation.[5] In addition, the guidelines recommend that all public safety first responders who respond to patients with chest pain and/or suspected cardiac arrest should be trained and equipped to provide early defibrillation with AEDs.

Ambulance Responders

EMS ambulances are staffed by a variety of different personnel throughout the United States. Most urban and suburban ambulances are staffed with paid or volunteer fire department, third-service EMS, private or hospital-based, and/or volunteer rescue squad personnel. Most EMS systems are "tiered," meaning that some of the ambulances are staffed and equipped at the basic life support (BLS) EMT level (which includes first aid, CPR, and early defibrillation with AEDs) and other units (either transporting or nontransporting) are staffed by paramedics or other intermediate-level EMTs who can, in addition to basic care, start intravenous drips, intubate, and administer medications. In some systems, advanced life support (ALS) providers can also perform 12-lead ECGs, provide external pacing for symptomatic bradycardia, and administer other advanced treatments. A minority of EMS systems provide only ALS ambulance service ("all-ALS" model). This has the theoretical advantage of providing the highest level of care to all patients and economic efficiency, but dilutes the individual paramedic's experience in managing difficult cases and doing procedures among a larger group of providers.[51,52]

Rural areas provide primarily BLS ambulance services, usually by volunteers supplemented by a relatively small number of ALS units. In some cases, paramedics or helicopter personnel respond to the scene ("ALS intercept") in addition to a BLS ambulance team to provide the higher level of service. Aeromedical services (helicopters, fixed-wing aircraft) are currently available throughout most of the United States for scene response and for interfacility transfer. Many communities use helicopter air ambulances to transport STEMI patients from noninterventional community hospitals to regional percutaneous coronary PCI centers.

| TABLE 4-2 • Attributes of Successful Law Enforcement AED Programs

- Ability to respond quickly and reliably to medical emergencies
- A supportive medical response culture
- Strong champions in the community and within the law enforcement agency who serve as program advocates
- Integration with the EMS system
- An effective, coordinated dispatch system
- A proactive, hands-on medical director
- A designated program coordinator
- Effective, competency-based initial and refresher training
- Familiarity with applicable laws and regulations and attention to liability concerns
- An effective, continuous quality-improvement program, including written policies and procedures, data collection, and analysis

From Mosesso J, Newman MM, Ornato JP, et al. Law enforcement agency defibrillation (LEA-D): Proceedings of the National Center for Early Defibrillation police AED issues forum. *Resuscitation* 2002;54(1):15–26, with permission.

Prehospital Assessment

STEMI is present in only 4% to 5% of EMS patients with chest pain.[53] Prehospital 12-lead ECG acquisition is critical for field assessment and triage to the nearest appropriate receiving facility.[54–60] Trained out-of-hospital care providers (paramedics and nurses) can identify STEMI accurately on a resting out-of-hospital 12-lead ECG in patients with chest pain using stringent inclusion criteria (i.e., ST elevation >0.1 mV in >2 adjacent precordial leads or >2 adjacent limb leads and with reciprocal depression), achieving a specificity of 91% to 100% and sensitivity of 71% to 97% compared with emergency physicians or cardiologists.[60–70] The International Liaison Committee on Resuscitation has concluded that "neither signs and symptoms nor cardiac markers alone are sufficiently sensitive to diagnose AMI or ischemia in the pre-hospital setting or the first 4-6 h in the ED. The 12-lead ECG in the ED and out-of-hospital settings is central to the initial triage of patients with possible ACS."[6]

 See Web site for AHA scientific statement on prehospital ECG and ACEP policy statement on prehospital 12-lead ECGs.

A number of respected national organizations (including the AHA, American College of Cardiology, National Association of EMS Physicians, and the National Heart Attack Alert Program) and the ACC/AHA STEMI guidelines strongly encourage EMS organizations to implement prehospital 12-lead ECG programs with appropriate medical oversight.[5,71] Despite these endorsements, only a minority of EMS systems currently have 12-lead ECG capability. The national paramedic training curriculum considers 12-lead ECG training as an "enhanced" rather than "core" skill.[71] In the National Registry of Myocardial Infarction (NRMI), a prehospital 12-lead ECG was recorded in fewer than 10% of STEMI patients.[60,72] A recent national survey reported that 67% of EMS systems in the 200 largest U.S. cities have some prehospital ECG equipment and capability.[73]

Acquisition of a high-quality 12-lead ECG is of paramount importance for the effective prehospital triage of patients with suspected ACS symptoms.[54,56,74] Most prehospital ECG devices currently in use throughout the United States are optional "add-on" modules that can be incorporated into a cardiac monitor/defibrillator rather than stand-alone machines. Such integrated devices now cost $9,000 to $25,000, but the price per unit will likely decrease as use of this technology becomes more commonplace.

 See Web site for ACC/AHA focused update guidelines on STEMI. <[2008—TK]>

Prehospital Pharmacologic Management

The AHA Acute Coronary Syndromes algorithm forms the basis for the prehospital treatment of patients with suspected STEMI in most EMS systems (Fig. 1-7).[2] This algorithm recommends empiric treatment of suspected STEMI patients with oxygen, ASA, nitroglycerin, and morphine sulfate if chest discomfort is unrelieved by nitrates.[2] EMS providers should also monitor vital signs and cardiac rhythm and be prepared to provide CPR and prompt defibrillation if necessary.[2]

Oxygen

The evidence for routine use of oxygen in ACS patients without evidence of hypoxemia is mixed. Maroko et al.[75] were able to demonstrate reduction in infarct size with administration of oxygen in an animal model during acute occlusion of the left anterior descending coronary artery. Madias et al.[76] demonstrated improvement in ischemic ECG changes in humans during AMI, but Rawles et al.[77] failed to show benefit in a controlled trial of oxygen in uncomplicated AMI patients.

However, in the absence of significant harm from the use of oxygen, the AHA guidelines on emergency cardiovascular care recommend administration of oxygen by EMS providers to all suspected ACS patients.[78] In addition, providers should titrate therapy based on oxygen saturation monitoring if the patient is hypoxemic (SaO_2 >90%).

Aspirin and Heparin

The ACC/STEMI guidelines express concern that advising the public to take an ASA in response to possible STEMI symptoms may be associated with patient delay in calling EMS, as was seen in the NIH-sponsored REACT trial.[5,33] Instead, the guidelines suggest that patients should focus on calling 911, which activates the EMS system, where they may receive instructions from emergency medical dispatchers to chew non-enteric coated ASA (162–325 mg) while emergency personnel are en route, or emergency personnel can give an ASA while transporting the patient to the hospital.[5] Alternatively, patients can be given ASA soon after hospital arrival.

Does earlier administration of ASA make a difference? Most paramedic protocols in the United States currently include a dose of chewable ASA (unless contraindicated) while en route to the hospital even though published data on the time dependency of ASA therapy are inconclusive. ISIS-2 was the first large, international, randomized clinical trial to document the mortality reduction with ASA alone or in combination with fibrinolysis (streptokinase), but there was no evidence that the beneficial effects of ASA were time dependent.[79] More recently, Friemark et al.[80] studied 1,200 fibrinolytic-treated STEMI patients and found that patients who received ASA early (before fibrinolytic drug administration, $n = 364$) versus late (after fibrinolytic drug administration, $n = 836$) had a lower mortality at 7 days (2.5% vs. 6.0%, $P = 0.01$), 30 days (3.3% vs. 7.3%, $P = 0.008$), and 1 year (5.0% vs. 10.6%, $P = 0.002$). Median time from symptom onset to initiation of ASA treatment was significantly shorter in early versus late users (1.6 vs. 3.5 hours; $P <0.001$). There were no significant differences between the two groups with respect to baseline clinical characteristics.

One possible explanation for the difference in these two studies is that ISIS-2[79] did not include use of heparin, while the latter study[80] randomized patients to either heparin or argatroban, a direct thrombin inhibitor. Theoretically, use of an antithrombin or direct thrombin inhibitor could be more effective early after MI onset because the thrombus is less organized. On this point, Zijlstra et al.[81] studied the angiographic data and 30-day clinical outcome of 1,702 STEMI patients treated with primary PCI; 860 received ASA and heparin before transport to the interventional hospital and 842 received ASA and heparin after interventional hospital arrival. TIMI-2 or -3 flow in the infarct-related artery was higher in the prehospital- versus hospital-treated group (31% vs. 20%, relative risk 0.65, 95% CI 0.55–0.78, $P <0.001$). Patients with TIMI-2 or -3 flow on the initial angiogram had a higher PCI success rate (94% vs. 89%, $P <0.001$), a smaller enzymatic infarct size, a higher left ventricular ejection fraction, and a lower 30-day mortality (1.6% vs. 3.4%, $P = 0.04$). The primary limitation of the study was that it was not randomized, although the results are likely valid since the authors were able to demonstrate no interaction between treatment effect and age, gender, MI location, ischemic time, or the presence of multivessel disease. Thus, although it is not possible to determine whether the apparent benefit from earlier combination ASA/heparin treatment is due to the ASA, heparin, or both, these findings raise the question of whether heparin, which is relatively inexpensive and easy to administer (particularly in low-molecular-weight form), should be added to prehospital EMS protocols for use on 12-lead ECG confirmed STEMI patients. If so, one minor practical issue is that paramedics are typically not trained to perform rectal examinations to check for occult blood, and it is not always possible to obtain adequate privacy until the patient is loaded onto the ambulance.

The AHA guidelines on emergency cardiovascular care recommend that EMS providers give the patient nonenteric coated ASA (160–325 mg) to chew if the patient has not taken ASA and has no history of ASA allergy or of recent gastrointestinal hemorrhage.[78] The ILCOR guidelines consider it reasonable for EMS providers to administer ASA because there is good evidence that it is safe and that the earlier ASA is given, the greater the reduction in risk of mortality.

Limited evidence from several very small studies suggests that the bioavailability and pharmacologic action of other formulations of ASA rectal, (soluble, IV [not available in the U.S.]) may be as effective as those of chewed tablets.[6]

The AHA guidelines on emergency cardiovascular care[78] and the ACC/AHA STEMI guidelines[5] recommend the use of heparin in STEMI, NSTEMI, and unstable angina patients after hospital arrival but do not offer any suggestions for prehospital administration. The ILCOR guidelines state that there is insufficient evidence to recommend for or against use of low-molecular-weight heparin in unstable angina or NSTEMI in the prehospital setting.[6] The same guidelines offer no recommendations on the prehospital use of unfractionated heparin or the use of low-molecular-weight heparin for STEMI patients.

Nitroglycerin and Morphine

The AHA guidelines on emergency cardiovascular care recommend administration of up to three nitroglycerin tablets (or spray) at 3- to 5-minute intervals for relief of ongoing chest discomfort in suspected STEMI patients if permitted by medical control and if the patient remains hemodynamically stable (systolic blood pressure >90 mm Hg or no less than 30 mm Hg below baseline, heart rate 50–100 bpm).[78] Held[82] reviewed results of seven randomized controlled trials of intravenous nitroglycerin. Overall, there were 51 deaths (12.5%) in the nitroglycerin group and 87 (20%) in the control group, yielding a 48% reduction in the odds of death ($P <0.001$; 95% CI, 25%–64%). There were five randomized trials of oral nitrates after AMI. In these trials, 11.8% of the patients in the nitrate group compared with 13.3% in the control group died, yielding a nonsignificant 12% reduction in the odds of death. If all trials of IV or oral nitrates are considered as a group, the reduction in the odds of death is 32% ($P <0.01$).

However, these results were dwarfed by the ISIS-4 trial, which randomized 58,050 STEMI patients in a 2 × 2 × 2 factorial study comparing oral captopril, oral controlled-release mononitrate, and intravenous magnesium sulfate with their respective placebo controls. In the long-acting mononitrate arm of the study, there was no significant reduction in 5-week mortality, either overall (2,129 [7.34%] mononitrate-allocated deaths vs. 2,190 [7.54%] placebo) or in any subgroup examined (including those receiving short-term nonstudy IV or oral nitrates at entry). Further follow-up did not indicate any later survival advantage. The only significant side effect of the mononitrate regimen studied was an increase of 15 (SD 2) per 1,000 in hypotension.[83]

Although IV morphine is commonly used for the treatment of chest pain in presenting ACS patients, its safety has not been evaluated. The CRUSADE initiative is a nonrandomized, retrospective, observational registry enrolling patients with non–ST-segment-elevation ACS to evaluate acute medications and interventions, in-hospital outcomes, and discharge treatments. CRUSADE investigators looked at data from 57,039 non–ST-segment-elevation ACS patients at 443 U.S. hospitals from January 2001 through

June 2003.[84] Outcomes were evaluated in patients receiving versus those not receiving morphine and between patients treated with morphine versus intravenous nitroglycerin. A total of 17,003 patients (29.8%) received morphine within 24 hours of presentation. Patients treated with morphine had a higher adjusted risk of death (OR 1.48; 95% CI, 1.33–1.64) than patients not treated with morphine. Patients treated with morphine also had a higher adjusted likelihood of death (OR 1.50; 95% CI, 1.26–1.78) compared with those receiving nitroglycerin. Utilizing a propensity score–matching method, the use of morphine was associated with increased in-hospital mortality (OR 1.41; 95% CI, 1.26–1.57). The increased risk of death in patients receiving morphine persisted across all measured subgroups. The authors concluded that (1) use of morphine either alone or in combination with nitroglycerin for patients presenting with non–ST-elevation ACS was associated with higher mortality even after risk adjustment and matching on propensity score for treatment, (2) their analysis raises concerns regarding the safety of using morphine in patients with non–ST-elevation ACS, and (3) there is need for a randomized trial to determine the safety of morphine use in patients with non-ST-elevation ACS.

Beta-Blockers

The 2004 ACC/AHA STEMI Guidelines recommend that "it is reasonable to administer intravenous beta-blockers promptly to STEMI patients without contraindications, especially if a tachyarrhythmia or hypertension is present," although "beta-blockers should not be administered to patients with frank cardiac failure evidenced by pulmonary vascular congestion or signs of a low-output state."[5] The 2004 European Society of Cardiology expert consensus document on beta-blockers gave a class I recommendation to the use of IV beta-blockers in patients with ischemic pain resistant to opiates, recurrent ischemia, and for the control of hypertension, tachycardia, and arrhythmias; it awarded a class II recommendation to limit infarct size.[85]

The basis for these recommendations was influenced strongly by clinical trials from the early 1980s, when reperfusion therapy was either not used or in its infancy.[86–90] A meta-analysis of 28 trials suggested that beta-blocker treatment of 1,000 patients would avoid 6 deaths, 6 reinfarctions, and 4 cardiac arrests.[89] A subsequent metaregression analysis found no mortality benefit with IV beta-blockers.[91] It has been difficult to show benefit from the use of IV beta-blocker treatment for STEMI patients in the recent era of reperfusion therapy.[90–93] More recently, there has even been evidence of harm from the use of intravenous beta blockade in STEMI patients. The Second Chinese Cardiac Study (CCS-2) randomly allocated 45,852 patients to receive metoprolol (up to 15 mg IV and then 200 mg orally daily) or matching placebo.[94,95] The two prespecified coprimary outcomes were (1) composite of death, reinfarction, or cardiac arrest; and (2) death from any cause during the scheduled treatment period. Neither of the coprimary outcomes was significantly reduced by allocation to metoprolol. For death, reinfarction, or cardiac arrest, 9.4% of

the metoprolol-treated patients had at least one such event compared with 9.9% of controls (OR 0.96, 95% CI 0.90–1.01; $P = 0.1$). For death alone, there were 7.7% deaths in the metoprolol group versus 7.8% in controls (OR 0.99, 0.92–1.05; $P = 0.69$). Allocation to metoprolol was associated with five fewer people having reinfarction (2.0% metoprolol vs. 2.5% placebo; OR 0.82, 0.72–0.92; $P = 0.001$) and five fewer having ventricular fibrillation (2.5% vs. 3.0%; OR 0.83, 0.75–0.93; $P = 0.001$) per 1,000 treated. These reductions were counterbalanced by 11 more per 1,000 developing cardiogenic shock (5.0% vs. 3.9%; OR 1.30, 1.19–1.41; $P < 0.00001$). The excess of cardiogenic shock was mainly during days 0 to 1 after admission, whereas the reductions in reinfarction and VF emerged more gradually.

The authors concluded that early beta-blocker therapy reduces the risks of reinfarction and VF but increases the risk of cardiogenic shock, especially during the first day or so after admission for STEMI. Following presentation of these results, a practice advisory was issued by the American College of Cardiology/American Heart Association/Agency for Healthcare Research and Quality/Centers for Medicare and Medicaid Services/Joint Commission on Accreditation of Healthcare Organizations questioning the use of IV beta-blockers followed by oral beta-blockers in the early stages of STEMI, especially in Killip class II and III heart failure patients (http://www.ahrq.gov/clinic/commitadvisory.htm). In a *Circulation* editorial, Bates suggests that it "may be time to remove routine intravenous beta-blocker therapy from our acute treatment protocols for STEMI and instead focus on initiating oral beta-blocker (and angiotensin-converting enzyme inhibitor) therapy the next day when hemodynamic stability has been established."

What does all this mean for prehospital providers? Although IV beta-blockers are relatively affordable and theoretically amenable to prehospital administration, the current evidence strongly suggests that they should not be given routinely to STEMI patients without careful evaluation by a physician knowledgeable about current indications and contraindications.

Prehospital Fibrinolysis

Prior to 1993, prehospital fibrinolysis was tested in a number of randomized trials (the majority conducted outside of the United States) and became the standard of care in several European countries. A meta-analysis of six trials involving 6,434 patients randomized to prehospital versus in-hospital fibrinolysis demonstrated a 58-minute average reduction in time to treatment, which was associated with a 17% relative risk reduction in mortality (1.7% absolute risk reduction).[96] Prehospital therapy was not associated with an increased risk of inappropriate therapy or compromised patient safety.

Despite the extensive, generally quite favorable experience with prehospital fibrinolysis worldwide,[64,74,96–130] it has not achieved popularity in the United States because of perceived lack of applicability of many studies to the design and function of the U.S. EMS and health care system, cost and logistics of providing fibrinolytics in the field, failure of the only NIH-sponsored, prospective, randomized clinical trial[74] to show convincing benefit, and medicolegal concerns.[131,132] The most relevant U.S. studies have been the NIH-sponsored Myocardial Infarction Triage and Intervention (MITI)[55] and ER-TIMI-19[133] trials.

MITI was a randomized clinical trial involving 19 hospitals and all paramedic systems in the Seattle metropolitan area.[55] A total of 360 patients with symptoms for ≤6 hours, no risk factors for serious bleeding, and STEMI on prehospital ECG were selected by paramedics and a remote physician for inclusion into the trial. The study population represented 4% of patients with chest pain who were screened and 21% of those with AMI. Patients were randomized to receive aspirin and tissue plasminogen activator (alteplase) initiated before or after hospital ED arrival. Intravenous heparin was given to both groups after ED arrival. Initiating treatment before hospital arrival decreased the interval from symptom onset to treatment from 110 to 77 minutes ($P <0.001$), but there were no significant differences in the composite score ($P = 0.64$), mortality (5.7% vs. 8.1%), ejection fraction (53% vs. 54%), or infarct size (6.1% vs. 6.5%). A secondary analysis of time to treatment and outcome showed that treatment initiated within 70 minutes of symptom onset was associated with better outcome (composite score, $P = 0.009$; mortality, 1.2% vs. 8.7%, $P = 0.04$; infarct size, 4.9% vs. 11.2%, $P <0.001$; and ejection fraction, 53% vs. 49%, $P = 0.03$) than later treatment.

The Early Retavase-Thrombolysis in Myocardial Infarction (ER-TIMI)-19 trial sought to determine the time that could be saved by prehospital initiation of bolus reteplase (rPA) by paramedics in 20 emergency medical systems in North America. A total of 315 STEMI patients were enrolled in this before and after comparison, nonrandomized feasibility study. The median time from EMS arrival to initiation of rPA was 31 minutes (25th–75th percentile, 24–37 minutes). The time from EMS arrival to in-hospital fibrinolytic for 630 control patients was 63 minutes (25th–75th percentile, 48–89 minutes), resulting in a 32-minute time savings ($P <0.0001$). By 30 minutes after first medical contact, 49% of study patients had received the first bolus of fibrinolytic compared with only 5% of controls ($P <0.0001$). In-hospital mortality was 4.7%. Intracranial hemorrhage occurred in 1.0%. The authors concluded that prehospital administration of rPA is a feasible approach to accelerating reperfusion in patients with STEMI.

There is some evidence that very early (i.e., ≤2 hours after STEMI symptom onset) fibrinolytic drug administration may have sufficient potency to dissolve fresh clot that the outcome may be better than that which can be achieved by transferring the patient to a PCI center. The CAPTIM study was conducted in France, where ambulances are staffed by physicians.[129] STEMI patients were randomized to receive prehospital thrombolysis with transfer to an interventional facility (and, if needed, PCI) versus primary PCI. Randomization within 2 hours ($n = 460$) or ≥2 hours ($n = 374$) after symptom onset had no impact on the effect of treatment on the 30-day combined primary endpoint of death, nonfatal reinfarction, and disabling stroke.

However, patients randomized <2 hours after symptom onset had a strong trend toward lower 30-day mortality with prehospital fibrinolysis compared with those randomized to primary PCI (2.2% vs. 5.7%, $P = 0.058$). Mortality was similar in patients randomized ≥2 hours (5.9% vs. 3.7%, $P = 0.47$). There was a significant interaction between treatment effect and delay with respect to 30-day mortality (hazard ratio 4.19; 95% CI, 1.033–17.004, $P = 0.045$). Among patients randomized in the first 2 hours, cardiogenic shock was less frequent with fibrinolytic therapy than with primary PCI (1.3% vs. 5.3%, $P = 0.032$), whereas rates were similar in patients randomized later. The authors concluded that prehospital fibrinolysis may be preferable to primary PCI for patients treated within 2 hours after symptom onset.

The AHA/ACC STEMI guidelines do not advocate a national policy of prehospital fibrinolytic therapy for the United States.[5] The guidelines suggest consideration of prehospital fibrinolysis in special settings in which physicians are present in the ambulance or prehospital transport times are ≥60 minutes in high-volume (≥25,000 runs/year) EMS systems. Other issues for EMS systems considering implementing prehospital fibrinolysis include the ability to transmit ECGs, paramedic initial and ongoing training in ECG interpretation and AMI treatment, online medical command, a medical director with training/experience in management of STEMI, and full-time paramedics. The ILCOR ACS guidelines state that it is safe and feasible for prehospital paramedics, nurses, or physicians to administer fibrinolytics to STEMI patients with no contraindications using an established protocol with adequate provisions for the diagnosis and treatment of STEMI and its complications, including strict treatment directives, fibrinolytic checklist, ECG acquisition and interpretation, defibrillators, experience in ACLS protocols, and the ability to communicate with medical control.[6]

Destination Protocols and Community Strategies

Fibrinolysis Versus PCI Reperfusion Strategies

Traditionally, most community protocols have directed EMS teams to bring chest pain patients to the nearest hospital, under the presumption that most hospitals could provide fibrinolysis if the patient were found to have a STEMI. In prehospital 12-lead ECG-equipped communities that permit transport of patients to both PCI-capable and non–PCI-capable receiving hospitals, paramedics often fill out a fibrinolytic "checklist" (Fig. 4-4) and relay the ECG and checklist findings to the receiving hospital.[53,55,59,134] This checklist helps to determine the presence of comorbid conditions for which fibrinolytic therapy may be contraindicated. Local protocols usually dictate the destination hospital for such patients.

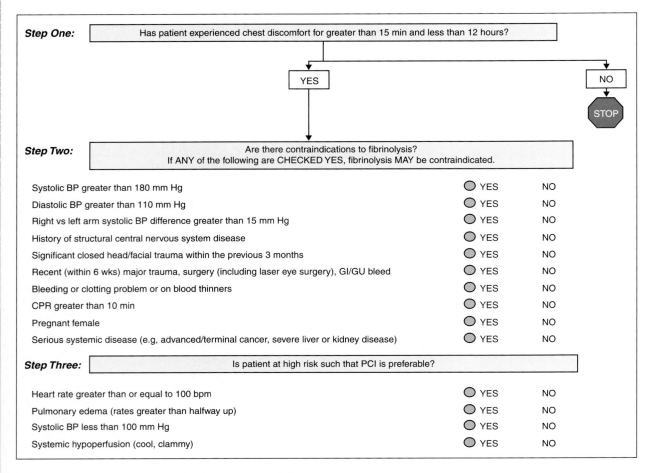

| FIGURE 4-4 • Reperfusion checklist for evaluation of the STEMI patient.

An increasing body of evidence suggests that a strategy of bringing patients directly to experienced PCI centers results in higher initial infarct artery patency and a lower mortality, reinfarction, and stroke rate than a strategy of primary fibrinolysis.[135] A meta-analysis of 23 randomized clinical trials suggests that the PCI strategy is superior to that of fibrinolysis as long as the time interval between when fibrinolysis could have been administered versus when infarct coronary artery balloon inflation occurs is ≤60 minutes.[135] PCI is preferable to fibrinolysis for patients who are at especially high risk of death (e.g., those with tachycardia [≥100 bpm]), hypotension (≤100 mm Hg), or signs of shock or pulmonary edema. The AHA/ACC STEMI guidelines recommend taking such patients directly to a PCI-capable receiving hospital.[5]

Many U.S. hospitals continue to use fibrinolysis as their primary reperfusion strategy with transfer to an interventional facility when needed for rescue. Others transfer patients more regularly for primary PCI, but National Registry of Myocardial Infarction (NRMI) published data on 4,278 patients transferred to 419 hospitals for primary PCI show a median initial hospital door-to-balloon time of 180 minutes, with only 4.2% of patients receiving reperfusion in <90 minutes, the benchmark recommended by national quality guidelines.[7]

In the DANAMI-2 study, the benefits of PCI (i.e., reduction in the reinfarction rate) were seen not only in patients who were brought directly to PCI centers but also in those who were transported to specialized interventional centers after bypassing closer hospitals or being transferred from them.[136] The median time from door of first hospital to balloon at second hospital was 108 minutes in patients transferred from a non-PCI to a PCI hospital. In a review of NRMI-3 and -4 data, Nallamothu et al.[7] found that the hospitals in the United States have longer time intervals to treatment than in Denmark. The median total door-to-balloon time was 180 minutes in patients transferred for PCI. Only 4.2% of those patients were treated within the AHA recommended 90 minutes. Not surprisingly, patients transferred in rural areas had the longest door-to-balloon times. Although hospitals in the United States are often challenged by longer transport times in rural areas and less organized systems of care than those in Europe, shorter transfer times for PCI are possible.

Facilitated PCI Strategy

A combined strategy of immediate fibrinolysis in the ambulance or ED followed by primary PCI could theoretically provide some early reperfusion with subsequent mechanical intervention to ensure complete, sustained reperfusion. Of the eight clinical trials that compared fibrinolysis with facilitated PCI, only the two most recent studies (GRACIA-1 and CAPITAL AMI) deserve mention, since the others did not involve "modern" PCI with its expanded arsenal of stents and glycoprotein IIb/IIIa inhibitors.[137] GRACIA-1, which randomized 500 STEMI patients who had received tissue plasminogen activator (t-PA) to either PCI within 24 hours or to a conservative ischemia-guided approach, showed a 1-year improvement in death/reinfarction/revascularization from 21% to 9% in the facilitated PCI group.[138] CAPITAL AMI enrolled 170 patients and showed a reduction in recurrent unstable ischemia at 6 months from 20.7% in a TNK-only group to 8.1% in the facilitated PCI group ($P = 0.03$).[139] Thus, there appears to be some modest benefit of facilitated PCI over fibrinolysis alone in the era of modern angioplasty.

Trials comparing facilitated PCI preceded by full- or half-dose fibrinolysis with primary PCI have been far less favorable. The largest and most recent ASSENT-4 trial randomized patients to PCI with or without full-dose tenecteplase with a primary endpoint of 90-day death, cardiogenic shock, or congestive heart failure.[140] The trial was stopped by the Data Safety Monitor Board because worse outcomes were observed in the facilitated PCI arm after investigators had randomized only 1,667 patients. Facilitated PCI patients had significantly higher rates of recurrent MI (6% vs. 4%; $P = 0.0279$), repeat target-vessel revascularization (7% vs. 3%; $P = 0.0041$), stroke (1.8% vs. 0%; $P < 0.0001$), and the combined endpoint of death, congestive heart failure, or shock (18% vs. 13%; relative risk 1.3, 95% CI 1.11–1.74; $P = 0.0045$).[140] Pending results of the ongoing FINESSE trial,[141] which is randomizing 3,000 primary PCI STEMI patients to abciximab plus reduced-dose reteplase, abciximab alone, or placebo, Borden and Faxon concluded in a recent review on facilitated PCI that "the ASSENT-4 trial raises serious concerns about continued use of facilitated PCI."[137]

Keeley et al.[142] published a quantitative review of randomized clinical trials comparing primary and facilitated PCI in STEMI patients. The facilitated approach resulted in more than double the number of patients with initial TIMI grade 3 flow compared with the primary approach (37% vs. 15%, OR 3.18, 95% CI 2.22–4.55). Final rates did not differ (89% vs. 88%; OR 1.19, 0.86–1.64). Significantly more patients assigned to the facilitated approach than those assigned to the primary approach died (5% vs. 3%; OR 1.38, 1.01–1.87), had higher nonfatal reinfarction rates (3% vs. 2%; OR 1.71, 1.16–2.51), and had higher urgent target-vessel revascularization rates (4% vs. 1%; OR 2.39, 1.23–4.66). The increased rates of adverse events seen with the facilitated approach were mainly in fibrinolytic therapy regimens rather than those involving platelet glycoprotein IIb/IIIa inhibitors. Facilitated intervention was associated with higher rates of major bleeding than was primary intervention (7% vs. 5%; OR 1.51, 1.10–2.08), hemorrhagic stroke (0.7% vs. 0.1%, $P = 0.0014$), and total stroke (1.1% vs. 0.3%, $P = 0.0008$). The authors concluded that facilitated PCI offers no benefit over primary PCI in STEMI patients and should not be used outside of randomized controlled trials. They also believe that fibrinolytic-based facilitated regimens should be avoided. The 2007 focused update of the ACC/AHA 2004 guidelines for the management of patients with ST-elevation MI recognized facilitated PCI with less than full-dose lytics as class IIB under limited clinical circumstances[5] (Table 4-3).

| TABLE 4-3 • Recommendations for Facilitated PCI

2004 STEMI Guideline Recommendation	2007 STEMI Focused Update Recommendation	Comments
	Class IIb	
Facilitated PCI might be performed as a reperfusion strategy in higher-risk patients when PCI is not immediately available and bleeding risk is low. *(Level of Evidence: B)*	Facilitated PCI using regimens other than full-dose fibrinolytic therapy might be considered as a reperfusion strategy when all of the following are present: a. Patients are at high risk, b. PCI is not immediately available within 90 minutes, and c. Bleeding risk is low (younger age, absence of poorly controlled hypertension, normal body weight). *(Level of Evidence: c)*	Modified recommendation (changed LOE and text)
	Class III	
	A planned reperfusion strategy using full-dose fibrinolytic therapy followed by immediate PCI may be harmful. *(Level of Evidence: B)*	New recommendation

LOE indicates level of evidence; PCI, percutaneous coronary intervention, and STEMI, ST-elevation myocardial infarction.

Community STEMI Programs and STEMI Systems of Care

There is increasing support for implementation of the "trauma center" model for STEMI patient care.[1,143] The AHA/ACC STEMI guidelines suggest that each community should develop a written plan for STEMI patient assessment, treatment, and triage by EMS providers, and system of STEMI patient care that incorporates PCI- and non–PCI-capable hospitals.[5] The plan should be developed with input from local EMS agencies, cardiologists, emergency physicians, hospitals, and others.[144] The plan should interface with that of neighboring communities and should include a requirement to track EMS and hospital performance using preestablished goals. There should be a written "destination protocol" that can guide EMS providers in determining where to transport suspected STEMI patients. The plan should designate regional PCI centers where STEMI patients can be treated promptly by experienced operators 24 hours a day, 7 days a week. EMS data should include sensitivity and specificity in 12-lead STEMI recognition as well as compliance with designated point-of-entry plan (including transport of non-STEMI cardiac patients to non-PCI hospitals). A quality improvement program must be established that identifies a neutral oversight authority (with representatives from non-PCI as well as PCI hospitals) to collect and analyze data and provide feedback to EMS and hospital providers.

Boston was the first large U.S. city to implement a comprehensive system of care in which STEMI patients identified by paramedics using prehospital 12-lead ECGs were transported only to designated centers that agree to use primary PCI as a dedicated reperfusion strategy in virtually all patients except in rare cases where it was clinically unwarranted.[145] Participating primary PCI centers collect and submit performance measure data to a central data coordinating center on all EMS- and non-EMS-transported STEMI patients. System oversight is provided by a steering committee (with representation from nine area hospitals and Boston EMS), which developed performance indicators and minimum standards based on nationally accepted guidelines. A central data coordinating center at Tufts–New England Medical Center receives and tabulates data from EMS and area hospitals, providing aggregated data reports. The reports are reviewed by an independent data and safety monitoring board (DSMB) composed of highly respected cardiologists and a statistician. Any hospital that does not meet preestablished quality treatment, time-to-treatment, and outcome goals for two successive 6-month periods, after discussion between the hospital and DSMB and review by the steering committee, is excluded from receiving EMS-transported STEMI patients for the next 6-month period.

Large regions of the state of Minnesota have also been organized into a STEMI triage and treatment network.[146–148] From March 2003 through May 2005, a total of 448 STEMI patients were transferred from 31 community hospitals by paramedic-staffed ambulance ($n = 149$) or paramedic/critical care nurse–staffed helicopter ($n = 299$) to the Minneapolis Heart Institute in Minneapolis for primary PCI. A standardized protocol and accompanying checklists were developed based on national guidelines. Community hospitals were required to transfer all patients with STEMI or new left bundle-branch block within 12 hours of symptom onset to the regional interventional center. A "level 1 MI protocol" was developed and used to specify the sequence of events, diagnostic tests, and treatments. Patients are preregistered by admitting personnel prior to hospital arrival, using a demographic form faxed from the referring hospital. Upon arrival at the primary PCI center, patients are admitted directly to the cardiac catheterization laboratory, bypassing the ED except in rare circumstances, as when two STEMI patients arrive simultaneously. Prompt verbal and written feedback is provided to the referring hospital physician and nursing staff and the time intervals, clinical and angiographic data, and clinical outcomes are entered into a database (including 1-month and 1-year follow-up phone calls). Time and outcome summary reports are sent to each community hospital on a quarterly basis.

Patient treatment times and outcomes have been superb with this regional STEMI care system. No STEMI patients were excluded from transfer, including those with cardiogenic shock (13.7%), cardiac arrest (9.9%), and the elderly (17% >80 years of age). No patient died during transport. After implementation, the median total door-to-balloon time was reduced from >3 hours before implementation of the regional system to 97 minutes for 11 participating hospitals located within <70 miles (zone 1).[146–148] The median total door-to-balloon time was 117 minutes using a facilitated PCI protocol in 17 participating hospitals located within <210 miles (zone 2) from the interventional center. The improvements in times to treatment were accompanied by low 30-day mortality rates of 4.3% in zone 1 and 3.4% in zone 2.

The common denominator of these two models is that they are based on a community system of care rather than centered on only one hospital. A third model is the Reperfusion of Acute Myocardial Infarction in Carolina Emergency Departments (RACE) project, which is a collaborative statewide effort to increase the rate and speed of coronary reperfusion through systematic changes in emergency care. The project is based upon the cooperation of EMS personnel, physicians, nurses, administrators, and payers from five regions and 68 hospitals throughout North Carolina. The recommendations of this project are based upon established national guidelines, published data, and the knowledge and experience of numerous individuals specializing in STEMI patient care. Detailed information about the program—including transfer criteria, protocols, training materials, and educational posters—is available on the North Carolina chapter of the American College of Cardiology website (http://www.nccacc.org/race.html).

The AHA/ACC STEMI guidelines recommend transport of STEMI patients directly to the closest regional PCI center if (1) the time interval from symptom onset to EMS arrival is >2 hours; (2) the time interval from symptom onset to EMS arrival is <2 hours and the transport time interval to the regional center is expected to be <30 minutes; or (3) a patient appears to be in cardiogenic shock or is developing evidence of severe congestive heart failure.[5] If the time interval from symptom onset to EMS arrival is <2 hours and the transport time interval to the nearest PCI center is expected to be >30 minutes, then the patient may benefit from fibrinolysis unless contraindicated (either prehospital or at the nearest non-PCI capable hospital). After fibrinolysis, such patients should be transferred to the nearest PCI center by ground ALS or aeromedical ambulance. Non-PCI hospitals that receive a STEMI patient by ambulance or identify STEMI in an ED "walk-in" patient should strongly consider immediate transfer of such a patient to a PCI center if it can be accomplished promptly based on the above guidelines. Otherwise the patient should be treated with fibrinolysis then transferred to a PCI hospital. Recent data suggest that the time interval in which the delay to PCI versus immediate fibrinolysis may still result in better outcomes is multifactorial, based on patient age, symptom duration, and infarct location.[149] The ACC/AHA 2004 Guidelines for the management of patients with ST-elevation MI recognized that PCI has further defined EMS goals as well as institutional goals based on whether transport is by EMS or the patient and whether the receiving facility is PCI-capable in relation to time goals (Fig. 4-5).[5]

The ILCOR ACS guidelines[6] state: "primary PCI is the preferred reperfusion strategy in STEMI with symptom duration >3 hours if a skilled team can perform primary PCI in ≤90 minutes after first medical contact with the patient or if there are contraindications to fibrinolysis. If the duration of symptoms is <3 hours, treatment is more time-sensitive, and the superiority of out-of-hospital fibrinolysis, immediate in-hospital fibrinolysis, or transfer for primary PCI is not established."

Developing an organized, community-based system of care for identifying, triaging, and treating STEMI patients is not without its challenges. Non-PCI hospitals may fear loss of revenue, as cardiac care is often a lifeline of a hospital's financial success. At first glance, it appears that there might be strong economic disincentives for non-PCI hospitals to participate in such a community program because cardiovascular care is often vital to hospital's financial success. Anderson et al.[150] have estimated that implementation of a prehospital triage strategy for patients with suspected STEMI would result in the diversion of 22% of patients with AMI from hospitals without PCI capability even if there was perfect specificity of prehospital triage. STEMI patients account for only a small percentage (4%–5%) of EMS patients with chest discomfort, but diminished prestige of non-PCI hospitals may draw additional non-STEMI cardiac patients away from them.[53] To survive, non-PCI hospitals will need to continue to receive non-STEMI cardiac patients and will need financial support through changes in reimbursement schemes and sharing of finances across systems including non-PCI and PCI hospitals.

The AHA's Acute MI Advisory Working Group has published recommendations on how to increase the number of STEMI patients who have timely access to primary PCI in the United States.[151] The group commissioned PriceWaterhouseCoopers to conduct national market research, interviewing a wide variety of key stakeholders (including patients, physicians, nurses, EMS representatives, community hospitals and primary PCI facilities, payers, and evaluation/outcomes organizations such as the Agency for Healthcare Research and Quality, the Food and Drug Administration, and the Joint Commission on Accreditation of Healthcare Organizations), to determine the desirability, feasibility, and potential effectiveness of establishing regional systems and/or centers of care for STEMI patients with a focus on whether and how this might improve patient access to quality care and outcomes. The researchers found that key stakeholders would support a national primary PCI certification program with the understanding that some nonprimary PCI hospitals would experience a modest decline in revenue. Jacobs et al.[152] summarized results of an AHA national stakeholder meeting in Boston from March 30 to April 1, 2006, to continue development of a more detailed plan for an ideal national system of STEMI patient care that emphasizes community organization. In such a system, hospitals implement protocols and procedures to ensure that both ambulatory and ambulance transported patients arriving at their ED with symptoms suspicious for STEMI or other acute coronary syndrome receive prompt evaluation, including performance and physician interpretation of a 12-lead ECG within 10 minutes of ED arrival. Interventional facilities with primary PCI capability implement a "cardiac alert" or "STEMI team" activation protocol that empowers emergency physicians to alert and activate the interventional team and laboratory immediately after a 12-lead ECG confirms that a STEMI is present on either an ED patient or one being transported to the ED by an EMS unit that has performed and/or transmitted a diagnostic-quality prehospital 12-lead ECG. Jacoby et al.[153] showed that a strategy that mandated the activation of a cardiac catheterization laboratory by the emergency physician without prior cardiology consultation for STEMI reduced door-to-balloon time from 118 to 89 minutes ($P = 0.039$) in an active community hospital in Bethlehem, PA.

EMS-transported, prehospital 12-lead ECG-confirmed STEMI patients arriving at primary PCI centers need not stop in the ED to receive interventions and pharmacologic therapies unless these are necessary and add value to the final outcome. A multidisciplinary team composed of emergency physicians, cardiologists, nurses, pharmacists, and other appropriate personnel should oversee a data-driven process of performance improvement that provides feedback to all participants and further modifies the system based on objective data.

Conclusions

Prehospital providers play a critical role in the identification, stabilization, treatment, and triage of ACS patients. Early identification of STEMI patients in need of highly time-dependent reperfusion therapy with appropriate triage to the nearest appropriate facility can literally be lifesaving. All communities should develop a regional STEMI plan that provides guidance and performance improvement oversight to medical and destination protocols.

PART ONE • ACUTE CORONARY SYNDROMES

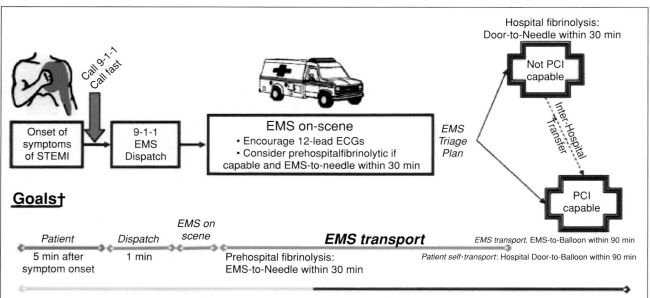

Goals†

Reperfusion in patients with STEMI can be accomplished by pharmacological (fibrinolysis) or catheter-based (primary PCI) approaches. The overarching goal is to **keep total ischemic time within 120 minutes** (ideally within 60 minutes) from symptom onset to initiation of reperfusion treatment. Within this context, the following are goals for the medical system* based on the mode of patient transportation and the capabilities of the receiving hospital:

Medical System Goals: EMS Transport (Recommended):
- If EMS has fibrinolytic capability and the patient qualifies for therapy, prehospital fibrinolysis should be started within 30 minutes of arrival of EMS on the scene.
- If EMS is not capable of administering prehospital fibrinolysis and the patient is transported to a non–PCI-capable hospital, the **door-to-needle** time should be within 30 minutes for patients for whom fibrinolysis is indicated.
- If EMS is not capable of administering prehospital fibrinolysis and the patient is transported to a PCI-capable hospital, the **EMS arrival-to-balloon** time should be within 90 minutes.
- If EMS takes the patient to a non–PCI-capable hospital, it is appropriate to consider emergency *interhospital transfer* of the patient to a PCI-capable hospital for mechanical revascularization if
  - There is a contraindication to fibrinolysis.
  - PCI can be initiated promptly within 90 minutes **from EMS arrival-to-balloon time at the PCI-capable hospital.**†
  - Fibrinolysis is administered and is unsuccessful (i.e., "rescue PCI").

Patient Self-Transport (Discouraged):
- If the patient arrives at a non–PCI-capable hospital, the **door-to-needle** time should be within 30 minutes of arrival at the emergency department.
- If the patient arrives at a PCI-capable hospital, the **door-to-balloon** time should be within 90 minutes.
- If the patient presents to a non–PCI-capable hospital, it is appropriate to consider emergency *interhospital transfer* of the patient to a PCI-capable hospital if
  - There is a contraindication to fibrinolysis.
  - PCI can be initiated within 90 minutes after the patient presented to the initial receiving hospital or within 60 minutes compared with when fibrinolysis with a fibrin-specific agent could be initiated at the initial receiving hospital.
  - Fibrinolysis is administered and is unsuccessful (i.e., "rescue PCI").

*The medical system goal is to facilitate rapid recognition and treatment of patients with STEMI so that **door-to-needle** (or **medical contact-to-needle**) for initiation of fibrinolytic therapy can be achieved within 30 minutes or **door-to-balloon** (or **medical contact-to-balloon**) for PCI can be achieved within 90 minutes. These goals should not be understood as "ideal" times but rather the longest times that should be considered acceptable for a given system. Systems that are able to achieve even more rapid times for treatment of patients with STEMI should be encouraged. Note "**medical contact**" is defined as "time of EMS arrival on scene" after the patient calls EMS/9-1-1 or "time of arrival at the emergency department door" (whether PCI-capable or non–PCI-capable hospital) when the patient transports himself/herself to the hospital.
†EMS Arrival→Transport to non–PCI-capable hospital→Arrival at non–PCI-capable hospital to transfer to PCI-capable hospital→Arrival at PCI-capable **hospital-to-balloon** time=90 minutes.
EMS indicates emergency medical system; PCI, percutaneous coronary intervention; and STEMI, ST-elevation myocardial infarction.
Modified with permission from (90) and from (15).

FIGURE 4-5 • Options for transportation of STEMI patients and initial reperfusion treatment goals.

References

1. Ornato JP. The ST–segment Elevation Myocardial Infarction Chain of Survival. *Circulation* 2007;116.
2. American Heart Association Emergency Cardiovascular Care Committee. 2005 American Heart Association Guidelines for Cardiopulmonary Resuscitation and Emergency Cardiovascular Care. *Circulation* 2005;112(24 Suppl):IV1–I203.
3. Braunwald E, Antman EM, Beasley JW, et al. ACC/AHA guidelines for the management of patients with unstable angina and non–ST-segment elevation myocardial infarction: executive summary and recommendations. A report of the American College of Cardiology/American Heart Association task force on practice guidelines (committee on the management of patients with unstable angina). *Circulation* 2000;102(10): 1193–1209.
4. Braunwald E, Antman EM, Beasley JW, et al. ACC/AHA guideline update for the management of patients with unstable angina and non–ST-segment elevation myocardial infarction—2002: summary article: a report of the American College of Cardiology/American Heart Association Task Force on Practice Guidelines (Committee on the Management of Patients With Unstable Angina). *Circulation* 2002;106(14):1893–1900.
5. Antman EM, Anbe DT, Armstrong PW, et al. ACC/AHA guidelines for the management of patients with ST-elevation myocardial infarction—executive summary: a report of the American College of Cardiology/American Heart Association Task Force on Practice Guidelines (Writing Committee to Revise the 1999 Guidelines for the Management of Patients With Acute Myocardial Infarction). *Circulation* 2004;110(5):588–636.
6. 2005 International Consensus on Cardiopulmonary Resuscitation and Emergency Cardiovascular Care Science with Treatment Recommendations. Part 5: Acute coronary syndromes. *Resuscitation* 2005;67(2–3):249–269.
7. Nallamothu BK, Bates ER, Herrin J, et al. Times to treatment in transfer patients undergoing primary percutaneous coronary intervention in the United States: National Registry of Myocardial Infarction (NRMI)-3/4 analysis. *Circulation* 2005; 111(6):761–767.
8. Goff DC Jr, Mitchell P, Finnegan J, et al. Knowledge of heart attack symptoms in 20 US communities. Results from the Rapid Early Action for Coronary Treatment Community Trial. *Prev Med* 2004;38(1):85–93.
9. Bleeker JK, Simoons ML, Erdman RA, et al. Patient and doctor delay in acute myocardial infarction: a study in Rotterdam, The Netherlands. *Br J Gen Pract* 1995;45(393):181–184.
10. Bleeker JK, Lamers LM, Leenders IM, et al. Psychological and knowledge factors related to delay of help-seeking by patients with acute myocardial infarction. *Psychother Psychosom* 1995;63(3–4): 151–158.
11. Goff DC Jr, Sellers DE, McGovern PG, et al. Knowledge of heart attack symptoms in a population survey in the United States: The REACT Trial. Rapid Early Action for Coronary Treatment. *Arch Intern Med* 1998;158(21):2329–2338.
12. Devon HA, Zerwic JJ. Symptoms of acute coronary syndromes: are there gender differences? A review of the literature. *Heart Lung* 2002;31(4):235–245.
13. Douglas PS, Ginsburg GS. The evaluation of chest pain in women. *N Engl J Med* 1996;334(20):1311–1315.
14. Sullivan AK, Holdright DR, Wright CA, et al. Chest pain in women: clinical, investigative, and prognostic features. *BMJ* 1994;308(6933):883–886.
15. Dempsey SJ, Dracup K, Moser DK. Women's decision to seek care for symptoms of acute myocardial infarction. *Heart Lung* 1995;24(6):444–456.
16. Peberdy MA, Ornato JP. Coronary artery disease in women. *Heart Dis Stroke* 1992;1(5):315–319.
17. Solomon CG, Lee TH, Cook EF, et al. Comparison of clinical presentation of acute myocardial infarction in patients older than 65 years of age to younger patients: the Multicenter Chest Pain Study experience. *Am J Cardiol* 1989;63(12):772–776.
18. Canto JG, Shlipak MG, Rogers WJ, et al. Prevalence, clinical characteristics, and mortality among patients with myocardial infarction presenting without chest pain. *JAMA* 2000;283(24): 3223–3229.
19. Christenson RH, Leino EV, Giugliano RP, et al. Usefulness of prodromal unstable angina pectoris in predicting better survival and smaller infarct size in acute myocardial infarction (The InTIME-II Prodromal Symptoms Substudy). *Am J Cardiol* 2003;92(5):598–600.
20. Bahr R, Christenson R, Farin H, et al. Prodromal symptoms of acute myocardial infarction: overview of evidence. *Md Med* 2001; (Suppl):49–59.
21. Bahr RD, Leino EV, Christenson RH. Prodromal unstable angina in acute myocardial infarction: prognostic value of short- and long-term outcome and predictor of infarct size. *Am Heart J* 2000;140(1):126–133.
22. Bahr RD. Prodromal symptoms of heart attacks. *J Am Coll Cardiol* 1992;20(3):751–752.
23. McSweeney JC, Cody M, O'Sullivan P, et al. Women's early warning symptoms of acute myocardial infarction. *Circulation* 2003;108(21):2619–2623.
24. Luepker RV, Raczynski JM, Osganian S, et al. Effect of a community intervention on patient delay and emergency medical service use in acute coronary heart disease: the Rapid Early Action for Coronary Treatment (REACT) Trial. *JAMA* 2000;284(1): 60–67.
25. Ho MT, Eisenberg MS, Litwin PE, et al. Delay between onset of chest pain and seeking medical care: the effect of public education. *Ann Emerg Med* 1989;18(7):727–731.
26. Herlitz J, Hartford M, Karlson BV, et al. Effect of a media campaign to reduce delay times for acute myocardial infarction on the burden of chest pain patients in the emergency department. *Cardiology* 1991;79(2):127–134.
27. Blohm MB, Hartford M, Karlson BW, et al. An evaluation of the results of media and educational campaigns designed to shorten the time taken by patients with acute myocardial infarction to decide to go to hospital. *Heart (British Cardiac Society)* 1996;76(5): 430–434.
28. Faxon D, Lenfant C. Timing is everything: Motivating patients to call 9-1-1 at onset of acute myocardial infarction. *Circulation* 2001;104(11):1210–1211.
29. Ornato JP, Hand MM. Warning signs of a heart attack. *Circulation* 2001;104(11):1212–1213.
30. Leslie WS, Urie A, Hooper J, et al. Delay in calling for help during myocardial infarction: reasons for the delay and subsequent pattern of accessing care. *Heart (British Cardiac Society)* 2000;84(2):137–141.
31. Dracup K, Alonzo AA, Atkins JM, et al. The physician's role in minimizing prehospital delay in patients at high risk for acute myocardial infarction: Recommendations from the National Heart Attack Alert Program. *Ann Intern Med* 1997;126(8):645–651.
32. Alonzo AA. The impact of the family and lay others on care-seeking during life-threatening episodes of suspected coronary artery disease. *Soc Sci Med* 1986;22(12):1297–1311.
33. Brown AL, Mann NC, Daya M, et al. Demographic, belief, and situational factors influencing the decision to utilize emergency medical services among chest pain patients. Rapid Early Action for Coronary Treatment (REACT) study. *Circulation* 2000;102(2): 173–178.
34. Becker L, Larsen MP, Eisenberg MS. Incidence of cardiac arrest during self-transport for chest pain. *Ann Emerg Med* 1996;28(6): 612–616.
35. Heward A, Damiani M, Hartley-Sharpe C. Does the use of the Advanced Medical Priority Dispatch System affect cardiac arrest detection? *Emerg Med J* 2004;21(1):115–118.
36. Flynn J, Archer F, Morgans A. Sensitivity and specificity of the medical priority dispatch system in detecting cardiac arrest emergency calls in Melbourne. *Prehosp Disast Med* 2006;21 (2 Suppl 2):72–76.
37. Moule P, Albarran JW. Automated external defibrillation as part BLS: implications for education and practice. *Resuscitation* 2002;54(3):223–230.
38. Aufderheide T, Stapleton ER, Hazinski MF, et al. *Heartsaver AED for the Lay Rescuer and First Responder*. Dallas: American Heart Association, 1999.
39. Swor RA, Boji B, Cynar M, et al. Bystander vs EMS first-responder CPR: initial rhythm and outcome in witnessed nonmonitored out-of-hospital cardiac arrest. *Acad Emerg Med* 1995;2(6):494–498.
40. Kaye W, Mancini ME, Giuliano KK, et al. Strengthening the in-hospital chain of survival with rapid defibrillation by first responders using automated external defibrillators: training and retention issues. *Ann Emerg Med* 1995;25(2):163–168.

41. Hoekstra J, Banks J, Martin D, et al. Effect of First-Responder automated defibrillation on time to therapeutic interventions during out-of-hospital cardiac arrest. *Ann Emerg Med* 1993;22:1247–1253.

42. White RD, Vukov LF, Bugliosi TF. Early defibrillation by police: initial experience with measurement of critical time intervals and patient outcome. *Ann Emerg Med* 1994;23(5):1009–1013.

43. White RD, Asplin BR, Bugliosi TF, et al. High discharge survival rate after out-of-hospital ventricular fibrillation with rapid defibrillation by police and paramedics. *Ann Emerg Med* 1996;28(5):480–485.

44. White RD, Hankins DG, Bugliosi TF. Seven years' experience with early defibrillation by police and paramedics in an emergency medical services system. *Resuscitation* 1998;39(3):145–151.

45. White RD, Bunch TJ, Hankins DG. Evolution of a community-wide early defibrillation programme experience over 13 years using police/fire personnel and paramedics as responders. *Resuscitation* 2005;65(3):279–283.

46. Myerburg RJ, Fenster J, Velez M, et al. Impact of community-wide police car deployment of automated external defibrillators on survival from out-of-hospital cardiac arrest. *Circulation* 2002;106(9):1058–1064.

47. Groh WJ, Newman MM, Beal PE, et al. Limited response to cardiac arrest by police equipped with automated external defibrillators: lack of survival benefit in suburban and rural Indiana—the police as responder automated defibrillation evaluation (PARADE). *Acad Emerg Med* 2001;8(4):324–330.

48. Sayre MR, Evans J, White LJ, et al. Providing automated external defibrillators to urban police officers in addition to a fire department rapid defibrillation program is not effective. *Resuscitation* 2005;66(2):189–196.

49. Groh WJ, Lowe MR, Overgaard AD, et al. Attitudes of law enforcement officers regarding automated external defibrillators. *Acad Emerg Med* 2002;9(7):751–753.

50. Mosesso J, Newman MM, Ornato JP, et al. Law enforcement agency defibrillation (LEA-D): Proceedings of the National Center for Early Defibrillation police AED issues forum. *Resuscitation* 2002;54(1):15–26.

51. Stout J, Pepe PE, Mosesso VN Jr. All-advanced life support vs tiered-response ambulance systems. *Prehosp Emerg Care* 2000;4(1):1–6.

52. Ornato JP, Racht EM, Fitch JJ, et al. The need for ALS in urban and suburban EMS systems. *Ann Emerg Med* 1990;19(12):1469–1470.

53. Weaver WD, Eisenberg MS, Martin JS, et al. Myocardial Infarction Triage and Intervention Project, phase I: patient characteristics and feasibility of prehospital initiation of thrombolytic therapy. *J Am Coll Cardiol* 1990;15(5):925–931.

54. Brainard AH, Froman P, Alarcon ME, et al. Physician attitudes about prehospital 12-lead ECGs in chest pain patients. *Prehosp Disast Med* 2002;17(1):33–37.

55. Weaver WD, Cerqueira M, Hallstrom AP, et al. Prehospital-initiated vs hospital-initiated thrombolytic therapy. The Myocardial Infarction Triage and Intervention Trial. *JAMA* 1993;270(10):1211–1216.

56. Kereiakes DJ, Weaver WD, Anderson JL, et al. Time delays in the diagnosis and treatment of acute myocardial infarction: a tale of eight cities. Report from the Pre-hospital Study Group and the Cincinnati Heart Project. *Am Heart J* 1990;120(4):773–780.

57. Kudenchuk PJ, Ho MT, Weaver WD, et al. Relative importance of emergency medical system transport and the prehospital electrocardiogram on reducing hospital time delay to therapy for acute myocardial infarction: a preliminary report from the Cincinnati Heart Project. *Am Heart J* 1992;123(4 Pt 1):835–840.

58. Racht EM. Prehospital 12-lead ECG. An evolving standard of care in EMS systems. *Emerg Med Serv* 2001;30(5):105–107.

59. Kudenchuk PJ, Maynard C, Cobb LA, et al. Utility of the prehospital electrocardiogram in diagnosing acute coronary syndromes: the Myocardial Infarction Triage and Intervention (MITI) Project. *J Am Coll Cardiol* 1998;32(1):17–27.

60. Canto JG, Rogers WJ, Bowlby LJ, et al. The prehospital electrocardiogram in acute myocardial infarction: is its full potential being realized? National Registry of Myocardial Infarction 2 Investigators. *J Am Coll Cardiol* 1997;29(3):498–505.

61. Ioannidis JP, Salem D, Chew PW, et al. Accuracy and clinical effect of out-of-hospital electrocardiography in the diagnosis of acute cardiac ischemia: a meta-analysis. *Ann Emerg Med* 2001;37(5):461–470.

62. Brinfield K. Identification of ST elevation AMI on prehospital 12 lead ECG; accuracy of unaided paramedic interpretation. *J Emerg Med* 1998;16:22S.

63. Foster DB, Dufendach JH, Barkdoll CM, et al. Prehospital recognition of AMI using independent nurse/paramedic 12-lead ECG evaluation: impact on in-hospital times to thrombolysis in a rural community hospital. *Am J Emerg Med* 1994;12(1):25–31.

64. Keeling P, Hughes D, Price L, et al. Safety and feasibility of prehospital thrombolysis carried out by paramedics. *BMJ* 2003;327(7405):27–28.

65. Aufderheide TP, Hendley GE, Woo J, et al. A prospective evaluation of prehospital 12-lead ECG application in chest pain patients. *J Electrocardiol* 1992;24 (Suppl):8–13.

66. Whitbread M, Leah V, Bell T, et al. Recognition of ST elevation by paramedics. *Emerg Med J* 2002;19(1):66–67.

67. Myers RB. Prehospital management of acute myocardial infarction: Electrocardiogram acquisition and interpretation, and thrombolysis by prehospital care providers. *Can J Cardiol* 1998;14(10):1231–1240.

68. Urban MJ, Edmondson DA, Aufderheide TP. Prehospital 12-lead ECG diagnostic programs. *Emerg Med Clin North Am* 2002;20(4):825–841.

69. Mant J, McManus RJ, Oakes RA, et al. Systematic review and modelling of the investigation of acute and chronic chest pain presenting in primary care. *Health Technol Assess* 2004;8(2):iii,1–158.

70. Lau J, Ioannidis JP, Balk EM, et al. Diagnosing acute cardiac ischemia in the emergency department: a systematic review of the accuracy and clinical effect of current technologies. *Ann Emerg Med* 2001;37(5):453–460.

71. Garvey JL, MacLeod BA, Sopko G, et al. Pre-hospital 12-lead electrocardiography programs: a call for implementation by emergency medical services systems providing advanced life support—National Heart Attack Alert Program (NHAAP) Coordinating Committee; National Heart, Lung, and Blood Institute (NHLBI); National Institutes of Health. *J Am Coll Cardiol* 2006;47(3):485–491.

72. Canto JG, Zalenski RJ, Ornato JP, et al. Use of emergency medical services in acute myocardial infarction and subsequent quality of care: Observations from the national registry of myocardial infarction 2. *Circulation* 2002;106(24):3018–3023.

73. Williams D, in collaboration with Fitch and Associates. 2004 JEMS 200 city survey. *J Emerg Med Serv* 2005;30:42–60.

74. Weaver W, Cerqueira M, Hallstrom A, et al. Prehospital-initiated vs hospital-initiated thrombolytic therapy: the Myocardial Infacrtion Triage and Intervention Trial (MITI). *JAMA* 1993;270:1203–1210.

75. Maroko PR, Radvany P, Braunwald E, et al. Reduction of infarct size by oxygen inhalation following acute coronary occlusion. *Circulation* 1975;52(3):360–368.

76. Madias JE, Madias NE, Hood WB Jr. Precordial ST-segment mapping. 2. Effects of oxygen inhalation on ischemic injury in patients with acute myocardial infarction. *Circulation* 1976;53(3): 411–417.

77. Rawles JM, Kenmure AC. Controlled trial of oxygen in uncomplicated myocardial infarction. *Br Med J* 1976;1(6018):1121–1123.

78. 2005 American Heart Association Guidelines for Cardiopulmonary Resuscitation and Emergency Cardiovascular Care. *Circulation* 2005;112(24 Suppl):IV1–IV203.

79. Randomised trial of intravenous streptokinase, oral aspirin, both, or neither among 17,187 cases of suspected acute myocardial infarction: ISIS-2. ISIS-2 (Second International Study of Infarct Survival) Collaborative Group. *Lancet* 1988;2(8607):349–360.

80. Freimark D, Matetzky S, Leor J, et al. Timing of aspirin administration as a determinant of survival of patients with acute myocardial infarction treated with thrombolysis. *Am J Cardiol* 2002;89(4):381–385.

81. Zijlstra F, Ernst N, De Boer M-J, et al. Influence of prehospital administration of aspirin and heparin on initial patency of the infarct-related artery in patients with acute ST elevation myocardial infarction. *J Am Coll Cardiol* 2002;39(11):1733–1737.

82. Held P. Effects of nitrates on mortality in acute myocardial infarction and in heart failure. *Br J Clin Pharmacol.* 1992;34(Suppl 1):25S–28S.

83. ISIS-4: a randomised factorial trial assessing early oral captopril, oral mononitrate, and intravenous magnesium sulphate in 58,050 patients with suspected acute myocardial infarction. ISIS-4 (Fourth International Study of Infarct Survival) Collaborative Group. *Lancet* 1995;345(8951):669–685.

84. Meine TJ, Roe MT, Chen AY, et al. Association of intravenous morphine use and outcomes in acute coronary syndromes: results from the CRUSADE Quality Improvement Initiative. *Am Heart J* 2005;149(6):1043–1049.

85. Lopez-Sendon J, Swedberg K, McMurray J, et al. Expert consensus document on beta-adrenergic receptor blockers. *Eur Heart J* 2004;25(15):1341–1362.

86. Hjalmarson A, Herlitz J, Holmberg S, et al. The Goteborg metoprolol trial. Effects on mortality and morbidity in acute myocardial infarction: Limitation of infarct size by beta-blockers and its potential role for prognosis. *Circulation* 1983;67(6 Pt 2):I26–I32.

87. Hjalmarson A, Herlitz J. Limitation of infarct size by beta-blockers and its potential role for prognosis. *Circulation* 1983;67 (6 Pt 2):I68–I71.

88. The MIAMI Trial Research Group. Metoprolol in acute myocardial infarction (MIAMI): a randomised placebo-controlled international trial. *Eur Heart J* 1985;6(3):199–226.

89. Randomised trial of intravenous atenolol among 16 027 cases of suspected acute myocardial infarction: ISIS-1. First International Study of Infarct Survival Collaborative Group. *Lancet* 1986;2(8498):57–66.

90. Bates ER. Role of intravenous beta-blockers in the treatment of ST-elevation myocardial infarction: of mice (dogs, pigs) and men. *Circulation* 2007;115(23):2904–2906.

91. Freemantle N, Cleland J, Young P, Mason J,et al. B-blockade after myocardial infarction: systematic review and meta regression analysis. *BMJ* 1999;318(7200):1730–1737.

92. Van de Werf F, Janssens L, Brzostek T, et al. Short-term effects of early intravenous treatment with a beta-adrenergic blocking agent or a specific bradycardiac agent in patients with acute myocardial infarction receiving thrombolytic therapy. *J Am Coll Cardiol* 1993;22(2):407–416.

93. Roberts R, Rogers WJ, Mueller HS, et al. Immediate versus deferred beta-blockade following thrombolytic therapy in patients with acute myocardial infarction. Results of the Thrombolysis in Myocardial Infarction (TIMI) II-B Study. *Circulation* 1991;83(2):422–437.

94. Rationale, design and organization of the Second Chinese Cardiac Study (CCS-2): a randomized trial of clopidogrel plus aspirin, and of metoprolol, among patients with suspected acute myocardial infarction. Second Chinese Cardiac Study (CCS-2) Collaborative Group. *J Cardiovasc Risk* 2000;7(6):435–441.

95. Chen ZM, Jiang LX, Chen YP, et al. Addition of clopidogrel to aspirin in 45,852 patients with acute myocardial infarction: randomised placebo-controlled trial. *Lancet* 2005;366(9497):1607–1621.

96. Morrison LJ, Verbeek PR, McDonald AC, et al. Mortality and prehospital thrombolysis for acute myocardial infarction: A meta-analysis. *JAMA* 2000;283(20):2686–2692.

97. Weiss AT, Fine DG, Applebaum D, et al. Prehospital coronary thrombolysis. A new strategy in acute myocardial infarction. *Chest* 1987;92(1):124–128.

98. Dubois-Rande JL, Herve C, Duval-Moulin AM, et al. Prehospital thrombolysis. Evaluation of preliminary experiences at Val-de-Marne. *Arch Mal Coeur Vaiss* 1989;82(12):1963–1966.

99. Roth A, Barbash GI, Hod H, et al. Should thrombolytic therapy be administered in the mobile intensive care unit in patients with evolving myocardial infarction? A pilot study. *J Am Coll Cardiol* 1990;15(5):932–936.

100. Schofer J, Buttner J, Geng G, et al. Prehospital thrombolysis in acute myocardial infarction. *Am J Cardiol* 1990;66(20):1429–1433.

101. Sherrid M, Greenberg H, Marsella R, et al. A pilot study of paramedic-administered, prehospital thrombolysis for acute myocardial infarction. *Clin Cardiol* 1990;13(6):421–424.

102. Prehospital thrombolysis in acute myocardial infarction: the Belgian eminase prehospital study (BEPS). BEPS Collaborative Group. *Eur Heart J* 1991;12(9):965–967.

103. Risenfors M, Gustavsson G, Ekstrom L, et al. Prehospital thrombolysis in suspected acute myocardial infarction: results from the TEAHAT Study. *J Intern Med Suppl* 1991;734:3–10.

104. Risenfors M, Herlitz J, Berg C-H, et al. Early treatment with thrombolysis and beta-blockade in suspected acute myocardial infarction: Results from the TEAHAT Study. *J Intern Med Suppl* 1991;229(734):35–42.

105. Aufderheide TP, Haselow WC, Hendley GE, et al. Feasibility of prehospital r-TPA therapy in chest pain patients. *Ann Emerg Med* 1992;21(4):379–383.

106. Bouten MJ, Simoons ML, Hartman JA, et al. Prehospital thrombolysis with alteplase (rt-PA) in acute myocardial infarction. *Eur Heart J* 1992;13(7):925–931.

107. Gallagher D, O'Rourke M, Healey J, et al. Paramedic-initiated, prehospital thrombolysis using urokinase in acute coronary occlusion (TICO 2). *Coron Artery Dis* 1992;3(7):605–609.

108. Forycki ZF, Schreiber P, Wagner J. Prehospital and hospital thrombolytic treatment in acute myocardial infarction with APSAC: Comparison of efficiency and safety. [German]. *Intensiv Notfallbehand* 1993;18(1):7–11.

109. Rawles J. Halving of mortality at 1 year by domiciliary thrombolysis in the Grampian Region Early Anistreplase Trial (GREAT). *J Am Coll Cardiol* 1994;23(1):1–5.

110. Weaver WD. Prehospital thrombolysis in myocardial infarction. *Hosp Pract* 1994;29(4):77–82, 85.

111. Rozenman Y, Gotsman MS, Weiss AT, et al. Early intravenous thrombolysis in acute myocardial infarction: the Jerusalem experience. *Int J Cardiol* 1995;49(Suppl):S21–S28.

112. Brouwer MA, Martin JS, Maynard C, et al. Influence of early prehospital thrombolysis on mortality and event-free survival (the Myocardial Infarction Triage and Intervention [MITI] Randomized Trial). MITI Project Investigators. *Am J Cardiol* 1996;78(5):497–502.

113. Casaccia M, Bertello F, De Bernardi A, et al. Prehospital management of acute myocardial infarct in an experimental metropolitan system of medical emergencies [in Italian]. *G Ital Cardiol* 1996;26(6):657–672.

114. Carlsson J, Schuster HP, Tebbe U. Prehospital thrombolytic therapy in acute myocardial infarction [in German]. *Anaesthesist* 1997;46(10):829–839.

115. Rawles JM. Quantification of the benefit of earlier thrombolytic therapy: five-year results of the Grampian Region Early Anistreplase Trial (GREAT). *J Am Coll Cardiol* 1997;30(5):1181–1186.

116. Rawles J, Sinclair C, Jennings K, et al. Audit of prehospital thrombolysis by general practitioners in peripheral practices in Grampian. *Heart (British Cardiac Society)* 1998;80(3):231–234.

117. Stern R, Arntz HR. Prehospital thrombolysis in acute myocardial infarction. *Eur J Emerg Med* 1998;5(4):471–479.

118. Cannon CP, Sayah AJ, Walls RM. Prehospital thrombolysis: An idea whose time has come. *Clin Cardiol* 1999;22(8 Suppl):IV-10–IV-19.

119. Arntz H-R. The role of prehospital thrombolysis in the treatment of acute myocardial infarction. *Wien Klin Wochenschr* 2000;112(1):1–6.

120. Arntz HR. Prehospital thrombolysis in acute myocardial infarction. *Intensivmed Notfallmed* 2000;37(1):53–61.

121. Cannon CP, Sayah AJ, Walls RM. ER TIMI-19: testing the reality of prehospital thrombolysis. *J Emerg Med* 2000;19(3 Suppl):21S–25S.

122. Cooke M. The case for prehospital thrombolysis in acute myocardial infarction. *Emerg Med J* 2000;12(3):190–197.

123. Arntz H-R. Prehospital thrombolysis in acute myocardial infarction. *Thromb Res* 2001;103(Suppl 1):S91–S96.

124. Brunner G, Brussee H. Experience with reteplase for prehospital thrombolysis of acute myocardial infarction – Results from the emergency medical system of the University of Graz. *J Kardiol* 2001;8(9):349–351.

125. Benger JR, Karlsten R, Eriksson B. Prehospital thrombolysis: lessons from Sweden and their application to the United Kingdom. *Emerg Med J* 2002;19(6):578–583.

126. Goldstein P, Assez N, Adriansen C, et al. Prehospital reperfusion strategies to optimize outcomes in acute myocardial infarction. *JEUR* 2003;16(3):132–141.

127. Lamfers EJ, Schut A, Hooghoudt TE, et al, Verheugt FW. Prehospital thrombolysis with reteplase: the Nijmegen/Rotterdam study. *Am Heart J* 2003;146(3):479–483.

128. Rawles J. GREAT: 10 year survival of patients with suspected acute myocardial infarction in a randomised comparison of pre-hospital and hospital thrombolysis. *Heart (British Cardiac Society)* 2003;89(5):563–564.

129. Steg PG, Bonnefoy E, Chabaud S, et al. Impact of time to treatment on mortality after prehospital fibrinolysis or primary angioplasty: data from the CAPTIM randomized clinical trial. *Circulation* 2003;108(23):2851–2856.

130. Puel J. Predictive clinical criteria of the efficacy of thrombolysis in a prehospital setting: The OPTIMAL study. *Arch Mal Coeur Vaiss-Pratique* 2004(Spec Iss):14.

131. Brugemann J, van der Meer J, de Graeff PA, et al. Logistical problems in prehospital thrombolysis. *Eur Heart J* 1992;13(6):787–788.

132. Ornato JP. The earliest thrombolytic treatment of acute myocardial infarction: ambulance or emergency department? *Clin Cardiol* 1990;13(8 Suppl 8):VIII27–VIII31.

133. Morrow DA, Antman EM, Sayah A, et al. Evaluation of the time saved by prehospital initiation of reteplase for ST-elevation myocardial infarction: results of The Early Retavase-Thrombolysis in Myocardial Infarction (ER-TIMI) 19 trial. *J Am Coll Cardiol* 2002;40(1):71–77.

134. Aufderheide TP, Keelan MH, Hendley GE, et al. Milwaukee Prehospital Chest Pain Project—phase I: feasibility and accuracy of prehospital thrombolytic candidate selection. *Am J Cardiol* 1992;69(12):991–996.

135. Keeley EC, Boura JA, Grines CL. Primary angioplasty versus intravenous thrombolytic therapy for acute myocardial infarction: a quantitative review of 23 randomised trials. *Lancet* 2003;361(9351):13–20.

136. Andersen HR, Nielsen TT, Rasmussen K, et al. A comparison of coronary angioplasty with fibrinolytic therapy in acute myocardial infarction. *N Engl J Med.* 2003;349(8):733–742.

137. Borden WB, Faxon DP. Facilitated percutaneous coronary intervention. *J Am Coll Cardiol* 2006;48(6):1120–1128.

138. Fernandez-Aviles F, Alonso JJ, Castro-Beiras A, et al. Routine invasive strategy within 24 hours of thrombolysis versus ischaemia-guided conservative approach for acute myocardial infarction with ST-segment elevation (GRACIA-1): a randomised controlled trial. *Lancet* 2004;364(9439):1045–1053.

139. Le May MR, Wells GA, Labinaz M, et al. Combined angioplasty and pharmacological intervention versus thrombolysis alone in acute myocardial infarction (CAPITAL AMI study). *J Am Coll Cardiol* 2005;46(3):417–424.

140. ASSENT-4 Investigators. Primary versus tenecteplase-facilitated percutaneous coronary intervention in patients with ST-segment elevation acute myocardial infarction (ASSENT-4 PCI): randomised trial. *Lancet* 2006;367(9510):569–578.

141. Ellis SG, Armstrong P, Betriu A, et al. Facilitated percutaneous coronary intervention versus primary percutaneous coronary intervention: design and rationale of the Facilitated Intervention with Enhanced Reperfusion Speed to Stop Events (FINESSE) trial. *Am Heart J* 2004;147(4):E16.

142. Keeley EC, Boura JA, Grines CL. Comparison of primary and facilitated percutaneous coronary interventions for ST-elevation myocardial infarction: quantitative review of randomised trials. *Lancet* 2006;367(9510):579–588.

143. Smalling RW, Giesler G. The level I cardiovascular center: is it time? *Am Heart Hosp J* 2003;1(2):170–174.

144. Moyer P, Ornato JP, Brady WJ Jr, et al. Development of systems of care for st-elevation myocardial infarction patients. the emergency medical services and emergency department perspective. *Circulation* 2007;116(2):e43–48.

145. Moyer P, Feldman J, Levine J, et al. Implications of the mechanical (PCI) vs thrombolytic controversy for ST segment elevation myocardial infarction on the organization of emergency medical services: the Boston EMS experience. *Crit Pathways Cardiol* 2004;3(2):53–61.

146. Henry T. Contemporary challenges in the management of acute myocardial infarction: ST-elevation myocardial infarction guidelines and the real world. *Am Heart J* 2006;151(6 Suppl):S11–S16.

147. Henry TD, Atkins JM, Cunningham MS, et al. ST-segment elevation myocardial infarction: recommendations on triage of patients to heart attack centers: is it time for a national policy for the treatment of ST-segment elevation myocardial infarction? *J Am Coll Cardiol* 2006;47(7):1339–1345.

148. Henry TD, Unger BT, Sharkey SW, et al. Design of a standardized system for transfer of patients with ST-elevation myocardial infarction for percutaneous coronary intervention. *Am Heart J* 2005;150(3):373–384.

149. Pinto DS, Kirtane AJ, Nallamothu BK, et al. Hospital delays in reperfusion for ST-elevation myocardial infarction: implications when selecting a reperfusion strategy. *Circulation* 2006;114(19):2019–2025.

150. Anderson PD, Mitchell PM, Rathlev NK, et al. Potential diversion rates associated with prehospital acute myocardial infarction triage strategies. *J Emerg Med* 2004;27(4):345–353.

151. Jacobs AK, Antman EM, Ellrodt G, et al. Recommendation to develop strategies to increase the number of ST-segment-elevation myocardial infarction patients with timely access to primary percutaneous coronary intervention. *Circulation* 2006;113(17):2152–2163.

152. Jacobs AK, Antman EM, Faxon DP, et al. Development of Systems of Care for ST-Elevation Myocardial Infarction Patients. Executive Summary. Endorsed by Aetna, the American Ambulance Association, the American Association of Critical-Care Nurses, the American College of Emergency Physicians, the Emergency Nurses Association, the National Association of Emergency Medical Technicians, the National Association of EMS Physicians, the National Association of State EMS Officials, the National EMS Information System Project, the National Rural Health Association, the Society for Cardiovascular Angiography and Interventions, the Society of Chest Pain Centers, and UnitedHealth Networks. *Circulation* 2007;116:217–230.

153. Jacoby J, Axelband J, Patterson J, et al. Cardiac cath lab activation by the emergency physician without prior consultation decreases door-to-balloon time. *J Invasive Cardiol* 2005;17(3):154–155.

Chapter 5
Emergency Department Management of Acute Coronary Syndromes

Charles V. Pollack Jr. and Richard L. Summers

The essential role of the acute care physician is to identify possible ACS patients in a timely fashion, initiate an immediate reperfusion strategy in patients with STEMI, risk-stratify other patients, initiate appropriate therapy and provide for timely specialty consultation as indicated. The challenge to a knowledgeable acute care physician is to individually apply the dearth of group-derived guidelines data to individual patients and orchestrate the necessary comprehensive interdisciplinary care that will largely determine outcome success in ACS.

- Management of the ACS patient beyond triage (see also Chapter 3)
- Updated AHA/ACC/ACEP guidelines and clinical policies, 2007
- Special considerations for reperfusion therapy: primary PCI and patient transfer
- A key consideration: systems of care and multidisciplinary cooperation and management

Profile of the ACS Patient

The term "acute coronary syndrome" (ACS) encompasses a spectrum of acute conditions punctuating the chronic atherosclerotic progression of coronary artery disease. These clinical syndromes include unstable angina, ST-segment-elevation myocardial infarction (STEMI, formerly termed Q-wave MI), and non–ST-elevation MI (NSTEMI, formerly termed non–Q-wave MI).[1] The diversity and variability of presentations within ACS reflect a pathophysiology that inherently is dynamic and progressive in nature. From the moment of plaque disruption (the typical initiating event of ACS), a platelet and coagulation cascade results in restriction of coronary blood flow that may ultimately be partial or complete, stable or dynamic. The essential role of the acute care physician is to identify the ACS patient in a timely fashion, initiate an immediate reperfusion strategy in patients with STEMI, risk-stratify other patients, and initiate appropriate risk-directed therapy and timely specialty consultation as indicated.

Due to the acute nature of the coronary event, the initial risk-stratification process typically takes place in the emergency department (ED) setting. Differentiation of acute coronary syndromes is critical from the emergency medicine perspective, as it relates to the "3 Ts" of emergency coronary care (triage, treatment, and timeliness of specialty consultation).

Initial Triage of the ACS Patient

Triage is the general process of prioritizing patients based on their need for immediate medical treatment and the estimate for benefit from possible interventions. For the ACS patient, triage also initiates empiric therapy and a risk-stratification process, with a primary focus on the STEMI patient because of the extremely time-sensitive nature of reperfusion therapy. The effectiveness of the initial triage is frequently the critical element determining the outcomes for these patients.

Patient Considerations

Patients who opt for emergency care begin their own triage when they consider their symptoms and choose a method of transport to the ED. There are still a significant number of patients who never seek medical attention for a possible coronary event. Many will delay medical attention for varied reasons. The significance of this fact is evident in the poor survival rates reported in those experiencing an out-of-hospital cardiac arrest.[2] Over the past few years, national campaigns and public education efforts have brought some improvement in symptom recognition and self-triage experience, but there has been little durable impact, and there are many difficult economic and cultural barriers to be overcome[3] (see also Chapter 4).

Emergency Medical Services

When a patient decides to seek medical attention for a suspected ACS event, emergency medical services (EMS), which include the ambulance and other prehospital services are utilized 25% to 53% of the time.[4,5] Although transport is usually a relatively small increment in overall time delay (Fig. 5-1), the responsiveness, assessment, performance of a 12-lead electrocardiogram (ECG) (when feasible), and transport by EMS to the destination hospital may be a highly significant component in determining time to treatment.

EMS determination of the initial destination facility of the patient is also an important aspect of EMS triage. Of the approximately 5,000 acute-care hospitals in the United States, 2,200 have cardiac catheterization laboratories and only 1,200 have the capability for percutaneous coronary angiography and intervention.[6,7] Some states have developed "cardiac zones," with well-defined destination proto-cols, for ambulance services to better assist in the appropriate triage of the ACS patient.[8]

Emergency Department Triage

The task of ED triage is one of the most difficult responsibilities in health care. Overcrowding and severe limitations in resources often result in extended waiting time during initial triage. This ED triage decision is usually made by an experienced nurse using limited information in a short time frame. Differentiating the ACS patient from one with noncardiac chest pain can be a major initial challenge. Since the timely treatment of the ACS patient is critical in determining outcome, the risk of delays to definitive care is important. To address these issues for the patient with acute chest pain, guidelines have been developed for the identification of ACS patients by ED registration clerks and triage nurses[9] (Table 5-1).

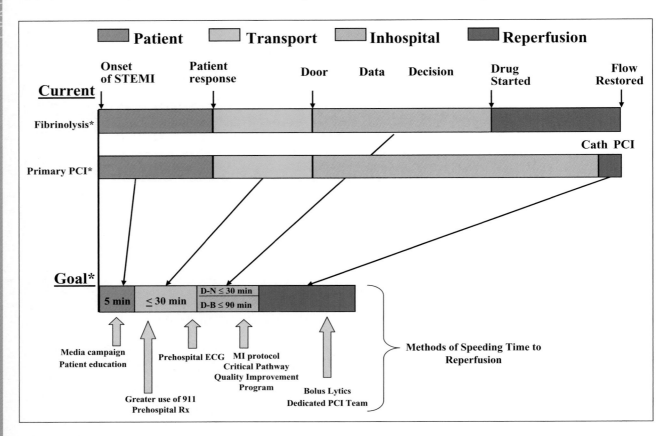

FIGURE 5-1 • Major components of potential time delay between onset of symptoms from ST-segment-elevation MI and restoration of flow in the infarct artery. Plotted sequentially from left to right are the time for patients to recognize symptoms and seek medical attention, transportation to the hospital, in-hospital decision making, and implementation of reperfusion strategy in time for restoration of flow once the reperfusion strategy has been initiated. The time to initiate fibrinolytic therapy is the "door-to-needle" (D–N) time; this is followed by the period of time required for pharmacologic restoration of flow. More time is required to move the patient to the catheterization laboratory for a percutaneous coronary interventional (PCI) procedure, referred to as the "door-to-balloon" (D–B) time, but restoration of flow in the epicardial infarct artery occurs promptly after PCI. At the bottom are shown a variety of methods for speeding the time to reperfusion along with the goals for the time intervals for the various components of the time delay. Cath, catheterization; PCI, percutaneous coronary intervention; min, minutes; ECG, electrocardiogram; MI, myocardial infarction; Rx, therapy. These bar graphs are meant to be semiquantitative and not to scale. (Modified with permission from Cannon et al. *J Thromb Thrombol* 1994;1:27–34 and ACC/AHA Guidelines for Management of Patients with ST-Segment Elevation MI.)

STEMI Priority

The STEMI patient has the most time-sensitive ACS condition, requiring reperfusion therapy as early as possible for best outcome.[10] Reperfusion therapy has been shown to decrease mortality[11] and infarct size,[12] and improves regional[13] and global left ventricular function.[14–16] For survivors of MI, the incidence and severity of heart failure is reduced with prompt reperfusion.[17,18] Therefore patients must be recognized as early as possible at the time of initial evaluation, whether outside the hospital or in the ED. Current guidelines from the American

| TABLE 5-1 • Guidelines for the Identification of ACS Patients by ED Registration Clerks or Triage Nurses

Registration/clerical staff
Patients with the following chief complaints require immediate assessment by the triage nurse and should be referred for further evaluation: • Chest pain, pressure, tightness, or heaviness; pain that radiates to neck, jaw, shoulders, back, or one or both arms • Indigestion or "heartburn;" nausea and/or vomiting associated with chest discomfort • Persistent shortness of breath • Weakness, dizziness, light-headedness, loss of consciousness
Triage nurse

Patients with the following symptoms and signs require immediate assessment by the triage nurse for the initiation of the ACS protocol:
• Chest pain or severe epigastric pain, nontraumatic in origin, with components typical of myocardial ischemia or MI:
  Central/substernal compression or crushing chest pain
  Pressure, tightness, heaviness, cramping, burning, aching sensation
  Unexplained indigestion, belching, epigastric pain
  Radiating pain in neck, jaw, shoulders, back, or one or both arms
• Associated dyspnea
• Associated nausea and/or vomiting
• Associated diaphoresis
 	
If these symptoms are present, obtain stat ECG.

Medical history
The triage nurse should take a brief, targeted, initial history with an assessment of current or past history of: • CABG, PCI, CAD, angina on effort, or MI • NTG use to relieve chest discomfort • Risk factors, including smoking, hyperlipidemia, hypertension, diabetes mellitus, family history, and cocaine or methamphetamine use • Regular and recent medication use The brief history must not delay entry into the ACS protocol.
Special considerations
• Women may present more frequently than men with atypical chest pain and symptoms. • Diabetic patients may have atypical presentations due to autonomic dysfunction. • Elderly patients may have atypical symptoms such as generalized weakness, stroke, syncope, or a change in mental status.

ACS, acute coronary syndrome; CABG, coronary artery bypass graft surgery; CAD, coronary artery disease; ECG, electrocardiogram; ED, emergency department; MI, myocardial infarction; NTG, nitroglycerin; PCI, percutaneous coronary intervention.
Source: Adapted from National Heart Attack Alert Program. Emergency Department: rapid identification and treatment of patients with acute myocardial infarction. NIH Publication No. 93-3278. Bethesda, MD: U.S. Department of Health and Human Services. U.S. Public Health Service. National Institutes of Health. National Heart, Lung and Blood Institute, September 1993.

College of Cardiology/American Heart Association for reperfusion therapy include a "door-to-needle" time of 30 minutes for fibrinolysis and a "door-to-balloon" time of 90 minutes for primary intervention. It should be realized that these time limits are not goals but the outside limits of timely reperfusion. Reperfusion should be accomplished as early as possible.

Unstable Angina and NSTEMI

Complete risk stratification of ACS patients based upon traditional risk factors, presenting symptoms, and physical findings alone has been shown to be insufficient. Prognosis and selection of treatment strategies for patients with unstable angina (UA)/NSTEMI require further risk stratification.[19] However, the 12-lead ECG is central to the triage and diagnosis of ACS and should be obtained rapidly and early in the risk-stratification process. The 12-lead ECG should be obtained within 10 minutes of ED arrival and interpreted by a senior physician knowledgeable in ECG interpretation and ACS triage protocols.[20,21] The presence of ST-segment elevation >1 mm in two anatomically contiguous leads consistent with injury has high specificity for STEMI and triggers the institutional reperfusion protocol. Some evidence supports the use of >2 mm in the anteroseptal leads, as this increases the specificity for anterior infarctions (see "Electrocardiography," below).[22] A new or presumably new bundle-branch block obscuring ST-segment analysis may also be indicative of STEMI (see "Electrocardiography," below).[23,24] If ischemic ST-segment depression or dynamic T-wave changes are found on the ECG, the patient may require aggressive anticoagulant (antiplatelet and antithrombotic) therapy.

In summary, triage personnel must maintain high vigilance and a low threshold for consideration of the possibility of ACS. In the absence of an obvious noncardiac cause for chest discomfort, rapid, triage for possible ACS should be initiated. This also requires that the triage nurse be experienced in recognizing patients with atypical symptoms, especially in women, the elderly, and diabetic patients.

Risk Stratification of the ACS Patient

Risk stratification is the process of categorizing patients according to the severity of their illness, potential for an adverse outcome, and the likelihood of incremental benefit from treatment (see also Chapter 1). The CRUSADE Investigators have evaluated mortality risk stratified by patient risk at presentation (low/intermediate/high), and found a convincing association between the number of guideline-recommended therapies used, patient risk, and mortality (Fig. 5-2). Diagnostic and therapeutic strategies are often linked to this categorization of patients and are tested to result in the best possible outcomes based upon the risk cohort. For example, the TIMI risk score evaluated in the Tactics (TACTICS-TIMI-18) trial identified patients at intermediate and high risk as benefiting disproportionately from an invasive as opposed to a conservative strategy (Fig. 5-3).[25]

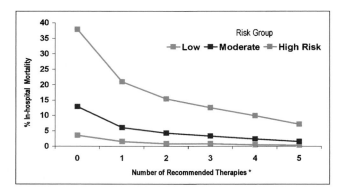

FIGURE 5-2 • Data from the CRUSADE Registry demonstrating the relationship of mortality to degree of risk (low/intermediate/high) and to number of guideline-recommended therapies within the degree of risk. Mortality rates by number of acute guideline-recommended therapies received by risk group.
Therapies = acute aspirin, acute beta blockers, acute heparin, GP IIb/IIIa inhibitors, cardiac catheterization <48 hours; Based on CRUSADE Risk Score.

For the potential ACS patient, risk stratification occurs at two parallel yet overlapping levels. First, patients can be stratified into diagnostic categories based on defined clinical, electrocardiographic, and laboratory criteria, which profile a provisional diagnosis (Fig. 5-4). In this scheme patients can also be categorized based upon the initial ECG diagnostic category as having STEMI, other ACS, or possible noncardiac disease, with each category having a separate, implicit potential for adverse outcome. Unfortunately, the selection of the appropriate diagnostic category is not always immediately evident upon arrival of the ACS patient to the ED. Hence, the majority of ACS risk stratification involves differentiating and categorizing the remainder of potential ACS patients (UA, NSTEMI, noncardiac). In this instance, integration of additional clinical

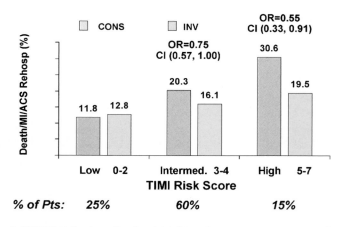

FIGURE 5-3 • Benefit of an initial invasive versus conservative risk strategy using the TIMI risk score in the TACTICS-TIMI 18 trial. Patients classified as intermediate to high risk benefited from an initial invasive strategy compared to those patients at low risk. (From Sabatine MS, Morrow DA, Giugliano RP, et al. *Circulation* 2004;109[7]:874–880, with permission.)

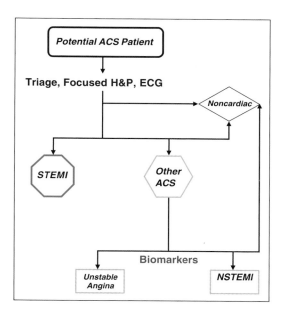

FIGURE 5-4 • Patients can be stratified into diagnostic categories that are based upon defined clinical, electrocardiographic, and laboratory criteria.

TABLE 5-2 • Thrombolysis in Myocardial Infarction (TIMI) Risk-Scoring System for UA/NSTEMI[a]

Historical Attributes	Points
Age ≥65 years	1
More than 3 typical CAD risk factors	1
Known CAD (stenosis >50%)	1
Aspirin use in the preceding 7 days	1
Presentation Attributes	**Points**
2 or more severe angina events in past 24 hours	1
ST segment elevation or depression >1 mm	1
Elevated cardiac biomarkers	1

[a]The arithmetic sum of positive findings relates to the likelihood of death, myocardial infarction, or urgent revascularization within 14 days.
Source: From Antman EM, Cohen M, Bernink PJ, et al. The TIMI risk score for unstable angina/non-ST elevation MI: A method for prognostication and therapeutic decision making. JAMA 2000;284(7):835–842.

criteria—described by Braunwald and prospectively validated—may assist in further risk stratification (see Chapter 1).

The usefulness of any risk-stratification scheme derives from how well the system links severity to a specific outcome. There have been numerous attempts at describing the potential risk of an adverse event for ACS patients by means of a scoring system. The most widely recognized of these systems is the TIMI risk score, which was derived from a large database of ACS patients and validated in several subsequent studies.[7,19,26, 27] A combination of historical and presentation attributes are combined to determine the risk score (Table 5-2). Patients with a score of 0 to 2 are considered at lower risk, while those with scores of 3 to 4 are in an intermediate risk category. A score of 5 to 7 indicates those patients expected to have the highest risk. The TIMI risk score was largely developed from a subgroup of patients at higher risk with either ST-segment depression, positive cardiac troponin, or both. A prospective validation of the system in the setting of unselected ED patients with chest pain revealed a more useful graded assessment of 30-day risk of mortality, MI, or the need for urgent revascularization in patients presenting with chest pain (Fig. 5-5).[28] A limitation in the overall TIMI risk scoring scheme is the paradox that a patient can have a positive troponin but a calculated TIMI risk score of only 1. While this rarely occurs, it does serve as a reminder that such scores are to be used as a supplement to knowledgeable clinical judgment and not a replacement for it.

Initial Clinical Evaluation

From the perspective of the emergency assessment of the ACS patient, there are three major tools integral to the initial risk-stratification process: a focused history and physical examination, the ECG, and serum cardiac biomarker determinations

(Fig. 5-4). These tools are the essential determinants for establishing a provisional diagnosis for patients with possible ACS. However, there are limitations to the sensitivity and specificity of each of these diagnostic elements, and it is important to interpret the results of these tests in the context of a patient considered to possibly be having an acute event. This requires a Bayesian approach to the evaluation of patients with possible ACS, in which tests are obtained and interpreted based upon a pretest probability assessment. In this way the final diagnostic conclusions are built upon a foundation of relevant clinical evidence and not solely the result of a spurious test abnormality. Indiscriminate testing, as with ECG and troponin ordering, can lead to erroneous conclusions as well as unnecessary treatments and advanced testing (i.e., coronary catheterization), all of which have inherent complication potentials, especially when patients with limited anticipation of benefit are subjected to interventions with potential harm. It is important to develop a realistic balance between concerns over missing an ACS event and the potential harm (and burdens on the health-care system) that overzealous testing can generate.

History and Physical Examination

The patient with ACS may present with a variety of symptoms—including chest discomfort, referred pain, nausea, vomiting, jaw pain, dyspnea, headache, and light-headedness. Typical stable angina is described as pain that is substernal, occurs on exertion, and is relieved with rest. Patients with these complaints have a greater likelihood of having ACS than patients with none of these features. However, in practice, the presentation is uncommonly classic, and the recognition of a

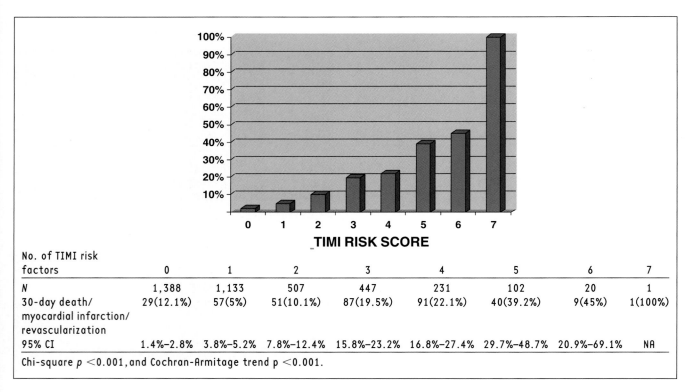

No. of TIMI risk factors	0	1	2	3	4	5	6	7
N	1,388	1,133	507	447	231	102	20	1
30-day death/ myocardial infarction/ revascularization	29(12.1%)	57(5%)	51(10.1%)	87(19.5%)	91(22.1%)	40(39.2%)	9(45%)	1(100%)
95% CI	1.4%–2.8%	3.8%–5.2%	7.8%–12.4%	15.8%–23.2%	16.8%–27.4%	29.7%–48.7%	20.9%–69.1%	NA

Chi-square *p* <0.001, and Cochran-Armitage trend p <0.001.

FIGURE 5-5 • Rates of mortality, myocardial infarction, and revascularization within 30 days of ED presentation in unselected patients with chest pain as related to the TIMI risk score. (From Pollack CV Jr et al. *Acad Emerg Med* 2006;13[1]:13–18, with permission.)

potential ACS patient from a constellation of symptoms can be difficult, requiring skill in the art of medical history taking.

It is extremely important to note that atypical symptoms (pleuritic pain, stabbing or sharp pain, etc.) do not necessarily exclude ACS. In the National Registry of Myocardial Infarction, 33% of patients diagnosed as having an MI did not present with chest pain.[30] Chest pain or discomfort descriptions may also be influenced by cultural or geographic settings and might differ from one gender or race to another.[31] A failure to recognize atypical symptoms could result in significant delays or failure to provide appropriate treatment.[32] Chest pain symptoms should probably never be used as the major or sole determining factor in the risk-stratification process. However, concerning symptoms may be combined with other information, such as predisposing risk factors in the context of a Bayesian approach, to further help make the assessment of overall associated risk.

A small subset of ACS patients may present with silent ischemia or "painless" MI and can be exceedingly difficult to identify unless there is a high degree of appropriate clinical suspicion.[33] This presentation has traditionally has been thought to be more likely in patients with diabetes. The "silent MI" hypothesis is based on the relatively high incidence of ischemic changes noted on screening ECGs in patients with diabetes. However, in a prospective observational study of 528 patients with symptoms suggestive of coronary artery disease on presentation to the ED of a cardiac referral center, the symptoms did not differ significantly in patients with or without diabetes.[34] The increased frequency of ischemic changes noted on screening ECGs in patients with diabetes may simply reflect their greater baseline prevalence of coronary artery disease.

The physical examination in patients with ACS is usually normal. However, clinical signs of left ventricular dysfunction (pulmonary rales, jugular venous distention, S3 gallop, hypotension, mitral regurgitation murmur, etc.) portend an increased risk of a poor outcome. Other physical findings—such as hypoxia, diaphoresis, or an appearance of a mottled skin—may indicate impaired circulation or shock arising from a primary cardiac event. An anxious or frightened appearance in an otherwise reasonable patient may also be a reflection of the severity of the condition. A finding of chest wall tenderness that reproduces the patient's symptom reduces the likelihood of an acute coronary event but should not, by itself, be considered indicative of a noncardiac cause.

CLINICAL CLASSIFICATION OF CHEST PAIN

Typical angina (definite)

1. Substernal chest discomfort with a characteristic quality and duration
2. Provoked by exertion or emotional stress
3. Relieved by rest or NTG

Atypical angina (probable)

Meets two of the above characteristics.

Noncardiac chest pain

Meets one or none of the typical anginal characteristics.

Source: Modified from Diamond GA. A clinically relevant classification of chest discomfort. *J Am Coll Cardiol* 1983;1(2 Pt 1):574–575, with permission.

See Web site for ACEP's clinical policy statement: "Critical Questions on Patients Suspected with MI."

Electrocardiography

The ECG provides information that helps to stratify the patient's risk of having ACS, establish the diagnosis, and determine the treatment strategy. Even with its noted limitations, the ECG remains the best and most facile tool for the early differentiation of patients with possible ACS. Its diagnostic accuracy is generally enhanced when the ECG is obtained in a patient with ongoing symptoms.[35] In the risk-stratification process, the ECG is most important in differentiating STEMI from the other possibilities. STEMI should be considered if there is J-point elevation (origin of the ST segment at its junction with the QRS complex) consistent with myocardial injury. ST-segment deviation is measured 0.04 to 0.06 seconds after the J point, and this defines a sensitivity and specificity for ischemia or injury.

Myocardial Injury (ST-Segment Elevation)

When there is an injury current of >1 mm in two anatomically contiguous leads, consideration for emergent reperfusion is required. Diagnostic criteria of >1 mm (0.1 mV) in leads V1 to V4 may have reduced specificity for patients with early repolarization, and some evidence supports the use of >2 mm in the anteroseptal leads as a preferable threshold.[21,22]

New or Presumably New Bundle-Branch Block

The development of a bundle-branch block (right or left) with STEMI increases mortality.[36] Patients with left bundle-branch block (LBBB) have a higher in-hospital mortality complicating STEMI,[37] and LBBB obscures the initial and terminal portion of the QRS complex, making identification of a typical injury current difficult. The GUSTO-1 investigators, however, proposed that patients with a LBBB having typical ischemic symptoms suggestive of MI and one of three ECG criteria be considered for reperfusion therapy. These criteria include ST elevation of ≥1 mm in leads with a positive QRS, ST-segment depression ≥1 mm in leads V1 to V3, and ST-segment elevation ≥5 mm in leads with a

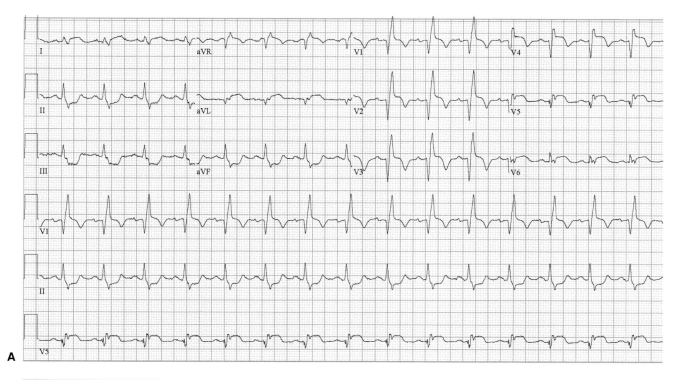

A

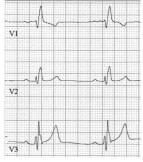

B

FIGURE 5-6 • **A.** 12-lead ECG with right bundle-branch block (RBBB) and ST-segment elevation consistent with acute myocardial infarction. There is elevation of the ST segment in precordial leads V1 to V6 and lateral leads 1 and aVL. **B.** For comparison, leads V1 to V3 from patient with RBBB and secondary repolarization changes without acute myocardial infarction.

negative QRS.[38,39] The determination of "new" left bundle-branch block is frequently difficult unless there is a readily available old ECG for comparison. When such evidence is lacking and the diagnosis is uncertain, percutaneous intervention (PCI) has been proposed as preferable to fibrinolytic therapy when PCI can be performed in a timely fashion.

Right bundle-branch block (RBBB) obscures only the terminal portion of the QRS complex; therefore identification of STEMI can be made by physicians experienced in the interpretation of the 12-lead ECG (Fig. 5-6).

ST-Segment Depression Consistent With High-Risk Unstable Angina/NSTEMI

Patients presenting with ischemic ST-segment depression also have an increased risk for major adverse cardiac events. In the TIMI IIIB registry of patients with unstable angina/non-Q wave MI, 60% of patients had no ECG changes and were at lower risk than those with 1-mm ST-segment depression, who had an 11% 1-year rate of death or nonfatal MI.[40] In this registry, patients with only 0.5-mm ST-segment depression had a similar prognosis. In this study T-wave inversion was not helpful, but other investigators have found that in patients suspected of ACS, T-wave inversion of >2 mm in leads with positive R waves or deep symmetric anterior T-wave inversion suggested acute ischemia.[41,42]

Nondiagnostic or Normal ECG

T-wave inversion ≤2 mm is nonspecific unless changes occur with chest discomfort and are dynamic. The ECG is currently our best but an imprecise tool for the early detection of ischemia, and as many as 10% of ACS patients may present with a normal ECG.[43] Therefore, a normal ECG should not be used to reliably exclude the diagnosis of ACS, especially among patients with a higher pretest probability of disease.

Finally, when the initial ECG is nondiagnostic or equivocal, ACC/AHA guidelines recommend repeating the ECG at 5- to 10-minute intervals (or using a continuous recording) if there is a high clinical index of suspicion for STEMI. In addition, a repeat ECG should be performed with recurrent chest discomfort and with resolution of symptoms. This may be a diagnostic opportunity for patients suspected of having ACS.

Biomarkers

Determinations of serum cardiac biomarkers play a central role in the diagnosis of acute MI (AMI) and in the differentiation of ACS subtypes. It is extremely important to understand the nuances and limitations of these tests if they are to be used effectively[44] (Fig. 5-7).

See Web site for ACC/AHA guidelines for unstable angina and NSTEMI: "Cardiac Biomarkers of Necrosis and the Redefinition of AMI."[45]

- Cardiac biomarkers should be measured in all patients who present with chest discomfort consistent with ACS.
- A cardiac-specific troponin is the preferred marker.
- Patients with negative biomarkers within 6 hours of pain onset should have repeat markers 8–12 hours later taking into consideration uncertainties present with timing exact onset of pain and the institutional norms for marker assays.

Myoglobin

Myoglobin is a low-molecular-weight protein that is present in both cardiac and skeletal muscle and may be detected in elevated levels in the serum as early as 2 hours after myocardial necrosis begins.[46] However, because of its poor cardiac specificity,[47] myoglobin should be used only in conjunction with other serum markers to confirm a diagnosis of MI. Myoglobin does have a high sensitivity, which makes it most

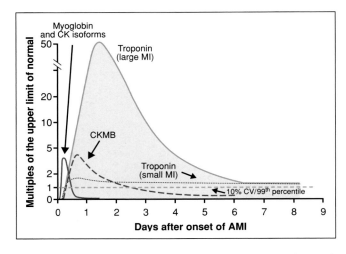

FIGURE 5-7 • Cardiac biomarkers and recommendations for serial measurement and diagnosis of myocardial infarction. The biomarkers are plotted showing the multiples of the cutoff for acute myocardial infarction (AMI) over time. The dashed horizontal line shows the upper limit of normal (ULN; defined as the 99th percentile from a normal reference population without myocardial necrosis; the coefficient of variation of the assay should be ≤10%). The earliest rising biomarkers are myoglobin and CK isoforms (leftmost curve). CK-MB (*dashed curve*) rises to a peak of two to five times the ULN and typically returns to the normal range within 2 to 3 days after AMI. The cardiac-specific troponins show small elevations above the ULN in small infarctions (e.g., as is often the case with NSTEMI) but rise to 20–50 times the ULN in the setting of large infarctions (e.g., as is typically the case in STEMI). The troponin levels may stay elevated above the ULN for 7 days or more after AMI. CK, creatine kinase; CK-MB, MB fraction of creatine kinase; CV, coefficient of variation; MI, myocardial infarction; NSTEMI, non–ST-elevation myocardial infarction; UA/NSTEMI, unstable angina/non–ST-elevation myocardial infarction. (Modified from Shapiro BP, Jaffe AS. Cardiac biomarkers. In: Murphy JG, Lloyd MA, editors. *Mayo Clinic Cardiology: Concise Textbook*. 3rd ed. Rochester, MN: Mayo Clinic Scientific Press and New York: Informa Healthcare USA, 2007:773–80. Used with permission of Mayo Foundation for Medical Education and Research.)

useful for excluding MI if the level is normal after the first few hours of symptom onset. From the perspective of the risk-stratification process, myoglobin levels should only enter in the decision-making process in low-risk patients who present very early in their symptomatic course, when more specific tests may still be normal.

CK and CK-MB

Creatine kinase (CK) is a ubiquitous enzyme that is found in striated muscle and tissues of the brain, kidney, lung, and gastrointestinal tract. This biomarker has low sensitivity and specificity for cardiac damage and may be commonly elevated in noncardiac conditions such as trauma, seizures, and hyperthermia. The CK-MB isoenzyme of CK is much more cardiac-specific than CK alone and may be useful in the early diagnosis of AMI.[47] CK-MB typically is detectable in the serum 4 to 6 hours after the onset of infarction, peaks in 12 to 24 hours, and normalizes in 2 to 3 days. Since some small percentage of CK-MB exists in noncardiac tissues, the ratio of CK-MB to CK >5% is usually used in conjunction with the total elevation of CK to determine the likelihood of a cardiac origin. Since elderly patients typically have less muscle mass, it is possible to see a rise in the ratio of CK-MB to CK even when the total CK is normal. These conditions and other comorbid states that might affect CK measurements have limited the specificity of the test, and its value has recently diminished in importance in the risk-stratification process. However, since CK and CK-MB values normalize in 2 to 3 days after an infarction and up to 1 week before troponin normalizes, CK and CK-MB can be useful for detecting a new MI in a returning ACS patient whose troponin has not yet normalized from a recent infarct.

CK-MB may be further characterized into subforms or isoforms. CK-MB2 is almost exclusively found in myocardial tissue, while CK-MB1 is more common in the plasma. Measurement of the isoforms of CK-MB greatly improves the specificity of the test. However, the CK-MB subform assay has not found widespread adoption.

Troponin

Of all the currently available cardiac biomarkers, the troponins have had the greatest impact on ACS risk stratification, and they are considered the preferred markers for the diagnosis of myocardial injury.[48] Troponins (T, I, C) are found in both striated and cardiac muscle, but the cardiac isoforms of troponin T and I differ structurally from those of skeletal muscle, and hence elevations of serum levels of these isoforms above normal are very specific for myocardial necrosis. Troponin I has been found to be slightly more specific than troponin T, mainly due to fewer false-positive errors, and therefore has been more commonly used over the past few years. There is a possibility of false-positive (for ACS) troponins (both I and T levels) in patients with renal disease, polymyositis, dermatomyositis, pulmonary embolism, congestive heart failure, or in those with positive rheumatoid factor or with heterophilic antibodies of a murine nature.[44] It is important that the clinician not presuppose that elevated troponins are falsely positive in these conditions, because these patients can also have an ongoing ACS event. Serial measurements should indicate a time-dependent increase in the levels of the troponin values if there is truly an acutely evolving cardiac event.

Troponin measurements are often used in the ED setting to help identify low-risk patients who may be sent home with close follow-up. The experimental evidence to support this widespread practice is not definitive and is very case-dependent. The cardiac troponins historically were measured upon admission to the ED and repeated every 4 to 6 hours for up to 12 hours or more.[49] At 12 hours, the sensitivity of troponin to discern myocardial injury is >90% in most studies, and many clinicians like to use this evidence to risk-stratify patients.[44,47,48,49] It is important to remember that troponins may never be elevated with unstable angina or ischemia without infarction by definition. These patients are also at risk of progression to MI or death. Hence, it is always necessary to consider this information only in the context of a sequential risk-stratification process and the complete patient profile. A provocative test such as a nuclear scan or exercise stress test should be considered to further risk-stratify this patient group.

Patients with a normal CK-MB level but an elevated troponin at low levels have traditionally been considered to have sustained minor myocardial damage or "myocardial leak." These patients have myocyte necrosis and are still at least at intermediate risk, so careful consideration should be given to their management. The cardiac troponins may remain elevated for up to 2 weeks after MI, which makes them useful as late markers of an ACS event. An elevated troponin level is also useful in the early identification of patients at increased risk for death. There is an increasing risk of morbidity and mortality that is directly related to the absolute serum troponin level. In those cases where CK-MB and troponin assay results are discordant, an elevated troponin portends a poorer prognosis.[50]

Other Biomarkers

The ideal biomarker for use in the risk-stratification process would be one that would appear in the serum within minutes of the onset of the cardiac event and stay elevated for at least 6 to 8 hours. This biomarker would also be very specific for the myocardium and be elevated in response to ischemia prior to the occurrence of infarction. No such biomarker currently exists, despite many forthcoming contenders. The only biomarker approved by the FDA for ischemia risk stratification is ischemia-modified albumin (IMA), detected by the albumin cobalt binding (ACB) test.[51] However, this marker lacks the specificity needed to rule-in ischemia and is relevant in ED risk stratification only as a rule-out tool in patients at very low risk. There is concern that a high false-positive rate may result in harmful treatments and the performance of testing in patients who might otherwise have been sent home. Most other "ischemia" biomarkers (C-reactive protein [CRP], fatty acid–binding protein [FABP] levels, etc.) are in actuality indicators only of an increased risk of atherosclerosis or inflammatory conditions that may be associated with plaque rupture. However, they do not directly indicate that the patient is presenting because of an acute ACS event. The appearance of a true ischemia biomarker with ready utility in the ED setting would be a revolutionary development in the early risk stratification of the potential ACS patient.

Adjunctive Tests

While it is most important to identify the ACS patient from the large number of patients who present to the ED with potential cardiac symptoms, it is often left to the ED physician ultimately to decide which patients can be safely sent home for an outpatient evaluation. The combination of results from the history, physical exam, ECG, and biomarker determinations are sometimes inadequate to allow for a safe and timely disposition. A number of adjunctive tests have been developed to improve the risk-stratification process. While these adjunctive studies have definitely improved the overall disposition decisions of these patients, their use is often limited by logistic complexities and time limitations within the ED framework.

Stress Testing

Based upon many years of outpatient experience, 12-lead ECG exercise testing has been introduced into the ED as a tool for risk stratification and the evaluation of patients presenting to the ED with possible ACS. Typically the process begins by identifying low-risk ACS patients with repeated negative or nonspecific ECG and serial cardiac biomarkers. If there is still some doubt about the state of these patients, provocative testing using a standardized exercise stress test can be used to determine their potential risk of developing an ischemic event if discharged. The length of time involved in the initial portion of the risk-stratification protocol usually results in this group of patients being admitted to the hospital telemetry floor or to some type of "chest pain unit." Clinical trials that have studied the practical implementation of these protocols have found that they effectively reduce the need for hospitalization of a significant number of patients without an increase in risk of mortality.[52] There is also evidence that this testing can be accurately performed and interpreted by physicians other than cardiologists who are trained and experienced in functional testing, making this approach even more resource-efficient if it can be accomplished in the ED.[53]

Computed Tomography Coronary Angiography

There has recently been a consideration of incorporating high-resolution coronary CT angiography (64-slice) into the evaluation of low-risk patients (TIMI score >2) presenting to the ED with chest pain.[54, 55] The advantage of this study over other methodologies lies in its ease and rapidity of use. Early studies suggest that using this technology may safely allow ED physicians to discharge low-risk patients with negative studies in a timely fashion and without an increased risk of mortality. However, there may currently be some limitations to the widespread adoption of this testing due to the cost of the special equipment used, expertise required to interpret the results, high radiation exposure, and clinical application. Newer imaging modalities are undergoing clinical validation and application at this time. Coronary CT angiography may have a particular utility in acute chest pain syndromes with an intermediate probability of disease, normal or nondiagnostic ECG, and negative cardiac biomarkers.[56]

Nuclear Imaging

A significant number of studies over the past two decades have examined the ability of early myocardial perfusion imaging (MPI) using technetium-99m sestamibi to risk-stratify potential ACS patients who present to the ED with nondiagnostic ECGs and negative cardiac biomarkers.[57] A positive test has been found to accurately identify patients at high risk for adverse cardiac outcomes, whereas a negative MPI identifies a very low-risk patient group.[57] Both rest and stress MPI studies (depending on the timing of the test after the termination of symptoms) are now considered important endpoints in the risk stratification of these patients.[57] Unfortunately, the availability of this testing is limited and resource-intensive in most hospitals, and the use of this testing has not resulted in more timely ED dispositions in most cases.

Selecting a Strategy and Initiating Treatment

The appropriate triage and risk stratification of patients presenting to the ED with symptoms suggestive of an acute coronary event remains a continuing challenge for the ED physician. A low threshold for admission has been the standard because of heightened concern for adverse patient outcomes and the litigation potential associated with the inadvertent discharge of a patient having an ischemic event. This trend toward caution has resulted in a system in which fewer than 30% of patients admitted for chest pain are ultimately determined to have ACS.[58] The costs and resource demands required by this inefficient practice are of great concern to many in the health care industry and government. In order to reduce unnecessary admissions while preserving patient safety, a number of protocols and strategies have been applied to the risk stratification of ED patients with chest pain syndrome. These strategies have evolved as new tests and methods have been developed.

The first charge of the ED physician is the early recognition of the STEMI patient, using ECG criteria to initiate timely treatment. After this group is identified, the next step is to differentiate the high-risk ACS patient (typically with NSTEMI or severe UA) from the remainder of the chest pain population. ECG changes indicative of ischemia, with or without a positive biomarker, may help to define this patient, but are not uniformly present. While it is presently uncertain what time frame is required to make this determination of high risk, it is intuitively evident that an early management strategy should result in improved outcomes. Identification of patients with variable levels of risk and appropriate application of strategies, resources, and evolving diagnostic modalities will improve both patient outcomes and resource utilization.

Despite all of the available diagnostic aids, ultimately the integration of clinical information and medical decision making will be the responsibility of the physician. This requires both experience and a broad-based knowledge of the disease process and the diagnostic tools used to differentiate the patient's condition. A systematic approach to patient evaluation should include a sequential risk prediction or probability assessment as performed by the clinician using the focused history, initial ECG, and cardiac biomarkers discussed above. Based upon the results of these tests and the pretest probability of ACS, further treatment or diagnosis is indicated. Patients with definite high-risk features should not undergo functional testing until stabilized. Others will have expeditious testing or appropriate designated follow-up based upon clinical assessment and exclusion of MI.

General Measures and Aspirin

Once patients are identified as having, or likely having, ACS, specific pharmacologic management should be initiated in a risk-appropriate fashion. Patients at higher presumed ACS risk should generally receive more intensive therapy. However, with escalation of therapy comes increased risk (e.g., anticoagulant-related bleeding). Therefore, treatment of ACS must be individualized for each patient and each presentation based on the balancing of potential efficacy with risk.

All patients without contraindications, even those with suspected ACS, should be given aspirin (ASA) as soon as possible after presentation. ASA acts as an antiplatelet agent and as such is considered in more detail below. Other general measures include routine telemetry monitoring (for rhythm disturbances and identification of ST-segment changes) and application of supplementary oxygen and pulse oximetry. Ischemia and its common clinical manifestation—chest pain—are treated with nitroglycerin, and with morphine if pain is unrelieved by nitrates and oxygen. Based upon data from the CRUSADE registry, a caution with the use of morphine has been introduced with the recent update (2007) of the ACC/AHA guidelines; its strength of recommendation was reduced to class IIa from class I.[59]

 See Web site for ACC/AHA guidelines for unstable angina and NSTEMI: "General Care."[45]

Nitrates

Nitroglycerin (NTG) reduces myocardial oxygen demand and improves myocardial oxygen delivery through peripheral and coronary vascular effects that reduce both preload and afterload. It is thought that NTG promotes not only the dilation of large coronary arteries but also collateral flow that may reach ischemic regions. NTG should be initially administered by sublingual tablets (0.4 mg) or spray, with up to three doses every 5 minutes. Absolute contraindications to NTG use include hypotension, obvious volume depletion, clinical or electrocardiographic concern for right ventricular ischemia/infarction, myocardial wall ischemia, or recent use of phosphodiesterase inhibitors (e.g. Viagra, Cialis, and Levitra) for erectile dysfunction.[45]

Nitrates can also be administered topically in patients without ongoing significant symptoms or risk of hemody-namic instability. NTG can be given intravenously to normotensive patients at an initial rate of 5 to 10 µg/min and then increased by 10 µg/min every 3 to 5 minutes until a symptomatic or blood pressure response is evident. However, blood pressure should generally not be reduced to <110 mm Hg in patients who were previously normotensive or to >25% below the starting mean arterial blood pressure if hypertension was present.

Side effects of nitrates include headache and hypotension. Tolerance to the drug may develop. It is thought that NTG alone does not exert a beneficial effect on mortality in ACS, but its salutary effects on ischemic symptoms and elevated blood pressure keep it firmly in the pharmacologic armamentarium for ACS patients with chest pain.[35]

Morphine Sulfate

In patients whose ischemic symptoms are incompletely relieved by nitrates, morphine sulfate (1–5 mg IV) is reasonable. Acting as both an analgesic and an anxiolytic, it also is a venodilator and therefore may lead to symptomatic benefit for patients with pulmonary congestion as well. Potential adverse effects include hypotension, pruritus, nausea and vomiting, and diminished respiratory drive.[45] There have been no randomized controlled trials to advise clinicians on the contribution of morphine to ACS outcomes or on optimal dosing regimens. Data from a contemporary registry, however, suggest that the use of morphine in NSTE ACS patients may actually increase short-term mortality, even after adjustment for risk and other medications.[59]

This being said, there are no good data regarding alternative analgesics for ACS pain either. In the presence of persistent pain despite nitrates, the emergency physician should:

1. Consider alternative diagnoses if there is no objective evidence of ischemia or infarction.
2. Consider administration of beta-blockers if not already given and there are no contraindications.
3. Initiate cardiology consultation for coronary angiography and PCI with pain refractory to initial management.

Morphine sulfate (1–5 mg IV) is reasonable for patients whose symptoms are not relieved despite NTG (e.g., after 3 serial sublingual NTG tablets) or whose symptoms recur despite adequate anti-ischemic therapy. A cautionary note on morphine use has been raised by data from a large observational registry. Patients in this registry receiving morphine (30%) had a higher adjusted likelihood of death, which persisted across all subgroups.[59] Although subject to uncontrolled selection biases, these results raise a safety concern and suggest the need for a randomized trial. Meanwhile, the writing committee has downgraded the recommendation for morphine use for uncontrolled ischemic chest discomfort from a class I to a class IIa (Updated 2007 ACC/AHA Guidelines Recommendations).

Beta-Adrenergic Blocking Agents

Beta-adrenergic blockers improved both morbidity and mortality in early ACS clinical trials, but an early mortality benefit was questioned in the reperfusion era in STEMI patients (see below). These drugs inhibit the effect of catecholamines on the myocardium, resulting in reduced cardiac work and oxygen consumption. They also reduce blood pressure and, by increasing the duration of diastole, improve coronary blood flow.

Oral beta-blockers should be administered early for ACS of all types unless contraindications are present. Beta-blockers may also be beneficial for NSTEMI. They should be given irrespective of the need for revascularization therapies (class I).

 See Web site for ACC/AHA focused guidelines update for STEMI: "beta-blockers."[45]

The above recommendations were largely based on studies evaluating IV beta blockade in patients receiving fibrinolytic therapy. In patients who receive fibrinolytic agents, IV beta-blockers decrease postinfarction ischemia and nonfatal AMI. A small but significant decrease in death and nonfatal infarction has been observed in patients treated with beta-blockers very soon after the onset of symtpoms.[65] In-hospital administration of beta blockers may reduce the size of the infarct, and mortality in patients who do not receive fibrinolytic therapy.[60] Beta-blockers also reduce the incidence of ventricular ectopy and fibrillation.[66]

These data were largely observed during clinical trials before the "reperfusion era." But subsequent studies and reviews did not find reductions in mortality.[67–69]

IV beta-blockers are often administered in the ED using a dose regimen from the Metoprolol in Acute Myocardial Infarction (MIAMI) trial.[70] To assess modern use, the Clopidogrel and Metoprolol in Myocardial Infarction Trial (COMMIT CCS2) trial studied the administration of the usual dosing—metoprolol 5 mg IV over 15 minutes.[71] In COMMIT CCS2 there was no benefit of early administration of IV beta-blockers (Fig. 5-8). An analysis of prespecified subgroups showed that about 10 lives per 1,000 were saved by a reduction in ventricular fibrillation (VF) and recurrent MI, but this benefit was offset by an increase in patient death from cardiogenic shock. Lives lost from cardiogenic shock increased with increasing Killip class, likely as a result of an increase in death from heart failure, since left ventricular dysfunction (LVD) increases with infarct size. For this reason careful attention should be given to treating patients with congestive heart failure. A tachycardia in these patients may be compensatory, as heart rate compensates for impaired and decreased stroke volume due to infarction.

UPDATED RECOMMENDATIONS FOR BETA-BLOCKING AGENTS (STEMI)

Recommendation for oral beta-adrenergic blockade early in STEMI (class I recommendation; level of evidence changed from A to B):

Oral beta blockade should be initiated within first 24 hours in STEMI to patients not at high risk[a] without any of the following:
- Signs of heart failure
- Evidence of low output state
- Increased risk for cardiogenic shock
- Other relative contraindications

Patients with early contraindication to beta blockade should be reevaluated for candidacy for secondary prevention before discharge.

Patients with moderate to severe heart failure should receive beta blockade as secondary prevention with a gradual titration scheme.

Recommendation for IV beta-adrenergic blockade early in STEMI (class II recommendation; level of evidence changed from A to B):

- Reasonable to administer IV beta blockade to patients who are *hypertensive* and who do not have
  - Signs of heart failure
  - Evidence of low-output state
  - Increased risk for cardiogenic shock
  - Other relative contraindications

IV Beta-adrenergic blockade class III (new 2007 recommendation)

IV beta blockade should not be administered to patients who have any of the following:
- Signs of heart failure
- Evidence of low-output state
- Risk factors for cardiogenic shock[a]
- Other relative contraindications: PR interval >0.24 second or higher AV block, active asthma, or reactive airway disease

---

[a]Risk factors for cardiogenic shock include
- Age >70 years
- SBP <120 mm Hg
- Heart rate >110/min or <60/min
- Delayed presentation

Updated Recommendations in STEMI Patients

Oral beta-blocker therapy should be initiated in the first 24 hours for STEMI patients who do not have any of the following: (1) signs of heart failure, (2) evidence of a low-output state, (3) increased risk for cardiogenic shock, or (4) other relative contraindications to beta blockade (PR interval >0.24 seconds, second- or third-degree heart block, active asthma, or reactive airway disease). For patients with severe hypertension, metoprolol may be given intravenously in 5-mg increments repeated every 5 minutes for a total initial dose of 15 mg in the absence of contraindications or clinical evidence of heart failure.

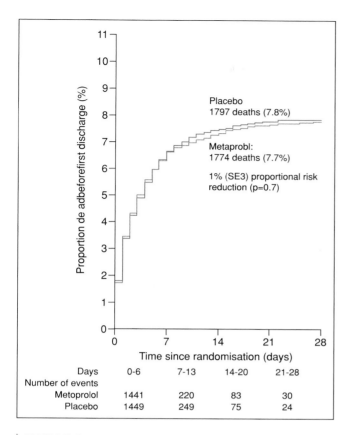

FIGURE 5-8 • Effects of metoprolol allocation on death before first discharge from hospital in the COMMITT CCS2 Trial. (Reprinted with permission from Chen ZM et al. *Lancet* 2005;366:1622–1632, with permission.)

Other Pharmacologic Measures

Angiotensin converting enzyme inhibitor (ACE-I) therapy has been shown to have a significant benefit in the chronic management of patients with coronary artery disease and left ventricular dysfunction (LVD).[45] In the acute ACS setting, this should be considered in patients with evidence of LVD, especially diabetic patients. ACE-I can also be used to control blood pressure not adequately responsive to nitrates and beta-blockers. However, they are usually administered after the patient has received reperfusion therapy (if STEMI) and is hemodynamically stable. In most instances, the initiation of ACE-I therapy is not a consideration in early ED management.

Calcium antagonists have a limited (if any) role in the early management of ACS, being useful primarily when hypertension is unresponsive to nitrates and beta blockers. Verapamil and diltiazem are the best choices in this class because they tend to slow the heart rate.[45]

Antiplatelet Therapy

Perhaps the best data for a long-term beneficial effect of drug treatment in ACS exists for aspirin (ASA). Its mechanism of action derives primarily from its irreversible inhibition of cyclo-oxygenase (COX-1) within platelets, which in turn prevents the formation of thromboxane A2 and diminishes platelet aggregation; ASA also likely exerts an additional (though less well defined) intravascular anti-inflammatory effect.[73] The benefit of ASA therapy is apparent early and persists with regular dosing.[74] Although the *optimal* dose of ASA has not been established in clinical trials, doses from 162 to 325 mg have generally been employed. Acute doses of >325 mg may reduce cardiac morbidity and mortality, but only with an increased risk of stroke; the currently recommended ED dose for ACS is 162 to 325 mg.[75] Nonenteric formulations should be used to promote rapid absorption and activity and a rectal suppository is available for patients intolerant of oral medications. IV ASA is not available in the U.S.

See Web site for ACC/AHA focused guidelines update for STEMI and UA/NSTEMI: "Antiplatelet and Anticoagulant Therapy."[45]

The 2007 focused update of the ACC/AHA 2004 STEMI guidelines recommend the administration of a proton-pump inhibitor if the patient has history of GI bleed or GI intolerance. Patients already anticoagulated with warfarin should receive ASA if suspected of having ACS unless there is concern for serious coagulopathy, because the antiplatelet effect of ASA is considered beneficial over and above anticoagulation.

The selection, use, and patient risk stratification for antiplatelet and anticoagulant therapy is complex. In addition, clinical trials and information continue to evolve. An institutional interdisciplinary guideline provides the best framework for health care providers and ED physicians to approach the initial and continuing care of individual patients.

Clopidogrel

Clopidogrel should be given to those patients with hypersensitivity or major gastrointestinal intolerance to ASA. This is rare in the ED, where the more typical approach would be to consider administration of clopidogrel *in addition to* ASA. Clopidogrel monotherapy was compared to ASA in the Clopidogrel versus Aspirin in Patients at Risk of Ischemic Events (CAPRIE) trial and was found to be at least as effective as the latter.[76] Nonetheless, clopidogrel is even more effective in combination with ASA, as shown in the Clopidogrel in Unstable Angina to Prevent Recurrent Events (CURE) trial, which randomized 12,562 patients with UA/NSTEMI either to ASA monotherapy or dual antiplatelet therapy with ASA plus clopidogrel (300-mg loading dose, followed by 75 mg/day for 3–12 months) and showed a reduction in ischemic and composite endpoints—including death, nonfatal MI, and stroke—favoring the combination arm.[77] Patients in the combination arm experienced significantly more major bleeding (3.7% vs. 2.7% in the ASA monotherapy group) and more minor bleeding but no excess of life-threatening bleeding. The net effect of adding clopidogrel to ASA was positive, and this has been supported by contemporary ACS registry data.[78] However, there are limitations of the CURE data for U.S. practice, in that invasive management was rare in the trial, platelet glycoprotein IIb/IIIa receptor inhibitors (GPIs) were only rarely used, and coronary artery bypass grafting (CABG)—for which the use of clopidogrel clearly increases bleeding risk—was not often performed. For those ACS patients in whom a noninterventional approach is planned, CURE provides very strong evidence for the addition of clopidogrel to ASA.

Data on patients enrolled in CURE who underwent percutaneous coronary intervention (PCI) were reported in a secondary observational substudy analysis called PCI-CURE.[79] In this group the addition of clopidogrel led to similar ischemic advantages as in the overall study. Overall there was a statistically significant 31% reduction in cardiovascular death or MI. An overall assessment of the strategy of preloading UA/NSTEMI patients with clopidogrel, managing them with PCI, and then continuing dual therapy for 1 year showed it to be both clinically reasonable and cost-effective.[80]

The optimal timing for a loading dose of clopidogrel in UA/NSTEMI management has not been determined. Although there is evidence for a benefit from the loading dose alone (there is a significant reduction in the composite of death, MI, and stroke evident within 24 hours),[81] loading with clopidogrel appears to also be associated with an increased bleeding risk among those patients going to CABG within 5 days of clopidogrel administration. Given this increased risk of bleeding at CABG and the difficulty in identifying early which patients will ultimately require CABG, enthusiasm for loading the drug prior to diagnostic angiography *performed expeditiously* has been limited. The longer the delay to angiography, the more benefit can be expected from early loading and daily administration. This approach was supported prospectively by the Clopidogrel for the Reduction of Events During Observation (CREDO) trial.[82]

Clopidogrel in STEMI—Updated Recommendations

Clopidogrel irreversibly inhibits the platelet adenosine diphosphate receptor (ADP), resulting in a reduction in platelet aggregation through a different mechanism than aspirin. Since the publication of ECC guidelines in 2005, several important clopidogrel studies have been published and reviewed by the ACC/AHA STEMI writing group; these document its efficacy for patients with STEMI. It was recently approved by the FDA for use in patients with STEMI, either with or without fibrinolytic therapy. Approval was based on results of the Clopidogrel as Adjunctive Reperfusion Therapy (CLARITY-TIMI 28) and COMMIT CCS-2 trials, which demonstrated increased efficacy of dual therapy with aspirin with no increase in intracerebral hemorrhage.

UPDATED RECOMMENDATIONS FOR CLOPIDOGREL

Patients undergoing reperfusion with *fibrinolytic agents and those not receiving reperfusion* should receive combination antiplatelet therapy with both aspirin and clopidogrel.

Recommendation for adjunctive use with fibrinolytics
- Clopidogrel 75 mg oral daily maintenance dose
- A loading dose of 300 mg was administered in CLARITY TIMI-28, but
  - Efficacy and safety not demonstrated in patients ≥75 years of age
  - Patients receiving bolus 4,000 IU heparin dose were excluded

Recommendation for adjunctive use without reperfusion
- Clopidogrel 75 mg oral daily maintenance dose
- A loading dose of 300 mg was administered in CLARITY TIMI-28, but
  - Efficacy and safety not demonstrated in patients ≥75 years of age
  - Patients receiving bolus 4,000 IU heparin dose were excluded

No recommendation for adjunctive use upstream from PCI

No recommendation was made for upstream use prior to PCI, but it was noted that clopidogrel appears to be beneficial when PCI is subsequently performed in patients receiving prior fibrinolytic therapy.

In patients up to 75 years of age with STEMI who are treated with fibrinolysis, aspirin, and heparin (low-molecular-weight heparin [LMWH] or unfractionated heparin [UFH]), a 300-mg oral loading dose of clopidogrel given at the time of initial management (followed by a 75-mg daily dose for up to 8 days in hospital) improved coronary artery patency and reduced major adverse cardiovascular events (MACE).[155] The COMMIT trial,[67] which included more than 45,000 patients, found that those receiving clopidogrel 75 mg had a highly significant 9% reduction in death, reinfarction, or stroke, corresponding to 9 fewer events per 1,000 patients treated for only about 2 weeks. There was also no increase in intracerebral hemorrhage. Based on these findings, providers should administer a 300-mg oral dose of clopidogrel to ED patients up to 75 years of age with STEMI who receive aspirin, anticoagulation, and fibrinolysis. The 2007 Focused Update of the ACC/AHA/SCAI PCI Guidelines[85] further recommend the administration of 600 mg clopidogrel as soon as possible to patients undergoing primary PCI. Clopidogrel should not be administered to patients in shock or those who may require urgent surgical procedures.

Anticoagulation

Anticoagulation is appropriate for patients deemed to be at intermediate or higher ACS ischemic risk. There are many options for anticoagulation in the upstream environment (prior to diagnostic angiography), including both indirect antithrombin agents (UFH, LMWH, and anti-Xa inhibitors) and direct antithrombins. The choice may be influenced by many issues, including (1) emergency physician preference, (2) cardiologist preference, (3) perceived level of ischemic risk, (4) concern for hemorrhagic risk, (5) likely duration of therapy prior to angiography and possible revascularization, and (6) logistic issues such as FDA labeling and institutional formularies. Clinical trials continue to evaluate therapies, and strategies are evolving with these agents. Extrapolation from clinical trials can be difficult, as these trials are often designed or executed in a fashion that makes uncertain (1) the equivalent potency of drugs being compared, (2) the impact of prerandomization anticoagulation therapy (often administered in the ED), (3) the inconsistency and impact of concomitant antiplatelet therapy, and (4) the inclusion and timing of revascularization procedures.

Unfractionated Heparin

UFH is an indirect antithrombin; that is, it requires a cofactor, the circulating protein antithrombin III (AT3). The AT3-UFH complex then can inactivate thrombin (factor IIa), factor IXa, and factor Xa. It prevents clot propagation but cannot fragment existing thrombi.[86] There are significant pharmacologic limitations to the use of UFH, notably its relatively poor bioavailability and interpatient variability in anticoagulant effect. Nonetheless, UFH has been used clinically in the management of ACS for decades. UFH use is supported by six relatively small placebo-controlled trials and four more trials that compared the combination of ASA and UFH to ASA alone.[35] The addition of ASA appears partially protective against "heparin rebound," in which ACS may recur after initial therapy and stabilization.[87,88]

When UFH is used in ACS, it is recommended that it be dosed according to patient weight (initial bolus 60 U/kg, max 4,000 U; then 12 U/kg/hr infusion, max 1,000 U/hr) and monitored by the activated partial thromboplastin time (aPTT) instead of by fixed dosing (e.g., 5,000 or 10,000 U bolus, then 1,000 U/hr). The target aPTT range is 60 to 80 seconds.[87] Because of the dual risks of bleeding from anticoagulation and development of heparin-induced antiplatelet antibodies, daily complete blood counts are recommended for patients receiving UFH therapy. The optimal duration of therapy with UFH has not been clearly established, but most of the trials that have evaluated it in UA/NSTEMI have continued treatment for 2 to 5 days. If necessary, the anticoagulant effect of UFH can be largely reversed with the parenteral administration of protamine sulfate.

Low-Molecular-Weight Heparins

LMWHs (e.g., enoxaparin and dalteparin) are the product of chemical or enzymatic depolymerization of UFH (e.g., enoxaparin and dalteparin). Enoxaparin and dalteparin are approved by the U.S. FDA for treatment of UA/NSTEMI and enoxaparin is approved for STEMI, but there are several other LWMHs in use worldwide with varying molecular weights. These agents, like the parent compound, require the presence of AT3 and therefore are also indirect antithrombins. However, the LMWH-AT3 complex is more effective at inactivating factor Xa than factor IIa. The molecular weight of the agent determines the anti-Xa:anti-IIa activity ratio, and this in turn seems to correlate to performance in clinical trials. Important advantages of LMWHs over UFH include substantially better bioavailability (owing to less avid binding to other proteins and cells), a longer half-life that allows once- or twice-daily subcutaneous dosing instead of a continuous intravenous infusion, and, in most patients, no need for ongoing monitoring of anticoagulation activity. When monitoring is required (as in patients with renal insufficiency or morbid obesity), the aPTT does not accurately reflect the extent of anticoagulation with LMWHs. However, measures of anti–factor Xa activity (limited laboratory availability at present) do directly correlate to the degree of anticoagulation provided by LMWHs and therefore may be used to assess for adequate dosing. The therapeutic range of anti–factor Xa activity in ACS is felt to be 0.3 to 0.7 U/mL.[87] While anti-IIa activity would seem more pertinent than anti-Xa activity in the ACS scenario, the latter remains an important therapeutic target. In the clotting cascade, factor Xa is an "amplifier," and the inhibition of a single molecule of Xa will suppress the generation of 50 molecules of thrombin (IIa).[35]

In the earliest trial of a LMWH agent in UA/NSTEMI, the combination of nadroparin and ASA resulted in better ischemic outcomes than UFH + ASA.[89] In the Fragmin (i.e., dalteparin) during Instability in coronary artery disease (FRISC) trial,[90] dalteparin was found to be essentially equivalent to UFH in patients with UA/NSTEMI. In this study, however, dalteparin was continued for 1 month or longer after admission; it therefore does not reflect current standard practice. In five of six trials comparing enoxaparin with UFH, the former was favored, with statistical significance driven primarily by a reduction in nonfatal MI. In the 2002 ACC/AHA UA/NSTEMI guidelines, enoxaparin was preferred over UFH for patients managed initially by a conservative strategy.[35] (This continues as a class IIa recommendation in the 2007 guidelines.) Enoxaparin and UFH are considered acceptable class I agents for patients initially managed with an early invasive strategy. However, the lack of ready monitoring of the anticoagulant effect of enoxaparin—from one perspective an advantage in that it reduces cost of care—has also limited its use in the interventional management of UA/NSTEMI, during which cardiologists often prefer to closely monitor aPTT (or its counterpart in the catheterization lab, the activated clotting time [ACT]), before inflating balloons, deploying stents, or removing sheaths. In at least one study it was shown that PCI can be performed safely, without additional monitoring, following administration of enoxaparin.[91]

This experience would argue in favor of a consistent anticoagulation approach from ED through the catheterization laboratory. The Efficacy and Safety of Subcutaneous Enoxaparin in Non-Q-wave Coronary Events (ESSENCE) and Thrombolysis in Myocardial Infarction (TIMI)–11B trials showed clear superiority of enoxaparin over UFH in the medical management setting.[92,93] However, there is still a lack of acceptance for LMWHs among some interventional cardiologists, and this may explain the transitioning of patients from LMWH to UFH during interventional procedures. A transition was shown in a posthoc analysis of the Superior Yield of the new Strategy of Enoxaparin, Revascularization and Glycoprotein IIb/IIIa inhibitors (SYNERGY) study[94] to be associated with an increased risk of bleeding. Given this increased risk of bleeding associated with switching patients from LMWH to UFH, decisions regarding initial antithrombotic therapy should be made in a thoughtful, prospective, and multidisciplinary fashion. Frequently used approaches such as withholding the morning dose of LMWH or waiting until 8 hours after the prior LMWH dose to start UFH have some intuitive appeal based on pharmacokinetics, but these strategies have not been prospectively validated.

The SYNERGY study compared 10,027 patients with *high-risk* UA/NSTEMI who were randomized to receive either enoxaparin or UFH in a setting where nearly all patients underwent angiography and 57% received adjunctive glycoprotein IIb/IIIa receptor inhibitors (GPIs). The two anticoagulants provided similar protection against death and MI at 30 days, but there were some signals (higher TIMI major bleeding rates but similar GUSTO severe bleeding and transfusion rates) suggesting an increased risk of bleeding with enoxaparin.[94] Based on these results, enoxaparin was felt to be an equivalent agent to UFH using an early invasive strategy.

The LMWHs are cleared by renal elimination and the dose should be adjusted according to the estimated creatinine clearance. Adjusting the dose according to the serum creatinine level alone is considered an inadequate approach. The creatinine clearance can be estimated in the ED according to the following formula:

$$\text{Estimated creatinine clearance in males} = \frac{(140 - \text{age in years}) \times (\text{weight in kg})}{72 \times \text{serum creatinine (mg/dl)}}$$

$$\text{Estimated creatinine clearance in females} = \frac{(140 - \text{age in years}) \times (\text{weight in kg}) \times 0.85}{72 \times \text{serum creatinine (mg/dl)}}$$

Although there is a lower incidence of heparin-induced thrombocytopenia with LMWH, both UFH and LMWH should be avoided if a patient has thrombocytopenia or a history of HIT. A direct thrombin inhibitor in this instance is recommended.

The typical dose of enoxaparin in UA/NSTEMI is 1 mg/kg subcutaneously every 12 hours. The dosing interval is extended to every 24 hours if the patient's creatinine clear-

ance is <30 mL/hr. The dose of dalteparin in UA/NSTEMI is 120 U/kg (up to a maximum 10,000 U) subcutaneously every 12 hours. Although dalteparin is also cleared by renal excretion, there is no specific recommendation in its U.S. package insert for dose adjustment in patients with renal insufficiency. The anticoagulant effect of LMWHs can be partially reversed with protamine sulfate, but in the face of frank hemorrhage, fresh frozen plasma and other blood products should also be given.

Direct Thrombin Inhibitors

Direct thrombin inhibitors bind to factor IIa and can inhibit both plasma and clot-bound thrombin. They are termed "direct" because their action does not require the interaction of AT3. The direct antithrombin agent bivalirudin was investigated in a small population of ACS patients in the Randomized Evaluation in PCI Linking Angiomax to Reduced Clinical Events (REPLACE)–2 trial[95,96] and in a large cohort of moderate and high-risk UA/NSTEMI patients in the Acute Catheterization and Urgent Intervention Triage Strategy (ACUITY) trial.[97] In each of these trials the combination of an indirect antithrombin agent with a GPI was compared with bivalirudin and either planned or provisional GPIs.[98–100] In both studies the use of bivalirudin was associated with noninferior ischemic outcomes and significantly improved rates of bleeding complications. Interpolation of these results into clinical practice is complicated by the broad range of risk levels of patients enrolled in the study, incomplete data on the use of thienopyridine before randomization, and the relatively short interval (compared with contemporary practice) between initiation of randomized therapy and diagnostic angiography. There was concern that the bivalirudin groups in both studies had higher rates of ischemic endpoints than standard therapy, albeit these were not statistically significant.

There was limited practice experience with bivalirudin outside the catheterization laboratory at the time this chapter was written. The ACC/AHA 2007 UA/NSTEMI guidelines recommend that UA/NSTEMI patients managed with upstream bivalirudin be also given at least 300 mg of clopidogrel at least 6 hours before the procedure. This regimen is an attractive option for anticoagulation in UA/NSTEMI patients at higher risk of bleeding complications (especially if they are being transitioned to the cath lab quickly) and in those in whom heparin-induced thrombocytopenia is a concern. The "upstream" dose of bivalirudin used for ACS patients in ACUITY—which at this writing is not FDA-approved—was an initial intravenous bolus of 0.1 mg/kg, followed by an infusion of 0.25 mg/kg/hr. Prior to PCI, patients received a second bolus of 0.5 mg/kg of bivalirudin, after which the infusion rate was increased to 1.25 mg/kg/hr. Patients with a creatinine clearance of <30 mL/min were excluded from the study.[97]

Although the direct thrombin inhibitors appear to be associated with significantly lower bleeding risk than that seen with indirect agents (e.g., heparin), bleeding complications may still occur. Protamine sulfate does not reverse the effect of bivalirudin. If significant hemorrhage occurs in a patient being treated with bivalirudin, the agent should be immediately discontinued and fresh frozen plasma as well as other blood products considered as indicated.

Anti-Xa Agents

Anticoagulation may also be achieved by inhibition of factor Xa, inhibiting the downstream production of factor IIa (thrombin). The anti-Xa agent fondaparinux, like UFH and conventional LWMHs, requires AT3 to bind to its target. Fondaparinux has no activity against thrombin that is already formed or that is produced after it is administered. The most contemporary experience with fondaparinux in the UA/NSTEMI patient was reported in the Organization to Assess Strategies for Ischaemic Syndromes (OASIS) –5 study.[101] In this large study, the control anticoagulation strategy was enoxaparin 1 mg/kg subcutaneously twice daily (once daily if creatinine clearance was <30 mL/min), with supplemental UFH at the time of PCI if intervention was initiated more than 6 hours after the last subcutaneous dose of enoxaparin. The study arm was fondaparinux 2.5 mg subcutaneously once daily, which was also supplemented with UFH at the time of PCI if more than 6 hours had elapsed since the previous dose. The addition of UFH for PCI was based on concern for catheter thrombosis with fondaparinux, which occurred infrequently but three times more often than with enoxaparin. Although ischemic efficacy between the two arms was equivalent at 9 days, patients in the fondaparinux arm experienced significantly fewer bleeding complications. Additionally, the fondaparinux cohort showed significantly lower mortality at 30 days and at 180 days than those on enoxaparin.[101]

The increased risk of bleeding seen in the enoxaparin arm of OASIS-5 has been attributed to (1) the lack of anti-IIa activity by fondaparinux, (2) the increased risk of bleeding associated with the combination of enoxaparin and UFH in PCI patients (SYNERGY), and (3) the extended duration (6 days) of enoxaparin use when compared with the ESSENCE and SYNERGY trials. The ACC/AHA 2007 UA/NSTEMI guidelines concluded that there is not enough evidence available from these trials to recommend a preferred regimen when an early, invasive strategy is used for UA/NSTEMI. More experience with these regimens is still needed. However, based on the available evidence from these trials and the large number of patients treated with an initial noninvasive or delayed invasive strategy, the evidence does suggest preference for an anticoagulant for patients treated with a noninvasive strategy in the order of fondaparinux, enoxaparin, and UFH (least preferred), using the specific regimens tested in these trials. Fondaparinux may prove useful in the medical management of UA/NSTEMI patients owing to the convenience in dosing and administration as well as its associated lower rate of bleeding complications, and it received a I-B recommendation in the 2007 ACC/AHA/NSTE ACS guidelines. Still, in patients in whom there is planned intervention, concern for catheter thrombosis militates against its use, leaving providers with a need to "switch" antithrombotic strategies in the midst of patient management, which involves the concern for increased risk of bleeding.[94] As in the case of bivalirudin, the anticoagulant effect of fondaparinux cannot be reversed with protamine sulfate.

Anticoagulation therapy is a cornerstone of UA/NSTEMI management. As noted previously, the choice of an agent must be individualized to the patient based on ischemic risk, bleeding risk, and expected course of therapy. Anticoagulation with UFH may now have a more limited role in UA/NSTEMI management, given the more recent data on other agents such as enoxaparin, fondaparinux, and bivalirudin.

Platelet Glycoprotein IIb/IIIa Receptor Antagonists

Intravenous platelet glycoprotein IIb/IIIa receptor inhibitors (GPIs) are recommended for upstream (prior to diagnostic angiography) therapy in UA/NSTEMI patients who have elevated troponin levels. In patients with UA/NSTEMI but normal troponin, GPIs are still indicated if there are dynamic ST-segment changes, especially among patients unlikely to undergo angiography within a few hours.

The GP IIb/IIIa receptor is ubiquitous on the surface of the activated platelet. Strands of fibrinogen link between GP IIb/IIIa receptors on adjacent platelets, helping to develop the platelet aggregates that ultimately lead to the blockage of coronary blood flow in ACS. Occupancy of at least 80% of these receptors results in potent antithrombotic activity.[102] Once a platelet has been activated, GPIs represent the only therapeutic option for blocking platelet aggregation in ACS.

There are two types of GPIs: the humanized murine antibody abciximab, which binds noncompetitively to the IIb/IIIa receptor, and the "small molecules" eptifibatide and tirofiban, which competitively inhibit the receptors by mimicking fibrinogen. The small-molecule drugs have relatively short half-lives, and platelet activity can be expected to return to normal within 4 to 8 hours after cessation of therapy; the effect of abciximab is much longer-lived, continuing to inhibit platelet aggregation for 24 to 48 hours after the infusion ends. There are only scant directly comparative data among these agents (with the notable exception of the Do Tirofiban and ReoPro Give Similar Efficacy [TARGET] trial[103]), but generally the data are best for abciximab in the PCI setting.

On the other hand, in the Global Use of Strategies To open Occluded coronary arteries (GUSTO)-IV ACS trial,[104] abciximab was found to afford inferior outcomes compared with placebo in the *medical* management of UA/NSTEMI; therefore, its use is indicated only among those patients receiving planned PCI within 24 hours.

However, there is clinical trial support for the upstream use of both eptifibatide (Platelet IIb/IIIa Underpinning the Receptor for Suppression of Unstable Ischemia Trial [PURSUIT][105]) and tirofiban (Platelet Receptor inhibition in Ischaemic Syndrome Management in Patients Limited by Unstable Signs and symptoms [PRISM-PLUS][106]) in high-risk UA/NSTEMI. The benefits afforded by eptifibatide or tirofiban appear to be especially significant among patients with an elevated troponin prior to catheterization.[35,84,107] Both drugs should be given with ASA and anticoagulation when not contraindicated. Studies have shown that LWMH and bivalirudin can be used in combination with GPIs, although the original studies used UFH. Eptifibatide is approved for use in UA/NSTEMI patients treated medically alone or with PCI. The recommended dosage of eptifibatide in patients with ACS and normal renal function is an intravenous bolus of 180 µg/kg as soon as possible, followed by a continuous infusion of 2 µg/kg/min until hospital discharge or until CABG, for a maximum of 72 hours among those receiving medical management alone or 18 to 24 hours post-PCI. In patients with an estimated creatinine clearance of <50 mL/min, the adjusted dose is an intravenous bolus of 180 µg/kg, immediately followed by a continuous infusion of 1 µg/kg/min.

Tirofiban is also approved for use in both the medical management of UA/NSTEMI as well as in those who undergo PCI. The labeled dose is a bolus of 0.4 µg/kg/min for 30 minutes, followed by 0.1 µg/kg/min through angiography, for 12 to 24 hours post-PCI, and for a maximum of 48 to 96 hours for those receiving medical management alone. Both doses should be halved in patients with a creatinine clearance of <30 mL/min.

An important meta-analysis of the benefit of GPIs in UA/NSTEMI suggested that an elevated troponin is likely the best indication for initiation of therapy.[85] This benefit is magnified in those patients who subsequently undergo PCI. Treatment with a GPI increases the risk of bleeding, although this is typically limited to mucocutaneous and vascular access sites. No trials have shown a statistically significant increase in the risk of intracranial bleeding. The ongoing Early Glycoprotein IIb/IIIa Inhibition in Non–ST-Segment Elevation Acute Coronary Syndrome (EARLY-ACS) trial plans to address the contemporary role of pre-catheterization GPI therapy.[108] Results are expected in 2008 or 2009.

In summary, the management and risk stratification of patients with UA/NSTEMI is complex and requires the integration of several clinical parameters by a thoughtful and knowledgeable physician. A general schematic of the risk-directed therapeutic approach to the early management of UA/NSTEMI is shown in Figure 5-9. The therapeutic agents used also require careful consideration and dosing regimens, and integration into risk-based strategies continues to evolve. The current recommendations for these agents are summarized in Table 5-3, from the Update ACC AHA 2007 Guidelines for the Management of UA/NSTEMI.

Reperfusion Therapy for STEMI

The primary initial objective in patients with STEMI is reperfusion of the myocardium subtended by the infarct-related artery (IRA). Historically, fibrinolytic therapy (called also thrombolytic therapy) was the first treatment modality to meet this goal. Early attempts combining fibrinolytic therapy and interventional management were abandoned when increased mortality was observed. But as methodology and equipment evolved, primary angioplasty became an alternative treatment, and so-called rescue angioplasty was applied in cases of fibrinolytic failure. Recent attempts to combine a pharmacologic approach (fibrinolytic, anticoagulant) with a catheter-based approach have largely been unimpressive, but investigation continues.

Fibrinolytic Therapy

Intravenous fibrinolytic therapy is indicated only in patients with ST-segment-elevation ACS or ST-segment depression that is believed representative of a posterior AMI. Use of fibrinolytic therapy in other patients (e.g., those with ST-segment depression or nondiagnostic ECGs) is contraindicated and may be harmful. Patients may benefit from fibrinolytic therapy for up to 12 hours after symptom onset, although risk-benefit analysis may identify those patients more likely to benefit as the time from onset of continuous persistent symptoms increases. Patients also should have no absolute contraindications and should be carefully evaluated when a relative contraindication exists (Table 5-4). Additionally, fibrinolysis may also be indicated in patients with any type of BBB (right, left, and atypical—new or old) thought to be obscuring ST-segment analysis in patients with clinical presentation *strongly suggestive* of AMI.[23,24,110–116]

Fibrinolytic therapy is a proven approach to reperfusion therapy in STEMI.[109,117] All of the fibrinolytic agents currently available and under investigation are plasminogen activators. They act by exposing, enzymatically, the active center of plasmin. Aspirin, beta-blockers for recurrent ischemia,[71] and nitrates for recurrent ischemic pain or hypertension with STEMI[118,130] remain mainstays of adjunctive pharmacologic therapy.[119] Recent data from the Clopidogrel and Metoprolol in Myocardial Infarction Trial/Second Chinese Cardiac Study (COMMIT/CCS-2)[120] suggest that oral beta-blocker management within 24 hours is effective and safer than early IV loading in most STEMI patients (see above). Intravenous dosing should still be considered in STEMI patients with severe hypertension, tachycardia without congestive heart failure or risk factors for cardiogenic shock, and ongoing ischemic pain. Blood pressure should be optimally controlled before administration of a fibrinolytic agent in order to reduce the risk of hemorrhagic stroke. The

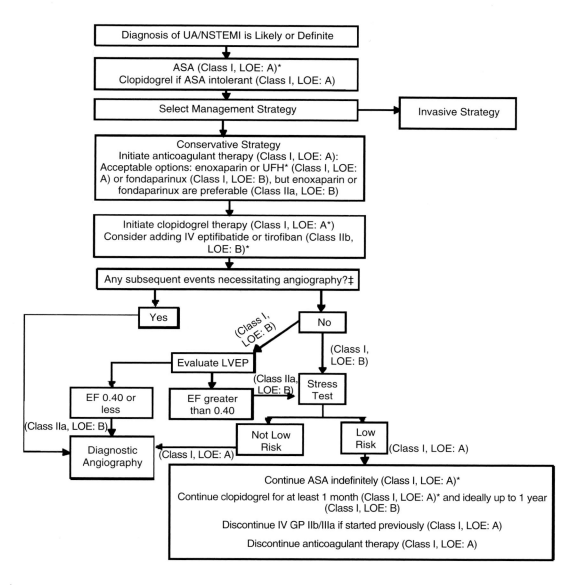

FIGURE 5-9 • Algorithm for patients with UA/NSTEMI managed by an initial conservative strategy. When multiple drugs are listed, they are in alphabetical order and not in order of preference. ‡Recurrent symptoms/ischemia, heart failure, serious arrhythmia. ASA, aspirin; EF, ejection fraction; GP, glycoprotein; IV, intravenous; LOE, level of evidence; LVEF, left ventricular ejection fraction; UA/NSTEMI, unstable angina/non–ST-elevation myocardial infarction; UFH, unfractionated heparin.

patient's initial blood pressure is a risk factor for intracerebral hemorrhage, and severe hypertension (SBP >180 mm Hg; DBP >110 mm Hg) is relative contraindication to fibrinolytics.[21]

The choice of fibrinolytic agent is often made at a hospital level, and treating physicians use whichever agent is in their protocol or formulary. Previous studies have shown both alteplase[121] and reteplase[122] (with UFH) to be superior to streptokinase, albeit with a slightly higher stroke risk. Tenecteplase offers similar efficacy, similar stroke rates, and fewer systemic mild-to-moderate bleeding complications than alteplase.[123]

Primary Percutaneous Intervention

Fibrinolytic agents reduce mortality from STEMI, and these benefits are durable over at least 10 years.[124,125] Recent data, however, suggest improved patient outcomes with primary percutaneous coronary intervention (PPCI) versus fibrinolysis.[126] In a quantitative review of 10 randomized trials involving 2,606 patients comparing PPCI with fibrinolytic therapy, Weaver et al. concluded that PPCI was associated with a significant improvement in all major short-term outcomes, including mortality at 30 days, nonfatal reinfarction, total incidence of stroke, and hemorrhagic stroke.[126] The

| TABLE 5-3 • Dosing Table for Antiplatelet and Anticoagulant Therapy in Patients With UA/NSTEMI

Drug[a]	Initial Medical Treatment	During PCI		After PCI	At Hospital Discharge
		Patient Received Initial Medical Treatment	Patient Did Not Receive Initial Medical Treatment		
Oral Antiplatelet Therapy					
Aspirin	162–325 mg nonenteric formulation, swallowed or chewed	No additional treatment	162–325 mg nonenteric formulation swallowed or chewed	162–325 mg daily should be given[b] for at least 1 month after BMS implantation, 3 months after SES implantation, and 6 months after PES implantation, after which chronic aspirin should be continued indefinitely at a dose of 75–162 mg	162–325 mg daily should be given[c] for at least 1 month after BMS implantation, 3 months after SES implantation, and 6 months after PES implantation, after which daily chronic aspirin should be continued indefinitely at a dose of 75–162 mg
Clopidogrel	LD of 300–600 mg PO, MD of 75 mg PO per day	A second LD of 300 mg PO may be given to supplement a prior LD of 300 mg	LD of 300–600 mg PO	For BMS: 75 mg daily for at least 1 month and ideally up to 1 year. For DES, 75 mg daily for at least 1 year (in patients who are not at high risk of bleeding) (See Fig. 5-11)	For BMS: 75 mg daily for at least 1 month and ideally up to 1 year. For DES, 75 mg daily for at least 1 year (in patients who are not at high risk of bleeding) (See Fig. 5-11)
Ticlopidine	LD of 500 mg PO, MD of 250 mg PO twice daily	No additional treatment	LD of 500 mg PO	MD of 250 mg PO twice daily (duration same as clopidogrel)	MD of 250 mg PO twice daily (duration same as clopidogrel)
Anticoagulants					
Bivalirudin	0.1 mg/kg bolus, 0.25 mg/kg/hr infusion	0.5 mg/kg bolus, increase infusion to 1.75 mg/kg/hr	0.75 mg/kg bolus, 1.75 mg/kg/hr infusion	No additional treatment or continue infusion for up to 4 hr	
Dalteparin	120 IU/kg SC every 12 hours (maximum 10,000 IU twice daily)[c]	IV GP IIb/IIIa planned: target ACT 200 sec using UFH No IV GP IIb/IIIa planned: target ACT 250–300 sec for HemoTec; 300–350 sec for Hemochron using UFH	IV GP IIb/IIIa planned: 60–70 IU/kg[d] of UFH No IV GP IIb/IIIa planned: 100–140 IU/kg of UFH	No additional treatment	

CHAPTER 5 • EMERGENCY DEPARTMENT MANAGEMENT | 83

PART ONE • ACUTE CORONARY SYNDROMES

Enoxaparin	LD of 30 mg IV bolus may be given[e] MD = 1 mg/kg SC every 12 hours[e]; extend dosing interval–1 mg/kg every 24 hr if estimated creatinine clearance <30 mL/min[e]	Last SC dose less than 8 hours: no additional therapy. Last SC dose >8 hr: 0.3 mg/kg IV bolus	0.5–0.75 mg/kg IV bolus	No additional treatment
Fondaparinux	2.5 mg SC once daily. Avoid for creatinine clearance <30 mL/min[e]	50–60 U/kg IV bolus of UFH is recommended by the OASIS 5 Investigators[f]	50–60 U/kg IV bolus of UFH is recommended by the OASIS 5 Investigators[f]	No additional treatment
Unfractionated heparin	LD of 60 U/kg (max 4,000 U) as IV bolus[e] MD of IV infusion of 12 U/kg/hr (max 1,000 U/hr)–maintain aPTT at 1.5–2.0 times control (approximately 50–70 s)[e]	IV GP IIb/IIIa planned: target ACT 200 s. No IV GP IIb/IIIa planned: target ACT 250–300 sec for HemoTec; 300–350 s for Hemochron	IV GP IIb/IIIa planned: 60–70 U/kg[d] No IV GP IIb/IIIa planned: 100–140 IU/Kg	No additional treatment
Intravenous Antiplatelet Therapy				
Abciximab	Not applicable	Not applicable	LD of 0.25 mg/kg IV bolus MD of 0.125 µg/kg/min (max 10 µg/min)	Continue MD infusion for 12 h
Eptifibatide	LD of IV bolus of 180 µg/kg MD of IV infusion of 2.0 µg/kg/min; reduce infusion by 50% in patients with estimated creatinine clearance <50 mL/min	Continue infusion	LD of IV bolus of 180 µg/kg followed 10 min later by second IV bolus of 180 µg/kg MD of 2.0 µg/kg/min; reduce infusion by 50% in patients with estimated creatinine clearance <50 mL/min	Continue MD infusion for 18–24 h

| TABLE 5-3 • Dosing Table for Antiplatelet and Anticoagulant Therapy in Patients With UA/NSTEMI (Continued)

Drug[a]	Initial Medical Treatment	During PCI		After PCI	At Hospital Discharge
		Patient Received Initial Medical Treatment	Patient Did Not Receive Initial Medical Treatment		
Intravenous Antiplatelet Therapy					
Tirofiban	LD of IV infusion of 0.4 µg/kg/min for 30 min MD of IV infusion of 0.1 µg/kg/min; reduce rate of infusion by 50% in patients with estimated creatinine clearance <30 mL/min	Continue infusion	LD of IV infusion of 0.4 µg/kg/min for 30 min MD of IV infusion of 0.1 µg/kg/min; reduce rate of infusion by 50% in patients with estimated creatinine clearance <30 mL/min	Continue MD infusion for 18–24 h	

[a]This list is in alphabetical order and is not meant to indicate a particular therapy preference.

[b]In patients in whom the physician is concerned about the risk of bleeding, a lower initial ASA dose after PCI of 75–162 mg/day is reasonable (Class IIa, LOE: C).

[c]Dalteparin was evaluated for management of patients with UA/NSTEMI in an era before the widespread use of important therapies such as stents, clopidogrel, and GP IIb/IIIa inhibitors. Its relative efficacy and safety in the contemporary management era is not well established.

[d]Some operators use <60 U/kg of UFH with GP IIb/IIIa blockade, although no clinical trial data exist to demonstrate the efficacy of doses below 60 U/kg in this setting.

[e]For patients managed by an initial conservative strategy, agents such as enoxaparin and fondaparinux offer the convenience advantage of SC administration compared with an intravenous infusion of UFH. They are also less likely to provoke heparin-induced thrombocytopenia than UFH. Available data suggest fondaparinux is associated with less bleeding than enoxaparin in conservatively managed patients using the regimens listed.

[f]Personal communication, OASIS-5 Investigators, July 7, 2006. Note that this regimen has not been rigorously tested in prospective randomized trials.

Additional considerations include the possibility that a conservatively managed patient may develop a need for PCI, in which case an intravenous bolus of 50–60 U/kg is recommended if fondaparinux was given for initial medical treatment; the safety of this drug combination is not well established. For conservatively managed patients in whom enoxaparin was the initial medical treatment, as noted in the table, additional intravenous enoxaparin is an acceptable option.

ACT, activated clotting time; BMS, bare metal stent; GP, glycoprotein; hr, hour; IU, international unit; IV, intravenous; LD, loading dose; MD, maintenance dose; PCI, percutaneous coronary intervention; PES, paclitaxel-eluting stent; PO, orally; SC, subcutaneous; SES, sirolimus-eluting stent; U, units; UA/NSTEMI, unstable angina/non–ST-elevation myocardial infarction; UFH, unfractionated heparin.

| TABLE 5-4 • Contraindications to Fibrinolytic Therapy

Absolute contraindications
• Any prior intracranial hemorrhage
• Known structural vascular or neoplastic lesion in the central nervous system
• Ischemic stroke within previous 3 months unless coincident with current STEMI
• Significant closed head injury or facial trauma within previous 3 months
• Suspected aortic dissection
• Active bleeding or bleeding diathesis (excluding menses)
Relative contraindications
• Diastolic blood pressure >110 mm Hg or systolic blood pressure >180 mm Hg on presentation
• History of severe, chronic, poorly controlled hypertension
• Prior ischemic stroke >3 months
• Dementia or other intracranial pathology not listed above
• Pregnancy
• Bleeding concerns: prolonged cardiopulmonary resuscitation, recent surgery, recent internal bleeding, active peptic ulcer disease, therapeutic anticoagulation

initial benefit of PPCI appears sustained for at least 6 to 18 months.[127,128] Keeley compared 23 trials and evaluated both short- and long-term clinical outcomes. Primary percutaneous transluminal coronary angioplasty (PTCA) was better than thrombolytic therapy at reducing overall short-term death (7% [$n = 270$] vs. 9% [$n = 360$]; $P = 0.0002$), death excluding the SHOCK trial data (5% [$n = 199$] vs. 7% [$n = 276$]; $P = 0.0003$), nonfatal reinfarction (3% [$n = 80$] vs. 7% [$n = 222$]; $P < 0.0001$), stroke (1% [$n = 30$] vs. 2% [$n = 64$]; $P = 0.0004$), and the combined endpoint of death, nonfatal reinfarction, and stroke (8% [$n = 253$] vs. 14% [$n = 442$]; $P < 0.0001$). The results seen with primary PTCA remained better than those seen with thrombolytic therapy during long-term follow-up and were independent of both the type of thrombolytic agent used, and whether or not the patient was transferred for PPCI[129] (Fig. 5-10).

These data suggest that, in appropriate patients, PPCI is the preferred reperfusion strategy. In practical terms, however, PPCI is not available in many facilities and may not be available in a timely manner around the clock even in specialized centers. In these patients, fibrinolytic therapy may be considered when STEMI is identified <6 hours after symptom onset and expected delay time from initial STEMI identification in the ED until PCI (i.e., balloon time) is >90 minutes. While acknowledging that particular patients may be better suited to either pharmacologic or mechanical reperfusion, the ACC/AHA guidelines for STEMI emphasize that the reperfusion method is probably less important than its speed of delivery.[130] The target times for reperfusion are 30 minutes from ED arrival to administration of a fibri-

nolytic or 90 minutes from ED arrival to balloon inflation in the cardiac catheterization laboratory.[130]

"Lytics Versus Lab": Selection of Reperfusion Strategy

It is clear that the prompt use of reperfusion therapy is associated with improved survival after STEMI.[131] STEMI patients presenting to a facility without the capability for expert, prompt intervention with primary PCI within 90 minutes of first medical contact should undergo fibrinolysis unless contraindicated (ACC/AHA STEMI guidelines, class I). Unfortunately pitfalls in reperfusion therapy persist, primarily among patients for whom PPCI is not available.[132–134] While the choice between fibrinolysis and PPCI can be discussed in an academic forum, *indecision* about the choice of reperfusion therapy should not deter physicians from using one or the other as quickly as possible for the individual patient. There are several issues pertinent to the selection of reperfusion therapy: (1) time since onset of symptoms, (2) risk (location) of the STEMI itself, (3) bleeding risk of the patient, and (4) time to expert PPCI capability.

Time from onset of symptoms, over and above time of presentation, is a key variable in the prognosis of STEMI. Regardless of the mode of reperfusion, the guiding concept is to minimize total ischemic time from onset of symptoms to reperfusion. Clearly the efficacy of fibrinolysis diminishes with time.[135] As its efficacy decreases, its risk of adverse events (primarily bleeding) remains steady, worsening the

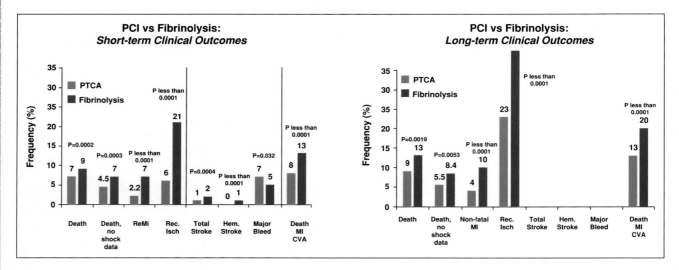

FIGURE 5-10 • Comparison of PPCI versus thrombolytic therapy for various endpoints shown. (Source: Modified from ACC/AHA 2004 STEMI Guidelines. Modified from original source, Keeley EC et al. *Lancet* 2003;361[9351]:13–20.)

risk–benefit ratio over time. However, fibrinolysis adminis-tered within the first hour or two after onset of STEMI symptoms may abort the MI and has a profound impact on mortality.[131,136,137] Herein lies the potential appeal of pre-hospital lysis,[138] which has traditionally enjoyed more popu-larity in Europe than in the United States. In contrast, the ability to produce a patent infarct artery is much less dependent on symptom duration in patients undergoing PPCI; some authors have, in fact, suggested that time to PPCI is important only in patients presenting in cardiogenic shock.[139] This does not hold beyond the original presenta-tion period, as the OAT study showed in 2006 that PCI 3 to 28 days after STEMI occurrence afforded no better out-comes than medical management alone in the patient with an occluded IRA who are now symptom-free.[140]

All STEMIs are not created equal. Anterior STEMI carries a much poorer prognosis than inferior or pure pos-terior MI. Patients who present in cardiogenic shock with STEMI are at higher risk still. Although there has been no prospective study that randomizes patients to a reperfusion strategy based on projected mortality at presentation, PPCI is thought to be more beneficial, the higher the initial risk.[141,142] Likewise, patients carry different bleeding risks, and, intuitively, the higher the patient's bleeding risk, the less desirable fibrinolytic therapy becomes as an option. The ACC/AHA STEMI guidelines suggest that fibrinolytic ther-apy is preferred over no reperfusion until the life-threaten-ing bleeding risk exceeds 4%.[130] There are formulas for making such calculations[143–145] (Fig. 5-11), but they have not been prospectively validated. When major bleeding is a risk, just as when fibrinolytic therapy is frankly contraindicated, PPCI is preferred to reperfusion therapy.

Perhaps the key issue in the choice between fibrinolysis and PPCI is the availability of, and transport time to a skilled PCI laboratory. When this option is available on site, time to balloon inflation is reduced and PCI is preferred over emergent transfer to another facility with additional delay.[146]

When a transfer protocol specifically for STEMI does not exist, this can create many unknowns for the emergency physician who, on behalf of the patient eligible for fibri-nolytics, must balance both the benefit and risk of immedi-ate fibrinolytic therapy with the benefit but possibly delayed onset of PPCI (see "Transfer for PCI," below). This situa-tion argues clearly for the creation of standard transfer agreements that facilitate the logistics of transfer of these critically ill patients. The DANAMI-2 trial (DANish trial in Acute Myocardial Infarction) found that patients treated at facilities without PPCI capability had better composite out-comes with transfer for PPCI within 2 hours of presentation than with lysis at the local hospital.[147] Whether these results could be duplicated in the United States is not known. The receiving catheterization lab will also optimally be experi-enced in managing STEMI. Studies have shown that volume of PPCI equates to better outcomes.[146]

In summary, (1) time to reperfusion is critical; (2) PPCI is always preferred over lysis when balloon inflation can occur within 90 minutes; (3) when PPCI is not readily avail-able and patients do not have contraindications to lysis (Table 5-4), lysis remains standard of care; and (4) confi-dence in lysis can be improved by initiating it as soon as pos-sible after symptom onset and in patients with no identifi-able untoward bleeding risk. Clinical circumstances that dictate whether fibrinolytic therapy or an invasive strategy is generally preferred are shown in Table 5-5.

Transfer for PCI

A special situation exists when patients present to facilities without PCI capabilities and patients are considered for transfer to a specialized tertiary care center. Updated guidelines recommend consideration of time from symp-tom onset and time to PCI in deciding this issue[148] (Antman Circulation 2008).[130] A detailed discussion is reviewed in the ACC/AHA practice guidelines and the

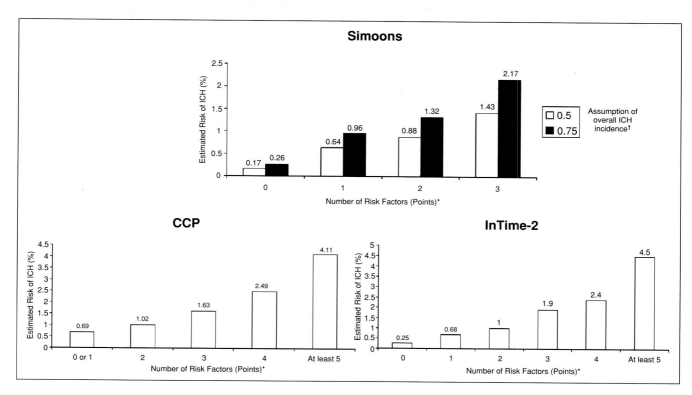

FIGURE 5-11 • Estimation of risk of ICH with fibrinolysis. ICH, intracranial hemorrhage; CCP, Cooperative Cardiovascular Project; InTIME-2, Intravenous nPA for treatment of Infarcting Myocardium Early-2; *The number of risk factors is the sum of the points based on the criteria shown in Table 13. †If the overall incidence of ICH is assumed to be 0.75%, patients without risk factors who receive streptokinase have a 0.26% probability of ICH. The risk is 0.96%, 1.32%, and 2.17% in patients with one, two, or three risk factors, respectively. (See Simoons et al.[144] for further discussion. See Brass et al.[143,145] for sources of CCP and InTime-2 data, respectively.)

TABLE 5-5 • Reperfusion Options and Steps for Assessing Strategies

STEP 1: Assess Time and Risk

Time since onset of symptoms

Risk of STEMI: anterior vs non-anterior

Risk of fibrinolysis

Time required for transport to a skilled PCI lab

STEP 2: Determine if Fibrinolysis or an Invasive Strategy is Preferred

If presentation is less than 3 hours and there is no delay to an invasive strategy, there is no preference for either strategy

Fibrinolysis is generally preferred if:	An Invasive Strategy is generally preferred if:

• *Early Presentation (less than or equal to 3 hours from symptom onset and delay to invasive strategy) (see below)*
• *Invasive Strategy is not an option*
  Catheterization lab occupied/not available
  Vascular access difficulties
  Lack of access to a skilled PCI lab
• *Delay to Invasive Strategy*
  Prolonged transport
  (Door-to-Balloon) – (Door-to-Needle) is greater than 1 hour
  Medical Contact-to-Balloon or Door-to-Balloon is greater than 90 minutes
	• *Skilled PCI lab available with surgical backup*
	  Medical Contact-to-Balloon or Door-to-Balloon is less than 90 minutes
	  (Door-to-Balloon) – (Door-to-Needle) is less than 1 hour
	• *High Risk from STEMI*
	  Cardiogenic shock
	  Killip class is greater than or equal to 3
	• *Contraindications to fibrinolysis including increased risk of bleeding and ICH*
	• *Late Presentation*
	  The symptom onset was greater than 3 hours ago
	• *Diagnosis of STEMI is in doubt*

American College of Emergency Physicians' (ACEP) Clinical Policy for Reperfusion Therapy.

See Web site for ACC/AHA guidelines for STEMI and ACEP clinical policy indications: "Reperfusion Therapy."

Facilitated PCI

Fibrinolytic therapy is still the major reperfusion modality worldwide and is discussed here as a standard-of-care alternative to PPCI. Attempts to combine these two strategies ("facilitated PCI") have resulted in equivocal or poorer patient outcomes[126,149–151]; consequently, the two techniques have come to be regarded as mutually exclusive except in cases where fibrinolytic therapy fails and "rescue" PCI is attempted as a lifesaving procedure or for myocardial salvage in high-risk patients. Clinical investigation continues to search for an anticoagulant that is an optimal upstream adjunct to PPCI.

See Web site for ACC/AHA guidelines for STEMI: "Facilitated PCI."

Adjunctive Reperfusion Therapy for STEMI

Aspirin and Unfractionated Heparin

In addition to basic medical therapy for STEMI in the patient undergoing fibrinolysis, anticoagulation and antiplatelet therapy should also be considered. The International Study Group randomized 20,891 patients who had received fibrinolytic treatment to a regimen that either did or did not include heparin.[152] Most patients also received ASA. A similar comparison was performed by the Third International Study of Infarct Survival (ISIS-3) Collaborative Group, in which half of a cohort of 41,299 fibrinolytic- and aspirin-treated patients were randomized to also receive heparin treatment.[153] In both trials, the heparin-treated patients showed nonsignificant reductions in the short-term risk of death and reinfarction. When data from both trials were combined, the effect of heparin on mortality was significant, but only during the period of actual heparin treatment.[153] After a period of 6 months, mortality rates were similar in the heparin and nonheparin groups.[152,154] Major bleeding complications were more frequent in the three-drug combination groups in both trials.[152,153]

Clopidogrel

Antiplatelet therapy in addition to ASA is also indicated in the fibrinolytic management of STEMI. In the Clopidogrel as Adjunctive Reperfusion Therapy—Thrombolysis In Myocardial Infarction (CLARITY-TIMI) –28 trial, addition of clopidogrel to standard fibrinolytic therapy (ASA plus fibrinolytic, with or without anticoagulation with UFH or LMWH) reduced ischemic complications and improved arterial patency following STEMI.[155] In this randomized, double-blind, placebo-controlled study that enrolled a total of 3,491 patients, clopidogrel (300-mg loading dose followed by 75 mg once daily) was associated with a 36% odds reduction compared with placebo for the primary endpoint of occluded infarct-related arteries on angiography or death or MI recurrence before angiography (which was performed 2 to 8 days after lysis). Clopidogrel treatment also led to a significant 20% reduction in major cardiovascular events (cardiovascular death, recurrent MI, or recurrent ischemia requiring urgent revascularization) within 30 days of presentation. There was no significant increase in the incidence of TIMI-defined major bleeding in the clopidogrel group (1.3% vs. 1.1% for placebo), and the rates of minor bleeding and intracranial hemorrhage were also similar. Of note, this contrasts with the increased incidence of bleeding events observed with the addition of a GPI to aspirin plus fibrinolytic therapy.[156–159] A substudy, PCI-CLARITY, showed that clopidogrel was also effective in reducing major cardiovascular events and did not increase the risk of bleeding in the 1,863 patients who underwent PCI after fibrinolysis.[160] Of note, these were elective PCI cases, not rescue or facilitated PCI. Enrollment in CLARITY was limited to patients under age 75 years, and this age limitation was included in the FDA label extension of Plavix in clopidogrel to STEMI patients treated with fibrinolysis.

Similarly positive results were reported when clopidogrel was added to ASA in the COMMIT/CCS-2 trial.[120] This placebo-controlled, randomized trial evaluated the effects of daily doses of clopidogrel 75 mg (there was no loading dose in this study) in 45,852 patients in China with the clinical or confirmed diagnosis of AMI who were receiving ASA 162 mg/day. Half the patients received fibrinolytic therapy, but PPCI was an exclusion criterion. After a mean follow-up period of 16 days, patients receiving clopidogrel showed a significant 9% reduction in the relative risk of the composite endpoint of death, reinfarction, or stroke compared with placebo. Additionally, there was also a significant 7% reduction in the single endpoint of all-cause mortality (7.5% vs. 8.1%). There was no significant increase in the combined risk of fatal hemorrhage, intracranial hemorrhage, or need for transfusion in the clopidogrel group, including those patients who received fibrinolytic therapy.[120] The combination of clopidogrel and ASA thus appears to represent an effective and safe adjunctive therapy in STEMI patients. While the CLARITY trial excluded patients >75 years of age, no such age limit was specified for COMMIT, and 26% of study participants were ≥70 years of age. This provides indirect assurance that clopidogrel (at least without a loading dose) is safe in elderly STEMI patients.

Low-Molecular-Weight Heparin

An alternative antithrombotic agent for STEMI patients undergoing fibrinolysis is the LMWH enoxaparin. The Assessment of the Safety and Efficacy of a New Thrombolytic (ASSENT) –3 trial compared the efficacy and safety of tenecteplase + enoxaparin with tenecteplase + unfractionated heparin in 6,095 patients with recent acute STEMI.[161] The enoxaparin-treated group showed a significant reduction in the combined endpoint of ischemic cardiovascular events (30-day mortality, in-hospital reinfarction, or refractory ischemia).[161] A third treatment group in this trial received half-dose tenecteplase, low-dose UFH, and abciximab. The overall efficacy and efficacy plus safety outcomes of this group were almost identical to those of the tenecteplase + enoxaparin group. However, ST-segment resolution was more rapid and complete with tenecteplase + abciximab and reinfarction was less frequent among patients with ≥70% ST resolution who were receiving tenecteplase + abciximab or tenecteplase + enoxaparin than in those treated with tenecteplase and UFH.[162] The incidences of thrombocytopenia, bleeding complications (total, major, and minor), and blood transfusions were higher in the abciximab group than the enoxaparin group.

Benefits were also observed for enoxaparin relative to UFH in the Enoxaparin and Thrombolysis Reperfusion for Acute Myocardial Infarction (ExTRACT) –TIMI-25 trial, which enrolled more than 20,000 STEMI patients undergoing fibrinolysis.[163] Compared with UFH, enoxaparin significantly reduced the relative risk of the primary endpoint, death or nonfatal recurrent MI at 30 days (–17%; $P < 0.001$). Enoxaparin was associated with a significantly increased incidence of major but nonfatal, non-stroke bleeding episodes relative to unfractionated heparin (2.1% vs. 1.4% of patients). Similar findings were revealed in a PCI substudy among the 4,676 patients in the ExTRACT-TIMI-25 trial who went on to receive PCI following fibrinolysis.[164] Enoxaparin reduced the risk of death or nonfatal MI by 23% relative to unfractionated heparin, and unlike the parent study, was *not* associated with an increased incidence of bleeding episodes (1.4% vs. 1.6% of patients with unfractionated heparin). The FDA-labeled dosing for enoxaparin in STEMI is as follows:

- Patients <75 years of age: 30-mg IV bolus, then 1 mg/kg every 12 hours until hospital discharge
- Patients ≥75 years of age: no IV enoxaparin, 0.75 mg/kg every 12 hours until hospital discharge
- Change dosing intervals for both groups to every 24 hours if creatinine clearance <30 mL/min

Fondaparinux, an indirect anti-Xa agent, has also shown utility in patients with STEMI.[165] The Sixth Organization to Assess Strategies in Acute Ischemic Syndromes (OASIS-6) trial showed that when initiated early and administered for up to 8 days in patients not undergoing primary PCI, fondaparinux was superior to initial treatment with placebo for the prevention of death or reinfarction. It was noninferior to UFH in medical and fibrinolytic STEMI management, but showed no benefit in patients undergoing PPCI. There was a tendency toward fewer severe hemorrhages for patients treated with fondaparinux compared with similar agents.

Glycoprotein IIb/IIIa Inhibitor Therapy

The results of the Strategies for Patency Enhancement in the Emergency Department (SPEED),[159] the Platelet Aggregation Receptor Antagonist Dose Investigation and Reperfusion Gain in Myocardial Infarction (PARADIGM),[158] and the GUSTO-V[156] studies have demonstrated the success of administering a GPI, in addition to ASA, in combination with reteplase, streptokinase, or tissue plasminogen activator (tPA) in patients with acute STEMI. These studies showed that satisfactory reperfusion is achieved more rapidly and in a higher percentage of patients if an additional antiplatelet agent is included in the treatment regimen. Addition of a GPI to aspirin plus fibrinolytic therapy is also associated with a significant reduction in the incidence of reinfarction within 7 days of the index event.[156,157] To date, however, the short-term benefits of combination fibrinolytic/GPI/ASA therapy have not been clearly associated with a decrease in mortality during follow-up periods of between 30 days and 1 year.[157–159] Furthermore, the addition of a GPI to ASA plus fibrinolytic therapy may increase the risk of bleeding events.[156–159]

More recent studies have shown that combining fibrinolytics with GPIs is no more effective than GPIs alone in patients referred for PPCI.[166,167] In the Bavarian Reperfusion Alternative Evaluation (BRAVE) trial, treatment with reteplase in combination with abciximab did not reduce infarct size, the primary endpoint, as compared to abciximab alone in patients referred for PCI.[166] The Addressing the Value of Facilitated Angioplasty After Combination Therapy or Eptifibatide Monotherapy in Acute Myocardial Infarction (ADVANCE MI) trial reported similar results.[168] In this study, compared with patients receiving eptifibatide alone, those treated with eptifibatide plus 50% of standard-dose tenecteplase had a higher incidence of death and new/worsening severe heart failure (primary endpoint) at 30 days both in the "as treated" (3% vs. 10%) and the "as randomized" (1% vs. 11%) groups, although definitive conclusions cannot be drawn owing to the small sample size. Interestingly, artery patency and myocardial tissue patency were improved with eptifibatide plus tenecteplase on pre-PCI angiography; however, bleeding complications were twofold higher in this treatment group.

Results from the Controlled Abciximab and Device Investigation to Lower Later Angioplasty Complications (CADILLAC) study showed that stenting with or without abciximab therapy was more effective than balloon angioplasty alone with or without abciximab in patients following an AMI.[168] At 6 months, the primary endpoint—a composite of death, reinfarction, disabling stroke, or revascularization of the target vessel—had occurred in 11.5% of patients after stenting and 10.2% after stenting and abciximab compared with 20% after angioplasty and 16.5% after angioplasty and abciximab ($P < 0.001$).

Multidisciplinary Collaboration: Key to Success in ACS Management

The massive medical literature pertaining to the diagnosis and management of ACS makes the task of developing a practical and cohesive practice pattern that is grounded in science nearly impossible. The ACC/AHA guidelines and ACEP clinical policy statements seek to provide an evidenced-based adjudication and synopsis of this information in the form of concise and weighted recommendations.[35,148,169] They also present a framework for best practices and a platform to encourage a consistency of care among all practicing clinicians. The challenge for the emergency clinician is to apply population evidence-based data to individual patients, taking into consideration local system requirements and protocols. An analysis of ACS patients in the large CRUSADE registry (UA/NSTEMI) has validated the practical application of the ACC/AHA UA/NSTEMI guidelines recommendations by demonstrating improvements in outcome measures, such as in-hospital mortality, when there is an adherence to the recommendations.[170] These provide an evidence-based comprehensive resource for the clinician.

In recent years it has become recognized that the process of delivering quality acute care must begin in the ED, particularly for disease states where time-sensitive management issues are imperative. The ED functional structure and care delivery processes that are most important in ensuring ACC/AHA guideline adherence have been shown to be mostly dependent upon the following factors:[171]

1. **Development of quality improvement initiatives that are supported by the hospital administration.** Through the support of hospital administration, these initiatives can cross traditional departmental boundaries and bring ancillary personnel such as pharmacists and nursing staff into the broader scope of patient care. The guidelines present the best framework for building and standardizing these efforts and provide a means for developing a hospital-wide consensus on the definitions of quality care.
2. **Strong, cohesive, and independent emergency medicine practice groups.** Since the initiation of quality care in the ED sets the tone for the entire management scheme of the ACS patient, it is important that the emergency physicians are committed to these quality initiatives. This level of interest in patient care beyond the confines of the ED requires that the emergency practitioners feel involved in the total functioning of the hospital and are a part of the institution's community of health care providers. Well-organized practice groups of dedicated emergency physicians are more likely to be involved in hospital committees and a part of the medical decision-making process.
3. **Collaboration between emergency physicians and other health-care providers.** Agreement on practice standards is critical for the smooth transitioning of care from the ED to the general hospital environment of the chest pain unit, cardiac catheterization laboratory, coronary care unit, and telemetry floor. Collaboration among specialties and departmental areas reduces medical errors and ensures expedient management. Care practices that place the patient's needs at the center of the process can be important in building a collaborative environment.
4. **Development of care pathways and protocols.** Perhaps the best way to develop consistency in clinical practice is to formulate management schemes that help direct the process of care. Such pathways are really the translation of the guidelines to practical patient care. These pathways often take into account the specific nuances of the institution (e.g., availability of cardiac catheterization) while trying to best maintain guideline adherence. When developed in conjunction with all health-care providers involved in the management of the ACS patient, these pathways and protocols also become a platform for ensuring collaboration. It is important to note that the specific algorithms within these protocols are based upon population studies and that the individual ACS patient might not necessarily fit into the described management scheme. Hence the protocols should never be considered as a blind "recipe" but rather as a guide for the clinician to apply evidence-based medicine to individual ACS patients in systems of care.
5. **Quality-improvement feedback and review.** Even if there are protocols and pathways, hospital administrative support, and good collaboration between specialties, monitoring and analysis of the actual care provided is required. When a quality-improvement initiative provides routine feedback to practitioners on the success of the implemented care processes, there is evidence that there is also an improved adherence to the guidelines.[172,173]

References

1. Kamineni R, Alpert JS. Acute coronary syndromes: initial evaluation and risk stratification. *Prog Cardiovasc Dis* 2004;46(5):379–392.
2. Kellermann AL, Hackman BB, Somes G. Predicting the outcome of unsuccessful prehospital advanced cardiac life support. *JAMA* 1993;270(12):1433–1436.
3. Cannon CP. Treatment algorithms and critical pathways for acute coronary syndromes. *Semin Vasc Med* 2003;3(4):425–432.
4. Brown SG, Galloway DM. Effect of ambulance 12-lead ECG recording on times to hospital reperfusion in acute myocardial infarction. *Med J Aust* 2000;172(2):81–84.
5. Canto JG, Zalenski RJ, Ornato JP, et al. Use of emergency medical services in acute myocardial infarction and subsequent quality of care: Observations from the national registry of myocardial infarction 2. *Circulation* 2002;106(24):3018–3023.
6. Jacobs AK, Antman EM, Ellrodt G, et al. Recommendation to develop strategies to increase the number of ST-segment-elevation myocardial infarction patients with timely access to primary percutaneous coronary intervention. *Circulation* 2006;113(17):2152–2163.
7. Jacobs AK. Regionalized care for patients with ST-elevation myocardial infarction: it's closer than you think. *Circulation* 2006;113(9):1159–1161.

8. Henry TD, Sharkey SW, Burke MN, et al. A regional system to provide timely access to percutaneous coronary intervention for ST-elevation myocardial infarction. *Circulation* 2007;116(7): 721–728.

9. Emergency department: rapid identification and treatment of patients with acute myocardial infarction. National Heart Attack Alert Program Coordinating Committee, 60 Minutes to Treatment Working Group. *Ann Emerg Med* 1994;23(2):311–329.

10. Weaver WD. Time to thrombolytic treatment: factors affecting delay and their influence on outcome. *J Am Coll Cardiol* 1995; 25(suppl)(7):3S–9S.

11. Brouwer MA, Martin JS, Maynard C, et al. Influence of early pre-hospital thrombolysis on mortality and event-free survival (the Myocardial Infarction Triage and Intervention [MITI] Randomized Trial). MITI Project Investigators. *Am J Cardiol* 1996;78(5):497–502.

12. Raitt MH, Maynard C, Wagner GS, et al. Relation between symptom duration before thrombolytic therapy and final myocardial infarct size. *Circulation* 1996;93(1):48–53.

13. Wackers FJ, Terrin ML, Kayden DS, et al. Quantitative radionuclide assessment of regional ventricular function after thrombolytic therapy for acute myocardial infarction: results of phase I Thrombolysis in Myocardial Infarction (TIMI) trial. *J Am Coll Cardiol* 1989;13(5):998–1005.

14. Res JC, Simoons ML, van der Wall EE, et al. Long term improvement in global left ventricular function after early thrombolytic treatment in acute myocardial infarction. Report of a randomised multicentre trial of intracoronary streptokinase in acute myocardial infarction. *Br Heart J* 1986;56(5):414–421.

15. Mathey DG, Sheehan FH, Schofer J, et al. Time from onset of symptoms to thrombolytic therapy: a major determinant of myocardial salvage in patients with acute transmural infarction. *J Am Coll Cardiol* 1985;6(3):518–525.

16. Serruys PW, Simoons ML, Suryapranata H, et al. Preservation of global and regional left ventricular function after early thrombolysis in acute myocardial infarction. *J Am Coll Cardiol* 1986;7(4): 729–742.

17. GUSTO-1 Investigators, Newby LK, Rutsch WR, et al. Time from symptom onset to treatment and outcomes after thrombolytic therapy. GUSTO-1 Investigators. *J Am Coll Cardiol* 1996;27(7):1646–1655.

18. Anderson JL, Karagounis LA, Califf RM. Metaanalysis of five reported studies on the relation of early coronary patency grades with mortality and outcomes after acute myocardial infarction. *Am J Cardiol* 1996;78(1):1–8.

19. Antman EM, Cohen M, Bernink PJ, et al. The TIMI risk score for unstable angina/non-ST elevation MI: A method for prognostication and therapeutic decision making. *JAMA* 2000;284(7): 835–842.

20. Antman EM, Anbe DT, Armstrong PW, et al. ACC/AHA guidelines for the management of patients with ST-elevation myocardial infarction—executive summary: a report of the American College of Cardiology/American Heart Association Task Force on Practice Guidelines (Writing Committee to Revise the 1999 Guidelines for the Management of Patients With Acute Myocardial Infarction). *Circulation* 2004;110(5):588–636.

21. Antman EM, Anbe DT, Armstrong PW, et al. ACC/AHA guidelines for the management of patients with ST-elevation myocardial infarction—executive summary. A report of the American College of Cardiology/American Heart Association Task Force on Practice Guidelines (Writing Committee to revise the 1999 guidelines for the management of patients with acute myocardial infarction). *J Am Coll Cardiol* 2004;44(3):671–719.

22. Menown IB, Mackenzie G, Adgey AA. Optimizing the initial 12-lead electrocardiographic diagnosis of acute myocardial infarction. *Eur Heart J* 2000;21(4):275–283.

23. Dubois C, Pierard LA, Smeets JP, et al. Short- and long-term prognostic importance of complete bundle-branch block complicating acute myocardial infarction. *Clin Cardiol* 1988;11(5):292–296.

24. Moreno AM, Alberola AG, Tomas JG, et al. Incidence and prognostic significance of right bundle branch block in patients with acute myocardial infarction receiving thrombolytic therapy. *Int J Cardiol* 1997;61(2):135–141.

25. Sabatine MS, Morrow DA, Giugliano RP, et al. Implications of upstream glycoprotein IIb/IIIa inhibition and coronary artery stenting in the invasive management of unstable angina/non-ST-elevation myocardial infarction: a comparison of the Thrombolysis In Myocardial Infarction (TIMI) IIIB trial and the Treat angina with Aggrastat and determine Cost of Therapy with Invasive or Conservative Strategy (TACTICS)-TIMI 18 trial. *Circulation* 2004;109(7):874–880.

26. Sabatine MS, Antman EM. The thrombolysis in myocardial infarction risk score in unstable angina/non-ST-segment elevation myocardial infarction. *J Am Coll Cardiol* 2003;41(4 Suppl S):89S–95S.

27. Bradshaw PJ, Ko DT, Newman AM, et al. Validation of the Thrombolysis In Myocardial Infarction (TIMI) risk index for predicting early mortality in a population-based cohort of STEMI and non-STEMI patients. *Can J Cardiol* 2007;23(1):51–56.

28. Pollack CV Jr, Sites FD, Shofer FS, et al. Application of the TIMI risk score for unstable angina and non-ST elevation acute coronary syndrome to an unselected emergency department chest pain population. *Acad Emerg Med* 2006;13(1):13–18.

29. Diamond GA. A clinically relevant classification of chest discomfort. *J Am Coll Cardiol* 1983;1(2 Pt 1):574–575.

30. Canto JG, Shlipak MG, Rogers WJ, et al. Prevalence, clinical characteristics, and mortality among patients with myocardial infarction presenting without chest pain. *JAMA* 2000;283(24): 3223–3229.

31. Summers RL, Cooper GJ, Carlton FB, et al. Prevalence of atypical chest pain descriptions in a population from the southern United States. *Am J Med Sci* 1999;318(3):142–145.

32. Summers RL, Cooper GJ, Woodward LH, et al. Association of atypical chest pain presentations by African Americans and the lack of utilization of reperfusion therapy. *Ethnicity Dis* 2001;11(3): 463–468.

33. Brieger D, Eagle KA, Goodman SG, et al. Acute coronary syndromes without chest pain, an underdiagnosed and undertreated high-risk group: insights from the Global Registry of Acute Coronary Events. *Chest* 2004;126(2):461–469.

34. Funk M, Naum JB, Milner KA, et al. Presentation and symptom predictors of coronary heart disease in patients with and without diabetes. *Am J Emerg Med* 2001;19(6):482–487.

35. Braunwald E, Antman EM, Beasley JW, et al. ACC/AHA 2002 guideline update for the management of patients with unstable angina and non-ST-segment elevation myocardial infarction—summary article: a report of the American College of Cardiology/American Heart Association task force on practice guidelines (Committee on the Management of Patients With Unstable Angina). *J Am Coll Cardiol* 2002;40(7):1366–1374.

36. Bogale N, Orn S, James M, et al. Usefulness of either or both left and right bundle branch block at baseline or during follow-up for predicting death in patients following acute myocardial infarction. *Am J Cardiol* 2007;99(5):647–650.

37. Guerrero M, Harjai K, Stone GW, et al. Comparison of the prognostic effect of left versus right versus no bundle branch block on presenting electrocardiogram in acute myocardial infarction patients treated with primary angioplasty in the primary angioplasty in myocardial infarction trials. *Am J Cardiol* 2005;96(4):482–488.

38. Sgarbossa EB, Pinski SL, Barbagelata A, et al. Electrocardiographic diagnosis of evolving acute myocardial infarction in the presence of left bundle-branch block. GUSTO-1 (Global Utilization of Streptokinase and Tissue Plasminogen Activator for Occluded Coronary Arteries) Investigators. *N Engl J Med* 1996;334(8):481–487.

39. Sgarbossa EB, Pinski SL, Wagner GS. Left bundle-branch block and the ECG in diagnosis of acute myocardial infarction. *JAMA* 1999;282(13):1224–1225.

40. Cannon CP, McCabe CH, Stone PH, et al. The electrocardiogram predicts one-year outcome of patients with unstable angina and non-Q wave myocardial infarction: results of the TIMI III Registry ECG Ancillary Study. Thrombolysis in Myocardial Ischemia. *J Am Coll Cardiol* 1997;30(1):133–140.

41. Haines DE, Raabe DS, Gundel WD, et al. Anatomic and prognostic significance of new T-wave inversion in unstable angina. *Am J Cardiol* 1983;52(1):14–18.

42. de Zwaan C, Bar FW, Janssen JH, et al. Angiographic and clinical characteristics of patients with unstable angina showing an ECG pattern indicating critical narrowing of the proximal LAD coronary artery. *Am Heart J* 1989;117(3):657–665.

43. Slater DK, Hlatky MA, Mark DB, et al. Outcome in suspected acute myocardial infarction with normal or minimally abnormal admission electrocardiographic findings. *Am J Cardiol* 1987;60(10):766–770.

44. McCullough PA, Nowak RM, Foreback C, et al. Performance of multiple cardiac biomarkers measured in the emergency department in patients with chronic kidney disease and chest pain. *Acad Emerg Med* 2002;9(12):1389–1396.

45. Anderson JL, Adams CD, Antman EM, et al. ACC/AHA 2007 guidelines for the management of patients with unstable angina/non ST-elevation myocardial infarction: a report of the American College of Cardiology/American Heart Association Task Force on Practice Guidelines (Writing Committee to Revise the 2002 Guidelines for the Management of Patients With Unstable Angina/Non ST-Elevation Myocardial Infarction): developed in collaboration with the American College of Emergency Physicians, the Society for Cardiovascular Angiography and Interventions, and the Society of Thoracic Surgeons: endorsed by the American Association of Cardiovascular and Pulmonary Rehabilitation and the Society for Academic Emergency Medicine. *Circulation* 2007;116(7): e148–e304.

46. Eggers KM, Oldgren J, Nordenskjold A, et al. Diagnostic value of serial measurement of cardiac markers in patients with chest pain: limited value of adding myoglobin to troponin I for exclusion of myocardial infarction. *Am Heart J* 2004;148(4):574–581.

47. de Winter RJ, Koster RW, Sturk A, et al. Value of myoglobin, troponin T, and CK-MB mass in ruling out an acute myocardial infarction in the emergency room. *Circulation* 1995;92(12): 3401–3407.

48. Jaffe AS, Ravkilde J, Roberts R, et al. It's time for a change to a troponin standard. *Circulation* 2000;102(11):1216–1220.

49. Fesmire FM, Hughes AD, Fody EP, et al. The Erlanger chest pain evaluation protocol: a one-year experience with serial 12-lead ECG monitoring, two-hour delta serum marker measurements, and selective nuclear stress testing to identify and exclude acute coronary syndromes. *Ann Emerg Med* 2002;40(6):584–594.

50. Newby LK, Roe MT, Chen AY, et al. Frequency and clinical implications of discordant creatine kinase-MB and troponin measurements in acute coronary syndromes. *J Am Coll Cardiol* 2006;47(2):312–318.

51. Peacock F, Morris DL, Anwaruddin S, et al. Meta-analysis of ischemia-modified albumin to rule out acute coronary syndromes in the emergency department. *Am Heart J* 2006;152(2):253–262.

52. Amsterdam EA, Kirk JD, Diercks DB, et al. Early exercise testing in the management of low risk patients in chest pain centers. *Progr Cardiovasc Dis* 2004;46(5):438–452.

53. Kirk JD, Turnipseed SD, Diercks DB, et al. Interpretation of immediate exercise treadmill test: interreader reliability between cardiologist and noncardiologist in a chest pain evaluation unit. *Ann Emerg Med* 2000;36(1):10–14.

54. Hollander JE, Litt HI, Chase M, et al. Computed tomography coronary angiography for rapid disposition of low-risk emergency department patients with chest pain syndromes. *Acad Emerg Med* 2007;14(2):112–116.

55. Gallagher MJ, Ross MA, Raff GL, et al. The diagnostic accuracy of 64-slice computed tomography coronary angiography compared with stress nuclear imaging in emergency department low-risk chest pain patients. *Ann Emerg Med* 2007;49(2):125–136.

56. Hendel RC, Patel MR, Kramer CM, et al. ACCF/ACR/SCCT/SCMR/ASNC/NASCI/SCAI/SIR 2006 appropriateness criteria for cardiac computed tomography and cardiac magnetic resonance imaging: a report of the American College of Cardiology Foundation Quality Strategic Directions Committee Appropriateness Criteria Working Group, American College of Radiology, Society of Cardiovascular Computed Tomography, Society for Cardiovascular Magnetic Resonance, American Society of Nuclear Cardiology, North American Society for Cardiac Imaging, Society for Cardiovascular Angiography and Interventions, and Society of Interventional Radiology. *J Am Coll Cardiol* 2006;48(7):1475–1497.

57. Kontos MC, Jesse RL, Schmidt KL, et al. Value of acute rest sestamibi perfusion imaging for evaluation of patients admitted to the emergency department with chest pain. *J Am Coll Cardiol* 1997;30(4):976–982.

58. Braunwald E. Unstable angina: diagnosis and management. Clinical practice guideline no. 10. Publication no. 94-0602. Rockville, Md: US Department of Health and Human Services, Public Health Service, Agency for Health Care Policy and Research, National Heart, Lung, and Blood Institute; 1994.

59. Meine TJ, Roe MT, Chen AY, et al. Association of intravenous morphine use and outcomes in acute coronary syndromes: results from the CRUSADE Quality Improvement Initiative. *Am Heart J* 2005;149(6):1043–1049.

60. Hjalmarson A, Herlitz J, Holmberg S, et al. The Göteborg metoprolol trial. Effects on mortality and morbidity in acute myocardial infarction. *Circulation* 1983;67(6 pt 2):I26–I32.

61. Hjalmarson A, Herlitz J. Limitation of infarct size by beta blockers and its potential role for prognosis. *Circulation* 1983;67(6 pt 2)(6 Pt 2):I68–I71.

62. The MIAMI Trial Research Group. Metoprolol in acute myocardial infarction (MIAMI): a randomised placebo-controlled international trial. *Eur Heart J* 1985;6(3):199–226.

63. Sleight P, Yusuf S, Peto R, et al. Early intravenous atenolol treatment in suspected acute myocardial infarction. *Acta Med Scand Suppl* 1981;210(Suppl 651):185–192.

64. Randomised trial of intravenous atenolol among 16 027 cases of suspected acute myocardial infarction: ISIS-1. First International Study of Infarct Survival Collaborative Group. *Lancet* 1986; 2(8498):57–66.

65. Roberts R, Rogers WJ, Mueller HS, et al. Immediate versus deferred beta-blockade following thrombolytic therapy in patients with acute myocardial infarction. Results of the Thrombolysis in Myocardial Infarction (TIMI) II-B Study. Circulation 1991;83(2): 422–37.

66. Chen ZM, Pan HC, Chen YP, et al. Early intravenous then oral metoprolol in 45,852 patients with acute myocardial infarction: Randomised placebo-controlled trial. *Lancet* 2005;366:1622–32.

67. Pfisterer M, Cox JL, Granger CB, et al. Atenolol use and clinical outcomes after thrombolysis for acute myocardial infarction: the GUSTO-I experience. Global Utilization of Streptokinase and TPA (alteplase) for Occluded Coronary Arteries. *J Am Coll Cardiol* 1998;32(3):634–640.

68. Freemantle N, Cleland J, Young P, et al. B-blockade after myocardial infarction: systematic review and meta regression analysis. *BMJ* 1999;318(7200):1730–1737.

69. Roberts R, Rogers WJ, Mueller HS, et al. Immediate versus deferred beta-blockade following thrombolytic therapy in patients with acute myocardial infarction. Results of the Thrombolysis in Myocardial Infarction (TIMI) II-B Study. *Circulation* 1991; 83(2):422–437.

70. Chen ZM, Pan HC, Chen YP, et al. Early intravenous then oral metoprolol in 45,852 patients with acute myocardial infarction: randomised placebo-controlled trial. *Lancet* 2005;366(9497): 1622–1632.

71. Metoprolol in acute myocardial infarction (MIAMI). A randomised placebo-controlled international trial. The MIAMI Trial Research Group. *Eur Heart J* 1985;6(3):199–226.

72. Nigam A, Wright RS, Allison TG, et al. Excess weight at time of presentation of myocardial infarction is associated with lower initial mortality risks but higher long-term risks including recurrent re-infarction and cardiac death. *Int J Cardiol* 2006;110(2): 153–159.

73. Ridker PM, Cushman M, Stampfer MJ, et al. Inflammation, aspirin, and the risk of cardiovascular disease in apparently healthy men. *N Engl J Med* 1997;336(14):973–979.

74. The RISC Group. Risk of myocardial infarction and death during treatment with low dose aspirin and intravenous heparin in men with unstable coronary artery disease. *Lancet* 1990;336(8719): 827–830.

75. Antithrombotic Trialists' Collaboration. Collaborative meta-analysis of randomised trials of antiplatelet therapy for prevention of death, myocardial infarction, and stroke in high risk patients. *BMJ (Clinical research ed)* 2002;324(7329):71–86.

76. CAPRIE Steering Committee. A randomised, blinded, trial of clopidogrel versus aspirin in patients at risk of ischaemic events (CAPRIE). *Lancet* 1996;348(9038):1329–1339.

77. Yusuf S, Zhao F, Mehta SR, et al. Effects of clopidogrel in addition to aspirin in patients with acute coronary syndromes without ST-segment elevation. *N Engl J Med* 2001;345(7):494–502.

78. Mehta RH, Roe MT, Mulgund J, et al. Acute clopidogrel use and outcomes in patients with non-ST-segment elevation acute coronary syndromes undergoing coronary artery bypass surgery. *J Am Coll Cardiol* 2006;48(2):281–286.

79. Mehta SR, Yusuf S, Peters RJ, et al. Effects of pretreatment with clopidogrel and aspirin followed by long-term therapy in patients undergoing percutaneous coronary intervention: the PCI-CURE study. *Lancet* 2001;358(9281):527–533.

80. Schleinitz MD, Heidenreich PA. A cost-effectiveness analysis of combination antiplatelet therapy for high-risk acute coronary syndromes: clopidogrel plus aspirin versus aspirin alone. *Ann Intern Med* 2005;142(4):251–259.

81. Yusuf S, Mehta SR, Zhao F, et al. Early and late effects of clopidogrel in patients with acute coronary syndromes. *Circulation* 2003;107(7):966–972.

82. Steinhubl SR, Berger PB, Mann JT III, et al. Early and sustained dual oral antiplatelet therapy following percutaneous coronary intervention: a randomized controlled trial. *JAMA* 2002;288 (19):2411–2420.

83. Mega JL, Morrow DA, Sabatine MS, et al. Correlation between the TIMI risk score and high-risk angiographic findings in non-ST-elevation acute coronary syndromes: observations from the Platelet Receptor Inhibition in Ischemic Syndrome Management in Patients Limited by Unstable Signs and Symptoms (PRISM-PLUS) trial. *Am Heart J* 2005;149(5):846–850.

84. Boersma E, Harrington RA, Moliterno DJ, et al. Platelet glycoprotein IIb/IIIa inhibitors in acute coronary syndromes: a meta-analysis of all major randomised clinical trials.[erratum appears in Lancet 2002 Jun 15;359(9323):2120]. *Lancet* 2002;359(9302):189–198.

85. King SB, Smith SC, Hirshfield LW. 2007 Focused Update of the ACC/AHA/SCAI 2005 Guideline Update for Percutaneous Coronary Intervention: a report of the American College of Cardiology/American Heart Association Task Force on Practice Guidelines: 2007 Writing Group to Review New Evidence and Update the ACC/AHA/SCAI 2005 Guideline Update for Percutaneous Coronary Intervention, Writing on Behalf of the 2005 Writing Committee. *Circulation* 2008;117:261–95.

86. Hirsh J. Heparin. *N Engl J Med* 1991;324(22):1565–1574.

87. Hirsh J, Raschke R. Heparin and low-molecular-weight heparin: the Seventh ACCP Conference on Antithrombotic and Thrombolytic Therapy. *Chest* 2004;126(3 Suppl):188S–203S.

88. Granger CB, Miller JM, Bovill EG, et al. Rebound increase in thrombin generation and activity after cessation of intravenous heparin in patients with acute coronary syndromes. *Circulation* 1995;91(7):1929–1935.

89. Alpert JS, Thygesen K, Antman E, et al. Myocardial infarction redefined—a consensus document of The Joint European Society of Cardiology/American College of Cardiology Committee for the redefinition of myocardial infarction. *J Am Coll Cardiol* 2000;36(3):959–969.

90. Fragmin during Instability in Coronary Artery Disease (FRISC) study group. Low-molecular-weight heparin during instability in coronary artery disease. *Lancet* 1996;347(9001):561–568.

91. Collet JP, Montalescot G, Lison L, et al. Percutaneous coronary intervention after subcutaneous enoxaparin pretreatment in patients with unstable angina pectoris. *Circulation* 2001;103(5):658–663.

92. Cohen M, Demers C, Gurfinkel EP, et al. A comparison of low-molecular-weight heparin with unfractionated heparin for unstable coronary artery disease. Efficacy and Safety of Subcutaneous Enoxaparin in Non-Q-Wave Coronary Events Study Group. *N Engl J Med* 1997;337(7):447–452.

93. Antman EM, McCabe CH, Gurfinkel EP, et al. Enoxaparin prevents death and cardiac ischemic events in unstable angina/non-Q-wave myocardial infarction. Results of the thrombolysis in myocardial infarction (TIMI) 11B trial. *Circulation* 1999;100(15): 1593–1601.

94. Ferguson JJ, Califf RM, Antman EM, et al. Enoxaparin vs unfractionated heparin in high-risk patients with non-ST-segment elevation acute coronary syndromes managed with an intended early invasive strategy: primary results of the SYNERGY randomized trial. *JAMA* 2004;292(1):45–54.

95. Antman EM. Should bivalirudin replace heparin during percutaneous coronary interventions? *JAMA* 2003;289(7):903–905.

96. Lincoff AM, Kleiman NS, Kereiakes DJ, et al. Long-term efficacy of bivalirudin and provisional glycoprotein IIb/IIIa blockade vs heparin and planned glycoprotein IIb/IIIa blockade during percutaneous coronary revascularization: REPLACE-2 randomized trial. *JAMA* 2004;292(6):696–703.

97. Stone GW, McLaurin BT, Cox DA, et al. Bivalirudin for patients with acute coronary syndromes. *N Engl J Med* 2006;355(21): 2203–2216.

98. Bittl JA, Chaitman BR, Feit F, et al. Bivalirudin versus heparin during coronary angioplasty for unstable or postinfarction angina: Final report reanalysis of the Bivalirudin Angioplasty Study. *Am Heart J* 2001;142(6):952–959.

99. Lincoff AM, Kleiman NS, Kottke-Marchant K, et al. Bivalirudin with planned or provisional abciximab versus low-dose heparin and abciximab during percutaneous coronary revascularization: results of the Comparison of Abciximab Complications with Hirulog for Ischemic Events Trial (CACHET). *Am Heart J* 2002;143(5):847–853.

100. Lincoff AM, Bittl JA, Kleiman NS, et al. Comparison of bivalirudin versus heparin during percutaneous coronary intervention (the Randomized Evaluation of PCI Linking Angiomax to Reduced Clinical Events [REPLACE]-1 trial). *Am J Cardiol* 2004;93(9):1092–1096.

101. Yusuf S, Mehta SR, Chrolavicius S, et al. Comparison of fondaparinux and enoxaparin in acute coronary syndromes. *N Engl J Med* 2006;354(14):1464–1476.

102. Coller BS. Monitoring platelet GP IIb/IIIa [corrected] antagonist therapy. *Circulation* 1997;96(11):3828–3832.

103. Topol EJ, Moliterno DJ, Herrmann HC, et al. Comparison of two platelet glycoprotein IIb/IIIa inhibitors, tirofiban and abciximab, for the prevention of ischemic events with percutaneous coronary revascularization. *N Engl J Med* 2001;344(25): 1888–1894.

104. Simoons ML. Effect of glycoprotein IIb/IIIa receptor blocker abciximab on outcome in patients with acute coronary syndromes without early coronary revascularisation: the GUSTO IV-ACS randomised trial. *Lancet* 2001;357(9272):1915–1924.

105. Platelet Glycoprotein IIb/IIIa in Unstable Angina: Receptor Suppression Using Integrilin Therapy. Inhibition of platelet glycoprotein IIb/IIIa with eptifibatide in patients with acute coronary syndromes. The PURSUIT Trial Investigators. *N Engl J Med* 1998;339(7):436–443.

106. Platelet Receptor Inhibition in Ischemic Syndrome Management (PRISM) Study Investigators. A comparison of aspirin plus tirofiban with aspirin plus heparin for unstable angina. *N Engl J Med* 1998;338(21):1498–1505.

107. Wu AH. A comparison of cardiac troponin T and cardiac troponin I in patients with acute coronary syndromes. *Coron Artery Dis* 1999;10(2):69–74.

108. Giugliano RP, Newby LK, Harrington RA, et al. The early glycoprotein IIb/IIIa inhibition in non-ST-segment elevation acute coronary syndrome (EARLY ACS) trial: a randomized placebo-controlled trial evaluating the clinical benefits of early front-loaded eptifibatide in the treatment of patients with non-ST-segment elevation acute coronary syndrome—study design and rationale. *Am Heart J* 2005;149(6):994–1002.

109. Indications for fibrinolytic therapy in suspected acute myocardial infarction: collaborative overview of early mortality and major morbidity results from all randomised trials of more than 1000 patients. Fibrinolytic Therapy Trialists' (FTT) Collaborative Group. *Lancet* 1994;343(8893):311–322.

110. Ricou F, Nicod P, Gilpin E, et al. Influence of right bundle branch block on short- and long-term survival after inferior wall Q-wave myocardial infarction. *Am J Cardiol* 1991;67(13):1143–1146.

111. Newby KH, Pisano E, Krucoff MW, et al. Incidence and clinical relevance of the occurrence of bundle-branch block in patients treated with thrombolytic therapy. *Circulation* 1996;94(10):2424–2428.

112. Melgarejo-Moreno A, Galcera-Tomas J, Garcia-Alberola A, et al. Incidence, clinical characteristics, and prognostic significance of right bundle-branch block in acute myocardial infarction: a study in the thrombolytic era. *Circulation* 1997;96(4):1139–1144.

113. Sgarbossa EB, Pinski SL, Topol EJ, et al. Acute myocardial infarction and complete bundle branch block at hospital admission: clinical characteristics and outcome in the thrombolytic era. GUSTO-I Investigators. Global Utilization of Streptokinase and t-PA [tissue-type plasminogen activator] for Occluded Coronary Arteries. *J Am Coll Cardiol* 1998;31(1):105–110.

114. Gunnarsson G, Eriksson P, Dellborg M. Bundle branch block and acute myocardial infarction. Treatment and outcome. *Scand Cardiovasc J* 2000;34(6):575–579.

115. Brilakis ES, Wright RS, Kopecky SL, et al. Bundle branch block as a predictor of long-term survival after acute myocardial infarction. *Am J Cardiol* 2001;88(3):205–209.

116. Go AS, Barron HV, Rundle AC, et al. Bundle-branch block and in-hospital mortality in acute myocardial infarction. National Registry of Myocardial Infarction 2 Investigators. *Ann Intern Med* 1998;129(9):690–697.

117. From GISSI-1 to GUSTO: ten years of clinical trials on thrombolysis. GISSI-3 Steering Committee. *Eur Heart J* 1994;15(9):1155–1157.

118. ISIS-4: a randomised factorial trial assessing early oral captopril, oral mononitrate, and intravenous magnesium sulphate in 58,050 patients with suspected acute myocardial infarction. ISIS-4 (Fourth International Study of Infarct Survival) Collaborative Group. *Lancet* 1995;345(8951):669–685.

119. Randomised trial of intravenous streptokinase, oral aspirin, both, or neither among 17,187 cases of suspected acute myocardial infarction: ISIS-2. ISIS-2 (Second International Study of Infarct Survival) Collaborative Group. *Lancet* 1988;2(8607):349–360.

120. Chen ZM, Jiang LX, Chen YP, et al. Addition of clopidogrel to aspirin in 45,852 patients with acute myocardial infarction: randomised placebo-controlled trial. *Lancet* 2005;366(9497):1607–1621.

121. The GUSTO investigators. An international randomized trial comparing four thrombolytic strategies for acute myocardial infarction. *N Engl J Med* 1993;329(10):673–682.

122. GUSTO III Investigators. A comparison of reteplase with alteplase for acute myocardial infarction. The Global Use of Strategies to Open Occluded Coronary Arteries (GUSTO III) Investigators. *N Engl J Med* 1997;337(16):1118–1123.

123. Assessment of the Safety and Efficacy of a New Thrombolytic Investigators. Single-bolus tenecteplase compared with front-loaded alteplase in acute myocardial infarction: the ASSENT-2 double-blind randomised trial. *Lancet* 1999;354(9180):716–722.

124. Baigent C, Collins R, Appleby P, et al. ISIS-2: 10 year survival among patients with suspected acute myocardial infarction in randomised comparison of intravenous streptokinase, oral aspirin, both, or neither. The ISIS-2 (Second International Study of Infarct Survival) Collaborative Group. *BMJ* 1998;316(7141):1337–1343.

125. Franzosi MG, Santoro E, De Vita C, et al. Ten-year follow-up of the first megatrial testing thrombolytic therapy in patients with acute myocardial infarction: results of the Gruppo Italiano per lo Studio della Sopravvivenza nell'Infarto-1 study. The GISSI Investigators. *Circulation* 1998;98(24):2659–2665.

126. Simoons ML, Arnold AE, Betriu A, et al. Thrombolysis with tissue plasminogen activator in acute myocardial infarction: no additional benefit from immediate percutaneous coronary angioplasty. *Lancet* 1988;1(8579):197–203.

127. Grines C, Patel A, Zijlstra F, et al. Primary coronary angioplasty compared with intravenous thrombolytic therapy for acute myocardial infarction: Six-month follow up and analysis of individual patient data from randomized trials. *Am Heart J* 2003;145(1):47–57.

128. Keeley EC, Cigarroa JE. Facilitated primary percutaneous transluminal coronary angioplasty for acute ST segment elevation myocardial infarction: rationale for reuniting pharmacologic and mechanical revascularization strategies. *Cardiol Rev* 2003;11(1):13–20.

129. Keeley EC, Boura JA, Grines CL. Primary angioplasty versus intravenous thrombolytic therapy for acute myocardial infarction: a quantitative review of 23 randomised trials. *Lancet* 2003;361(9351):13–20.

130. Antman EM, Hand M, Armstrong PW, et al. 2007 Focused update of the ACC/AHA 2004 Guidelines for the Management of Patients With ST-Elevation Myocardial Infarction. A report of the American College of Cardiology/American Heart Association Task Force on Practice Guidelines. *Circulation* 2007.

131. Fibrinolytic Therapy Trialists' (FTT) Collaborative Group. Indications for fibrinolytic therapy in suspected acute myocardial infarction: collaborative overview of early mortality and major morbidity results from all randomised trials of more than 1000 patients. *Lancet* 1994;343(8893):311–322.

132. Eagle KA, Goodman SG, Avezum A, et al. Practice variation and missed opportunities for reperfusion in ST-segment-elevation myocardial infarction: findings from the Global Registry of Acute Coronary Events (GRACE). *Lancet* 2002;359(9304):373–377.

133. Weaver WD, Simes RJ, Betriu A, et al. Comparison of primary coronary angioplasty and intravenous thrombolytic therapy for acute myocardial infarction: a quantitative review [published correction appears in *JAMA* 1998;279:1876]. *JAMA* 1997;278(23):2093–2098.

134. Hasdai D, Behar S, Wallentin L, et al. A prospective survey of the characteristics, treatments and outcomes of patients with acute coronary syndromes in Europe and the Mediterranean basin; the Euro Heart Survey of Acute Coronary Syndromes (Euro Heart Survey ACS). *Eur Heart J* 2002;23(15):1190–1201.

135. Zeymer U, Tebbe U, Essen R, et al. Influence of time to treatment on early infarct-related artery patency after different thrombolytic regimens. ALKK-Study Group. *Am Heart J* 1999;137(1):34–38.

136. Weaver WD, Cerqueira M, Hallstrom AP, et al. Prehospital-initiated vs hospital-initiated thrombolytic therapy. The Myocardial Infarction Triage and Intervention Trial. *JAMA* 1993;270(10):1211–1216.

137. Steg PG, Bonnefoy E, Chabaud S, et al. Comparison of A, Prehospital Thrombolysis In acute Myocardial infarction I. Impact of time to treatment on mortality after prehospital fibrinolysis or primary angioplasty: data from the CAPTIM randomized clinical trial. *Circulation* 2003;108(23):2851–2856.

138. Morrison LJ, Verbeek PR, McDonald AC, et al. Mortality and prehospital thrombolysis for acute myocardial infarction: A meta-analysis. *JAMA* 2000;283(20):2686–2692.

139. Brodie BR, Stuckey TD, Muncy DB, et al. Importance of time-to-reperfusion in patients with acute myocardial infarction with and without cardiogenic shock treated with primary percutaneous coronary intervention. *Am Heart J* 2003;145(4):708–715.

140. Hochman JS, Lamas GA, Buller CE, et al. Coronary intervention for persistent occlusion after myocardial infarction. *N Engl J Med* 2006;355(23):2395–2407.

141. Kent DM, Schmid CH, Lau J, et al. Is primary angioplasty for some as good as primary angioplasty for all? *J Gen Intern Med* 2002;17(12):887–894.

142. Hochman JS, Sleeper LA, White HD, et al. One-year survival following early revascularization for cardiogenic shock. *JAMA* 2001;285(2):190–192.

143. Intravenous NPA for the treatment of infarcting myocardium early; InTIME-II, a double-blind comparison of single-bolus lanoteplase vs accelerated alteplase for the treatment of patients with acute myocardial infarction. *Eur Heart J* 2000;21(24):2005–2013.

144. Simoons ML, Maggioni AP, Knatterud G, et al. Individual risk assessment for intracranial haemorrhage during thrombolytic therapy. *Lancet* 1993;342(8886–8887):1523–1528.

145. Brass LM, Lichtman JH, Wang Y, et al. Intracranial hemorrhage associated with thrombolytic therapy for elderly patients with acute myocardial infarction: results from the Cooperative Cardiovascular Project. *Stroke* 2000;31(8):1802–1811.

146. Magid DJ, Calonge BN, Rumsfeld JS, et al. Relation between hospital primary angioplasty volume and mortality for patients with acute MI treated with primary angioplasty vs thrombolytic therapy. *JAMA* 2000;284(24):3131–3138.

147. Andersen HR, Nielsen TT, Rasmussen K, et al. A comparison of coronary angioplasty with fibrinolytic therapy in acute myocardial infarction. *N Engl J Med* 2003;349(8):733–742.

148. Fesmire FM, Brady WJ, Hahn S, et al. Clinical policy: indications for reperfusion therapy in emergency department patients with suspected acute myocardial infarction. American College of Emergency Physicians Clinical Policies Subcommittee (Writing Committee) on Reperfusion Therapy in Emergency Department Patients with Suspected Acute Myocardial Infarction. *Ann Emerg Med* 2006;48(4):358–383.

149. The TIMI Study Group. Comparison of invasive and conservative strategies after treatment with intravenous tissue plasminogen activator in acute myocardial infarction: results of the Thrombolysis in Myocardial Infarction (TIMI) phase II trial. *N Engl J Med* 1989;320(10):618–627.

150. O'Neill WW, Weintraub R, Grines CL, et al. A prospective, placebo-controlled, randomized trial of intravenous streptokinase and angioplasty versus lone angioplasty therapy of acute myocardial infarction. *Circulation* 1992;86(6):1710–1717.

151. Primary versus tenecteplase-facilitated percutaneous coronary intervention in patients with ST-segment elevation acute myocardial infarction (ASSENT-4 PCI): randomised trial. *Lancet* 2006;367(9510):569–578.

152. The International Study Group. In-hospital mortality and clinical course of 20,891 patients with suspected acute myocardial infarction randomised between alteplase and streptokinase with or without heparin. *Lancet* 1990;336(8707):71–75.

153. ISIS-3 (Third International Study of Infarct Survival) Collaborative Group. ISIS-3: a randomised comparison of streptokinase vs tissue plasminogen activator vs anistreplase and of aspirin plus heparin vs aspirin alone among 41,299 cases of suspected acute myocardial infarction. *Lancet* 1992;339(8796):753–770.

154. GISSI-2 Trial Investigators. Six-month survival in 20,891 patients with acute myocardial infarction randomized between alteplase and streptokinase with or without heparin. GISSI-2 and International Study Group. Gruppo Italiano per lo Studio della Sopravvivenza nell'Infarto. *Eur Heart J* 1992;13(12):1692–1697.

155. Sabatine MS, Cannon CP, Gibson CM, et al. Addition of clopidogrel to aspirin and fibrinolytic therapy for myocardial infarction with ST-segment elevation. *N Engl J Med* 2005;352(12):1179–1189.

156. Topol EJ. Reperfusion therapy for acute myocardial infarction with fibrinolytic therapy or combination reduced fibrinolytic therapy and platelet glycoprotein IIb/IIIa inhibition: the GUSTO V randomised trial. *Lancet* 2001;357(9272):1905–1914.

157. Lincoff AM, Califf RM, Van de Werf F, et al. Mortality at 1 year with combination platelet glycoprotein IIb/IIIa inhibition and reduced-dose fibrinolytic therapy vs conventional fibrinolytic therapy for acute myocardial infarction: GUSTO V randomized trial. *JAMA* 2002;288(17):2130–2135.

158. PARADIGM Investigators. Combining thrombolysis with the platelet glycoprotein IIb/IIIa inhibitor lamifiban: results of the Platelet Aggregation Receptor Antagonist Dose Investigation and Reperfusion Gain in Myocardial Infarction (PARADIGM) trial. *J Am Coll Cardiol* 1998;32(7):2003–2010.

159. Strategies for Patency Enhancement in the Emergency Department (SPEED) Group. Trial of abciximab with and without low-dose reteplase for acute myocardial infarction. *Circulation* 2000;101(24):2788–2794.

160. Sabatine MS, Cannon CP, Gibson CM, et al. Effect of clopidogrel pretreatment before percutaneous coronary intervention in patients with ST-elevation myocardial infarction treated with fibrinolytics: the PCI-CLARITY study. *JAMA* 2005;294(10):1224–1232.

161. ASSENT-3 Trial Investigators. Efficacy and safety of tenecteplase in combination with enoxaparin, abciximab, or unfractionated heparin: the ASSENT-3 randomised trial in acute myocardial infarction. *Lancet* 2001;358(9282):605–613.

162. Armstrong PW, Wagner G, Goodman SG, et al. ST segment resolution in ASSENT 3: insights into the role of three different treatment strategies for acute myocardial infarction. *Eur Heart J* 2003;24(16):1515–1522.

163. Antman EM, Morrow DA, McCabe CH, et al. Enoxaparin versus unfractionated heparin with fibrinolysis for ST-elevation myocardial infarction. *N Engl J Med* 2006;354(14):1477–1488.

164. Gibson CM, Cannon CP, Murphy SA, et al. Relationship of the TIMI myocardial perfusion grades, flow grades, frame count, and percutaneous coronary intervention to long-term outcomes after thrombolytic administration in acute myocardial infarction. *Circulation* 2002;105(16):1909–1913.

165. Yusuf S, Mehta SR, Chrolavicius S, et al. Effects of fondaparinux on mortality and reinfarction in patients with acute ST-segment elevation myocardial infarction: the OASIS-6 randomized trial. *JAMA* 2006;295(13):1519–1530.

166. Kastrati A, Mehilli J, Schlotterbeck K, et al. Early administration of reteplase plus abciximab vs abciximab alone in patients with acute myocardial infarction referred for percutaneous coronary intervention: a randomized controlled trial. *JAMA* 2004;291(8):947–954.

167. ADdressing the Value of facilitated ANgioplasty after Combination therapy or Eptifibatide monotherapy in acute Myocardial Infarction (ADVANCE MI) Trial Investigators. Facilitated percutaneous coronary intervention for acute ST-segment elevation myocardial infarction: results from the prematurely terminated ADdressing the Value of facilitated ANgioplasty after Combination therapy or Eptifibatide monotherapy in acute Myocardial Infarction (ADVANCE MI) trial. *Am Heart J* 2005;150(1):116–122.

168. Stone GW, Grines CL, Cox DA, et al. Comparison of angioplasty with stenting, with or without abciximab, in acute myocardial infarction. *N Engl J Med* 2002;346(13):957–966.

169. Fesmire FM, Decker WW, Diercks DB, et al. Clinical policy: critical issues in the evaluation and management of adult patients with non-ST-segment elevation acute coronary syndromes. *Ann Emerg Med* 2006;48(3):270–301.

170. Peterson ED, Roe MT, Mulgund J, et al. Association between hospital process performance and outcomes among patients with acute coronary syndromes. *JAMA* 2006;295(16):1912–1920.

171. Mehta RH, Newby LK, Patel Y, et al. The impact of emergency department structure and care processes in delivering care for non-ST-segment elevation acute coronary syndromes. *Am Heart J* 2006;152(4):648–660.

172. Roe MT, Ohman EM, Pollack CV Jr, et al. Changing the model of care for patients with acute coronary syndromes. *Am Heart J* 2003;146(4):605–612.

173. Mehta RH, Roe MT, Chen AY, et al. Recent trends in the care of patients with non-ST-segment elevation acute coronary syndromes: insights from the CRUSADE initiative. *Arch Intern Med* 2006;166(18):2027–2034.

174. Nallamothu BK, Bates ER. Percutaneous coronary intervention versus fibrinolytic therapy in acute myocardial infarction: is timing (almost) everything? *Am J Cardiol* 2003;92(7):824–826.

Chapter 6
Heart Failure and Acute Pulmonary Edema in the Emergency Department

W. Frank Peacock

HF is a syndrome, and no single test defines the diagnosis. At initial presentation, it may be difficult to accurately diagnose HF, and integration of clinical and laboratory parameters may be necessary to refine diagnosis and prognosis. In one primary care study, the initial diagnosis was falsely positive in over 50%. When symptoms attributed to heart failure develop and are mild to moderate, annual mortality is 5% to 10%; if symptoms are severe, annual mortality increases to 30% to 40%.

- Diagnostic considerations in acute heart failure
- Initial differential diagnosis using B-type natriuretic peptide (BNP) and N-terminal proBNP (NTproBNP)
- Therapy considerations for diuretic therapy, vasodilator therapy, and noninvasive positive pressure ventilation
- Risk stratification for discharge and short-stay management

Introduction

The United States is currently experiencing a heart failure (HF) epidemic. With 4.7 million cases and approximately 550,000 new patients each year,[1] HF represents the single greatest expense for the Centers of Medicare and Medicaid Studies (CMS). Although HF can occur at any age, it is primarily a disease of the aged. While less than 1% of Americans <50 years of age carry a HF diagnosis, the prevalence doubles each decade until, by the age of 80 years, nearly 10% carry the diagnosis. Among those >65 years, HF is the most common cause of hospitalization,[1] accounting for nearly 1 million annual hospitalizations. Furthermore, HF is a disease of recidivism, with up to 60% of patients discharged with HF being rehospitalized within 6 months due to recurrent decompensation.[2] As demographic trends predict, the population over age 65 will double in the next 30 years; therefore, the impact of HF is expected to increase significantly as well. Estimated to exceed $27 billion dollars, the current annual U.S. costs for HF care approximately double that of any cancer diagnoses.[2]

Prognosis

The diagnosis of HF is associated with a very poor long-term prognosis. Once diagnosed with HF, the annual death rate is 18.7%.[2] After the development of symptoms, 2-year mortality approximates 35%; over the following 6 years, this increases to 80% for men and 65% for women.[1] Outcome is predicted by symptom severity. When symptoms attributed to heart failure develop and are rated as mild to moderate, annual mortality is 5% to 10%. However, if symptoms are considered severe, annual mortality increases to 30% to 40%. Finally, after an episode of pulmonary edema, only half survive a year; if diagnosed with cardiogenic shock, as many as 85% die within 7 days.[2]

The New York Heart Association (NYHA) HF classification is a commonly used prognostic scale and is reported in the majority of published HF studies. Although it is limited by excluding asymptomatic HF and has poor sensitivity and high interobserver variability, it is a strong mortality predictor. Once a

PREVALENCE OF HF BY SEX AND AGE (NHANES: 1999–2004)

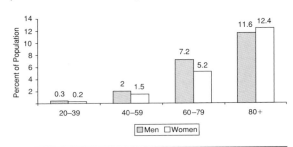

Source: NCHS and NHLBI.

96

| TABLE 6-1 • Heart Failure Classifications and Stages

NYHA Class	ACC/AHA Class	Stage	Patient Description
	A	High risk for developing LVD	Hypertension, coronary artery disease, diabetes mellitus, family history of cardiomyopathy
I	B	Asymptomatic LVD	Previous MI or LV systolic dysfunction, asymptomatic valvular disease, no limitations of physical activity
II and III	C	Symptomatic LVD	Known structural heart disease, reduced exercise tolerance, shortness of breath and fatigue with ADL
IV	D	Refractory end-stage heart failure	Marked symptoms at rest despite maximal medical therapy

ACC/AHA, American College of Cardiology/American Heart Association; ADL, activities of daily living; LV, left ventricular; LVD, left ventricle dysfunction; MI, myocardial infarction; NYHA, New York Heart Association.

patient is determined to be NYHA class IV, 1-year mortality exceeds 50%. The newer American Heart Association (AHA) scale includes risk factors as an integral part of the rating system, thus recognizing the fact that earlier intervention has the greatest potential for morbidity and mortality reduction (see Table 6-1).[3]

Pathophysiology

Heart failure may present acutely because of pump dysfunction occurring in the setting of myocardial infarction. In this scenario, loss of a critical amount of functional myocardium results in immediate symptoms. If symptomatic hypotension exists, as a result of inadequate perfusion, cardiogenic shock is diagnosed (see Chapter 7). Heart failure may present precipitously as acute pulmonary edema (APE). Also referred to as acute heart failure syndrome, pulmonary edema is the final manifestation of a reflexively increased systemic vascular resistance (SVR) having the effect of a rapidly decreasing cardiac output (CO) as a compromised myocardium is unable to match the increased workload. By this mechanism, even small elevations of blood pressure (BP) can result in a decreased CO. Decreasing CO triggers further increases in SVR, which worsens the downward spiral. APE can present rapidly with severe symptoms, and if the elevated SVR is not promptly reversed, death or respiratory failure/arrest may result.

Heart failure may also manifest insidiously as the final consequence of pathologic neurohormonal and hemodynamic reflexes initiated by myocardial injury or stress. Threats to CO trigger a neurohormonally mediated cascade that includes activation of the renin-angiotensin-aldosterone system and the sympathetic nervous system. Levels of norepinephrine, vasopressin, endothelin (a potent vasoconstrictor), and tissue necrosis factor are increased. Although not available clinically, the levels of these hormones directly correlate with HF mortality. The clinical consequences of neurohormonal activation are sodium and water retention and increased SVR. These mechanisms may maintain BP and perfusion, but at the cost of increased myocardial workload, wall tension, and myocardial oxygen demand. While some patients are initially asymptomatic, the mechanisms for cardiac remodeling, the final pathologic stage, are in place. "Remodeling" refers to a change in size, shape, and function of the left ventricle (LV) in response to damage or stress. The process is an attempt to compensate for a decline in LV function. Ultimately, the results of remodeling determine future hemodynamics and therapies.

Systolic versus Diastolic Heart Failure

Myocardial wall tension is described by the law of LaPlace as the product of pressure (afterload) and the ventricular radius. Increased tension is believed to be the stimulus for cardiac remodeling. Initially, myocytes hypertrophy or die (apoptosis) and form scar tissue. The dominant response determines HF type. Thus, HF represents the common final pathway of myocardial injury, which may be the result of many different pathologies (Table 6-2).

HF is classified as systolic or diastolic by the measurement of ejection fraction (EF), which is normally 55%–75%. Determining the etiology for diastolic dysfunction is rarely an ED task, but the workup may be initiated in observation or an acute care unit. *Systolic dysfunction*, defined as an EF <45%, is most commonly from ischemic heart disease, but other etiologies in order of frequency include hypertension, cardiomyopathies, valvular heart disease, and myocarditis.[4] Mechanistically, the ventricle has difficulty ejecting blood. Impaired contractility leads to increased intracardiac volumes, with pressure and *afterload sensitivity*. With circulatory stress (e.g., walking), failure to improve contractility, despite increasing venous return, results in increased cardiac pressures, pulmonary congestion, and edema.

TABLE 6-2 • Common Causes of Heart Failure and Pulmonary Edema

Myocardial Ischemia: Acute and Chronic
Valvular Dysfunction
  Endocarditis
  Prosthetic valve malfunction
  Aortic valve disease
    Stenosis or insufficiency
  Mitral valve disease
    Stenosis, regurgitation
    Papillary muscle dysfunction
    Ruptured chordae tendinea
Other causes of left ventricular outflow obstruction
  Supravalvular aortic stenosis
  Membranous subvalvular aortic stenosis
Cardiomyopathy
  Hypertrophic cardiomyopathy
  Dilated or restrictive
Acquired cardiomyopathy
  Toxic: alcohol, cocaine, doxorubicin
  Metabolic: thyrotoxicosis, myxedema
  Myocarditis: radiation, infection
Constrictive pericarditis
Cardiac tamponade
Systemic hypertension
Miscellaneous
  Anemia
  Cardiac dysrhythmias

TABLE 6-3 • Diastolic HF Etiologies[a]

Restrictive Cardiomyopathy
  (e.g. Cardiac amyloidosis)
Constrictive pericarditis
Ischemic Heart disease
  Post-infarction scarring/remodeling
Hypertrophic Heart disease
  Hypertrophic cardiomyopathy
  Chronic hypertension
  Aortic Stenosis
Mitral or tricuspid stenosis

[a]Grossman W. Diastolic dysfunction in congestive heart failure. NEJM 1991;325:1557-64.

In *diastolic HF*, also referred to as preserved systolic function, contractile function is preserved and the EF is normal or higher. The main pathology is impaired ventricular relaxation, causing an abnormal relation between diastolic pressure and volume. This results in a LV that has difficulty receiving blood. Decreased LV compliance necessitates higher atrial pressures to ensure adequate diastolic LV filling and results in *preload sensitivity*. The frequency of diastolic dysfunction increases with age, and is more common in elderly women. Chronic hypertension and LV hypertrophy are often responsible for this condition (see Table 6-3). Coronary artery disease also contributes, as diastolic dysfunction is an early event in the ischemic cascade.

As many as 30% to 50% of elderly HF patients have circulatory congestion on the basis of diastolic dysfunction.[5] Treatment for volume overload, the most common ED presentation, is the same irrespective of EF. However, because patients with diastolic dysfunction are preload-dependent, excessive diuresis or venodilation may exacerbate the underlying deficit in ventricular filling and cause hypotension. After hemodynamics are stabilized and congestion resolved, treatment of diastolic dysfunction requires consideration of

the underlying etiology. Determining HF type is difficult from the history and physical examination; consequently an echocardiogram is usually necessary and recommended as an initial diagnostic step. A combination of diastolic BP $\geq$105 mm Hg and the absence of jugular venous distention (JVD) has a specificity of 100% but only a 30% sensitivity for indicating preserved LV contractility.[6]

Some differentiate left- from right-sided HF. Isolated left-sided HF is associated with dyspnea, fatigue, weakness, cough, paroxysmal nocturnal dyspnea, and orthopnea in the absence of peripheral edema, JVD, or hepatojugular reflux. Right-sided HF typically includes peripheral edema, JVD, right-upper-quadrant pain, and hepatojugular reflex without pulmonary symptoms. When abnormal pressure and chamber volumes exist, they will eventually be reflected to the contralateral side. Thus, untreated or poorly controlled left-sided HF will contribute to the genesis of right heart failure and is the most common cause. With isolated right-sided HF (e.g., right ventricular infarct), left-sided HF is less likely but can eventually occur. This traditional distinction of right versus left HF, although often mentioned, does not have great bearing on the ED management, as volume overload is addressed uniformly regardless of the underlying dysfunction. The right-left distinction has greatest applicability when there is suspicion of valvular heart disease or right ventricular infarction.

High-output HF can occur when the normally intact myocardium is unable to meet excess functional demands. These instances are relatively uncommon but include anemia, thyrotoxicosis, large atrioventricular shunts, beriberi, and Paget's disease of the bone. The appropriate treatment for these conditions is symptomatic while addressing the causative pathology.

Diagnosis

HF is a syndrome, and no single test defines the diagnosis. Thus, at initial presentation, it may be difficult to accurately

TABLE 6-4 • Framingham Criteria for the Diagnosis of Heart Failure

Major Criteria	Minor Criteria
Paroxysmal nocturnal dyspnea	Bilateral extremity edema
Neck vein distention	Night cough
Rales	Dyspnea on exertion
Radiographic cardiomegaly	Hepatomegaly
Acute pulmonary edema	Pleural effusion
S3 gallop	Vital capacity reduce by one-third
Increased venous pressure (>16 cm H$_2$O)	Tachycardia (≥120)
Positive Abdominal Jugular Reflux (AJR)	

diagnose HF. In one primary care study, the initial diagnosis was falsely positive in over 50% of cases. Reasons for misdiagnosis were attributed to obesity, unsuspected cardiac ischemia, and exacerbation of pulmonary disease.[7] Gender also contributes to diagnostic errors. Rates of an initially correct HF diagnosis are reported as low as 18% in women and 36% in men.[7,8] In the 1,500-patient Breathing Not Properly study, based on history and physical alone, the ED HF diagnosis was correct in 74%.[9]

Consideration of established criteria may assist in making a diagnosis. The Framingham criteria,[10,11] using history and physical findings, require at least one major and two minor criteria for a HF diagnosis (see Table 6-4). The Boston criteria (see Table 6-5) add chest x-ray (CXR) to the history and exam.[12] More points give higher probabilities for HF. A score ≥4 correlates with a pulmonary artery occlusion pressure (PaoP) ≥12 mm Hg and has a sensitivity and specificity of 90% and 85%, respectively. These diagnostic criteria are validated but have limited predictive capability when the patient is asymptomatic.

History and Physical Examination

An acute pulmonary edema presentation is typically characterized by severe respiratory distress. Additionally, relative hypertension and cool diaphoretic skin are common. Auscultation will identify rales, which may exist over most of the lung fields. JVD is often marked, but the presence of peripheral edema is variable. The acute HF syndrome can be challenging to diagnose. It occurs in a population of patients at risk for many comorbidities, and errors in diagnosis are further compounded by a lack of more definitive testing available in real time (e.g., echocardiography). In the post-NP assay era, the ED HF misdiagnosis rate is reported as 18%.[9] Errors still occur because neither history nor physical examination are completely accurate in diagnosing HF[13,14] (Table 6-6).

The physical finding most suggestive of an elevated pulmonary capillary wedge pressure (PCWP) is the S3, which has a specificity of 99%. However, using a stethoscope for detection, its sensitivity is only 20%.[13,14] Newer technology utilizing digital microphone detection obtained at the time of ECG performance provides sensitivity and specificity of 40% and 90%, respectively. When detected in patients suspected of having heart failure, the presence of an S3 should raise concern, as outcomes are markedly worsened, including a doubling of 90-day mortality. In similar patients, JVD has a specificity of 94% and a sensitivity of 39% for identifying patients with an elevated PCWP. In other studies, reported confounders impeding a correct HF diagnosis include obesity, deconditioning, and female sex.[13]

TABLE 6-5 • Boston Criteria for the Diagnosis of Heart Failure

History	Points	Chest X-Ray	Points	Physical Exam	Points
Dyspnea at rest	4	Alveolar pulmonary edema	4	HR 91–110 bpm	1
Orthopnea	4	Interstitial pulmonary edema	3	HR >110 bpm	2
Paroxysmal nocturnal dyspnea	3	Bilateral pleural effusions	3	JVD >6 cm H$_2$O	2
Dyspnea while walking	2	Cardiothoracic ratio >0.5	3	JVD and edema or hepatomegaly	3
Dyspnea while climbing stairs	1	Kerley A lines	2	Basilar rales	1
				Rales >basilar	2
				Wheezing	3
				S3 gallop	3

Each category (history, physical examination and chest x-ray) can have a maximum score of 4 points (12 total for score). Heart failure is considered definite with a score of 8–12 points, possible with 5–7 points, and unlikely with 4 or less points.

TABLE 6-6 • Sensitivity of History and Physical Findings for a Diagnosis of Heart Failure

Variable	Sensitivity	Specificity	Accuracy
Hx of HF	62	94	80
Dyspnea	56	53	54
Orthopnea	47	88	72
Rales	56	80	70
S3	20	99	66
Jugular venous distention	39	94	72
Edema	67	68	68

Chest Radiography

Although the diagnostic "gold standard" for HF is echocardiography,[15] the lack of technologic and performance expertise limits its use for this purpose in most EDs (see Chapter 8 Ultrasonography in ED). Thus other measures are required. Chest radiographs (CXR) are easily obtained but are insensitive for evaluating cardiopulmonary status. While a normal CXR does not exclude abnormal LV function, it can help eliminate other diagnoses in the differential (e.g., pneumonia). The radiographic findings of left-side HF are, in descending order of frequency, dilated upper lobe vessels, cardiomegaly, interstitial edema, enlarged pulmonary artery, pleural effusion, alveolar edema, prominent superior vena cava, and Kerley lines.[16] Because acute abnormalities lag the clinical appearance by up to 6 hours, CXR should not necessarily delay therapy.

With at least 75% of HF presentations having a prior diagnosis of HF, chronic HF presentations are common in the ED. In this population the CXR signs of congestion have unreliable sensitivity, specificity, and predictive value in identifying patients with high PCWP.[17] Radiographic pulmonary congestion is absent in 53% of patients with mild to moderately elevated PCWP (16–29 mm Hg) and in 39% of those with markedly elevated PCWP (>30 mm Hg).[17] Cardiomegaly can assist in a diagnosis of HF. However, while a cardiothoracic ratio >60% is associated with increased 5-year mortality, the CXR can be insensitive for this finding owing to intrathoracic cardiac rotation. In fact, in a study of echocardiographically proven cardiomegaly, 22% of patients had a normal cardiothoracic ratio.[18]

CXR technique affects its performance. Pleural effusions can be missed, especially if obtained with the patient supine. The sensitivity, specificity, and accuracy of the supine CXR were 67%, 70%, and 67%, respectively.[19] Although the portable CXR is commonly used in the ED, its sensitivity for HF is poor. When HF symptoms were rated as mild, only the finding of dilated upper lobe vessels was reported in more than 60% of patients.

Despite its limitations, the ED CXR is helpful because it is noninvasive and relatively inexpensive and can be performed rapidly, even at the bedside. The frequency with which the CXR reveals findings of HF increases with HF severity. With severe HF symptoms, the CXR finding consistent with HF occurred in at least two-thirds of patients.[16] The radiographic exceptions were Kerley lines and a prominent vena cava, present in only 11% and 44% respectively. The diagnosis of HF is reassuringly less likely in the absence of any CXR findings of HF or significant abnormalities in vital signs and pulse oximetry.

 See Web site for ACEP policy statement on acute heart failure syndromes: Natriuretic Peptides

Natriuretic Peptide Assay

Natriuretic peptides (NPs) are the endogenous counterregulatory arm to the pathologic neurohormonal activation that occurs in HF. Four types are recognized: atrial NP, primarily secreted from the atria; B-type NP (BNP), secreted mainly from the cardiac ventricle; CNP, localized in the endothelium; and DNP, possibly of renal origin. NPs result in vasodilation, natriuresis, decreased endothelin, and inhibition of both the renin-angiotensin-aldosterone system and the sympathetic nervous system. BNP is the only NP for which an assay is currently available for clinical use in the ED. Because elevated levels of neurohormones portend a worse prognosis in HF, their attenuation provides the theoretical basis for most therapies proven to delay HF morbidity and mortality. These include treatment with angiotensin converting enzyme inhibitors (ACEIs), angiotensin receptor blockers (ARBs), aldosterone antagonists, beta-blockers, and nesiritide.

B-type natriuretic peptide (BNP), discovered approximately 20 years ago and available for less than a decade as an assay, has become the one of the most common ED tests for the evaluation of suspected acute decompensated HF (ADHF). BNP measurement offers improved diagnostic accuracy in the setting of suspected HF. Synthesized as pre-proBNP in the myocyte as a response to elevated ventricular pressure or volume stimulus, it is cleaved by the enzyme corin into active BNP and biologically inert N-terminal proBNP (NTproBNP) fragments. BNP is stored in membrane granules.[20] Once released, its half-life is approximately 22 minutes. It is cleared by a C receptor, neutral endopeptidases,[21] and to some extent by the kidney.[22] NTproBNP undergoes predominately renal elimination, and has a half-life of about 2 hours.

Both proteins are available to be measured clinically. They are elevated in relation to NYHA HF class (Fig. 6-1).[23]

Addition of a single BNP or NT proBNP measurement can improve the diagnostic accuracy for acute heart failure compared to clinical judgment alone.

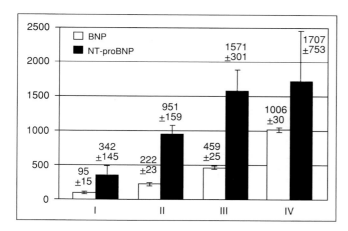

FIGURE 6-1 • BNP vs. NYHA HF class. (From McCullough PA et al. *Rev Cardiovasc Med* 2003;4:72–80, with permission.)

To obtain both good sensitivity and specificity, natriuretic peptide (NP) measurement must be considered in the context of both a low and high cutpoint. Measures beneath the low cutpoint provide excellent sensitivity and may help exclude a HF diagnosis, and levels above the high cutpoint provide strong specificity, such that a HF diagnosis contributing to the clinical presentation should be considered likely. Thus a gray zone between cutpoints remains and constitutes an area of diagnostic uncertainty. Results of NP testing in the gray zone include conditions resulting in non-HF ventricular strain or pressure overload; e.g., primary pulmonary hypertension, pulmonary embolus, myocardial infarction.

The BNP assay has a range of 0 to 5,000 pg/mL, while the range of the NTproBNP assay is 0 to 35,000 pg/mL. Low and high cutpoints are seen in Table 6-7. If the patient is >75 years of age, per the manufacturer, NTproBNP requires correction. Despite sharing a common synthetic pathway, no consistent relationship between these molecules has been described, so measures of BNP cannot be converted to NTproBNP or vice versa.

NP interpretation requires consideration of the clinical scenario. Besides non-HF conditions known to cause NP elevations into the gray zone, higher levels than clinically predicted are reported in patients with renal failure or insuf-

ficiency.[24,25] Conversely, BNP levels may be lower than clinically anticipated in two scenarios: (1) despite rapid release, BNP levels may lag by 1 hour or more in the setting of an acute presentation and (2) obesity results in lower BNP concentrations than suggested by the clinical presentation[26] (Fig. 6-2).

Finally, patients with chronic HF may have persistently elevated BNP levels, thus requiring consideration of their baseline dry weight BNP to accurately diagnose new symptoms. Although not well studied, in the setting of chronic elevation, changes exceeding 40% to 50% of baseline are considered clinically relevant.

BNP measurement has also demonstrated economic consequence if unavailable in the ED. The Basel trial was a prospective blinded evaluation of BNP in ED patients presenting with dyspnea managed with and without BNP results. BNP testing resulted in a 3.1-day decrease in subsequent length of stay (13.7 vs. 10.6 days) compared with patients in the blinded cohort.[27]

Beyond diagnosis, several studies describe the prognostic value of ED BNP testing, identifying a population of patients in whom more aggressive therapy or follow-up may be warranted. In the ED, BNP levels >480 pg/mL are associated with a 40% rate of death or HF rehospitalization within the next 6 months versus only 3% if levels were <230 pg/mL.[28] In another analysis of hospitalized HF patients, those with an initial BNP >1,740 pg/mL had an acute mortality of 6%, versus only 1.9% if <430 pg/mL[29] (Fig. 6-3).

Bioimpedance Measurement

Bioimpedance measurement has been used to aid in the diagnosis and management of patients presenting to the ED with dyspnea and suspected heart failure.[30] A noninvasive test that can be performed in the ED, at the bedside, and within minutes of presentation, this technology provides accurate measures of thoracic water content and cardiac output. In a prospective blinded study of patients presenting to the ED with dyspnea, physician knowledge of bioimpedance data resulted in a changed diagnosis in 13% of cases (95% CI 7%–22%), and a change in therapy in 39% (95% CI 29%–50%).

| TABLE 6-7 • Natriuretic Peptide Cutpoints for Clinical Decision Making

	Low Cutpoint (HF unlikely) LR− = 0.1	High Cutpoint (HF likely) LR+ = 6	Adjustments
BNP	100 pg/mL[39] Sensitivity 90% NPV 89%	500 pg/mL[85,86] Specificity PPV 90%[14]	Per package insert: <100 pg/mL HF unlikely
NTproBNP	300 pg/mL[87] Sensitivity 99% NPV 99%	900–1,000 pg/mL[87] Specificity 85% PPV 76%	Per package insert: If age >75 years, cutpoint is 450 pg/mL if age <75 years, cutpoint is 125 pg/mL

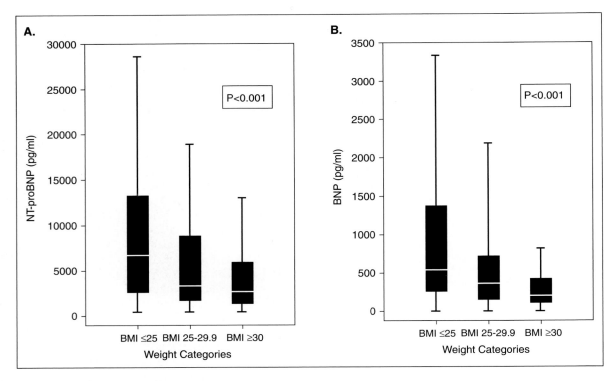

FIGURE 6-2 • NP levels vs. body mass index. (From Krauser P et al. *Am Heart J* 2005;149:744–750, with permission).

Differential Diagnosis

Differentiating HF from other causes of dyspnea is challenging. The differential diagnosis of patients presenting with potential HF (Table 6-8) is confounded by the fact that there are many HF mimics, and these mimics may actually lead to HF or worsen existing HF (Table 6-9). This includes acute myocardial infarction, which must also be considered as a potential cause of a HF exacerbation. A common confounder is coexisting obstructive pulmonary disease. Severe hypertension and peripheral vasoconstriction suggest an acute HF syndrome even in the setting of audible wheezing. Pneumonia and pulmonary embolus can also mimic or exacerbate HF. History and physical examination can help in differentiation, but the CXR and NP assay results may be misleading in the setting of chronic HF. Prior medical records may assist. Edema is seen in HF but is nonspecific, as is noted in hypoproteinemic states, hepatic or renal failure, and vascular diseases.

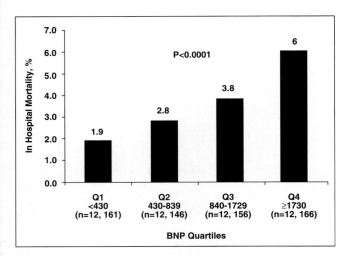

FIGURE 6-3 • Admission BNP vs. acute mortality in decompensated heart failure. (From Fonarow GC, Peacock WF, Phillips CO, et al for the ADHERE Scientific Advisory Committee and Investigators. *J Am Coll Cardiol* 2007;49:1943–1950, with permission.)

Treatment and Stabilization

General Measures

The initial approach is driven by presentation acuity, volume status, and systemic perfusion. If stability is questionable, airway management supersedes all other processes, with therapeutic and diagnostic interventions occurring simultaneously. This is in contrast to the less severely symptomatic patient whose evaluation may be performed in a more step-

| TABLE 6-8 • Differential Diagnoses for Heart Failure

Dyspneic states
Asthma exacerbation
Chronic obstructive pulmonary disease exacerbation
Pleural effusion
Pneumonia or other pulmonary infection
Pneumothorax
Pulmonary embolus
Physical deconditioning or obesity

Fluid-retentive states
Dependent edema or deep venous thrombosis
Hypoproteinemia
Liver failure or cirrhosis
Portal vein thrombosis
Renal failure or nephrotic syndrome

Impaired cardiac output states
Acute myocardial infarction
Acute valvular insufficiency
Drug overdose/effect
Dysrhythmias
Pericardial tamponade
Tension hydro- or pneumothorax
High-output state
Sepsis
Anemia
Thyroid dysfunction

| TABLE 6-9 • Precipitants of an Acute Heart Failure Syndrome

Noncompliance
Excess salt[a]
Medication noncompliance[a]

Cardiac causes
New arrhythmia
Rapid atrial fibrillation
Acute coronary syndrome
Uncontrolled hypertension

Iatrogenic
Use of calcium-channel blocker, beta-blocker, or non steroidal anti-inflammatory drugs
Inappropriate therapy reduction
Antiarrhythmic agents within 48 hours

Noncardiac causes
Exacerbation of comorbidity (e.g., chronic obstructive pulmonary disease)
Pulmonary embolus

Volume overload
Renal failure (especially missed dialysis)[a]

[a]Very common.

wise progression. Initial stabilization is directed at ensuring and maintaining airway control as well as adequate ventilation. Supplemental oxygen use may be guided by pulse oximetry. As the acute risk of hypoxia exceeds that of hypercarbia, O_2 should not be withheld for fear of CO_2 retention. Arterial blood gas measurements can be helpful in the criti-

See Web site for ACEP policy statement on acute heart failure syndromes: Noninvasive Positive Pressure Ventilation

cally ill and where CO_2 retention is a possibility. Endotracheal intubation with mechanical ventilation is indicated if stability is unclear.
Noninvasive positive pressure ventilation (NIV) may stabilize or improve airway concerns in patients with acute pulmonary edema. For NIV, close monitoring, hemodynamic stability, anatomy providing a face-mask seal, and cooperation by the patient are required. NIV is performed by face mask as continuous positive airway pressure (CPAP) or by a nasal or face mask in a biphasic (BiPAP) mode, with separately controlled inspiratory and expiratory cycles. Which technique is best is unclear. One report included higher rates of myocardial infarction in patients receiving BiPAP,[31] but sub-

sequent studies disputed this association of BiPAP with acute myocardial infarction. In comprehensive meta-analysis reviewing CPAP and BiPAP,[30a,31,31a] no significant difference between CPAP or BiPAP was found in terms of efficacy or safety; recommendations did not favor one or the other. However NIV is the only ED therapy that has been noted to improve early mortality in patients with cardiogenic pulmonary edema.

The American College of Emergency Physicians (ACEP) guidelines[32] for acute HF recommend the use of 5- to 10-mm Hg CPAP. In a pooled analysis of 494 patients, NIV combined with standard therapy reduced hospital mortality (RR 0.61; 95% CI 0.41, 0.91) and suggested NIV was associated with decreased endotracheal intubation (RR 0.43; 95% CI 0.21, 0.87).[31a]

Use of 5 to 10 mm Hg CPAP by nasal or face mask in patients with acute heart failure without hypotension or needing emergent intubation can improve heart rate, respiration, and blood pressure, and may reduce need for intubation and possibly mortality.

Standard initial ED measures include cardiac monitoring, pulse oximetry, 12-lead ECG, intravenous access, and frequent vital sign assessments, CXR, complete blood cell count, electrolytes, BNP level, and cardiac markers. Coronary artery disease is one of the most common underlying conditions associated with HF. As myocardial ischemia may precipitate acute HF, an ECG is needed shortly after presentation. Changes suggestive of MI should prompt immediate cardiology consultation and the evaluation of reperfusion therapy candidacy. The ECG also assists in evaluating cardiac arrhythmia, electrolyte abnormality (e.g., hyperkalemia), drug toxicity (e.g., digoxin toxicity), and prognosis. Abnormal Q waves in dilated cardiomyopathy, QRS duration >0.12 ms, or left bundle-branch block predicts increased 5-year mortality.[33] While the patient is in the ED, continuous cardiac monitoring is needed to help exclude arrhythmia as a cause of HF exacerbation and allow the early detection of arrhythmias resulting from potassium shifts that may occur during stabilization. As many as 14% of ED patients presenting with acute HF will ultimately rule in for myocardial infarction by necrosis markers.[34] If acute myocardial infarction is suspected, emergent reperfusion therapy is considered.

TREATMENT HIGHLIGHTS

- Intravenous nitrate therapy is beneficial in patients with acute heart failure, especially when combined with low-dose diuretic therapy.
- ACEI therapy is may be used in the absence of acute myocardial infarction, but patients should be monitored carefully for first-dose hypotension and hemodynamic instability.
- Nesiritide is considered second-line therapy.
- Diuretic therapy should be combined with IV nitrates.
- Aggressive diuretic therapy is unlikely to prevent the need for intubation and may worsen renal function, a marker of increased long-term mortality.

Other laboratory considerations include liver enzymes in the face of hepatomegaly, which may exclude etiologies other than passive congestion. In the presence of widened anion gap acidosis, an elevated lactate level may help confirm cardiogenic shock. Measurement of drug levels (e.g., digoxin) and screening for drugs of abuse should be individualized for each patient. A serum magnesium level should be considered with arrhythmia or severe hypokalemia. A urinary drainage catheter may also be necessary to monitor fluid status in the severely ill or, if urine output is sufficient, to improve the patient's ability to rest.

Acute Pulmonary Edema

The failing heart can be very sensitive to afterload increases. In some, systolic BP as low as 150 mm Hg can precipitate pulmonary edema. Prompt recognition and treatment to decrease afterload may avoid the need for the escalation of therapy, including endotracheal intubation. As long as there is adequate blood pressure to support vasodilation, an initial approach may include repeated administration of sublingual nitroglycerin (NTG), 0.4 mg, at rates of up to one per minute, until intravenous NTG (0.2–0.4 µg/kg/min) can be started, BP declines, or symptoms improve. Intravenous

NTG is titrated rapidly upward (to 200 µg/min) until BP is controlled. If nitroglycerin is ineffective at decreasing blood pressure and clinical improvement is not achieved, conversion to IV nitroprusside may be necessary. Nesiritide may be considered as an alternative to NTG in selected patients, but it is not recommended as a first-line agent by ACEP Clinical Policy because of the current uncertainty regarding its safety.

The critical endpoint is rapidly lowering left ventricular filling pressure to prevent the need for endotracheal intubation. Intravenous vasodilators should be administered as soon as vascular access is established. The use of ACEIs to achieve vasodilation is controversial, as data are limited. Recommendations for their use are limited in the absence of large randomized clinical trials. Successful management of BP and filling pressures by vasodilation is evidenced by marked improvement in respiratory status long before any significant diuresis occurs.

 See Web site for ACEP policy statement on acute heart failure syndromes: Vasodilator and Diuretic Therapy

Acute heart failure is a heterogenous disease, and it is important to understand that not all AHF is secondary to volume overload. Volume reduction with diuretics ultimately lowers BP and cardiac filling pressures. However, aggressive diuretic monotherapy will rarely prevent the requirement for endotracheal intubation compared with aggressive vasodilation. IV furosemide or bumetanide are the preferred diuretics in the setting of acute pulmonary edema (Table 6-10). Ethacrynic acid is used if there is a serious sulfa allergy. These diuretics share the parameters of rapid onset; diuresis can begin 10 to 15 minutes after IV furosemide. If urine output is inadequate 20 to 30 minutes after administration, the diuretic dose is typically increased and repeated. Although diuretics are not without complications, the emergency physician has few options for volume reduction. An increasing body of literature suggests that diuretic-induced azotemia is associated with acute mortality. Thus, for loop diuretics, the smallest effective dose is preferred.

Morphine (2–5 mg IV) has been used historically as a venodilator and sedative. However, there is minimal evidence to support this effect or its safety. In the era of safe and efficacious vasodilators, the role of morphine must be questioned.

Contraindications and Complications of Vasodilation

Excessive vasodilation has the potential to result in symptomatic hypotension, and a number of pathologic conditions

| TABLE 6-10 • Treatment Options for Congestive Heart Failure

Diuretics for Heart Failure			
Diuretic	Dose (IV)	Effect (see text for comments regarding the rapidity of diuresis)	Complications
Furosemide	No prior use: 40 mg IVP If prior use: give usual PO dose as IV bolus If no effect by 20–30 min: double the dose and readminister	Diuresis starts within 15–20 minutes Duration of action is 4–6 h	Hypokalemia, hypomagnesemia hyperuricemia, hypovolemia Ototoxicity, prerenal azotemia, sulfa allergy
Bumetanide	1–3 mg	Diuresis starts within 10 min Peak action at 60 min	Same as above
Vasodilators for Acute Heart Failure			
Vasodilator	Dose	Titration Endpoint	Complications
SL NTG	0.4 mg, q1–5min	Blood pressure	Hypotension, headache
IV NTG	0.2–0.4 μg/kg/min (starting dose) More than 3 μg/kg/min may be required	Symptoms	Hypotension, headache
Nitroprussside	0.3 μg/kg/min (starting dose), 10 μg/kg/min (maximum)	Blood pressure Symptoms	Hypotension, cyanide toxicity, ? coronary steal Thiocyanate toxicity
Nesiritide	2 μg/kg bolus, then infusion of 0.01 μg/kg/min, 0.03 μg/kg/min (maximum)	Titration usually unnecessary	Hypotension
Morphine	2–5 mg IV, q3–5min	Blood pressure Respiratory rate Symptoms	Respiratory depression Hypotension Altered mental status

IVP, intravenous push; NTG, nitroglycerin; SL, sublingual.

increase the risk of hypotension (Table 6-11). Physiologically, these are the flow limiting preload-dependent states. Additionally, the potential for misdiagnosis must be considered. In the VMAC trial,[35] of 489 AHF patients receiving nitroglycerin or nesiritide, only 1% and 0.5%, respectively, developed symptomatic hypotension within 3 hours of initiation of the vasodilator infusion. Since nearly 1 in 5 patients ultimately found to have ADHF will be initially misdiagnosed in the ED or prehospital arena, the rate of misdiagnosis markedly exceeds that of vasodilator-induced hypotension. Although the rate of symptomatic hypotension resulting from vasodilator use in patients presenting with a HF mimic is unknown (e.g., pulmonary embolus, pneumonia, sepsis, etc.), this cohort would be expected to become hypotensive if treated with a vasodilator. Therefore, in the face of symptomatic hypotension after vasodilation, the clinician must consider the probability that a misdiagnosis is numerically much more likely than a primary drug effect. Clinicians should consider the possibility of misdiagnosis regardless of the development of hypotension on nitrates. In the setting of hypotension following vasodilator administration, the drug should be terminated immediately, ACS and cardiogenic shock should be considered, and a small fluid bolus should be administered if additional intervention is required.

Hypertrophic cardiomyopathy (HCM) is a contraindication to vasodilation. Combined with acute pulmonary edema, HCM is very difficult to manage. Increases in cardiac contractility or heart rate increases the dynamic outflow obstruction of HCM, and conditions of decreased preload or

| TABLE 6-11 • Causes of Hypotension After Vasodilator Use

Excessive vasodilation
Hypertrophic obstructive cardiomyopathy
Intravascular volume depletion
Right ventricular infarction
Cardiogenic shock/myocardial infarction
Aortic stenosis
Anaphylaxis
Unsuspected sepsis

afterload also worsen the obstructive gradient. Therapy is aimed at decreasing the outflow gradient by slowing heart rate and cardiac contractility. Although this can be accomplished with intravenous beta-blockers, it is best done in the intensive care unit (ICU) with hemodynamic guidance. If there is coexistent shock in the setting of HCM, phenylephrine (40–100 µg/min IV) may be the preferred pressor, as it results in peripheral vasoconstriction without increasing cardiac contractility.

Acute Heart Failure Syndrome

While patients may have relatively stable vital signs, adequate oxygenation, and ventilation, significant signs and symptoms are common (e.g., shortness of breath, orthopnea, jugular venous distention, rales, and possibly an S3). The majority of these patients will require supplementary oxygen, BP control, and diuresis. Selecting optimal treatment requires determining peripheral perfusion status and estimating the degree of pulmonary congestion. Vasoconstricted patients may benefit from vasodilators and those with congestion may benefit from diuretics. The most common presentation of ED HF is the vasoconstricted and congested patient. For these patients, combination therapy with vasodilators and diuretics may generate the best outcomes.

Stable Heart Failure

Very large blinded randomized controlled trials provide evidence-based data for managing stable systolic HF in an outpatient setting. The principal drugs are ACEIs or ARBs, hydralazine and nitrates, beta-blockers, diuretics, digoxin, aldosterone antagonists and spironolactone. The general treatment strategy focuses on maintaining the lowest possible BP while preserving mentation, ambulation, and adequate urination. Although treatment for many diseases is symptom-based, the neurohormonal antagonism needs of HF patients typically requires that they receive chronic therapy as long as there are no contraindications. Thus ACEIs and beta-blockers are often prescribed, even in the setting of stable disease and minimal symptoms. The focus on neurohormonal antagonism is a major management shift, as previously the relief of congestion with diuretics was the main thrust of therapy.

Details of Pharmacotherapy
Diuretics

Loop diuretics are generally prescribed for pulmonary edema and in acute HF syndromes. Diuretics may improve the effects of ACEIs by decreasing intravascular volume. Most ED HF patients will require intravenous dosing of diuretics, as bowel wall edema may prevent proper gastrointestinal absorption. Dosing is guided by symptoms and prior usage (Table 6-9). Once pulmonary congestion is resolved, a fixed maintenance dose may be considered to prevent recurrence. However, because diuretics do not provide any mortality benefit, they are not used as monotherapy.[15]

By promoting the excretion of free water and sodium, loop diuretics are effective except in patients with severe renal dysfunction (e.g., creatinine clearance <5 mL/min). This is in contrast to distal tubule diuretics (thiazides, metolazone, and potassium-sparing agents), which are less effective at sodium and free water clearance and lose their utility at moderate levels of renal dysfunction (creatinine clearance <40 mL/min).[15]

Furosemide is inexpensive and effective. If bumetanide is used, 1 mg has equivalent potency to 40 mg of furosemide.[36] Torsemide is also used with 10 mg reccommended as the initial dose. Some patients require the addition of a thiazide diuretic (e.g., metolazone) for efficacy. Metolazone (5–20 mg PO daily) should be given 30 minutes prior to furosemide. Combination therapy derives its benefits by acting at different nephron sites. Ethacrynic acid is the only loop diuretic that can be used if there is a significant sulfa allergy.

Aggressive diuresis can cause severe hypokalemia; therefore potassium levels must be monitored closely. An increasing QT interval may suggest hypocalcemia, hypokalemia, or hypomagnesemia. Furosemide ototoxicity is rare but can occur if used with aminoglycoside antibiotics. Potassium-sparing diuretics (e.g., spironolactone) are usually reserved for NYHA class III and IV HF.

Urinary output requires monitoring. With greater symptoms or decreased response, intravenous diuretic dosing may be doubled and repeated in 20 to 60 minutes as needed. Adequate urine output should exceed 500 mL by 2 hours unless the creatinine exceeds 2.5 mg/dL, when output goals are halved.[37] Prognosis is associated with diuretic response. Inadequate diuresis in the setting of acute pulmonary edema is associated with a fourfold increase in mortality.[38] Diuretic resistance may be overcome by IV dosing, use of multiple diuretics, or by agents that increase renal blood flow (e.g., dobutamine).[1,39]

In outpatients, diuretic use is guided by daily measured body weight. Patients taking diuretics should limit their salt intake to less than 3–4 g daily. Agents that antagonize diuretic action including the nonsteroidal anti-inflammatory drugs and cyclooxygenase-2 inhibitors are discouraged.

Vasodilators

Vasodilators are also indicated for pulmonary edema and an acute HF syndrome. Common IV vasodilators are NTG, nitroprusside, and nesiritide (Table 6-10). Because all may exert significant hypotensive effects, they are not recommended if there are signs of cardiogenic shock (hypoperfusion or symptomatic hypotension). Before their use, the physician should auscultate for murmurs and inquire about the presence of HCM or aortic stenosis, as these patients are more susceptible to developing hypotension with vasodilator use.

Nitroglycerin

Nitroglycerin can be beneficial in HF if there is adequate BP and particularly if there is hypertension. A short-acting, rapid-onset, systemic arterial and venous dilator, NTG decreases mean arterial pressure by reducing afterload and preload. As a coronary vasodilator, it may also decrease myocardial ischemia and thus improve cardiac function. NTG is administered intravenously, sublingually, or transdermally. In the setting of vasoconstriction, transdermal NTG would be anticipated to be less efficacious than other routes of administration. Intravenous NTG is initiated at 0.2 to 0.4 μg/kg/min (10–30 μg/min), rapidly increased by increments of 5 to 10 μg/min, and titrated to BP and symptomatic improvement. High doses may be required in the acute setting. Headache and abdominal pain are frequent complaints with the use of NTG, but acetaminophen is usually adequate therapy. Methemoglobinemia has been reported with use of high doses of NTG. After 24 hours of administration, a nitrate-free interval is required to attenuate tachyphylaxis to the drug.

Nitroprusside

If further afterload reduction is required (i.e., continued high systemic vascular resistance usually evidenced by persistently elevated BP despite NTG doses >200 μg), IV nitroprusside may be used. A more potent arterial vasodilator than NTG, its hemodynamic effects include decreased BP and LV filling pressure and increased CO. The initial dose is usually 0.3 μg/kg/min; it is titrated upwards every 5 to 10 minutes based on BP and clinical response. The major complication associated with nitroprusside is hypotension. Long-term use (many hours to days at a high dose) is associated with cyanide toxicity, especially with coexisting renal failure.

Nesiritide

Like endogenously produced BNP, nesiritide has acute beneficial hemodynamic, renal, and neurohormonal effects. Nesiritide produces vasodilation of veins, arteries, and coronaries resulting in a rapid decrease in right atrial pressure, pulmonary artery pressure, PCWP, SVR, and mean arterial pressure. This results in increased stroke volume and CO.[40] Although more expensive, nesiritide demonstrated better PCWP decrease, clinical improvement, and less dyspnea by 24 hours than low-dose NTG. It is unclear whether nesiritide is better than high-dose NTG therapy. Complications from nesiritide are similar to those with NTG, but with less headache and abdominal pain.[35] Nesiritide does not need to be delayed while awaiting cardiac marker results, as a small pilot study suggested better outcomes compared to NTG in HF patients with concurrent non–ST-segment-elevation MI or an ACS.[41]

Nesiritide has modest diuretic and natriuretic properties that increase urinary sodium and volume but without increased urinary potassium or creatinine clearance.[42] From a neurohormonal perspective, it antagonizes the renin-angiotensin-aldosterone axis and the sympathetic nervous system, resulting in decreases of the pathologic elevations of neurohormones in HF.[43]

In the past 5 years, two meta-analyses[44,45] suggested the renal impairment and mortality risk of nesiritide. Since those publications, two multicenter prospective, blinded, randomized, standard therapy– and placebo-controlled trials of patients with nonacute heart failure have been completed. The NAPA trial[46] evaluated renal outcomes in 272 patients with an EF ≤40% who underwent open heart surgery. In this trial, nesiritide exerted a protective renal effect, with the greatest benefit in those at the highest risk of renal injury. FUSION II evaluated mortality in 911 HF outpatients receiving nesiritide once or twice per week for 12 weeks and found no difference in mortality outcomes between the nesiritide and control cohorts.[47]

Nesiritide may be used in acute HF syndrome without cardiogenic shock and concurrently with ACEI, beta-blockers, and diuretics. Recommended dosing is an initial bolus of 2 μg/kg, followed by an IV infusion of 0.01 μg/kg/min. The most common complication is dose-dependent hypotension, with an overall rate of 4%.[48] As described previously, ACEP Clinical Policy states that nesiritide may be considered as an alternative to NTG, but it is not recommended as a first-line agent among patients with acute HF syndrome owing to the current uncertainty regarding its safety in this setting.

Other Heart Failure Drugs

Angiotensin Converting Enzyme Inhibitors

Angiotensin II (AII) has deleterious effects in HF, including vasoconstriction, aldosterone secretion, and activation of the sympathetic nervous system. It also contributes to vascular hypertrophy.[49] ACEIs prevent the conversion of AI to AII. ACE also degrades bradykinin, a mediator of anaphylaxis. Increased bradykinin is proposed as the cause of some of the benefits and complications of ACEI therapy.

Because ACEIs improve symptoms, and decrease both mortality and hospitalizations,[15,50–52] all HF patients should be on an ACEI before hospital discharge unless contraindicated (Table 6-12). Enalapril decreases 1-year mortality in class IV HF by 31% and in classes II and III HF by 16%.[50] For mortality reduction, ACEIs are equivalent to ARBs and better than the combination of hydralazine and isosorbide dinitrate.

ACEI–induced angioedema results from increased bradykinin. In angioedema, emergent anaphylaxis treatment may be necessary, and all ACEIs should be permanently discontinued. Cough can complicate ACEI therapy but should prompt a search for other causes (e.g., infection) before it is considered a side effect. If caused by an ACEI, the cough will stop within 14 days of drug cessation. However, if this side

TABLE 6-12 • Contraindications to the Use of ACEIs and Beta-Blockers

ACEI Contraindications	
Vital signs	Hemodynamic instability Systemic hypotension (SBP <80 mm Hg, especially in ambulatory patients)
Lab	Hyperkalemia Progressive azotemia (creatinine >3 mg/dL, or increasing)
Intolerance	Severe cough Angioedema
Other	Bilateral renal artery stenosis Pregnancy
Beta-blocker Contraindications	
Unstable	Inotropic therapy or cardiogenic shock Unstable hemodynamics, or congested and requiring IV diuresis (most ED patients) Symptomatic bradycardia Class IV stable HF (therapy should be provided by HF specialist)
Cardiac	Advanced heart block Severe conduction system disease (unless protected by a pacemaker)
Underlying disease	Acute vascular insufficiency or worsening claudication/rest pain Severe bronchospastic airway disease

ACE, angiotensin converting enzyme; HF, heart failure; SBP, systolic blood pressure.

effect is not severe, education of the benefits and encouragement to continue the ACEI may be appropriate. Hydralazine/isosorbide should be considered in patients unable to take ACEIs or ARBs.

ACEIs may cause hypotension, so their use may be held during aggressive diuresis (Table 6-12). Hyponatremia suggests renin-angiotensin-aldosterone system activation and may predict ACEI-induced hypotension. Mild azotemia during ACEI use is tolerated as long as the patient does not have bilateral renal artery stenosis, oliguria, or a creatinine >3 mg/dL. Potassium and renal function monitoring are required when ACEIs are started.

In general, low doses are started and titrated upward, but even low doses of ACEIs reduce mortality.[2,15] Because they inhibit neurohormonal pathways, ACEIs may take weeks to months to exert symptomatic benefit. Even in the absence of symptomatic improvement, ACEI therapy should be continued for its long-term effects on LV remodeling and mortality.[2,15]

ACEI Alternative: Angiotensin Receptor Blockers

Angiotension II (AII) is detrimental in HF. However, despite ACE inhibition, its synthesis continues by other pathways. Angiotensin II promotes aldosterone release, LV remodeling (including apoptosis), arterial vasoconstriction, and renal damage. ARBs block AII at its receptor, providing effective AII inhibition but leaving the ACE pathway intact. Intact ACE allows bradykinin degradation and complications from its accumulation (e.g., cough, anaphylaxis) to be reduced. Studies of ARBs have not demonstrated lower morbidity or mortality compared with ACEIs.[53,54] Cough and angioedema are reported less frequently with ARBs, and ARBs should replace ACEIs when ACEI is not tolerated or contraindicated. The 2,548-patient CHARM trial[55] evaluated the addition of candesartan to a guideline-recommended dose of ACEI and found that their combined use improves outcomes in HF patients.

ACEI Alternative: Hydralazine/Isosorbide Dinitrate

The combination of hydralazine and isosorbide dinitrate decreases preload and afterload and achieves protective effects against ventricular remodeling; these reduce mortality when compared with placebo.[2,15] However, enalapril-treated patients have better long-term outcomes.[2,15] Therefore, when an ARB intolerance exists, the combination of hydralazine and isosorbide dinitrate is recommended.[15,56] Since the beneficial effect of the hydralazine/isosorbide dinitrate combination is less than that of the ACEIs, such combination therapy should generally be reserved as a second-line strategy when the patient has failed therapy with ACEIs[57,58] or has an elevated serum potassium or creatinine level. There is no evidence to support the use of either agent alone. Complications include drug-induced lupus, hypotension, gastrointestinal complaints, and headache.

Recently, race-based therapy has reported marked mortality reduction with the use of hydralazine/isosorbide dinitrate when added to standard therapy in blacks.[59] In the black population with decreased renin-angiotensin activity, the addition of 75 mg of hydralazine and 40 mg of isosorbide dinitrate three times daily, added to standard care, resulted in an additional 43% mortality reduction (HR 0.57, $P = 0.01$), a 33% reduction in rehospitalizations ($P = 0.001$), and improved quality of life ($P = 0.02$).[60] Although not well represented in guidelines as yet, the mortality benefit appears to be of sufficient magnitude to warrant the addition of hydralazine/isosorbide dinitrate in black patients with HF.

Beta-Blockers

Elevated serum norepinephrine levels occurring in HF contribute to myocardial hypertrophy, afterload increases, and coronary vasoconstriction; they are also associated with increased mortality. Since beta-blockers reduce sympathetic nervous system activity, they are used in HF to reduce mortality and improve symptoms, with treatment effects comparable to those of some ACEIs.[59,61–63] Metoprolol decreases 1-year mortality as much as 34% in class II and III chronic HF[60] and decreases sudden death by 41%. Other studies have shown benefit in NYHA classes II, III, and IV HF.[15]

Beta-blockers are unlikely to be initiated in the acute setting except to control rate-related HF, as they are generally reserved for stable patients. All HF patients are considered for beta-blockers except as listed in Table 6-12.

Patients on maintenance beta-blockers presenting in an acutely volume-overloaded state represent a difficult management problem. Discontinuation of the beta-blocker may result in deterioration from beta-blocker withdrawal, but higher doses may compromise blood pressure. An appropriate compromise may be a short course of an intravenous inotrope (e.g., milrinone) to support hemodynamics while stabilizing with intravenous diuretics and vasodilators. This usually requires cardiology consultation. In the presence of hypoperfusion or pulmonary edema, beta-blockers may be temporarily stopped.

Digoxin

This alkaloid inhibits myocardial cellular membrane sodium–potassium ATPase and is recommended for control of ventricular response in atrial fibrillation.[15] However, in patients with chronic HF and atrial fibrillation, beta-blockers may be more effective. Digoxin is considered if therapy with ACEIs, beta-blockers, and diuretics fail to control HF symptoms. Digoxin is started at 0.125 mg/day orally. Using the highest tolerable dose is no longer recommended.

Except in those patients with atrial fibrillation, digoxin is not used unless the patient requires an agent in addition to ACEIs, nitrates, and diuretics. There are no data to recommend the use of digoxin in patients with asymptomatic reduction of LVEF except in those with atrial fibrillation. Levels need close monitoring in the elderly, in patients with renal insufficiency, and in those with electrolyte abnormalities. Toxicity results in cardiac arrhythmia (heart block and ectopic rhythms), nausea, vomiting, visual disturbances, disorientation, and confusion. Levels associated with toxicity are >2 ng/mL. However, digoxin toxicity may occur at lower serum levels if concurrent hypokalemia or hypomagnesemia is present. Quinidine, verapamil, spironolactone, flecainide, propafenone, and amiodarone all increase digoxin levels. If any of these medications are added, digoxin dosing should be decreased.

Spironolactone

Aldosterone has negative cardiac effects independent of AII. Use of an aldosterone antagonist (e.g., spironolactone) decreases mortality by about 30% in classes III and IV HF.[64] Spironolactone is not recommended in patients with NYHA class I or II HF. Patients with classes III and IV HF may receive 12.5 to 25 mg daily in addition to routine loop diuretics.[15,64] Adverse effects include hyperkalemia and gynecomastia. Spironolactone is recommended in symptomatic patients refractory to ACEI, beta-blockers, digoxin, and diuretic therapies. Contraindications to spironolactone include creatinine levels above 2.5 mg/dL or potassium levels above 5 mEq/L. The potassium level should be checked 1 week after starting or changing the dose. In general, spironolactone is not initiated from the ED.

Morphine Sulfate

Morphine may be used to treat acute pulmonary edema, as it is promoted as a vasodilator and sedative. Given that there is scant data supporting any significant hemodynamic effect of morphine in HF, no safety data, and the existence of newer agents with documented safety and efficacy profiles, morphine's routine use should be questioned. Morphine may reduce anxiety and help relieve the chest pain of AMI. The initial dose of morphine in HF is typically 2 to 5 mg IV; it is then titrated to clinical effect. Because morphine is a respiratory and central nervous system depressant, it should be avoided in patients with diminished respiratory effort or altered sensorium. If morphine is to be used, its antagonist, naloxone, should be available. Complications with morphine include hypotension, hypoventilation, sedation, nausea, and vomiting.

Anticoagulation: Chronic Therapy

Thromboembolic risk in the clinically stable HF outpatient is low, estimated at 1% to 3% per year, but is greatest in those with the lowest EF.[65,66] Warfarin is sometimes used in HF, but there are limited data to guide a precise approach.[15] Most investigators recommend warfarin for patients with atrial fibrillation, a LV thrombus, or prior embolic event.

Anticoagulation: Inpatient Therapy

HF inpatients are at significant risk of deep venous thrombosis (DVT). In one study, 40 mg of subcutaneous enoxaparin daily decreased venographically documented DVT from 14.9% to 5.5%.[39] While this therapy can be initiated in the ED, empiric DVT prophylaxis must be balanced against the risk of complications associated with anticoagulant use.

Drugs to Be Avoided in Heart Failure

Calcium-Channel Blockers

Since short-term use of calcium-channel blockers with negative inotropic effects may result in pulmonary edema and cardiogenic shock and long-term use may increase the risk of worsening HF and death,[67–71] their use is not recommended in systolic HF. The adverse effects of calcium-channel blockers are attributed to their negative inotropic effect. Although amlodipine has no clear mortality effect, it may be considered for compelling clinical reasons (e.g., as an antianginal agent despite maximal therapy with nitrates and beta-blockers).

Nonsteroidal Anti-Inflammatory Drugs

Nonsteroidal anti-inflammatory drugs should be avoided in HF as they inhibit the effects of diuretics and ACEIs and can worsen cardiac and renal function.[15] The routine use of aspirin for CAD prophylaxis, in patients with HF that are being concurrently treated with ACEI is controversial.

Antiarrhythmics

Since HF patients are sensitive to the proarrhythmic and cardiodepressant effects of antiarrhythmics and because their use does not prevent sudden cardiac death,[72,73] suppression of asymptomatic ventricular arrhythmias usually is unnecessary. Class I antiarrhythmics (e.g., quinidine, procainamide, and flecainide) should not be used in HF except for emergency treatment of life-threatening ventricular arrhythmias.[15,73,74] Amiodarone does not increase the risk of sudden death[75,76] and is preferred for atrial arrhythmias.[15] However, due to its chronic toxicity, amiodarone is not recommended for chronic use to prevent sudden death in patients already treated with mortality-reducing drugs (ACEIs or beta-blockers).[15]

Complications of Heart Failure

Sudden Death or Ventricular Arrhythmias

HF is the greatest risk factor for sudden death. In HF, ventricular arrhythmias are common. With dilated cardiomyopathy, 95% of patients have PVCs, and nonsustained ventricular tachycardia (VT) occurs in about one-third of patients. Syncope, resuscitation after cardiac arrest, sustained VT, symptomatic nonsustained VT, and ventricular fibrillation (VF) should prompt consideration of internal cardioverter-defibrillator (ICD) placement. Sudden death increases proportionally to both decreased EF and HF severity.[78] It occurs in 10% to 40% of patients[77–79] and is due to VF or VT in 50%. Pump failure is the terminal event in 50% of HF. The remainder die when hypotension or bradycardia progresses to pulseless electrical activity.[80]

Risk Stratification

Risk stratification is an important process in the setting of suspected acute coronary syndromes, and proper interventions in response to investigations have reasonably well-defined algorithms. Although a number of definitive measures exist, AHF does not have as extensive of a data set as ACS, and therefore risk stratification is more difficult.

After the diagnosis of AHF has been determined, patients can be divided into those with low- versus high-risk predictors of adverse outcomes. Those with low-risk predictors will be anticipated to have fewer adverse outcomes, receive less aggressive therapy, be considered for shorter hospitalizations, and may possibly be admitted to an observation unit. Those at high risk for adverse events should receive more aggressive therapy and possibly be considered for IV vasoactive therapy in an intensive care environment.

Two studies have evaluated the low-risk population. The first, by Diercks,[81] evaluated a number of parameters among ED patients at presentation to determine the best markers of successful therapy. Low risk was defined as discharge within 24 hours and no death or repeat hospitalization within 30 days. Parameters predicting low risk were a negative troponin and an initial systolic blood pressure >160 mm Hg. Using similar methodology, Burkhardt et al.[82] identified predictors of short-stay failure. They reported that a BUN at ED presentation >30 mg/dL was associated with an increased probability of hospitalization for >24 hours.

At the other extreme of risk stratification are parameters identifying a high risk of acute mortality. In an analysis of over 80,000 patients[83] from the ADHERE registry, an elevated BUN was the greatest acute mortality predictor. If the BUN was >43 mg/dL, acute mortality was nearly 9%, compared with only 2.8% if it was <43 mg/dL. Furthermore, the combination of a systolic BP <115 mm Hg and high BUN was associated with an in-hospital mortality over 15%. Finally, the addition of a creatinine >2.75 mg/dL, resulted in an in-hospital mortality rate more than 22%.

Using the above criteria of low- and high-risk patients, a simple risk-stratification tool can be applied to determine which patients are more appropriate candidates for admis-

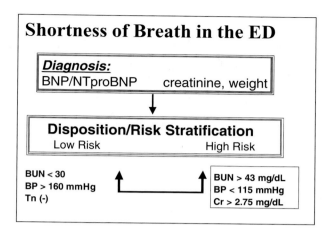

FIGURE 6-4 • Risk stratification for emergency department patients with acute dyspnea/shortness of breath in the ED.

sion to a short-stay unit versus which have a mortality risk of sufficient magnitude that more aggressive care and monitoring are warranted (Fig. 6-4).

Disposition

Acute Pulmonary Edema

Most patients with acute pulmonary edema unresponsive to initial therapy are likely to require ICU admission. A subset of initially severely hypertensive patients will improve greatly while still in the ED. For these patients, if the hypertension is controlled and dyspnea resolved, admission to a non-ICU monitored bed may be feasible. In more stable patients, the choice of medication may determine disposition. Relatively stable and improving patients receiving IV NTG or nesiritide may be managed in a telemetry unit. Those patients who appear less stable, without improvement, or who require frequent intravenous medication adjustments should be admitted to an ICU. This disposition decision also depends on the underlying etiology of the HF. Because even transient hypertension can result in a recurrence of hemodynamic decompensation, close monitoring is needed.

Acute Heart Failure Syndrome

These patients usually require hospital admission, vasodilator therapy, intravenous diuresis, adjustment of oral medications, and correction of any of the reversible causes of HF decompensation. If the clinical scenario suggests ACS, ICU admission is warranted.

All patients with new-onset HF, poor social support, hypoxemia, hypercarbia, concurrent infection, respiratory distress, syncope, or symptomatic hypotension typically require admission to the hospital.

Although candidates for discharge home from the ED represent only a minority of ED patients, they are those with mild symptoms secondary to a clearly correctable precipitant (e.g., medication noncompliance) who are likely to comply with outpatient follow-up; whose symptoms resolve with ED therapy; who have normal laboratory analyses, chest radiographs, and ECGs; and whose social situation is strong. Patients with more significant symptoms or inadequate responses to therapy warrant hospital admission.

Observation, Acute Care, and Short-Stay Unit

Intensive HF management with vasodilators and diuretics has beneficial effects in preventing inpatient hospitalizations and decreasing repeat admissions.[37,84] Protocol-driven therapy improves outcomes as compared with non-protocol management and ensures that the many multidisciplinary interactions required for successful HF management occur in a timely fashion.[37] It is important that patients entered into an intensive regimen of diuretics be properly selected. HF management guidelines are listed in Tables 6-13 and 6-14, respectively.[84] Suggested guidelines

TABLE 6-13 • Observation/Acute Care/Short-Stay Unit Heart Failure Protocol Entry Guidelines[a]

History
- Orthopnea
- Dyspnea on exertion
- Paroxysmal nocturnal dyspnea
- Shortness of breath
- Swelling of legs or abdomen
- Weight gain

Physical examination
- Jugular venous distention
- Hepatojugular reflux
- S3/S4
- Inspiratory rales
- Peripheral edema

Chest radiograph
- Cardiomegaly
- Pulmonary vascular congestion
- Kerley B lines
- Pulmonary edema
- Pleural effusion

Laboratory
- B-type natriuretic peptide >100 pg/mL

[a] Must have at least one from each category.

| TABLE 6-14 • Exclusion Criteria for HF Management in a Short Stay/Observation Unit[a]

Hemodynamic instability
  Unstable vital signs (BP >220/120 mm Hg, RR >25, HR >130 bpm)
  Unstable airway or needing >4 L/min nasal cannula O_2 for SaO_2 >90%
  Requiring continuous vasoactive medication (e.g., nitroglycerin, nitroprusside, dobutamine, or milrinone) except nesiritide
  Evidence of cardiogenic shock (systolic BP <90 mm Hg, altered mental status, peripheral vasoconstriction)
  Clinically significant arrhythmia (e.g., nonsustained VT not due to electrolyte imbalance)
Signs of acute coronary syndrome (ECG change or cardiac marker elevation)
Chronic renal failure requiring dialysis
Complex decompensation (underlying precipitant is not clearly cardiac or volume-related)
Multiple comorbidities
Acute mental status abnormality

ECG, electrocardiogram; HR, heart rate; RR, respiratory rate; Sao2, arterial oxygen saturation; VT, ventricular tachycardia.
[a]Any one positive result excludes the patient from the heart failure protocol and suggests inpatient management.

for disposition from the observation/acute-care unit are listed in Table 6-15.

Discharge Home

Patients treated for heart failure who are ultimately discharged from the ED or observation unit require outpatient follow-up by a physician knowledgeable in the management of HF. Social service evaluation may be needed to ensure medication compliance, dietary education, and reenforcement of smoking cessation instructions. Patient education is important, as patients with knowledge of the components of a sodium-restricted diet have 30% fewer rehospitalizations, and smoking cessation has the same mortality effect as the best medication therapies.[50]

| TABLE 6-15 • Discharge Guidelines from Observation/Acute Care/Short-Stay Units

Patients not meeting all of the following criteria should be considered for inpatient treatment:[a]
  Patient reports subjective improvement
  Ambulatory, without long-suffering orthostasis
  Resting HR <100 bpm
  Systolic BP >80 mm Hg
  Net urine output >1,000 mL and no new decrease in urine output <30 mL/hr (or <0.5 mL/kg/hr)
  Room air Sao2 >90% (unless on home O_2)
  All CK-MB <8.8 ng/mL, and troponin T <0.1 μg/L
  No ischemic-type chest pain
  No new clinically significant arrhythmia
  Stable electrolyte profile

CK-MB, muscle and brain types of creatine kinase; HR, heart rate; Sao₂, arterial oxygen saturation.
[a]Except as appropriate in the end-stage palliative-care cohort.

References

1. Massie BM, Shah NB. Evolving trends in epidemiologic factors of heart failure: rationale for preventative strategies and comprehensive disease management. *Am Heart J* 1997;133:703.

2. American Heart Association. *Heart Disease and Stroke Statistics: 2005 Update.* Dallas: American Heart Association, 2005.

3. Hunt SA, Baker D, Chin MH, et al. American College of Cardiology/American Heart Association. ACC/AHA guidelines for the evaluation and management of chronic heart failure in the adult: executive summary. A report of the American College of Cardiology/American Heart Association Task Force on Practice Guidelines (committee to revise the 1995 guidelines for the Evaluation and Management of Heart Failure). *J Am Coll Cardiol* 2001;38:2101.

4. Studies of left ventricular dysfunction (SOLVD)—rationale, design and methods: two trials that evaluate the effect of enalapril in patients with reduced ejection fraction. *Am J Cardiol* 1990; 66(3): 315–322.

5. Rich MW. Epidemiology, pathophysiology, and etiology of congestive heart failure in older adults. *J Am Geriatr Soc* 1997;45:968.

6. Ghali JK, Kadakia S, Cooper RS, et al. Bedside diagnosis of preserved versus impaired left ventricular systolic function in heart failure. *Am J Cardiol* 1991;67:1002–1006.

7. Remes J, Miettinen H, Reunanen A, et al. Validity of clinical diagnosis of heart failure in primary health care. *Eur Heart J* 1991;12: 315–321.

8. Francis CM, Caruana L, Kearney P, et al. Open access echocardiography in management of heart failure in the community. *BMJ* 1995;310(6980):634–636.

9. Maisel AS, Krishnaswamy P, Nowak RM, et al. Rapid measurement of B-type natriuretic peptide in the emergency diagnosis of heart failure. *N Engl J Med* 2002;347:161.

10. McKee PA, Castelli WP, McNamara PM, et al. The natural history of congestive heart failure: the Framingham study. *N Engl J Med* 1971;285:1441–1446.

11. Ho KKL, Anderson KM, Kannel WB, et al. Congestive heart failure/myocardial responses/valvular heart disease: survival after the onset of congestive heart failure in Framingham heart study subjects. *Circulation* 1993; 88(1):107–115.

12. Marantz PR, Kaplan MC, Alderman MH. Clinical diagnosis of congestive heart failure in patients with acute dyspnea. *Chest* 1990; 97(4):776–781.

13. Dao Q, Krishnaswamy P, Kazanegra R, et al. Utility of B-type natriuretic peptide in the diagnosis of congestive heart failure in an urgent-care setting. *J Am Coll Cardiol* 2001;37:379.

14. Remes J, Miettinen H, Reunanen A, et al. Validity of clinical diagnosis of heart failure in primary health care. *Eur Heart J* 1991; 12:15.

15. Packer M, Cohn JN. Consensus recommendations for the management of chronic heart failure. *Am J Cardiol* 1999;83:1A.

16. Chait A, Cohen HE, Meltzer LE, et al. The bedside chest radiograph in the evaluation of incipient heart failure. *Radiology* 1972;105:563.

17. Chakko S, Woska D, Marinez H, et al. Clinical, radiographic, and hemodynamic correlations in chronic congestive heart failure: conflicting results may lead to inappropriate care. *Am J Med* 1991;90:353.

18. Kono T, Suwa M, Hanada H, et al. Clinical significance of normal cardiac silhouette in dilated cardiomyopathy—evaluation based upon echocardiography and magnetic resonance imaging. *Jpn Circ J* 1992;56:359.

19. Ruskin JA, Gurney JW, Thorsen MK, et al. Detection of pleural effusions on supine chest radiographs. *AJR* 1987;148:681.

20. Nakao K, Mukoyama M, Hosoda K, et al. Biosynthesis, secretion, and receptor selectivity of human brain natriuretic peptide. *Can J Physiol Pharmacol* 1991;59:1500–1506.

21. Lainchbury JG, Richards AM, Nicholls MG, et al. Brain natriuretic peptide and neutral endopeptidase inhibition in left ventricular impairment. *J Clin Endocrinol Metab* 1999;84:723–729.

22. Mair J, Thomas S, Puschendorf B. Natriuretic peptides in assessment of left-ventricular dysfunction. *Scand J Clin Invest* 1999; 59(suppl 230):132–142.

23. McCullough PA, Omland T, Maisel AS. B-type natriuretic peptides: a diagnostic breakthrough for clinicians. *Rev Cardiovasc Med* 2003;4:72–80.

24. McCullough PA, Duc P, Omland T, et al and the Breathing Not Properly Multinational Study Investigators. B-type natriuretic peptide and renal function in the diagnosis of heart failure: an analysis from the Breathing Not Properly Multinational Study. *Am J Kidney Dis* 2003;41(3):571–579.

25. Vickery S, Price CP, John RI, et al. B-type natriuretic peptide (BNP) and amino-terminal proBNP in patients with CKD: Relationship to renal function and left ventricular hypertrophy. *Am J Kidney Dis* 2005;46:610–620.

26. Krauser P, Lloyd-Jones DM, Chae CU, et al. Effect of body mass index on natriuretic peptide levels in patients with acute congestive heart failure: A ProBNP Investigation of Dyspnea in the Emergency Department (PRIDE) substudy. *Am Heart J* 2005;149:744–750.

27. Mueller C, Scholer A, Laule-Kilian K, et al. Use of B-type natriuretic peptide in the evaluation and management of acute dyspnea. *N Engl J Med* 2004;350:647–654.

28. Harrison A, Morrison LK, Krishnaswamy P, et al. B-type natriuretic peptide predict future cardiac events in patients presenting to the emergency department with dyspnea. *Ann Emerg Med* 2002;39:131.

29. Fonarow GC, Peacock WF, Phillips CO, et al. Admission B-type natriuretic peptide levels and in-hospital mortality in acute decompensated heart failure. *J Am Coll Cardiol* 2007;49:1943–1950.

30. Peacock WF, Summers RL, Vogel J, et al. Impact of impedance cardiography on diagnosis and therapy of emergent dyspnea: the ED-IMPACT Trial. *Acad Emerg Med* 2006;13(4):365–371.

30a. Masip J, Betbese AJ, Paez J, et al. Non-invasive pressure support ventilation versus conventional oxygen therapy in acute cardiogenic pulmonary oedema: a randomised trial. *Lancet* 2000;356:2126–2132.

31. Mehta S, Jay GD, Woolard RH, et al. Randomized, prospective trial of bilevel versus continuous positive airway pressure in acute pulmonary edema. *Crit Care Med* 1997;25:620–628.

31a. Collins SP, Mielniczuk LM, Whittingham HA, et al. The use of noninvasive ventilation in emergency department: a systematic review. *Ann Emerg Med* 2006;48:260–269.

32. Silvers SM, Howell JM, Kosowsky JM, et al. Clinical policy: critical issues in the evaluation and management of adult patients presenting to the emergency department with acute heart failure syndromes. *Ann Emerg Med* 2007;49:627–669.

33. Koga Y, Wada T, Toshima H, et al. Prognostic significance of electrocardiographic findings in patients with dilated cardiomyopathy. *Heart Ves* 1993;8:37–41.

34. Peacock WF, Emerman CL, Doleh, M, et al. A retrospective review: the incidence of non-ST segment elevation MI in emergency department patients presenting with decompensated heart failure. *Congest Heart Failure* 2003;9(6):303–308.

35. VMAC Investigators. Intravenous nesiritide vs. nitroglycerin for treatment of decompensated congestive heart failure: a randomized controlled trial. *JAMA* 2002;287:1531.

36. Bumetadine, in *1998 Physician's Desk Reference.* Montvale, NJ: Medical Economics Company, 1998:2441–2443.

37. Peacock WF IV, Remer EE, Aponte J, et al. Effective observation unit treatment of decompensated heart failure. *Congest Heart Failure* 2002;8:68.

38. Le Conte P, Coutant V, N'Guyen JM, et al. Prognostic factors in acute cardiogenic pulmonary edema. *Am J Emerg Med* 1999;17:329.

39. Turpie AG. Thrombosis prophylaxis in the acutely ill medical patient: insights from the prophylaxis in MEDical patients with ENOXaparin (MEDENOX) trial. *Am J Cardiol* 2000;86:48M.

40. Abraham WT, Lowes BD, Ferguson DA, et al. Systemic hemodynamic, neurohormonal, and renal effects of a steady-state infusion of human brain natriuretic peptide in patients with hemodynamically decompensated heart failure. *J Cardiac Failure* 1998;4:37.

41. Peacock WF, Emerman CL, Young J. Nesiritide in congestive heart failure associated with acute coronary syndromes: a pilot study of safety and efficacy. *J Cardiac Failure* 2004;10(2):120–125.

42. Marcus LS, Hart D, Packer M, et al. Hemodynamic and renal excretory effects of human brain natriuretic peptide infusion in patients with congestive heart failure. A double-blind, placebo controlled, randomized crossover trial. *Circulation* 1996;94:3184–3189.

43. Yoshimura M, Yasue H, Ogawa H. Pathophysiological significance and clinical application of ANP and BNP in patients with heart failure. *Can J Physiol Pharmacol* 2001;79:730–735.

44. Sackner-Bernstein JD, Skopicki HA, Aaronson KD. Risk of worsening renal function with nesiritide in patients with acutely decompensated heart failure. *Circulation* 2005;111:1487–1491.

45. Sackner-Bernstein JD, Kowalski M, Fox M. Short-term risk of death after treatment with nesiritide for decompensated heart failure: a pooled analysis of randomized controlled trials. *JAMA* 2005;293(15):1900–1905.

46. Mentzer RM, Oz MC, Sladen RN, et al on behalf of the NAPA Investigators. Effects of perioperative nesiritide in patients with left ventricular dysfunction undergoing cardiac surgery: the NAPA trial. *J Am Coll Cardiol* 2007;49(6):716–726.

47. Yancy CW, Krum H, Massie BM, et al, the FUSION II Investigators. The Second Follow-up Serial Infusions of Nesiritide (FUSION II) trial for advanced heart failure: study rationale and design. *Am Heart J* 2007;153(4):478–484.

48. Colucci WS, Elkayam U, Horton DP, et al. for the Nesiritide Study Group. Intravenous nesiritide, a natriuretic peptide, in the treatment of decompensated congestive heart failure. *N Engl J Med* 2000;343:246–253.

49. Francis G, Cohn J, for the V-HeFT VA Cooperative Studies Group. Plasma norepinephrine, plasma renin activity and congestive heart failure. *Circulation* 1993;87:41–48.

50. SOLVD Investigators. Effect of enalapril on survival in patients with reduced ventricular ejection fraction and congestive heart failure. *N Engl J Med* 1991;325:293.

51. Cohn JN, Johnson G, Ziesche S, et al. A comparison of enalapril with hydralazine-isosorbide dinitrate in the treatment of chronic congestive heart failure. *N Engl J Med* 1991;325:303–310.

52. The CONSENSUS Trial Study Group. Effects of enalapril on mortality in severe congestive heart failure: results of the Cooperative North Scandinavian Enalapril Survival Study (CONSENSUS). *N Engl J Med* 1987;315:1429–1435.

53. McKelvie R, Yusuf S, Pericak D, et al. Comparison of candesartan, enalapril, and their combination in congestive heart failure: Randomized Evaluation of Strategies for Left Ventricular Dysfunction (RESOLVD pilot study) (abstract). *Eur Heart J* 1998;19(Suppl):133.

54. Pitt B, Segal R, Martinez FA, et al on behalf of Elite Study Investigators. Randomized trial of losartan versus captopril in patients over 65 with heart failure (Evaluation of Losartan in the Elderly Study, ELITE). *Lancet* 1997;349:747–752.

55. McMurray JJ, Young JB, Dunlap ME, et al. CHARM Investigators. Relationship of dose of background angiotensin-converting enzyme inhibitor to the benefits of candesartan in the Candesartan in Heart failure: Assessment of Reduction in Mortality and morbidity (CHARM)-Added trial. *Am Heart J* 2006;151(5):985–991.

56. ACC/AHA Task Force. Guidelines for the evaluation and management of heart failure: report of the American College of Cardiology/American Heart Association task force on practice guidelines (Committee of Evaluation and Management of Heart Failure). *Circulation* 1995;92:2764–2784.

57. Cohn JN, Johnson G, Ziesche S, et al. A comparison of enalapril with hydralazine-isosorbide dinitrate in the treatment of chronic congestive heart failure. *N Engl J Med* 1991;325:303–310.

58. Cohn JN, Archibald DG, Ziesche S, et al. Effect of vasodilator therapy on mortality in chronic congestive heart failure: results of the Veterans Administration Cooperative Study. *N Engl J Med* 1986;314:1547–1552.

59. Tsuyuki RT, Yusuf S, Rouleau JL, et al. Combination neurohormonal blockade with ACE inhibitors, Angiotensin II antagonists and beta-blockers in patients with congestive heart failure: design of the Randomized Evaluation of Strategies for Left Ventricular Dysfunction (RESOLVD) Pilot Study. *Can J Cardiol* 1997;13:1166–1174.

60. MERIT-HF Study Group. Effect of metoprolol CR/XL in chronic heart failure: metoprolol CR/XL randomized intervention trial in congestive heart failure. *Lancet* 1999;353:2001.

61. Colucci WS, Packer M, Bristow MR, et al. For the U.S. Carvedilol Study Group. Carvedilol inhibits clinical progression in patients with mild symptoms of heart failure. *Circulation* 1996;94:2800–2806.

62. CIBIS Investigators and Committees. A randomized trial of β-blockade in heart failure: the Cardiac Insufficiency Bisoprolol Study (CIBIS). *Circulation* 1994;90:1765–1767.

63. Bristow MR, Gilbert EM, Abraham WT, et al For the MOCHA Investigators. Carvedilol produces dose-related improvements in left ventricular function and survival in subjects with chronic heart failure. *Circulation* 1996;94:2807–2816.

64. RALES Study Investigators. The effect of spironolactone on morbidity and mortality in patients with severe heart failure. *N Engl J Med* 1999;341:709.

65. Cioffi G, Pozzoli M, Forni G, et al. Systemic thromboembolism in chronic heart failure. A prospective study in 406 patients. *Eur Heart J* 1996;17:1381–1389.

66. Baker DW, Wright RF. Management of heart failure. IV. Anticoagulation for patients with heart failure due to left ventricular systolic dysfunction. *JAMA* 1994;272:1614–1618.

67. Elkayam U, Weber L, McKay C, et al. Spectrum of acute hemodynamic effects of nifedipine in severe congestive heart failure. *Am J Cardiol* 1985;56:560–566.

68. Barjon JN, Rouleau JL, Bichet D, et al. Chronic renal and neurohumoral effects of the calcium entry blocker nisoldipine in patients with congestive heart failure. *J Am Coll Cardiol* 1987;9:622–530.

69. Elkayam U, Amin J, Mehra A, et al. A prospective, randomized, double-blind, crossover study to compare the efficacy and safety of chronic nifedipine therapy with that of isosorbide dinitrate and their combination in the treatment of chronic congestive heart failure. *Circulation* 1990;82:1954–1961.

70. Goldstein RE, Boccuzzi SJ, Cruess D, et al. Diltiazem increase late-onset congestive heart failure in post-infarction patients with early reduction in ejection fraction. The Adverse Experience Committee and the Multicenter Diltiazem Post-infarction Research Group. *Circulation* 1991;83:52–60.

71. Advisory Council to Improve Outcomes Nationwide in Heart Failure. Packer M, Cohn JN, eds. Consensus recommendations for the management of chronic heart failure. *Am J Cardiol* 1999; 83:54A.

72. The Cardiac Arrhythmia Suppression Trial (CAST) Investigators. Preliminary report: effect of encainide and flecainide on mortality in a randomized trial of arrhythmia suppression after myocardial infarction. *N Engl J Med* 1989;321:406–412.

73. The Cardiac Arrhythmia Suppression Trial II Investigators. Effect of antiarrhythmic agent moricizine on survival after myocardial infarction. *N Engl J Med* 1992;327:227–233.

74. Doval HC, Nul DR, Grancelli HO, et al for Grupo de Estudio de la Sobrevida en la Insuficiencia Cardiaca en Argentina (GESICA). Randomised trial of low-dose amiodarone in severe congestive heart failure. *Lancet* 1994;344:493–498.

75. Doval HC, Nul DR, Grancelli HO, et al for Grupo de Estudio de la Sobrevida en la Insuficiencia Cardiaca en Argentina (GESICA). Randomised trial of low-dose amiodarone in severe congestive heart failure. *Lancet* 1994;344:493–498.

76. Singh SN, Fletcher RD, Fisher SG, et al for the Survival Trial of Antiarrhythmic Therapy in Congestive Heart Failure. Amiodarone in patients with congestive heart failure and asymptomatic ventricular arrhythmias. *N Engl J Med* 1995;333:77–82.

77. Hobbs RE, Czerska MD. Congestive heart failure. Current and future strategies to decrease mortality. *Postgrad Med* 1994;96:167–172.

78. Batsford WP, Mickleborough LL, Elefteriades JA. Ventricular arrhythmias in heart failure. *Cardiol Clin* 1995;13:87–91.

79. Stevenson WG, Stevenson LW, Middlekauff HR, et al. Sudden death prevention in patients with advanced ventricular dysfunction. *Circulation* 1993; 88(6):2953–2961.

80. The SOLVD Investigators. Effect of enalapril on survival in patients with reduced left ventricular ejection fractions and congestive heart failure. *N Engl J Med* 1991;325:293–202.

81. Diercks DB, Kirk JD, Peacock WF, et al. Identification of emergency department patients with decompensated heart failure at low risk for adverse events and prolonged hospitalization. *J Cardiac Failure* 2004;10(Suppl 4):S118.

82. Burkhardt J, Peacock WF, Emerman CL. Elevation in blood urea nitrogen predicts a lower discharge rate from the observation unit. *Ann Emerg Med* 2004;44(Suppl 4):S99.

83. Fonarow GC, Heywood JT, Heidenreich PA, et al. Risk stratification for in-hospital mortality in acutely decompensated heart failure: classification and regression tree analysis. *JAMA* 2005;293(5):572–580.

84. Peacock WF IV, Albert NM. Observation unit management of heart failure. *Emerg Med Clin North Am* 2001;19:209.

85. Silver MA, Maisel A, Yancy CW, et al. BNP Consensus Panel 2004: A clinical approach for the diagnostic, prognostic, screening, treatment monitoring, and therapeutic roles of natriuretic peptides in cardiovascular disease. *Congest Heart Fail* 2004;10(5):S3.

86. Peacock WF. The B-type natriuretic peptide assay: a rapid test for heart failure. *Cleve Clin J Med* 2002;69:243.

87. Januzzi JL Jr, Camargo CA, Anwaruddin S, et al. The N-terminal Pro-BNP Investigation of Dyspnea in the Emergency Department (PRIDE) study. *Am J Cardiol* 2005;95:948–954.

Chapter 7
Cardiogenic Shock Complicating Acute Coronary Syndromes

John M. Field

Patients with cardiogenic shock and STEMI should be primarily transported or secondarily transferred (with a door-to-departure time of within 30 minutes) to facilities capable of invasive strategies such as insertion of an intra-aortic balloon pump (IABP), percutaneous coronary intervention (PCI), and coronary artery bypass grafting (CABG). Recent trial data have shown an improved prognosis for survivors of cardiogenic shock who benefit from an early invasive strategy. Thus an aggressive approach to achieve early and complete reperfusion of the infarct related artery (IRA), to prevent or correct mechanical complications of MI, and to provide pharmacologic and mechanical interventions to favorably influence early infarct remodeling are warranted in patients with cardiogenic shock or at high-risk for this complication.

- The incidence of cardiogenic shock had largely remained unchanged but appears to be decreasing in parallel with increasing rates of primary PCI for STEMI. And mortality is now, in the modern era, ~50% below historical levels of 80% to 90%.
- Right ventricular (RV) shock (usually found in association with inferior wall MI) has a high mortality rate, similar to that of left ventricular (LV) shock.
- An invasive strategy is recommended for patients <75 years of age; carefully selected patients age ≥75 can also receive aggressive early revascularization. If heart failure and shock develop after hospital admission or if shock develops within the first 36 hours of onset of MI, the patient should undergo diagnostic angiography and PCI or CABG if possible.

This chapter describes complications of acute coronary syndromes (ACS): shock, pulmonary edema, and hypotension. The first section discusses a general approach to the patient presenting with undifferentiated hypotension (see also Chapter 8). The second section summarizes the pathophysiology and treatment of cardiogenic shock associated with ST-segment elevation myocardial infarction (STEMI) and other ACS, emphasizing therapy unique to these patients. The last section reviews the algorithm for acute pulmonary edema, hypotension, and shock and details the initial evaluation and stabilization of any patient with pulmonary edema and shock or hypertensive urgency. It also contains more information about treatment decisions based on the initial response to therapy.

 See Web site for AHA/ACC Guidelines for Management of Cardiogenic Shock[1]

Epidemiology

Cardiogenic shock remains the leading in-hospital cause of mortality. In general, cardiogenic shock is due to decreased systemic cardiac output in the presence of adequate intravascular volume, resulting in tissue ischemia and cellular hypoxia. In 75% of patients with STEMI, cardiogenic shock is most often caused by extensive MI. But while cardiogenic shock may be secondary to a large STEMI, it can also be due to NSTEMI and potentially reversible conditions such as mechanical complications of MI or multivessel disease with reversible ischemia in the non–infarct-related arteries.

Historically, during the advent of the reperfusion era, the incidence of cardiogenic shock remained unchanged at about 7.5% and prognosis was poor, with in-hospital mortality exceeding 77%.[2] The incidence of cardiogenic shock in large trials of fibrinolysis is variable but has also ranged from 4% to 7%.[3–5] Overall, the prognosis of patients with cardiogenic shock has largely remained unchanged. However, recent data indicate that survivors of cardiogenic shock may have a reasonable and improved prognosis. In a 6-year follow-up of the SHOCK trial,[6] long-term survival was 62.4% in the revascularized group and 44.4% in the aggressively managed medical group. Thus, an aggressive approach—to achieve early and complete reperfusion of the IRA, prevent or correct mechanical complications of MI, and provide pharmacologic and mechanical interventions to favorably influence early infarct remodeling—is warranted.[7-9]

Hypotension and Shock

Hypotension is defined as a systolic blood pressure <90 mm Hg or an acute fall in blood pressure ≥30 mm Hg from baseline in previously hypertensive patients.[1] In patients with MI, hypotension can be due to other causes in addition to impaired ventricular function. In considering the differential diagnosis of hypotension and shock even in patients with MI, secondary causes that may complicate management should be kept in mind. For example, these may include bleeding from procedures or anticoagulation, sepsis, and inadequate volume or preload conditions.

Shock is a clinical condition characterized by a sustained and significant reduction in blood flow and oxygen delivery to organs and tissues. It is important to realize that shock and low blood pressure, although related, are not the same. In basic terms, shock is a condition in which tissue oxygenation (and cellular ventilation and nutrition) is inadequate for demand.

Patients frequently present with shock and no immediately obvious etiology (i.e., undifferentiated shock). Blood pressure alone can be misleading or "normal" for a variety of reasons. Hence the diagnosis of shock is a clinical one characterized by several of the following findings:

- Clinically ill appearance or altered mental status
- Low blood pressure (defined as a systolic blood pressure [SBP] <80 to 90 mm Hg)
- Tachycardia (heart rate >100)
- Tachypnea (respiratory rate >22 breaths/min or $PaCO_2$ <32 mm Hg)
- Systemic acidosis (serum lactate >4 mmol/L)
- Decreased urine output (<0.5 mL/kg/hr)

Differential Diagnosis of Shock

Not all of these criteria may be present. For example, patients on beta-blockers may not have tachycardia. In early shock, blood pressure may be normal or only slightly low because of excess adrenergic drive, and it may not drop significantly until late in the process.

The clinician can use provisional etiologic mechanisms to characterize shock and to identify the appropriate initial focus of therapy:

- Arrhythmic shock → antiarrhythmic therapy
- Hypovolemic shock → volume therapy
- Cardiogenic shock → reperfusion for STEMI; support of ventricular function
- Distributive shock → vasoactive drug therapy

An etiologic approach to shock often oversimplifies the problem. Any patient with severe or sustained shock will likely require some support of heart rate and rhythm, titration of fluid therapy to optimize intravascular volume, support of ventricular function, and manipulation of vascular resistance and distribution of blood flow. All patients with severe or sustained shock will have some myocardial failure or even necrosis. In fact, patients in intensive care units (ICUs) with elevation of troponin in the absence of coronary artery disease have a worse prognosis.[10,11]

Determinants of Cardiac Output

Low cardiac output from any cause impairs oxygen delivery and respiration at the cellular level. A more detailed diagnostic approach that defines the variable of cardiac output and allows for a more targeted approach to therapy is often required. Three variables determine cardiac output and distribution of blood to the periphery: stroke volume (ventricular function), heart rate (rhythm), and vascular resistance (systemic).

Arterial Pressure = **cardiac output**
$\times$ total (systemic) vascular resistance

Cardiac output = stroke volume $\times$ heart rate

Determinants of cardiac function and other variables influencing cardiac output are complex; but one major determinant relevant to the initial assessment is the volume loading conditions of the heart. At normal volume loading conditions and in the absence of pathologic conditions, cardiac output is optimal at rest. When cardiac output falls, compensatory mechanisms are activated to maintain cardiac output. Historically, it was taught that these mechanisms in cardiogenic shock included an increase in heart and peripheral systemic vascular resistance. New data however suggest that cardiogenic shock may be heterogeneous and in some cases resemble a systemic inflammatory state (see below).

If the diagnosis or etiology of shock is unclear, a pulmonary arterial catheter can measure filling pressures (central venous and pulmonary capillary wedge pressures) and cardiac output and calculate systemic vascular resistance. With three variables, there are 27 possible hemodynamic combinations, so interpretation can be complex. But three general hemodynamic subdivisions allow better diagnostic accuracy (Table 7-1). It should be remembered that insertion of a pulmonary artery (PA) catheter is a diagnostic and not a therapeutic procedure, with associated complications. In most patients, clinical assessment of filling pressure (central venous pressure, rales) and clinical circumstances are diagnostic and sufficient.

An individualized approach to the use of a PA catheter is recommended by the American College of Cardiology (ACC)/American Heart Association (AHA) guidelines.[12] There has been a decline in PA catheter use and controversy concerning an association with poor outcome,[13] but no association has been shown in patients with MI and cardiogenic shock.[14]

TABLE 7-1 • Hemodynamic Parameters in the Three Major Categories of Shock[a]

Hypovolemic	Cardiogenic	Vasogenic
Low CVP/PCWP	High CVP/PCWP	Low CVP/PCWP
Low CO	Low CO	High CO
High SVR	High SVR	Low SVR

[a]In **hypovolemic shock**, filling pressure (central venous pressure [CVP], pulmonary capillary wedge pressure [PCWP]) is low, reducing cardiac output. In an attempt to compensate and maintain arterial pressure, systemic vascular resistance (SVR) increases. In **cardiogenic shock**, impaired and cardiac output is low, raising filling pressures (CVP, PCWP) and decreasing cardiac output. Because cardiac output is low, SVR also increases to maintain arterial pressure. In **vasogenic shock**, as seen in sepsis, for example, vasodilation occurs, lowering SVR. This vasodilation causes a fall in vascular volume, and cardiac output increases in an attempt to compensate and "fill the tank." (CVP estimates right atrial pressure, and PCWP estimates left atrial pressure. CO indicates cardiac output.)

Cardiogenic Shock Complicating Acute Myocardial Infarction

Cardiogenic shock is described as inadequate organ perfusion resulting from depressed cardiac function in the presence of normal intravascular volume. Infarction of 40% or more of the LV myocardium in acute STEMI usually results in cardiogenic shock and death. Although the mortality rate of cardiogenic shock has decreased in selected recent trials, death rates have averaged 50% to 70%.[4] The overall incidence had not declined appreciably[15,16] until recently, with increasing use of revascularization, especially primary PCI, in both the United States and Europe.[17–19]

Risk factors for the development of cardiogenic shock with MI include advancing age, anterior MI, prior MI or angina, multivessel coronary artery disease, new bundle-branch block with MI, or prior heart failure.[20] Mortality varies according to demographic, clinical, and hemodynamic parameters. These include age, clinical signs of poor peripheral perfusion, anoxic/hypoxic brain damage, and left ventricular ejection fraction. Of these, hemodynamic factors are associated with short- but not long-term prognosis.

Cardiogenic Shock in NSTEMI Acute Coronary Syndrome

It should also be appreciated that shock can occur in patients with non–ST-elevation MI (NSTEMI), and even a small or modest infarct can cause hemodynamic instability if prior MI or LV dysfunction is present at the time of recurrent ACS. The SHOCK trial found that approximately 17% of all cardiogenic shock complicating MI was associated with NSTEMI. Patients with NSTEMI are significantly older

and have more prior MI, heart failure, and three-vessel disease. They also have more comorbidities—including renal dysfunction, bypass surgery, and peripheral vascular disease—than patients with STEMI.[5,21] The Global Use of Strategies to Open Occluded Coronary Arteries (GUSTO)-II and PURSUIT trials found that cardiogenic shock occurs in up to 5% of patients with NSTEMI and that mortality rates are >60%.[5,22]

Pathophysiology and Hemodynamics of Cardiogenic Shock

MI may result in hemodynamic instability and congestive heart failure (CHF). As described above, cardiogenic shock classically has been defined as a "pump" problem due to "massive" heart attack. In this context, cardiac output and ventricular ejection fraction fall due to severe left ventricular dysfunction. Heart rate increases to compensate for the fall in stroke volume in a reflex compensatory effort to maintain cardiac output. If the patient survives initially, ventricular dilation and remodeling occur over days to months, resulting in an increase in end-diastolic volume (increased ventricular *preload*), which may help to maintain stroke volume despite the fall in ejection fraction.

In cardiogenic shock, the degree of myocardial dysfunction is often severe. But in many case this severe impairment of contractility does not lead to shock, and LV ejection fraction (LVEF) may only be moderately depressed.[23] In the SHOCK trial, mean ejection fraction was ~30%.[24] In addition, LVEF is similar in the acute phase and 2 weeks later, when shock has resolved in survivors. Approximately half of patients with cardiogenic shock have small or normal LV size representing failure of an adaptive mechanism of acute dilation to maintain stroke volume early in MI.[25] Paradoxically, reduced ejection fraction and ventricular dilation are prognostic indicators of increased survival in septic shock syndrome.[26]

Iatrogenic Cardiac Shock

The majority of patients with cardiogenic shock following MI develop shock after the first 24 hours. In some patients at high risk for cardiogenic shock, medications contribute to the development of shock, including beta-blocking agents, angiotensin converting enzyme inhibitors (ACEIs), and other vasodilators such as nitrates and morphine[27–30] (Fig. 7-1).

In acute pulmonary edema, intravascular volume is redistributed to the extravascular pulmonary interstitial space in the lungs. A tachycardia may be largely compensatory for depressed myocardial function and tenuous intravascular volume. Beta-blocking agents may decrease heart rate diminishing stroke volume and vasodilators or diuretics may further redistribute blood volume or cause a poorly tolerated diuresis, precipitating a low output state. Low-dose diuretics should be initially used and nitrates added cautiously. Noninvasive positive-pressure ventilation may be useful if tolerated. IV ACEIs are contraindicated early in MI. Oral ACEIs should be

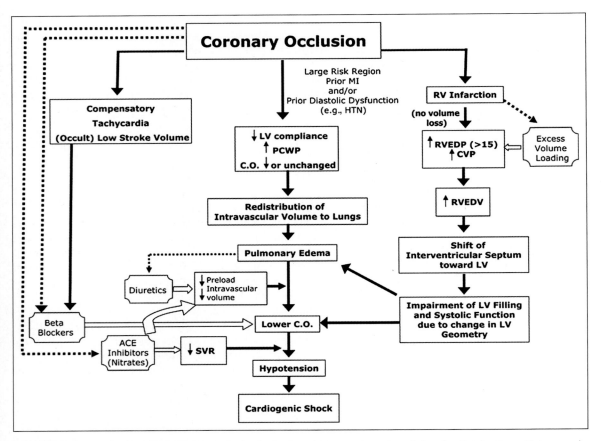

FIGURE 7-1 • Pathophysiology of iatrogenic shock. Acute pulmonary edema is a state of redistribution of intravascular volume into extracellular space in the lungs (center pathway). When hemodynamic stability is tenuous, the additional decrease in plasma volume caused by diuretics in patients without prior heart failure may induce shock. Tachycardia is often compensatory for lower stroke volume but is not appreciated as such (left-sided pathway). Treatment with beta-blockade lowers heart rate and stroke volume, leading to shock. Decompensation may also occur when patients who are reliant on compensatory vasoconstriction are aggressively treated with angiotensin-converting enzyme inhibitors, particularly intravenously and very early before they have hemodynamically stabilized. Nitrates would be expected to have a similar effect but did not in the only systematic study, which used oral low-dose treatment. Volume expansion may be deleterious when used to excess or when RV filling pressure is already elevated, because the RV may become volume overloaded with shift of the septum, causing impairment in LV filling and contraction (right-sided pathway). CVP, central venous pressure; HTN, hypertension; PCWP, pulmonary capillary wedge pressure; RVEDP, RV end-diastolic pressure; RVEDV, RV end-diastolic volume. (From Reynolds HR, Hochman JS. *Circulation* 2008;117[5]:686–697, with permission.)

deferred until patients are hemodynamically stable. In ISIS-4, the only significant side effect of captopril was hypotension.[28] In this trial, patients who developed hypotension were at increased risk for the development of cardiogenic shock and tended to have lower blood pressures and higher heart rates.

It is important to note that MI may lead to pulmonary edema without the development of shock. An initial effect of ischemia is a decrease in LV compliance, and pulmonary edema initially may mimic diastolic heart failure.

Beta-Blockade and Heart Failure—Updated Guidelines

As noted, tachycardia may help maintain cardiac output despite the fall in ejection fraction and stroke volume. But all compensatory changes are likely to increase myocardial oxygen consumption. They can worsen ischemia in viable or dis-

tant myocardium and extend the infarct area. In patients without acute heart failure, a reduction in heart rate with beta-blockade improves outcome mainly by decreasing episodes of fatal ventricular fibrillation. Blockade of excess sympathetic and neurohumoral stimulation reduces myocardial oxygen consumption. But in compensatory tachycardia, beta-blockade can be life-threatening, as in cardiogenic shock or severe heart failure, when the stroke volume is critically dependent on the tachycardia (Fig. 7-2) (see Chapter 5).

Hemodynamic Parameters of Cardiogenic Shock

When LV end-diastolic pressure increases substantially (>25–30 mm Hg), interstitial and then pulmonary edema develops. If RV end-diastolic pressure increases, peripheral

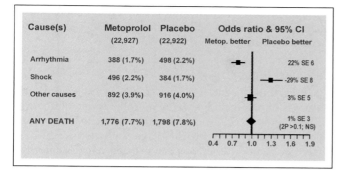

FIGURE 7-2 • Effects of metoprolol on death before discharge from hospital. A beneficial effect on reduction in deaths due to arrhythmia was negated by an offsetting increase in patients dying from cardiogenic shock. These deaths occurred primarily during the first day of admission. (Modified from Chen ZM, Pan HC, Chen YP, et al. *Lancet* 2005;366[9497]:1622–1632, with permission.)

CLASSIC HEMODYNAMIC DEFINITION OF CARDIOGENIC SHOCK

Cardiogenic shock is defined[31] as SBP ≤90 mm Hg for ≥1 hour that is

- Not responsive to fluid administration alone
- Secondary to cardiac dysfunction
- Associated with signs of hypoperfusion or a cardiac index ≤2.2 L/min per m2 and a pulmonary capillary wedge pressure >18 mm Hg

Changing the Paradigm of Cardiogenic Shock

The changes described above for cardiogenic shock result from severe depression of myocardial contractility due to MI. Cardiogenic shock remains the leading cause of in-hospital mortality from MI. In the SHOCK trial, the classic assumption that acute reduction in CO leads to compensatory vasoconstriction was not present in all patients, and a subgroup of patients was identified with low SVR.[32] These findings and new insights suggest that an inflammatory response and inappropriate vasodilation may play a role in these patients.[33] (Fig. 7-3).

In the SHOCK trial, sepsis was suspected in 18% of patients. Approximately three fourths of these patients developed positive blood cultures.[34] Inappropriate vasodilation as part of systemic inflammatory response syndrome (SIRS) may

edema will be observed. A fall in cardiac output also triggers an adrenergic response, producing tachycardia and peripheral vasoregulatory changes that try to redistribute blood flow. Constriction of arteries to the skin, kidneys, and gut redistributes blood flow away from these tissues to maintain blood flow to the brain and heart. But this systemic vasoconstriction may create increased LV *afterload*, impeding LV ejection. As cardiac output continues to fall, hypotension and lactic acidosis develop. This combination of pulmonary edema with signs of inadequate systemic perfusion is the hallmark of cardiogenic shock.

The patient with LV dysfunction classically has been described as one with a cardiac index (cardiac output corrected for body surface area) ≤2.2 L/min/m², PCWP >18 mm Hg, and SBP <90 mm Hg. When the cardiac index falls to 2.2 L/min/m² and SBP falls to 90 mm Hg, frank signs of poor peripheral perfusion are usually present.

See Web site for Cardiogenic Shock Complicating Acute Myocardial Infarction: Expanding the Paradigm

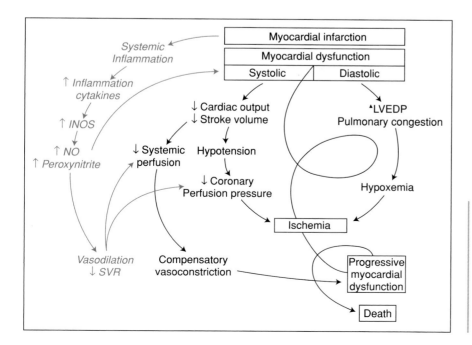

FIGURE 7-3 • Classic shock paradigm, as illustrated by S. Hollenberg, is shown in black. The influence of the inflammatory response syndrome initiated by a large MI is illustrated in red. LVEDP indicates left ventricular end-diastolic pressure. (From Hochman JS. Cardiogenic shock complicating acute myocardial infarction: expanding the paradigm. *Circulation* 2003;107:2998–3002, with permission.)

impair perfusion of the gut, enabling transmigration of bacteria. SIRS is more common with increasing duration of shock.[35] Investigation of inflammatory markers and mediators of SIRS may provide further targets for therapeutic intervention.

Treatment of Cardiogenic Shock Associated With Acute Myocardial Infarction

The mortality rate and occurrence of death from cardiogenic shock has been variably reported. In patients with persistent ST-segment elevation, failure of fibrinolytic therapy or persistent occlusion of an IRA after attempted primary PCI shock develops with a median time of 10 to 12 hours and most within 48 hours of infarction.[3,5,36,37]

General Measures

Initial therapy for LV dysfunction *without* shock includes oxygen administration, IV administration of nitrates to reduce cardiac preload and afterload, and diuresis. Morphine is an excellent adjunctive agent if the STEMI patient has continuing ischemia. If SBP is <100 mm Hg, nitrates and morphine should be used with caution if at all. When SBP is <90 mm Hg, they are contraindicated. In a recent registry study, however, the use of morphine sulfate in unstable angina (UA)/NSTEMI patients was *associated* with excess mortality.[27] In these patients, the ACC/AHA 2007 focused STEMI updates/guidelines have recommended caution and reduced morphine administration from a class I to a class IIa recommendation for UA/NSTEMI patients. One potential mechanism for harm includes a reduction in coronary perfusion pressures and coronary flow in patients with marginal mean arterial pressure required for maintaining flow in partially occluded arteries.

Volume Replacement

As noted above, hypotension may be due to causes other than LV power failure. Hypovolemia is a common occurrence and may be due to diaphoresis and vomiting, use of vasodilators, and hemorrhage due to fibrinolytic therapy, anticoagulation, or bleeding from procedures. Therefore, *cautious and appropriate* volume loading in patients without clinically significant pulmonary edema is recommended as part of the initial strategy for those who become hypotensive.

Vasoactive Drugs

If the patient presents or becomes markedly hypotensive, avoid or discontinue vasodilators and administer vasoactive drugs based on SBP to increase arterial tone (vasopressors), improve blood pressure, and redistribute cardiac output. If the patient does not respond to these initial therapies, be prepared to perform additional diagnostic studies, initiate advanced hemodynamic monitoring, and provide advanced

therapies. In selected patients, mechanical circulatory assistance with intra-aortic balloon counterpulsation is an effective adjunct with reperfusion therapy (Fig. 7-4).

Echocardiography

The differential diagnosis of shock includes mechanical complications of MI, including acute mitral regurgitation due to papillary muscle rupture or dysfunction, ventricular septal defect, subacute left ventricular free wall rupture, and RV infarction. Echocardiography can provide valuable information to guide therapy in patients with undifferentiated shock and in those with cardiogenic shock. Echocardiography should be performed early and can be done at the bedside in the emergency department (see Chapter 8).

Intra-aortic Balloon Counterpulsation

IABP has long been used as adjunctive mechanical therapy to treat cardiogenic shock and response predicts a better outcome.[38] IABP may be especially beneficial as a bridge to reperfusion therapy. If personnel and time are available during preparation for transport, IABP placement may help to stabilize the patient before and during transfer to a PCI-capable facility with cardiac surgical availability.

DeWood first reported in a small study in 1980 that reperfusion and counterpulsation within 16 to 18 hours from the onset of symptoms in patients with cardiogenic shock led to a lower mortality rate.[39] Investigators in the TAMI trial observed that patients treated with IABP had improved outcomes.[40] And large registry data also suggest that IABP could be beneficial in patients treated with fibrinolytic therapy.[41] It has been postulated that use of an IABP can stabilize patients with cardiogenic shock for transfer and that the use of IABP would be a useful adjunct in maintaining patency after fibrinolysis reducing infarct artery reocclusion.[42,43] However, there is only one randomized trial of IABP in patients receiving fibrinolytic therapy. While this trial was incomplete due to lack of randomization, it did show a reduction in mortality in patients randomized to treatment with IABP.[44]

Reperfusion Therapy

With increasing use of both fibrinolytic therapy and PCI, controversy arose over which strategy was the better method of reperfusion. Multiple investigators in small trials reported reduced mortality in patients with cardiogenic shock and AMI who received IABP treatment followed by cardiac catheterization and revascularization with PCI or CABG (when anatomy was suitable).[43, 47] The GUSTO-I investigators reported that mortality was lower in patients with cardiogenic shock treated with an aggressive PCI strategy than in similar patients given fibrinolytic therapy,[8] and investigators have reported higher survival rates for cardiogenic shock patients who undergo mechanical revascularization instead of fibrinolysis.[45] In a large registry of patients with shock, mortality was lower in AMI patients who received early revascularization with either PCI or CABG.[46] In the U.S. Second National Registry of Myocardial Infarction, the mortality rate in patients with AMI and shock was lower in those treated with PCI as a primary strategy than in those treated with fibrinolytics.[45]

The best method and timing of revascularization as well as optimal therapy for shock was a topic of controversy until evaluated and resolved by the randomized, controlled SHOCK trial.[24] This study compared early revascularization using IABP plus PCI or CABG with early medical stabilization using fibrinolytic therapy. Mortality at 6 months and at 1 year of follow-up was significantly lower in the early revascularization group than in the early medical therapy group (number needed to treat was approximately 8 at both time points). Follow-up data through 6 years are now available from this randomized trial.[6] Almost two thirds of hospital survivors with cardiogenic shock who were treated with early revascularization were alive 6 years later. A strategy of early revascularization resulted in a 13.2% absolute and a 67% relative improvement in 6-year survival compared with initial medical stabilization.

Fibrinolytic therapy is less effective but is indicated if PCI is not available or a delay in transfer for PCI is expected. Figure 7-4 gives recommendations for reperfusion therapy when cardiogenic shock complicates AMI.

Transfer and Destination Hospital Protocols

Current ACC/AHA guidelines recommend that patients who arrive in cardiogenic shock (15%) or who develop cardiogenic shock (85%) be transferred to a regional tertiary care facility with revascularization capabilities and personnel experienced in caring for these individuals. Ideally, patients at high risk for developing cardiogenic shock could be diverted or transferred to these facilities for expectant care and management.

In hospitals without interventional capabilities or an on-site intervention team, reperfusion therapy with fibrinolytics should be initiated unless timely transfer to an experienced facility can be accomplished rapidly with an estimated door-to-balloon time of 90 minutes or less. If the patient fails to reperfuse with fibrinolytics, is not eligible for fibrinolytic therapy, remains clinically unstable, or has persistent shock and CHF, they should be rapidly transferred for coronary angiography and PCI (or CABG). A door-to-departure time of 30 minutes or less should be achieved. This level of efficiency will require predetermined transfer protocols, policies, and commitment of personnel and emergency medical services (EMS).

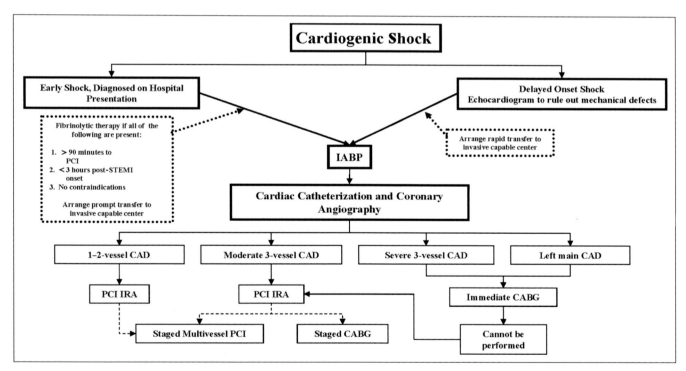

FIGURE 7-4 • Recommendations for initial reperfusion therapy when cardiogenic shock complicates STEMI. Early mechanical revascularization with PCI/CABG is a Class I recommendation for candidates less than 75 years of age with ST elevation or LBBB who develop shock less than 36 hours from STEMI, and in whom revascularization can be performed within 18 hours of shock, and a Class IIa recommendation for patients 75 years of age or older with the same criteria. 85% of shock cases are diagnosed after initial therapy for STEMI, but most patients develop shock within 24 hours. IABP is recommended when shock is not quickly reversed with pharmacologic therapy, as a stabilizing measure for patients who are candidates for further invasive care. Dashed lines indicate that the procedure should be performed in patients with specific indications only. Recommendations for staged CABG and PCI are discussed in the text, as are definitions of moderate and severe 3-vessel CAD. CABG indicates coronary artery bypass graft surgery; CAD, coronary artery disease; IABP, intra-aortic balloon pump; IRA, infarct-related artery; LBBB, left bundle branch block; MI, myocardial infarction; PCI, percutaneous coronary intervention. (Modified from Hochman JS, *Circulation* 2003;107:2998–3002, with permission.)

Prehospital Recommendations

When possible, identify and transfer patients with shock, at high risk for mortality or severe LV dysfunction with signs of shock, pulmonary congestion, heart rate >100 *and* SBP <100 mm Hg to a facility capable of performing cardiac catheterization and rapid revascularization (PCI or CABG). The use of prehospital electrocardiograms, treatment, and destination hospital protocols will facilitate this ideal goal and eliminate an intermediate and time-consuming way point for those patients possibly requiring PCI or surgical revascularization in an appropriate facility.

Cardiogenic Shock in the Elderly

As the population ages and life expectancy increases, the number of elderly patients presenting with AMI can be expected to increase as well. Mortality from MI also increases with age, in part due to accompanying comorbidities and less well tolerated complications from therapy and procedures. The AHA statistical update shows that men and women >65 years of age constitute the single largest age group experiencing MI (Fig. 7-5).[48] Longitudinal data in the Worcester, Massachusetts, registry suggests that patients >75 years of age now account for 40% or more of heart attack admissions. Therefore, an increasing number of patients >75 will become candidates for revascularization procedures now and as the population ages and the prevalence of coronary heart disease increases.

In 2004, the ACC/AHA Committee on Management of Acute Myocardial Infarction updated prior guidelines, and PCI remained a class I recommendation for patients with ACS and shock who were <75 years old but class IIa for patients ≥75 years of age, largely based upon the SHOCK trial results noting no benefit in patients in this age group. However, only 56

patients ≥75 years of age were enrolled, and of this group only 12 patients actually underwent PCI. These differences could be due to the play of chance or baseline differences.[49] Since the SHOCK registry did not detect this difference suggesting a selection bias by physicians, practice guidelines indicated that functional status and comorbidities be taken into account.

The current recommendations from the updated ACC/AHA STEMI guidelines[1] are as follows:

A strategy of coronary angiography with intent to perform PCI is reasonable in patients ≥75 years of age who received fibrinolytic therapy and are in cardiogenic shock provided that they are candidates for reperfusion.

Right Ventricular Shock

RV shock occurs in only about 5% of cases of cardiogenic shock due to MI.[50] In the majority of persons the right coronary artery supplies blood to the inferior wall and right ventricle (Fig. 7-6). When a thrombus occludes the right coronary

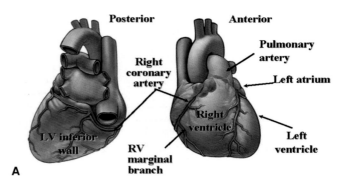

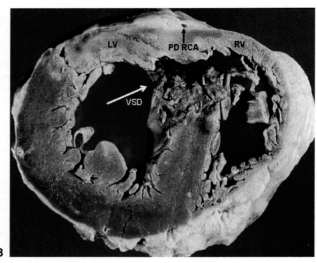

FIGURE 7-6 • **A.** Schematic anatomy of the heart, showing the right coronary artery and RV marginal branch, which supplies blood to the right ventricle. **B.** A thrombus occluding the right coronary artery proximal to the RV marginal branch causes infarction of the inferior and posterior walls of the heart (if not supplied by the circumflex coronary artery) and the right ventricle. RV, right ventricle; LV, left ventricle; VSD, ventricular septal defect; PD RCA, posterior descending coronary artery branch of right coronary artery.

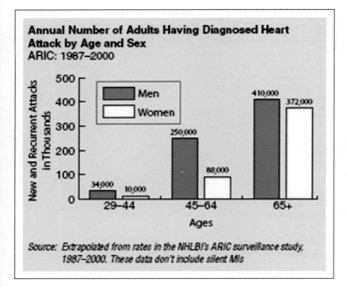

FIGURE 7-5 • Number of men and women having a diagnosed heart attack by age category. As the population ages and life span increase, men and women >65 years of age constitute the single largest group. (Source: AHA 2007 Statistical Update.)

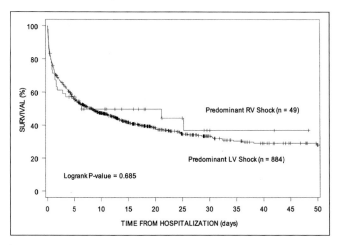

FIGURE 7-7 • In-hospital survival curves for patients with predominant right ventricular (RV) and left ventricular (LV) shock truncated at 50 days. (From Jacobs AK et al. *J Am Coll Cardiol* 2003;41:1273–1279, with permission.)

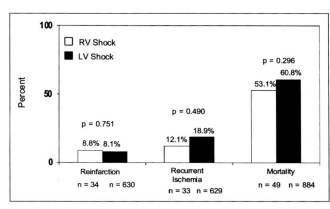

FIGURE 7-8 • In-hospital outcomes in patients with predominant right ventricular (RV) and left ventricular (LV) shock. (From Jacobs AK et al. *J Am Coll Cardiol* 2003;41:1273–1279, with permission.)

artery, ischemia and infarction of the right ventricle occur, causing RV dysfunction. The RV marginal branch is involved in about one third of patients with inferior infarction, and in half of these patients occlusion is hemodynamically significant.[51,52] The RV is fairly resistant to infarction; most acute dysfunction is due to ischemic but viable myocardium. Infarction of the RV has a favorable long-term prognosis, but hemodynamic infarction of the RV at the time of infarction more than doubles mortality. In fact, mortality from RV infarction rivals that from LV infarction (Fig. 7-7), with a similar occurrence of reinfarction, recurrent ischemia, and mortality (Fig. 7-8).

The SHOCK Registry evaluated 933 patients in cardiogenic shock due to predominant RV (*n* = 49) or LV failure (*n* = 884). Patients with predominant RV shock were younger and had a lower prevalence of previous MI and multivessel disease. Despite the younger age, lower rate of anterior MI, and higher prevalence of single-vessel coronary

disease in patients with RV shock and the similar benefit they receive from revascularization, mortality in these patients was unexpectedly high, similar to that in patients with LV shock.[50]

Patients with RV shock have difficulty filling the lungs and returning blood to the left heart. Only a small area of myocardium may be involved (inferior and posterior walls, e.g., Fig. 7-6), and shock usually stems from inadequate filling of the left ventricle, which is due to RV dysfunction. In patients with an inferior wall MI, RV involvement should be suspected and a right-sided 12-lead ECG performed. A 1-mm ST-segment elevation in lead V4 is 88% sensitive and 78% specific for RV involvement (Fig. 7-9).[53]

Clinical findings are different in RV and LV shock. Lungs may be relatively clear because of the inability of the RV to pump blood to the pulmonary vasculature and the absence of LV dysfunction, causing increased pulmonary capillary pressures. Paradoxically, neck veins may be distended

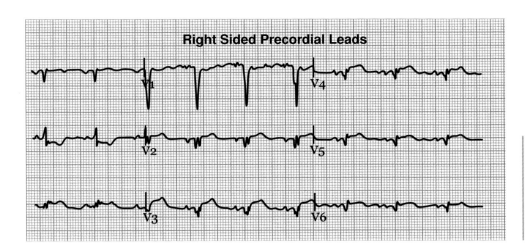

FIGURE 7-9 • Right-sided 12-lead ECG showing junctional ST-segment elevation in leads over the right ventricle. Lead V4R has 1-mm ST-segment elevation. This elevation is 88% sensitive and 78% specific for right ventricular involvement.

because of high RA pressures. The triad of clear lungs, elevated jugular venous distention, and hypotension is present in only about 25% of patients.[51]

Both RV and LV cardiogenic shock require emergent reperfusion. Medical management is different for each type. Vasodilators and low filling pressures are to be avoided in RV shock. The impaired RV requires optimal preload. The optimal RV filling pressure in the setting of RV dysfunction and shock is variable. An RV end-diastolic pressure of 10 to 15 mm Hg is associated with better RV output than are higher or lower pressures.[54]

Treatments that decrease preload—including nitrates, morphine, diuretics, and ACE inhibitors—may increase mortality and should be avoided. Optimal preload should be achieved with cautious and monitored volume replacement. Initially 1 to 2 L of fluid may be required. This should be given in a 250- to 500-mL bolus, and vital signs and clinical assessment should be serially evaluated. The rapid and injudicious administration of large amounts of fluid without clinical benefit should also be avoided, because high pressures and large amounts of volume will further impair RV

function and recovery. In patients with multivessel involvement or prior MI, significant LV dysfunction may require additional measures, such as IABP support. When initial measures do not improve hemodynamics, inotropic support of the right ventricle with dobutamine may be beneficial and mechanical complications of RV infarction should be evaluated (Figure 7-6B).[55,56] Dopamine can be added to augment arterial perfusion pressure if indicated.

The Acute Pulmonary Edema, Hypotension, and Shock Algorithm

The acute pulmonary edema, hypotension, and shock algorithm (Fig. 7-10) illustrates the management of patients who present with these complications of AMI. Based on clinical assessment and judgment, some of these

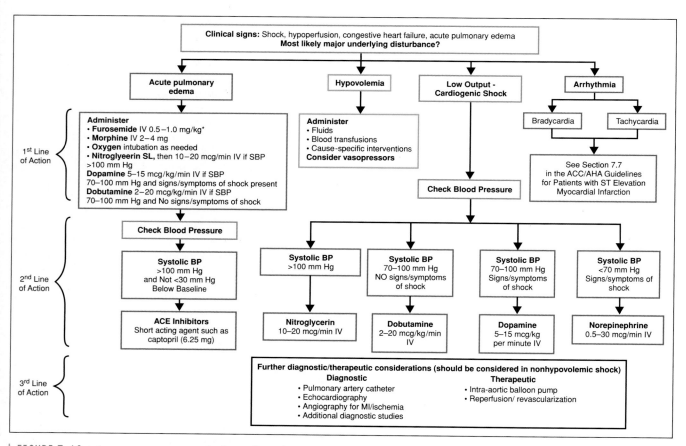

FIGURE 7-10 • Emergency management of complicated STEMI. The emergency management of patients with cardiogenic shock, acute pulmonary edema, or both is outlined. Give *furosemide <0.5 mg/kg for new onset acute pulmonary edema without hypovolemia; 1 mg/kg for acute or chronic volume overload or renal insufficiency. Nesiritide has not been studied adequately in patients with STEMI. Combinations of medications (e.g., dobutamine and dopamine) may be used. (Modified from Antman EM, Anbe DT, Armstrong PW, et al. ACC/AHA guidelines for the management of patients with ST-elevation myocardial infarction: a report of the American College of Cardiology/American Heart Association Task Force on Practice Guidelines.

recommendations will also be applicable to patients without MI or applicable during the early evaluation for ACS. The management of CHF and pulmonary edema in the ED is specifically addressed in Chapter 6. There is a paucity of randomized trials addressing the management of acutely decompensated heart failure.

Clinical Signs

Shock and pulmonary edema are medical emergencies. Signs of shock include inadequate tissue perfusion (diminished peripheral pulses, cool extremities, delayed capillary refill, decreased urine output, and lactic acidosis). With CHF, signs of systemic and pulmonary venous congestion are present. Pulmonary edema produces tachypnea, labored respirations, rales, dyspnea, cyanosis, and hypoxemia. Frothy sputum may also be present. Providers should identify these conditions and begin treatment as soon as possible. As noted above, in RV shock the lungs are clear unless significant or preexisting LV dysfunction is present.

First-Line Actions

If signs of acute pulmonary edema are present, proceed with first-line actions if *low blood pressure and shock are absent*:

- Supplementary oxygen and NIV/intubation as needed
- Nitroglycerin SL, then IV
- Furosemide IV 0.5 to 1 mg/kg
- Morphine IV 2 to 4 mg

If the patient's blood pressure is adequate, help the patient sit upright with the legs dependent. This position increases lung volume and vital capacity, diminishes the work of breathing, and decreases venous return to the heart. Administer morphine to dilate veins and arteries and to reduce cardiac preload and afterload.

Provide oxygen, establish IV access, and begin cardiac monitoring. Monitor oxyhemoglobin saturation with pulse oximetry, although results may be inaccurate and misleading if peripheral perfusion is poor. Oxyhemoglobin saturation does not provide information about hemoglobin concentration, oxygen content, ventilation, or acid–base status. Additional laboratory studies are ordered to evaluate any significant comorbidity or complicating factors, such as anemia, renal dysfunction, or electrolyte imbalance.

Oxygen and Possible Intubation

Deliver oxygen at high flow rates, starting at 5 or 6 L/min by mask. Nonrebreathing masks with reservoir bags can provide oxygen concentrations of 90% to near 100%. A bag-mask may be used to provide assisted ventilation if the patient's ventilation is inadequate. If the patient is breathing spontaneously, consider continuous positive airway pressure by mask (BiPAP).

Be prepared to intubate the patient who has significant respiratory distress or respiratory failure. A need for intuba-

tion is particularly likely in situations that indicate progressive or imminent respiratory failure despite initial measures:

- PaO_2 cannot be maintained above 60 mm Hg despite 100% oxygen.
- Signs of cerebral hypoxia (e.g., lethargy or confusion) develop.
- PCO_2 increases progressively.
- Respiratory acidosis develops.

Always verify successful intubation using both clinical confirmation and a device. Pulmonary edema should not interfere with detection of exhaled CO_2 in the trachea, but if copious respiratory secretions are present, an esophageal detector device may fail to reinflate despite correct placement of the tube in the trachea. This failure may lead to the inaccurate conclusion that the tube is in the esophagus when it is accurately placed in the trachea.

Nitroglycerin

If SBP is adequate (usually >90–100 mm Hg) and the patient has no serious signs or symptoms of shock, then IV nitroglycerin is the drug of choice for acute pulmonary edema. Nitroglycerin reduces pulmonary congestion by dilating the venous capacitance vessels, reducing preload. It also dilates systemic arteries, decreasing systemic vascular resistance. This effect can reduce afterload and increase cardiac output.

Nitroglycerin may initially be administered by sublingual tablets, oral spray (isosorbide oral spray is an acceptable alternative), or the IV route. A standard 0.4-mg tablet can be given every 5 to 10 minutes provided that SBP remains >90 to 100 mm Hg and the patient has no clinical signs of tissue hypoperfusion (shock).

Nitroglycerin is contraindicated in hypotensive patients with signs of shock. Typically these patients cannot tolerate vasodilatation because of impaired cardiac output. They cannot compensate for the nitrate-induced tachycardia with increased stroke volume, which is one reason why tachycardia is a contraindication to nitroglycerin. Patients with RV infarction are preload-dependent. Nitrates are also contraindicated in patients who have used a phosphodiesterase inhibitor within the previous 24 hours (tadalafil within 48 hours). In these patients nitroglycerin can cause severe hypotension refractory to vasopressors. Use nitroglycerin with caution (if at all) if the patient has an inferior wall AMI with possible RV involvement. Patients with RV dysfunction are very dependent on maintenance of RV filling pressures to maintain cardiac output and blood pressure.

Furosemide

Furosemide has long been a mainstay in the treatment of acute pulmonary edema. It has a biphasic action. First, within approximately 5 minutes, it causes an immediate decrease in venous tone and an increase in venous capacitance. These changes lead to a fall in LV filling pressure (preload) that may improve clinical symptoms. Second, furosemide produces diuresis within 5 to 10 minutes of IV administration. The diuresis need not be marked to be effective. If the patient is not already taking furosemide, a small titrated dose is given as a slow IV bolus over 1 to 2 minutes. If the response to this dose is inadequate after about 20 minutes, a bolus of 2 mg/kg is administered. If the patient is already taking oral furosemide, a clinical rule of thumb is to administer an initial dose that is twice the daily oral dose. If no effect occurs within about 20 minutes, double the initial dose. Higher doses may be required if the patient has massive fluid retention, refractory heart failure, or renal insufficiency. Use caution in patients who may be volume-dependent or who are at high risk for cardiogenic shock (see above). Recommendations for initial dosing are as follows:

- Administer furosemide <0.5 mg/kg IV bolus for new onset acute pulmonary edema without hypovolemia. Use caution in patients who are at high risk for cardiogenic shock or who may be preload-dependent.
- Give 0.5–1.0 mg/kg for acute or chronic volume overload.
- Give 1 mg/kg to patients with underlying renal insufficiency.

Clinical trials have been conducted with nesiritide, a recombinant human brain natriuretic peptide, in patients hospitalized with decompensated CHF. Compared with placebo and "standard therapy," nesiritide was associated with improved hemodynamic function, decreased dyspnea and fatigue, and better global clinical status.[57]

Morphine Sulfate

Morphine sulfate remains a part of the therapy for acute pulmonary edema, although some question its effectiveness, especially in place of nitrates outside the hospital.[58] Morphine dilates the capacitance vessels of the peripheral venous bed. This dilatation reduces venous return to the central circulation and diminishes ventricular preload. Morphine also reduces afterload by causing mild arterial vasodilatation. It also has a sedative effect. More effective vasodilators are now available, so morphine is considered an acceptable adjunct rather than a drug of choice for acute pulmonary edema. Use with caution in NSTEMI patients and those who are at high risk for cardiogenic shock or who may be preload-dependent.[27]

Agents to Optimize Initial Blood Pressure

First-line actions also include the administration of agents to optimize blood pressure. Patients with acute pulmonary edema have excess adrenergic drive, and many have preexisting hypertension. These patients can present with high blood pressures or accelerated hypertension. Often treatment of the pulmonary edema itself will resolve high blood pressure. But initial therapy may include the use of IV nitroglycerin as an antihypertensive agent as well as a venodilator. Nitrates will reduce both preload and afterload to achieve this goal. In these patients the goal is to reduce blood pressure by no more than 30 mm Hg below the presentation blood pressure by titration of nitrates. IV nitroglycerin is initiated at 10 mcg/min and titrated to this target goal. As mentioned, patients may respond to initial therapy with resolution of their elevated blood pressure, decreasing or eliminating the need for IV nitrates. Use caution to avoid precipitating hypotension, because this may aggravate cardiac ischemia or precipitate organ ischemia in other vascular beds (e.g., brain, kidneys, or gut).

Second-Line Actions

Patients who respond to first-line actions for pulmonary edema may not require additional therapy unless otherwise indicated (ACEIs). If additional therapy is indicated, second-line actions are based on the patient's SBP and clinical response.

Patients Not in Shock With SBP >100 mm Hg

If SBP is >100 mm Hg and not <30 mm Hg below baseline, an ACEI is given to reduce afterload and attenuate LV remodeling in STEMI patients. ACEIs are generally administered after reperfusion therapy has been achieved and the patient is hemodynamically stable. Other agents can be used as indicated and tailored to the patient's clinical profile.

Nitrates can be continued with the precautions noted under first-line actions. Tachyphylaxis (tolerance) to nitrates occurs in about 24 hours, so other agents are considered once the patient is stable. Avoid long-acting and topical preparations in hemodynamically unstable or potentially unstable patients. Avoid use of nitroglycerin in patients who have taken phosphodiesterase inhitors within the previous 24 hours (48 hours with tildalafil) with hypotension (SBP <90 mm Hg), with extreme bradycardia (heart rate <50), or with tachycardia. Use with caution in patients with an inferior wall AMI with possible RV involvement. Nitroprusside is an alternative drug to treat hypertension.

IV nitroglycerin may be initiated at a rate of 10 mcg/min through continuous infusion with nonabsorbing tubing. Increase by 5 to 10 mcg every 3 to 5 minutes until a symptom or blood pressure response is noted. If no response is seen at 20 μg/min, incremental increases of 10 μg/min and later 20 μg/min can be used. As the symptoms and signs of acute pulmonary edema or cardiac ischemia begin to resolve, there is no need to continue upward titration of nitroglycerin simply to obtain a fall in blood pressure. When blood pressure reduction is a therapeutic goal, reduce the dosage when the blood pressure begins to fall. Frequently recommended limits for blood pressure reduction are 10% of baseline level in normotensive patients and 30% (or 30 mm Hg below baseline) in hypertensive patients.

Patients with SBP <100 mm Hg

If SBP is between 70 and 100 mm Hg and signs of shock *are* present, a dopamine infusion is recommended. If SBP is 70 to 100 mm Hg and the patient has *no signs of shock*, a dobutamine infusion is recommended as an inotropic agent to improve cardiac output or distribution of blood flow.

Third-Line Actions

Although called third-line actions, these diagnostic and therapeutic considerations or interventions may occur concurrently with first- and second-line actions. For example, reperfusion in patients with pulmonary edema and STEMI is pursued without delay while treatment is initiated. An ECG is obtained within 10 minutes of presentation in patients with pulmonary edema to assess STEMI as a cause or complication. Any reversible or complicating conditions are identified and treated if possible. For example, mechanical complications of MI occur as the second leading cause of in-hospital mortality. Patients with acute mitral regurgitation due to rupture of a papillary muscle or chorda are surgical emergencies. The use of echocardiography in the ICU or ED on an emergent basis can identify these patients early. Patients at bed rest and those with heart failure are at increased risk for pulmonary embolism. An ED and hospital plan for rapid activation of cardiology and ancillary personnel and for IABP should be in place. Hospitals without the capability for IABP, PCI, or cardiac surgery should also have an action plan to mobilize personnel and equipment for rapid transfer of STEMI patients to facilities with these capabilities.

Summary

Cardiogenic shock occurs in 5% to 7% of patients with AMI and carries a high mortality and poor in-hospital prognosis. Patients with or at high risk for cardiogenic shock should be taken primarily or transferred urgently to regional interventional facilities for expert care and aggressive management. Since the majority of patients with cardiogenic shock have a large MI early, complete and expedient reperfusion is necessary to improve prognosis. When a delay in transfer is anticipated prolonging reperfusion with primary PCI, fibrinolytic therapy should be administered in eligible patients. If it can be performed in a timely manner, IABP can help to stabilize patients hemodynamically until reperfusion can be achieved. Medications that impair LV function or potentially reduce blood pressure further (e.g., beta-blocking agents, nitrates, ACE-inhibitor therapy) should be discontinued or avoided.

See Web site for Cardiogenic Shock: Current Concepts and Improving Outcomes

Acknowledgment

The author would like to recognize and thank Judith Hochman, MD, for her permission to use and incorporate material from her excellent clinician updates and reviews in the American Heart Association journal *Circulation*.[33,59]

References

1. Antman EM, Anbe DT, Armstrong PW, et al. ACC/AHA guidelines for the management of patients with ST-elevation myocardial infarction—executive summary. A report of the American College of Cardiology/American Heart Association Task Force on Practice Guidelines (Writing Committee to revise the 1999 guidelines for the management of patients with acute myocardial infarction). *J Am Coll Cardiol* 2004;44(3):671–719.
2. Goldberg RJ, Gore JM, Alpert JS, et al. Cardiogenic shock after acute myocardial infarction: incidence and mortality from a community-wide perspective, 1975 to 1988. *N Engl J Med* 1991;325(16): 1117–1122.
3. Holmes DR Jr, Bates ER, Kleiman NS, et al. Contemporary reperfusion therapy for cardiogenic shock: the GUSTO-I trial experience. The GUSTO-I Investigators. Global Utilization of Streptokinase and Tissue Plasminogen Activator for Occluded Coronary Arteries. *J Am Coll Cardiol* 1995;26(3):668–674.
4. GUSTO Investigators, Hasdai D, Holmes DR Jr, Califf RM, et al. Cardiogenic shock complicating acute myocardial infarction: predictors of death. GUSTO Investigators. Global Utilization of Streptokinase and Tissue-Plasminogen Activator for Occluded Coronary Arteries. *Am Heart J* 1999;138(1 Pt 1):21–31.
5. Holmes DR Jr, Berger PB, Hochman JS, et al. Cardiogenic shock in patients with acute ischemic syndromes with and without ST-segment elevation. *Circulation* 1999;100(20):2067–2073.
6. Hochman JS, Sleeper LA, Webb JG, et al. Early revascularization and long-term survival in cardiogenic shock complicating acute myocardial infarction. *JAMA* 2006;295(21):2511–2515.
7. Bengtson JR, Kaplan AJ, Pieper KS, et al. Prognosis in cardiogenic shock after acute myocardial infarction in the interventional era. *J Am Coll Cardiol* 1992;20(7):1482–1489.
8. Berger PB, Holmes DR Jr, Stebbins AL, et al. Impact of an aggressive invasive catheterization and revascularization strategy on mortality in patients with cardiogenic shock in the Global Utilization of Streptokinase and Tissue Plasminogen Activator for Occluded Coronary Arteries (GUSTO-I) trial. An observational study. *Circulation* 1997;96(1):122–127.
9. Brodie BR, Stone GW, Morice M-C, et al. Importance of time to reperfusion on outcomes with primary coronary angioplasty for acute myocardial infarction (Results from the Stent Primary Angioplasty in Myocardial Infarction Trial). *Am J Cardiol* 2001;88(10):1085–1090.
10. Lim W, Qushmaq I, Devereaux PJ, et al. Elevated cardiac troponin measurements in critically ill patients. *Arch Intern Med* 2006;166(22): 2446–2454.
11. Klein Gunnewiek JM, van de Leur JJ. Elevated troponin T concentrations in critically ill patients. *Intens Care Med* 2003;29(12): 2317–2322.
12. Antman EM, Anbe DT, Armstrong PW, et al. ACC/AHA guidelines for the management of patients with ST-elevation myocardial infarction–executive summary. A report of the American College of Cardiology/American Heart Association Task Force on Practice Guidelines (Writing Committee to revise the 1999 guidelines for the management of patients with acute myocardial infarction). *J Am Coll Cardiol*. 2004;44(3):671–719.
13. Connors AF Jr, Speroff T, Dawson NV, et al. The effectiveness of right heart catheterization in the initial care of critically ill patients. SUPPORT Investigators. *JAMA* 1996;276(11):889–897.
14. Cohen MG, Kelly RV, Kong DF, et al. Pulmonary artery catheterization in acute coronary syndromes: insights from the GUSTO IIb and GUSTO III trials. *Am J Med* 2005;118(5):482–488.
15. Goldberg RJ, Samad NA, Yarzebski J, et al. Temporal trends in cardiogenic shock complicating acute myocardial infarction. *N Engl J Med* 1999;340(15):1162–1168.
16. Goldberg RJ, Gore JM, Alpert JS, et al. Cardiogenic shock after acute myocardial infarction. Incidence and mortality from a community-wide perspective, 1975 to 1988. *N Engl J Med* 1991;325(16): 1117–1122.
17. Fox KA, Anderson FA Jr, Dabbous OH, et al. Intervention in acute coronary syndromes: do patients undergo intervention on the basis of their risk characteristics? The Global Registry of Acute Coronary Events (GRACE). *Heart* 2007;93(2):177–182.
18. Babaev A, Frederick PD, Pasta DJ, et al. Trends in management and outcomes of patients with acute myocardial infarction complicated by cardiogenic shock. *JAMA* 2005;294(4):448–454.
19. Zeymer U, Vogt A, Zahn R, et al. Predictors of in-hospital mortality in 1333 patients with acute myocardial infarction complicated by cardiogenic shock treated with primary percutaneous coronary intervention (PCI); Results of the primary PCI registry of the Arbeitsgemeinschaft Leitende Kardiologische Krankenhausarzte (ALKK). *Eur Heart J* 2004;25(4):322–328.
20. Lindholm MG, Kober L, Boesgaard S, et al. Cardiogenic shock complicating acute myocardial infarction; prognostic impact of early and late shock development. *Eur Heart J* 2003;24(3):258–265.
21. Jacobs AK, French JK, Col J, et al. Cardiogenic shock with non-ST-segment elevation myocardial infarction: a report from the SHOCK Trial Registry. SHould we emergently revascularize

Occluded coronaries for Cardiogenic shocK? *J Am Coll Cardiol* 2000;36(3 Suppl A):1091–1096.

22. Inhibition of platelet glycoprotein IIb/IIIa with eptifibatide in patients with acute coronary syndromes. The PURSUIT Trial Investigators. Platelet Glycoprotein IIb/IIIa in Unstable Angina: Receptor Suppression Using Integrilin Therapy. *N Engl J Med* 1998;339(7):436–443.

23. Bennett KM, Hernandez AF, Chen AY, et al. Heart failure with preserved left ventricular systolic function among patients with non-ST-segment elevation acute coronary syndromes. *Am J Cardiol* 2007;99(10):1351–1356.

24. Hochman JS, Sleeper LA, Godfrey E, et al. SHould we emergently revascularize Occluded Coronaries for cardiogenic shocK: an international randomized trial of emergency PTCA/CABG-trial design. The SHOCK Trial Study Group. *Am Heart J* 1999;137(2):313–321.

25. Picard MH, Davidoff R, Sleeper LA, et al. Echocardiographic predictors of survival and response to early revascularization in cardiogenic shock. *Circulation* 2003;107(2):279–284.

26. Parrillo JE, Burch C, Shelhamer JH, Parker MM, et al. A circulating myocardial depressant substance in humans with septic shock. Septic shock patients with a reduced ejection fraction have a circulating factor that depresses in vitro myocardial cell performance. *J Clin Invest* 1985;76(4):1539–1553.

27. Meine TJ, Roe MT, Chen AY, et al. Association of intravenous morphine use and outcomes in acute coronary syndromes: results from the CRUSADE Quality Improvement Initiative. *Am Heart J* 2005;149(6):1043–1049.

28. ISIS-4: a randomised factorial trial assessing early oral captopril, oral mononitrate, and intravenous magnesium sulphate in 58,050 patients with suspected acute myocardial infarction. ISIS-4 (Fourth International Study of Infarct Survival) Collaborative Group. *Lancet* 1995;345(8951):669–685.

29. ACE Inhibitor MI Collaborative Group. Indications for ACE inhibitors in the early treatment of acute myocardial infarction: systematic overview of individual data from 100,000 patients in randomized trials. ACE Inhibitor Myocardial Infarction Collaborative Group. *Circulation* 1998;97(22):2202–2212.

30. Chen ZM, Pan HC, Chen YP, et al. Early intravenous then oral metoprolol in 45,852 patients with acute myocardial infarction: randomised placebo-controlled trial. *Lancet* 2005;366(9497):1622–1632.

31. Hasdai D, Topol EJ, Califf RM, et al. Cardiogenic shock complicating acute coronary syndromes. *Lancet* 2000;356(9231):749–756.

32. Menon V, Slater JN, White HD, et al. Acute myocardial infarction complicated by systemic hypoperfusion without hypotension: report of the SHOCK trial registry. *Am J Med* 2000;108(5):374–380.

33. Hochman JS. Cardiogenic shock complicating acute myocardial infarction: expanding the paradigm. *Circulation* 2003;107(24):2998–3002.

34. Kohsaka S, Menon V, Lowe AM, et al. Systemic inflammatory response syndrome after acute myocardial infarction complicated by cardiogenic shock. *Arch Intern Med* 2005;165(14):1643–1650.

35. Brunkhorst FM, Clark AL, Forycki ZF, et al. Pyrexia, procalcitonin, immune activation and survival in cardiogenic shock: the potential importance of bacterial translocation. *Int J Cardiol* 1999;72(1):3–10.

36. Brodie BR, Stuckey TD, Hansen CJ, et al. Timing and mechanism of death determined clinically after primary angioplasty for acute myocardial infarction. *Am J Cardiol* 1997;79(12):1586–1591.

37. Berrocal DH, Cohen MG, Spinetta AD, et al. Early reperfusion and late clinical outcomes in patients presenting with acute myocardial infarction randomly assigned to primary percutaneous coronary intervention or streptokinase. *Am Heart J* 2003;146(6):E22.

38. Ramanathan K CJ, Harkness SM, French JK, et al. Reversal of systemic hypoperfusion following intra aortic balloon pumping is associated with improved 30-day survival independent of early revascularization in cardiogenic shock complicating myocardial infarction. *Circulation* 2003;108 (Suppl I):I–672.

39. DeWood MA, Notske RN, Hensley GR, et al. Intraaortic balloon counterpulsation with and without reperfusion for myocardial infarction shock. *Circulation* 1980;61(6):1105–1112.

40. Ohman EM, Califf RM, George BS, et al. The use of intraaortic balloon pumping as an adjunct to reperfusion therapy in acute myocardial infarction. The Thrombolysis and Angioplasty in Myocardial Infarction (TAMI) Study Group. *Am Heart J* 1991;121(Pt 1)(3):895–901.

41. Barron HV, Every NR, Parsons LS, et al. The use of intra-aortic balloon counterpulsation in patients with cardiogenic shock complicating acute myocardial infarction: data from the national registry of myocardial infarction 2. *Am Heart J* 2001;141(6):933–939.

42. Bates ER, Stomel RJ, Hochman JS, et al. The use of intraaortic balloon counterpulsation as an adjunct to reperfusion therapy in cardiogenic shock. *Int J Cardiol* 1998;65(suppl 1):S37–S42.

43. Ohman EM, Califf RM, Topol EJ, et al. Intra-aortic balloon pumping: Benefits after thrombolytic therapy. *Cardiol Board Rev* 1991; 8(11):41–56.

44. Ohman EM, Nanas J, Stomel RJ, et al. Thrombolysis and counterpulsation to improve survival in myocardial infarction complicated by hypotension and suspected cardiogenic shock or heart failure: results of the TACTICS Trial. *J Thromb Thrombolysis* 2005;19(1):33–39.

45. Tiefenbrunn AJ, Chandra NC, French WJ, et al. Clinical experience with primary percutaneous transluminal coronary angioplasty compared with alteplase (recombinant tissue-type plasminogen activator) in patients with acute myocardial infarction: a report from the Second National Registry of Myocardial Infarction (NRMI-2). *J Am Coll Cardiol* 1998;31(6):1240–1245.

46. Lee L, Erbel R, Brown TM, et al. Multicenter registry of angioplasty therapy of cardiogenic shock: initial and long-term survival. *J Am Coll Cardiol* 1991;17(3):599–603.

47. Grines CL. Aggressive intervention for myocardial infarction: angioplasty, stents, and intra-aortic balloon pumping. *Am J Cardiol* 1996;78(3A):29–34.

48. Furman MI, Dauerman HL, Goldberg RJ, et al. Twenty-two year (1975 to 1997) trends in the incidence, in-hospital and long-term case fatality rates from initial Q-wave and non-Q-wave myocardial infarction: a multi-hospital, community-wide perspective. *J Am Coll Cardiol*. 2001;37(6):1571–1580.

49. Dzavik V, Sleeper LA, Picard MH, et al. Outcome of patients aged > or =75 years in the SHould we emergently revascularize Occluded Coronaries in cardiogenic shocK (SHOCK) trial: do elderly patients with acute myocardial infarction complicated by cardiogenic shock respond differently to emergent revascularization? *Am Heart J* 2005;149(6):1128–1134.

50. Jacobs AK, Leopold JA, Bates E, et al. Cardiogenic shock caused by right ventricular infarction: a report from the SHOCK registry. *J Am Coll Cardiol* 2003;41(8):1273–1279.

51. Berger PB, Ryan TJ. Inferior myocardial infarction: high-risk subgroups. *Circulation* 1990;81(2):401–411.

52. Zehender M, Kasper W, Kauder E, et al. Right ventricular infarction as an independent predictor of prognosis after acute inferior myocardial infarction. *N Engl J Med* 1993;328(14):981–988.

53. Robalino BD, Whitlow PL, Underwood DA, et al. Electrocardiographic manifestations of right ventricular infarction. *Am Heart J*. 1989;118(1):138–144.

54. Berisha S, Kastrati A, Goda A, et al. Optimal value of filling pressure in the right side of the heart in acute right ventricular infarction. *Br Heart J* 1990;63(2):98–102.

55. Francis GS, Sharma B, Hodges M. Comparative hemodynamic effects of dopamine and dobutamine in patients with acute cardiogenic circulatory collapse. *Am Heart J* 1982;103(6):995–1000.

56. Iqbal MZ, Liebson PR. Counterpulsation and dobutamine. Their use in treatment of cardiogenic shock due to right ventricular infarct. *Arch Intern Med* 1981;141(2):247–249.

57. Colucci WS, Elkayam U, Horton DP, et al. Intravenous nesiritide, a natriuretic peptide, in the treatment of decompensated congestive heart failure. Nesiritide Study Group. *N Engl J Med* 2000; 343(4):246–253.

58. Mosesso VN, Jr., Dunford J, Blackwell T, Griswell JK. Prehospital therapy for acute congestive heart failure: state of the art. *Prehosp Emerg Care*. 2003;7(1):13–23.

59. Reynolds HR, Hochman JS. Cardiogenic shock: current concepts and improving outcomes. *Circulation* 2008;117(5):686–697.

60. Antman EM, Braunwald E. In: *Harrison's Principles Internal Medicine*. New York: McGraw-Hill; 2001.

61. Guidelines 2000 for cardiopulmonary resuscitation and emergency cardiovascular care. Part 7: the era of reperfusion. Section 1: acute coronary syndromes (acute myocardial infarction). The American Heart Association in collaboration with the International Liaison Committee on Resuscitation. *Circulation* 2000;102(8 Suppl):I172–I203.

Chapter 8
Ultrasonography in Emergency Cardiovascular Care

Anthony J. Dean and Sarah A. Stahmer

Ultrasonography is rapidly available, noninvasive, and can be performed at the bedside in the emergency department. When performed by trained and skilled individuals, it can speed diagnosis in the critically ill or arrested patient, allowing for targeted interventions.

- Use in undifferentiated hypotension
- An adjunct to assessment and triage of chest pain and dyspnea
- An aid to central access to the circulation
- Rapid assessment for correctable causes of pulseless electrical activity

Introduction

Evaluation and management of the critically ill often necessitates rapid interventions initiated on the basis of a brief and limited assessment. Occasionally the history and physical examination are unequivocal; but for many patients with hemodynamic instability, the clinical evaluation is not diagnostic. The ultrasound evaluation in this setting will be directed to obtaining immediate anatomic and pathophysiologic data about the patient's condition and response to therapeutic interventions. Cardiac assessment may include evaluation of function, chamber size, valves, and the pericardial space. The inferior vena cava (IVC) may provide information about volume status. The lungs and pleura can be checked for consolidations, effusions, and pneumothorax. The peritoneal cavity may be evaluated for hemorrhage, aortic disease, or gross visceral abnormalities. Each of these studies may be repeated, performed once only, or not at all, depending on the clinical scenario and the patient's condition and course. Ultrasound will also be used in guiding invasive procedures.

In order to put this wide range of sonographic applications in context, the material in this chapter is presented through clinical scenarios. These are centered around four cardinal syndromes of the critically ill:

1. Shock/unexplained hypotension/circulatory collapse
2. Chest pain
3. Shortness of breath/respiratory insufficiency
4. Cardiac arrest

While technical aspects of some applications are discussed in detail, this chapter is not intended as a

See Web site for ACEP policy statement on use of ultrasound imaging by emergency physicians, ACC/AHA clinical competence statement on echocardiography.

tutorial on sonography. For such information, the reader is directed to specialty-specific educational resources.

Bedside Ultrasound in the Evaluation of Undifferentiated Hypotension: Clinical Scenario

A 52-year-old man with end-stage renal disease who was last dialyzed the previous day presents with 6 hours' severe chest pain, productive cough, shortness of breath, and subjective chills. He has a history of heavy smoking, hypertension, atrial fibrillation, and myocardial infarction. He is unable to provide a list of his medications. The patient appears diaphoretic and anxious, with pale extremities. BP 106/70, HR 82, RR 22, and oral temperature 100°F (37.8°C) (rectal temperature pending). His lungs reveal distant breath sounds with rhonchi. His heart sounds are also distant but regular, with a systolic murmur.

Indications for Sonography

The commonest mechanisms of shock are hypovolemic, cardiac, distributive, and mechanical. Current concepts of "septic" and "neurogenic" shock, both of which used to be considered as separate categories, are now recognized as special cases in which one or more of the first three are concurrent in a single patient. Thus the shock of sepsis (in varying combinations) may result from hypovolemia (secondary to dehydration and vasodilation), myocardial depression, and distributive mechanisms (secondary to vasodilation and microcirculatory dysregulation). Similarly, neurogenic shock arises from a combination of neurally mediated vasodilation and microcirculatory dysregulation, often compounded by bradycardia. Mechanical causes of shock [e.g., cardiac tamponade, tension pneumothorax, or massive pulmonary embolus (PE)] are especially important to consider in the sonographic evaluation of pulseless electrical activity because they may be readily treatable.

This patient with chronic hypertension almost certainly is relatively hypotensive. Potential causes in this patient would include infection with distributive shock and/or hypovolemic shock, myocardial infarction with cardiogenic shock, pericarditis with tamponade, and aortic dissection. In the evaluation and management of hypotension, invasive monitoring by central venous and pulmonary artery catheters has been the mainstay of diagnostic information about volume status, cardiac output and central venous oxygen saturation. However, invasive monitoring has associated risks and complications, and its clinical validity continues to be debated. In addition, central venous access requires allocation of precious time and human resources.

Focused, limited, clinician-performed bedside ultrasonography is noninvasive and can be rapidly deployed in a patient without invasive monitoring devices. It is directed to determining the type of the patient's shock, its severity, and, where possible, its cause. Several causes (e.g., infarction, pneumothorax, and massive PE) are discussed elsewhere in this chapter. The following discussion focuses on the utility of ultrasound in determining the type of the patient's shock and its severity, both of which form the basis of initial treatment decisions, including the choice between volume resuscitation, diuretics, or neither and the use of pressors of cardiac inotropes. In addition to guiding immediate fluid management, bedside sonography assesses cardiac function and the pericardial space.

Intravascular Volume Assessment

Volume assessment can be accomplished by evaluating the heart and inferior vena cava (IVC). An extensive body of literature describes a relationship between the sonographic appearance of the IVC and both intravascular volume and cardiac filling pressures.[1-5] Assessment of the IVC is made both qualitatively (shape) and quantitatively (absolute size and collapse index). There is strong evidence that in a given patient, increasing intravascular volume will result in both an expanding IVC diameter and diminishing the percent variation in diameter related to the respiratory cycle (collapse index). Decreasing intravascular volume will have the opposite effects.[1,3,4,4a,6] In healthy volunteers at rest, the expiratory diameter ranges from 15 to 20 mm and the inspiratory diameter from 0 to 14 mm.[1,3] Since a wide range of normal and abnormal values for these parameters has been reported in the variety of patient groups and clinical settings where it has been investigated, it is likely that absolute, universally applicable cutoffs do not exist.[3,7] This is consistent with the physiologic role of the IVC as a capacitance vessel that can buffer fluctuations of hydration. Thus the clinician should become familiar with the spectrum of IVC findings encountered in normovolemic patients and use this as a basis for the recognition of patients at extremes with either grossly distended or grossly underfilled cavae.

The absolute measurement of the IVC is often made at the maximal diameter (atrial contraction) in expiration, although some have used inspiratory diameters, and many studies do not specify. As noted, a range of "normal" IVC diameters has been reported, with those in the cardiology literature frequently larger than those in studies made of previously healthy patients with acute illnesses. This may be due to a higher prevalence of heart disease among patients in echocardiographic studies, many of whom require chronically elevated preload. The consensus that emerges is that an adequate central venous pressure (CVP) (for hearts not depending on increased preload) can be predicted by an IVC diameter of greater than 10 to 12 mm.[4] Young, conditioned athletes will normally have significantly larger IVC.[8] With an IVC diameter below 5 mm, abnormally low CVP becomes increasingly likely.

The IVC collapse index (IVC-CI) is defined by the following equation:

$$IVC\text{-}CI = (IVCD\text{-}exp - IVCD\text{-}insp) / IVCD\text{-}exp$$

See Figure 8-1.

> **Ultrasonography in Emergency Cardiovascular Care Videos**
>
> See Web site for video clips 8-1 to 8-28, called out in text below.

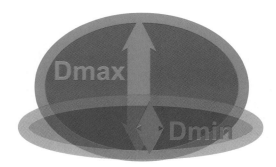

FIGURE 8-1 • IVC D_{max} and D_{min} should be measured during expiration and inspiration, respectively. They do not refer to beat-to-beat variation of IVC diameter.

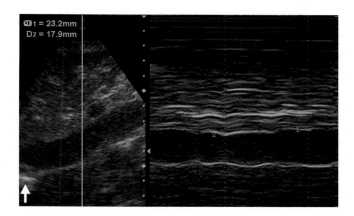

FIGURE 8-2 • A longitudinal view of a well-filled IVC with a minimal (inspiratory) diameter of 17.9 mm. The M-mode reading is slightly more caudad than usually described (the *arrow* indicates the diaphragm), but this is unlikely to be of significance in this case, since the vessel can be seen to be without taper. Note the beat to beat variation throughout the respiratory cycle.

Where IVCD-insp is the IVC diameter in inspiration and IVCD-exp is the IVC diameter in expiration (see Figs. 8-2 and 8-3 and **Video Clip 8-1**). Again, precise cutoffs between abnormal and normal are not available. However, the closer that the IVC-CI approaches either 0% or 100%, the more likely that the patient is volume overloaded or depleted, respectively.[9-11] IVC-CI in normal healthy volunteers has been reported in the range of 25% to 75%.[1,3] In hypovolemic patients with slit-like IVCs it is sometimes necessary to give primary consideration to the absolute IVC diameter over IVC-CI. For example, a patient with a maximum IVCD-exp of 4 mm that collapses to a minimum IVCD-insp of 2 mm is volume-depleted regardless of the normal IVC-CI of 50%. Positive-pressure ventilation, by reversing the usual pressure changes through the respiratory cycle, might be expected to undermine the utility of IVC-CI assessment.[5,10,12-15] Studies have not been consistent on this subject, although several have confirmed that maximal IVC diameter will be found in inspi-

ration in ventilated patients.[12,13] These studies also suggest that the collapse index in ventilated patients is much lower than that commonly encountered in unvented patients, so that any IVC-CI >10% to 20% may be an indicator of fluid-responsive shock.[12,13] The lack of consensus and the findings of these reports suggest that caution is needed in interpretation of IVC findings in ventilated patients.

Several slightly different techniques for IVC-CI measurement have been described, using either normal respirations or a forced sniff (both difficult to standardize). Measurements are often made in diastole (i.e., the moment when the IVC is smallest in the cardiac beat-to-beat cycle) and taken just inferior (1–3 cm) to the junction of the hepatic veins. The traditional window has been subxiphoid, although recent reports have suggested that equivalent results can be obtained using a right intercostal view with the liver as a sonographic window.[16,17] This approach is highly useful, since many critically ill patients may have the subxiphoid view obscured by bowel gas or dressings.[18] In addition, transducer placement in the epigastrium could theoretically cause artifactual narrowing of the IVC by probe pressure—a concern that is obviated by intercostal probe placement. Longitudinal and transverse planes are equivalent for measurement of the IVC.[19] However, each plane has intrinsic advantages and disadvantages, many of which are mutually complementary, so that experienced sonographers usually perform assessment in both planes. This allows for a qualitative estimate of the size and dynamics of the IVC, which, with experience, often gives a better sense of intravascular volume than a raw number (see **Video Clip 8-2**).

The commonest and most serious pitfall in IVC evaluation is the misidentification of the vessel. Experienced sonologists are familiar with cases in which all the elongated fluid-filled structures in the upper abdomen (aorta most commonly, but also gallbladder, hepatic veins, portal vein, and pleural effusions) have been mistaken for the vein. This is especially likely to occur in cases where severe hypovolemia renders the slit-like IVC almost invisible (see Fig. 8-4 and **Video Clip 8-3**).

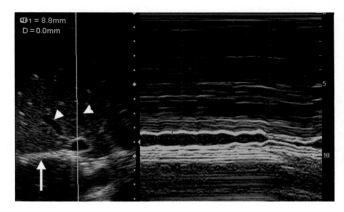

FIGURE 8-3 • A transverse view of a dehydrated patient with a 100% IVC collapse index. Two hepatic veins can be seen in close proximity (*arrowheads*), as well as a transverse view of the diaphragm (*arrow*).

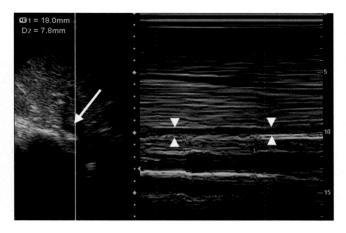

FIGURE 8-4 • This figure demonstrates a classic pitfall of overlooking the IVC (*arrow* in B-mode, *arrowheads* in M-mode on right of image) when it is small, and instead measuring the aorta (shown also in Video Clip 8-3). The IVC often appears to overlie the aorta in the intercostal window, as in this case. Misidentification can be avoided by positively identifying both vessels in every patient.

Color-flow may help in elucidation, but more often a reliable evaluation IVC depends on the following:

1. Positive identification of both aorta and IVC in the transverse plane
2. Positive identification of the IVC entering the right atrium (longitudinal and transverse planes)
3. Experience and familiarity with the technique

IVC-CI measurements are expected to be less reliable in ventilated patients, as previously noted. Positive-pressure ventilation, by creating a gradient between thoracic and abdominal compartments, is also likely to result in an artifactually dilated IVC. In such patients a well-filled IVC should be interpreted with caution, and an IVC <12 mm is highly likely to be a sign of intravascular hypovolemia.[14,15] Overestimation of intravascular volume status may also occur with any condition that impedes forward flow through the right heart. These include tricuspid regurgitation or stenosis, pulmonic stenosis, pulmonary hypertension (including hemodynamically significant pulmonary embolism; see above), right ventricular infarct, or severe left-sided failure. Young, healthy athletes have large and dilated IVCs, so that a "mildly collapsed" IVC in such a patient might represent a state of significant hypovolemia.[8] Underestimation of intravascular volume will occur with extrinsic compression of the IVC. Tense ascites, which is usually clinically apparent, is a common cause.[20] Hepatomegaly and retroperitoneal lymph nodes are less common but usually sonographically evident in the longitudinal view.

Cardiac Function

Several studies have shown that bedside ultrasonography provides estimates of ejection fraction (EF) that correlate as closely with the reading of an experienced echocardiologist as do the readings of two echocardiologists compared with one another.[21–26] For the purposes of clinical decision making with an acutely ill patient, EF can be divided into four broad categories: "abnormally high" (>75%), "normal" (50%–75%), "moderately depressed" (30%–50%), and "severely depressed" (<30%) (see Video Clips 8-4, and 8-5a and b, 8-6, 8-7a and b, and 8-8). "Abnormally high" EF suggests intravascular hypovolemia with an underfilled heart, although it can also be seen with hypertrophic cardiomyopathy. This finding should be correlated with the findings of the IVC evaluation. An exam showing severely depressed myocardial contractility will mandate caution in the administration of fluids and may prompt consideration of diuresis if the heart is severely dilated as well as the initiation of inotropic therapy, early percutaneous transluminal coronary angioplasty (PTCA), and/or placement of an intra-aortic balloon pump (IABP). Conversely, demonstration of mildly depressed, normal, or hyperdynamic cardiac function excludes acute myocardial dysfunction as a primary cause of hypotension. Caution should be observed in ascribing hypotension to moderately depressed contractility, since these patients usually have chronic and compensated cardiomyopathy, so that acute hypotension usually betokens an acute and unrelated process such as sepsis or dehydration.

Cardiac Tamponade

Common nonsurgical causes of tamponade include neoplastic, idiopathic, and uremic effusions.[27] Many pericardial effusions are clinically silent until they cause symptoms of tamponade, the physical findings of which (pulsus paradoxus and Beck's triad) are unreliable and late findings.[27–31] Fortunately, ultrasonography accurately detects pericardial fluid and identifies findings of tamponade early. Various categorizations of effusion have been proposed. That of the European Society of Echocardiography distinguishes "small" (often physiologic, <10 mm maximal thickness in diastole), "moderate" (10–20 mm maximal thickness in diastole), "large" (>20 mm maximal thickness), and "very large" (>20 mm maximal thickness with cardiac compression).[27] The problem with this classification system is that it is most applicable to patients with long-standing or slowly evolving pericardial effusions. Rapidly forming pericardial effusions can cause tamponade physiology with circumferential effusions of less than 10 mm, especially in patients with cardiomyopathy dependent on high filling pressures.[32,33] Thus, in assessing an acutely unstable patient without the benefit of prior studies or known cardiac history, the clinician may be better served by the categories of "noncircumferential/physiologic" (see Fig. 8-5 and Video Clip 8-9); "circumferential, <10 mm maximal thickness" (see Fig. 8-6 and Video Clip 8-6); and "circumferential, >10 mm maximal thickness" (see Fig. 8-7 and Video Clip 8-10), with a further determination made in each case as to the presence or absence of tamponade (Fig. 8-8 and Video Clips 8-11 and 8-12).

Tamponade occurs when the intrapericardial pressure equals or exceeds diastolic filling pressures. The more rapid the accumulation of pericardial fluid, the smaller the volume necessary to cause tamponade.[27,32,33] Intrapericardial pressure can rise abruptly with the acute accumulation of as little as 80 to 200 mL of fluid.[32] Right ventricular diastolic

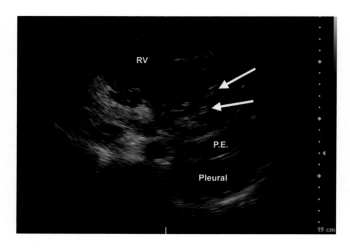

FIGURE 8-5 • This parasternal short axis view shows a non-circumferential pericardial effusion (P.E.) with a pleural effusion behind it. The slightly thickened mitral valve leaflets in their characteristic location are indicated by arrows. (RV, right ventricle).

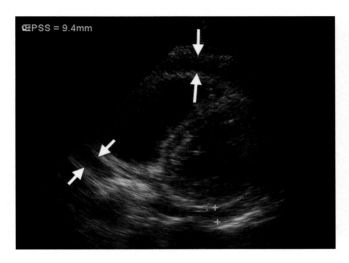

FIGURE 8-6 • This parasternal short axis view shows a moderate circumferential effusion (*arrows*) with measured thickness of 9.4 mm.

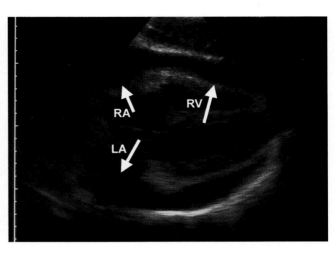

FIGURE 8-8 • Assessment of tamponade should be done dynamically, however this subxiphoid image caught in diastole shows collapse of right atrial (RA), left atrial (LA), and right ventricular (RV) walls.

collapse (RVDC) has been shown to be the most accurate finding in tamponade (Fig. 8-8 and Video Clips 8-11 and 8-12).[34,35] Right atrial collapse is more sensitive but less specific.[35,36] Left ventricular collapse may also occur.[35,37] Subxiphoid and apical four-chamber windows provide good views of the right heart, although the former may be easier to obtain. If cineloop is available, a good image should be obtained, frozen, and the motion of the right ventricular free wall carefully reviewed frame by frame, since RVDC may be fleeting in the tachycardic heart.

False-positive diagnoses of pericardial effusions have been caused by misidentification of epicardial fat, pleural

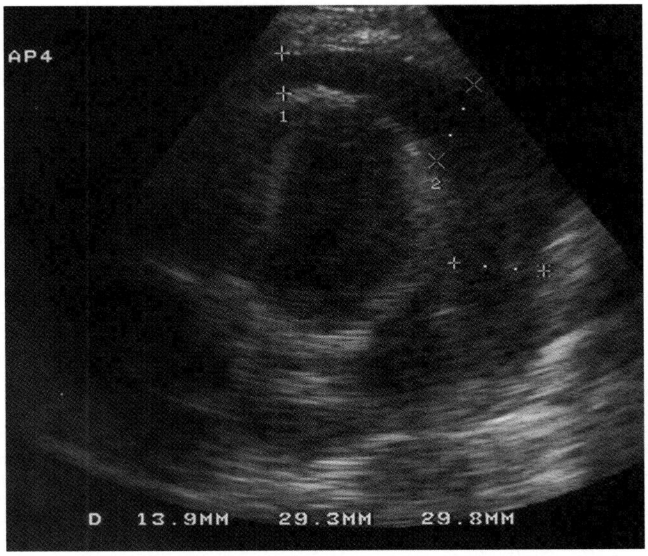

FIGURE 8-7 • This apical four chamber view in a patient with chronic liver failure shows a massive circumferential effusion of up to more than 3 cm in thickness.

effusions, and vessels posterior to the heart (e.g., descending aorta, pulmonary vessels, or coronary sinus).[38] Epicardial fat is noncircumferential, localized, has an irregular outline, tends to lie along the paths of the coronary vessels (interventricular and interatrial grooves), and with optimal gain adjustment demonstrates internal echoes (see Video Clip 8-13). In contrast to effusions it usually gets thinner towards the apex. The distinction between pericardial and pleural fluid can be made by the conforming shape of the pericardial sac. Such an apparently obvious distinction may be challenging in the setting of an unstable patient with limited time, suboptimal cardiac windows, and poor patient positioning. Efforts should be made to image the fluid in the axillary or scapular lines, looking for the characteristic wedge shape of pleural fluid in the costophrenic sulci. In parasternal views, pericardial fluid will appear anterior to the descending aorta, while pleural fluid will appear to be surrounding or posterior to it (Video Clip 8-14). The descending aorta itself can be mistaken for pericardial fluid when seen longitudinally, but its tubular structure should be apparent in an orthogonal plane (Video Clips 8-15a and b).

Severe hypovolemia can also cause diastolic ventricular collapse, but other clinical findings usually clarify the situation.[33,39] If there is any doubt, the IVC should be checked, and if it is not plethoric and with minimal or no respiratory collapse, tamponade is excluded. Conversely, tamponade may occur without RVDC in conditions causing elevated right heart pressures (e.g., pulmonary hypertension).[36] The "sniff test" may help to identify tamponade in this setting: the IVC should collapse by 50% or more of its diameter with sudden inspiration, but will fail to do so with tamponade. Absence of IVC collapse with "sniff" is highly sensitive for tamponade, but since it occurs in many other conditions, it is very nonspecific.

Acutely clotting blood (usually in traumatic tamponade) may be mistaken for thickened myocardium, although gain

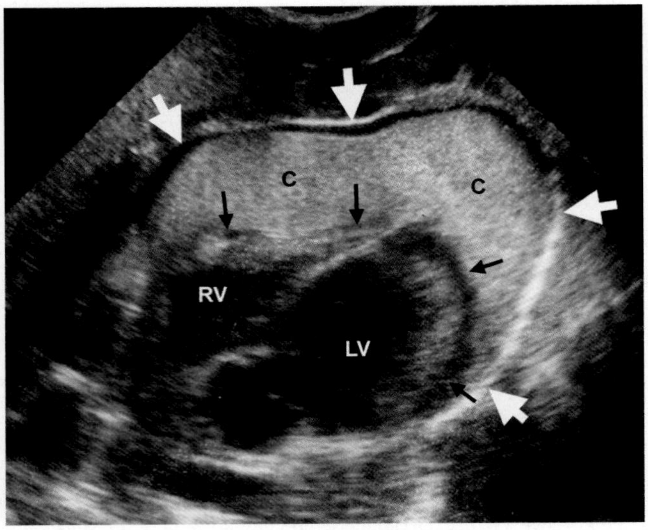

FIGURE 8-9 • This ultrasound taken less than 15 minutes after thoracic trauma caused PEA arrest from tamponade shows a thick layer of already clotted blood (C) between the epicardium (*black arrows*) and the pericardium (*white arrows*), with a thin layer of (*black*) unclotted blood below the anterior pericardium. (RV, right ventricle; LV, left ventricle).

optimization reveals heterogeneous echodensities reflecting blood at different stages of thrombosis (Fig. 8-9).[40] While there are a number of echocardiographic findings that, considered in isolation, can be misleading, their significance is usually clarified by consideration of the clinical context (Fig. 8-8).

Bedside Ultrasound in the Evaluation of Acute Chest Pain: Clinical Scenario

A 76-year-old presents to the ED complaining of approximately 2 hours' midsternal pressure and shortness of breath. He has no prior cardiac history. At one point he felt as if he were going to "pass out." He smokes and has mild hypertension. His vital signs reveal a BP of 148/88 mm Hg, a pulse of 88, and a pulse oximetry of 98%. His exam is remarkable only for his anxiety, discomfort, and pallor. His electrocardiogram (ECG) with ongoing symptoms shows a sinus rhythm with left ventricular hypertrophy (LVH) and nonspecific ST-T wave abnormalities. The patient has no prior ECGs for comparison.

Indications for Sonography

In view of the multiple risk factors, this patient's symptoms are probably due to acute coronary syndrome (ACS). Other, less likely causes of chest pain include aortic dissection, pulmonary embolism, spontaneous pneumothorax, and pneu-

monia. The latter three are discussed in the section on the evaluation of acute dyspnea. This section considers the use of bedside ultrasound in the evaluation of acute ischemia and dissection.

Assessment of Cardiac Ischemia

Several studies have evaluated the ability of echocardiography to stratify patients presenting with acute chest pain according to their risk for cardiac events.[41–43] The overall predictive value of a positive echocardiogram (identification of wall motion abnormalities) varies with disease prevalence in the study population. In studies where the observed cardiac event rate is high, the predictive value of a positive study is 90% or greater.[44–47] Conversely, the absence of wall motion abnormalities predicts that the likelihood of infarct or active ischemia is low but not so low as to reliably exclude the presence of acute ischemia with negative predictive value (NPV) ranging from 57% to 93%. In groups of low-risk patients with overall event rates of less than 20%, a positive echocardiogram is less predictive of subsequent cardiac events, with positive predictive value (PPV) ranging from 34% to 44%.[41,42,48] In this group, the absence of regional wall motion abnormalities identifies low-risk patients, with an NPV of 93% to 98%. Although reassuring, this may still not be sufficient to allow safe discharge from the ED. Thus, a resting echocardiogram cannot be used alone as the basis for decisions about the disposition of patients with possible ischemic chest pain.

The American College of Cardiology (ACC)/American Heart Association (AHA) guidelines on the clinical use of echocardiography give the diagnosis of suspected acute ischemia or infarction a class I recommendation for patients with suspected acute myocardial ischemia when baseline ECG and laboratory markers are nondiagnostic and when the study can be performed during pain or within minutes of its abatement.[49,50] The studies of transthoracic echocardiography (TTE) in the evaluation of chest pain were performed and interpreted by trained echocardiologists with American Society of Echocardiography level 3 training, a requirement that, given the complexity of wall motion analysis, is unlikely to change. These conditions are met only at the minority of institutions in which echocardiologists are available on a stat basis for image interpretation at all times.[51]

TTE is directed to the detection of segmental wall motion abnormalities, which occur at the onset of myocardial ischemia and may precede clinical symptoms and ECG changes. The location of these abnormalities correlates well with the vessel involved and will reflect changes in regional perfusion in response to therapy.[52,53] In addition to the challenge of performing the test prior to the resolution of symptoms, there are several factors that limit the utility of echocardiography in the setting of acute ischemia. Segmental wall motion abnormalities are not specific for acute ischemia, since they can also be caused by myocarditis and cardiomyopathies as well as scarring from prior myocardial infarction. In addition to ischemia, paradoxical motion of the septum can be due to conduction abnormalities, right ventricular (RV) pressure, and volume overload and can also be a sequela of sternotomy. Evaluation of wall motion is particularly dependent on image quality and precisely obtained scanning planes. This frequently limits its usefulness in technically challenging patients, including those with chest wall deformities, obesity, and lung disease. The variety of impediments to wall motion assessment makes it one of the most challenging skills in echocardiography.[54]

Most of the studies on this topic have used unenhanced TTE. Advances in sonographic technology—such as harmonic imaging, tissue characterization, and use of myocardial contrast agents—improve the overall image quality and possibly the predictive value for ischemic events.[55–60] More recent studies have found improved performance when myocardial contrast is used to enhance visualization of the ventricular cavity and assess overall myocardial perfusion. The contrast agents used are microbubbles, which have a distinct echogenicity and perfuse not only the ventricular cavity but also the myocardium. Studies using myocardial contrast to identify segmental wall motion abnormalities and myocardial perfusion demonstrate greater diagnostic accuracy than using unenhanced 2D echo.[55–58]

The impact of echocardiography in the assessment of patients with chest pain has not been studied in large-scale prospective trials. Smaller studies have suggested that the benefits include confirmation of clinical impression, especially among patients at low risk for cardiac disease, and identification of nonischemic cardiac conditions including critical aortic stenosis, hypertrophic cardiomyopathy, and pericardial disease as well as noncardiac diagnoses such as hemodynamically significant PE and aortic dissection. While sonographic evaluation of the heart by echocardiologists may be useful in the management of a patient with undifferentiated chest pain, there are currently no large-scale studies describing the impact of bedside ultrasound in this setting. At this time, the role of noncardiologist, clinician-performed bedside TTE in the evaluation of acute chest pain is not certain.

Aortic Dissection

Although one of the less common causes of undifferentiated chest pain, aortic dissection needs to be considered due to its life-threatening nature and the fact that if it is unrecognized, anticoagulation could be catastrophic. TTE for the diagnosis of aortic dissection was first described in 1972.[61] Since then, studies have suggested a sensitivity of 67% to 80% and a specificity of 99% to 100% using the identification of an undulating intimal flap by TTE or transabdominal ultrasound (Fig. 8-10A and B and Video Clip 8-16).[62–63] Thus, in cases with a low pretest probability of dissection, ultrasound can be used to screen for disease and confirm the clinical impression, usually in favor of an alternative diagnosis. In cases where the index of suspicion is high, ultrasound cannot reliably exclude the presence of disease. Some patients may have a pericardial effusion as a clue to the presence of a proximal dissection. To reliably exclude dissection in patients at high risk,

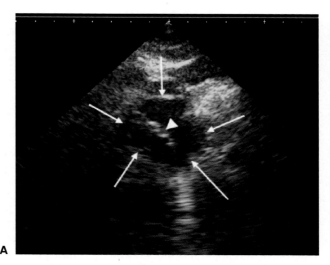

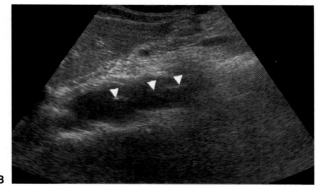

FIGURE 8-10 • **A.** A suprasternal transverse image of the aortic arch (outlined by *arrows*). **B.** The intimal flap (*arrowheads*, both images) can be seen extending into the abdominal aorta (longitudinal view).

either a transesophageal echocardiogram (TEE) or an alternative imaging modality such as CT or MRI will be necessary.

Bedside Ultrasound in the Evaluation of Unexplained Dyspnea: Clinical Scenario

A 58-year-old woman presents to the ED with progressive shortness of breath, productive cough, and chest heaviness. She is 5 feet 2 inches tall and weighs 100 kg. She is unable to give a detailed history, but her medications include oral hypoglycemics, antihypertensives, bronchodilators, and steroids. She states she has home oxygen at night and has had problems with "fluid round the heart." Her HR is 118, her BP 112/56, her respiratory rate 30, and she speaks in short, broken sentences. Her breath sounds are distant, with rhonchi and possible scattered rales. Her heart sounds are distant, with a 3/6 systolic murmur in the precordium. Her ECG shows sinus tachycardia with low voltages and non-specific ST-T-wave abnormalities. A portable chest radiograph of poor quality suggests bilateral pleural effusions, and shows no pneumothorax.

Indications for Sonography

Several potentially critical disease processes could be causing the symptoms of this patient. These include ACS, congestive heart failure (CHF)/acute pulmonary edema, cardiac tamponade, PE, pneumonia, massive pleural effusions, and pneumothorax. Each of these entities has described sonographic findings, some of which are sensitive and specific; others are less reliably and consistently found. Bedside ultrasound may also guide therapy. Both pulmonary edema and ACS may be caused by, or be the cause of, mitral regurgitation. The patient's murmur may be due to critical aortic stenosis. Management will vary depending on whether the patient has a hypertrophic left ventricle with an ejection fraction of 75%, or an effaced and dilated one with an EF of 10%, or obvious regions of focal wall motion abnormality. Furthermore, the interventions needed to treat some of the diagnoses in this patient's differential are contraindicated and potentially harmful for others: volume resuscitation, which is needed if this patient has pneumonia and incipient sepsis, would be deleterious if the patient has CHF. Similarly, the anticoagulation that is called for in PE or ACS would be contraindicated if the patient has a large pericardial effusion with or without tamponade.

Congestive Heart Failure

In most cases, the emergent diagnosis and management of pulmonary edema can be made on clinical grounds without the assistance of ultrasound. However an ultrasound evaluation of mild heart failure or previously unrecognized heart disease in patients presenting solely with undifferentiated dyspnea may lead to the recognition of an unsuspected cardiac etiology such as peripartum cardiomyopathy or viral myocarditis.

Several sonographic parameters are used in routine echocardiography to identify, measure, and detect aspects of cardiac failure. These include diastolic filling velocities, waveforms, pressures, and volumes, assessed on both the right and left side of the heart. Cardiac output, tissue Doppler waveforms, EF, pulmonary artery pressures, and the IVC are also evaluated. Many of these echocardiographic findings require both time and skills that are not available to most clinician sonographers performing bedside ultrasonography on the critically ill. Of this list, EF has been most extensively studied in bedside sonography, and is most likely to be of use in the first minutes or hours of an acute episode of CHF.

As previously noted, qualitative estimates of EF by non-cardiologists can categorize a patient's cardiac function as "normal" (50%–75%), "moderately depressed" (30%–50%), and "severely depressed" (<30%) (see **Video Clips 8-4, 8-5a and b, 8-6, 8-7a and b, and 8-8**).[21–26] In critically ill patients, accurate assessment of EF is possible even when

the exam is abbreviated by limitations of time or lack of access to cardiac windows.[57] Two other parameters that can be readily assessed in a focused bedside evaluation for CHF but which, at this time, have not been widely used by intensivist sonologists are mitral valve (MV) inflow velocity and septal velocity measured by tissue Doppler imaging (TDI). Both measurements are made using an apical four-chamber view. The inflow velocity is measured at the tips of the MV and in normal health shows a dual positive deflection due to passive filling in early diastole ("E wave"), followed by a second, smaller, late-diastolic deflection caused by atrial contraction ("A wave") (Fig. 8-11A). With decreased myocardial compliance, which is often the result of diastolic dysfunction, there is reversal of the usual E/A

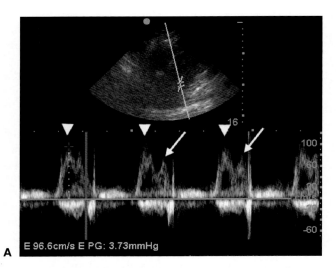

E 96.6cm/s E PG: 3.73mmHg

A

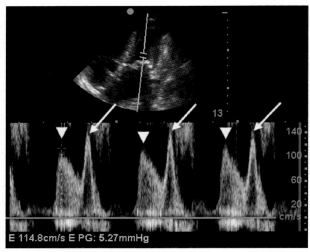

E 114.8cm/s E PG: 5.27mmHg

B

FIGURE 8-11 • **A** and **B.** E (*arrowheads*) and A wave (*diagonal arrows*) inflow patterns. **A.** A normal patient in whom E/A is >1. **B.** Diastolic dysfunction is suggested by the E/A ratio of <1. At the top of parts A and B, B-mode apical four-chamber views (seen more clearly in B) are seen showing the Doppler path (*long line*) and gate (*parallel transverse lines*), with flow angle correction (seen only in A; see text).

ratio >1, resulting in an E/A <1 (Fig. 8-11B). With increasing left atrial pressure (LAP) and diminishing effect of the atrial kick, there is "pseudonormalization," with the E/A returning to >1. This can progress to "late stage" dysfunction, when very high LAP causes E>>A.

One of the ways that pseudonormalization can be recognized is by the use of TDI, a feature found on an increasing number of bedside ultrasound machines. This technology applies Doppler principles traditionally used to measure blood flow to the motion of solid tissues. The tissue Doppler gate is placed on the septum (or lateral wall) adjacent to the MV annulus, and a waveform is recorded. Like the MV inflow waveform, the waveform of the normal septum shows a dual deflection in diastole. The first deflection is known as the "e′ ("E prime") wave" (Fig. 8-12). The ratio E/e′ is then calculated. Normal LV filling pressures and intravascular volume are reflected by E/e′<8; increased left ventricular filling pressures by an E/e′>15.[63-66] Values between 8 and 15 are of indeterminate significance. The use of Doppler and TDI in the hands of nonechocardiologists has not been widely reported.[67] However, the relative speed and simplicity of the test make it likely that this technique will be of use to intensivist bedside sonographers, especially in patients with dilated IVCs, which might be clinically suspected of being due to factors other than fluid overload, such as pulmonary hypertension and right heart failure or severe tricuspid insufficiency.

In patients with clinical failure, an assessment of gross cardiac size and wall thickness may also be helpful. Nomograms based on gender, age, and habitus have been developed but are unlikely to be accessible in caring for a critically ill patient. The range of normal end-diastolic dimensions (measured from septum to posterior free wall at the level of the mitral leaflets) is 35 to 60 mm.[68] Normal diastolic LV wall thickness (measured on the septum or posterior free wall at the level of the distal mitral leaflets) ranges from 8 to 12.5 mm.[68] Low ventricular volumes and thickened ventricular walls in the setting of failure suggest hypertrophy and luseotropic failure. Conversely, a dilated ventricle with effaced ventricular walls suggests likely primary forward failure. Focal wall motion abnormalities may suggest unrecognized cardiac ischemia.

Pulmonary Embolus

PE sufficient to cause hemodynamic instability results in gross, readily identifiable echocardiographic abnormalities.[69-73] Several parameters that can be readily assessed by a bedside clinician sonographer have been used, including right ventricular (RV) to LV dimension ratio, intracardiac thrombus, septal wall flattening, abnormal septal wall motion, and loss of the normal IVC collapse index.[73] Other sonographic findings, such as tricuspid regurgitant peak flow velocities and pulmonary artery hypertension, require time-consuming color-flow and spectral Doppler analysis that is beyond the expertise of most critical care bedside sonographers.[74] Reports of the accuracy of echocardiography in the evaluation of stable patients with PE are inconsistent, so that this modality should be used only to exclude PE in patients with hemodynamic instability. The following discussion focuses on this group.

The normal RV end-diastolic dimension, measured at the tips of the tricuspid leaflets in the apical four-chamber view (or subxiphoid if that is not possible) should be less than 27 mm.[75] This RV dimension will be exceeded in hemodynamically significant PE as well as many other causes of cardiac dilatation. Another index of RV enlargement—which can be obtained without the time-consuming process of caliper measurement does not require the memorization of arbitrary numbers and will not be falsely positive in the case of global dilated cardiomyopathy—is the right-to-left ventricular ratio, usually estimated at end-diastole. This is normally <60%. In patients with acute PE, the ratio is almost always >100% (see Video Clips 8-17a and b and 8-18, and 8-19).[76] Chronic pulmonary hypertension also causes RV dilation but is likely to be accompanied by a thickened ventricular wall, whereas in PE the RV wall is effaced (<7 mm).[74] RV infarct and PE may cause similar clinical, hemodynamic, and sonographic findings, including ventricular distention with a thin, hypokinetic RV free wall, septal flattening, and paradoxical septal motion.[74,77-79] Usually the distinction between RV infarction and acute PE can be made clinically and by ECG. Paradoxical septal motion occurs when acute pulmonary arterial occlusion (from PE) results in reversal of the normal pressure relationships between the left and right heart. With acute pulmonary artery occlusion, RV preload and afterload rapidly rise, while the underfilled LV generates progressively lower perfusion pressures. This results in abnormal contraction of the septal wall towards the RV in systole and relaxation of the septal wall towards the LV in diastole (see Video Clip 8-18 and 8-19). TR distinguishes the

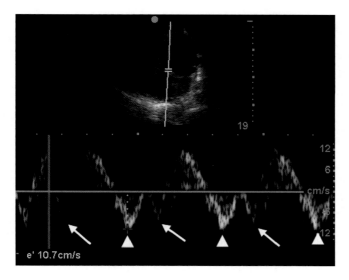

FIGURE 8-12 • Motion of the septum is away from the transducer in diastole, so that the waveform of its motion is represented in a negative direction. The e′ waves are indicated by arrowheads. The a′ waves, which are frequently not clearly seen, are indicated by diagonal arrows.

high-pressure overload state of acute PE from the low pressure overload state of RV infarction in which TR is uncommon.[75] This is identified by placing color flow on the mitral valve in the apical four-chamber view (Video Clip 8-17b). In one series, tricuspid regurgitation (TR) occurred in 99% of the 60 patients with acute PE.[75] A low (<50%) IVC collapse index has also been used as a marker for acute PE, but with inconsistent results.[71,73,74,80] The technique for this measurement is described in detail above (see "Bedside Ultrasound in the Evaluation of Undifferentiated Hypotension").

Sonographic Evaluation of the Lung

An increasing number of studies have described the role of ultrasound in the evaluation of pulmonary conditions. Two sonographic findings in particular may be of utility in the initial evaluation of the critically ill. The first is the finding of pleural-based, comet-tail artifacts (also known as "lung rockets"), which are associated with "wet lung" conditions including pulmonary edema and acute respiratory distress syndrome as well as chronic parenchymal lung diseases.[80a,81–86] The comet-tail artifacts are thought to arise from subpleural air pockets surrounded by thickened edematous interstitial tissue, giving rise to intense reverberation artifacts arising from the pleural line (Fig. 8-13 and Video Clip 8-20; compare with Video Clip 8-22).[80a,82,83,87,88]

The ultrasound exam is performed by placing the probe in the rib spaces of the anterior and lateral chest. The probe may be oriented either parallel or perpendicular to the ribs; but for less experienced sonographers, it may be easier to use the latter, because the rib shadows serve as landmarks for the pleural line. In the supine patient, each rib space is evaluated in the midclavicular line from the clavicle to the diaphragm. On the left, if the cardiac silhouette is encountered, the lower rib spaces may be examined in the anterior axillary line.

Since precise criteria for a positive test are not established, clinical judgment is required in interpreting the findings of ultrasound, but studies have consistently indicated that increasing numbers of comet tails are increasingly predictive of wet lung and that ultrasound is more accurate than clinical exam alone.[80a,81,84,86,88] Some authors state that the test is positive if more than one comet tail is found per rib space in the anterior chest, although patients with conditions associated with pulmonary or pleural scarring (such as chronic obstructive pulmonary disease) are often found to have scattered lung rockets without evidence of abnormal lung water.[84]

Ultrasound can also be used to evaluate for atelectasis and pulmonary consolidation, both of which cause the lung to transmit ultrasound like a solid organ, giving the sonographic appearance of "hepatization" (see Video Clip 8-21).[89] The sensitivity and specificity of this finding have not been prospectively evaluated.

Pneumothorax

In normal expanded lung, the contiguous parietal and visceral pleura can be identified with real-time ultrasound as a

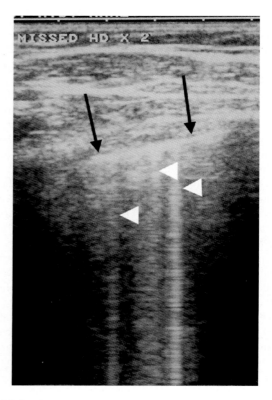

FIGURE 8-13 • Multiple comet tails (*white arrowheads*) can be seen arising from the pleura (*black arrows*) in this patient with end-stage renal disease who had missed hemodialysis for several days and presented with acute congestive heart failure.

shimmering motion in a plane parallel with the skin. This is referred to as "lung sliding" or "pleural sliding" (see Video Clip 8-22). With pneumothorax, the parietal pleural line can still be seen parallel with the skin immediately below the ribs; but in the absence of an apposed visceral pleura, lung sliding is absent. This is the primary criterion for the sonographic diagnosis of pneumothorax (see Video Clip 8-23).[90] An additional criterion is the "lung point sign," also known as the "leading edge sign."[91] This is seen if the transition between collapsed and fully expanded lung occurs immediately under the probe. It is sonographically recognized by the pleural line demonstrating zones both with and without pleural sliding that shift back and forth reciprocally. The "lung point" refers to the transition between these zones. Since the lung point sign can occur only if the pneumothorax is small and the transition zone happens to occur within the sonographic window, it is found in the minority of cases (see Video Clip 8-24). Demonstration of the presence of pulmonary artifacts, specifically lung rockets as noted above, confirms the presence of lung sliding and thus rules out pneumothorax under the probe.[92]

False-positive pleural evaluations can be caused by pleural scarring, adhesions, or extremely effaced visceral pleurae (as in bullous emphysema, for example). They may also occur if the patient is splinting or has poor ventilatory volumes for other reasons. While it can be extremely helpful to compare the two sides of the chest, this must be done with caution, especially if lung sliding is not clearly seen on either side: in one series, pneumothorax was missed on one or both sides in 12 of the 13 cases of bilateral pneumothorax.[93] An important technical component in the evaluation of the pleura is avoidance of motion between the probe and the patient's skin or chest wall, which can give rise to the artifactual appearance of pleural sliding (see **Video Clips 8-23 and 8-24**). To avoid this, the sonographer should anchor the transducer to the chest using the fingertips of the scanning hand.

Larger prospective series on this topic have found that ultrasonography has a sensitivity of 50% to 60% and specificity of 99% compared with CT of the chest. When the patient is supine, chest radiography is compared to the same reference standard; the sensitivity is halved to 20% to 30%, with the same high specificity.[54,94] It is extremely rare that chest radiography identifies a pneumothorax that is missed on bedside ultrasound.[95]

Pleural Effusion and Thoracentesis

In the normal chest, the interface between the air-filled lung and the visceral pleura is highly reflective. Beneath the pleural line, the sonographic signal of normal lung appears as a uniform pattern of bright echoes (see **Video Clip 8-22**). Free fluid within the pleural space will appear as an anechoic area bounded by the visceral and parietal pleurae and inferiorly (if it is not loculated) by the brightly echogenic diaphragm. Atelectatic lung may be seen floating within the pleural fluid, moving with respiration (Fig. 8-14 and **Video Clip 8-25**). Echogenic material within the pleural fluid may be due to strands of fibrin, partially fibrinolysed blood, or pus, depending on the underlying etiology. Acute hemorrhage into an effusion and empyema may result in a fluid–fluid level. In effusions due to chronic inflammatory conditions or malignancy, the fluid may be loculated or contain septations. Ultrasound-guided thoracentesis is discussed in the section on procedures, below.

Bedside Ultrasound in the Management of Cardiac Arrest: Clinical Scenario

A 55-year-old woman collapsed at home after complaining for several hours of chest pain and difficulty breathing. The patient's daughter called fire-rescue and started cardiopulmonary resuscitation (CPR). The medics arrived within 10 minutes to find the patient apneic and pulseless, with a wide complex rhythm of 60 bpm. She was intubated, given epinephrine, and transported to the nearest ED with continued CPR. On arrival, after a primary assessment, bedside ultrasonography was performed, revealing a hypokinetic heart beating at 50 bpm. There

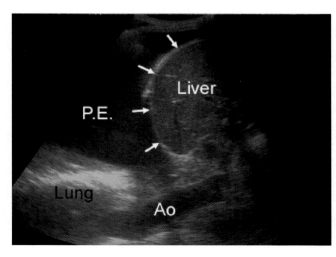

FIGURE 8-14 • A large pleural effusion (P.E.) is seen as a dark area superior to the diaphragm (*arrows*). The echoic lung transmits enough ultrasound waves to permit visualization of the descending aorta (Ao), indicating either atelectasis or consolidation. The thickness of the chest wall to the parietal pleura should be measured prior to thoracentesis.

was no pericardial effusion. Chamber sizes and right-to-left ventricular ratios were within normal limits. The IVC was adequately filled, and a search for a reversible cause of pulseless electrical activity (PEA) was initiated. A venous blood sample was sent for blood gas and electrolyte analysis. Atropine was administered, followed by a transcutaneous pacemaker, both without effect. Preparations were made for a transvenous pacemaker. Since ultrasound had excluded asystole, tamponade, and massive hypovolemia, the abdomen was examined for alternative causes of the patient's state of PEA. No free fluid or abdominal aortic aneurysm was identified, but severe bilateral hydronephrosis and a large pelvic mass were noted. A presumptive diagnosis of obstructive nephropathy with resultant hyperkalemia was entertained. The patient was treated with calcium, insulin, and D50 with an increase in heart rate, narrowing of the QRS complexes, and stabilization of vital signs. The results of the venous blood gas confirmed the diagnosis with a potassium of 8.9 meq/L. The patient was transferred to the intensive care unit, where she made a full neurologic recovery.

Indications for Sonography

The applications previously discussed in this chapter relate to diseases that, untreated, can ultimately lead to death. Thus, in evaluating cardiac arrest, any of these applications may be needed if such diseases are suspected. The initial ultrasonographic approach is similar to that for unexplained hypotension, since, even if one of the common shock states is not the primary cause of the patient's arrest, optimization of intravascular volume and cardiac function are prerequisites for successful resuscitation. As this case demonstrates, ultrasound may also provide unanticipated but vital clues to the etiology of arrest by providing information about the visceral organs.[96] In arrest, ultrasonography can also be used to guide invasive procedures (considered in detail below) and to confirm cardiac death.

Pulseless Electrical Activity

American and European resuscitation guidelines emphasize the need for early identification of treatable causes of cardiac arrest.[97–99] If a primary dysrhythmia is identified, this should be treated immediately as recommended by Advanced Cardiovascular Life Support (ACLS) algorithms.[100] However, if the patient is found to be in PEA arrest, bedside sonography is unique in its ability to diagnose many of the reversible causes of this condition immediately (see Table 8-1). Although these diagnoses may sometimes be suggested by the clinical context, in most cases the history and physical exam are either extremely limited or absent.

Studies describing ultrasonography in cardiac arrest have focused on its use in the differentiation of PEA from

cardiac standstill and on the prognosis of such patients.[101–105] The finding shared by these studies of varied design and enrollment is that absence of cardiac activity in out-of-hospital and in-hospital arrest victims makes survival to hospital discharge exceedingly unlikely. Patients with cardiac activity also have an extremely poor prognosis, although a proportion do survive to hospital admission. At the time of writing, most studies have either not investigated the broader use of bedside ultrasound in the diagnosis of reversible causes of PEA or have included an extremely small proportion of arrest patients with such diagnoses. Thus it is not known whether bedside sonography actually improves the outcome of patients in cardiac arrest. However, this literature suggests that some cardiac activity is a necessary condition for the possibility of successful management of a "treatable cause" of arrest or PEA. Beyond the mere identification of cardiac activity, the AHA mandate of a search for treatable causes is met by the ability of ultrasound to identify many of these disease processes. There are several reports describing both applications of ultrasound in patients with PEA arrest.[96,104–108] Conversely, the absence of cardiac activity, especially with the presence

TABLE 8-1 • Sonographic Findings in Pulseless Electrical Activity

Sonographic Findings	Interpretation	Potentially Reversible Etiologies	Intervention
Hypercontractile, empty ventricles with EF>75% and possible end-systolic collapse. Slit-like IVC. Max IVC diameter <9 mm. IVC-CI >75% (see text)	Underfilled ventricle, hypovolemia	Intravascular hypovolemia	Volume replacement. Search for sources of bleeding
RV >LV. Paradoxical septal motion. Dilated IVC with blunted respiratory variation	Pulmonary hypertension (acute)	Pulmonary embolism	Fluids, consider lytic therapy
Pericardial effusion, RV collapse. Dilated IVC with blunted respiratory variation	Pericardial tamponade	Myocardial rupture, malignancy, infectious	Pericardiocentesis
Grossly hypocontractile ventricles. Dilated IVC with blunted respiratory variation	Cardiogenic shock. End-stage cardiomyopathy	AMI. Consider toxic and metabolic causes: CCB and BB overdose, hyperkalemia, etc.	Inotropic therapy, IABP, PTCA
No wall movement, regular cardiac rhythm	Cardiac standstill. Electromechanical dissociation	Massive MI. Electrolyte (hyperkalemia)	Specific therapies

AMI, acute myocardial infarction; BB, beta-blocker; CCB, calcium channel blocker; IABP, intra-aortic balloon pump; IVC, inferior vena cava; IVC-CI, inferior vena cava collapse index; LV, left ventricle; PTCA, percutaneous transluminal coronary angioplasty; RV, right ventricle.

of intracardiac thrombus, may guide the termination resuscitative efforts following ACLS guidelines, thus minimizing the unnecessary expenditure of health-care resources (Video Clip 8-26a and b).[105]

The risks and costs of routine performance of ultrasound in PEA arrest are minimal, although a potential drawback is the interruption of CPR while the study is performed. In the patient who has a witnessed arrest in the presence of health-care providers, sonography can be performed as part of the initial "look, listen, and feel" assessment. For the majority of patients, resuscitative efforts are well under way by the time they can be assessed sonographically, and interruptions in CPR should be minimal.[98] In a manikin study, Breitkreutz evaluated sonography performed by a dedicated rescuer as part of a resuscitation algorithm after a minimum of five cycles of high-quality CPR.[108] The ultrasound exam was done in 5 seconds or less using the subxiphoid window, and the quality of the CPR was compared with a standard approach without ultrasound. They found that sonography did not affect no-flow intervals and that adherence to recommended CPR cycles was actually improved. The authors demonstrated that this algorithm can be taught in an 8-hour course, which includes acquisition of images within the 5-second time frame and accurate interpretation of 5-second video clips of normal and pathologic conditions, including pericardial effusion, asystole, hypovolemia, and reduced LV function.

Bedside Ultrasound as an Adjunct to Invasive Procedures

Indications for Ultrasound

Many invasive procedures are performed in the resuscitation of the critically ill. Ultrasound has been described as an adjunct in the performance of almost all of them, including peripheral and central venous access and thora-, pericardio- , and paracentesis. While some of these techniques are beyond the scope of this chapter, the *prima facie* validity of the concept that an invasive procedure would be safer with visual guidance than without it means that several of these techniques have not been evaluated by randomized prospective trials and that such trials may never be undertaken. It is probable that the use of ultrasound as an adjunct in invasive procedures will continue to grow as sonography becomes more widespread and clinician sonographers gain skill and experience. The following discussion focuses on those procedures that at this time are commonly performed with the ultrasound guidance.

Central Line Placement

With increasing focus on health-care safety and the reduction of medical errors, ultrasound guidance for central vein cannulation has been recommended by the U.S. Department of Health and Human Services. In a report prepared in 2001 by the Agency for Health Care Research and Quality, ultrasound guidance for central vein cannulation was listed as one of the 11 most highly rated safety practices.[109] This report was based on a meta-analysis of all prospective studies in the English language medical literature on this topic. A similar review, coming to similar conclusions, was published by the National Institute for Clinical Excellence (NICE) in 2003.[110] There has been some debate over these recommendations, and implementation 6 years later is far from universal.[111,112] However, the increasing availability of inexpensive ultrasound equipment, the intuitive advantages of direct visualization, and the difficulty of attaining the experience required for expertise in the landmark technique are likely to make ultrasonography increasingly widely used for central venous access.

Placement of a central line in an unstable patient may be compromised by hypotension, other ongoing resuscitative efforts, and the patient's inability to cooperate. Bedside ultrasound has been shown to improve the likelihood of successful central vein cannulation and to reduce the number of complications. These advantages are likely to be compounded in unstable patients as well as those with poor anatomic landmarks, prior failed attempts at blind cannulation, and prior central lines.

The primary role of ultrasound in central vein cannulation is to locate the vessel, ensure patency, and document placement of the catheter within the lumen. Whether the actual cannulation of the vein is observed sonographically is up to the individual practitioner. Typically one will watch for evidence of the needle's proximity to the vein, which will cause the vein to indent. As the vein is entered, it will briefly collapse and then rapidly rebound once cannulated. At this point blood will be aspirated into the syringe and the catheter placement continues "blindly." Prior to actually using the catheter for infusion, it should be visualized within the lumen of the vessel. Central vein localization and cannulation can be readily accomplished using either transverse or longitudinal imaging planes. More experienced sonographers find the longitudinal view allows for more accurate localization of the needle tip.

Internal Jugular Vein

Cannulation of the internal jugular vein, when performed under sonographic guidance, has been shown to require fewer attempts and is less likely to be complicated by carotid puncture, brachial plexus injury, or hematoma.[113–116] The relationship between the internal jugular vein and the carotid artery is highly variable and changes with head rotation, which often causes the vein to lie directly anterior to the artery. Knowledge of the patient's anatomy prior to puncture reduces the chance of inadvertent carotid puncture.[117,118] In addition to locating the vessel, ultrasound can be used to identify its depth, size, and patency and to show changes in response to Valsalva and Trendelenburg.

Unless precluded by clinical circumstances, every attempt should be made to position the patient in Trendelenburg. The internal jugular vein and carotid artery will appear as relatively superficial structures. When viewed in the transverse plane, the internal jugular vein is a thin-walled ovoid anechoic structure anterior and lateral to the carotid artery, which, unless the patient is in full arrest, will collapse much more easily than the artery (Fig. 8-15A and B). The entire course of the vein and artery in the neck should be reviewed and the optimal head position and the most convenient location for cannulation chosen.

Femoral Vein

As with cannulation of the internal jugular vein, the use of sonographic guidance in femoral vein catheterization leads to a greater chance of success and fewer complications compared with standard landmark-guided technique.[119,120] Hilty found that in patients undergoing CPR, ultrasound-guided femoral venous access had a success rate of 90%, with no arterial punctures, compared with rates of 65% success and a 20% femoral artery puncture in patients using the traditional landmark technique.[120]

When viewed in the transverse plane, the femoral artery and vein will appear as superficial anechoic circular structures. High in the femoral triangle, the vein is found in its traditionally described location, medial to the artery.

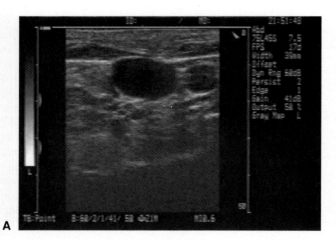

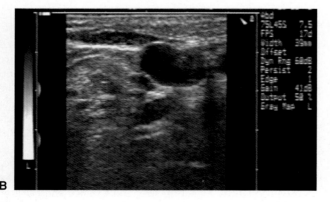

FIGURE 8-15 • **A.** In this transverse view the beam of the ultrasound intersects the carotid artery and the internal jugular vein in a transverse plane. **B.** As the needle approaches the vein, it will indent the vein. An alternative approach is to image the vein in the longitudinal view. The potential benefits include minimizing the risk of puncture of the posterior wall.

However, within centimeters of the inguinal crease, it travels posterior to the artery, precluding direct access. The vein can usually be recognized by it location, its thinner walls, its compressibility, and its larger size (the last two are unreliable in cardiac arrest). All central veins are subject to venous pulsations, so this finding should be used with caution in distinguishing it from the artery, especially in patients undergoing CPR, where pulsations will be seen primarily in the vein.[121] The vessel's size can be increased by reverse Trendelenburg or applied inguinal pressure proximal to the intended site of cannulation.

Subclavian Vein

The subclavian vein (SCV) is a commonly used site for central venous access during resuscitative efforts because the anatomic landmarks are clear, the vein is tethered by musculoskeletal structures, and access can be performed without interruption of airway management or CPR. The procedure is not without complications, including arterial puncture and pneumothorax. The benefits of ultrasound guidance in SCV catheterization are not as clear cut as those in accessing the internal jugular vein, although some studies have shown that sonographic guidance improves the likelihood of successful placement, reduces the number of attempts needed, and decreases complications, including arterial puncture, hematoma, pneumothorax, and catheter malposition.[110,122]

The SCV can be visualized by using either a supra- or infraclavicular window. If the supraclavicular approach is used, the ultrasound probe is placed parallel to and above the clavicle. The internal jugular vein is identified and then followed down to where it joins the subclavian vein. When the infraclavicular approach is planned, the probe is placed parallel and inferior to the most lateral aspect of the clavicle (Fig. 8-16A and B). The SCV usually lies anterior to the artery in this plane and can be identified by typical venous features of respiratory variation, thin wall, dilation with Valsalva, and compressibility.

Both approaches to the subclavian may be limited by the size of available linear array transducers, since a wider probe (e.g., 5–7 cm) may preclude simultaneous visualization and access to the skin for the procedure. If a narrower-footprint transducer is not available, many experienced clinicians will access the distal axillary vein, lateral to the deltopectoral groove.

Pericardiocentesis

The role of bedside sonography in the management of patients with suspected pericardial effusion is to establish the diagnosis and directly visualize placement of the aspirating needle or catheter within the pericardial sac. Prior to the use of sonography, aspiration of the pericardial sac was usually performed as a last resort effort in patients with PEA. The traditional approach involves a blind stick from the subxiphoid region through the left lobe of the liver. This technique is associated with a variety of complications, including liver injury, lung puncture, pneumothorax, and laceration of the myocardium or coronary vessels. Over the past decade, ultrasound guidance has become standard in

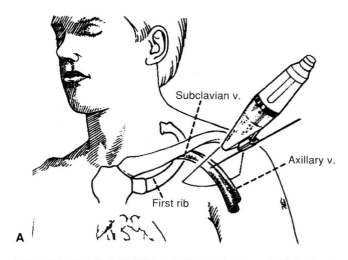

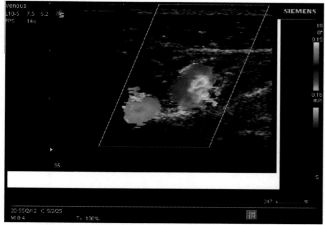

FIGURE 8-16 • **A.** To visualize the subclavian artery and vein, the probe is placed transversely just below the distal clavicle. **B.** The artery will appear as a small, noncompressible vessel with pulsatile flow if color flow Doppler is used. The adjacent vein, which is usually located above the artery, will be thin-walled and readily collapse under pressure. In this image, color-flow enhancement clearly identifies the vein (*blue*) and the artery (*red*).

the aspiration of pericardial effusion in the stable patient and is often performed at the bedside as a temporizing measure prior to definitive management.[102,123–125] In the critically ill, the indication is usually massive effusion or tamponade. With the advent of bedside ultrasonography, this procedure is not indicated unless a pericardial effusion is identified.

The best window is that which identifies a direct needle path to the effusion. Ideally this path should be short and removed from the liver, lungs, and myocardium. Except in patients with advanced emphysema, it is extremely unusual to have difficulty establishing a direct sonographic and procedural pathway to large pericardial effusions from the parasternal rib spaces of the anterior chest wall. Thus, except in unusual circumstances, ultrasound guided pericardiocentesis employs a direct transthoracic approach rather than the traditional subxiphoid transhepatic method, with

much lower complication rates and higher success rates.[123,126,127]

The patient is placed with the head of the bed slightly elevated, in a semidecubitus position on the left side to maximize cardiac contact with the chest wall. The rib space where the effusion is thickest and most directly accessible below the probe is located. Ideally, a site more than 5 cm from the left sternal border is found to avoid the internal mammary artery. The sonographer analyzes and memorizes the planned angle and direction of the pericardiocentesis needle. The needle is directed along the predetermined trajectory into the pericardial sac. Real-time sonographic information can be obtained from an adjacent window, but this is rarely practical in the management of critically ill patients.

If pericardial drainage is not successful or stops, the location of the catheter can be checked by direct visualization or by use of a bedside sonographic contrast agent. This can be created by squirting 5 to 10 mL of saline back and forth between two partly filled syringes by way of a three-way stopcock. This aerated solution is then introduced through the catheter. If it is in the correct location, the contrast agent will be seen entering the pericardium (**Video Clip 8-27**).

Complications of ultrasound-guided pericardiocentesis in large series are very rare.[123,128,129] They include hemothorax, pneumothorax, bacterial pericarditis, and failure of drainage. A technique using a probe-mounted needle has also been shown to be equally successful, but such equipment is often unavailable in critical care settings.[130]

Thoracentesis

The use of ultrasound to guide aspiration is routine in the management of pleural effusions. Complications including pneumothorax, dry aspiration, inadvertent liver or splenic lacerations, and subcutaneous hemorrhage. These are reduced when the procedure is performed under sonographic guidance.[131,132] In addition, ultrasound can distinguish between tissue masses, fluid, and loculations in cases where these cannot be distinguished on chest radiography.

The optimal position for thoracentesis is with the patient seated comfortably with the arms supported by a table and the back exposed to the physician.[133] In most cases where there are no loculations, this will allow the effusion to collect in the most dependent space in the thorax: the posterior costophrenic sulcus. If the patient is unable to sit, the procedure can be performed supine, although this makes it technically more challenging and precludes an evaluation of the posterior costophrenic sulcus. A site should be located at the point of greatest depth of the effusion and where there is a surrounding area free of overlying lung and diaphragm throughout the respiratory cycle. Thoracentesis should probably be avoided if the depth of the effusion is <15 mm from the parietal to the visceral pleura throughout the respiratory cycle and if the effusion does not extend at least one rib space above and below the site of needle entry. Scanning through transverse and longitudinal planes around the site of the planned thoracentesis should be performed to identify nearby lung, heart, and diaphragm.

For larger effusions, pleurocentesis can be performed as a two-step procedure. In the first step, the site is identified by ultrasound, the distance between the skin surface and the parietal pleura is measured so that the distance to which the needle will have to be inserted is known, and the skin is marked, with care that mobile skin folds are not displaced by the ultrasound probe. The patient should be kept still while the area is prepped and draped and standard sterile thoracentesis is accomplished, usually within 1 minute. If the fluid pocket is small, a one-step technique is used in which the chest wall is punctured with real-time guidance from the ultrasound probe, protected by a sterile cover and located immediately adjacent to the thoracentesis needle.

Transvenous Pacemaker Insertion

Transvenous cardiac pacing is often required for the patient with symptomatic bradycardia or heart block for whom transcutaneous pacing fails to provide consistent capture or is poorly tolerated by the patient. Under optimal conditions, forward flow will float the catheter into the right ventricle and ensure contact with the right ventricular wall, conditions that may not be met in patients who are hemodynamically compromised or who require emergent pacing. Success rates for blind transvenous pacemaker insertion with capture of the heart are highly variable, ranging from 10% to 90%. Bedside sonography can readily demonstrate the passage of the pacing wire into the right ventricle, confirm contact with the right ventricular myocardium, and verify successful capture of the ventricle. Pacing catheter wires are highly reflective of sound waves and appear as bright linear echoes within the heart (Video Clip 8-28). The pacing wire can be tracked passing into the right ventricle and maneuvered under direct visualization into the ventricular apex. Myocardial capture is demonstrated sonographically as rhythmic contractions of the heart at the paced rate. Complications of pacemaker placement, including malposition and septal perforation, can also be identified by ultrasound.[134–137]

Assessment of Capture by Transthoracic Pacemaker

Although application of a transthoracic pacemaker is relatively straightforward, it may be difficult to ascertain whether there is ventricular capture. The large currents generated by the pacemaker and skeletal muscle contraction may make rhythm strips difficult to interpret. Additionally, many devices have special damping circuits that make the pacer spikes hard to identify. Ultrasound can confirm capture by identifying ventricular contractions occurring at the paced rate. This can be tested by monitoring cardiac activity in response to changes of rate and output (Video Clip 8-29). Studies describing the role of ultrasound in this setting are small but demon-

strate that the sonographic impression of capture correlates with hemodynamic improvement.[138]

Issues of Training and Skill Acquisition

As this chapter demonstrates, clinicians have found uses for a wide range of ultrasound applications in their resuscitation of the critically ill. Common to all these applications is that they are *limited in scope* and *focused* by the need to answer specific clinical questions. Despite these limitations, clinician-performed bedside ultrasonography, like the history and physical exam, is an operator-dependent diagnostic modality that can be mastered only through a combination of training and experience. For this reason, training and practice guidelines for bedside ultrasonography have been developed by the specialty societies of the clinicians who use it.

See Web site for ACEP Clinical Policy on Ultrasound Guidelines. ASE/ACC policy statement on echocardiography in emergency medicine.

Ultrasound assessment of the heart has traditionally been the purview of echocardiologists. As noted in the discussion of chest pain above, American Society of Echocardiography (ASE) level 2 and 3 echocardiographic studies exceed most of the focused limited questions being asked during resuscitation and require expertise and experience beyond that available to most general intensivists.[139] Furthermore, echocardiologists with these skills are rarely available around the clock to perform or interpret such exams.[51] As noted previously, studies have shown that bedside ultrasonography significantly enhances the ability of a clinician, regardless of specialty or level of training, to evaluate and treat patients.[54,93,140–144] Although a complete echocardiographic examination may provide additional information about the patient's condition, this information is likely to be moot until the patient's condition has stabilized.[139] The training necessary for this level of sonographic evaluation has been a topic of debate between and within specialty societies.[145–148] The ASE considers that the most basic sonographic evaluation of the heart (level I) requires 3 months of training, including 75 exams performed and an additional 75 exams interpreted.[149] Whether these training requirements are appropriate for clinicians in emergency or critical care fields continues to be scrutinized by those specialty societies as they develop training and practice guidelines tailored to their practice domains.[147,150–154]

Training programs in bedside ultrasonography typically start with cognitive and visual pattern-recognition skills. Since clinician sonographers cannot rely on technicians to obtain their images, they require practical training in "knobology" and the acquisition of images. This psychomotor skill can be attained only by physical practice and experience, so that proctored hands-on training sessions are required, usually as part of a basic training course.[154-155] This is followed by a period of monitored practice. The scope and length of training programs as well as methods for assessing competence continue to be debated.[155] It is likely that as resuscitation techniques evolve, so too will the clinical and sonographic skills needed to support them. These will mandate evolving skill sets and training. With this in mind, the clinician sonographer, regardless of experience, is always aware of the focused limited nature of the bedside ultrasonographic examination and, in equivocal cases, of the need for more definitive testing, often by imaging specialists.

Acknowledgment

The authors would like to express their gratitude to James N. Kirkpatrick for assistance in the preparation of parts of this manuscript.

References

1. Ando Y, Yanagiba S, Asano Y. The inferior vena cava diameter as a marker of dry weight in chronic hemodialyzed patients. *Artif Organs* 1995;19(12):1237–1242.

2. Cheriex E, Leunissen M, Janssen J, et al. Echography of the inferior vena cava is a simple and reliable tool for estimation of "dry weight" in haemodialysis patients. *Nephrol Dial Transpl* 1989;4: 563–568.

3. Lyon M, Blaivas M, Brannam L. Sonographic measurement of the inferior vena cava as a marker of blood loss. *Am J Emerg Med* 2005; 23:45–50.

4. Yanagawa Y, Nishi K, Sakamoto T, et al. Early diagnosis of hypovolemic shock by sonographic measurement of inferior vena cava in trauma patients. *J Trauma* 2005;58:825–829.

4a. Yanagiba S, Ando Y, Kusano E, et al. Utility of the inferior vena cava diameter as a marker of dry weight in nonoliguric hemodialyzed patients. *ASAIO Journal*. 2001;47(5):528–32.

5. Carr BG, Dean AJ, Everett WW, et al. Intensivist bedside ultrasound (INBU) for volume assessment in the intensive care unit: a pilot study. *J Trauma* 2007;63(3):495–502.

6. Kusaba T, Yamaguchi K, Oda H. Echocardiography of the inferior vena cava for estimating fluid removal from patients undergoing hemodialysis. *Jpn J Nephrol* 1996;38:119–123.

7. Capomolla S, Febo O, Caporotondi A, et al. Non-invasive estimation of right atrial pressure by combined Doppler echocardiographic measurements of the inferior vena cava in patients with congestive heart failure. *Ital Heart J* 2000;1(10): 684–690.

8. Goldhammer E, Mesnick N, Abinader EG, et al. Dilated inferior vena cava: a common echocardiographic finding in highly trained elite athletes. *J Am Soc Echocardiogr* 1999;12(11):988–993.

9. Kircher B, Himelman R, Schiller N. Noninvasive estimation of right atrial pressure from the inspiratory collapse of the IVC. *Am J Cardiol* 1990;66:493–496.

10. Mitaka C, Nagura T, Sakanishi N, et al. Two-dimensional echocardiographic evaluation of inferior vena cava, right ventricle, and left ventricle during positive-pressure ventilation with varying levels of positive end-expiratory pressure. *Crit Care Med* 1989;17(3): 205–210.

11. Jeffrey RB Jr, Federle MP. The collapsed inferior vena cava: CT evidence of hypovolemia. *Am J Roentgenol* 1988;150(2):431–432.

12. Barbier C, Loubieres Y, Schmit C, et al. Respiratory changes in inferior vena cava diameter are helpful in predicting fluid responsiveness in ventilated septic patients. *Intens Care Med* 2004; 30:1740–1746.

13. Feissel M, Michard F, Faller JP, et al. The respiratory variation in inferior vena cava diameter as a guide to fluid therapy. *Intens Care Med* 2004;30:1834–1837.

14. Jue J, Chung W, Schiller NB. Does inferior vena cava size predict right atrial pressures in patients receiving mechanical ventilation? *J Am Soc Echocardiogr* 1992;5:613–619.

15. Bendjelid K, Romand J, Walder B, et al. Correlation between measured inferior vena cava diameter and right atrial pressure depends on the echocardiographic method used in patients who are mechanically ventilated. *J Am Soc Echocardiogr* 2002;15:944–949.

16. Hayden G, Everett W, Mark D, et al. The right intercostal window in bedside ultrasonography for IVC measurements is an alternative to traditional subxiphoid views. *Ann Emerg Med* 2007;50(3): S67.

17. Hayden G, Everett W, Mark G, et al. The right intercostal window for IVC measurement in critically ill patients is an alternative to subxiphoid views. *Acad Emerg Med* 2007;14:S102.

18. Kazmers A, Groehn H, Meeker C. Duplex examination of the inferior vena cava. *Am Surg* 2000;66(10):986–989.

19. Hayden, G, Everett W, Mark, D, et al. Transverse and longitudinal inferior vena cava measurements are equally accurate and useful. *Ann Emerg Med* 2007;50(3):S68.

20. Wachsburg RH. Narrowing of the upper abdominal inferior vena cava in patients with elevated intraabdminal pressure: sonographic observations. *Journal of Ultrasound in Medicine*. 2000; 19(3):217–222.

21. Amico AF, Lichtenberg GS, Reisner SA, et al. Superiority of visual versus computerized echocardiographic estimation of radionuclide left ventricular ejection fraction. *Am Heart J* 1989; 118(6):1259–1265.

22. Pershad J, Myers S, Plouman C, et al. Bedside limited echocardiography by the emergency physician is accurate during evaluation of the critically ill patient. *Pediatrics* 2004;114:e667–e671.

23. Moore CL, Rose GA, Tayal VS. Determination of left ventricular function by emergency physician echocardiography of hypotensive patients. *Academic Emergency Medicine*. 2002;9(3):186–193.

24. Randazzo MR, Snoey ER, Levitt MA, et al. Accuracy of emergency physician assessment of left ventricular ejection fraction and central venous pressure using echocardiography. *Acad Emerg Med* 2003;10:973–977.

25. Kimura BJ, Amundson SA, Willis CL, et al. Usefulness of a handheld ultrasound device for bedside examination of left ventricular function. *Am J Cardiol* 2002;90(9):1038–1039.

26. McGowan JH, Cleland JG. Reliability of reporting left ventricular systolic function by echocardiography: a systematic review of 3 methods. *Am Heart J* 2003;146(3):388–397.

27. Maisch B, Seferovi PM, Risti AD, et al. Task Force on the Diagnosis and Management of Pericardial Diseases of the European Society of Cardiology. Guidelines on the diagnosis and management of pericardial diseases executive summary; The Task Force on the Diagnosis and Management of Pericardial Diseases of the European Society of Cardiology. *Eur Heart J* 2004;25(7): 587–610.

28. Calhoon JH, Hoffman TH, Trinkle JK, et al. Management of blunt rupture of the heart. *J Trauma* 1986;26(6):495–502.

29. Levine MJ, Lorell BH, Diver DJ, et al. Implications of echocardiographically assisted diagnosis of pericardial tamponade in contemporary medical patients: detection before hemodynamic embarrassment. *J Am Coll Cardiol* 1991;17(1):59–65.

30. Blaivas M, Graham S, Lambert MJ. Impending cardiac tamponade, an unseen danger? *Am J Emerg Med* 2000;18(3):339–340.

31. Guberman BA, Fowler NO, Engel PJ, et al. Cardiac tamponade in medical patients. *Circulation* 1981;64(3):633–640.

32. Lorell B. Pericardial diseases. In Braunwald E, ed. *Heart Disease: A Textbook Of Cardiovascular Medicine*, 5th ed. Philadelphia: Saunders, 1997.

33. Spodick DH. Pathophysiology of cardiac tamponade. *Chest* 1998; 113(5):1372–1378.

34. Armstrong WF, Schilt BF, Helper DJ, et al. Diastolic collapse of the right ventricle with cardiac tamponade: an echocardiographic study. *Circulation* 1982;65:1491–1496.

35. Singh S, Wann LS, Schuchard GH, et al. Right ventricular and right atrial collapse in patients with cardiac tamponade—a combined

echocardiographic and hemodynamic study. *Circulation* 1984; 70(6):966–971.

36. Chandraratna PA. Echocardiography and Doppler ultrasound in the evaluation of pericardial disease. *Circulation* 1991;84(3 Suppl I):I-303–110.

37. Conrad SA, Byrnes TJ. Diastolic collapse of the left and right ventricles in cardiac tamponade. *Am Heart J* 1988;115(2):475–478.

38. Blaivas M, DeBehnke D, Phelan MB. Potential errors in the diagnosis of pericardial effusion on trauma ultrasound for penetrating injuries. *Acad Emerg Med* 2000;7:1261–1266.

39. Sagrista-Sauleda J, Angel J, Sambola A, et al. Low-pressure cardiac tamponade: clinical and hemodynamic profile. *Circulation* 2006; 114(9):945–952.

40. Choo MH, Chia BL, Chia FK, et al. Penetrating cardiac injury evaluated by two-dimensional echocardiography. *Am Heart J* 1984;108(2):417–420.

41. Sabia P, Afrookteh A, Touchstone DA, et al. Value of regional wall motion abnormality in the emergency room diagnosis of acute myocardial infarction. A prospective study using two-dimensional echocardiography. *Circulation* 1991;4:I85–I92.

42. Kontos MC, Arrowood JA, Paulsen WHJ, et al. Early echocardiography can predict cardiac events in emergency department patients with chest pain. *Ann Emerg Med* 1998;31:550–557.

43. Levitt MA, Promes SB, Bullock S, et al. Combined cardiac marker approach with adjunct two-dimensional echocardiography to diagnose acute myocardial infarction in the emergency department. *Ann Emerg Med* 1996;27:1–7.

44. Peels CH, Visser CA, Kupper AJ, et al. Usefulness of two-dimensional echocardiography for immediate detection of myocardial ischemia in the emergency room. *American Journal of Cardiology* 1990;65(11):687–691.

45. Mohler ER, Ryan T, Segar DS, et al. Clinical utility of troponin T levels and echocardiography in the emergency department. *Am Heart J* 1998;135:253–260.

46. Sasaki H, Charuzi Y, Beeder C, et al. Utility of echocardiography for the early assessment of patients with nondiagnostic chest pain. *Am Heart J* 1986;12:494–497.

47. Horowitz RS, Morganroth J, Parrotto C, et al. Immediate diagnosis of acute myocardial infarction by two-dimensional echocardiography. *Circulation* 1982;65(2):323–329.

47a. Horowitz RS, Morganroth J. Immediate detection of early high-risk patients with acute myocardial infarction using two-dimensional echocardiographic evaluation of left ventricular regional wall motion abnormalities. *American Heart Journal* 1982;103(5): 814–822.

48. Kontos MC, Arrowood JA, Jesse RL, et al. Comparison between 2-dimensional echocardiography and myocardial imaging in the emergency department in patients with possible myocardial ischemia. *Am Heart J* 1998;136:724–733.

49. Braunwald E, Antman EM, Beasley JW, et al. American College of Cardiology. American Heart Association. Committee on the Management of Patients With Unstable Angina. ACC/AHA 2002 guideline update for the management of patients with unstable angina and non–ST-segment elevation myocardial infarction—summary article: a report of the American College of Cardiology/American Heart Association task force on practice guidelines (Committee on the Management of Patients With Unstable Angina). *J Am Coll Cardiol* 2002;40(7):1366–1374.

50. Cheitlin MD, Armstrong WF, Aurigemma GP, et al. ACC/AHA/ASE 2003 guideline update for the clinical application of echocardiography—summary article: a report of the American College of Cardiology/American Heart Association Task Force on Practice Guidelines (ACC/AHA/ASE Committee to Update the 1997 Guidelines for the Clinical Application of Echocardiography). *J Am Coll Cardiol* 2003;42(5):954–970.

51. Beaulieu Y. Bedside echocardiography in the assessment of the critically ill. *Crit Care Med* 2007;35(5 Suppl):S235–S249.

52. Hauser AM, Gangadharan V, Ramos RG, et al. Sequence of mechanical, electrocardiographic and clinical effects of repeated coronary artery occlusion in human beings: echocardiographic observations during coronary angioplasty. *J Am Coll Cardiol* 1985;5:193–197.

53. Lundgren C, Bourdillon PD, Dillon JC, et al. Comparison of contrast angiography and two-dimensional echocardiography for the evaluation of left ventricular regional wall motion abnormalities after acute myocardial infarction. *Am J Cardiol* 1990;65: 1071–1077.

54. Kobal SL, Atar S, Siegel RJ. Hand-carried ultrasound improves the bedside cardiovascular examination. *Chest* 2004;126(3):693–701.

55. Lewis WR. Echocardiography in the evaluation of patients in chest pain units. *Cardiol Clin* 2005;23(4):531–539.

56. Hickman M, Swinburn JM, Senior R. Wall thickening assessment with tissue harmonic echocardiography results in improved risk stratification for patients with non–ST-segment elevation acute chest pain. *Eur J Echocardiogr* 2004;5:142–148.

57. Kaul S, Senior R, Firschke C, et al. Incremental value of cardiac imaging in patients presenting to the emergency department with chest pain and without ST-segment elevation: a multicenter study. *Am Heart J* 2004;148(1):129–136.

58. Korosoglou G, Labadze N, Hansen A, et al. Usefulness of real-time myocardial perfusion imaging in the evaluation of patients with first time chest pain. *Am J Cardiol* 2004;94:1225–1231.

59. Mulvagh SL, DeMaria AN, Feinstein SB, et al. Contrast echocardiography: current and future applications. *J Am Soc Echocardiogr* 2000;13(4): 331–342.

60. Kalvaitis S, Kaul S, Tong KL, et al. Effect of time delay on the diagnostic use of contrast echocardiography in patients presenting to the emergency department with chest pain and no S-T segment elevation. *J Am Soc Echocardiogr* 2006;19(12): 1488–1493.

61. Millward DK, Robinson NJ, Craige E. Dissecting aortic aneurysm diagnosed by echocardiography in a patient with rupture of the aneurysm into the right atrium; rare cause for continuous murmur. *American Journal of Cardiology* 1972;30(4):427–431.

62. Cobbs BW Jr, Nicholson WJ. Diagnosis of dissecting aortic aneurysm with suprasternal echocardiography. *Am J Cardiol* 1980;45(1):183–184.

63. Victor MF, Mintz GS, Kotler MN, et al. Two dimensional echocardiographic diagnosis of aortic dissection. *Am J Cardiol* 1981;48(6):1155–1159.

63a. Nagueh SF, Middleton KJ, Kopelen HA, et al. Doppler tissue imaging: a noninvasive technique for evaluation of left ventricular relaxation and estimation of filling pressures. *J Am Coll Cardiol* 1997;30(6):1527–1533.

64. Nagueh SF, Lakkis NM, Middleton KJ, et al. Doppler estimation of left ventricular filling pressures in patients with hypertrophic cardiomyopathy. *Circulation* 1999;99(2):254–261.

65. Ommen SR, Nishimura RA, Appleton CP, et al. Clinical utility of Doppler echocardiography and tissue Doppler imaging in the estimation of left ventricular filling pressures: a comparative simultaneous Doppler-catheterization study. *Circulation* 2000;102(15): 1788–1794.

66. Kasner M, Westermann D, Steendijk P, et al. Utility of Doppler echocardiography and tissue Doppler imaging in the estimation of diastolic function in heart failure with normal ejection fraction: a comparative Doppler-conductance catheterization study. *Circulation* 2007;116(6):637–647.

67. Dean A, Hayden G, Mark D, et al. Bedside ultrasonography assessment of mitral valve inflow velocity and tissue Doppler are similar to echocardiology measurements. *Acad Emerg Med* 2007; 14:S101–S102.

68. Oh JK, Seward JB, Tajik AJ, et al, eds. *The Echo Manual*, 2nd ed. Philadelphia: Lippincott Williams & Wilkins, 1999, appendix.

69. Torbicki A. Imaging venous thromboembolism with emphasis on ultrasound, chest CT, angiography and echocardiography. *Thromb Haemost* 1999;82(2):907–912.

70. Frazee BW, Snoey ER. Diagnostic role of ED ultrasound in deep venous thrombosis and pulmonary embolism. *Am J Emerg Med* 1999;17(3):271–278.

71. Rudoni RR, Jackson RE, Godfrey GW, et al. Use of two-dimensional echocardiography in the diagnosis of pulmonary embolus. *J Emerg Med* 1998;16(1):5–8.

72. Lualdi JC, Goldhaber SZ. Right ventricular dysfunction after acute pulmonary embolism: pathophysiologic factors, detection, and therapeutic implications. *Am Heart J* 1995;130:1276–1282.

73. Weston MJ, Wilde P. Echocardiographic diagnosis of massive pulmonary embolism. *Br J Radiol* 1989;62(740):751–753.

74. Grifoni S, Olivotto I, Cecchini P, et al. Utility of an integrated clinical, echocardiographic, and venous ultrasonographic

approach for triage of patients with suspected pulmonary embolism. *Am J Cardiol* 1998;82(10):1230–1235.

75. Cheriex EC, Sreeram N, Eussen YF, et al. Cross sectional Doppler echocardiography as the initial technique for the diagnosis of acute pulmonary embolism. *Br Heart J* 1994;72(1):52–57.

76. Kasper W, Meinertz T, Kersting F, et al. Echocardiography in assessing acute pulmonary hypertension due to pulmonary embolism. *Am J Cardiol* 1980;45(3):567–572.

77. Goldberger JJ, Himelman RB, Wolfe CL, et al. Right ventricular infarction: recognition and assessment of its hemodynamic significance by two-dimensional echocardiography. *J Am Soc Echocardiogr* 1991;4(2):140–146.

78. Sharkey SW, Shelley W, Carlyle PF, et al. M-mode and two-dimensional echocardiographic analysis of the septum in experimental right ventricular infarction: correlation with hemodynamic alterations. *Am Heart J* 1985;110(6):1210–1218.

79. Kinch JW, Ryan TJ. Right ventricular infarction. *N Engl J Med* 1994;330(17):1211–1217.

80. Steiner P, Lund GK, Debatin JF, et al. Acute pulmonary embolism: value of transthoracic and transesophageal echocardiography in comparison with helical CT. *AJD* 1996;167:931–936.

80a. Agricola E, Bove T, Oppizzi M, et al. Ultrasound comet-tail images: a marker of pulmonary edema: a comparative study with wedge pressure and extravascular lung water. *Chest* 2005;127(5):1690–1695.

81. Bedetti G, Gargani L, Corbisiero A, et al. Evaluation of ultrasound lung comets by hand-held echocardiography. *Cardiovasc Ultrasound* 2006;4:34.

82. Soldati G, Rossi M. "Wet" and "dry" lungs: a useful sonographic distinction. *Crit Care* 1999;3(Suppl 1):124–125.

83. Lichtenstein D, Meziere G, Biderman P, et al. The comet-tail artifact. An ultrasound sign of alveolar-interstitial syndrome. *Am J Respir Crit Care Med* 1997;156(5):1640–1646.

84. Lichtenstein D, Goldstein I, Mourgeon E, et al. Comparative diagnostic performances of auscultation, chest radiography, and lung ultrasonography in acute respiratory distress syndrome. *Anesthesiology* 2004;100(1):9–15.

85. Volpicelli G, Mussa A, Garofalo G, et al. Bedside lung ultrasound in the assessment of alveolar–interstitial syndrome. *Am J Emerg Med* 2006;24(6):689–696.

86. Reissig A, Kroegel C. Transthoracic sonography of diffuse parenchymal lung disease: the role of comet tail artifacts. *J Ultrasound Med* 2003;22(2):173–180.

87. Jambrik Z, Monti S, Coppola V, et al. Usefulness of ultrasound lung comets as a nonradiologic sign of extravascular lung water. *Am J Cardiol* 2004;93(10):1265–1270.

88. Picano E, Frassi F, Agricola E, et al. Ultrasound lung comets: a clinically useful sign of extravascular lung water. *J Am Soc Echocardiogr* 2006;19(3):356–363.

89. Lichtenstein DA, Lascols N, Meziere G, et al. Ultrasound diagnosis of alveolar consolidation in the critically ill. *Intens Care Med* 2004;30(2):276–281.

90. Lichtenstein DA, Menu Y. A bedside ultrasound sign ruling out pneumothorax in the critically ill: lung sliding. *Chest* 1995;108:1345–1348.

91. Lichtenstein D, Meziere G, Biderman P, et al. The "lung point": an ultrasound sign specific to pneumothorax. *Intens Care Med* 2000;26(10):1434–1440.

92. Lichtenstein D, Meziere G, Biderman P, et al. The comet-tail artifact: an ultrasound sign ruling out pneumothorax. *Intens Care Med* 1999;25:383–388.

93. Kirkpatrick AW, Sirois M, Laupland KB, et al. Hand-held thoracic sonography for detecting post-traumatic pneumothoraces: the Extended Focused Assessment with Sonography for Trauma (EFAST). *J Trauma Inj Infect Crit Care* 2004;57(2):288–295.

94. Dean A. Ultrasound evaluation of the thorax as a component of the focused assessment with sonography in trauma. *Acad Emerg Med* 2007;14:e6.

95. Ball CG, Kirkpatrick AW, Laupland KB, et al. Factors related to the failure of radiographic recognition of occult posttraumatic pneumothoraces. *Am J Surg* 2005;189(5):541–546.

96. Hendrickson RG, Dean AJ, Costantino TG. A novel use of ultrasound in pulseless electrical activity: the diagnosis of an acute abdominal aortic aneurysm rupture. *J Emerg Med* 2001;21(2):141–144.

97. Nolan JP, Deakin CD, Soar J, et al. European Resuscitation Council guidelines for resuscitation 2005: Section 4. Adult advanced life support. *Resuscitation* 2005;67(Suppl 1):S39–S86.

98. Hazinski MF, Nadkarni VM, Hickey RW, et al. Major changes in the 2005 AHA Guidelines for CPR and ECC: reaching the tipping point for change. *Circulation* 2005;112(24 Suppl):IV206–IV211.

99. AHA/ECC Guidelines 2000 for cardiopulmonary resuscitation and emergency cardiovascular care. *Circulation* 2000;102(Suppl 1):I150–I152.

100. Cummins RO, ed. *ACLS Provider Manual.* Dallas: American Heart Association, 2001:201.

101. Niendorff DF. Rapid cardiac ultrasound of inpatients suffering PEA arrest performed by nonexpert sonographers. *Resuscitation* 2005; 67(1): 81–87.

102. Blaivas M, Fox JC. Outcome of cardiac arrest patients found to have cardiac standstill on the bedside emergency department echocardiogram. *Acad Emerg Med* 2001;8(6):616–621.

103. Salen P, O'Connor R, Sierzenski P, et al. Can cardiac sonography and capnography be used independently and in combination to predict resuscitation outcomes? *Acad Emerg Med* 2001;8(6):610–615.

104. Salen P, Melniker L, Chooljian C, et al. Does the presence or absence of sonographically identified cardiac activity predict resuscitation outcomes of cardiac arrest patients? *Am J Emerg Med* 2005;23(4):459–462.

105. Varriale P, Maldonado JM. Echocardiographic observations during in-hospital cardiopulmonary resuscitation. *Crit Care Med* 1997;25(10):1717 –1720.

106. Tayal VS, Kline JA. Emergency echocardiography to detect pericardial effusion in patients in PEA and near PEA states. *Resuscitation* 2003;59:315–318.

107. Bocka JJ, Overton DT, Hauser A. Electromechanical dissociation in human beings: an echocardiographic evaluation. *Ann Emerg Med* 1988;17:450–452.

108. Breitkreutz R, Walcher F, Seeger FH. Focused echocardiographic evaluation in resuscitation management: concept of an advanced life support-conformed algorithm. *Crit Care Med* 2007; 35(5 Suppl): S150–S161.

109. Rothschild JM. Ultrasound guidance of central vein catheterization: making health care safer: a critical analysis of patient safety practices (Agency for Healthcare Research and Quality Web site). Publication No. 01-E058. Available at http://www.ahrq.gov/clinic/ptsafety.

110. Calvert N, Hind D, McWilliams RG, et al. The effectiveness and cost-effectiveness of ultrasound locating devices for central venous access: a systematic review and economic evaluation. *Health Technol Assess* (Winchester, UK). 2003;7(12):1–84.

111. Muhm M. Ultrasound guided central venous access.[editorial; see comment]. *BMJ* 2002;325(7377):1373–1374.

112. Chalmers N. Ultrasound guided central venous access. NICE has taken sledgehammer to crack nut. *BMJ* 2003;326(7391):712.

113. Denys BG, Uretsky BF, Reddy PS. Ultrasound-assisted cannulation of the internal jugular vein. A prospective comparison to the external landmark-guided technique. *Circulation* 1993;87:1557.

114. Leung J, Duffy M, Finckh A, et al. Real-time ultrasound guided internal jugular vein catheterization in emergency department increases success rate and reduces complications: a prospective study. *Ann Emerg Med* 2006;48:540.

115. Hrics P, Wilber S, Blanda M, et al. Ultrasound-assisted internal jugular vein catheterization in the ED. *Am J Emerg Med* 1998;16:401.

116. Milling TJ, Rose M, Briggs WM, et al. Randomized, controlled clinical trial of point of care limited ultrasonography assistance of central venous cannulation: The Third Sonography Outcomes Assessment Program (SOAP-3) trial. *Crit Care Med* 2005;33: 1764.

117. Denys BG, Uretsky BF. Anatomical variations of internal jugular vein location: impact on central venous access. *Crit Care Med* 1991;19:1516.

118. Troianos CA, Kuwik RJ, Pasqual JR, et al. Internal jugular vein and carotid artery anatomic relation as determined by ultrasonography. *Anesthesiology* 1996;85:43.

119. Kwon TH, Kim YL, Cho DK. Ultrasound-guided cannulation of the femoral vein for acute haemodialysis. *Nephrol Dial Transplant* 1997;12:1009.

120. Hilty WM, Hudson PA, Levitt MA, et al. Real-time ultrasound-guided femoral vein catheterization during cardiopulmonary resuscitation. *Emerg Med Ann* 1997;29:331.

121. Coletti RH, Hartjen B, Gozdziewski S, et al. Origin of canine femoral pulses during standard CPR. *Crit Care Med* 1983;11:218.

122. Gualtieri E, Deppe SA, Sipperly ME, et al. Subclavian venous catheterization: greater success rate for less experienced operators using ultrasound guidance. *Crit Care Med* 1995;23:692.

123. Tsang TS, Freeman WK, Sinak LJ, et al. Echocardiographically guided pericardiocentesis: evolution and state-of-the-art technique. *Mayo Clin Proc* 1998;73(7):647–652.

124. Mandavia DP, Hoffner RJ, Mahaney K, et al. Bedside echocardiography by emergency physicians. *Ann Emerg Med* 2001;38:377.

125. Mazurek B, Jehle D, Martin M. Emergency department echocardiography in the diagnosis and therapy of cardiac tamponade. *J Emerg Med* 1991;9:27.

126. Salem K, Mulji A, Lonn E. Echocardiographically guided pericardiocentesis: the gold standard for the management of pericardial effusion and cardiac tamponade. *Can J Cardiol* 1999; 15(11):1251–1255.

127. Caspari G, Bartel T, Mohlenkamp S, et al. Contrast medium echocardiography–assisted pericardial drainage. *Herz* 2000; 25(8):755–760.

128. Callahan JA, Seward JB, Nishimura RA, et al. Two-dimensional echocardiographically guided pericardiocentesis: experience in 117 consecutive patients. *Am J Cardiol* 1985;55(4):476–479.

129. Susini G, Pepi M, Sisillo E, et al. Percutaneous pericardiocentesis versus subxiphoid pericardiotomy in cardiac tamponade due to postoperative pericardial effusion. *J Cardiothorac Vasc Anesth* 1993;7(2):178–183.

130. Maggiolini S, Bozzano A, Russo P, et al. Echocardiography-guided pericardiocentesis with probe-mounted needle: report of 53 cases. *J Am Soc Echocardiogr* 2001;14(8):821–824.

131. Diacon AH, Brutsche MH, Soler M. Accuracy of pleural puncture sites: a prospective comparison of clinical examination with ultrasound. *Chest* 2003;123(2):436–441.

132. Mayo PH, Goltz HR, Tafreshi M, et al. Safety of ultrasound-guided thoracentesis in patients receiving mechanical ventilation. *Chest* 2004;125(3):1059–1062.

133. Mayo PH, Doelken P. Pleural ultrasonography. *Clin Chest Med* 2006;27(2):215–227.

134. Meier B, Felner JM. Two-dimensional echocardiographic evaluation of intracardiac transvenous pacemaker leads. *J Clin Ultrasound* 1982;10:421–425.

135. Aguilera PA, Durham BA, Riley DA. Emergency transvenous cardiac pacing placement using ultrasound guidance. *Ann Emerg Med* 2000;36:224–227.

136. Syverud S, Dalsey W, Hedges J, et al. Radiographic assessment of transvenous pacemaker placement during CPR. *Ann Emerg Med* 1986;15:131–137.

137. Macedo W Jr, Sturmann K, Kim JM, et al. Ultrasonographic guidance of transvenous pacemaker insertion in the emergency department: a report of three cases. *J Emerg Med* 1999;17(3):491–496.

138. Holger JS, Minnigan HJ, Lamon RP, et al. The utility of ultrasound to determine ventricular external cardiac pacing. *Am J Emerg Med* 2001;19:134–136.

139. Goodkin GM, Spevack DM, Tunick PA, et al. How useful is hand-carried bedside echocardiography in critically ill patients? *J Am Coll Cardiol* 2001;37(8):2019–2022.

140. Fedson S, Neithardt G, Thomas P, et al. Unsuspected clinically important findings detected with a small portable ultrasound device in patients admitted to a general medicine service. *J Am Soc Echocardiogr* 2003;16(9):901–905.

141. Kronzon I. The hand-carried ultrasound revolution. *Echocardiography* 2003;20(5):453–454.

142. Mark DG, Ku BS, Carr BG, et al. Directed bedside transthoracic echocardiography: preferred cardiac window for left ventricular ejection fraction estimation in critically ill patients. *Am J Emerg Med* 2007;25(8):894–900.

143. DeCara JM, Lang RM, Koch R, et al. The use of small personal ultrasound devices by internists without formal training in echocardiography. *Eur J Echocardiogr* 2003;4(2):141–147.

144. Manasia AR, Nagaraj HM, Kodali RB, et al. Feasibility and potential clinical utility of goal-directed transthoracic echocardiography performed by noncardiologist intensivists using a small hand-carried device (SonoHeart) in critically ill patients. *J Cardiothorac Vasc Anesth* 2005;19(2):155–159.

145. Stewart WJ, Douglas PS, Sagar K, et al. Echocardiography in emergency medicine: a policy statement by the American Society of Echocardiography and the American College of Cardiology. Task Force on Echocardiography in Emergency Medicine of the American Society of Echocardiography and the Echocardiography and Technology and Practice Executive Committees of the American College of Cardiology. *J Am Coll Cardiol* 1999;33(2):586–588.

146. Krause RS. Echocardiography in emergency medicine: A policy statement by the American Society of Echocardiology and the American College of Cardiology. *Journal of American Society of Echocardiography* 1999;12(7):607–608.

147. Beaulieu Y. Specific skill set and goals of focused echocardiography for critical care clinicians. *Crit Care Med* 2007;35(5 Suppl): S144–149.

148. Seward JB, Douglas PS, Erbet R, et al. Hand-carried cardiac ultrasound (HCU) device: Recommendations regarding new technology. A report from the Echocardiography Task Force on New Technology of the Nomenclature and Standards Committee of the American Society of Echocardiography. *J Am Soc Echocardiogr* 2002;15:369–373.

149. Quinones MA, Douglas PS, Foster E, et al. American Society of Echocardiography. Society of Cardiovascular Anesthesiologists. Society of Pediatric Echocardiography. ACC/AHA clinical competence statement on echocardiography: a report of the American College of Cardiology/American Heart Association/American College of Physicians–American Society of Internal Medicine Task Force on clinical competence. *J Am Soc Echocardiogr* 2003;16(4):379–402.

150. Neri L, Storti E, Lichtenstein D. Toward an ultrasound curriculum for critical care medicine. *Crit Care Med* 2007;35(5 Suppl): S290–S304.

151. Mazraeshahi RM, Farmer JC, Porembka DT. A suggested curriculum in echocardiography for critical care physicians. *Crit Care Med* 2007;35(8 Suppl):S431–S433.

152. Langlois Sle P. Focused ultrasound training for clinicians. *Crit Care Med* 2007;35(5 Suppl):S138–143.

153. American College of Emergency Physicians. Emergency ultrasound imaging criteria compendium. American College of Emergency Physicians. *Ann Emerg Med* 2006;48(4):487–510.

154. American College of Emergency Physicians. ACEP emergency ultrasound guidelines–2001. *Ann Emerg Med* 2001;38(4): 470–481.

155. Nair, Siu SC, Sloggett CE, Biclar L, et al. The assessment of technical and interpretative proficiency in echocardiography. *J Am Soc Echocardiogr* 2006;19(7):924–931.

Basic Life Support

Chapter 9
Pathophysiology of Cardiac Arrest

Karl B. Kern

The mechanism of blood-flow generation during cardiopulmonary resuscitation (CPR) is complex and depends on body habitus, the duration of CPR and the CPR technique utilized. Cardiac compression predominates as the mechanism early in CPR, with the thoracic pump mechanism more predominant as time progresses.

- Current concepts of the physiology of blood flow during CPR and their clinical implications
- Coronary perfusion pressure as a major determinant of resuscitation outcome
- Mechanisms for optimizing coronary perfusion pressure during CPR
- Cardiac dysfunction and the CPR stunned myocardium: implications for management as part of the post–circulatory arrest syndrome

Introduction

Cardiac arrest causes the complete cessation of forward blood flow, with resultant global ischemia affecting the entire organism. Various tissues have different tolerances to such global ischemia, but all will eventually succumb if blood flow is not restored in a timely fashion. The most prominent injuries occur in the central nervous system, which initially responds to ischemia with loss of consciousness after only 7 to 10 seconds of an circulatory arrest. Likewise, once the myocardial cells become globally ischemic, cellular function, including contraction, stops; if blood flow is not restored, myocytes begin to autoinfarct. The duration of no blood flow is crucial in these responses; hence the importance of CPR for restoring at least some modicum of flow during cardiac arrest. CPR restores only a portion of normal blood flow previously generated by a contracting heart. Nonetheless, such support is crucial for the survival of both the central nervous system and the myocardium.

The Mechanism of Blood Flow During CPR

The mechanism of blood flow produced during CPR has been a controversial and debated topic for several decades. Just how blood flow is produced became an important issue in trying to determine the optimal external chest compression rate. In 1977, Taylor and colleagues suggested that within the range of 40 to 80 compressions per minute, the *duration* of chest compression was more important than the *rate* of compression.[1] This ratio of the duration of compression to decompression is the "duty cycle." A duty cycle of 50% (50% of the time the chest is compressed and 50% decompressed, generally by passive recoil) with 60 compressions per minute was initially thought optimal. In opposition to this concept, investigators at Duke University found that a higher chest compression rate produced better blood flow during closed chest CPR, up to a maximum rate of 140 compressions per minute.[2] Above a compression rate of 140/min, the relaxation or diastolic period for coronary filling is compromised to the point where total myocardial blood flow diminishes. In recognition of these findings, the National Conference on CPR in 1985 recommended increasing the chest compressions to 80 to 100/min.[3]

Cardiac or Thoracic Pump Mechanism?

Physicians and scientists alike have assumed that external chest compression produces temporary blood flow by compressing the heart between the sternum and the vertebral column.

Physicians and scientists alike have assumed that external chest compression produces temporary blood flow by compressing the heart, similar to the manner of open chest internal cardiac massage, with the heart being squeezed between the sternum and the vertebral column. Indeed, a famous illustration by Frank Netter suggests such a mechanism, with the heart being squeezed between the sternum and the vertebral column and competent, functional valves directing the resultant blood flow out the aortic valve and to the body. It has been assumed that with such cardiac compression and competent mitral and aortic valves, blood moved in an antegrade fashion from the left ventricle into the aorta. This widely held concept was challenged in the late 1970s and early 1980s.[4] Some investigators felt that the concept of cardiac compression and competent valvular function was inconsistent with the number of observations during resuscitation. They noted that when sternal compression was performed in a patient with a flail chest, no arterial blood pressure was recorded until the chest was bound to prevent paradoxical expansion.[5] They also observed that patients with severe chronic obstructive pulmonary disease with marked increases in their anterior–posterior chest diameter and relatively small hearts could nonetheless be resuscitated by sternal compression. Finally, they observed that during conventional CPR, the compression cycle that followed ventilation often resulted in an increased blood pressure and carotid blood flow. To them, these observations appeared inconsistent with direct cardiac compression from external chest compression, and a new potential mechanism for blood-flow generation during CPR was developed. The "thoracic pump" mechanism of blood-flow generation suggested that forward blood flow occurring during CPR was due to an increase in intrathoracic pressure compared with extrathoracic pressure. This theory was also supported by the work of Criley et al. on "cough CPR."[6]

Cough Cardiopulmonary Resuscitation

Cough CPR consists of having a patient with a recent onset of asystole or ventricular fibrillation forcefully cough every second.[7] Since no hands are placed on the patient, this is an excellent example of the power of the thoracic pump mechanism to produce blood flow during CPR. If the patient coughs forcefully every second, significant aortic systolic pressures can occur. These pressures are often enough to perfuse the brain and consciousness can be preserved. The obvious disadvantage of this technique is that it must be initiated before unconsciousness occurs. Cough CPR has been most successfully employed in the cardiac catheterization suite, where Criley et al. have reported examples of patients sustaining consciousness for up to 40 seconds after the onset of ventricular fibrillation.[6] Although some lay publications have touted this technique as a way to perform CPR on oneself, cough CPR has generally failed to meet its initial expectations outside the cardiac catheterization laboratory.[8]

The Thoracic Pump Mechanism

An important rediscovery was that blood pressures in the aorta and right atrium were often similar during external chest compressions. This observation was initially reported by Weal and Rockwell-Jackson in 1962 but at the time received little attention.[9] Nearly two decades later, investigators at Johns Hopkins noted that during external chest compressions, central venous and aortic pressures were often similar; indeed, pressures in all cardiac chambers and the intrapleural space were nearly equal. If the cardiac compression mechanism is responsible for blood flow during CPR, the fluid-filled systems of the heart and great vessels must contain a pressure gradient across a resistance for the production of forward blood flow. Under the normal physiology occurring during sinus rhythm, there is a large pressure gradient involving the aorta, right atrium, and central venous systems. The lack of such a gradient during external chest compression suggests the heart is not functioning strictly as a pump but that the entire thorax was indeed the pump.[10]

In contrast to the intrathoracic structures with similar pressures, the investigators at Johns Hopkins found a significant pressure difference between the extrathoracic carotid artery and the intrathoracic cardiac chambers and the right atrium and the extrathoracic jugular veins. This pressure gradient was thought to be responsible for producing the forward cerebral blood flow. It is at this time that Criley et al. demonstrated that the jugular venous valves were operative during cough CPR.[11] Indeed, early anatomists had also appreciated the presence of internal jugular venous valves and had described them in the 1950s.[12]

Further supports for the theory that increases in intrathoracic pressure create forward blood flow during external chest compression came in the 1980s from echocardiographic studies of clinical CPR.[13–14] Two different two-dimensional echocardiographic studies performed late in a protracted resuscitation effort, showed that the mitral valve was not competent and did not close in a consistent fashion and that the left ventricular internal diameter was not deformed with chest compressions.[13–14] These findings suggest that increased intrathoracic pressure in some patients, not cardiac compression, accounted for forward blood flow during chest compressions.

Nonetheless, cardiac compression does occur in some humans.[5] In a few patients studied at Johns Hopkins, central venous pressures were significantly lower than arterial pressure during external chest compression, indicating a pressure gradient and the possibility that in these patients a cardiac compression mechanism for blood flow during CPR was possible.

Based on this new theory for blood-flow generation during external chest compression, the investigators at Purdue University attempted to apply this concept to improving alternative techniques to conventional CPR. The group explored two basic strategies, simultaneous chest compression and ventilation, as well as abdominal binding.[15] Increased intrathoracic pressure could be obtained by clamping the endotracheal tube during chest compressions; however, the initial increase in pressure and flow dissipated rapidly, secondary to the inhibition of venous return by high intrathoracic pressure. Maintaining inflated lungs during external chest compressions, these investigators found significant increases in arterial pressure and carotid flow over those observed with conventional CPR.[10] Of particular interest, in their experimental model large animals (i.e., canines), treatment with simultaneous high-pressure ventilation and chest compressions produced significant systolic flows in the carotid arteries. However, the same was not true in smaller dogs.[16] In the smaller dogs, cardiac compression evidently occurs with relatively good blood-flow generation, and the addition of simultaneous high-pressure ventilation did not appear to improve these hemodynamics. However, in large animals, in which cardiac compression plays a smaller role, if any, the addition of simultaneous ventilation clearly improved the peripheral circulation during CPR.[10] Abdominal binding was shown by Redding et al. to improve hemodynamics during CPR.[17] Unfortunately, further investigations of this technique reported increases in liver lacerations secondary to the abdominal binding, and the technique fell out of favor. It was also noted that abdominal binding had a detrimental effect on coronary perfusion pressure by the consistent increase in right atrial pressure both in systole and diastole.

The ultimate test for the presence and efficacy of the "thoracic pump mechanism" as employed using simultaneous chest compressions and high-pressure ventilation with or without abdominal binding is its effect on survival. In an effort to evaluate this effect on survival, simultaneous chest compression and ventilation CPR with abdominal binding was compared with standard CPR in a laboratory experiment at the University of Arizona.[18] Survival in the control group of canines receiving standard CPR was 5 out of 6, whereas none of the 6 animals undergoing simultaneous chest compression and high-pressure ventilation had return of spontaneous circulation in spite of intensive efforts.[18] A clinical trial with simultaneous compression–ventilation CPR was also performed.[19] This clinical study enrolled nearly a thousand patients in an out-of-hospital cardiac arrest trial where ambulance staff were randomly assigned to use simultaneous compression–ventilation CPR or conventional CPR. Both hospital admission and survival to discharge were greater in the conventional CPR group than in the experimental group receiving simultaneous compression–ventilation CPR ($P \leq 0.01$). In the subset of adult patients with nontraumatic witnessed cardiac arrest, survival was 35% of 337 versus 23% of 365 ($P \leq 0.001$). These two studies have dampened enthusiasm for simultaneous chest compression–ventilation CPR, and this technique is not currently recommended.

Other investigators were less convinced about the importance of the thoracic pump mechanism for blood-flow generation during resuscitation efforts. Rankin and colleagues at Duke University were convinced, from their own clinical experience, that rapid chest compression rates were more effective than slower rates and that this reflected a cardiac compression mechanism for blood-flow generation. These investigators studied the effects of varying manual chest compression rates, force, and durations in large chronically instrumented dogs.[2,20] In their model, they found that the relative contribution of thoracic pump and direct cardiac compression mechanisms to blood flow varied depending on the method of CPR being performed. During high-impulse (increased frequency) CPR, direct cardiac compression seems to be the predominant mechanism, while during low-momentum compression techniques, the thoracic pump mechanism seemed to predominate. At the same time, new echocardiographic experimental studies by Weil et al. supported the cardiac/vascular compression theory of CPR-generated blood flow.[21] In fact, echocardiographic studies in anesthetized minipigs demonstrated incompetent cardiac valve motion with a clear change in left ventricular dimensions during the early phases of cardiac arrest with closed-chest CPR. The investigators interpreted these data as further evidence for direct cardiac compression in the early phases of cardiac arrest and resuscitation efforts. Since that time, additional transesophageal echocardiographic studies in experimental models of cardiac arrest[22] and clinical cases[23] have also shown left ventricular compression in competent mitral valve function, again suggesting a cardiac compression mechanism for blood flow.

Current Concepts on Blood Flow During CPR

As in most disagreements, there appears to be truth on both sides of this controversy. Cardiac compression clearly occurs at times, while the thoracic pump mechanism for blood-flow generation during CPR also appears to be operational, particularly later in the resuscitation effort. Open-chest cardiac massage and high-impulse closed-chest compression in small subjects undoubtedly produce blood flow predominantly by cardiac or vascular compression. Whereas cough and "vest CPR" forms of CPR, both of which produce very little thoracic compression, but rather large fluctuations in intrathoracic pressure, appear to produce blood flow via the thoracic pump mechanism.

The authors examined this at the University of Arizona using our large database of experimental CPR studies. On subjects undergoing open-chest cardiac compression, the authors observed that there is a large difference between the aortic and right atrial systolic pressures. In contrast, the authors found little or no difference in systolic pressure between the aorta and right atrium in experimental subjects in whom blood is generated by the thoracic pump mechanism during vest CPR. This led to the conclusion that the absolute difference between aortic and right atrial systolic pressure, which we termed the systolic pressure gradient, could actually indicate the mechanism of blood flow in real time. The authors reviewed 63 experiments using a variety of CPR techniques and animal sizes. Each underwent 3 minutes of untreated ventricular fibrillation and then one of the five different types of CPR was initiated. Systolic pressure gradients between the aortic and right atrium were measured at 1, 7, and 17 minutes of the resuscitation effort.[24] The systolic pressure gradient was greatest during open-chest cardiac massage (true cardiac compression), intermediate with external mechanical or manual standard CPR, and lowest with CPR performed with a vest apparatus (predominantly thoracic pump). With open-chest cardiac massage, this gradient was 60 to 65 mm Hg; with standard CPR in small animals, it was 28 to 30 mm Hg; and in larger animals, it was 15 to 20 mm Hg. With vest CPR, the gradient was only 2 to 5 mm Hg. In this particular series, it was also noted that 24-hour survival was greatest in those animals where cardiac compression mechanisms seemed to be the predominant mechanism of blood-flow generation. This is of interest in light of a report from Deshmukh and associates using 2D echocardiography to evaluate eight minipigs during CPR.[21] They found aortic and mitral valves demonstrating competency (not wide open with constant leakage) during the first 5 minutes of CPR in all animals. In the three successfully resuscitated animals, valve competency persisted for the full 12 minutes of CPR.

It appears that the mechanism of blood flow during CPR can vary accorded to the CPR technique utilized and the duration of cardiac arrest.

It appears that the mechanism of blood flow during cardiopulmonary resuscitation can vary accorded to the CPR

technique utilized. Cardiac/vascular compression is greatest with open-chest cardiac massage or high-impulse CPR, particularly in smaller subjects, while it is lowest with cough CPR or vest CPR. The mechanism of blood-flow generation also seems to vary with the duration of CPR efforts. Cardiac compression predominates as the mechanism early in CPR, with the thoracic pump mechanism more predominant as time progresses. This is consistent with the reported clinical echocardiographic reports noted earlier.[13,14,23] In summary, the mechanism of blood-flow generation during CPR depends on body habitus, the duration of CPR, and the CPR technique utilized. Both mechanisms appear feasible and are probably present in each subject resuscitated.

Importance of Coronary Perfusion Pressure

"The basic problem, then, in resuscitations seems to us to be that of securing some means of some infusion—a coronary pressure, approximately amounting to 30 to 40 mm Hg."

Experimental work in resuscitation research in the 1970s and 1980s seemingly focused on the physiologic mechanisms for creating systemic blood flow during closed-chest resuscitation.[25,26] During that era, the importance of blood flow to sustain the myocardium and central nervous system during CPR became evident. Using microsphere techniques to measure blood flow, investigators found that regional perfusion of vital organs occurs with closed-chest compression CPR, but at substantially lower levels than during normal sinus rhythm.[27–29] Central nervous system flows average about 30% of normal with good anteroposterior chest compressions. Myocardial blood flows achieved with external chest compressions average even less, generally only 10% to 20% of normal. Peripheral perfusion is almost nonexistent during CPR. Nevertheless, good CPR efforts can temporarily provide at least some perfusion to the myocardium and cerebrum until more definitive treatment (i.e., defibrillation) can be accomplished.

Myocardial perfusion during cardiac arrest can be estimated by measuring "coronary perfusion pressure" during the resuscitation effort. This perfusion pressure gradient correlates well with resultant cerebral and myocardial blood flows generated with CPR, and with the subsequent possibility of successful defibrillation and resuscitation.[27,28]

Determinants of Coronary Perfusion Pressure During Cardiopulmonary Resuscitation

Adequate Perfusion Pressure

The importance of an adequate perfusion pressure for successful resuscitation was first described by Crile and Dolley in 1906.[30] While studying means of reversing cardiorespiratory arrest in dogs and cats asphyxiated with the anesthetics of that time (chloroform and ether), they noted that "the basic problem, then, in resuscitations seems to us to be that of securing some means of some infusion—a coronary pressure, approximately amounting to 30 to 40 mm Hg." This concept was further developed through the work of Redding and Pearson.[17,31–33] These investigators showed that when aortic diastolic pressure during resuscitation was ≥40 mm Hg, animals could be successfully revived from cardiac arrest; but this was not possible if that level of diastolic pressure was not achieved. From their early work they deduced that the mechanism of action for epinephrine and other alpha-adrenergic agonists during cardiac arrest was to cause peripheral vasoconstriction, which raised the central aortic diastolic pressure and thereby increased coronary perfusion. Otto and coworkers confirmed this mechanism. By using selective blockade, these investigators evaluated the role of the alpha- and beta-adrenergic receptors during resuscitation. Animals that were blocked with the former had difficulty in responding to epinephrine (i.e., diastolic aortic pressure did not increase and they were not resuscitated). In contrast, those that were blocked with the latter were successfully resuscitated and exhibited peripheral vasoconstriction with elevated aortic diastolic pressures in response to adrenergic agonists.[34–36]

Perfusion Pressure Gradient

Other investigators have confirmed not only the importance of a perfusion pressure (i.e., the aortic diastolic pressure) but also of a defined perfusion pressure gradient, which included a "downstream" pressure from the myocardial venous system acting as an impedance to forward flow. Voorhees et al.—measuring regional blood flow to the brain, heart, and other peripheral tissues—noted that the arteriovenous gradient was important during the compression phase of CPR for cerebral blood flow and postulated that the same arteriovenous gradient during the relaxation component of CPR was important for myocardial blood flow.[37] Both Niemann et al.[38] and Ditchey et al.[39] suggested that coronary perfusion during CPR results from the difference in mean pressure of the aorta and that of the right atrium. Ditchey et al. found that coronary blood flow during CPR was a linear function of the pressure difference generated across the coronary circulation (i.e., the mean pressure difference between the ascending aortic and right atrial pressures).[39]

Measurement of Coronary Perfusion Pressure

No standard method for measuring coronary perfusion pressure during CPR has been agreed upon. Some investigators have suggested subtracting the middiastolic right atrial pressure from simultaneously obtained middiastolic aortic pressure,[18,27] whereas others have suggested that coronary perfusion pressure be obtained by measuring the peak positive diastolic pressure gradient between the aorta and the right atrium.[40] Another approach has been to calculate the coro-

nary perfusion pressure gradient by subtracting the mean right atrial diastolic pressure from the mean diastolic aortic pressure.[28,29] To address this uncertainty, the Utstein-style guidelines for reporting laboratory CPR research specify that the point just before compression be used as the reference point for measurement of coronary perfusion pressure. This point was selected because it is easily identified and more likely to be consistent among investigators.[41] Nonetheless, multiple techniques for calculating coronary perfusion pressure during CPR are still in use. See ILCOR Utstein-style Guidelines for reporting laboratory data.

An interesting alternative for calculating coronary perfusion pressure by measuring the integrated area under the aortic diastolic pressure minus the right atrial diastolic pressure curves during each minute of CPR was reported by investigators at the University of Arizona.[42] This technique was developed to account for the effect of interrupting chest compression/relaxation cycles during the resuscitation effort. Since chest compression/relaxation cycles (i.e., the relaxation phase specifically) are responsible for generating blood flow to the heart, a decrease in delivered chest compression cycles can markedly decrease the total amount of myocardial perfusion generated with the resuscitation effort. Calculating coronary perfusion pressure in the usual fashion (end-diastolic aortic minus right atrial pressures) does not account for periods of chest compression interruptions. A more accurate method is to use the integrated area coronary perfusion pressure (iCPP) over each minute. The effect of chest compressions interruptions—for example, for rescue breathing—on coronary perfusion pressure becomes readily apparent, typically resulting in a 40% decrease in cumulative coronary perfusion (Fig. 9-1A, B).

Clinical Implications

Interruption of chest compression/relaxation has direct effects on the amount of coronary perfusion pressure generated during the period of consecutive compression cycles (15/min previously and 30/min currently). We found that at the beginning of each cycle of 15, the first 5 to 10 compressions/relaxations are "building up" the coronary perfusion gradient and that it is not optimal until at least one third of the series is completed.[43] Then with cessation of chest compressions/relaxations, this diastolic gradient falls off rapidly, often returning to near zero within 5 seconds. When chest compressions do resume, the coronary perfusion gradient must be rebuilt, usually starting from near zero (Fig. 9-2).

Does antegrade coronary flow occur during the compression phase or only during the relaxation phase of CPR? Schleien et al. suggested that forward coronary flow may occur during the compression phase of CPR when epinephrine infusions are used because of a net positive pressure gradient from the aorta to the right atrium even during the compression phase. They concluded that the diastolic gradient as an index of coronary blood flow during CPR may be incomplete.[44] Subsequent work has shown that many methods of CPR routinely generate some degree of pressure difference from the aorta to the right atrium during the

PART TWO • BASIC LIFE SUPPORT

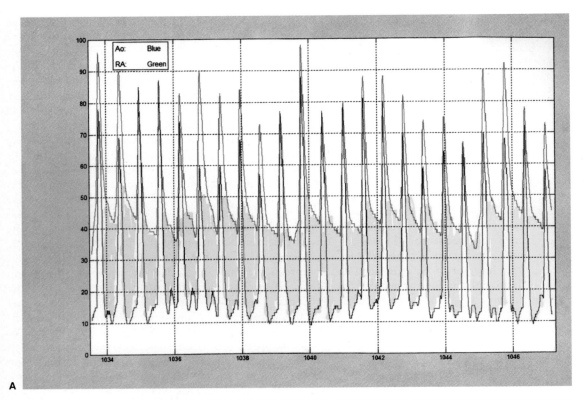

A

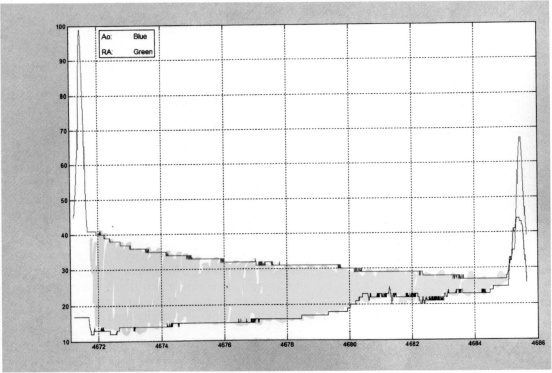

B

FIGURE 9-1 • Aortic and right atrial pressure tracings demonstrating the coronary perfusion pressure gradient during the relaxation phase of chest compressions. Note the marked difference in cumulative area under the curve (*yellow*) for coronary perfusion pressure (CPP) when continuous chest compressions **(A)** are done versus interrupted chest compressions, in this case interrupted for ventilations **(B)**. Each panel illustrates aortic and right atrial pressure data during 13.5 seconds of CPR. Area under the curve (yellow) measurement of "integrated CPP" was 59,223 mm Hg★dt seconds in A (continuous chest compressions) and 35,737 mm Hg★dt seconds in B (interrupted chest compressions). This calculates to a 40% decrease in the integrated area CPP (iCPP) with the interrupted chest compressions.

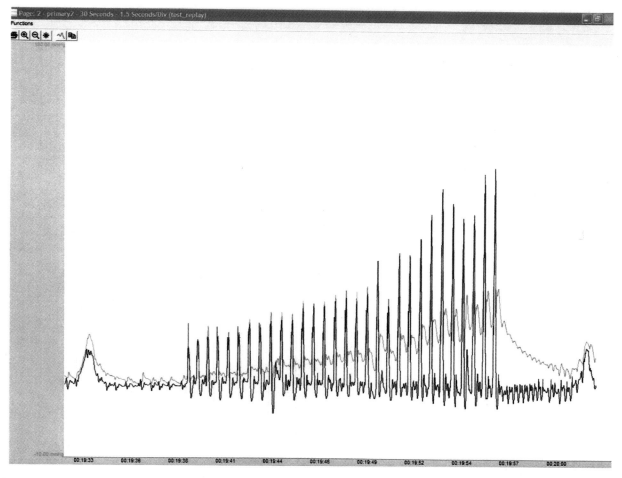

FIGURE 9-2 • Aortic and right atrial pressure tracings demonstrating the coronary perfusion pressure gradient during the relaxation phase of chest compressions. Note the rapid fall off in the diastolic gradient with the cessation of chest compressions, and the time required to "rebuild" a maximal CPP after such interruption.

compression phase, either positive or negative; hence the potential for antegrade or retrograde coronary blood flow exists during chest compression or CPR systole. Total "net" flow during CPR may require consideration of the entire cardiac cycle (the compression phase and the relaxation phase). This hypothesis has been tested using an intracoronary Doppler flow catheter to determine the relationship between systolic or compression phase coronary perfusion pressure as well as diastolic or relaxation-phase coronary perfusion and the direction of coronary blood flow in the proximal left anterior coronary artery.[45] Retrograde coronary artery blood flow (flow from the left main coronary artery back into the ascending aorta) occurred routinely during the compression phase of manual CPR, regardless of the measured pressure gradient from the aorta to the right atrium. Even in circumstances where the aortic pressure exceeded right atrial pressure during compressions, no antegrade coronary blood flow occurred. Rather, such antegrade coronary blood flow occurred exclusively during the relaxation phase of chest compression and correlated only with a positive "diastolic" or relaxation-phase perfusion pressure gradient between the aorta and the right atrium. The greater

the gradient, the greater the antegrade coronary blood-flow velocity produced. Positive systolic coronary perfusion gradients occurring during the compression phase do not significantly improve antegrade blood flow and, indeed, can be associated with significant amounts of retrograde coronary flow. Hence diastolic perfusion pressure gradients account for the vast majority of cases of myocardial perfusion.

Myocardial Blood Flow and Coronary Perfusion Pressure During Cardiopulmonary Resuscitation

Aortic and right atrial pressures can be easily measured in the experimental laboratory but require great effort in the clinical setting. During the relaxation phase of chest compressions, aortic pressure largely depends upon intrinsic arterial tone. Right atrial pressure during the relaxation phase of

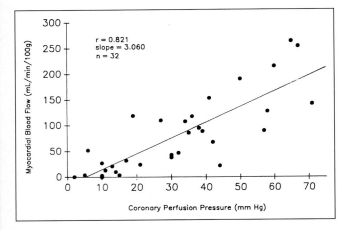

FIGURE 9-3 • Left ventricular myocardial blood flow during CPR increases as the coronary perfusion pressure increases. (From Kern KB, Lancaster LD, Goldman S, et al. *Am Heart J* 1990;120:324–333. © Elsevier 1990, with permission.)

CPR is largely determined by central venous return and venous capacitance. A significant correlation has been established between coronary perfusion pressure and simultaneously measured myocardial blood flow during CPR.[27–29,46] Correlation coefficients vary from 0.82 to 0.89. Ralston et al. found a correlation coefficient of 0.89 in dogs where no epinephrine was used and of 0.85 when epinephrine was used.[27] Using epinephrine, Michael et al. found a correlation coefficient of 0.84[28] and Halperin et al., from the same laboratory at Johns Hopkins, found a correlation coefficient with multiple forms of CPR of 0.88.[29] Finally, Kern et al. reported a correlation coefficient of 0.82 between the coronary perfusion pressure achieved and the resultant myocardial blood flow to the anterior left ventricular wall (Fig. 9-3).[46]

The generally low coronary perfusion pressures generated with standard CPR (10 to 20 mm Hg) produce only small amounts of myocardial blood flow. With a coronary perfusion pressure of 10 to 20 mm Hg, Ralston et al. found left ventricular flows of 15 to 20 mL/min/100 g.[27] Michael et al. found flows of 5 to 40 mL/min/100 g,[28] Halperin et al. found flows of 5 to 25 mL/min/100 g,[29] and Taylor et al. found flows of 10 to 15 mL/min/100 g.[47] However, these studies also demonstrated that if perfusion pressures are in the range of 40 to 60 mm Hg, excellent myocardial blood flow levels can result. Such perfusion pressure gradients produce myocardial blood flows of 40 to 200 mL/min/kg.[27–29,46]

Myocardial Blood Flow and Coronary Artery Stenosis

All of this previously described work correlating myocardial blood flow and coronary perfusion pressure was performed on experimental animals with normal coronary arteries and normal left ventricular function. To examine the effect of coronary artery lesions on the relationship between coronary perfusion pressure and myocardial blood flow during

CPR, investigators at the University of Arizona evaluated a closed-chest porcine model of fixed artificial coronary artery stenoses.[46] In a closed-chest model with minimal collateral circulation, coronary artery lesions were found to have major effects on regional myocardial blood flow measured during CPR. Coronary stenoses greatly decrease the amount of distal coronary blood flow for any given coronary perfusion pressure produced. As expected, where few collateral vessels exist, complete coronary occlusion results in negligible distal myocardial perfusion, regardless of the coronary perfusion pressure. Where patent 33% diameter stenoses existed, myocardial blood flow measured during CPR continued to show a high correlation with coronary perfusion pressure, albeit with less myocardial blood flow for every increment in coronary perfusion pressure. With coronary perfusion pressure of 30 to 60 mm Hg, coronary stenosis resulted in an approximate 50% reduction in distal blood flow. For any given coronary perfusion pressure generated with CPR, a significant reduction in myocardial blood flow distal to the stenosis was seen. Therefore, even minimal or previously considered "insignificant" coronary lesions may have a profound effect on distal myocardial blood flow during the performance of CPR.[48]

Resuscitation Duration

Coronary perfusion pressure declines with lengthy resuscitation efforts.[49] The highest pressure gradients and the greatest myocardial perfusion occur during the first minutes of resuscitation. This decline occurs from the gradual loss of arterial tone and increase in right heart pressures.

The effect of "no-flow time" (period of cardiac arrest without support where no blood flow is being generated) on subsequent coronary perfusion pressure generated during CPR was studied by Duggal et al.[50] They found no particular compromise in what level of coronary perfusion pressure could be generated after extending the downtime from 9 minutes to 15 minutes of untreated ventricular fibrillation. However, they did note that the previously established threshold levels of coronary perfusion pressure for resuscitability were not valid after the longer downtimes (i.e., a higher coronary perfusion pressure was needed after lengthy "downtimes" to ensure successful outcome).

Coronary Perfusion Pressure, Resuscitation, and Survival

Coronary perfusion pressure correlates with myocardial blood flow during CPR but has also been shown to be predictive of successful resuscitation (i.e., restoration of spontaneous circulation [ROSC], short-term outcome, and long-term survival). Both Ralston et al.[27] and Michael et al.[28] showed that increased coronary perfusion pressure produced not only increased myocardial blood flow but also better outcomes. Other experimental studies have confirmed the predictive value of the myocardial perfusion gradient and longer-term survival rates up to 7 days.[27–29,51] The use of coronary perfusion pressure to monitor the effectiveness of resuscitation makes it attractive for use in clinical cardiac arrest.

Over the last two decades there have been more than 200 patients who had coronary perfusion pressure measured during the performance of CPR.[52–61] Important lessons have been learned. It is feasible to measure coronary perfusion pressure in victims of clinical cardiac arrest. The necessary instrumentation, including cannulation of the ascending aorta and right atrium, can be accomplished safely even during resuscitation efforts. Usually, however, by the time the pressure-measuring catheters are in place, the patient is relatively late in the course of cardiac arrest. In most cases, the information obtained so late is not useful for making any survival enhancing changes. Occasionally, cardiac arrest occurs in patients who already have a pulmonary artery catheter or an arterial line. Such patients can more easily be monitored for coronary perfusion pressure during CPR by the appropriate use of these pressures.

The majority of measurements obtained during clinical cardiac arrest demonstrate very poor coronary perfusion pressures. The mean coronary perfusion pressures reported in human series range from zero to 15 mm Hg. Consistent with these low values, most humans monitored for coronary perfusion pressure during CPR have not survived. However, some data exist for survivors. McDonald[53] reported that 1 of his 12 patients survived. That patient had the highest coronary perfusion pressure from his series (16 mm Hg). Paradis et al.[59] reported on 100 patients, of whom 24 had return of spontaneous circulation. When coronary perfusion pressures between survivors and nonsurvivors were compared, there was a statistically significant difference in initial and maximal coronary perfusion pressure measurements. Patients without return of spontaneous circulation had a mean initial coronary perfusion pressure of 2 mm Hg; those in whom spontaneous circulation returned had mean initial perfusion pressure of 13 mm Hg. Likewise, maximal coronary perfusion pressures were significantly different between the two groups: 8 mm Hg versus 26 mm Hg. This series in particular substantiates the experimental data from animal models, showing that coronary perfusion pressure can be a predictor of the return of spontaneous circulation. Paradis et al. noted that in patients with prolonged cardiac arrest, coronary perfusion pressure was a better predictor of resuscitation outcome than was aortic pressure alone.[59] A coronary perfusion pressure of 15 mm Hg appeared to be the minimum required to obtain successful return of spontaneous circulation.

After Restoration of Spontaneous Circulation

Once spontaneous circulation is restored a new challenge arises. Many times the lack of blood flow during untreated cardiac arrest and the resultant reperfusion can result in a postresuscitation syndrome. The myocardium is especially vulnerable. Postresuscitation myocardial dysfunction has become increasingly recognized as a major contributor to the poor long-term outcome results with current resuscitation efforts. Both systolic and diastolic left ventricular abnormalities are readily identified following successful resuscitation. The global myocardial stunning seen during this period can be severe and unless supported can lead to death. Although the exact mechanism of postresuscitation global myocardial dysfunction is not yet known, a number of factors that contribute have been identified, as well as several potential treatment strategies (see also Chapter 29).

Postresuscitation myocardial dysfunction has become increasingly recognized as a major contributor to the poor long-term outcome results with current resuscitation efforts.

Experimental evidence of the postresuscitation syndrome was first reported in detail by University of Pittsburgh resuscitation researchers.[62] In their experimental canine model of prolonged cardiac arrest and resuscitation, they found elevated myocardial filling pressures with decreased cardiac outputs postresuscitation.

Weil and colleagues at the Institute for Critical Care Medicine have shown, in isolated perfused hearts of Sprague-Dawley rats, decreases in myocardial contractile function and left ventricular compliance following resuscitation from ventricular fibrillation cardiac arrest.[63] Further studies by this group in a large animal porcine model of cardiac arrest revealed similar findings.[64] Pressure-volume relationships postresuscitation showed strikingly reduced myocardial contractility accompanied by decreased stroke volume and ejection fraction.

The University of Arizona Resuscitation Research Group studied invasive and noninvasive measurements of ventricular function before and after 10 or 15 minutes of untreated cardiac arrest in a swine model of ventricular fibrillation and subsequent resuscitation.[65] Left ventricular ejection fraction showed a significant reduction 30 minutes after resuscitation, which progressively worsened through the first 5 hours postresuscitation. Partial recovery was seen by 24 hours, and full recovery was seen by 48 hours. The systolic left ventricular dysfunction was a diffuse, global process with wall motion abnormalities seen in all ventricular walls. Hemodynamic changes seen after resuscitation included a dramatic rise in left ventricular end-diastolic pressure, a fall in cardiac output, and an increase in isovolumic relaxation time ("tau"). These changes demonstrate significant diastolic left ventricular dysfunction as well as the systolic dysfunction seen by the angiographic measurements.

Transthoracic echocardiographic studies showed similar results, with diminished systolic ventricular function and diminished diastolic ventricular function postresuscitation.

This was the first report in an *in vivo* model of cardiac arrest to elucidate the time course of left ventricular systolic and diastolic dysfunction after successful CPR. Maximal dysfunction was seen at 6 hours, with partial resolution by 24 hours and full recovery by 48 hours, indicating a true "stunning" phenomenon.

Clinical Evidence for Postresuscitation Myocardial Dysfunction

Clinical reports and studies have recently collaborated the experimental evidence for postresuscitation myocardial dysfunction. Several case reports of global left ventricular failure after successful resuscitation from prolonged cardiac arrest of different etiologies have appeared in the literature.[66–68]

Investigators in Paris reported on a series of successfully resuscitated out-of-hospital cardiac arrest victims, approximately half of whom developed myocardial dysfunction.[6] Among 148 consecutive patients admitted after successful resuscitation from out-of-hospital cardiac arrest, 73 (49%) developed myocardial failure manifested as hypotension and shock. Those who developed myocardial dysfunction had significantly lower ejection fractions at initial testing (presumably worse left ventricular function prior to cardiac arrest), significantly longer basic life support efforts, more defibrillation shocks, and more epinephrine administered. All of these features suggest a more difficult and longer resuscitation effort before circulation was restored.

Similar to the experimental data, these clinical investigators found that the left ventricular dysfunction or shock was generally transient, indicating global myocardial stunning rather than permanent scarring. At 8 hours postresuscitation, the average cardiac index postresuscitation among the 73 patients who developed shock was 2.1 L/min/m^2 (range 1.4–2.9). This improved to 3.2 L/min/m^2 (range 2.7–4.2) by 24 hours and to 3.8 L/min/m$^($ (range 3.0–4.5) by 72 hours. However, although most postresuscitation shock was reversible, not all improved. Nearly 20% (14 of 73) shock patients did not improve and subsequently died of persistent shock. Early death from multiple organ failure was associated with a persistently low cardiac index at 24 hours (2.6 L/min/m^2 [range 2.3–3.0] vs. 3.3 L/min/m^2 [range 2.9–4.3]; $P < 0.003$).

Mechanism of Postresuscitation Myocardial Dysfunction

The mechanism of postresuscitation myocardial dysfunction remains unknown. A number of factors have been identified that affect postresuscitation myocardial function.

Epinephrine, a commonly used medication during advanced cardiac life support (ACLS), has been shown to significantly worsen postresuscitation myocardial dysfunction.[70] It appears that the increase in systemic afterload following epinephrine administration is responsible for its worsening of postresuscitation myocardial dysfunction. In some cases, the postresuscitation stunned left ventricle may be unable to tolerate the substantially increased systemic vascular resistance persisting after the use of epinephrine during the resuscitation, resulting in overt failure of both systolic and diastolic pumping function.

Buffer therapy combined with standard adrenergic vasoconstrictors during CPR has resulted in even greater impairment of postresuscitation myocardial dysfunction and a decrease in survival.[71]

Another factor that appears to worsen myocardial dysfunction postresuscitation is defibrillation. Weil and colleagues, using their established cardiac arrest rodent model, showed that high-energy defibrillation produced more severe left ventricular postresuscitation dysfunction and shorter duration of survival than low-energy defibrillation.[72] These same investigators have shown, in a porcine cardiac arrest model, that biphasic waveform defibrillation significantly reduces the severity of postresuscitation myocardial dysfunction compared with escalating monophasic energy defibrillation.[73,74]

The most significant factor for developing postresuscitation myocardial dysfunction is the duration of the resuscitation effort. Data from both experimental laboratories and clinical trials have consistently shown a correlation between prolonged resuscitation effort and the development of postresuscitation myocardial dysfunction. In work at the University of Arizona, left ventricular ejection fraction and pulmonary artery wedge pressure were both significantly worse postresuscitation after 15 minutes of ventricular fibrillation compared with only 10 minutes of ventricular fibrillation.[65] Investigators at the Institute of Critical Care Medicine in Palm Springs, CA, found lower ejection fractions at 2 hours postresuscitation with increasing time of cardiac arrest. Laurent et al., in their clinical series, also identified length of resuscitation effort as a major determinant for the development of post–cardiac arrest myocardial stunning.[69]

Potential Treatments for Postresuscitation Myocardial Dysfunction

Several specific therapies have been explored for postresuscitation myocardial dysfunction. Transient use of a beta-adrenergic agonist has worked well in other conditions where global stunning is seen, as after heart transplantation. Previous studies have shown this agent to be a significant inotrope capable of enhancing left ventricular function, including increasing left ventricular dP/dt and cardiac output.[75]

We studied the effect of dobutamine infusions begun 15 minutes after resuscitation compared to no treatment in the postresuscitation period.[76] The marked deterioration in systolic and diastolic left ventricular function postresuscitation seen in the control animals was ameliorated in the dobutamine-treated animals. Left ventricular ejection fraction fell from a prearrest 58% ± 3% to 25% ± 3% at 5 hours postresuscitation in the control group but remained unchanged in the dobutamine (10 µg/kg/min) group (52% ± 1% prearrest and 55 ± 3% at 5 hours postresuscitation). Measurement of isovolumic relaxation of the left ventricle (tau) demonstrated a similar benefit of the dobutamine infusion for overcoming postresuscitation diastolic dysfunction. Left ventricular end-diastolic pressure rose significantly in the control group but not in the dobutamine group when prearrest and 5-hour data were compared. However, heart rate rose significantly in the dobutamine-treated group. Average heart rate at 30 minutes postresuscitation in animals treated with 10 µg/kg/min of dobutamine was 190 ± 12 bpm, as opposed to 134 ± 8 bpm in the control group ($P < 0.05$). Heart rate response was significantly less with a lower dose (5 µg/kg/min), while left ventricular ejection fraction continued to be better than in the untreated controls.

Weil, Tang, and coworkers have explored the possibility that ischemic preconditioning, whether by short periods of precedent ventricular fibrillation or by chemically induced preconditioning using a potassium ATP channel opener, could influence postresuscitation left ventricular stunning.[77] The potassium ATP channel activator significantly lowered coronary perfusion pressure during CPR but also resulted in a reduction of postresuscitation myocardial dysfunction with an increase in postresuscitation survival.

Finally, this same group has found improved postresuscitation function and better neurologically normal survival after the administration of 21-aminosteroids during CPR.[78] These compounds have been shown to minimize reperfusion injury mediated by the liberation of free radicals. None of these treatments are yet proven in clinical trials.

Summary

The pathophysiology of cardiac arrest includes the generalized global ischemia associated with total cessation of forward blood flow. Timely initiation of CPR, including defibrillation for ventricular fibrillation, is essential to limit long-term sequelae, particularly damage to the myocardium and central nervous system.

Crucial to providing adequate forward blood flow to the heart and brain is the coronary perfusion pressure generated during the resuscitation effort. Many circulatory adjuncts for resuscitation have been developed to enhance the production of an adequate coronary perfusion pressure in an effort to improve long-term survival after cardiac arrest (see Chapter 10).

Once spontaneous circulation has been restored, attention must be given to the potential of developing postresuscitation myocardial dysfunction. If this is recognized and supported, improved survival can be achieved.

References

1. Taylor GJ, Tucker WM, Greene HL, et al. Importance of prolonged compression duration during cardiopulmonary resuscitation in man. *N Engl J Med* 1977;296:1515–1517.
2. Maier GW, Tyson GS, Olsen CO, et al. The physiology of external cardiac massage. High impulse cardiopulmonary resuscitation. *Circulation* 1984;70:86–101.
3. Standards and guidelines for cardiopulmonary resuscitation (CPR) and emergency cardiac care (ECC). National Academy of Sciences–National Research Council. *JAMA* 1986;255:2905–2989.
4. Criley JM, Niemann JT, Rosborough JP, et al. The heart as a conduit in CPR. *Crit Care Med* 1981;9:373–374.
5. Weisfeldt ML, Chandra N, Tsitlik JE. New attempts to improve blood flow during CPR. In: Schluger J, Lyon AF, eds. *CPR in Emergency Cardiac Care: Looking into the Future.* New York: EM Books, 1980:29

6. Criley JM, Blaufuss AH, Kissel GL. Cough-induced cardiac compression. *JAMA* 1976;236:1246–1250.
7. Criley JM. Cough CPR. In Shugar J, Lyon AF, eds. *CPR in Emergency Cardiac Care: Look into the Future.* New York: EM Books, 1980:47.
8. http://www.americanheart.org/presenter.jhtml?identifier=4535
9. Weale FE, Rockwell-Jackson RL. Efficiency of cardiac massage. *Lancet* 1962;1:990.
10. Chandra N, Weisfeldt ML, Tsitlik JE, et al. Augmentation of carotid flow during cardiopulmonary resuscitation (CPR) in the dog by simultaneous compression and ventilation with high airway pressure. *Am J Cardiol* 1979;48:1053–1063.
11. Neimann JT, Rosborough JP, Hausknect M, et al. Blood flow without cardiac compression during closed chest cardiac pulmonary resuscitation. *Crit Care Med* 1981;9:380–381.
12. Weathersby HT. The valves of the axillary, subclavian and internal jugular vein. *Anat Rec* 1956;124:379.
13. Werner JA, Greene JL, Janko C, et al. Visualization of cardiac valve motion in man during external chest compressions using 2-dimensional echocardiography: implications regarding the mechanism of blood flow. *Circulation* 1981;63:1417–1421.
14. Rich S, Wix HL, Shapiro EP. Clinical assessment of heart chamber size and valve motion during cardiopulmonary resuscitation by 2-D echocardiography. *Am Heart J* 1981;102:368–373.
15. Babbs CF, Tacker WA, Paris RJ, et al. Cardiopulmonary resuscitation with simultaneous compression and ventilation at higher airway pressure in four animal models. *Crit Care Med* 1982;10:501–504.
16. Redding JS, Haines RR, Thomas JD. "Old" and "new" CPR manually performed in dogs. *Crit Care Med* 1981;9:386–387.
17. Redding JS. Abdominal compression in cardiopulmonary resuscitation. *Anesth Analg* 1971;50:668–675.
18. Sanders AB, Ewy GA, Alverness C, et al. Failure of one method of simultaneous chest compression, ventilation, and abdominal binding during cardiopulmonary resuscitation. *Crit Care Med* 1982;10:509–513.
19. Krischer JP, Fine EG, Weisfeldt ML, et al. Comparison of prehospital conventional and simultaneous compression–ventilation cardiopulmonary resuscitation. *Crit Care Med* 1989;17:1263–1269.
20. Olsen CO, Tyson GS, Maier GW, et al. Diminished stroke volume during inspiration: a reverse thoracic pump. *Circulation* 1985;72:668–679.
21. Deshmukh HG, Weil MH, Rackow EC. Echocardiographic observations during cardiopulmonary resuscitation: a preliminary report. *Crit Care Med* 1985;13:904–906.
22. Feneley MP, Maier GW, Jaynor JW, et al. Sequence of mitral valve motion in transmitral blood flow during manual cardiopulmonary resuscitation in dogs. *Circulation* 1987;76:363–375.
23. Higano ST, Oh JK, Ewy GA, et al. The mechanism of blood flow during closed chest cardiac massage in humans: transesophageal echocardiographic observations. *Mayo Clin Proc* 1990;65:1432–1440.
24. Raessler KL, Kern KB, Sanders AB, et al. Aortic and right atrial systolic pressures as an indicator of the mechanism of blood flow during CPR. *Am Heart J* 1988;115:1021–1029.
25. Rudikoff MT, Maughan WL, Effron M, et al. Mechanism of blood flow during cardiopulmonary resuscitation. *Circulation* 1980;61:345–352.
26. Gazmuri RJ, Becker J. Cardiac resuscitation: the search for hemodynamically more effective methods. *Chest* 1997;111:712–723.
27. Ralston SH, Voorhees WD, Babbs CF. Intrapulmonary epinephrine during prolonged cardiopulmonary resuscitation: improved regional blood flow and resuscitation in dogs. *Ann Emerg Med* 1984;13:79–86.
28. Michael JR, Guerci AD, Koehler RC, et al. Mechanism by which epinephrine augments cerebral and myocardial perfusion during cardiopulmonary resuscitation in dogs. *Circulation* 1984;69:822–835.
29. Halperin HR, Tsitlik JE, Guerci AD, et al. Determinants of blood flow to vital organs during cardiopulmonary resuscitation in dogs. *Circulation* 1986;73:539–550.
30. Crile G, Dolley DH. Experimental research into resuscitation of dogs killed by anesthetics and asphyxia. *J Exp Med* 1906;8:713–738.
31. Redding JS, Pearson JW. Evaluation of drugs for cardiac resuscitation. *Anesthesiology* 1963;24:203–207.
32. Pearson JW, Redding JS. Influence of peripheral vascular tone on cardiac resuscitation. *Anesth Analg* 1976;44:746–752.
33. Redding JS, Pearson JW. Resuscitation from ventricular fibrillation. *JAMA* 1968;203:255–260.

34. Yakaitis RW, Otto CW, Blitt CD. Relative importance of alpha and beta adrenergic receptors during resuscitation. *Crit Care Med* 1979;7:293–296.

35. Otto CW, Yakaitis RW, Blitt CD. Mechanism of action of epinephrine and resuscitation from asphyxia arrest. *Crit Care Med* 1981;9:364–366.

36. Otto CW, Yakaitis RW, Redding JS, et al. Comparison of dopamine, dobutamine, and epinephrine in CPR. *Crit Care Med* 1981;9:366.

37. Voorhees WD, Babbs CF, Tacker WA. Regional blood flow during cardiopulmonary resuscitation in dogs. *Crit Care Med* 1980;8:134–136.

38. Niemann JT, Rosborough JP, Ung S, et al. Coronary perfusion pressure during experimental cardiopulmonary resuscitation. *Ann Emerg Med* 1982;11:127–131.

39. Ditchey RV, Winkler JV, Rhodes CA. Relative lack of coronary blood flow during closed-chest resuscitation in dogs. *Circulation* 1982;66:297–302.

40. Niemann JT, Rosborough JP, Niskanen RA, et al. Mechanical "cough" cardiopulmonary resuscitation during cardiac arrest in dogs. *Am J Cardiol* 1985;55:199–204.

41. Idris AH, Becker LB, Ornato JP, et al. Utstein-style guidelines for uniform reporting of laboratory CPR research. *Circulation* 1996;94: 2324–2336.

42. Berg RA, Sanders AB, Kern KB, et al. Adverse hemodynamic effects of interrupting chest compressions for rescue breathing during cardiopulmonary resuscitation for ventricular fibrillation cardiac arrest. *Circulation* 2001;104:2465–2470.

43. Kern KB, Hilwig RW, Berg RA, et al. Efficacy of chest compression-only BLS CPR in the presence of an occluded airway. *Resuscitation* 1998;39:179–188.

44. Schleien CL, Dean JM, Koehler RC, et al. Effect of epinephrine on cerebral and myocardial perfusion in an infant animal preparation of cardiopulmonary resuscitation. *Circulation* 1986;73:809–817.

45. Kern KB, Hilwig R, Ewy GA. Retrograde coronary blood flow during cardiopulmonary resuscitation in swine: intracoronary Doppler evaluation. *Am Heart J* 1994;128:490–499.

46. Kern KB, Lancaster L, Goldman S, et al. The effect of coronary artery lesions on the relationship between coronary perfusion pressure and myocardial flow during cardiopulmonary resuscitation in pigs. *Am Heart J* 1990;120:324–333.

47. Taylor RB, Brown CG, Bridges T, et al. A model for regional blood flow measurements during cardiopulmonary resuscitation in a swine model. *Resuscitation* 1988;16:107–118.

48. Kern KB, Ewy GA. Minimal coronary stenoses and left ventricular blood flow during CPR. *Ann Emerg Med* 1992;21:1066–1072.

49. Sharff JA, Pantley G, Noel E. Effect of time on regional organ perfusion during two methods of cardiopulmonary resuscitation. *Ann Emerg Med* 1984;13:649–656.

50. Duggal C, Weil MH, Tang W, et al. Effect of arrest time on the hemodynamic efficacy of precordial compression. *Crit Care Med* 1995;23:1233–1236.

51. Kern KB, Sanders AB, Badylak SF, et al. Long term survival with open-chest cardiac massage after ineffective closed-chest compression in a canine model. *Circulation* 1987;75:498–503.

52. Sanders AB, Ogle M, Ewy GA. Coronary perfusion pressure during cardiopulmonary resuscitation. *Am J Emerg Med* 1985;3:11–14.

53. McDonald JL. Effect of interposed abdominal compression during CPR on central arterial and venous pressures. *Am J Emerg Med* 1985;3:156–159.

54. Martin GB, Garden DL, Nowak RM, et al. Aortic and right atrial pressures during standard and simultaneous compression and ventilation CPR in human beings. *Ann Emerg Med* 1986;15:125–130.

55. Howard M, Carrubba C, Foss F, et al. Interposed abdominal compressions CPR: its effects on parameters of coronary perfusion in human subjects. *Ann Emerg Med* 1987;16:253–259.

56. Swenson RD, Weaver WD, Niskanen RA, et al. Hemodynamics in humans during conventional and experimental methods of cardiopulmonary resuscitation. *Circulation* 1988;78:630–639.

57. Lewinter JR, Carden DL, Nowak RM, et al. CPR dependent consciousness: evidence for cardiac compression causing forward flow. *Ann Emerg Med* 1989;18:1111–1115.

58. Paradis NA, Martin GB, Goetting MG, et al. Simultaneous aortic, jugular bulb, and right atrial pressures during cardiopulmonary resuscitation in humans. *Circulation* 1989;80:361–368.

59. Paradis NA, Martin GB, Rivers EP, et al. Coronary perfusion pressure and return of spontaneous circulation in human cardiopulmonary resuscitation. *JAMA* 1990;263:1106–1113.

60. Halperin HR, Tsitlik JE, Gelfand M, et al. A preliminary study of cardiopulmonary resuscitation by circumferential compression of the chest with use of a pneumatic vest. *N Engl J Med* 1993;329: 762–768.

61. Timerman S, Cardoso LF, Ramires JAF, et al. Improved hemodynamic performance with a novel chest compression device during treatment of in-hospital cardiac arrest. *Resuscitation* 2004;63: 273–280.

62. Cerchiari EL, Safar P, Klein E, et al. The cardiovascular postresuscitation syndrome. *Resuscitation* 1993;25:9–33.

63. Tang W, Weil MH, Sun S, et al. Progressive myocardial dysfunction after cardiac resuscitation. *Crit Care Med* 1993;21: 1046–1050.

64. Gazmuri RJ, Weil MH, Bisera J, et al. Myocardial dysfunction after successful resuscitation from cardiac arrest. *Crit Care Med* 1996;24:992–1000.

65. Kern KB, Hilwig RW, Rhee KH, et al. Myocardial dysfunction after resuscitation from cardiac arrest: An example of global myocardial stunning. *J Am Coll Cardiol* 1996;28:232–240.

66. Ascher EK, Stauffer JCE, Gaasch WH. Coronary artery spasm, cardiac arrest, transient electrocardiographic Q waves and stunned myocardium in cocaine-associated acute myocardial infarction. *Am J Cardiol* 1988;61:939–941.

67. Deantonio HJ, Kaul S, Lerman BB. Reversible myocardial depression in survivors of cardiac arrest. *PACE* 1990;13:982–985.

68. Bashir R, Padder FA, Khan FA. Myocardial stunning following respiratory arrest. *Chest* 1995;108:1459–1460.

69. Laurent I, Spaulding C, Monchi M, et al. Transient shock after successful resuscitation: clinical evidence for post-cardiac arrest myocardial stunning. *J Am Coll Cardiol* 2000;35(Suppl A):399A.

70. Tang W, Weil MH, Sun S, et al. Epinephrine increases the severity of postresuscitation myocardial dysfunction. *Circulation* 1995;92:3089–3093.

71. Sun S, Weil MH, Tang W, et al. Combined effects of buffer and adrenergic agents on postresuscitation myocardial function. *J Pharm Exp Ther* 1999;291:773–777.

72. Xie J, Weil MH, Sun S, et al. High-energy defibrillation increases the severity of postresuscitation myocardial dysfunction. *Circulation* 1997;96:683–688.

73. Tang W, Weil MH, Sun S, et al. The effects of biphasic and conventional monophasic defibrillation on post resuscitation myocardial dysfunction. *J Am Coll Cardiol* 1999;34:815–822.

74. Tang W, Weil MH, Sun S. Low energy biphasic waveform defibrillation reduces the severity of post resuscitation myocardial dysfunction. *Crit Care Med* 2000;(suppl):28:N222–N224.

75. LeJemtel TH, Katz SD, Scortichini D. Myocardial contractility and the effects of dobutamine on cardiac pump function. In: Chatterjee K, ed. *Dobutamine: A Ten-Year Review*. Indianapolis, IN: Eli Lilly, 1989:69–79.

76. Kern KB, Hilwig RW, Berg RA, et al. Postresuscitation left ventricular systolic and diastolic dysfunction: Treatment with dobutamine. *Circulation* 1997;95:2610–2613.

77. Tang W, Weil MH, Sun S, et al. K_{ATP} channel activation reduces the severity of postresuscitation myocardial dysfunction. *Am J Physiol Heart Circ Physiol* 2000;279:H1609–H1615.

78. Kamohara T, Weil MH, Tang W, et al. Improved function and survival after administration of 21-aminosteroids during CPR (abstract). *Circulation* 2000;102:II-571.

Chapter 10
Circulatory Adjuncts to Improve Coronary Perfusion Pressure

Karl B. Kern

Standard cardiopulmonary resuscitation (CPR) alone often fails to produce enough coronary perfusion pressure for successful resuscitation. The difficulty of achieving optimal coronary perfusion pressure and the early onset of rescuer fatigue with standard manual CPR has been a strong motivation for the development of numerous circulatory adjuncts in hope of achieving greater coronary perfusion pressures.

- ■ Rescuer fatigue and implications for successful resuscitation outcome
- ■ Circulatory adjuncts and CPR alternatives as methods and strategies to optimize coronary perfusion pressure (CPP) during prolonged CPR
- ■ Any interruption in effective chest compression decreases the chance for survival; pauses and interruptions in chest compressions should be minimized, e.g., time for defibrillation, rhythm, and pulse checks.

Improving Coronary Perfusion Pressure: Use of Circulatory Adjuncts

CPP correlates with myocardial blood flow and myocardial blood flow correlates with resuscitation success; hence the greater the CPP, the more likely a successful outcome. However, standard CPR alone often fails to produce enough CPP for successful resuscitation. Increasing the force of manual chest compressions to produce greater CPP is not without potential problems (Fig. 10-1). The use of excessive force in chest compressions may result in severe and even life-threatening injury. In an animal model (without coronary lesions) of cardiac arrest, a myocardial perfusion pressure of 30 mm Hg appears to be ideal for ensuring long-term survival without a high degree of CPR injury. More forceful chest compressions to increase perfusion pressure above 30 mm Hg resulted in CPR-induced trauma and a reduced rate of 24-hour survival.[1] In this series, animals that died from CPR-induced injury had a mean perfusion pressure of 39 mm Hg, whereas those that survived for 24 hours had a mean perfusion pressure of 29 mm Hg. These results suggest that CPP measured during CPR may not only be useful as a guide to predict successful defibrillation and return of spontaneous circulation but can also be used to avoid unnecessary injury when optimal levels have already been achieved.

Although effective or good CPR is associated with a better outcome, the ability to perform such CPR appears to be time-dependent, i.e., the longer CPR is performed, the less likely it is that compressions will remain effective in terms of sternal displacement or rate per minute. This phenomenon has been demonstrated in a number of CPR manikins, where recordings of the chest compression rate and depth are obtained.[2–5] A study by Ochoa et al. perhaps demonstrates this time effect most dramatically.[3] These authors evaluated the influence of rescuer fatigue on the quality of chest compressions and the influence of gender, age, weight, and height on the reduction of quality CPR. Thirty-eight health care professionals performed chest compressions on a recording manikin for 5 consecutive minutes. A marked decline in depth of sternal displacement was observed as early as the second minute of the trial, and the mean time to fatigue, as verbalized by the participants, was just over 3 minutes.

The difficulty of achieving optimal CPP and the early onset of rescuer fatigue with standard manual CPR has been a strong motivation for the development of numerous circulatory adjuncts in the hope of achieving greater CPPs and thereby improved outcome with resuscitation efforts.

Interposed Abdominal Compression CPR

Interposed abdominal compression CPR (IAC-CPR) is a method of manual basic life support where abdominal

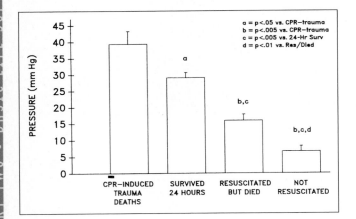

FIGURE 10-1 • Mean coronary perfusion pressure during CPR for those not resuscitated, resuscitated but not surviving, 24-hour survivors, and those suffering CPR-induced traumatic deaths. Note that the highest CPPs were among those suffering the traumatic injuries. (From Kern KB, Ewy GA, Voorhees WD, et al. *Resuscitation* 1988;16:246, with permission. © Elsevier 1988.)

pressure is applied over the midabdomen (midway between the xiphoid process and the umbilicus) with two hands from a second rescuer during the relaxation phase of chest compressions (Fig. 10-2). Investigators at Purdue University reported the hemodynamic advantages of intermittent abdominal compression during CPR.[6] Follow-up studies at Purdue verified improvement in CPP with the use of interposed abdominal compression CPR.[7] Two other reports examined the use of this

form of CPR in experimental models, one of which did not find improvement[8] and one of which did.[9] Three clinical reports have been published concerning the use of IAC-CPR in human subjects where coronary perfusion was measured. One patient reportedly had an increase in CPP.[10] In a separate series, 6 patients had no significant increase[11] and, in the largest series of 14 patients, IAC had inconsistent effects on the CPP.[12] Despite these hemodynamic inconsistencies, four clinical trials[13] comparing IAC-CPR and standard CPR demonstrated greater rates of initial successful resuscitation and a trend toward an increased survival rate to hospital discharge in the IAC-CPR group, including two in-hospital randomized trials.[14,15] The first found statistically greater rates of return of spontaneous circulation (ROSC), 24-hour survival, and survival to discharge in 48 of 103 patients randomized to IAC-CPR compared with standard CPR.[14] The other trial (from the same investigators and institution) found significantly more ROSC and 24-hour survival with IAC-CPR compared with standard CPR in patients with initial rhythms of asystole or pulseless electrical activity during their in-hospital cardiac arrests.[15] Pooled data from these two separate randomized trials showed a 24-hour survival benefit for IAC-CPR (33% vs. 13%). One pediatric case report[16] described intra-abdominal trauma, but none of the adult trials have found an increased incidence of CPR-induced trauma. Per the recommendations from International Liaison Committee on Resuscitation (ILCOR), IAC-CPR may be considered for in-hospital resuscitations when sufficient trained personnel are available (class IIb), but there is no convincing evidence that it is superior for out-of-hospital resuscitation; it is therefore not recommended for in that setting.

High-Frequency (Rapid Compression Rate) CPR

Whether done manually or mechanically, rapid chest compressions (>100/min) can improve CPP and other measures of resuscitation hemodynamics.[17–19] However, no clinical studies have shown improved outcome with this technique. Currently this alternative CPR method is given a class indeterminate rating by ILCOR.

Mechanical Piston Devices

Mechanical piston devices typically compress the sternum by a gas-powered piston, the prototype being the Thumper (Fig. 10-3). Experimental studies examining resuscitation hemodynamics achieved with such mechanical piston devices have found mixed results.[20,21] One prospective randomized clinical trial and two crossover-design clinical trials have found increased end-tidal carbon dioxide or mean arterial pressure compared to standard manual CPR.[20,22,23] The recognized advantage of such devices is in sustaining resuscitation efforts where manual chest compressions may not

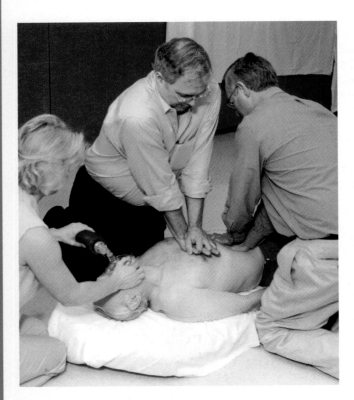

FIGURE 10-2 • Multirescuer performance of interposed abdominal compression (IAC) CPR.

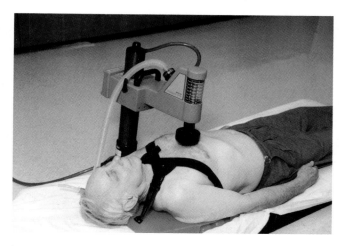

FIGURE 10-3 • Mechanical piston (Thumper) CPR.

be feasible, i.e., during transport, etc. (the ILCOR recommendation for such an indication is IIb). No long-term survival benefit had yet been shown.

LUCAS CPR

Another mechanical piston variation, the Lund University Cardiopulmonary Assist System (LUCAS), is also currently being evaluated. This device incorporates a gas-driven piston combined with active decompression (Fig. 10-4).

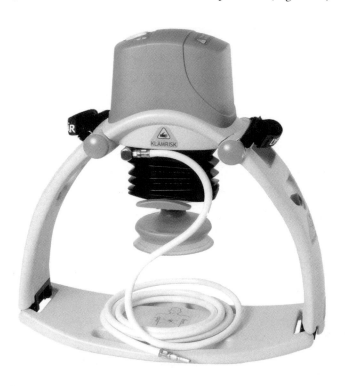

FIGURE 10-4 • LUCAS mechanical CPR device (Jolife AB; distributed by Medtronic).

LUCAS CPR produces greater perfusion pressures and resuscitation rates in experimental animals than a standard, commercially available pneumatic piston device.[24] Numerous case reports suggest that this device can support adequate circulation during cardiac arrest for substantial periods.[25,26] Like the load distributing board (LDB), LUCAS CPR has not been evaluated by ILCOR to date.

Simultaneous Ventilation–Compression CPR

Based on the theory of the thoracic pump generating blood flow during resuscitation efforts, this technique was found to provide increased peak aortic pressures ("systolic") and carotid blood flows.[27] It is performed using an altered Thumper mechanical compressor and ventilator, where each time the piston compresses the chest, a simultaneous ventilation is also administered. Experimental evidence was mixed,[27,28] and in an out-of-hospital study in Dade County, Florida, SVC-CPR failed to improve outcome; indeed, outcome was worse than with standard CPR (hospital discharge: 49 of 337 or 14.5% in the control group and 28 of 365 or 7.7% in the SVC-CPR group; P <0.001).[29] This alternative form of CPR is not currently recommended.

Active Compression–Decompression CPR

Active compression–decompression CPR (ACD-CPR) uses a handheld "suction cup" device applied to the anterior sternum. ACD-CPR pulls the anterior chest outward during the relaxation or release phase of chest compressions (Fig. 10-5). In contrast, standard CPR allows passive thoracic recoil

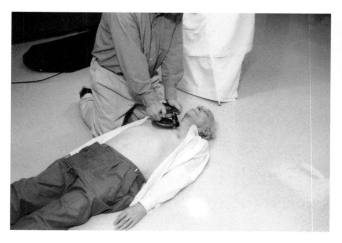

FIGURE 10-5 • Active compression-decompression (ACD) CPR with CardioPump (Ambu Inc.).

between compressions. The active "diastolic" component of ACD-CPR generates an increased negative intrathoracic pressure resulting in a lower diastolic right atrial pressure and a greater CPP.[30] Several reports in experimental models have shown improved diastolic or relaxation-phase CPP with the use of active compression–decompression CPR when compared to standard CPR.[31] Clinical trials with this device have shown conflicting results regarding outcome benefits when compared with standard CPR. The most positive results were seen in Paris, where 1-year survival rates were significantly better with ACD-CPR (17 of 373, or 5%) than with standard CPR (7 of 377, or 2%).[32] Another clinical trial, in Canada,[33] did not show such a benefit. A meta-analysis of 12 clinical trials (n = 4,165 out-of-hospital patients and n = 826 in-hospital patients) failed to show any survival benefit for ACD-CPR.[34] Rigorous training and frequent changing of rescuers when performing ACD-CPR are important factors in achieving good results with this alternative resuscitation technique. Some studies have shown an increase in rib fractures with this technique. ILCOR has given this alternative technique the same IIb recommendation as that given to IAC-CPR.

Impedance Threshold Valve

The impedance threshold valve (ITV) is a true adjunct rather than alternative form of CPR. It can be used with standard CPR or a variety of the other alternative forms listed in this section. A majority of the experimental work with this valve has occurred in combination with ACD-CPR or standard CPR. This valve limits air entry back into the lungs during chest recoil, thereby increasing the negative thoracic pressure within the thorax and theoretically increasing venous return (Fig. 10-6).[30] The valve has been modified through time and now is called the ResQ POD. It has been studied attached to the end to an endotracheal tube but also with a bag-valve face mask.[35–37] Experimental studies have shown improved hemodynamics, blood flows, and outcomes.[38] Two randomized trials of out-of-hospital cardiac arrest victims (n = 610) compared ACD-CPR plus the ITV versus standard CPR and found improved ROSC and 24-hour survival rates.[39,40] One out-of-hospital study in humans (n = 230) combining the ITV with standard CPR showed improved systolic pressures but not CPPs; however, it did result in improved rates of admission to hospital for those with pulseless electrical activity.[17,41] This adjunct has been given the highest recommendation (IIa) by ILCOR for improving hemodynamics and short-term survival.

Vest CPR and Load-Distributing-Band CPR

Circumferential compression of the thorax with an inflatable vest-like garment was described in the 1980s and tested in small, selected clinical populations in the late 1980s and

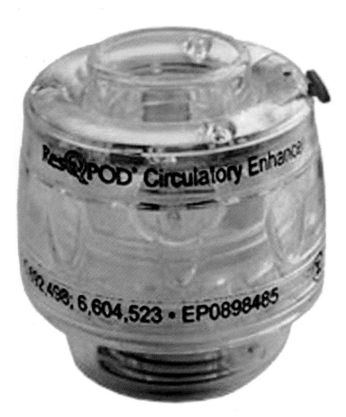

FIGURE 10-6 • Latest rendition of the impedance threshold valve (ITV, now called the ResQ. Pod.)

early 1990s.[17,42] This device was designed to maximally exploit the concept of a "thoracic pump" as the driving force for blood flow during chest compressions. Vest CPR has increased CPP in experimental cardiac arrest models and in patients. However, the device was logistically difficult to incorporate into clinical resuscitation owing to the size of the power source. Based upon the success seen with the circumferential vest but realizing the need for a more compact power source, redesign and experimentation led to substantial revisions and reintroduction of a thoracic compression band device (AutoPulse, Revivant Inc., Sunnyvale, CA). The load-distributing band (LDB) is a semicircumferential chest-compression device composed of a pneumatically actuated constricting band and backboard (Fig. 10-7). The band, applied over the anterior chest, is rhythmically tightened and released, resulting in a decrease in thoracic dimension or size of about 20%. Experimental animal and clinical studies indicate that the device produces greater CPPs than those measured during chest compression performed with a mechanical, pneumatic piston device.[1,43] An early clinical trial demonstrated a greater rate of return of spontaneous circulation treated with the device when compared with a historical control group who received conventional, manual CPR.[44] Two recent clinical trials have found opposite results. An out-of-hospital randomized trial found no significant difference in the primary endpoint of survival to 4 hours (158 of 554, or 28.5%, with the LDB versus 153 of 517, or 29.5%; P = 0.74), but survival to discharge was 32 of 554 (5.8%, versus 51 of 517, or 9.9%; P = 0.06) and the study was

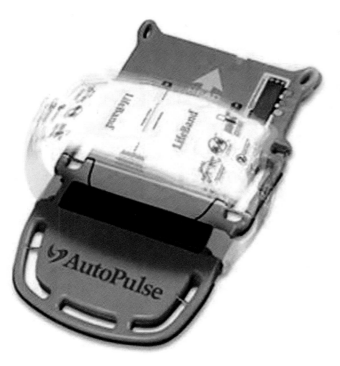

| FIGURE 10-7 • Auto pulse mechanical CPR device (Zoll Medical).

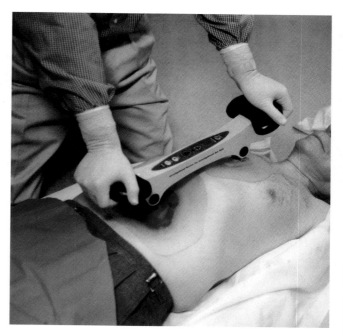

| FIGURE 10-8 • Phased thoracic-abdominal compression-decompression CPR device (prototype: LifeStick, Datascope Inc.).

stopped prematurely by the data and safety monitoring board for safety concerns.[45] A concurrently published "before and after" (nonrandomized) clinical trial found substantially increased rates of survival to discharge compared with standard CPR (28 of 284, or 9.7%, versus 14 of 499, or 2.9%; adjusted OR = 2.27).[46] This technology has not been formally evaluated by ILCOR.

Phased Thoracic-Abdominal Compression–Decompression CPR

Phased thoracic–abdominal compression–decompression (PTACD) CPR combines the concepts of interposed abdominal counterpulsation (IAC–CPR) and active compression–decompression (ACD-CPR). Using a single rescuer handheld device with adherent pads over the chest and abdomen, one performs a somewhat rocking motion, which compresses the chest while actively decompressing the abdomen; then it compresses the abdomen while actively decompressing the chest (Fig. 10-8). One experimental study has shown improved hemodynamics, including CPP, compared with standard CPR,[47] and another showed that a 5:1 ratio of compression to ventilation optimized PTACD-CPR.[48] Only one clinical report has been completed to date, and it also showed improved hemodynamics with PTACD-CPR.[49] No formal evaluation has yet been done by ILCOR.

Open-Chest CPR

Open-chest cardiac massage (OCCM) or invasive CPR has probably the most data of all these circulatory adjuncts and has shown the greatest ability to improve CPP.[50] Numerous studies have shown improvement in hemodynamics, specifically CPP, with the institution of open-chest cardiac massage.[51–56] Typically these increases are not merely the improvements of 10 or 15 mm Hg reported with other adjuncts but as much as 40 to 50 mm Hg!

A particularly clinically relevant investigation of open-chest resuscitation illustrated how and when such should be considered after failure of closed-chest resuscitation efforts.[53] Invasive forms of resuscitation often have dramatic effects on CPP; but, because of morbidity associated with an invasive approach, these treatment options are often instituted late in the course of resuscitation. In this experimental model with closed-chest CPR efforts for periods varying between 15 and 25 minutes, Sanders et al. found that aggressive intervention with open-chest cardiac massage could improve CPP substantially above that achieved with continued closed-chest compressions, but successful resuscitation was not achieved if such therapy was instituted beyond 15 minutes of cardiac arrest. These data indicate that improvements in CPP may not translate into improved survival if they come too late in the course of resuscitation therapy.

In another series of experimental animals undergoing open-chest cardiac massage after a limited period of ineffective closed-chest compressions, tremendous improvements in mean CPP were seen compared with continued closed-chest efforts (65 vs. 19 mm Hg). The animals that had improved CPP during CPR were not only resuscitated more easily and survived 24 hours but also had a better rate of 7-day survival.[51] Thus it appears that even during a relatively short period of CPR, CPP can be used to predict long-term 7-day survival. Clinical trials of OCCM have shown that when it is instituted after 30 minutes of unsuccessful closed-chest compressions, it does not improve outcome.[57] But in another human study where OCCM was applied earlier, it did improve both CPP and ROSC.[58] ILCOR recommends OCCM for penetrating chest trauma associated with cardiac arrest and if considered after a period of limited (<15 minutes) unsuccessful closed chest efforts, but not as a "last-ditch effort."

Other Invasive Circulatory Adjuncts

Partial Cardiopulmonary Bypass

Several other alternative invasive circulatory adjuncts exist that do not require a full thoracotomy. Most studied is "femorofemoral" bypass. This emergency device consists of a cardiopulmonary bypass machine that can be rapidly inserted using femoral artery and femoral vein access. The venous catheter must still be placed at the inferior vena cava–right atrium junction, but the procedure does not require opening the thorax. Animal models of cardiac arrest have shown improved hemodynamics and survival with the use of cardiopulmonary bypass, but most have not included the difficulty of insertion in their protocols.[59–62] Numerous case reports and several small series of nonrandomized experience have been reported.[63–65] Some refractory cardiac arrests have been successfully treated with such a device, but most commonly these result from catastrophic complications in the catheterization suite, where, if the patient is stabilized, definitive treatment can be accomplished (i.e., coronary artery bypass surgery) with good long-term results.[66–76] Some have suggested the use of such devices in the emergency department for refractory cardiac arrest, but there the long-term results are less encouraging.[68] There is a growing interest in similar "rescue" application of extracorporeal membrane circulation (ECMO).[69]

Minimally Invasive Direct Cardiac Massage

Another alternative is "minimally invasive direct cardiac massage," where, through a fifth intercostal anterior axillary line thoracostomy incision, a collapsible umbrella-like device is inserted directly to the pericardial surface (Fig. 10-9A). The umbrella is then opened and rhythmic direct

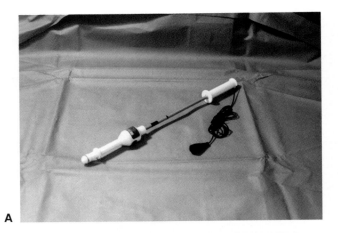

A

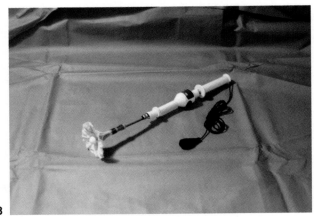

B

FIGURE 10-9 • **A.** Minimally invasive direct cardiac massage device in the insertion configuration. **B.** Minimally invasive direct cardiac massage device in the pumping configuration, with the collapsible umbrella opened, and as it would appear against the epicardial surface of the heart.

compressions of the heart are performed (Fig. 10-9B). Experimental studies have shown improved CPP and cerebral blood flows with this approach compared with standard CPR.[70] A limited clinical series from out-of-hospital cardiac arrests treated by ambulances staffed by physicians found improved resuscitation-generated hemodynamics as well.[71] A randomized clinical trial for out-of-hospital cardiac arrest was unfortunately prematurely halted for lack of funding.

Balloon Occlusion of the Aorta

Finally, balloon occlusion of the aorta (using an inflated intra-aortic balloon pump, or IABP) has shown improved hemodynamics in both experimental models and limited clinical case reports.[72,73] Insertion of an IABP after cardiac arrest occurs is not recommended, but if such a device is already in place, the balloon can be inflated and left inflated during the resuscitation efforts in order to improve myocardial and cerebral perfusion.

References

1. Kern KB, Ewy GA, Voorhees WD, et al. Myocardial perfusion pressure: a predictor of 24-hour survival during prolonged cardiac arrest in dogs. *Resuscitation* 1988;16:241–250.
2. Hightower D, Thomas SH, Stone CK, et al. Decay in quality of closed-chest compressions over time. *Ann Emerg Med* 1995;26:300–303.
3. Ochoa FJ, Ramalle-Gomara E, Lisa V, et al. The effect of rescuer fatigue on the quality of chest compressions. *Resuscitation* 1998;37:149–152.
4. Ashton A, McClusky A, Gwinnutt CL, et al. Effect of rescuer fatigue on performance of continuous external chest compressions over 3 min. *Resuscitation* 2002;55:151–155.
5. Baubin M, Schirmer M, Nogler M, et al. Rescuer's work capacity and duration of cardiopulmonary resuscitation. *Resuscitation* 1996;33:135–139.
6. Ralston SH, Babbs CF, Niebauer MJ. Cardiopulmonary resuscitation with interposed abdominal compression in dogs. *Anesth Analg* 1982;61:645–651.
7. Voorhees WD, Niebauer MJ, Babbs CF. Improved oxygen delivery during cardiopulmonary resuscitation with interposed abdominal compressions. *Ann Emerg Med* 1983;12:128–135.
8. Kern KB, Carter AB, Showen RL, et al. Twenty-four hour survival in a canine model of cardiac arrest comparing three methods of manual cardiopulmonary resuscitation. *J Am Coll Cardiol* 1986;7:859–867.
9. Lindner KH, Ahnefeld FW, Bowdler IM. Cardiopulmonary resuscitation with interposed abdominal compression after asphyxia or fibrillatory cardiac arrest in pigs. *Anesthesiology* 1990;72:675–681.
10. Berryman CR, Phillips GM. Interposed abdominal compression CPR in human subjects. *Ann Emerg Med* 1984;13:226–229.
11. McDonald JL. Effect of interposed abdominal compression during CPR on central arterial and venous pressures. *Am J Emerg Med* 1985;3:156–159.
12. Howard M, Carrubba C, Foss F, et al. Interposed abdominal compressions CPR: its effects on parameters of coronary perfusion in human subjects. *Ann Emerg Med* 1987;16:253–259.
13. Babbs CF. Interposed abdominal compression CPR: a comprehensive evidence based review. *Resuscitation* 2003;59:71–82.
14. Sack JB, Kesselbrenner MB, Bregman D. Survival from in-hospital cardiac arrest with interposed abdominal compression during cardiopulmonary resuscitation. *JAMA* 1992;267:379–385.
15. Sack JB, Kesselbrenner MB, Jarrad A. Interposed abdominal compression–cardiopulmonary resuscitation and resuscitation outcome during asystole and electromechanical dissociation. *Circulation* 1992;86:1692–1700.
16. Waldman PJ, Walters BL, Grunau CF. Pancreatic injury associated with interposed abdominal compressions in pediatric cardiopulmonary resuscitation. *Am J Emerg Med* 1984;2:143–146.
17. Lewinter JR, Carden DL, Nowak RM, et al. CPR dependent consciousness: evidence for cardiac compression causing forward flow. *Ann Emerg Med* 1989;18:1111–1115.
18. Kern KB, Sanders AB, Raife J, et al. A study of chest compression rates during cardiopulmonary resuscitation in humans: the importance of rate-directed chest compressions. *Arch Intern Med* 1992;152:146–149.
19. Ornato JP, Gonzalez ER, Garnett AR, et al. Effect of cardiopulmonary resuscitation compression rate on end-tidal carbon dioxide concentration and arterial pressure in man. *Crit Care Med* 1988;16:241–245.
20. McDonald JL. Systolic and mean arterial pressure during manual and mechanical CPR in humans. *Crit Care Med* 1981;9:382–383.
21. Kern KB, Carter AB, Showen RL, et al. Comparison of mechanical techniques of cardiopulmonary resuscitation: survival and neurological outcome in dogs. *Am J Emerg Med* 1987;5:190–195. [Published erratum in *Am J Emerg Med* 1987;5:304]
22. Dickinson ET, Verdile VP, Schneider RM, et al. Effectiveness of mechanical versus manual chest compressions in out-of-hospital cardiac arrest resuscitation: a pilot study. *Am J Emerg Med* 1998;16:289–292.
23. Ward KR, Menegazzi JJ, Zelenak RR, et al. A comparison of chest compressions between mechanical and manual CPR by monitoring end-tidal PCO2 during human cardiac arrest. *Ann Emerg Med* 1993;22:669–674.
24. Steen S, Liao Q, Pierre L, et al. Evaluation of LUCAS, a new device for automatic mechanical compression and active decompression resuscitation. *Resuscitation* 2002;55:285–299.
25. Holmstrom P, Boyd J, Sorsa M, et al. A case of hypothermic cardiac arrest treated with an external chest compression device (LUCAS) during transport to re-warming. *Resuscitation* 2005;67:139–141.
26. Wik L, Kiil S. Use of an automatic chest compression device (LUCAS) as a bridge to establishing cardiopulmonary bypass for a patient with hypothermic cardiac arrest. *Resuscitation* 2005;66:391–394.
27. Chandra N, Weisfeldt ML, Tsitlik JE, et al. Augmentation of carotid flow during cardiopulmonary resuscitation (CPR) in the dog by simultaneous compression and ventilation with high airway pressure. *Am J Cardiol* 1979;48:1053–1063.
28. Sanders AB, Ewy GA, Alverness C, et al. Failure of one method of simultaneous chest compression, ventilation, and abdominal binding during cardiopulmonary resuscitation. *Crit Care Med* 1982;10:509–513.
29. Krischer JP, Fine EG, Weisfeldt ML, et al. Comparison of prehospital conventional and simultaneous compression–ventilation cardiopulmonary resuscitation. *Crit Care Med* 1989;17:1263–1269.
30. Lurie K. Mechanical devices for cardiopulmonary resuscitation. An update. *Emerg Med Clin North Am* 2002;20:771–784.
31. Mauer D, Wolcke B, Dick W. Alternative methods of mechanical cardiopulmonary resuscitation. *Resuscitation* 2000;44:81–85.
32. Plaisance P, Lurie KG, Vicaut E, et al. A comparison of standard cardiopulmonary resuscitation and active compression–decompression resuscitation for out-of-hospital cardiac arrest. French Active Compression–Decompression Cardiopulmonary Resuscitation Study Group. *N Engl J Med* 1999;341:569–575.
33. Steill I, H'ebert P, Well G, et al. The Ontario trial of active compression–decompression cardiopulmonary resuscitation for in-hospital and prehospital cardiac arrest. *JAMA* 1996;275:1417–1423.
34. Lafuente-Laufente C, Melero-Bascones M. Active chest compression–decompression for cardiopulmonary resuscitation. *Cochrane Database Syst Rev* 2004;CD002751.
35. Plaisance P, Lurie KG, Payen D. Inspiratory impedance during active-compression–decompression cardiopulmonary resuscitation: a randomized evaluation in patients in cardiac arrest. *Circulation* 2000;101:989–994.
36. Plaisance P, Soleil C, Lurie KG, et al. Use of an inspiratory impedance threshold device on a face mask and endotracheal tube to reduce intrathoracic pressures during the decompression phase of active-decompression cardiopulmonary resuscitation. *Crit Care Med* 2005;33:990–994.
37. Wolcke BB, Mauer DK, Schoefmann MF, et al. Comparison of standard cardiopulmonary resuscitation versus the combination of active compression–decompression cardiopulmonary resuscitation and an inspiratory impedance threshold device for out-of-hospital cardiac arrest. *Circulation* 2003;108:2201–2205.
38. Lurie KG, Mulligan KA, McKnite S, et al. Optimizing standard cardiopulmonary resuscitation with an inspiratory impedance valve. *Chest* 1998;113:1084–1090.
39. Plaisance P, Lurie KG, Vicaut E, et al. Evaluation of an impedance threshold device in patients receiving active compression–decompression cardiopulmonary resuscitation for out-of-hospital cardiac arrest. *Resuscitation* 2004;61:265–271.
40. Pirrallo RG, Aufdeheide TP, Provo TA, et al. Effect of an inspiratory impedance threshold device on hemodynamics during conventional manual cardiopulmonary resuscitation. *Resuscitation* 2005;66:13–20.
41. Aufderheide TP, Pirrallo RG, Provo TA, et al. Clinical evaluation of an inspiratory impedance threshold device during standard cardiopulmonary resuscitation in patients with out-of-hospital cardiac arrest. *Crit Care Med* 2005;33:734–740.
42. Timerman S, Cardoso LF, Ramires JAF, et al. Improved hemodynamic performance with a novel chest compression device during treatment of in-hospital cardiac arrest. *Resuscitation* 2004;273–280.
43. Halperin HR, Paradis N, Ornato JP, et al. Cardiopulmonary resuscitation with a novel chest compression device in a porcine model of cardiac arrest. *J Am Coll Cardiol* 2004;44:2214–2220.
44. Casner M, Andersen D, Isaacs M. The impact of a new CPR assist device on rate of return of spontaneous circulation in out-of-hospital cardiac arrest. *Prehosp Emerg Care* 2005;9:61–67.

45. Hallstrom A, Rea TD, Sayre MR, et al. Manual chest compression vs use of an automated chest compression device during resuscitation following out-of-hospital cardiac arrest. *JAMA* 2006;295:2620–2628.

46. Ong MEH, Ornato JP, Edwards DP, et al. Use of an automated, load-distributing band chest compression device for out-of-hospital cardiac arrest resuscitation. *JAMA* 2006;295:2629–2637.

47. Tang W, Weil MH, Schock RB, et al. Phased chest and abdominal compression–decompression: a new option for cardiopulmonary resuscitation. *Circulation* 1997;95:1335–1340.

48. Kern KB, Hilwig RW, Berg RA, et al. Optimizing ventilation in conjunction with phased chest and abdominal compression–decompression (Lifestick) resuscitation. *Resuscitation* 2002;52: 91–100.

49. Arntz HR, Agrawal R, Richter H, et al. Phased chest and abdominal compression–decompression versus conventional cardiopulmonary resuscitation in out-of-hospital cardiac arrest. *Circulation* 2001;104:768–772.

50. Alzaga-Fernandez AG, Varon J. Open-chest cardiopulmonary resuscitation: past, present and future. *Resuscitation* 2005;64:149–156.

51. Sanders AB, Ogle M, Ewy GA. Coronary perfusion pressure during cardiopulmonary resuscitation. *Am J Emerg Med* 1985;3:11–14.

52. Sanders AB, Kern KB, Ewy GA, et al. Improved resuscitation from cardiac arrest with open-chest massage. *Ann Emerg Med* 1984;13: 672–675.

53. Sanders AB, Kern KB, Atlas M, et al. Importance of the duration of inadequate coronary perfusion pressure on resuscitation from cardiac arrest. *J Am Coll Cardiol* 1985;6:113–118.

54. Bircher N, Safar P. Cerebral perfusion during cardiopulmonary resuscitation. *Crit Care Med* 1985;13:185–190.

55. Bircher N, Safar P, Stewart R. A comparison of standard, "MAST"-augmented and open-chest CPR in dogs. *Crit Care Med* 1980;8: 147–152.

56. Bircher N, Safar P. Manual open-chest cardiopulmonary resuscitation. *Ann Emerg Med* 1984;13:770–773.

57. Geehr EC, Lewis FR, Auerbach PS. Failure of open-heart massage to improve survival after prehospital nontraumatic cardiac arrest (letter). *N Engl J Med* 1986;314:1189–1190.

58. Takino M, Okada Y. The optimum timing of resuscitative thoracotomy for non-traumatic out-of-hospital cardiac arrest. *Resuscitation* 1993;26:69–74.

59. Martin GB, Nowak RM, Carden DL, et al. Cardiopulmonary bypass vs CPR as treatment for prolonged canine cardiopulmonary arrest. *Ann Emerg Med* 1987;16:628–636.

60. Levine R, Gorayeb M, Safar P, et al. Cardiopulmonary bypass after cardiac arrest and prolonged closed-chest CPR in dogs. *Ann Emerg Med* 1987;16:620–627.

61. Angelos MG, Gaddis ML, Gaddis GM, et al. Improved survival and reduced myocardial necrosis with cardiopulmonary bypass reperfusion in a canine model of coronary occlusion and cardiac arrest. *Ann Emerg Med* 1990;19:1122–1128.

62. Safar P, Abramson NS, Angelos M, et al. Emergency cardiopulmonary bypass for resuscitation from prolonged cardiac arrest. *Am J Emerg Med* 1990;8:55–67.

63. Hartz R, LoCicero J, Sanders AB Jr., et al. Clinical experience with portable cardiopulmonary bypass in cardiac arrest patients. *Ann Thorac Surg* 1990;50:437–441.

64. Rousou JA, Engelman RM, Flack JE III, et al. Emergency cardiopulmonary bypass in the cardiac surgical unit can be a lifesaving measure in postoperative cardiac arrest. *Circulation* 1994;90(Suppl II):280–284.

65. Martin GB, Rivers EP, Paradis NA, et al. Emergency department cardiopulmonary bypass in the treatment of human cardiac arrest. *Chest* 1998;113:743–751.

66. Shawl FA, Domanski MJ, Wish MH, et al. Emergency cardiopulmonary bypass support in patients with cardiac arrest in the catheterization laboratory. *Cathet Cardiovasc Diagn* 1990.;19:8–12.

67. Overlie PA. Emergency use of portable cardiopulmonary bypass. *Cathet Cardiovasc Diagn* 1990;20:27–31.

68. Nagao K, Hayashi N, Kanmatsuse K, et al. Cardipulmonary cerebral resuscitation using emergency cardiopulmonary bypass, coronary reperfusion therapy, and mild hypothermia in patients with cardiac arrest outside the hospital. *J Am Coll Cardiol* 2000;36:776–783.

69. Younger JG, Schreiner RJ, Swaniker F, et al. Extracorporeal resuscitation of cardiac arrest. *Acad Emerg Med* 1999;6:700–707.

70. Paiva EF, Kern KB, Hilwig RW, et al. Minimally invasive direct cardiac massage versus closed-chest cardiopulmonary resuscitation in a porcine model of prolonged ventricular fibrillation cardiac arrest. *Resuscitation* 2000;47:287–299.

71. Rozenberg A, Incagnoli P, Delpech P, et al. Prehospital use of minimally invasive direct cardiac massage (MID-CM): a pilot study. *Resuscitation* 2001;50:257–262.

72. Paradis NA, Rose MI, Gawryl MS. Selective aortic perfusion and oxygenation: an effective adjunct to external chest compression-based cardiopulmonary resuscitation. *J Am Coll Cardiol* 1994;23:497–504.

73. Tang W, Weil MH, Noc M, et al. Augmented efficacy of external CPR by intermittent occlusion of the ascending aorta. *Circulation* 1993;88:1916–1921.

74. Cerchiari EL, Safar P, Klein E, et al. The cardiovascular post-resuscitation syndrome. *Resuscitation* 1993;25:9–33.

75. Tang W, Weil MH, Sun S, et al. Progressive myocardial dysfunction after cardiac resuscitation. *Crit Care Med* 1993;21:1046–1050.

76. Gazmuri RJ, Weil MH, Bisera J, et al. Myocardial dysfunction after successful resuscitation from cardiac arrest. *Crit Care Med* 1996;24: 992–1000.

Chapter 11
Basic Life Support: Science to Survival

Michael R. Sayre and Diana M. Cave

Strong medical leadership can dramatically increase survival rate from cardiac arrest in any community. There is emerging evidence that improving basic life support (BLS) care can have a dramatic impact on survival. In almost all communities with improved out-of-hospital arrest survival, the communities and emergency medical services (EMS) systems optimized the BLS provided by their professional rescuers. Innovative strategies for delivering BLS employed now in a few communities may offer additional opportunities for further increasing survival from out-of-hospital cardiac arrest.

- Excellent BLS is essential for optimizing chances of survival.
- Advanced cardiac life support (ACLS) is effective only if high-quality CPR is consistently and continuously delivered.
- Any interruption in effective chest compression decreases the chance for survival; therefore, pauses and interruptions in chest compressions should be minimized (e.g., time for defibrillation, rhythm, and pulse checks).

Introduction and Overview of CPR

One beautiful fall afternoon, a college student left his calculus class for home. As he crossed the quad near the art building, he suddenly collapsed. Another student saw him fall and called 911. A nurse stopped and began vigorous chest compressions. A fire engine equipped with a defibrillator responded from the firehouse a mile away and was on the scene about 6 minutes after the onset of the student's ventricular fibrillation. The emergency medical technicians on the fire truck took over CPR, quickly applied the defibrillator, analyzed, gave a single shock, and immediately resumed chest compressions. Within a minute, the victim developed a pulse. He remained in a coma, was intubated, and was brought to the University Hospital emergency department, where hypothermia therapy was begun. Three days later, the 70-year-old retired engineer, college student and patient was sitting up in his hospital bed working on differential equations and waiting for placement of an implantable defibrillator.

What Is Basic Life Support?

During a resuscitation attempt, the victim's survival depends on the circulation of oxygenated blood to the brain and the heart muscle. CPR takes on the function of the heart and lungs through the delivery of external chest compression and positive-pressure ventilation.

The skills are considered "basic" in that little or no equipment is required and nearly anyone can learn them. However, "basic" does not mean unimportant. With excellent CPR, the victim's chance of survival is dramatically increased, and advanced interventions such as drug therapy will not be effective without excellent CPR.

BLS training includes essential lifesaving skills that do not require medical training for proficiency. Most BLS courses include training in the recognition of cardiac arrest, delivery of CPR for adults and children, use of an automated external defibrillator, and opening of an airway obstructed by a foreign body.

This chapter introduces the reader to the science of BLS for victims of sudden cardiac arrest. The focus of BLS is on the integration of BLS skills to enhance the emergency response system and facilitate delivery of early advanced care.

The Challenge

Common Disease

As noted in the section on the epidemiology of sudden cardiac arrest (SCA) (see Chapter 2), more than 310,000 Americans develop SCA each year in and out of the hospital. The most common initial rhythms are pulseless ventricular tachycardia (VT), with degeneration to ventricular fibrillation (VF) or primary VF. In most cases there is a delay of several minutes for help to arrive. By the time rescuers apply a defibrillator, <40% of events outside the hospital and <25% of events in the hospital will still involve VF/VT. For all patients with cardiac arrest, early effective CPR is essential.

Research Evidence Limited

Despite the large number of victims of SCA, the scientific basis for BLS interventions is largely extrapolated from animal models of cardiac arrest. Most animal studies evaluate only short-term outcomes, such as return of spontaneous circulation or survival for 60 minutes. Only a few studies measure neurologic outcome following the event, as providing intensive care to a pig is expensive.

The conduct of human studies of BLS is quite challenging. It is impossible to blind rescuers to the type of CPR they are providing, and randomization is also difficult because there is no time at the onset of the cardiac arrest to perform a randomization procedure. Thus many human research studies use a before–after design, with its attendant limitations, which include the introduction of Hawthorne effects and a need to consider the effect of evolving medical knowledge, which can render some aspects of patient care incomparable. The few clinical trials using concurrent controls often employ a cluster randomization process in which the ambulance is randomized to an intervention or control group. Other studies evaluate interventions by comparing outcomes in a community implementing the intervention with outcomes in a control community.

Research in SCA also faces additional challenges regarding the need to conduct it in an ethical manner that also complies with state and federal laws and regulations.[1,2] While this is possible, the endeavor should not be underestimated and can be quite complex.[3,4]

Despite the challenge in conducting research, new strategies for improving survival have been studied and implemented and cardiac arrest outcomes are improving. Significant recent changes in BLS, described below, have helped to advance the care of SCA victims.

Good Outcomes Possible

In many communities around the world, survival rates from out-of-hospital cardiac arrest remain abysmally low.[5] There is emerging evidence that improvements in BLS care can have a dramatic impact on survival.[6]

A few communities deliver a higher level of BLS care than is typical. Most have paid careful attention to optimizing the BLS provided by their professional rescuers, and some have achieved dramatic results.

Rochester, Minnesota

Beginning in the early 1990s, Roger White, the medical director for the Rochester, Minnesota, EMS system, led an effort to shorten the time interval from collapse to defibrillation. The local police department, working closely with the paramedic

service, actively embraced the plan to add automated external defibrillators (AEDs) to its system. In 1998, the fire department also added AEDs, and the time interval from a 911 call to delivery of the first shock averaged about 6.5 minutes. As a result, the survival rate to hospital discharge for patients presenting in ventricular fibrillation is now about 40%.[7]

Seattle/King County

Physicians from the University of Washington guided efforts to respond to out-of-hospital cardiac arrest in Seattle and King County, Washington, beginning in the late 1960s. Today both systems have established excellent outcomes, with survival rates to hospital discharge for patients presenting in VF >30%.[8] In early 2005, the King County program implemented a modified approach to CPR+AED use which maximized chest compressions while still using a 15:2 compression-to-ventilation ratio.[6] The time during which the patient was without chest compressions declined after the protocol change. For example, the mean time interval from delivery of the first shock to resumption of chest compressions decreased from 28 to 7 seconds. Under this approach, survival to hospital discharge for patients with witnessed collapse and a presenting rhythm of ventricular fibrillation rose from 33% to 46%.[6]

Dense Public Spaces

Some of the best survival rates from ventricular fibrillation occur in high-population settings in which people are out and about. Following implementation of public AED programs at the airports in Chicago, hospital discharge survival rates reported for victims with VF rose to 56%.[9] In Las Vegas casinos, after implementation of AED programs, survival rates to hospital discharge for patients with VF and a witnessed collapse were similar, at 59%.[10] At the Melbourne Cricket Ground, a large public stadium, survival rates to hospital discharge for patients with VF were an astounding 71%.[11] The key to these high discharge survival rates was achieving a time interval from collapse to first shock of <3 minutes.

Hospitals

A report from the National Registry of CPR, a database of cardiac arrests occurring in hospitals across the United States, evaluated outcomes for patients with VF.[12] The survival rate to hospital discharge among hospitalized patients found in VF/VT was similar to out-of hospital rates for SCA victims in Seattle at 34%.[12] More than 30% of the hospitalized patients had a time from collapse to defibrillation exceeding 2 minutes. Many people would be surprised to learn that they would be defibrillated more quickly in an airport or casino than in some parts of a hospital.

The Chain of Survival

The "chain of survival" (Fig. 11-1) is used as a metaphor for creating systems to successfully resuscitate victims of SCA.[13] If any of the links in the chain are brittle, then the SCA

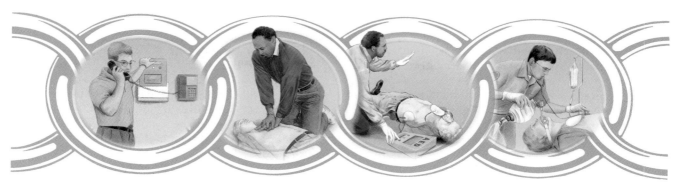

| FIGURE 11-1 • The "chain of survival."

victim will die. Most depictions of the chain of survival show four links, the first three of which are BLS interventions. They are:

- Early recognition of the emergency and activation of EMS.
- Early bystander CPR to double the victim's chance of survival from VF SCA.
- Early defibrillation: CPR plus defibrillation within 3 minutes of collapse can produce survival rates as high as 75%.
- Early ACLS delivered by experienced health care professionals.

Evidence Supporting Links in the Chain

Quicker response by trained responders clearly improves the victim's chance of survival. Depending on the presence of bystander CPR, patient characteristics, and other factors, each minute of delay in the arrival of emergency medical services decreases the victim's chance of survival by between 10% and 30%.[14]

Changing the EMS system to shorten response time intervals can improve survival at a reasonable cost.[15] Measurement is essential to improvement. A common characteristic of EMS systems with excellent survival rates is a long-established commitment to tracking victims of cardiac arrest to hospital discharge. In addition, several key process variables should be measured, including presence of a witness, initiation of CPR by a lay-rescuer, the initial cardiac rhythm, and response time points.

CPR initiated by citizens at the scene of the cardiac arrest doubles survival rates.[16] Rates of bystander CPR vary considerably among different communities: Ontario, 15%[17]; Los Angeles, 28%[18]; Denmark, 28%[19]; Melbourne, 36%[20]; Arizona, 37%[21]; and Seattle, 43%.[22] Many communities could easily begin to improve survival rates by teaching and encouraging more citizens to do CPR.

Optimizing the quality of CPR given by the EMS system is also important to improving survival.[6] Education in CPR has been shown to improve the quality of the CPR provided to patients.[23] Software for defibrillators is available that can help rescuers provide better CPR by providing immediate feedback.[24]

Interestingly, evidence demonstrating the impact of early ACLS on survival from cardiac arrest is far weaker.[25] For example, in a regression analysis involving five EMS systems, the time to arrival for the first responders was strongly predictive of survival, while the time to arrival for the second-tier paramedic service was not related to survival.[26] While patients with VF benefit most from excellent BLS, there are survivors of cardiac arrest whose initial rhythm was pulseless electrical activity (PEA) or asystole. Most likely advanced interventions, such as medications and airway control, are beneficial for these individuals and can save some lives.

EMS System

The details of the EMS system design have a major influence on the rates of survival for out-of-hospital cardiac arrest. New York, Los Angeles, and Seattle all have EMS systems based in the fire department. In each city, fire engines staffed with firefighters trained in CPR and the use of AEDs provide a first response that is backed up with ambulances staffed by two paramedics. Survival to hospital discharge for patients found in ventricular fibrillation is 33% in Seattle,[26] 6.9% in Los Angeles,[18] and 5.3% in New York.[27]

In Seattle, the time interval from the 911 call to arrival of the first vehicle at the scene is 5.0 minutes. In New York in 1994, the time was 9.9 minutes; and in Los Angeles in 2004, it was 7.2 minutes.[18,27] The longer response times noted in some cities account in part for their poor survival rates for patients who have experienced cardiac arrest. Yet other factors also contribute to reduced survival rates.

Role of Bystanders

Assistance from bystanders at the scene of the emergency is critical to helping the victim survive. If someone hears or sees the victim collapse, the victim's chance of survival is dramatically increased. If someone also starts CPR, the chance of survival is doubled. In certain locations with AEDs readily available, application of an AED also doubles survival. These effects of bystander CPR and AED use are synergistic.

Community leaders can enhance the role of bystanders. In locations where AEDs are widely available, the person who takes the emergency medical call can help those at the scene locate and retrieve the closest AED. In a few communities, innovative approaches are adding a "zero response" layer to the EMS system and mobilizing additional volunteer responders to the emergency. Short of providing an AED in every home, strategies like these are the only realistic way to shorten response time to <3 minutes.

Traditional CPR training takes 2 to 4 hours. An abbreviated self-instructional video course focusing on the skills of adult CPR takes <30 minutes and is as effective as a traditional instructor-led course.[28] Most of the skills learned from the video course can be retained for at least 3 months.[29]

BLS and AED Training in School Teaching CPR in schools is attractive because the students are available, and they often become enthusiastic about spreading the knowledge to others older than themselves. Children as young as 9 years of age can learn CPR methods, but they are not able to compress the chest to adult standards until they are about 13 years old.[30] Computer-based virtual reality simulators are attractive for introducing CPR because they are cost-effective to use with large numbers of people and they seem to be moderately effective in teaching CPR skills.[31,32]

Schoolchildren can be used as vectors to reach adults who would otherwise not learn CPR. In Denmark, 35,002 personal training manikins were distributed to seventh-grade students who each then trained an additional two or three people at home.[19] Bystander CPR rates during out-of-hospital cardiac arrest in Denmark subsequently increased from 25.0% to 27.9%, a non–statistically significant difference.

In Norway, 4% of the population learned CPR in <1 month. Personal training manikins were distributed to 62,000 seventh-graders, reaching 99% of the seventh-grade students in the country.[33] The children then trained an additional 118,000 parents and family members.

If a similar program were developed for the United States, 4.2 million seventh graders would learn CPR and could then teach an additional 8 million family members and friends every year. After 5 years, 21 million seventh-graders would have learned CPR. Given that many families have more than one child, about 25 million family and friends would learn CPR from the children, and 20% of the population would have learned how to do CPR.

Emergency Medical Dispatch

Emergency medical dispatch systems should provide telephone instructions for chest compressions that can remind those previously trained to begin chest compressions and encourage those who have never been trained.[34] Dispatchers are successful in identifying that the victim needs CPR between 40% and 70% of the time.[35–37] Even with dispatcher instructions, many rescuers are unable or unwilling to perform CPR.[38] Ongoing research may help improve question scripts so as to assist potential helpers identify symptoms indicating the need for CPR, such as the presence of agonal breathing.[39]

Shortening EMS Response Time

A shortened EMS response time increases survival from SCA. There is a quick drop in survival between minutes 1 and 5, which begins to level off after 6 minutes.[14] This suggests that the traditional goal of an 8-minute response from 911 call to arrival at the scene by EMS is inadequate.

Motivated EMS systems in some larger cities like Seattle, suburban areas like King County, Washington, and smaller cities like Rochester, Minnesota, are able to achieve mean response intervals <6 minutes.[6,26,40] This effort requires accurate measurement of all stages of the response time, and rigorous examination of data in search of opportunities to save 20 to 30 seconds. In a community of 500,000 people with a mean response time of 6 minutes, a decrease to 5.5 minutes would result in at least three lives saved from ventricular fibrillation cardiac arrest each year.[14]

Irreducible Response Times

Even in the best systems, survival from VF cardiac arrest does not exceed 50%.[6,7] Yet in a few circumscribed locations such as large stadiums survival rates as high as 70% have been reported.[11] If the collapse to defibrillation interval can be shortened to <3 minutes, much higher survival is possible.

In any EMS system, there is a certain amount of overhead associated with the EMS response. In most cities, the emergency medical dispatch (EMD) system consumes between 60 and 120 seconds in identifying the nature of the emergency, confirming the location of the victim, selecting responders, and notifying the selected responders about the cardiac arrest. Unless the responders are already in their vehicles on the street, most will need another 60 seconds to get to their vehicles and leave the station. Once they arrive at the location of the cardiac arrest, they will need a minimum of 60 seconds to retrieve equipment from the back of the truck, access the building, and locate the victim.

In a best-case scenario with a zero-minute drive time, more than 3 minutes will already have elapsed before the responders reach the victim. Since it is impractical to put a fire station on every city block, other strategies are needed to increase survival rates.

Public-Access Defibrillation (PAD) (see Chapter 13)

One strategy for shortening the time interval from collapse to defibrillation is placing AEDs in public locations. In a randomized trial, this approach doubled survival for SCA events in nonresidential locations.[41] That trial was recently confirmed with a meta-analysis of the impact public access defibrillators.[42]

Members of the public can learn CPR and AED skills in a 30-minute course with good retention for up to 6 months.[43] Successful programs use these trained volunteers with regular planned and practiced response. They can be assisted by just-in-time volunteers. The Chicago airport program achieved its high survival rate in part because rescuers who were not trained members of the program used a publicly visible AED without waiting for a trained rescuer to arrive.[9]

A key consideration is that the AEDs be placed in public locations with the most potential impact. Extended-care nursing facilities have a relatively high incidence of cardiac arrest, but most still do not have AEDs.[44,45] Schools have a relatively low incidence of cardiac arrest, but their high public visibility may have added benefits such as saving relatively young victims with many years of potential life and teaching young people about AEDs as part of a school-based CPR training initiative.[46]

CPR training provided to lay-volunteers in PAD programs is also likely to have a positive impact on survival, as less than half of the patients found in cardiac arrest in public settings have a shockable rhythm.[41] In addition, a perfusing rhythm is present less than half the time at 60 seconds following a defibrillation attempt.[47] Continuing CPR for several minutes is likely to be beneficial in restoring substrate and oxygen to the ischemic myocardium, a condition necessary for the heart to circulate blood effectively.[48]

Zero-Tier Responders

A number of approaches involving adding more responders to cardiac arrest calls have been aimed at shortening the time to first defibrillation. These additional responders are typically volunteers, identified prior to the event, who agree to respond to suspected cardiac arrest victims.

A PAD program in Maastrict, the Netherlands, has located AEDs on poles in residential areas and near automated teller machines (ATMs) at banks. ATM locations were selected because they are well lit and often well known to nearby residents. When a cardiac arrest event occurs, nearby volunteer rescuers are notified via a text message sent to their mobile phones that gives the locations of the cardiac arrest victim and the closest AED.

A program in Cypress Creek, Texas, uses off-duty police, firefighters, EMS personnel, and medical volunteers who have been provided with AEDs, which they keep with them at home or in their personal vehicles. When a cardiac arrest occurs near the residence of a volunteer, the emergency dispatcher also pages that volunteer to respond. Preliminary information from that system suggests that the time from call to first shock has decreased. In addition, those rescuers can provide CPR when no shock is indicated.

Geographic clustering of cardiac arrest events has been described in several communities.[49,50] Computer software running at 911 call centers can be programmed to include a map layer with the locations of known AEDs. With this system in place, the call taker can accurately locate the closest AED, which may, for example, be across the street at a bank. A rescuer may be able to retrieve that AED before EMS can arrive. This would be similar to the system in use in Maastrict, but it would use an untrained bystander rather than a trained volunteer.

Additional innovative approaches must be developed and funded to deploy AEDs and CPR effectively in suburban and urban areas and achieve the goal of providing early defibrillation to a substantial proportion of VF victims. In any system, responders will have the greatest impact when they can provide excellent BLS based on compelling science.

Major Recent Changes in BLS Recommendations

See Web site for AHA 2005 Guidelines for Cardiopulmonary Resuscitation and Emergency Cardiovascular Care, Part 4.

Major revisions in the approach to BLS occurred in 2005. With newer technology came the realization that CPR was performed much less effectively in the real world than it was in the laboratory.[51–53] Additional emphasis was placed on providing many more chest compressions by changing the compression to ventilation ratio to 30:2, using a single shock for VF rather than three stacked shocks, eliminating frequent pulse and rhythm checks, and immediately resuming compressions following a defibrillatory shock. Training courses from the most basic to advanced levels were revised to help ensure that students changed behavior and performed CPR of much better quality. This approach seems to be improving survival dramatically.[6,54,55]

Almost all health care professionals have learned how to perform CPR, yet few truly understand the physiology and scientific evidence that determine the recommendations for CPR. The significant changes in 2005—including the compression–ventilation ratio of 30:2, providing a period of CPR prior to defibrillation, and giving a single shock—all have significant evidence to justify their implementation.

Compression–Ventilation Ratio (See also Chapter 15)

No human data have identified a single optimal compression–ventilation ratio for victims of all ages. Traditional CPR has been complicated to perform. Students often fail to master essential skills during CPR training courses, and long-term retention is poor.[56,57] Simplification of training should lead to increased use of CPR by those near the victim.[58] Teaching a single compression–ventilation ratio for all cardiac arrest victims would be preferable if it was supported by available scientific evidence.

Interruptions in chest compressions of only a few seconds rapidly lower blood flow to the heart and brain and decrease survival rates from cardiac arrest.[59] Even with optimal CPR, pulmonary blood flow is only about 25% of normal, and the minute volume needed to maintain a normal ventilation–perfusion ratio during CPR is lower still.[60] In addition, each positive-pressure breath given elevates venous and intracranial pressure, decreasing venous return to the right side of the heart and further worsening cerebral blood flow.[61]

Delivery of rescue breaths by lone lay-rescuers switching between administering compressions, providing two "quick" breaths, and resuming compressions led to a mean 16-second interruption in chest compressions.[62,63]

When rescuers had been taught using the 2000 CPR guidelines, the poor quality of chest compressions plus long pauses in compressions with excessive ventilation rates severely reduced coronary and cerebral blood flow and dramatically diminished the likelihood of a successful resuscitation attempt.[61,64]

With the development of defibrillators that can measure the quality of CPR, researchers learned that nurses, physicians, and paramedics gave an inadequate number of compressions, did not push hard enough, interrupted compressions frequently, provided excessive ventilations particularly when victims were intubated, and did not allow full chest recoil.[51–53,61]

Major change in the approach to providing CPR was clearly needed. The challenge was to meet the educational need of simplification while providing acceptable CPR techniques for the multiple ages of victims and etiologies of cardiac arrest.

A number of options were considered. Continuous chest compressions alone are at least as good as traditional CPR in animal models of cardiac arrest for the first several minutes of VF SCA.[65,66] In models of cardiac arrest, pulmonary blood flow and minute ventilation match better at compression–ventilation ratios >15:2.[66,67] Other compression–ventilation ratios, such as 100:2 or 50:2, were evaluated as well.

One major concern about teaching chest compressions without rescue breathing to lay-rescuers is the possible negative impact on cardiac arrest patients who are not in VF or whose arrest is prolonged. Ventilations are necessary for patients with asphyxial etiology of arrest, which includes most pediatric patients and those who have submersion injury as well as all cardiac arrest victims after the first few minutes.[68–70]

In view of the lack of evidence that lay-rescuers would be able to determine the etiology of a cardiac arrest, a simplified compression–ventilation ratio was recommended for all single rescuers regardless of the age of the patient or the etiology of the event. With the goal of increasing the number of chest compressions delivered while recognizing the need for ventilation for some cardiac arrest victims, expert consensus settled on a universal compression–ventilation ratio of 30:2 for all *lone* rescuers of victims older than newborns. Choosing a single 30:2 ratio accomplished the goal of easing training in all lay-rescuer courses.

A different compression–ventilation ratio of 15:2 remained for two-rescuer CPR for infants and children, with the realization that this added training complexity for health care providers. Because pauses in compressions to give breaths are shorter with two rescuers,[71] there was not enough evidence to recommend fewer breaths for children, given their higher prevalence of asphyxial arrest.

The change from a 15:2 to a 30:2 compression–ventilation ratio in early 2006 is having a positive impact. Chest compression counts have increased significantly during training and in actual resuscitation attempts, and systems are beginning to report increased survival rates.[6,23,54,55,72–74]

Compression First Versus Shock First for VF SCA

Cobb and colleagues noted that survival from ventricular fibrillation cardiac arrest did not improve following the introduction of a first-responder AED program in Seattle in the early 1990s.[8] They contemplated animal models of cardiac arrest showing that hearts that have been fibrillating for more than several minutes are unlikely to resume effective cardiac output immediately following a defibrillatory shock unless there is a period of coronary perfusion to provide oxygen and substrate and remove of waste.[75,76] They implemented a 90-second period of 5:1 CPR prior to attempting defibrillation, which resulted in an increase in survival from out-of-hospital VF arrest from 24% to 30%.[8] See also sidebar Chapter 13.

A randomized trial of 3 minutes of 5:1 CPR prior to defibrillation in Norway showed no impact overall; but in a post hoc subgroup analysis, CPR before defibrillation did show improvements in survival rates when the interval between the call to the EMS system and delivery of the initial shock was 4 to 5 minutes or longer.[77] A second randomized trial in Perth, Australia, showed equivalent survival rates when either 90 seconds of 5:1 CPR or defibrillation was performed first for any interval between an EMS call and the delivery of shock.[78] Despite a high bystander-administered CPR rate (55%), survival from VF arrest in Perth was only about 4% to 5%, perhaps in part due to a long mean response interval of 9 minutes.

With the additional emphasis on quantity and quality of CPR and also with the change from three stacked shocks to one shock, the role of CPR prior to defibrillation remains unclear. Animal research confirms that the quality of chest compressions is key to successful implementation of a strategy of delaying defibrillation to prime the pump with CPR first.[79] If CPR is of high quality, then providing 90 to 180 seconds of continuous compressions or 30:2 CPR prior to defibrillation likely has a larger benefit on the cardiac myocytes than 5:1 CPR, with its many pauses in compressions, as was used in the Seattle, Norwegian, and Australian studies. On the other hand, minimizing the pauses in compressions prior to and following administration of a shock may diminish the negative impact of attempting a single shock very early in the resuscitation attempt. At the time of this writing, the Resuscitation Outcomes Consortium is engaged in a large, multicenter trial comparing early with later defibrillation. This may provide a more definitive answer prior to the planned 2010 revision of the Emergency Cardiovascular Care (ECC) guidelines.

When the collapse-to-shock time is short, <4 minutes, excellent survival rates are obtained by defibrillating as quickly as possible.[9,11,40,80] In most cases response intervals inside a hospital are <4 minutes, and immediate defibrillation is preferred.[12] Given the available evidence, a reasonable option for treatment of VF outside the hospital is for EMS rescuers to provide five cycles of 30:2 CPR (about 2 minutes) before attempting defibrillation when EMS responders did not witness the arrest. EMS system medical directors would do well to recommend a standard approach so that all members of the resuscitation team clearly know what to do at the time of the event.

One-Shock Versus Three-Shock Sequence for Attempted Defibrillation

For many years, the ECC guidelines recommended a series of up to three shocks, without interposed chest compressions, for the treatment of VF.[81] In 2005, the ECC guidelines implemented a major change by recommending a single shock rather than up to three.[82] Evidence emerging since the 2005 change supports this recommendation.[6,54,83,84]

Almost all defibrillators sold today no longer employ the old monophasic electrical waveform. Biphasic-waveform defibrillators have a first shock efficacy (defined as termination of VF at 5 seconds after the shock) above 90%, while monophasic-waveform defibrillators have a first-shock efficacy of about 60%.[85,86] Thus VF is likely to be eliminated with a single shock from a biphasic defibrillator. If one biphasic shock fails to eliminate VF, a second shock is often not effective either. Immediate resumption of effective chest compressions likely has greater value in improving the condition of cardiac myocytes than a second shock.

Following successful termination of VF of >1 or 2 minutes in duration, almost all victims demonstrate a nonperfusing rhythm for up to several minutes.[47,48,87] The treatment for such rhythms is immediate chest compressions. AEDs manufactured prior to 2006 required between 29 to 37 seconds to analyze the postshock rhythm and then provide a recommendation to begin CPR, resulting in long delays to beginning chest compressions.[87,88] This prolonged interruption in chest compressions is unnecessary when, more than 90% of the time, the victim is unlikely to have persistent VF.

There is compelling evidence that minimizing the pauses in compressions prior to and following a defibrillation attempt dramatically improves the likelihood that the victim will develop a perfusing heart rhythm.[6,88–90] Rescuers should resume chest compressions immediately after attempted defibrillation. They should not interrupt chest compressions to evaluate rhythm or pulse until after five cycles of 30:2 CPR. This approach may be modified if invasive hemodynamic monitoring shows resumption of spontaneous circulation or if the victim requests discontinuation of CPR.

Priorities in BLS and ACLS

Team Leader and Team Concept

Successful resuscitation leaders use the resuscitation team effectively. Setting priorities for the resuscitation is the responsibility of the team leader. CPR and early defibrillation come first; drug administration is a lower priority. After ensuring that excellent CPR is being given and accomplishing defibrillation if the victim is in VF, team leaders can ask for intravenous access, consider drug therapy, and insert an advanced airway. At all times, the team leader must ensure that ACLS interventions are performed with minimal interruption of CPR, especially chest compressions.

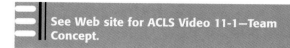
See Web site for ACLS Video 11-1—Team Concept.

Integration of CPR and Defibrillation

High-quality CPR is important both before and after shock delivery. CPR should be provided with minimal interruptions until a defibrillator is ready to give a shock. The pause in compressions to deliver the shock should be quite short, ideally <5 seconds. Many victims demonstrate asystole or PEA for several minutes after defibrillation, and good CPR can help convert these rhythms to a perfusing rhythm.[47] Rhythm checks should be brief, <10 seconds, and performed infrequently.

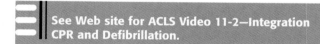
See Web site for ACLS Video 11-2—Integration CPR and Defibrillation.

Integration of CPR and ACLS Interventions

The AHA 2005 Emergency Cardiovascular Care (ECC) recommendations pointed out that the timing of drug delivery is less important than the need to minimize interruptions in chest compressions.[82] Needed medications can be administered when the rhythm is checked. The training approach taught in earlier ACLS courses led to too many interruptions in chest compressions.

Insertion of an advanced airway may also lead to interruption in CPR. The team leader must consider the risks (e.g., interruption in circulation) and benefits (e.g., ease of ventilation) of inserting an advanced airway during a resuscitation attempt. In balancing the risks and benefits, the team leader should consider the etiology of the arrest, the condition of the patient, and the operator's expertise in airway control. Often the best course is to defer insertion of an advanced airway until the patient fails to respond to initial CPR and defibrillation attempts or until the patient demonstrates a return of spontaneous circulation.

A Walk Through the BLS Health Care Provider and Lay-Provider Algorithms

The steps of BLS and CPR consist of a series of sequential assessments and actions, which are illustrated in the BLS algorithms for the health care provider and the lay-provider (Fig. 11-2). The AHA 2005 guidelines for CPR and ECC

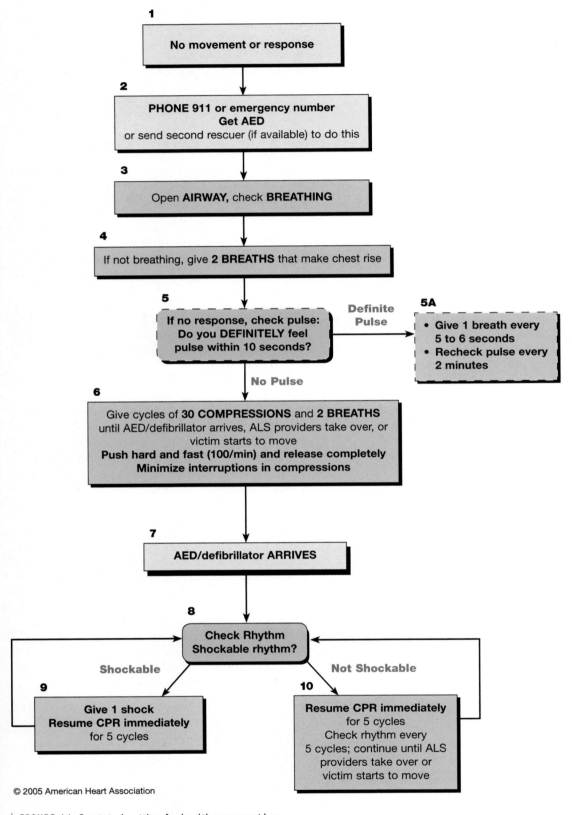

© 2005 American Heart Association

| FIGURE 11-2 • BLS algorithm for health care providers.

simplified the BLS algorithms to facilitate learning, retention, and performance of the steps of CPR. A universal compression–ventilation ratio of 30:2 is now recommended for all lone CPR rescuers regardless of the age of the victim. The guidelines for lay-rescuers were simplified to encourage prompt action in administering aid to an unresponsive victim and to decrease some of the fear reported by many lay-rescuers related to administering CPR.[91]

The box numbers in the following section refer to the corresponding boxes in the adult BLS health care provider algorithm. Differences between this algorithm and that for lay-providers are discussed below.

Check for Response

The first step in addressing the needs of the victim is to determine if the victim is responsive (Fig. 11-2, Box 1, and Fig. 11-3). This assessment begins the instant the rescuer finds the victim and notes the victim's need for assistance. Does the victim appear to be alert and moving or is he or she lying still? Is the victim speaking, coughing, or breathing? Are there other bystanders in close proximity who can help provide aid to the victim?

If the victim appears unresponsive, the rescuer should tap the victim and ask, "Are you all right?" If the victim responds but is injured, the rescuer should call 911 and then return to the victim until EMS arrives at the scene. If the patient does not respond, the rescuer should immediately shout for help.

Activate the EMS System

If more than one rescuer is present at the scene of an emergency with an unresponsive victim, several actions can occur

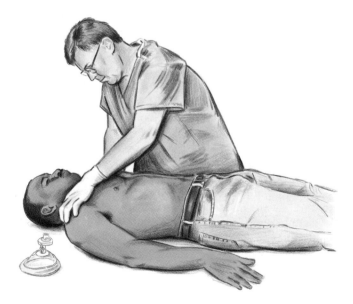

| FIGURE 11-3 • Check for response.

simultaneously. One bystander should be specifically instructed to call 911 to contact EMS and stay on the phone with the EMS dispatcher to provide information or receive instructions (Fig. 11-2, Box 2, and Fig. 11-4). Another rescuer can be directed to obtain the nearest AED. One or more of the trained rescuers can start the steps of CPR. However, if a lone rescuer finds an unresponsive victim, the sequence for activating EMS differs between the health care provider and lay-responder. The response is based on the rescuer's level of training and the ability of the rescuer to determine the primary reason for the victim's collapse.

Activate EMS: Health Care Provider

The lone health care provider will need to determine the most likely etiology of the victim's collapse before deciding the appropriate sequence for activating EMS—phone first or phone fast.[92] If the victim suddenly collapses, the rescuer should consider the primary etiology to be cardiac regardless of the victim's age. Sudden collapse signals that a lethal arrhythmia is likely present, which may require a shock. In this instance, the goal is to activate EMS as quickly as possible or phone first, to ensure that a defibrillator is on the way, retrieve an AED if available, and return to the victim to provide CPR and defibrillation. If the lone health care provider determines that the most likely etiology of the victim's collapse is asphyxial in nature, the rescuer will deliver five cycles or about 2 minutes of 30 compressions and two ventilations of CPR first, then pausing CPR to activate EMS and get the AED. The rescuer should then return to the victim to provide CPR and defibrillation as indicated until more advanced care arrives.

Activate EMS: Lay-Responders

The lay-responder is not taught to differentiate the etiology of the victim's collapse. The lay-rescuer's response is based on the victim's age and not the nature of the victim's arrest. For the unresponsive adult victim, the lay-rescuer should activate EMS and get an AED (if available). The lay-rescuer should then return to the patient and begin the steps of CPR, administering five cycles of 30 compressions and two ventilations and using the AED when appropriate. Because the primary cause of a cardiac arrest in infants and children is more often asphyxial, the lone lay-responder should provide the unresponsive pediatric victim with five cycles (or about 2 minutes) of 30 compressions and two ventilations. The lay-rescuer should then activate EMS, get the AED, and provide CPR and defibrillation as indicated.

> See Web site for BLS Video 11-3—Initial BLS: Unresponsiveness—Activate EMS.

Open the Airway and Check Breathing

CPR is most effective if the victim is in the supine position on a hard surface. If the victim has collapsed and is in a side or prone position, it will be necessary to roll the victim into

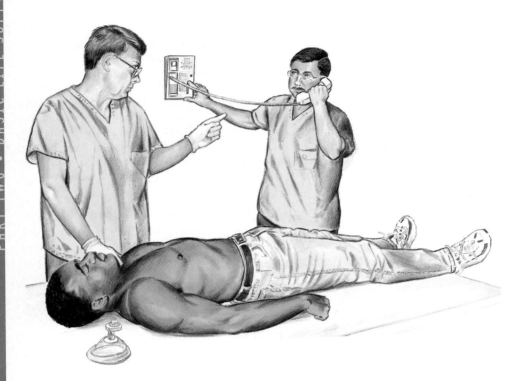

FIGURE 11-4 • Activate the EMS system.

a supine position (Fig. 11-2, Box 3, and Fig. 11-5). Because approximately 2% of blunt trauma victims have an associated injury of the cervical spine, the victim should be positioned carefully while maintaining spinal precautions.[93] In certain situations, as during spinal surgery, it may be impossible to move the patient into a supine position. If this is the case, the health care provider may proceed with CPR with the patient in the prone position. The prone position CPR technique is discussed later in this chapter. Once the patient is positioned and on a hard surface, the rescuer should open the airway and assess for breathing (see also Chapter 16).

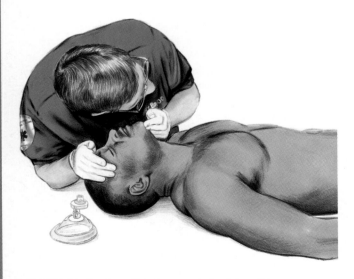

FIGURE 11-5 • Open the airway and check breathing.

Open the Airway: Health Care Provider

In an unconscious, unresponsive victim, the tongue will sometimes fall back against the larynx, causing a partial or complete airway obstruction. Two techniques are described for health care providers to relieve the obstruction in an unresponsive patient. First, if there is no evidence the victim sustained head or neck trauma, a health care provider should use the head tilt–chin lift maneuver to open the airway (Fig. 11-6). This technique was developed using unconscious, paralyzed adult volunteers in an operating room setting and has not been specifically studied with victims of cardiac arrest;[94] however, case studies and radiographic evidence have proven it to be an effective airway management technique.[95–97]

The second method for opening and maintaining a patent airway in an unresponsive victim is the jaw-thrust maneuver. This technique is reserved for health care providers because it is sometimes difficult to do and may result in excessive spinal movement if performed incorrectly.[97] It is estimated that 2% of blunt trauma victims have associated cervical spine trauma. If the victim has moderate to severe head injury and/or a Glasgow Coma Scale score of <8, the incidence of associated cervical spine trauma is approximately 6%. Therefore, the health care provider must be instructed in the appropriate technique for performing a jaw-thrust while maintaining cervical spine precautions for the victim.[93,98,99] If the jaw-thrust technique fails to open the airway and allow for adequate ventilation during CPR or if the health care provider is unable to perform the jaw-thrust maneuver for any reason, the head tilt–chin-lift maneuver should be used to open and maintain a patent airway.

Manual restriction of spinal motion is preferred over a cervical collar for a cardiac arrest victim with suspected

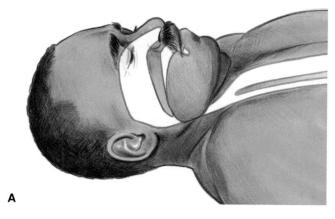

A

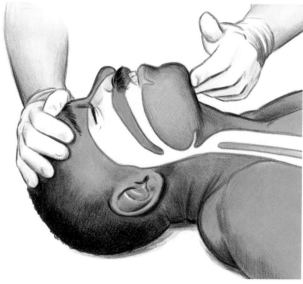

B

FIGURE 11-6 • Open the airway—the head tilt–chin lift maneuver for health care providers.

spinal injury.[100–104] Cervical collars and other immobilization devices may interfere with airway management and have been shown to increase intracranial pressure in a victim with a head injury.[105–108] Spine immobilization devices, such as cervical collars, are necessary during transport because of the potential for increased movement and additional injury.

Open the Airway: Lay-Rescuer

The head-tilt–chin-lift maneuver is the only technique taught to lay-rescuers to open the airway in unresponsive victims. The jaw-thrust technique is no longer recommended for lay-rescuers because it is difficult to learn and perform correctly. It is also difficult for the lay-provider to maintain the jaw-thrust position and ventilate the patient. If performed incorrectly, it may cause spinal movement and possibly more injury to the victim.

Check Breathing

Both the lay-rescuer and health care provider should look, listen, and feel for breathing while maintaining the victim's

open airway (Fig. 11-7). The assessment for the presence or absence of breathing should take between 5 and 10 seconds. If the victim is not adequately breathing, the rescuer should provide two breaths over 1 second for each breath. The rescuer should provide enough volume to see the chest rise. Lay-rescuers who are untrained in CPR or not confident in their ability to provide rescue breaths should begin continuous chest compressions.

Both professional and lay-rescuers may be unable to accurately determine the presence of normal breathing in unresponsive victims because of agonal gasps. Agonal gasps are a brainstem response to hypoxemia and often occur in the first few minutes following SCA; they indicate that the victim is in cardiac arrest.[109–111] Because agonal gasps are often mistaken for an effective breathing pattern, one of the goals of instruction is to make it clear to the lay-rescuer that CPR is indicated when such gasps are present.

Give Rescue Breaths

The recommendation for rescue breathing is the same for the lay-rescuer and the health care provider. Once it is determined that the victim is unresponsive and not breathing, the rescuer should give two breaths over 1 second each, with enough volume to produce visual chest rise without overinflating the chest. Give one breath every 5 to 6 seconds if the victim has a pulse present and only ventilatory support is needed. The purpose of ventilation is to provide adequate oxygenation, but researchers have yet to determine the optimal tidal volume, rescue ventilation rate, and inspired oxygen concentration levels (see Fig. 11-2, Boxes 4 and 5A).

During the initial minutes of an SCA from VF, rescue breaths are probably not as important as chest compressions.[64] Because the metabolic rate is greatly decreased during a cardiac arrest, the oxygen level in the blood remains high for the first several minutes. In early cardiac arrest, myocardial and cerebral hypoxia result more from the

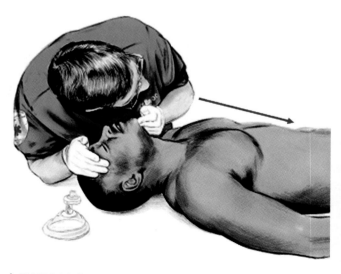

FIGURE 11-7 • Check breathing—look, listen, and feel for breathing while maintaining the victim's open airway.

absence of cardiac output than from the actual level of saturated oxygen in the blood. Some studies of patients with normal perfusion suggest that a tidal volume of 8 to 10 mL/kg maintains normal oxygenation and elimination of CO_2.[112] Although cardiac compressions provide only about 25% to 33% of the normal blood flow, a lower than normal tidal volume and respiratory rate can maintain effective oxygenation and ventilation during CPR.[113,114]

Ventilation tidal volumes of approximately 500 to 600 mL (6–7 mL/kg) during CPR are sufficient. Blood flow to the lungs is substantially reduced during CPR, thus lower ventilation rates and tidal volumes are needed to maintain an adequate ventilation/perfusion ratio.[115] Studies have demonstrated that rescuers have a tendency to deliver ventilations too frequently and with too much tidal volume.[61] Hyperventilation is harmful to the victim because it increases intrathoracic pressure, decreases venous return to the heart, and diminishes cardiac output and survival.[61]

Gastric inflation commonly occurs when breaths are delivered with excessive force or too much tidal volume and exceed the lower esophageal sphincter tone. Risk of gastric inflation is increased by high proximal airway pressure and decreased opening pressure of the lower esophageal sphincter.[61,115] Gastric inflation can result in stomach distention, regurgitation, and aspiration of the stomach contents into the lungs.[116] The rescuer should avoid delivering breaths that are too large or too forceful. To minimize the potential for gastric inflation and its complications, deliver each breath to patients with or without an advanced airway over 1 second and deliver a tidal volume that is sufficient to produce a visible chest rise.

The 2005 ECC guidelines greatly simplified the recommendations for tidal volumes, respiratory rates, and breath delivery intervals for health care providers during one- and two-rescuer CPR.[82] Rescuers are encouraged to give two rescue breaths over 1 second each and avoid delays between breaths and compressions. The goal is for the rescuer to provide the two ventilations in approximately 7 seconds during one-person CPR and within 4 seconds during two-rescuer CPR. Regardless of the ventilation delivery method (mouth-to-mouth/mask or bag mask with or without supplementary oxygen), the rescuer should provide enough tidal volume to produce visible chest rise. An observational study of trained BLS providers demonstrated that they were able to detect "adequate" chest rise in anesthetized, intubated, paralyzed adult patients with a tidal volume of approximately 400 mL.[115] A tidal volume of 500 to 600 mL is recommended during CPR because it is likely that this is the minimal volume required to produce chest rise in a victim with no advanced airway (e.g., endotracheal tube, Combitube, laryngeal mask airway [LMA]) in place.

Once an advanced airway is in place during two-person CPR, the ventilation rate is reduced to 8 to 10 breaths per minute without attempting to synchronize breaths between compressions. Chest compressions are constant, without pauses for ventilation, at a rate of approximately 100 compressions per minute.

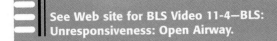

See Web site for BLS Video 11-4—BLS: Unresponsiveness: Open Airway.

Mouth-to-Mouth Rescue Breathing

When no other means of providing ventilation is available, mouth-to-mouth rescue breathing is a safe and effective technique for providing oxygen and ventilation to a victim who is not breathing[117,118] (Fig. 11-8). The exhaled air from the rescuer contains about 17% oxygen and 4% carbon dioxide, yet that is sufficient to provide adequate oxygenation because of the greatly reduced pulmonary blood flow during CPR.[119] To perform mouth-to-mouth rescue breathing, open the victim's airway using the head-tilt–chin-lift or jaw-thrust method, pinch the victim's nose closed, and create an airtight mouth-to-mouth seal. Give the victim two consecutive breaths. Each breath should be given over 1 second. The rescuer should take a regular breath to provide just enough ventilation to cause the victim's chest to rise. Rescuers are encouraged to breathe normally, because deep breathing may cause the rescuer to become light-headed or dizzy.[120] Deep breaths administered forcefully to the victim contribute to gastric inflation and thus increase the risk of the victim vomiting. An improperly opened airway is the most common cause of ventilation difficulty for the rescuer. If the victim's chest fails to rise with the first breath, the rescuer should reposition the victim's head and attempt a second rescue breath.

Many health care providers and lay-rescuers express a reluctance to perform mouth-to-mouth ventilation because of a perceived risk of disease transmission, although the risk of acquiring an infection by giving mouth-to-mouth ventilations is quite low.[118,121,122] However, if rescuers are unwilling or unable to provide mouth-to-mouth ventilations during a cardiac arrest, chest compressions alone should be administered. (See Hands Off Chest Compression Only below.)

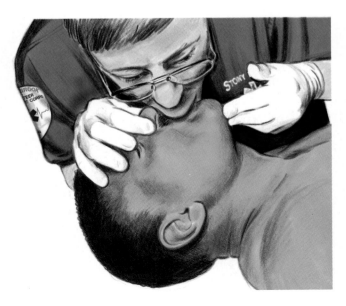

| FIGURE 11-8 • Mouth-to-mouth ventilation.

Mouth-to–Barrier Device Breathing

While the barrier device reduces the direct contact between the rescuer and the victim, it may not reduce the risk of infection transmission.[118] Some barrier devices actually impede airflow, making it more difficult to ventilate the victim.[123,124] A face shield is a plastic sheet that creates a barrier between the victim and the rescuer. It provides minimal protection against infection but can be used safely and effectively in lieu of direct mouth-to-mouth contact. Responders using a face shield should switch to a face mask or a bag-mask device as soon as an alternative is available.[125] A face mask with a one-way valve provides more protection for the rescuer while still providing an effective method of ventilation. The one-way valve directs the rescuer's breath into the patient but diverts the patient's exhaled air away from the rescuer, thus reducing the risk to the rescuer of contracting a respiratory infection[125] (see Fig. 11-9).

Mouth-to-Nose and Mouth-to-Stoma Ventilation

There are occasions where it may be impossible to provide ventilation through the patient's mouth. Facial trauma, dental trauma, facial hair, or water rescue may make it impossible to create a seal around the mouth and provide adequate ventilations. A series of case studies demonstrates that mouth-to-nose ventilation is a safe and effective alternative method to ventilate a patient when a mouth seal cannot be achieved.[126]

Patients with a surgical tracheotomy, postlaryngectomy patients, or other patients with a tracheal stoma will require mouth-to-stoma rescue ventilation. There is no published evidence on the safety, effectiveness, or feasibility of mouth-to-stoma ventilation. If available, a pediatric face mask can also be used to ventilate the patient by creating an airtight seal over the stoma with the mask. The study supporting this practice found that a pediatric face mask worked better than a standard ventilation mask for providing ventilatory support for these patients.[127]

Ventilation with Bag and Mask

Bag-mask ventilation is a technique that requires considerable skill and practice and is, therefore, reserved to the health care provider; it is not considered a lay-rescuer skill.[128] Bag-mask ventilation is most effective when it is provided by two trained and experienced rescuers. One rescuer opens the airway and seals the mask to the face while the other squeezes the bag. Both rescuers watch for visible chest rise. Because of the difficulty with mask placement and maintaining a seal, this mode of ventilation should be used sparingly by a lone rescuer (Figs. 11-10 and 11-11).

> See Web site for BLS Video 11-5—Initial BLS: Ventilation with Bag-Mask Device.

The rescuer should use an adult (1–2-L) bag to deliver a tidal volume of 500 to 600 mL, sufficient to achieve visible chest rise. If a good face seal is maintained, this tidal volume can usually be achieved by squeezing a 1-L adult bag by one-half to two-thirds its total volume. The rescuers should deliver cycles of 30 compressions and two ventilations with the bag-mask if the patient does not have an advanced airway in place. The rescuer providing compressions may pause very briefly to allow the ventilation rescuer to deliver two breaths. The total ventilation time for two-rescuer CPR using a bag-mask device should not exceed 4 seconds. If an oxygen reservoir is attached to the bag-mask device, 100% oxygen can be delivered with a flow rate set between 12 and 15 L/min.

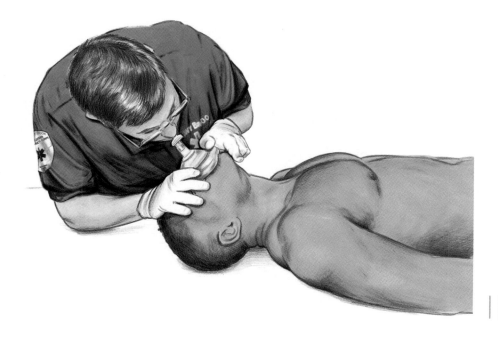

FIGURE 11-9 • Mouth-to-mask ventilation.

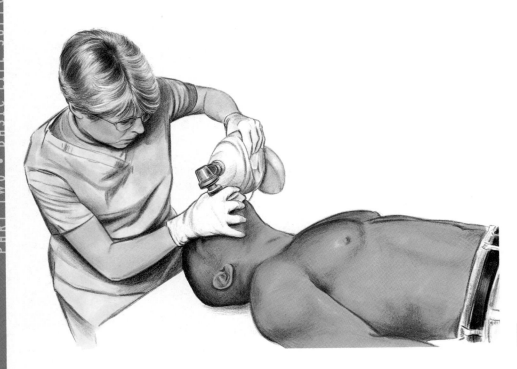

FIGURE 11-10 • One-person bag-mask ventilation.

It is within the scope of practice for many BLS practitioners (i.e., EMT Basic) to insert advanced airway devices, such as the LMA and the Combitube. These devices do not require direct visualization of the vocal cords for proper insertion or placement and may be preferred over the bag-mask device alone. They may be considered an acceptable alternative to the bag-mask device for health care providers well trained in their use.

Ventilation With an Advanced Airway

Once an advanced airway is in place (ET Tube, Combitube, or LMA), compressions and ventilations are no longer delivered in a synchronous manner or in cycles of 30:2. Instead, continuous chest compressions are delivered at a rate of 100 per minute without pauses for ventilation. Ventilations are provided at a rate of 8 to 10 breaths

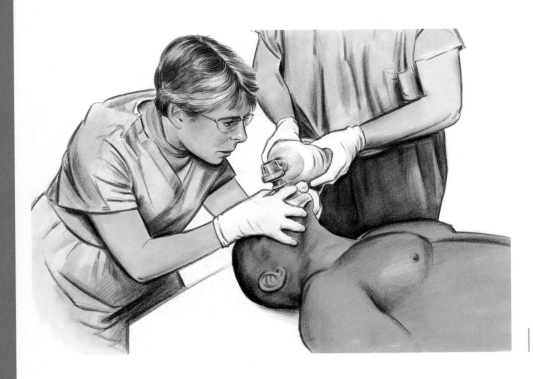

FIGURE 11-11 • Two-person bag-mask ventilation.

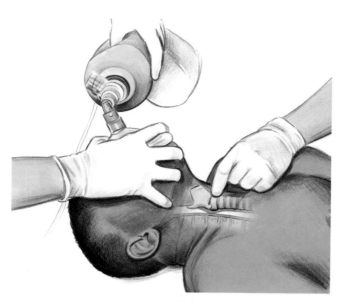

| FIGURE 11-12 • Cricoid pressure.

per minute. The two rescuers should change compressor and ventilator roles approximately every 2 minutes to prevent compressor fatigue and deterioration in the quality and rate of chest compressions. When multiple rescuers are present, they should rotate the compressor role about every 2 minutes.

Excessive ventilations, >12 per minute, lead to increased intrathoracic pressure, reduced venous return, and decreased coronary and cerebral perfusion pressure.[59,61,129] Rescuers should avoid excessive ventilation by giving the recommended breaths per minute and limiting tidal volume to achieve chest rise. To avoid decreasing cardiac output, it is critically important that ventilations not exceed 8 to 10 breaths per minute.

Cricoid Pressure

Cricoid pressure is a technique used during resuscitation, before an advanced airway is established, to prevent gastric inflation secondary to ventilation (Fig. 11-12). Cricoid pressure is important because it reduces the risk of passive regurgitation and aspiration, which can occur secondary to ventilatory support.[130,131] This technique requires a third rescuer who is dedicated to holding consistent pressure while the other rescuers perform compressions and ventilations until the advanced airway is placed. Downward pressure is applied to the victim's cricoid cartilage, which pushes the trachea posteriorly, thus compressing the esophagus between the trachea and the cervical vertebrae. Cricoid pressure should be used only in unresponsive victims; it is painful and may induce cough or gagging in a responsive patient. Since the trachea is more pliable in infants and children, the rescuer should be cautious and avoid excessive pressure that may obstruct the trachea and decrease ventilation.[132]

 See Web site for BLS Video 11-6— Initial BLS: Cricoid Pressure.

Pulse Check (for Health Care Providers)

As part of the Emergency Cardiovascular Care Guidelines 2000, the American Heart Association deleted the pulse check in lay-provider training and greatly de-emphasized it in training for health care providers as a means of assessing circulation.[81] Studies found that lay-rescuers identified a pulse in 10% of pulseless victims (poor sensitivity for cardiac arrest) and stated that there was no pulse present in 40% of victims with a pulse (poor specificity).[109,110] There is no evidence to support the lay-provider's assessment of signs of circulation by checking for breathing, coughing, or movement as being a superior method for detecting circulation in lieu of a pulse check.[47] Therefore, the lay-rescuer will be taught to assess for responsiveness and breathing. If the victim is unresponsive and not breathing, the lay-rescuer will begin CPR. Situations occur when a victim is unresponsive and apneic but still has a pulse. Since the lay-provider does not check for a pulse under this circumstance, chest compressions will be initiated anyway. Because there have been very few post-CPR–related injuries reported in the literature, it is felt that the risk for harm to the patient is low. More harm is done when CPR is not initiated when needed because of an error in assessing for the victim's pulse (Fig. 11-2, Box 5).

Health care providers also have difficulty determining if a pulse is present and may spend an excessive amount of time assessing for a pulse. This causes untoward delays in the initiation of chest compressions and may contribute to the victim's demise.[109,133] Owing to these concerns, the health care provider should take no more than 10 seconds to assess for a pulse. If the health care provider is unable to determine whether the victim has a pulse within 10 seconds, chest compressions should be initiated.

Rescue Breathing Without Chest Compressions

If the unresponsive victim is not breathing spontaneously but still has a pulse, the health care provider should deliver ventilatory support at a rate of 10 to 12 breaths per minute or about 1 breath every 5 to 6 seconds (Fig. 11-2, Box 5A). As with CPR, each rescue breath should be delivered over 1 second, with just enough volume to produce visible chest rise. For the infant or child with a perfusing rhythm but no breathing, give one breath every 3 to 5 seconds for a total of 12 to 20 breaths per minute.

Chest Compressions

Chest compressions are rhythmic applications of pressure over the lower half of the sternum given to a victim in cardiopulmonary arrest (Fig. 11-2, Box 6, and Fig. 11-13). The

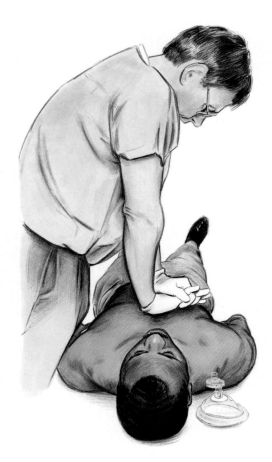

| FIGURE 11-13 • Chest compressions.

desired.[136,137] Various "CPR-friendly" deflatable mattresses have been studied; they do not provide an adequate surface on which to perform chest compressions.[138,139]

To give "effective" chest compressions, the rescuer must "push hard and fast." Compressions for the adult victim are given on the lower portion of the sternum, at the nipple line, at a depth of 1½ to 2 inches (4–5 cm), which is about 15% to 20% of the anteroposterior diameter of an adult chest.[140] A force of <50 kg is sufficient to achieve the recommended compression depth in most victims of cardiac arrest.[141] Compression depth for infants and children should be one-third to one-half the total anteroposterior diameter of the chest. Studies conducted in both in-hospital and out-of-hospital settings with health care providers have demonstrated that chest compressions were of insufficient depth approximately 40% of the time.[51,53]

The compression rate for all victims regardless of age is about 100 compressions per minute. Pauses in chest compressions for ventilations or other interventions should be kept to a minimum. The chest should be allowed to recoil completely after each compression. Chest recoil allows venous blood return to the heart. Study findings demonstrate that as rescuers become fatigued, they are less likely to allow for full recoil, thus reducing the depth and rate of their compressions.[142,143] For this reason, training should focus on the importance of alternating the compressor rescuer every 2 minutes with each five cycles of 30:2 CPR. The rescuer should provide a duty cycle of equal compression and relaxation times.

See Web site for BLS Video 11-7—Initial BLS: Chest Compressions.

The rescuer should compress the lower half of the victim's sternum in the center of the chest, between the nipples. The hand position used to deliver CPR compressions varies with the age of the patient.[144] For the adult victim, the rescuer should place the heel of one hand on the sternum in the center (middle) of the chest between the nipples and then place the heel of the second hand on top of the first, so that the hands are overlapped and parallel.[144–146] Either hand may be on top.[147] The health care provider may use a two-thumb encircling hands chest compression technique for infant compressions (<1 year of age). For a child in cardiac arrest, the rescuer may use the hand position described for adults or the heel of one hand. The hand position used for the child will depend mainly on the size of the child and the size and strength of the rescuer.

The sternum should be depressed approximately 1½ to 2 inches in the adult victim (approximately 4–5 cm) and then allowed to return to its normal position. Achieving a compression depth of at least 1.5 inches for the 30 seconds prior to defibrillation improves the efficacy of the shock.[90] Compressing the chest >2 inches is contraindicated, as it can be harmful. Studies in animals indicate that with excessive compression depth, significant chest wall injury occurs, which leads to the loss of spontaneous recoil. Therefore, venous return is diminished and cardiac return falls.[148,149]

goal is to mimic the beat of the heart and circulate oxygenated blood to the brain and heart. This action prolongs the victim's life until cardiac function can be restored through defibrillation or other interventions. Compressions create blood flow by increasing intrathoracic pressure and directly compressing the heart. Under the best conditions, properly performed chest compressions can produce systolic arterial pressure peaks of 60 to 80 mm Hg; however, diastolic pressure remains low and mean arterial pressure in the carotid artery seldom exceeds 40 mm Hg.[112] Chest compressions increase the likelihood that the heart will respond to a defibrillatory shock, particularly for victims of VF SCA if the first shock is delivered >4 minutes after the initial collapse.[6,8,53,134]

Since it is extremely difficult to perform randomized controlled clinical trials on humans to assess the effect of CPR variables such as compression rates, compression–ventilation ratios, no-flow time, duty cycles, chest recoil, and ventilation rates, much of the research knowledge is derived from animal models. Despite the dearth of human subject research on CPR mechanics, there are a few key principles that have been demonstrated to improve outcomes for victims of SCA.

To maximize the effectiveness of compressions, the victim should lie supine on a hard surface such as the floor, with the rescuer kneeling beside the victim's chest.[135] If the victim is in a hospital bed, a "CPR board" should be placed under the patient to simulate a hard surface, although there is some evidence that these boards are not as effective as

Compression–Ventilation Ratio

The 2005 AHA guidelines for CPR and ECC support a single compression–ventilation ratio of 30:2 for rescuers providing one-person CPR for a victim of any age—infant, child, or adult. While there was not a single human study to support this recommendation, it was nevertheless supported by the consensus of experts. The goal of this recommendation is to increase the number of compressions delivered over 1 minute while decreasing the likelihood of hyperventilation and frequent disruptions to provide ventilations. The uniform compression–ventilation ratio simplifies CPR instruction, making the skill easier for providers to learn and remember. Recently published information demonstrates that this recommendation is scientifically sound and has proven to increase cerebral blood flow while also increasing the number of compressions delivered per minute.[60]

For adult victims of cardiac arrest, the compression–ventilation ratio remains at 30:2, regardless of one rescuer or two, until an advanced airway is placed. Once an advanced airway device is in place, chest compressions are delivered continuously at a rate of 100 compressions per minute. Ventilations are asynchronous with compressions and delivered at 8 to 10 breaths per minute.

The ventilation–compression ratio of 30:2 is consistent with pediatric single-rescuer recommendations as well. However, once an additional rescuer arrives on the scene, infant and child CPR should be delivered at a rate of 15 compressions to 2 rescue breaths. The two rescuers should change compressor and ventilator roles every 10 cycles of 15:2, or approximately every 2 minutes, for the pediatric victim to prevent compressor fatigue and deterioration in quality and rate of chest compressions.[90] When multiple rescuers are present, they should rotate the compressor role about every 2 minutes.

Defibrillation and CPR

Anyone can be trained to provide defibrillation (Fig. 11-2, Boxes 7–10, and Fig. 11-14). Most survivors of SCA present in VF, and survival rates are highest when bystanders immediately begin CPR and defibrillation occurs within 3 minutes.[16] Immediate defibrillation is the treatment of choice for VF of short duration, such as witnessed SCA. Minimizing pauses before and after defibrillation increases the likelihood of return of spontaneous circulation.

Generally a patient who needs CPR should have a resuscitation attempt without being moved unless he or she is in a dangerous environment or in need of surgical intervention. CPR interruptions are fewer and quality better when the resuscitation is conducted on a stationary victim.[150]

See Web site for BLS Video 11-8—Initial BLS: Defibrillation.

Team Concept: Integration of Basic and Advanced Life Support

When initial BLS, including defibrillation when indicated, does not restore effective circulation, survival is in question. At this point, continued high-quality BLS, including effective high-quality chest compressions is critical to survival. With the arrival of advanced life support, high-quality BLS is essential for optimal outcome. Advanced life support should be provided with minimal interruption in chest compressions for defibrillation and advanced airway insertion when indicated. The team leader is responsible for monitoring the effectiveness of BLS, ensuring that provider fatigue does not occur and integrating advance life support interventions.

See Web site for BLS/ACLS Video 11-9—Integration BLS with ACLS Team Leader.

New Developments Since 2005

CPR Quality Feedback

Just prior to the development of the 2005 ECC guidelines, engineers developed technology to accurately measure the quality of CPR while it is administered to victims of cardiac arrest. Application of the defibrillators with the capability of measuring CPR quality demonstrated that many patients in and out of the hospital received chest compressions that were too shallow, too slow, with long pauses, and without allowing full chest recoil.[51,53,151] Since providing feedback in classroom settings is often ineffective in changing behavior, providing immediate feedback on the quality of CPR during the resuscitation is an attractive concept that might improve outcomes.[152]

In many animal laboratory experiments, manual chest compressions are guided by a metronome to help ensure the consistency of compressions. Often the technician providing chest compressions also can see an arterial pressure waveform, which is usually used to ensure an adequate compression depth.[153] This concept was tested for human cardiac arrest victims more than 15 years ago, and it worked, as the end-tidal CO_2 value almost doubled with metronome guidance.[154] Use of a commercial version of a metronome with a pressure sensor to estimate the depth of chest compressions increases the rate and depth of compressions given to manikins.[155] As of this writing, no studies have demonstrated improvement in clinical outcomes with the use of a metronome device.

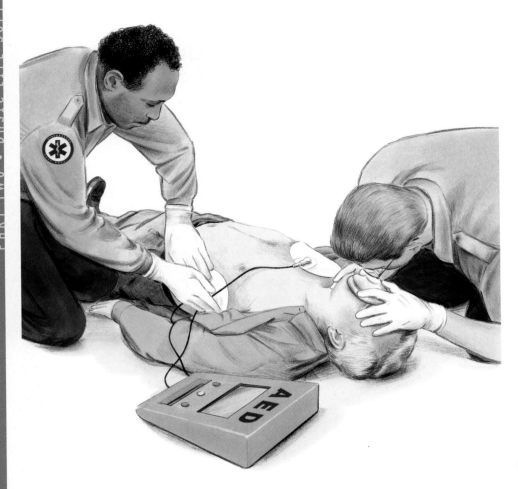

| FIGURE 11-14 • Defibrillation.

Biomedical engineers recently developed new defibrillators with the addition of a pressure sensor pad that is placed in the center of the victim's chest during CPR. The rescuer presses on the pad and the computer in the defibrillator calculates the rate, depth, and duration of compressions.[156] With the addition of continuous capnography or thoracic electrical impedance measurement, ventilation rate is calculated.[157,158] The thoracic impedance measurement technology can be used to detect resumption of spontaneous cardiac output.[159] The defibrillator displays a real-time graphic showing each compression with a target range for depth of compression. If compressions are outside of the depth or rate range for more than a few seconds, the defibrillator prompts the rescuer with an audible suggestion for improvement.[24]

A prospective cohort study of this technology demonstrated that CPR quality improved.[24] Compressions were too shallow 71% of the time at baseline compared with 41% when feedback was given.[24] Survival was poor in the EMS systems conducting the experiment (3%) and was not improved when feedback was given (4%). Similar results were obtained during a study in the hospital.[160]

Hands-Only CPR

Some CPR is much better than no CPR.[161] Yet even when an SCA is witnessed, often no one begins any CPR until professional help arrives.

Likely one barrier to the performance of CPR is aversion to mouth-to-mouth breathing. In surveys asking about attitudes on CPR, many rescuers express reluctance to give mouth-to-mouth ventilations when they do not know the victim.[121,162] On the other hand, lay-rescuers interviewed following attempted resuscitation from cardiac arrest uncommonly indicated that reluctance to give mouth-to-mouth ventilation inhibited their performance of CPR.[91] They were much more likely to cite panic and feeling incompetent at reasons for not acting.[91]

Hands-only CPR is easier to learn and perform than traditional CPR. Perhaps simplifying CPR education for lay-rescuers by teaching only chest compressions would empower action. There are fewer skills to learn and potential rescuers may feel more competent during an actual resuscitation attempt.[163]

Animal models of cardiac arrest as well as some human data suggest that rescue breathing is of little benefit and might actually be detrimental during the first 5 minutes of cardiac arrest due to VF.[34,64,65,164–167] At the onset of the cardiac arrest, the victim's lungs are filled with air containing oxygen from the last breath taken prior to the cardiac arrest. In addition, there is a store of oxygenated hemoglobin in the arterial blood.[168] If the airway is open, patients will often take agonal breaths, which have a clinically significant tidal volume.[169–171] There may also be some passive movement of air with chest recoil during CPR.[166,172]

Finally, continuous chest compressions without additional ventilation will maintain a similar amount of myocardial oxygen delivery as chest compression with rescue breathing for several minutes.[59] Opposing animal evidence suggests that a few ventilations are needed during cardiac arrest in pigs to prevent an increase in pulmonary vascular resistance.

During the time when a 5:1 compression–ventilation ratio was taught to lay-rescuers, observational studies showed that survival was improved with compressions alone compared to no CPR but was highest with compressions and ventilation.[173,174] A randomized trial of emergency medical dispatcher CPR instructions showed a trend toward higher survival with compression-only instructions compared to instructions in compressions and breathing.[34]

The relative value of ventilation may be different for health care providers than for lay-rescuers. Professional rescuers can provide ventilation using equipment such as a bag-mask device with a much shorter pause in compressions to provide ventilation. In two prospective studies, EMS crews were taught to perform continuous chest compressions with some passive insufflation of oxygen for the first 6 minutes of the resuscitation attempt. Survival to hospital discharge was higher following the implementation of continuous compressions when compared with historical controls using 15:2 CPR.[84,175]

Knowledge of the optimal way to employ hands-only CPR is now emerging. The strongest human evidence suggests that hands-only CPR performed by lay-rescuers for victims of sudden collapse is at least as good and may be superior to traditional CPR using 15:2 ratio (see Table 11-1).[34,176–178] Most children and some adults with cardiac arrest do benefit from immediate institution of rescue breathing with chest compressions (e.g., in cases of submersion injury).[69]

At this point, it is not clear whether the lay-public will be able to accurately identify the likely etiology of the cardiac arrest. Submersion injury is a relatively uncommon event, accounting for about 1% of attempted resuscitations.[179] There is likely some trade-off between widespread lay-rescuer training in hands-only CPR with loss of skill in rescue breathing. However, most patients with cardiac arrest regardless of etiology do not get any bystander CPR. There is evidence that chest compressions alone are better than nothing, even for cardiac arrest of asphyxial etiology.[69]

Hands Off Chest Compression Only

See Web site for AHA Scientific Statement: Chest Compression Only CPR

The American Heart Association recently reviewed the science for initially performing chest compression only CPR.[161] The scientific statement notes that all victims of cardiac arrest should receive, at a minimum, high-quality chest compressions (ie, chest compressions of adequate rate and depth with minimal interruptions).

To support that goal and save more lives, the AHA ECC Committee also recommended in an _adult having sudden collapse trained or untrained bystanders should activate their community emergency medical response system (eg, call 911) and provide high-quality chest compressions by pushing hard and fast in the center of the chest, minimizing interruptions (Class I):_

- If a bystander is not trained in CPR, then the bystander should provide hands-only CPR (Class IIa). The rescuer should continue hands-only CPR until an automated external defibrillator arrives and is ready for use or EMS providers take over care of the victim.
- If a bystander was previously trained in CPR and is confident in his or her ability to provide rescue breaths with minimal interruptions in chest compressions, then the bystander should provide either conventional CPR using a 30:2 compression-to ventilation ratio (Class IIa) or hands only CPR (Class IIa). The rescuer should continue CPR until an automated external defibrillator arrives and

| TABLE 11-1 • Comparison of Studies on Hands-Only CPR for Victims of Out-of-Hospital Cardiac Arrest

Study	Study Population	Time Period	Endpoint	No CPR (*N* % with 1° endpoint)	Compressions and Rescue Breathing	Compressions Alone
SOS-Kanto[176]	Witnessed adults in Tokyo, Japan	9/2002 to 12/2003	Good neurologic function at 30 days	2,917 2%	712 4%	439 6%
Iwami[177]	Witnessed adults, cardiac etiology, in Osaka, Japan	5/1998 to 4/2003	Survival at 1 year	3,550 2.1%	783 3.6%	544 3.5%
Bohm[178]	All cardiac arrests among 70% of population of Sweden	1990–2005	Survival at 30 days	NA	8,209 7.2%	1,145 6.7%

is ready for use or EMS providers take over care of the victim.

- If the bystander was previously trained in CPR but is not confident in his or her ability to provide conventional CPR including high-quality chest compressions (ie, compressions of adequate rate and depth with minimal interruptions) with rescue breaths, then the bystander should give hands-only CPR (Class IIa). The rescuer should continue hands-only CPR until an automated external defibrillator arrives and is ready for use or EMS providers take over the care of the victim.

Alternative Approaches to Standard CPR

"Cough" CPR

By vigorous and continuous coughing, an awake patient with VF/pulseless VT may be able to maintain a normal systolic blood pressure. Cough CPR was initially reported in awake monitored patients who developed VF or VT in the cardiac catheterization lab.[180] It has been reported that consciousness could be maintained for about 30 seconds while VF persists. Coughing could be useful under carefully coached circumstances with the patient on a heart monitor awaiting defibrillation.[181] Despite information widely circulated in a chain e-mail on the Internet, "cough" CPR has no role in lay-rescuer CPR.[182]

Prone CPR

When the prone victim of cardiac arrest cannot be rolled over quickly to a supine position (e.g., during a surgical procedure), rescuers may provide CPR while the patient remains prone, particularly when an advanced airway is already in place.[183] Two small crossover studies with a total of 17 recently dead patients documented higher blood pressure during CPR in the prone position when compared with standard CPR.[184,185] A review of prone CPR used for intubated hospitalized patients documented survival to discharge in 10 of 22 patients.[183]

Over-the-Head CPR

At times, limited space, as in airplanes and other locations, makes improvisation in CPR technique mandatory.[186] One intriguing option allows a single rescuer to perform chest compressions and mask ventilation from a single position. In over-the-head CPR, the victim is on the floor and the rescuer kneels with his legs placed on either side of the victim's head while facing the victim's feet. The rescuer performs chest compressions by leaning forward with elbows locked and hands placed in the center of the victim's chest. Ventilations can subsequently be given by sitting back com-

fortably while using a bag-mask.[186] In a simulated arrest situation using a recording manikin, the quality of CPR was similar between over-the-head CPR and standard CPR.[135,186,187]

Key Points

Physicians responsible for resuscitation teams should remember the following:

- Excellent BLS is essential for optimizing chances of survival.
- Advanced life support is effective only if good CPR is consistently and continuously delivered.
- Pauses in compression around defibrillation should be minimized.

Strong medical leadership can dramatically increase survival rates from cardiac arrest in any community. Paying attention to small details in the skills of BLS during resuscitation will save the lives of persons experiencing cardiac arrest.

References

1. Nichol G, Huszti E, Rokosh J, et al. Impact of informed consent requirements on cardiac arrest research in the United States: exception from consent or from research? *Resuscitation* 2004;62(1):3–23.
2. Halperin H, Paradis N, Mosesso V Jr, et al. Recommendations for implementation of community consultation and public disclosure under the food and drug administration's "exception from informed consent requirements for emergency research": a special report from the American Heart Association Emergency Cardiovascular Care Committee and Council on Cardiopulmonary, Perioperative and Critical Care: Endorsed by the American College of Emergency Physicians and the Society for Academic Emergency Medicine. *Circulation* 2007;116(16):1855–1863.
3. Mosesso VN Jr, Brown LH, Greene HL, et al. Conducting research using the emergency exception from informed consent: the Public Access Defibrillation (PAD) trial experience. *Resuscitation* 2004;61(1):29–36.
4. Morris MC, Mechem CC, Berg RA, et al. Impact of the privacy rule on the study of out-of-hospital pediatric cardiac arrest. *Prehosp Emerg Care* 2007;11(3):272–277.
5. Becker LB, Ostrander MP, Barrett J, et al. Outcome of CPR in a large metropolitan area—where are the survivors? *Ann Emerg Med* 1991;20(4):355–361.
6. Rea TD, Helbock M, Perry S, et al. Increasing use of cardiopulmonary resuscitation during out-of-hospital ventricular fibrillation arrest: survival implications of guideline changes. *Circulation* 2006;114(25):2760–2765.
7. White RD, Bunch TJ, Hankins DG. Evolution of a community-wide early defibrillation programme experience over 13 years using police/fire personnel and paramedics as responders. *Resuscitation* 2005;65(3):279–283.
8. Cobb LA, Fahrenbruch CE, Walsh TR, et al. Influence of cardiopulmonary resuscitation prior to defibrillation in patients with out-of-hospital ventricular fibrillation. *JAMA* 1999;281(13):1182–1188.
9. Caffrey SL, Willoughby PJ, Pepe PE, et al. Public use of automated external defibrillators. *N Engl J Med* 2002;347(16):1242–1247.
10. Valenzuela TD, Roe DJ, Nichol G, et al. Outcomes of rapid defibrillation by security officers after cardiac arrest in casinos. *N Engl J Med* 2000;343(17):1206–1209.

11. Wassertheil J, Keane G, Fisher N, et al. Cardiac arrest outcomes at the Melbourne Cricket Ground and shrine of remembrance using a tiered response strategy—a forerunner to public access defibrillation. *Resuscitation* 2000;44(2):97–104.

12. Chan PS, Krumholz HM, Nichol G, et al . Delayed time to defibrillation after in-hospital cardiac arrest. *N Engl J Med* 2008; 358(1):9–17.

13. Cummins RO, Ornato JP, Thies WH, et al. Improving survival from SCA: the "chain of survival" concept. A statement for health professionals from the Advanced Cardiac Life Support Subcommittee and the Emergency Cardiac Care Committee, American Heart Association. *Circulation* 1991;83(5):1832–1847.

14. De Maio VJ, Stiell IG, Wells GA, et al. Optimal defibrillation response intervals for maximum out-of-hospital cardiac arrest survival rates. *Ann Emerg Med* 2003;42(2):242–250.

15. Stiell IG, Wells GA, Field BJ, et al. Improved out-of-hospital cardiac arrest survival through the inexpensive optimization of an existing defibrillation program: OPALS study phase II. Ontario Prehospital Advanced Life Support. *JAMA* 1999;281(13):1175–1181.

16. Abella BS, Aufderheide TP, Eigel B, et al. Reducing barriers for implementation of bystander-initiated cardiopulmonary resuscitation: a scientific statement from the American Heart Association for healthcare providers, policymakers, and community leaders regarding the effectiveness of cardiopulmonary resuscitation. *Circulation* 2008;117(5):704–709.

17. Stiell IG, Wells GA, DeMaio VJ, et al. Modifiable factors associated with improved cardiac arrest survival in a multicenter basic life support/defibrillation system: OPALS Study Phase I results. Ontario Prehospital Advanced Life Support. *Ann Emerg Med* 1999;33(1):44–50.

18. Eckstein M, Stratton SJ, Chan LS. Cardiac arrest resuscitation evaluation in Los Angeles: CARE-LA. *Ann Emerg Med* 2005;45(5):504–509.

19. Isbye DL, Rasmussen LS, Ringsted C, et al. Disseminating cardiopulmonary resuscitation training by distributing 35,000 personal manikins among school children. *Circulation* 2007;116(12): 1380–1385.

20. Fridman M, Barnes V, Whyman A, et al. A model of survival following pre-hospital cardiac arrest based on the Victorian Ambulance Cardiac Arrest Register. *Resuscitation* 2007;75(2): 311–322.

21. Vadeboncoeur T, Bobrow BJ, Clark L, et al. The Save Hearts in Arizona Registry and Education (SHARE) program: who is performing CPR and where are they doing it? *Resuscitation* 2007;75(1):68–75.

22. Kim F, Olsufka M, Longstreth WT Jr, et al. Pilot randomized clinical trial of prehospital induction of mild hypothermia in out-of-hospital cardiac arrest patients with a rapid infusion of 4°C normal saline. *Circulation* 2007;115(24):3064–3070.

23. Hostler D, Rittenberger JC, Roth R, et al. Increased chest compression to ventilation ratio improves delivery of CPR. *Resuscitation* 2007;74(3):446–452.

24. Kramer-Johansen J, Myklebust H, Wik L, et al. Quality of out-of-hospital cardiopulmonary resuscitation with real time automated feedback: a prospective interventional study. *Resuscitation* 2006;71(3):283–292.

25. Stiell IG, Wells GA, Field B, et al. Advanced cardiac life support in out-of-hospital cardiac arrest. *N Engl J Med* 2004;351(7): 647–656.

26. Hallstrom A, Rea TD, Sayre MR, et al. Manual chest compression vs use of an automated chest compression device during resuscitation following out-of-hospital cardiac arrest: a randomized trial. *JAMA* 2006;295(22):2620–2628.

27. Lombardi G, Gallagher J, Gennis P. Outcome of out-of-hospital cardiac arrest in New York City. The Pre-Hospital Arrest Survival Evaluation (PHASE) study. *JAMA* 1994;271(9):678–683.

28. Einspruch EL, Lynch B, Aufderheide TP, et al. Retention of CPR skills learned in a traditional AHA Heartsaver course versus 30-min video self-training: a controlled randomized study. *Resuscitation* 2007;74(3):476–486.

29. Isbye DL, Meyhoff CS, Lippert FK, et al. Skill retention in adults and in children 3 months after basic life support training using a simple personal resuscitation manikin. *Resuscitation* 2007;74(2):296–302.

30. Jones I, Whitfield R, Colquhoun M, et al. At what age can schoolchildren provide effective chest compressions? An observational study from the Heartstart UK schools training programme. *BMJ* 2007;334(7605):1201.

31. Youngblood P, Hedman L, Creutzfeld J, et al. Virtual worlds for teaching the new CPR to high school students. *Stud Health Technol Inform* 2007;125:515–519.

32. Creutzfeldt J, Hedman L, Medin C, et al. Implementing virtual worlds for systematic training of prehospital CPR in medical school. *Stud Health Technol Inform* 2007;125:82–84.

33. Lorem T, Palm A, Wik L. Abstract 2228: Schoolchildren As Ambassadors Of CPR—A Model For Mass Training Of Lay Rescuers? *Circulation* 2007;116(16 MeetingAbstracts):II-485.

34. Hallstrom A, Cobb L, Johnson E, et al. Cardiopulmonary resuscitation by chest compression alone or with mouth-to-mouth ventilation. *N Engl J Med* 2000;342(21):1546–1553.

35. Bohm K, Rosenqvist M, Hollenberg J, et al. Dispatcher-assisted telephone-guided cardiopulmonary resuscitation: an underused lifesaving system. *Eur J Emerg Med* 2007;14(5):256–259.

36. Vaillancourt C, Verma A, Trickett J, et al. Evaluating the effectiveness of dispatch-assisted cardiopulmonary resuscitation instructions. *Acad Emerg Med* 2007;14(10):877–883.

37. Cairns KJ, Hamilton AJ, Marshall AH, et al. The obstacles to maximising the impact of public access defibrillation: an assessment of the dispatch mechanism for out of hospital cardiac arrest. *Heart* 2007;94(3):349–353.

38. Lerner EB, Sayre MR, Brice JH, et al. Cardiac arrest patients rarely receive chest compressions before ambulance arrival despite the availability of pre-arrival CPR instructions. *Resuscitation* 2008;77(1):51–56.

39. Dias JA, Brown TB, Saini D, et al . Simplified dispatch-assisted CPR instructions outperform standard protocol. *Resuscitation* 2007;72(1):108–114.

40. Bunch TJ, White RD, Gersh BJ, et al. Long-term outcomes of out-of-hospital cardiac arrest after successful early defibrillation. *N Engl J Med* 2003;348(26):2626–2633.

41. Hallstrom AP, Ornato JP, Weisfeldt M, et al. Public-access defibrillation and survival after out-of-hospital cardiac arrest. *N Engl J Med* 2004;351(7):637–646.

42. Sanna T, La Torre G, de Waure C, et al. Cardiopulmonary resuscitation alone vs. cardiopulmonary resuscitation plus automated external defibrillator use by non-healthcare professionals: A meta-analysis on 1583 cases of out-of-hospital cardiac arrest. *Resuscitation* 2008;76(2):226–232.

43. Roppolo LP, Pepe PE, Campbell L, et al. Prospective, randomized trial of the effectiveness and retention of 30-min layperson training for cardiopulmonary resuscitation and automated external defibrillators: the American Airlines Study. *Resuscitation* 2007;74(2):276–285.

44. Shah MN, Fairbanks RJ, Lerner EB. Cardiac arrests in skilled nursing facilities: continuing room for improvement? *J Am Med Dir Assoc* 2007;8(3 Suppl 2):e27–e31.

45. Fisher J, Anzalone B, McGhee J, et al. Lack of early defibrillation capability and automated external defibrillators in nursing homes. *J Am Med Dir Assoc* 2007;8(6):413–415.

46. Lotfi K, White L, Rea T, et al. Cardiac arrest in schools. *Circulation* 2007;116(12):1374–1379.

47. Carpenter J, Rea TD, Murray JA, et al. Defibrillation waveform and post-shock rhythm in out-of-hospital ventricular fibrillation cardiac arrest. *Resuscitation* 2003;59(2):189–196.

48. White RD, Russell JK. Refibrillation, resuscitation and survival in out-of-hospital sudden cardiac arrest victims treated with biphasic automated external defibrillators. *Resuscitation* 2002;55(1):17–23.

49. Ong ME, Tan EH, Yan X, et al. An observational study describing the geographic-time distribution of cardiac arrests in Singapore: what is the utility of geographic information systems for planning public access defibrillation? (PADS phase I). *Resuscitation* 2008;76(3):388–396.

50. Lerner EB, Fairbanks RJ, Shah MN. Identification of out-of-hospital cardiac arrest clusters using a geographic information system. *Acad Emerg Med* 2005;12(1):81–84.

51. Abella BS, Alvarado JP, Myklebust H, et al. Quality of cardiopulmonary resuscitation during in-hospital cardiac arrest. *JAMA* 2005;293(3):305–310.

52. Abella BS, Sandbo N, Vassilatos P, et al. Chest compression rates during cardiopulmonary resuscitation are suboptimal: a prospective

study during in-hospital cardiac arrest. *Circulation* 2005;111(4): 428–434.

53. Wik L, Kramer-Johansen J, Myklebust H, et al. Quality of cardiopulmonary resuscitation during out-of-hospital cardiac arrest. *JAMA* 2005;293(3):299–304.

54. Fales W, Farrell R. Impact of new resuscitation guidelines on out-of-hospital cardiac arrest survival (abstract). *Acad Emerg Med* 2007;14(5S):S157.

55. Aufderheide TP, Birnbaum M, Lick C, et al. A tale of seven EMS systems: an impedance threshold device and improved CPR techniques double survival rates after out-of-hospital cardiac arrest (abstract 64). *Circulation* 2007;116(16 MeetingAbstracts): II-936–II-937.

56. Kaye W, Mancini ME. Retention of cardiopulmonary resuscitation skills by physicians, registered nurses, and the general public. *Crit Care Med* 1986;14(7):620–622.

57. Brennan RT, Braslow A. Skill mastery in public CPR classes. *Am J Emerg Med* 1998;16(7):653–657.

58. Chamberlain DA, Hazinski MF. Education in resuscitation: an ILCOR symposium: Utstein Abbey: Stavanger, Norway: June 22–24, 2001. *Circulation* 2003;108(20):2575–2594.

59. Berg RA, Sanders AB, Kern KB, et al. Adverse hemodynamic effects of interrupting chest compressions for rescue breathing during cardiopulmonary resuscitation for ventricular fibrillation cardiac arrest. *Circulation* 2001;104(20):2465–2470.

60. Yannopoulos D, Aufderheide TP, Gabrielli A, et al. Clinical and hemodynamic comparison of 15:2 and 30:2 compression-to-ventilation ratios for cardiopulmonary resuscitation. *Crit Care Med* 2006;34(5):1444–1449.

61. Aufderheide TP, Sigurdsson G, Pirrallo RG, et al. Hyper-ventilation-induced hypotension during cardiopulmonary resuscitation. *Circulation* 2004;109(16):1960–1965.

62. Assar D, Chamberlain D, Colquhoun M, et al. Randomised controlled trials of staged teaching for basic life support. 1. Skill acquisition at bronze stage. *Resuscitation* 2000;45(1):7–15.

63. Heidenreich JW, Higdon TA, Kern KB, et al. Single-rescuer cardiopulmonary resuscitation: "two quick breaths"—an oxymoron. *Resuscitation* 2004;62(3):283–289.

64. Kern KB, Hilwig RW, Berg RA, et al. Importance of continuous chest compressions during cardiopulmonary resuscitation: improved outcome during a simulated single lay-rescuer scenario. *Circulation* 2002;105(5):645–649.

65. Ewy GA, Zuercher M, Hilwig RW, et al. Improved neurological outcome with continuous chest compressions compared with 30:2 compressions-to-ventilations cardiopulmonary resuscitation in a realistic swine model of out-of-hospital cardiac arrest. *Circulation* 2007;116(22):2525–2530.

66. Sanders AB, Kern KB, Berg RA, et al. Survival and neurologic outcome after cardiopulmonary resuscitation with four different chest compression-ventilation ratios. *Ann Emerg Med* 2002;40(6): 553–562.

67. Babbs CF, Kern KB. Optimum compression to ventilation ratios in CPR under realistic, practical conditions: a physiological and mathematical analysis. *Resuscitation* 2002;54(2):147–157.

68. Berg RA, Hilwig RW, Kern KB, et al. Simulated mouth-to-mouth ventilation and chest compressions (bystander cardiopulmonary resuscitation) improves outcome in a swine model of prehospital pediatric asphyxial cardiac arrest. *Crit Care Med* 1999; 27(9):1893–1899.

69. Berg RA, Hilwig RW, Kern KB, et al. "Bystander" chest compressions and assisted ventilation independently improve outcome from piglet asphyxial pulseless "cardiac arrest." *Circulation* 2000;101(14):1743–1748.

70. Idris AH, Becker LB, Fuerst RS, et al. Effect of ventilation on resuscitation in an animal model of cardiac arrest. *Circulation* 1994;90(6):3063–3069.

71. Odegaard S, Pillgram M, Berg NE, et al. Time used for ventilation in two-rescuer CPR with a bag-valve-mask device during out-of-hospital cardiac arrest. *Resuscitation* 2008;77(1):57–62.

72. Deschilder K, De Vos R, Stockman W. The effect on quality of chest compressions and exhaustion of a compression–ventilation ratio of 30:2 versus 15:2 during cardiopulmonary resuscitation—a randomised trial. *Resuscitation* 2007;74(1):113–118.

73. Ødegaard S, Saether E, Steen PA, et al. Quality of lay person CPR performance with compression: ventilation ratios 15:2, 30:2

or continuous chest compressions without ventilations on manikins. *Resuscitation* 2006;71(3):335–340.

74. Olasveengen TM, Wik L, Kramer-Johansen J, et al. Is CPR quality improving? A retrospective study of out-of-hospital cardiac arrest. *Resuscitation* 2007;75(2):260–266.

75. Niemann JT, Cairns CB, Sharma J, et al. Treatment of prolonged ventricular fibrillation. Immediate countershock versus high-dose epinephrine and CPR preceding countershock. *Circulation* 1992;85(1):281–287.

76. Berg RA, Hilwig RW, Ewy GA, et al. Precountershock cardiopulmonary resuscitation improves initial response to defibrillation from prolonged ventricular fibrillation: a randomized, controlled swine study. *Crit Care Med* 2004;32(6):1352–1357.

77. Wik L, Hansen TB, Fylling F, et al. Delaying defibrillation to give basic cardiopulmonary resuscitation to patients with out-of-hospital ventricular fibrillation: a randomized trial. *JAMA* 2003;289(11):1389–1395.

78. Jacobs IG, Finn JC, Oxer HF, et al. CPR before defibrillation in out-of-hospital cardiac arrest: a randomized trial. *Emerg Med Australas* 2005;17(1):39–45.

79. Ristagno G, Tang W, Chang YT, et al. The quality of chest compressions during cardiopulmonary resuscitation overrides importance of timing of defibrillation. *Chest* 2007;132(1):70–75.

80. Valenzuela TD, Kern KB, Clark LL, et al. Interruptions of chest compressions during emergency medical systems resuscitation. *Circulation* 2005;112(9):1259–1265.

81. Guidelines 2000 for cardiopulmonary resuscitation and emergency cardiovascular care. Part 3: adult basic life support. The American Heart Association in collaboration with the International Liaison Committee on Resuscitation. *Circulation* 2000;102(8 Suppl):I22–I59.

82. 2005 American Heart Association guidelines for cardiopulmonary resuscitation and emergency cardiovascular care. Part 4: Adult basic life support. *Circulation* 2005;112(24 Suppl): IV19–IV34.

83. Tang W, Snyder D, Wang J, et al. One-shock versus three-shock defibrillation protocol significantly improves outcome in a porcine model of prolonged ventricular fibrillation cardiac arrest. *Circulation* 2006;113(23):2683–2689.

84. Bobrow BJ, Vadeboncoeur TF, Clark L, et al. Statewide out-of-hospital cardiac arrest survival improves after widespread implementation of cardiocerebral resuscitation (abstract 1). *Circulation* 2007;116(16 Meeting Abstracts):II-923.

85. White RD, Blackwell TH, Russell JK, et al. Transthoracic impedance does not affect defibrillation, resuscitation or survival in patients with out-of-hospital cardiac arrest treated with a non-escalating biphasic waveform defibrillator. *Resuscitation* 2005; 64(1):63–69.

86. Morrison LJ, Dorian P, Long J, et al. Out-of-hospital cardiac arrest rectilinear biphasic to monophasic damped sine defibrillation waveforms with advanced life support intervention trial (ORBIT). *Resuscitation* 2005;66(2):149–157.

87. Rea TD, Shah S, Kudenchuk PJ, et al. Automated external defibrillators: to what extent does the algorithm delay CPR? *Ann Emerg Med* 2005;46(2):132–141.

88. Yu T, Weil MH, Tang W, et al. Adverse outcomes of interrupted precordial compression during automated defibrillation. *Circulation* 2002;106(3):368–372.

89. Berg RA, Hilwig RW, Kern KB, et al. Automated external defibrillation versus manual defibrillation for prolonged ventricular fibrillation: lethal delays of chest compressions before and after countershocks. *Ann Emerg Med* 2003;42(4):458–467.

90. Edelson DP, Abella BS, Kramer-Johansen J, et al. Effects of compression depth and pre-shock pauses predict defibrillation failure during cardiac arrest. *Resuscitation* 2006;71(2):137–145.

91. Swor R, Khan I, Domeier R, et al. CPR training and CPR performance: do CPR-trained bystanders perform CPR? *Acad Emerg Med* 2006;13(6):596–601.

92. Hazinski MF. Is pediatric resuscitation unique? Relative merits of early CPR and ventilation versus early defibrillation for young victims of prehospital cardiac arrest. *Ann Emerg Med* 1995;25(4): 540–543.

93. Demetriades D, Charalambides K, Chahwan S, et al. Nonskeletal cervical spine injuries: epidemiology and diagnostic pitfalls. *J Trauma* 2000;48(4):724–727.

94. Guildner CW. Resuscitation—opening the airway. A comparative study of techniques for opening an airway obstructed by the tongue. *J Am Coll Emerg Physicians* 1976;5(8):588–590.

95. Greene DG, Elam JO, Dobkin AB, et al. Cinefluorographic study of hyperextension of the neck and upper airway patency. *JAMA* 1961;176:570–573.

96. Ruben HM, Elam JO, Ruben AM, et al. Investigation of upper airway problems in resuscitation. 1. Studies of pharyngeal x-rays and performance by laymen. *Anesthesiology* 1961;22:271–279.

97. Elam JO, Greene DG, Schneider MA, et al. Head-tilt method of oral resuscitation. *JAMA* 1960;172:812–815.

98. Hackl W, Hausberger K, Sailer R, et al. Prevalence of cervical spine injuries in patients with facial trauma. *Oral Surg Oral Med Oral Pathol Oral Radiol Endod* 2001;92(4):370–376.

99. Holly LT, Kelly DF, Counelis GJ, et al. Cervical spine trauma associated with moderate and severe head injury: incidence, risk factors, and injury characteristics. *J Neurosurg* 2002;96(3 Suppl):285–291.

100. Majernick TG, Bieniek R, Houston JB, et al. Cervical spine movement during orotracheal intubation. *Ann Emerg Med* 1986; 15(4):417–420.

101. Lennarson PJ, Smith DW, Sawin PD, et al. Cervical spinal motion during intubation: efficacy of stabilization maneuvers in the setting of complete segmental instability. *J Neurosurg* 2001;94(2 Suppl):265–270.

102. Heath KJ. The effect of laryngoscopy of different cervical spine immobilisation techniques. *Anaesthesia* 1994;49(10):843–845.

103. Hastings RH, Wood PR. Head extension and laryngeal view during laryngoscopy with cervical spine stabilization maneuvers. *Anesthesiology* 1994;80(4):825–831.

104. Gerling MC, Davis DP, Hamilton RS, et al. Effects of cervical spine immobilization technique and laryngoscope blade selection on an unstable cervical spine in a cadaver model of intubation. *Ann Emerg Med* 2000;36(4):293–300.

105. Davies G, Deakin C, Wilson A. The effect of a rigid collar on intracranial pressure. *Injury* 1996;27(9):647–649.

106. Kolb JC, Summers RL, Galli RL. Cervical collar-induced changes in intracranial pressure. *Am J Emerg Med* 1999;17(2):135–137.

107. Mobbs RJ, Stoodley MA, Fuller J. Effect of cervical hard collar on intracranial pressure after head injury. *ANZ J Surg* 2002;72(6): 389–391.

108. Wechsler B, Kim H, Hunter J. Trampolines, children, and strokes. *Am J Phys Med Rehabil* 2001;80(8):608–613.

109. Eberle B, Dick WF, Schneider T, et al. Checking the carotid pulse check: diagnostic accuracy of first responders in patients with and without a pulse. *Resuscitation* 1996;33(2):107–116.

110. Bahr J, Klingler H, Panzer W, et al. Skills of lay people in checking the carotid pulse. *Resuscitation* 1997;35(1):23–26.

111. Ruppert M, Reith MW, Widmann JH, et al. Checking for breathing: evaluation of the diagnostic capability of emergency medical services personnel, physicians, medical students, and medical laypersons. *Ann Emerg Med* 1999;34(6):720–729.

112. Paradis NA, Martin GB, Goetting MG, et al. Simultaneous aortic, jugular bulb, and right atrial pressures during cardiopulmonary resuscitation in humans. Insights into mechanisms. *Circulation* 1989;80(2):361–368.

113. Dorph E, Wik L, Steen PA. Arterial blood gases with 700 ml tidal volumes during out-of-hospital CPR. *Resuscitation* 2004;61(1):23–27.

114. Winkler M, Mauritz W, Hackl W, et al. Effects of half the tidal volume during cardiopulmonary resuscitation on acid-base balance and haemodynamics in pigs. *Eur J Emerg Med* 1998;5(2):201–206.

115. Baskett P, Nolan J, Parr M. Tidal volumes which are perceived to be adequate for resuscitation. *Resuscitation* 1996;31(3):231–234.

116. Garnett AR, Ornato JP, Gonzalez ER, et al. End-tidal carbon dioxide monitoring during cardiopulmonary resuscitation. *JAMA* 1987;257(4):512–515.

117. Safar P, Escarraga LA, Elam JO. A comparison of the mouth-to-mouth and mouth-to-airway methods of artificial respiration with the chest-pressure arm-lift methods. *N Engl J Med* 1958;258(14): 671–677.

118. Mejicano GC, Maki DG. Infections acquired during cardiopulmonary resuscitation: estimating the risk and defining strategies for prevention. *Ann Intern Med* 1998;129(10):813–828.

119. Eisenburger P, Funk GC, Burda G, et al. Gas concentrations in expired air during basic life support using different ratios of compression to ventilation. *Resuscitation* 2007;73(1):115–122.

120. Thierbach AR, Piepho T, Kunde M, et al. Two-rescuer CPR results in hyperventilation in the ventilating rescuer. *Resuscitation* 2005;65(2):185–190.

121. Ornato JP, Hallagan LF, McMahan SB, et al. Attitudes of BCLS instructors about mouth-to-mouth resuscitation during the AIDS epidemic. *Ann Emerg Med* 1990;19(2):151–156.

122. Brenner BE, Van DC, Cheng D, et al. Determinants of reluctance to perform CPR among residents and applicants: the impact of experience on helping behavior. *Resuscitation* 1997;35(3):203–211.

123. Terndrup TE, Warner DA. Infant ventilation and oxygenation by basic life support providers: comparison of methods. *Prehosp Disaster Med* 1992;7(1):35–40.

124. Hess D, Ness C, Oppel A, et al. Evaluation of mouth-to-mask ventilation devices. *Respir Care* 1989;34(3):191–195.

125. Simmons M, Deao D, Moon L, et al. Bench evaluation: three face-shield CPR barrier devices. *Respir Care* 1995;40(6): 618–623.

126. Ruben H. The immediate treatment of respiratory failure. *Br J Anaesth* 1964;36:542–549.

127. Bhalla RK, Corrigan A, Roland NJ. Comparison of two face masks used to deliver early ventilation to laryngectomized patients. *Ear Nose Throat J* 2004;83(6):414, 416.

128. Elling R, Politis J. An evaluation of emergency medical technicians' ability to use manual ventilation devices. *Ann Emerg Med* 1983;12(12):765–768.

129. Dorph E, Wik L, Stromme TA, et al. Oxygen delivery and return of spontaneous circulation with ventilation:compression ratio 2:30 versus chest compressions only CPR in pigs. *Resuscitation* 2004;60(3):309–318.

130. Salem MR, Sellick BA, Elam JO. The historical background of cricoid pressure in anesthesia and resuscitation. *Anesth Analg* 1974;53(2):230–232.

131. Petito SP, Russell WJ. The prevention of gastric inflation—a neglected benefit of cricoid pressure. *Anaesth Intens Care* 1988;16(2): 139–143.

132. Hartsilver EL, Vanner RG. Airway obstruction with cricoid pressure. *Anaesthesia* 2000;55(3):208–211.

133. Moule P. Checking the carotid pulse: diagnostic accuracy in students of the healthcare professions. *Resuscitation* 2000;44(3): 195–201.

134. Stiell I, Nichol G, Wells G, et al. Health-related quality of life is better for cardiac arrest survivors who received citizen cardiopulmonary resuscitation. *Circulation* 2003;108(16):1939–1944.

135. Handley AJ, Handley JA. Performing chest compressions in a confined space. *Resuscitation* 2004;61(1):55–61.

136. Andersen LO, Isbye DL, Rasmussen LS. Increasing compression depth during manikin CPR using a simple backboard. *Acta Anaesthesiol Scand* 2007;51(6):747–750.

137. Perkins GD, Smith CM, Augre C, et al. Effects of a backboard, bed height, and operator position on compression depth during simulated resuscitation. *Intens Care Med* 2006;32(10):1632–1635.

138. Perkins GD, Benny R, Giles S, et al. Do different mattresses affect the quality of cardiopulmonary resuscitation? *Intens Care Med* 2003;29(12):2330–2335.

139. Tweed M, Tweed C, Perkins GD. The effect of differing support surfaces on the efficacy of chest compressions using a resuscitation manikin model. *Resuscitation* 2001;51(2):179–183.

140. Pickard A, Darby M, Soar J. Radiological assessment of the adult chest: implications for chest compressions. *Resuscitation* 2006;71(3): 387–390.

141. Tomlinson AE, Nysaether J, Kramer-Johansen J, et al. Compression force-depth relationship during out-of-hospital cardiopulmonary resuscitation. *Resuscitation* 2007;72(3):364–370.

142. Heidenreich JW, Berg RA, Higdon TA, et al. Rescuer fatigue: standard versus continuous chest-compression cardiopulmonary resuscitation. *Acad Emerg Med* 2006;13(10):1020–1026.

143. Odegaard S, Kramer-Johansen J, Bromley A, et al. Chest compressions by ambulance personnel on chests with variable stiffness: abilities and attitudes. *Resuscitation* 2007;74(1):127–134.

144. Handley AJ. Teaching hand placement for chest compression—a simpler technique. *Resuscitation* 2002;53(1):29–36.

145. Liberman M, Lavoie A, Mulder D, et al. Cardiopulmonary resuscitation: errors made by pre-hospital emergency medical personnel. *Resuscitation* 1999;42(1):47–55.

146. Kundra P, Dey S, Ravishankar M. Role of dominant hand position during external cardiac compression. *Br J Anaesth* 2000;84(4):491–493.

147. Nikandish R, Shahbazi S, Golabi S, et al. Role of dominant versus non-dominant hand position during uninterrupted chest compression CPR by novice rescuers: a randomized double-blind crossover study. *Resuscitation* 2008;76(2):256–260.

148. Aufderheide TP, Pirrallo RG, Yannopoulos D, et al. Incomplete chest wall decompression: a clinical evaluation of CPR performance by EMS personnel and assessment of alternative manual chest compression-decompression techniques. *Resuscitation* 2005;64(3):353–362.

149. Yannopoulos D, McKnite S, Aufderheide TP, et al. Effects of incomplete chest wall decompression during cardiopulmonary resuscitation on coronary and cerebral perfusion pressures in a porcine model of cardiac arrest. *Resuscitation* 2005;64(3):363–372.

150. Kim JA, Vogel D, Guimond G, et al. A randomized, controlled comparison of cardiopulmonary resuscitation performed on the floor and on a moving ambulance stretcher. *Prehosp Emerg Care* 2006;10(1):68–70.

151. Aufderheide TP, Lurie KG. Death by hyperventilation: a common and life-threatening problem during cardiopulmonary resuscitation. *Crit Care Med* 2004;32(9 Suppl):S345–S351.

152. Olasveengen TM, Tomlinson AE, Wik L, et al. A failed attempt to improve quality of out-of-hospital CPR through performance evaluation. *Prehosp Emerg Care* 2007;11(4):427–433.

153. Barsan WG, Levy RC. Experimental design for study of cardiopulmonary resuscitation in dogs. *Ann Emerg Med* 1981;10(3):135–137.

154. Kern KB, Sanders AB, Raife J, et al. A study of chest compression rates during cardiopulmonary resuscitation in humans. The importance of rate-directed chest compressions. *Arch Intern Med* 1992;152(1):145–149.

155. Beckers SK, Skorning MH, Fries M, et al. CPREzy improves performance of external chest compressions in simulated cardiac arrest. *Resuscitation* 2007;72(1):100–107.

156. Aase SO, Myklebust H. Compression depth estimation for CPR quality assessment using DSP on accelerometer signals. *IEEE Trans Biomed Eng* 2002;49(3):263–268.

157. Pellis T, Bisera J, Tang W, et al. Expanding automatic external defibrillators to include automated detection of cardiac, respiratory, and cardiorespiratory arrest. *Crit Care Med* 2002;30(4 Suppl):S176–S178.

158. Losert H, Risdal M, Sterz F, et al. Thoracic impedance changes measured via defibrillator pads can monitor ventilation in critically ill patients and during cardiopulmonary resuscitation. *Crit Care Med* 2006;34(9):2399–2405.

159. Losert H, Risdal M, Sterz F, et al. Thoracic-impedance changes measured via defibrillator pads can monitor signs of circulation. *Resuscitation* 2007;73(2):221–228.

160. Abella BS, Edelson DP, Kim S, et al. CPR quality improvement during in-hospital cardiac arrest using a real-time audiovisual feedback system. *Resuscitation* 2007;73(1):54–61.

161. Sayre MR, Berg RA, Cave DM, et al. Hands-only (compression-only) cardiopulmonary resuscitation: a call to action for bystander response to adults who experience out-of-hospital sudden cardiac arrest. A Science Advisory for the public from the American Heart Association Emergency Cardiovascular Care Committee. *Circulation* 2008;117(16):2162–2167.

162. Hew P, Brenner B, Kaufman J. Reluctance of paramedics and emergency medical technicians to perform mouth-to-mouth resuscitation. *J Emerg Med* 1997;15(3):279–284.

163. Ewy GA. Continuous-chest-compression cardiopulmonary resuscitation for cardiac arrest. *Circulation* 2007;116(25):2894–2896.

164. Berg RA, Kern KB, Sanders AB, et al. Bystander cardiopulmonary resuscitation. Is ventilation necessary? *Circulation* 1993;88(4 Pt 1):1907–1915.

165. Chandra NC, Gruben KG, Tsitlik JE, et al. Observations of ventilation during resuscitation in a canine model. *Circulation* 1994;90(6):3070–3075.

166. Tang W, Weil MH, Sun S, et al. Cardiopulmonary resuscitation by precordial compression but without mechanical ventilation. *Am J Respir Crit Care Med* 1994;150(6 Pt 1):1709–1713.

167. Berg RA, Wilcoxson D, Hilwig RW, et al. The need for ventilatory support during bystander CPR. *Ann Emerg Med* 1995;26(3):342–350.

168. Tucker KJ, Idris AH, Wenzel V, et al. Changes in arterial and mixed venous blood gases during untreated ventricular fibrillation and cardiopulmonary resuscitation. *Resuscitation* 1994;28(2):137–141.

169. Berg RA, Kern KB, Hilwig RW, et al. Assisted ventilation does not improve outcome in a porcine model of single-rescuer bystander cardiopulmonary resuscitation. *Circulation* 1997;95(6):1635–1641.

170. Kern KB, Hilwig RW, Berg RA, et al. Efficacy of chest compression-only BLS CPR in the presence of an occluded airway. *Resuscitation* 1998;39(3):179–188.

171. Eisenberg MS. Incidence and significance of gasping or agonal respirations in cardiac arrest patients. *Curr Opin Crit Care* 2006;12(3):204–206.

172. Hayes MM, Ewy GA, Anavy ND, et al. Continuous passive oxygen insufflation results in a similar outcome to positive pressure ventilation in a swine model of out-of-hospital ventricular fibrillation. *Resuscitation* 2007;74(2):357–365.

173. Waalewijn RA, Tijssen JG, Koster RW. Bystander initiated actions in out-of-hospital cardiopulmonary resuscitation: results from the Amsterdam Resuscitation Study (ARRESUST). *Resuscitation* 2001;50(3):273–279.

174. Van Hoeyweghen RJ, Bossaert LL, Mullie A, et al. Quality and efficiency of bystander CPR. Belgian Cerebral Resuscitation Study Group. *Resuscitation* 1993;26(1):47–52.

175. Kellum MJ, Kennedy KW, Ewy GA. Cardiocerebral resuscitation improves survival of patients with out-of-hospital cardiac arrest. *Am J Med* 2006;119(4):335–340.

176. Cardiopulmonary resuscitation by bystanders with chest compression only (SOS-KANTO): an observational study. *Lancet* 2007;369(9565):920–926.

177. Iwami T, Kawamura T, Hiraide A, et al. Effectiveness of bystander-initiated cardiac-only resuscitation for patients with out-of-hospital cardiac arrest. *Circulation* 2007;116(25):2900–2907.

178. Bohm K, Rosenqvist M, Herlitz J, et al. Survival is similar after standard treatment and chest compression only in out-of-hospital bystander cardiopulmonary resuscitation. *Circulation* 2007;116(25):2908–2912.

179. Claesson A, Svensson L, Silfverstolpe J, et al. Characteristics and outcome among patients suffering out-of-hospital cardiac arrest due to drowning. *Resuscitation* 2008;76(3):381–387.

180. Criley JM, Blaufuss AH, Kissel GL. Cough-induced cardiac compression. Self-administered from of cardiopulmonary resuscitation. *JAMA* 1976;236(11):1246–1250.

181. Girsky MJ, Criley JM. Cough cardiopulmonary resuscitation revisited. *Circulation* 2006;114(15):e530–e531.

182. American Heart Association. Cough CPR. 10/2007. Available at: http://www.americanheart.org/presenter.jhtml?identifier=4535. Accessed January 16, 2008.

183. Brown J, Rogers J, Soar J. Cardiac arrest during surgery and ventilation in the prone position: a case report and systematic review. *Resuscitation* 2001;50(2):233–238.

184. Mazer SP, Weisfeldt M, Bai D, et al. Reverse CPR: a pilot study of CPR in the prone position. *Resuscitation* 2003;57(3):279–285.

185. Wei J, Tung D, Sue SH, et al. Cardiopulmonary resuscitation in prone position: a simplified method for outpatients. *J Chin Med Assoc* 2006;69(5):202–206.

186. Bollig G, Steen PA, Wik L. Standard versus over-the-head cardiopulmonary resuscitation during simulated advanced life support. *Prehosp Emerg Care* 2007;11(4):443–447.

187. Perkins GD, Stephenson BT, Smith CM, et al. A comparison between over-the-head and standard cardiopulmonary resuscitation. *Resuscitation* 2004;61(2):155–161.

Three

Defibrillation

Chapter 12
Restoring Life: The Story of Human Defibrillation and Modern CPR

Mark E. Silverman

I tried an electric shock directed through the chest to the spine of the back, and not without success; for suddenly it [the bird] rose up and…walked about quietly on its feet.

- Efforts to revive the apparent dead with electricity date back over 230 years; however, it is only since the 1960s that defibrillation has become a clinical reality.
- The first recorded use of an electrical jolt for resuscitation is a 1774 report by the Royal Humane Society for the Apparently Dead in London in which a limp child was stimulated back to life.
- The first portable "defibrillator," using discharging rods attached to a Leiden jar capacitor, was reported in "An Essay on the Recovery of the Apparently Dead" by Charles Kite in London in 1788.
- The need for a universal defibrillator became a research priority in the early twentieth century, when the electrification of homes was accompanied by accidental electrocutions of the public and the company linemen who were up on the poles installing the circuits.
- The first successful human defibrillation was performed in 1947 by Claude Beck. Beck was operating on a 14-year-old boy whose heart went into arrest. After cardiac massage and drugs failed, Beck summoned a defibrillator from his experimental laboratory and defibrillated the patient, with a satisfying outcome.

Introduction

The restoration of life to the apparently dead is one of the great stories in medicine. This dream became universally possible with the invention of the defibrillator in the mid-20th century.[1-3] The story begins in 1672 in Germany, where Otto von Guerike found that a glass globe containing sulfur became charged when rubbed. He had discovered static electricity, which would be harnessed within a glass jar in the next century to deliver powerful shocks. The Leyden jar, invented by Pieter van Musschenbroek in the Netherlands in 1746, provided the first electrical storage device. This corked glass jar, with a central brass rod lined with tinfoil, stored static electricity, which could be released as strong shocks. It soon became popular for scientific, medical, and amusement purposes (Fig. 12-1).

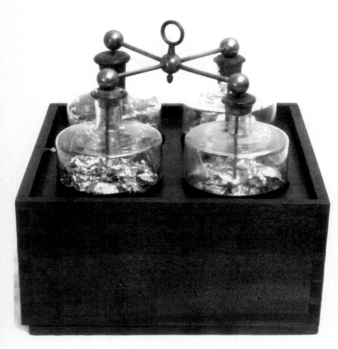

FIGURE 12-1 • A Leyden jar capacitor with discharging rods. (Courtesy of the Baaken Library.)

Early Attempts to Apply Electrical Shocks for Resuscitation

One of the first to experiment with electrical resuscitation was Peter Christian Abildgaard, a Danish physician and veterinarian with a special interest in electricity.[4] Abildgaard had observed that animals and men killed by lightning showed little internal damage to explain their death. In 1775, he performed experiments on hens, using shocks from 10 Leyden jars to kill the bird then reviving it from "swooning" with a second shock. He commented: "I tried an electric shock directed through the chest to the spine of the back, and not without success; for suddenly it rose up and . . . walked about quietly on its feet."

In the 18th and 19th centuries, sudden death was often due to drowning, asphyxiation, and lightning.[2,5] Rescue societies, originating as the Dutch Humane Society in Amsterdam in 1767 and spreading from there to other port cities in Europe, London, and America, organized volunteer resuscitative attempts and reported some early anecdotal success using heat, friction, spirits, smelling salts, fumigation with tobacco smoke instilled in the rectum, and artificial respiration with a bellows. Their enthusiastic efforts were among the first to counteract entrenched concepts about the inevitability of death and to foster important research in this area.[1,2]

The first recorded use of an electrical jolt for resuscitation is described in a 1774 report by the Royal Humane Society for the Apparently Dead in London, where a limp child was stimulated back to life.[5] This success inaugurated the regular application of electricity for such purposes. John Hunter of London, the great comparative anatomist, commented in1776: "Electricity has been known to be of service and should be tried when other methods have failed. It is probably the only method we have of immediately stimulating the heart."[6]

The first portable "defibrillator," using discharging rods attached to a Leyden jar capacitor, was reported in "An Essay on the Recovery of the Apparently Dead" by Charles Kite of London in 1788 (Fig. 12-2). Kite studied records from several hundred cases of drowning and noted that the "recovery of the apparently dead is the length of time that elapses before the proper remedies can be applied." He also recommended endotracheal intubation.[2]

In 1809, Allan Burns of Glasgow was recommending the universal application of electricity for sudden death: "Where however, the cessation of vital action is very complete, and continues long, we ought to inflate the lungs, and pass electric shocks through the chest; the practitioner ought never, if the death has been sudden, and the person not very far advanced in life, to despair of success, 'til he has unequivocal signs of real death."[7] Alexandro Volta's famous dispute with Galvani led to the 1799 invention of the earliest battery, the voltaic pile. This was incorporated into the "reanimation" chair of Richard Reece in about 1820, with the battery attached to the proximal end of a metallic tube inserted into the esophagus of the individual to be revived.[2] The

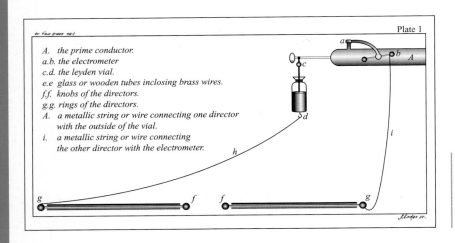

A. the prime conductor.
a.b. the electrometer
c.d. the leyden vial.
e.e glass or wooden tubes inclosing brass wires.
f.f. knobs of the directors.
g.g. rings of the directors.
A. a metallic string or wire connecting one director with the outside of the vial.
i. a metallic string or wire connecting the other director with the electrometer.

FIGURE 12-2 • Earliest defibrillator, used by Charles Kite in 1788. The Leyden jar (d) is suspended from the prime conductor (A) and both are connected to directors (f), which are placed on the patient. (Courtesy of the Baaken Library.)

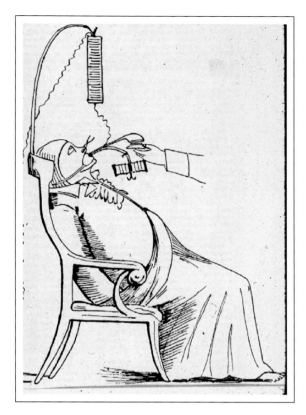

FIGURE 12-3 • Reanimation chair of 1820. A metallic tube is inserted into the throat and connected to a voltaic battery hanging above. The dangling wire is touched to the body. (Courtesy of the Baaken Library and Museum, Minneapolis.)

instructions read "In every case of suspended animation, endeavor to restore the functions of the lungs and heart. To accomplish this, extend the patient's body on the moveable back of the reanimation chair . . . an assistant should be preparing the Pensile Galvanic Pile . . . . Having attached the galvanic pile to the top of the chair, one of the wires is to be applied to the tube passing down the gullet, whilst the other is to be successively made to touch different parts of the external surface of the body, particularly about the regions of the heart"[2] (Fig. 12-3).

The Experimental Production and Significance of Ventricular Fibrillation

Ventricular fibrillation was first induced in animals by M. Hoffa and Carl Ludwig in 1850.[8] It was not understood as a cause of sudden death in humans until the experiments conducted by John MacWilliam, a professor at Aberdeen, Scotland, in 1885–1887[9–14] (Fig. 12-4). MacWilliam offered experimental proof that "fibrillar contraction" was the cause of sudden death. In 1889, he argued that "sudden cardiac

failure does not usually take the form of a simple ventricular standstill in diastole....It assumes, on the contrary, the form of a violent, though irregular and inco-ordinated, manifestation of ventricular energy. Instead of quiescence, there is a tumultuous activity, irregular in its character and wholly ineffective as regards its results."[13] He explained that a variety of pathologic conditions could predispose to ventricular fibrillation, including "degenerative changes of a fatty or fibroid nature in the muscular walls" and "diseased conditions...of the coronary arteries." MacWilliam also used cardiac compression, artificial resuscitation, and drugs to resuscitate the hearts.

In 1899, Jean Louis Prevost and Frederic Battelli, physiologists in Geneva, Switzerland, induced ventricular fibrillation by passing a weak (40 volt) current through an exposed dog heart or through the chest.[15] This was reversed with a repeat, stronger (240–4800 volt) alternating and direct current "countershock." Their important work, mostly overlooked until 1930, would eventually become crucial to the development of the modern defibrillator by Kouwenhoven.[1,2,9] Prevost and Battelli also learned that internal cardiac massage was required to preserve the heart if the second shock was delayed.

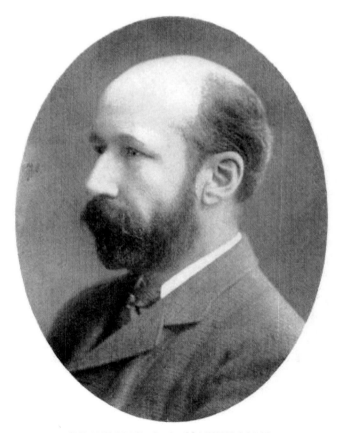

PROFESSOR J. A. MACWILLIAM.

FIGURE 12-4 • John MacWilliam. (Courtesy of Mr. A. Adam, Honorary Librarian, The Royal Infirmary, Foresterhill, Aberdeen, Scotland.)

Augustus Hoffman recorded the first human electrocardiogram of ventricular fibrillation in 1911, thereby confirming the hypothesis of MacWilliam 22 years earlier.[9,15] In the same year, A. G. Levy and Thomas Lewis documented that ventricular fibrillation was the mechanism of death from chloroform anesthesia. Lewis commented in 1915: "It is a remarkable fact that practically every form of irregularity, which has been produced experimentally in the mammalian heart, has now been recorded frequently in clinical cases. But there is one notable exception . . . Why is fibrillation of the ventricles so uncommon an experience? For a good reason: fibrillation of the ventricles is incompatible with existence...If it occurs in man, it is responsible for unexpected and sudden death."[16]

Critical Period for Defibrillation: Recognition of Hypoxia

Cardiac and cerebral hypoxia remained an insurmountable barrier outside of the laboratory setting. Carl Wiggers at Western Reserve University, the leading American cardiac physiologist, studied experimental myocardial infarction and ventricular fibrillation starting in the 1930s.[9,17,18] He developed his own defibrillator, first used in 1937, based on Kouwenhoven's work at Johns Hopkins. He advocated cardiac massage preceding the shock. In 1940, Carl Wiggers commented on "the race with time," saying: "Although the problem of reviving human fibrillating hearts must not be considered hopeless, we must not yet allow ourselves and others to expect too much in a practical way from our present methods until the next fundamental forward step is taken, viz. provision of oxygen for the fibrillating ventricle by methods other than massage."[17] He also voiced concern that shocking the heart with a 110-volt household alternating current through external electrodes might cause further damage to a heart in temporary standstill, endanger the rescuer, or increase recurrence of ventricular fibrillation in patients with coronary disease.

The Development of the Defibrillator; Integration With Cardiopulmonary Resuscitation

The need for a universal defibrillator became a research priority in the early 20th century, when the electrification of homes was accompanied by accidental electrocutions of the public and the company linemen who were up on the poles installing the circuits.[2,6,9] In 1926, Consolidated Edison of New York in collaboration with Simon Flexner and the

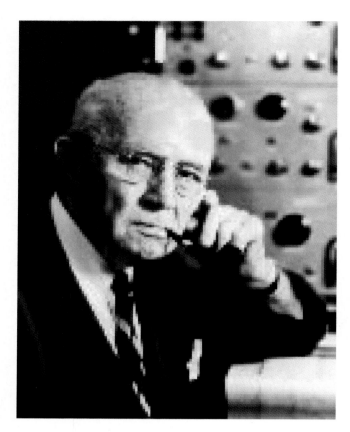

FIGURE 12-5 • William B. Kouwenhoven. Johns Hopkins University engineer who developed the portable defibrillator. (Courtesy of the National Library of Medicine.)

Rockefeller Institute offered a $10,000 award to develop a device for closed-chest defibrillation. Donald Hooker, William B. Kouwenhoven (Fig. 12-5), an electrical engineer, and their associates at Johns Hopkins Hospital were directed by physiologist W. H. Howell to investigate the effect of electrical current on the body, work they initiated in 1928.[19] First, they showed that ventricular fibrillation could easily be induced by small shocks of electricity. These studies, confirming the work of Prevost and Battelli, eventually led to their development of an open-chest alternating current defibrillator. However, successful defibrillation, which they reported in 1933, was confined to a 2-minute window of opportunity. In 1951, they were challenged to develop a practical closed-chest defibrillator. Their work, carried out over 40 years, culminated in the development of open- and closed-chest AC and DC defibrillators and a biphasic model, the forerunners of modern equipment[19] (Fig. 12-6). Their original defibrillator, weighing 280 pounds, was first utilized on a hospitalized patient in March 1957; their first portable defibrillator, a 50-pound device, was finally ready for service in 1963. The biphasic device delivered 166 joules and could be powered by a 6-volt battery or connected to the battery of a power company truck.[19]

The Kouwenhoven team also introduced closed-chest massage. They had serendipitously observed that "When

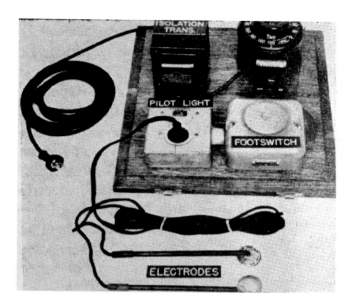

FIGURE 12-6 • Hopkins closed-chest AC defibrillator. Developed at Johns Hopkins University and first used on a patient in 1957. (Courtesy of the Annals of Internal Medicine and the Alan Mason Chesney Medical Archives of the Johns Hopkins Medical Institutions.)

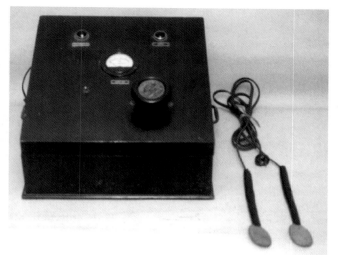

FIGURE 12-7 • Defibrillator used by Claude Beck in the operating room. (Courtesy of the Baaken Library.)

the electrodes were placed on the chest, there was a marked rise in the femoral arterial blood pressure." Further testing led to the technique of closed-chest massage, which they reported in 1960.[20] Mouth-to-mouth ventilation was shown to be effective by Peter Safar in 1958.[21] By the early 1960s, the three essential components of modern cardiopulmonary resuscitation (CPR)—maintenance of ventilation, chest massage, and closed-chest defibrillation —were finally in place for universal adoption. This would soon begin in coronary care units and emergency departments and then eventually spread throughout the hospital wards during the 1960s.

The First Successful Human Defibrillation and Coronary Care

The first successful human defibrillation was performed in 1947 by Claude Beck. Beck was an innovative though controversial professor of surgery at Western Reserve University.[22,23] Blaming himself for the death of a boy who had died from ventricular fibrillation during surgery in 1934, Beck researched intraoperative cardiac arrest, working with Carl Wiggers. They constructed an alternating current internal defibrillator based on the work of Kouwenhoven. In 1937, Beck presented a motion picture to the American Surgical Association showing how to ventilate the lungs and defibrillate the heart in dogs. Like Wiggers, he emphasized manual massage of the heart before shocking. His efforts were unsuccessful in five hospitalized patients over the next 10 years.

In 1947, Beck was operating on a 14-year-old boy whose heart arrested. After cardiac massage and drugs failed, Beck summoned a defibrillator from his experimental laboratory and defibrillated the patient, with a satisfying outcome[24] (Fig. 12-7). Between 1947 and 1955, open-chest defibrillation was accomplished in a few operating rooms. In 1955, a physician with coronary disease "fell over with a fatal heart attack" immediately outside Western Reserve University Hospital. He received an open chest shock and survived.[26] An opportune promoter, Beck took pictures of the clothed patient during the arrest to prove that it occurred outside the hospital! Until then, a cardiac arrest from coronary disease was assumed to be due to an acute heart attack and to be irreversible. After all, why would the heart restart? Even if it did, why would it not just lapse back into fibrillation again? Beck felt otherwise, eloquently stating: "The death factor in coronary artery disease is often small and reversible. It is comparable to turning the ignition switch in an automobile or to stopping and starting the pendulum of a clock. The heart wants to beat, and often it needs only a second chance."[25] Indeed, the resuscitated physician lived 28 more years, to age 93. Beck's inspiration—"hearts [are] too good to die," and his tireless campaigning and monthly CPR courses for 17 years on its behalf, helped to inaugurate a new era in cardiology, one that would eventually lead to coronary care units in 1962 and the universal application of CPR, first by professionals and eventually by the public. Beck anticipated this in 1956, saying "Any intelligent man or woman can be taught to do resuscitation. A medical or nursing degree is not a prerequisite to learn resuscitation, nor is it impossible to provide resuscitation kits to be opened for the emergency; these could be located in selected areas . . . .The veil of mystery is being lifted from heart conditions, and the dead are being brought back to life."[24] His concept of teaching lay people to do resuscitation, which he had started in 1963, proved highly controversial, including claims that Beck was playing God. Indeed, resuscitation was not recommended by the American Heart Association until 1973.

Cardioversion of Ventricular Tachycardia and Supraventricular Arrhythmias

Closed-chest defibrillation, electrical conversion of ventricular tachycardia, and cardioversion of atrial tachyarrhythmias were still to come. Paul Zoll and his colleagues at Beth Israel Hospital in Boston pioneered many advances in the electrical control of the heart rhythm, including the closed-chest approach.[2,26] In 1952, Zoll showed that external electrical stimuli to the chest of dogs and two patients was "a simple, effective and apparently safe means . . . of arousing the heart from ventricular standstill." He suggested the possibility of defibrillating the human heart and then stimulating it with an external pacemaker until an unaided rhythm resumed.[27] This concept was developed by Zoll into the use of temporary transvenous and transcutaneous pacing as well as the method for permanent implanted pacemakers. In 1956, Zoll was the first to report terminating ventricular fibrillation by closed-chest shock in four patients.[28] By 1960, he could claim success in an additional eight patients.

Prior to the early 1960s, treatment of sustained ventricular tachycardia depended upon the intravenous infusion of quinidine or procainamide—two antiarrhythmic drugs fraught with serious side effects and unpredictable efficacy. External countershock for ventricular tachycardia was first performed in Boston in 1960.[29] In 1962, Zoll published his experience using external, alternating current "countershock" in ill patients with prolonged rapid ventricular and supraventricular tachycardias that were unresponsive to drugs. His rationale was that "The deteriorating clinical condition of these [first] seven patients with the threat of imminent death impelled us to this new clinical application of external countershock." This was successful in seven of eight patients but was attended with some complications, including ventricular fibrillation and standstill, and it required these desperately ill patients to undergo general anesthesia.[30] The solution would be direct current shocks synchronized with the QRS, thus avoiding the vulnerable period. This would be accomplished by Bernard Lown at the Peter Bent Brigham Hospital, who developed a direct current cardioverter-defibrillator and showed that atrial fibrillation could be safely shocked back to sinus rhythm.[31] After other reports on the successful conversion of ventricular tachycardia with direct current shocks[18,19] and the introduction of lidocaine in 1963 and amiodarone in 1979, intravenous quinidine and procainamide became increasingly outmoded and are rarely used today.

A mobile coronary care unit, providing rapid response and on-the-scene defibrillation, was initiated by J. Frank Pantridge and John Geddes at the Royal Victory Hospital in Belfast in 1966.[2] They realized that the majority of deaths occurred before the patient could be admitted to a coronary care unit. By 1969, they reported a success rate of 87% in 50 patients when resuscitation was begun within 4 minutes of cardiac arrest.

Automatic Defibrillators

The automatic implantable defibrillator (ICD) was developed in the 1970s at Sinai Hospital in Baltimore. This remarkable idea occurred to Michel Mirosky, an Israeli working in a hospital near Tel Aviv, whose mentor suffered recurrent bouts of ventricular tachycardia and died in 1966.[32] No one believed that this miniaturization was possible; however, Mirosky was undaunted, and with the engineering assistance of Morton Mower in Baltimore, triumphed over seemingly impossible obstacles. Their first device was implanted February 1980 and received approval from the FDA in 1985.[32] Since then, the implanted defibrillator has become progressively smaller, more easily implanted with improved transvenous lead systems, and increasingly sophisticated. The ICD is now fully accepted as an incredible technologic advance that improves long-term survival compared with antiarrhythmic medications in patients who have been successfully resuscitated from cardiac arrest and when implanted as primary prevention in those with severely impaired ventricular function. (Fig. 12-7) (The Antiarrhytymics versus Implantable Defibrillators (AVID) Investigators. A comparison of antiarrhythmic drug therapy with implantable defibrillators in patients resuscitated from near-fatal ventricular arrhythmias. (Fig. 12-8).[39]

Automated External Defibrillators

Automated "smart" external defibrillators (AEDs), designed to be safely operated by an untrained bystander, were first produced in 1979 and have a 96% to 100% sensitivity for detecting ventricular fibrillation and a specificity of close to 100% in avoiding false shocks. The concept of public access to defibrillation—"Even a child could do it"—has been endorsed by the American Heart Association and was funded by Congress in June 2002.[33] Weighing <5 pounds and increasingly affordable, AEDs could significantly improve out-of-hospital cardiac arrest survival from VF from 5% to more than 50% in highly organized systems.[33,34]

Final Comment

Efforts to revive the apparent dead with electricity date back over 230 years; however, it is only since the 1960s that defib-

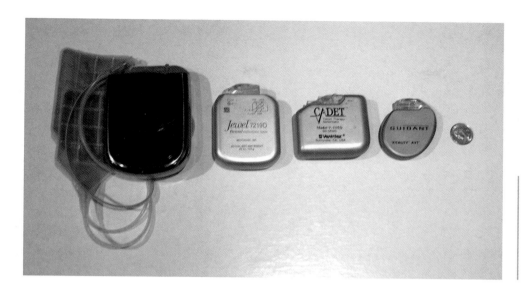

FIGURE 12-8 • Series of implantable defibrillators showing decreasing size from an early model on the left (with patches to attach to the ventricle) to a current model on the right. A quarter is shown for comparison. (Personal collection.)

rillation has become a clinical reality. The defibrillator of Kouwenhoven has evolved into an easily portable device that delivers biphasic current with low-energy waveforms that can deliver more current to high-impedance chests and lessen myocardial injury. It is estimated that 166,000 out-of-hospital cardiac arrests occur annually in the United States, or about one arrest every 3 minutes. Of these, it is estimated that 20% to 38% are due to ventricular fibrillation or ventricular tachycardia and as such, readily treatable with shock.[35] With the increasing availability of lower-cost, user-friendly AEDs and advances in implantable defibrillators, it is imaginable that such devices may become as commonplace in public facilities and higher-risk households as a fire extinguisher and as a cellular telephone in at-risk patients with serious heart disease.[36–38]

Acknowledgements

I appreciate the invaluable assistance of the librarians of the Sauls Memorial Library, Piedmont Hospital, and the secretarial work of Stacie Stepney.

References

1. Silverman ME. Hearts are too good to die for. *The Pharos*, Spring 2005.
2. Eisenberg MS. *Life in the Balance*. New York: Oxford University Press, 1997.
3. Cooper JA, Cooper JD, Cooper JM. Cardiopulmonary resuscitation: history, current practice, and future direction. *Circulation* 2006;114:2839–2849.
4. Drisol TE, Ratnoff OD, Nygaard OF. The remarkable Dr. Abilgaard and countershock. *Ann Intern Med* 1975;83:878–882.
5. Lee RV. Cardiopulmonary resuscitation in the eighteenth century. *J Hist Med* 1972; 27:418–413.
6. Eisenberg MS. Charles Kite's essay on the recovery of the apparently dead: the first scientific study of sudden death. *Ann Emerg Med* 1994;23:1049–1053.
7. Burns A. *Observations on Some of the Most Frequent and Important Diseases of the Heart; Aneurism of the Thoracic Aorta; on Preternatural Pulsation in the Epigastric Region: and on the Unusual Origin and Distribution of some of the large Arteries of the Human Body*. Edinburgh: Thomas Bryce and Co, John Murray, and J Callow, 1809.
8. Burch GE, dePasquale NP. *A History of Electrocardiography*. Chicago: Year Book, 1964.
9. Fye WB. Ventricular fibrillation and defibrillation: historical perspectives with emphasis on the contributions of John MacWilliam, Carl Wiggers, and William Kouwenhoven. *Circulation* 1985;71:858–865.
10. Silverman ME, Fye B. John A. MacWilliams: Scottish pioneer of cardiac electrophysiology. *Clin Cardiol* 2006;29:90–92.
11. de Silva, RA. John MacWilliam, evolutionary biology, and sudden cardiac death. *J Am Coll Cardiol* 1989;14:1843–1849.
12. MacWilliam JA. Fibrillar contraction of the heart. *J Physiol* 1887;8:296–310.
13. MacWilliam JA. Cardiac failure and sudden death. *Br Med J* 1889;1:6–8.
14. MacWilliam JA. Some applications of physiology to medicine. Ventricular fibrillation and sudden death. *Br Med J* 1923;2:215–227.
15. Prevost JL, Battelli F. La mort par les courants électriques. *J Physiol* 1899;1:399–412.
16. Lewis T. *Lectures on the Heart*. New York: Huebner, 1915.
17. Wiggers CJ. The physiologic basis for cardiac resuscitation from ventricular fibrillation-method for serial defibrillation. *Am Heart J* 1940;28:413–422.
18. Wiggers, CJ. The mechanism and nature of ventricular fibrillation. *Am Heart J* 1940;20:399–412.
19. Kouwenhoven WB. The development of the defibrillator. *Ann Intern Med* 1969;71:449–458.
20. Kouwenhoven WB, Jude JR, Knickerbocker GG. Closed-chest cardiac massage. *JAMA* 1960;173:94–97.
21. Safar P, Escarraga LA, Elam JO. A comparison of the mouth-to-mouth and mouth-to-airway methods of artificial respiration with the chest-pressure arm-lift methods. *N Engl J Med* 1958;258:671–677.
22. Timmerman S. Hearts too good to die: Claude S. Beck's contributions to life-saving. *J Hist Soc* 2001;14:108–131.
23. Beck CS, Keininger DS. Reversal of deaths in good hearts. *J Cardiovasc Surg* 1962;357–375.
24. Beck CS, Pritchard WH, Feil HS. Ventricular fibrillation of long duration abolished by electric shock. *JAMA* 1947;135:985–986.
25. Beck CS, Weckesser EC, Barry FM. Fatal heart attack and successful defibrillation: new concepts in coronary artery disease. *JAMA* 1956;161:434–436.
26. Abelman WH. Paul M Zoll and electrical stimulation on the human heart. *Clin Cardiol* 1986;9:131–135.
27. Zoll PM, Paul MH, Linenthal AJ, et al. The effects of external electric currents on the heart. *Circulation* 1956;14:745–756.

28. Zoll PM, Linenthal AJ, Gibson W, et al. Termination of ventricular fibrillation in man by externally applied electric countershock. *N Engl J Med* 1956;254:727–732.

29. Alexander S, Kleiger R, Lown B. Use of external electric countershock in the treatment of ventricular tachycardia. *JAMA* 1961;177:98–100.

30. Zoll PM, Linenthal AJ. Termination of refractory tachycardia by external countershock. *Circulation* 1962;25:596–603.

31. Lown B, Amarasingham R, Neuman J. New method for terminating cardiac arrhythmias: Use of synchronized capacitor discharge. *JAMA* 1962;182:548–555.

32. Kastor JA. Michel Mirowski and the automatic implantable defibrillator. *Am J Cardiol* 1989;63:977–982.

33. Hazinski MF, Idris AH, Kerber RE, et al. Lay rescuer automated external defibrillator ("public access defibrillation") programs: lessons learned from an international multicenter trial. *Circulation* 2005;111:3336–3340.

34. Hallstrom A, Ornata JP. Public-access defibrillation and survival after out-of-hospital cardiac arrest. *N Eng J Med* 2004;351:637–656.

35. American Heart Association Statistics Committee and Stroke Statistics Subcommittee. Heart disease and stroke statistics—2008 update. *Circulation* 2008;17:e25–146.

36. Adgey AA, Spence MS, Walsh SJ. Theory and practice of defibrillation: (2) defibrillation for ventricular fibrillation. *Heart* 2005;91:118–125.

37. Sado DM, Deakin CD. How good is your defibrillation technique? *J R Soc Med* 2005;98:3–6.

38. Cooper JA, Cooper JD, Cooper JM. Cardiopulmonary resuscitation: history, current practice, and future direction. *Circulation* 2006;114:2839–2849.

39. Bardy GH, Lee KL, Mark DB, et al. Amiodarone or an implantable cardioverter-defibrillator for congestive heart failure. *N Engl J Med* 2005;252:225–37.

Chapter 13
Defibrillation: Practice

Vincent N. Mosesso Jr. and Cheryl Rickens

Defibrillation has a pivotal place in the management of pulseless cardiac arrest. Delivering an electrical shock to the heart is the sine qua non for the reversal of ventricular fibrillation (VF) and is often necessary for unstable ventricular tachycardia. Defibrillation remains the only therapy that directly reverses VF. However, there is an evolving understanding of the importance of adjunctive therapies to improve the myocardial metabolic state and the time-sensitive nature of defibrillation.

- Defibrillation (delivery of an electric shock through the heart) is necessary for eradication of the lethal arrhythmia VF.
- In general, the earlier defibrillation occurs, the higher the likelihood of survival from VF.
- In cases of prolonged VF, a brief period of cardiopulmonary resuscitation (CPR) improves the likelihood of successful defibrillation.
- Defibrillators (both manual and automated) and providers must be maintained in a state of readiness.

Introduction

Defibrillation has a pivotal place in the management of pulseless cardiac arrest. Delivering an electrical shock to the heart is the *sine qua non* for the reversal of VF and is often necessary for unstable ventricular tachycardia. While "defibrillation" literally means "the reversal or absence of fibrillation," the term is commonly used to refer to the delivery of an electric shock in an attempt to terminate the fatal arrhythmia. Electrical defibrillation is intended to eradicate all active electrical current by depolarizing a critical mass of myocardium. Defibrillation literally stuns the heart, with the hope that a normal pacemaker site will then be able to regain control of the cardiac conducting system. Defibrillation remains the only therapy that directly reverses VF, although we are gaining an evolving understanding of the importance of adjunctive therapies to improve the myocardial metabolic state at the time of defibrillation. So while the concept of early defibrillation is still an important principle of management, guidelines now and in the future will address the timing of defibrillation for different patient populations and the integration of CPR and other therapies with defibrillatory shocks.

The Concept of "Early" Defibrillation

Early defibrillation is critical to survival from sudden cardiac arrest (SCA) for several reasons:

1. The most frequent initial rhythm in witnessed SCA is ventricular fibrillation.
2. The treatment for VF is electrical defibrillation.
3. The probability of successful defibrillation diminishes rapidly over time.
4. VF tends to deteriorate to asystole within a few minutes.[1]

Several studies have documented the effects of time to defibrillation and the effects of bystander CPR on survival from SCA. For every minute that passes between collapse and defibrillation, survival rates from witnessed VF SCA decrease 7% to 10% if no CPR is provided.[1] When bystander CPR is provided, the decrease in survival rates is more gradual and averages 3% to 4% per minute from collapse to defibrillation.[1,2] CPR can double[1-3] or triple[4] survival from witnessed SCA at any interval to defibrillation.

If bystanders provide immediate CPR, many adults in VF can survive with intact neurologic function, especially if defibrillation is performed within about 5 minutes after SCA.[5,6] CPR prolongs the window of time during which defibrillation will be effective[7-9] and provides a small amount of blood flow that may maintain some oxygen and substrate delivery to the heart and brain.[10] CPR alone, however, is unlikely to eliminate VF and restore a perfusing rhythm.

Nearly all neurologically intact survivors, who in some studies number more than 90% of survivors, have a ventricular tachyarrhythmia that was treated by early defibrillation.[10-15] In a subgroup of SCD patients, it appears from studies in which Holter monitors were used that a ventricular tachyarrhythmia is the initial rhythm disturbance in up to 85% of persons with sudden, out-of-hospital, nontraumatic cardiac arrest.[16] These studies are biased somewhat because they examined patients with underlying heart disease; the majority took antiarrhythmic drugs at the time of the study. Ventricular tachycardia is frequently short-lived and converts rapidly to VF, from

201

which the only hope for successful resuscitation lies in early defibrillation. The proportion of patients with VF also declines with each passing minute as more and more patients deteriorate into asystole, from which successful resuscitation is extremely unlikely. Some 4 to 8 minutes after collapse, approximately 50% of patients are still in VF.[1,2,17] In addition, the incidence of VF as the initial presenting arrhythmia in out-of-hospital cardiac arrest is declining. Patients without VF as the cause for their arrest have a lower probability of survival, potentially due to a different pathophysiology of cardiac arrest and the ineffectiveness (or lack) of current resuscitation techniques.

Survival rates from cardiac arrest can be remarkably high if the event is witnessed. For example, when people in supervised cardiac rehabilitation programs suffer a witnessed cardiac arrest, defibrillation is usually performed within minutes. In studies of cardiac arrest in this setting, 90 of 101 victims (89%) were resuscitated.[18–20] No other studies with a defined out-of-hospital population have observed survival rates this high. Adult patients in VF may survive neurologically intact even if defibrillation is performed as late as 6 to 10 minutes after arrest. When defibrillation is delayed, the critical factor determining survival is whether on-site bystanders perform effective CPR while waiting for the defibrillator.[3,6,20–22]

The interaction between early defibrillation and early CPR is displayed graphically in Fig. 13-1. This figure illustrates the probability of survival in relation to the intervals from collapse to first shock and from collapse to start of CPR. It clearly illustrates that the sooner CPR is started and the sooner the defibrillator arrives, the better the outcome. It also shows how starting CPR early changes the slope of the defibrillation survival curve and "buys time" for the defibrillator to arrive.

Development of Early Defibrillation Programs

More than 20 years ago, several communities with no advanced life support (ALS) services evaluated adding pre-

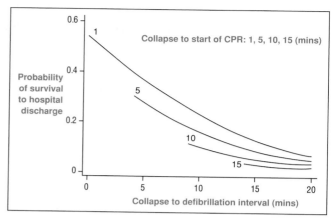

FIGURE 13-1 • Effect of collapse-to-CPR interval and collapse-to-defibrillation interval on survival to hospital discharge. The graph displays the probability of survival to hospital discharge in relation to four intervals from collapse to start of CPR (1, 5, 10, and 15 minutes) and collapse to defibrillation (5, 10, 15, and 20 minutes). To determine the probability of survival for an individual patient, identify the curve indicating the interval from collapse to CPR and then identify the point on that curve that corresponds to the interval from collapse to defibrillation (see horizontal axis). The probability of survival is then indicated on the vertical axis. Based on data from King County, Washington ($N = 1667$ witnessed VT/VF arrests),[1] and Tucson, Arizona ($N = 205$ witnessed VT/VF arrests).[2] (Adapted from Valenzuela TD, Roe DJ, Cretin S, et al. Estimating effectiveness of cardiac arrest interventions: a logistic regression survival model. *Circulation* 1997; 96[10]:3308–3313, with permission.)

hospital defibrillation. Invariably these "before and after" studies showed improved survival rates for cardiac arrest patients when the community added any type of program that resulted in earlier defibrillation (Table 13-1). Impressive results were reported from early studies in King County, Washington, where the odds ratio for improved survival (comparing survival after versus before the addition of an early defibrillation program) was 3.7,[23] and rural Iowa, where the odds ratio was 6.3.[24] Evidence continued to accumulate during the 1980s; investigators reported

| TABLE 13-1 • Effectiveness of Early Defibrillation Programs by Community

Location	% Survival Before Early Defibrillation	% Survival After Early Defibrillation	Odds Ratio for Improved Survival
King County, Washington	7%(4/56)	26%(10/38)	3.7
Iowa	3%(1/31)	19%(12/64)	6.3
Southeast Minnesota	4%(1/27)	17%(6/36)	4.3
Northeast Minnesota	2%(3/118)	10%(8/81)	5.0
Wisconsin	4%(32/893)	11%(33/304)	3.3

Values are percent surviving and, in parentheses, how many patients had ventricular fibrillation. (From Cummins RO. From concept to standard-of-care? Review of the clinical experience with automated external defibrillators. *Ann Emerg Med* 1989;18(12):1269–1275, with permission.)

| TABLE 13-2 • Survival to Hospital Discharge From Cardiac Arrest by System Type: Data From 29 Locations[a]

System Type	Survival: All Rhythms (%)	Weighted Average (%)	Survival: Ventricular Fibrillation (%)	Weighted Average (%)
EMT only	2–9	5	3–20	12
EMT-D	4–19	10	6–26	16
Paramedic	7–18	10	13–30	17
EMT/paramedic	4–26	17	23–33	26
EMT-D/paramedic	13–18	17	27–29	29

EMT, emergency medical technician; EMT-D, emergency medical technician-defibrillation.
[a]Values are the range of survival rates for all rhythms and ventricular fibrillation and the weighted average of each range.
From Eisenberg MS, Horwood BT, Cummins RO, et al. Cardiac arrest and resuscitation: a tale of 29 cities. *Ann Emerg Med* 1990;19(2):179–186, with permission.

positive odds ratios of 4.3 for improved survival in rural communities of southeastern Minnesota,[25] 5.0 in northeastern Minnesota,[26,27] and 2.8 in Wisconsin.

When the survival rates were examined not by community but by the type of system deployed across larger geographic areas, that same pattern emerged: the system organized to get the defibrillator there the fastest—independent of the arrival of personnel to perform endotracheal intuba-

tion and provide IV medications—achieved better survival rates (Table 13-2).

Figure 13-2 illustrates this same concept in a different way. The figure compares survival among victims who receive different interventions ("links in the chain") at different intervals.

In the earliest programs, EMTs with additional training used a manual defibrillator. Subsequently, personnel at the

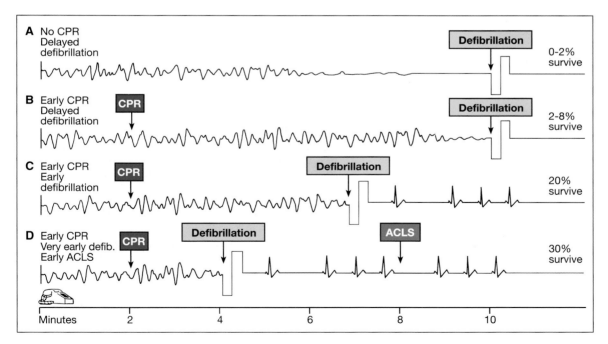

FIGURE 13-2 • Estimated rates of survival to hospital discharge for patients with witnessed VF arrest based on the presence or absence of chain-of-survival links. **A.** No bystander CPR; defibrillation performed by Advanced Cardiac Life Support (ACLS) personnel, who arrive 10 minutes after call to 911. **B.** Bystander CPR at 2 minutes; defibrillation at 10 minutes after call to 911. **C.** Bystander CPR at 2 minutes; defibrillation at 7 minutes after call to 911 by EMT-D. **D.** Bystander CPR at 2 minutes; public access defibrillation at 4 minutes after call to 911; ACLS interventions start at 8 minutes. Estimates are based on a large number of published studies, which were collectively reviewed by Eisenberg et al. (Adapted from Eisenberg MS, Horwood BT, Cummins RO, et al. Cardiac arrest and resuscitation: a tale of 29 cities. *Ann Emerg Med* 1990;19[2]:179–186; Eisenberg MS, Cummins RO, Damon S, et al. Survival rates from out-of-hospital cardiac arrest: recommendations for uniform definitions and data to report. *Ann Emerg Med* 1990;19[11]:1249–1259.)

first-responder level, such as firefighters, were trained and equipped with automated external defibrillators (AEDs). In 1989, a study of AED use by firefighter first responders in King County, Washington, found that this strategy improved the calculated survival among patients in VF from 19% to 30%.[31] This study catalyzed the deployment of AEDs among firefighter first responders in many other parts of the country and served to establish the legitimacy and value of this technology.

While firefighters are often available to serve as first responders in urban areas, most suburban communities do not have this resource. In these communities, police officers often fulfill this role. In the 1990s, studies in two locations demonstrated the feasibility of police providing early defibrillation. A study from Rochester, Minnesota, reported a remarkable survival rate of 45% after police were equipped with AEDs (shock was provided by EMS or police officers depending on who arrived first).[32] In suburbs of Pittsburgh, Pennsylvania, survival was improved nearly 10-fold if police performed defibrillation when they arrived before EMS rather than waiting for EMS

personnel (survival to hospital discharge was 26% versus 3%, $P = 0.027$).[33] This study also found that police officers were able to use the devices effectively with minimal errors and that the devices rarely malfunctioned.[34] A national survey of law enforcement agencies (LEAs) found that 80% routinely respond to medical emergencies and that 39% of these deploy AEDs.[35] This is a significant increase compared with a prior survey in the late 1990s, which found that only about 3% of LEAs were equipped with AEDs.[36]

For optimal effectiveness, defibrillation should be provided within about 5 minutes of collapse, a narrow therapeutic window that has been termed "the electrical phase of cardiac arrest"[37] (see sidebar). Unfortunately, first responders and EMS personnel usually cannot respond to the location of a cardiac arrest victim rapidly enough to provide defibrillation within this time frame. That goal can be achieved on a consistent basis only through the availability of on-site defibrillators and their use by willing on-site rescuers. Several programs and studies have evaluated this concept, commonly referred to as public-access defibrillation (PAD).

OPTIMAL TIMING FOR IMMEDIATE DEFIBRILLATION

The Three-Phase Model of Cardiac Arrest and New Recommendations

Successful Defibrillation from the Metabolic Perspective

Successful defibrillation depends on the electrical and metabolic state of the myocardium, the amount of myocardial damage that occurs during hypoxic arrest, the prior functional state of the heart, and the cause of VF. From a metabolic perspective VF depletes more of the cardiac energy stores—adenosine triphosphate (ATP)—per minute than does normal sinus rhythm. Prolonged VF will exhaust the energy stores of ATP in the myocardium, particularly in the cardiac pacemaker cells. The longer VF persists, the greater the myocardial deterioration as energy stores become exhausted. In a heart stunned into electrical silence by a defibrillatory shock, no spontaneous contractions will resume if the fibrillating myocardium has consumed all its energy stores. When ATP is depleted and cellular functions are disrupted, shocks are more likely to convert VF to asystole than to a spontaneous rhythm because no "fuel" remains to support spontaneous depolarization in the pacemaker tissues or the contracting myocardium. With depleted reserves of energy, any postshock *asystole* or *agonal rhythms* will be permanent, not temporary.

Delayed Defibrillation

For this reason, VF of short duration is much more likely to respond to a shock delivered soon after VF starts. An important objective for resuscitation and any effort to improve outcome is to shorten the interval between the onset of VF and the first shock. In *Emergency Cardiovascular Care (ECC) Guidelines 2000*, the American Heart Association (AHA) recommended that all patients who have a VF arrest out of hospital receive shocks in <5 minutes; a goal for patients who have an in-hospital VF arrest is <3minutes.

Cobb et al.[6] noted, however, that as more Seattle first responders were equipped with AEDs, survival rates from SCA unexpectedly fell. The investigators attributed this decline to a

reduced emphasis on CPR when defibrillation is delayed, and there is growing evidence to support this view. When VF causes cardiac arrest, three general phases of arrest occur: an electrical phase, a circulatory phase, and a metabolic phase (Figure).[37] Whether a shock is delivered immediately (during the early electrical phase) or after a brief period of CPR, later during the circulatory phase, may be one explanation for this observation. During the circulatory phase, a brief period of CPR may "prime the pump" and provide a small but important period of oxygen and energy substrate.

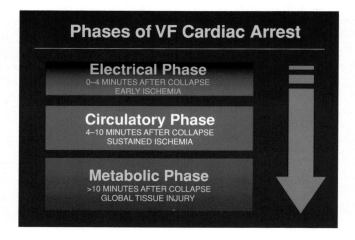

When cardiac arrest occurs due to VF, three phases can be proposed: an initial electrical phase, when early defibrillation is critical; a circulatory phase, when perfusion pressure to the heart and brain assume increasing importance; and a metabolic phase, when cellular damage and inflammatory and metabolic mediators of injury are present. (Adapted from Weisfeldt ML, Becker LB. Resuscitation after cardiac arrest: a 3-phase time-sensitive model. *JAMA* 2002;288[23]:3035–3038, with permission.)

Early Defibrillation Programs

See Web site for ACEP Policy Early Defibrillation Programs; Public Training in Early Defibrillation

Casinos

An innovative program implemented in casinos demonstrated the benefit of AED use by on-site responders. Security personnel were trained to use AEDs, which were deployed throughout the premises close enough to facilitate their use within 3 minutes of collapse. The average time interval from collapse to shock was 4.4 ± 2.9 minutes. The survival rate was 74% among patients shocked within 3 minutes and 49% among those shocked after more than 3 minutes.[38]

Commercial Aircraft

One venue where the need for defibrillation by on-site personnel was quite obvious was commercial aircraft. Qantas Airlines pioneered this concept by placing AEDs on their planes and training flight attendants in CPR and AED use.[39] American Airlines reported that over a 2-year period, 200 (191 on aircraft and 9 in terminals) arrests occurred.[40] The Federal Aviation Administration has now mandated that all aircraft staffed with at least one flight attendant must be equipped with an AED.

Another early PAD program was implemented at the Chicago airports. AEDs were deployed so that they were within a 90-second walk of each other. Over 3,000 airport workers were trained in CPR and AED use. Among 21 persons who experienced nontraumatic cardiac arrest, 18 were in VF and 11 (61%) survived. In five of these cases, persons who had no training or experience in the use of AEDs and no official duty to respond used the AED.[40a] This study suggested there is benefit in deploying AEDs in high-volume venues and making AEDs available for use by the general public.

Current Concepts

On-Site Rescuers with Defibrillator

If the collapse is witnessed, a defibrillator is present, and someone onsite is willing to use it, defibrillation should be administered as soon as the defibrillator is ready. The efficacy of on-site AED use is now supported by two large multicenter studies. The Public Access Defibrillation Trial compared outcomes between two on-site responder strategies at 1,000 locations through 20 different centers across the United States and Canada.[41] Both strategies included development of a response plan and training of designated

responders in CPR. Half of the sites were randomized to also have training in AED use and placement of on-site AEDs. Study sites comprised a range of settings, including office buildings, multiresidential units, and shopping malls selected to have an expected likelihood of one cardiac arrest per year. Survival was double in the AED arm. Interestingly, VF was the initial rhythm in 59% of victims at the AED sites; this is higher than what has been recently reported in some EMS-based cardiac arrest studies.

Surveillance data reported from the Resuscitation Outcomes Consortium (ROC) funded by the National Institutes of Health found that on-site AED use doubled the likelihood of survival after controlling for associated risk factors. This study looked at 10,663 patients with cardiac arrest treated by EMS at the 11 ROC sites. Overall survival to hospital discharge was 7%; this improved to 9% with bystander CPR and to 36% with bystander CPR and bystander AED use. Unfortunately only about 30% of patients received bystander CPR and only 2.4% bystander AED.[42]

Likely scenarios for defibrillation by on-site rescuers include AED use by lay-bystanders at a public location and use of an automated or manual defibrillator by health care personnel in a hospital or clinic.

Emergency Responders

There is mounting evidence from both animal and human research to suggest that resuscitation will be more successful if chest compressions are performed for a brief period prior to defibrillation for patients with longer than a brief period of VF (>5 minutes or so) (see Sidebar 13-1 above).[6] The period of chest compressions is believed to improve the metabolic state of the myocardium and, therefore, make the heart more amenable to defibrillation and to resumption of an organized cardiac rhythm with mechanical contraction. Thus, when rescuers must respond to the victim from off site, particularly when the response interval is >5 minutes, it may be beneficial to provide 90 to 180 seconds of chest compressions prior to attempting defibrillation.[5,6]

See Web site for AHA Guidelines for Cardiopulmonary Resuscitation and Emergency Cardiovascular Care—Electrical Therapies, Part V.

The AHA ECC 2005 guidelines suggest that EMS personnel may administer about 5 cycles (roughly 2 minutes) of CPR before checking the ECG rhythm and attempting defibrillation in treating an out-of-hospital cardiac arrest they did not witness. This recommendation is supported by two clinical studies of adult out-of-hospital VF SCAs. In those studies, when EMS call-to-arrival intervals were 4 to 5 minutes or longer, victims who received 1.5 to 3 minutes of CPR before defibrillation showed an increased rate of initial resuscitation, survival to hospital discharge, and 1-year survival when compared with those who received immediate defibrillation for VF SCA.[5,6] One randomized study, however, found no benefit to CPR before defibrillation for SCAs not witnessed by a paramedic.[43] There is no evidence to provide a current recommendation for CPR before defibrillation for in-hospital cardiac arrest. A large-scale, multicenter, randomized comparison of the two treatment strategies (immediate shock versus shock preceded by a defined period of CPR) is currently under way and may provide the basis for future treatment recommendations.

Defibrillators

Manual

Manual defibrillators are designed for use by health care providers with training in cardiac rhythm recognition and management. The device has a screen for visualization of the rhythm, often with the capability for viewing multiple leads. The operator sets the energy level, initiates charging of the capacitor, and manually triggers the delivery of current. Most devices allow shock delivery through both handheld paddles and self-adherent pads (see "Paddles Versus Pads," below). Manual devices usually have the capability to provide synchronized cardioversion, defibrillation (unsynchronized cardioversion), and transcutaneous pacing. Further, they may incorporate other monitoring capabilities, including noninvasive and invasive blood pressure measurement, pulse oximetry, and capnography. Some can also be used in an automated mode for defibrillation.

Automated External Defibrillators

Automated external defibrillators (AEDs) are sophisticated, reliable computerized devices that use voice and visual prompts to guide lay-rescuers and health care providers to safely defibrillate persons in VF, as demonstrated in many clinical trials.[24,33,38,40,44–54]

These portable devices are able to analyze the ECG rhythm, determine the presence of predetermined rhythms eligible for shock therapy, advise the user when such a rhythm is present, and deliver a defibrillation shock (Fig. 13-3). The ECG signal is input through two large self-adhesive pads that attach to the patient's chest wall and connect to the AED with a several-foot-long cable; these pads also serve to deliver the shock. AEDs have microprocessors that analyze multiple features of the surface ECG signal, including frequency, amplitude, and some integration of frequency and amplitude, such as slope or wave morphology. Filters check for QRS-like signals, radio transmission, or 50- or 60-cycle interference as well as loose electrodes and poor electrode contact. Some devices are able to detect patient movement and, when this is detected, interrupt further rhythm analysis and shock delivery. The shock delivery function

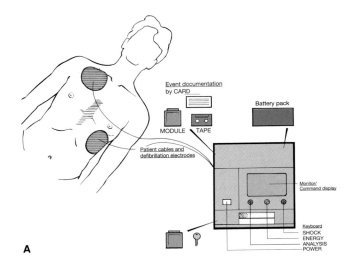

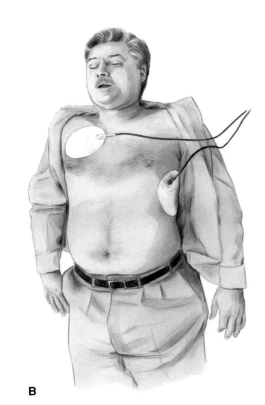

FIGURE 13-3 • Schematic drawing of automated external defibrillator and its attachments to patient.

comprises a capacitor which is charged when an appropriate rhythm is detected. The energy source is typically a removable battery, either rechargeable or, more commonly, a long-life nonrechargeable type such as a lithium-based battery. In some models, the energy level of first and subsequent shocks is programmable in advance but not adjustable by the provider at the time of use, as it is with manual defibrillators.

AEDs use proprietary algorithms developed through the analysis of many ECG recordings to determine if a particular rhythm should be shocked. "Shockable" rhythms include VF and wide-complex, rapid tachycardia. At least one brand will advise shock of narrow-complex tachycardia with a prespecified rate threshold, but this function can be disabled. All other rhythms are referred to as "nonshockable;" when these are detected, the user is directed to begin (or resume) CPR.

AEDs have been tested extensively, both *in vitro* against libraries of recorded cardiac rhythms[55] and clinically in many field trials in adults[56,57] and children.[58–61] They are extremely accurate in rhythm analysis, even in the presence of electromagnetic fields.[62,63] While early models were noted to in rare instances shock inappropriately,[64] in recent studies, sensitivity for VF is over 90% and specificity at or near 100%.[34,41,65]

AEDs come in a variety of models with varying levels of capabilities, complexity, and ruggedness. All are designed to be easy to use and provide voice and visual prompts to guide the user. The original models and some current models are designed with the premise that trained persons will use them, so prompts are more limited and may include jargon. Many of the newer models are designed with simpler-to-understand but more detailed instructions, such that even untrained laypeople can use them successfully.

Prototype devices were used in two recent clinical trials that recorded information about the frequency and depth of chest compressions during CPR.[66,67] This suggests that in the future, AEDs may be able prompt rescuers to improve CPR technique in real time based on actual rescuer performance.

Automated External Defibrillator Operation

After confirming that the victim is likely in cardiac arrest (unresponsive, lack of normal breathing) and calling 911, the main steps in using an AED include the following:

1. Turn the device on (mechanism varies by model) and follow prompts.
2. Place electrode pads on patient's bare chest (see Fig. 13-3) and attach cable to device if necessary.
3. Push "Analyze" button if necessary. Many devices will begin rhythm analysis automatically as soon as an adequate ECG signal is detected. No one should touch or move the patient during analysis.
4. Push "Shock" button if so prompted, or begin CPR if no shock is advised. Note that fully automated devices will deliver shock after warning without user action. No one should be touching the patient during shock delivery, although recent evidence suggests that there is minimal risk of shock to a gloved rescuer should there be such contact while performing CPR.[68]

Fully Versus Semiautomated If a shockable rhythm is determined to be present, a fully automated AED will automatically charge and fire, while a semiautomated unit will prompt the operator to push a button for shock delivery to occur. The advantage to the fully automated device is that it may decrease operator delays in shock delivery once the device is ready to shock; the disadvantage expressed by some is that the user does not have control of shock delivery, such as if someone were to be touching the patient or in the rare instance that the patient were to regain signs of life.

Device Maintenance and Readiness

Defibrillators fall into the category of items that are used rarely or relatively infrequently but must be available and ready for immediate use when needed. Therefore, it is essential that a process be in place to assure that every defibrillator (whether manual or automated, whether in hospital or at a public location) is both present where it is supposed to be and is in a state of operational readiness. Most AEDs have an automated daily self-check function that confirms such items as residual battery power and the presence and, in some cases, intactness of pads. The "ready indicator," easily visible on the AED, should be checked daily. Less frequently, typically monthly, many AEDs also do a more comprehensive check, including charge circuitry and capacitor testing. A manual check of every AED should also be performed at some regular interval (e.g., monthly or quarterly) to assure that battery or pads do not need to be replaced and that the device is otherwise intact. For both manual and automated defibrillators, the manufacturer's recommendations should be reviewed and, if it is decided to deviate from these, this should be noted and explained in writing.

Implanted Cardiac Defibrillators (*See also* Chapter 24)

Indications and General Operation

Implantable cardioverter-defibrillators (ICDs) are now indicated for secondary prevention in most patients with a history of sudden cardiac arrest or hemodynamically significant ventricular arrhythmias and as primary prevention in those with New York Heart Association class II or III heart failure and ejection fraction <35%, prior myocardial infarction with systolic dysfunction (ejection fraction <35%), or other high-risk factors for VF or tachycardia (Fig. 13-4).[69–70a] ICDs can automatically detect cardiac arrhythmias and deliver programmable energy shocks directly to the myocardium, repeated if necessary, usually through a transvenous lead in the right ventricle. Modern implanted devices have the capability to also do both anti-tachycardic and bradycardic pacing. The generator boxes are usually implanted subcutaneously in the left infraclavicular area of the chest wall but may also be right infraclavicular or in the abdominal wall.

See Web site for ACC/AHA/ESC Guidelines for Management of Patients with VA and the Prevention of SCD[69]

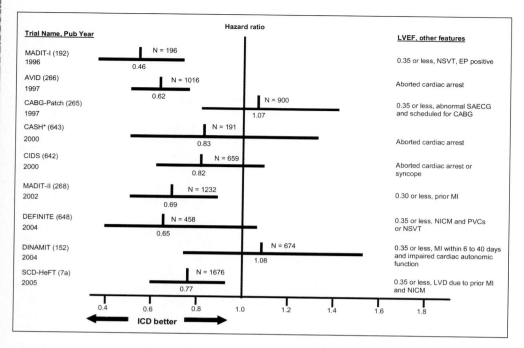

FIGURE 13-4 • Major implantable cardioverter-defibrillator (ICD) trials. Hazard ratios (*vertical line*) and 95% confidence intervals (*horizontal lines*) for death from any cause in the ICD group compared with the non-ICD group. CABG, coronary artery bypass grafting; EP, electrophysiologic study; LVD, left ventricular dysfunction; LVEF, left ventricular ejection fraction; MI, myocardial infarction; N, number of patients; NICM, nonischemic cardiomyopathy; NSVT, nonsustained ventricular tachycardia; PVCs, premature ventricular complexes; SAECG, signal-averaged electrocardiogram.

Interaction with Defibrillation and AICDs (*See also* Chapter 24)

Defibrillation Procedural Considerations

Shock Delivery Based on Fibrillation Waveform Analysis

Several retrospective case series, animal studies, and theoretical models[68–84] suggest that it is possible to predict the success of attempted defibrillation by analyzing the VF waveform (Fig. 13-5). These studies have evaluated a variety of waveform characteristics, including frequency, amplitude, and nonlinear measures and combinations of these. If prospective studies can demonstrate that any of these measures reliably predicts shock success, such a measure could be used clinically to determine the timing of shock delivery. For example, if an unfavorable reading were obtained, the patient in VF could be treated with CPR and medications before shock. This might not only improve the likelihood of successful defibrillation but also reduce the number of

shocks likely to fail and the coinciding exposure to potential injury.

At present there is insufficient evidence to recommend for or against analysis of VF ECG characteristics to determine timing of defibrillation. At issue is whether analysis of the VF waveform is useful in predicting therapeutic outcome and modifying therapy prospectively. Potential applications include prediction of shock success, selection of appropriate waveform type, and optimization of timing of defibrillation relative to CPR and medication delivery.

Coordination with Chest Compressions

Chest compressions should be provided until the instant of shock delivery, taking care to assure that no one is touching the patient when the shock is delivered, and then resumed immediately after shock delivery for about 2 minutes before assessing rhythm or pulse (or signs of life).[84a] At that time, a pulse check is performed after manual defibrillation only if an organized rhythm is present. If an AED is used, each analysis resulting in either a "shock" or "no shock" advisory is followed by 2 minutes of CPR before re-analysis until Advanced Life Support (ALS) providers arrive (and manual assessment of the rhythm is possible) or the victim shows obvious signs of life.

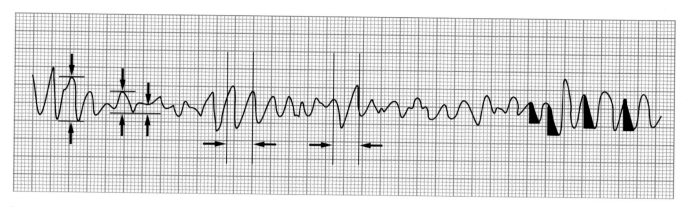

FIGURE 13-5 • Features of a surface electrocardiogram recorded on a monitor strip, which can be used to analyze ventricular fibrillation. Vertical arrows indicate amplitude, horizontal arrows indicate rate or frequency, and black wedges indicate morphology.

A variety of studies have reported detrimental effects of pauses between chest compressions and delivery of shock. Animal studies have shown that frequent or long interruptions in chest compressions for rhythm analysis[85,86] or rescue breathing[87,88] were associated with postresuscitation myocardial dysfunction and reduced survival rates. Secondary analyses of two randomized trials[89,90] showed that interruption in chest compressions was associated with a decreased probability of conversion of VF. Analyses of VF waveform characteristics predictive of shock success have documented that the shorter the time between a chest compression and delivery of a shock, the more likely the shock will be successful.[68,69] Reduction in the interval from compression to shock delivery by even a few seconds can increase the probability of shock success.[89] Concern that chest compressions might provoke recurrent VF in the presence of a postshock organized rhythm does not appear to be warranted.[91]

Single Versus Stacked Shocks

At the time of the 2005 International Liaison Committee on Resuscitation (ILCOR) Consensus Conference, no published human or animal studies were found that compared a one-shock protocol with a three-stacked-shock protocol for treatment of VF cardiac arrest. The rhythm analysis for a three-shock sequence performed by commercially available AEDs resulted in delays of up to 37 seconds between the first shock and the first postshock compression.[85] This long delay in providing chest compressions is difficult to justify in light of the first-shock efficacy of >90% reported by current biphasic defibrillators.[92–96] If the first shock fails to eliminate VF, the incremental benefit of immediate additional shocks is low, and resumption of CPR is likely to confer a greater value than another shock.[97] When this reasoning is considered with the data from animal studies documenting harmful effects from interruptions of chest compressions, the approach of one shock at a time seems most reasonable.

Thus the AHA ECC 2005 guidelines recommend that when VF/pulseless ventricular tachycardia (VT) is present,

the rescuer should deliver one shock and then immediately resume CPR, beginning with chest compressions. There should be no delay in resuming compressions to check rhythm or assess for pulse unless the patient exhibits spontaneous movement or breathing. Compressions should continue right up until the time of shock delivery, with the defibrillator charged and pads or paddles in place before stopping compressions. Health care providers must practice efficient coordination between CPR and defibrillation.

Electrodes (Pads and Paddles)

Electrode Size

In general, the larger the electrode, the lower the impedance. But too large an electrode can result in inadequate contact with the chest or a large portion of the current traversing extracardiac pathways and missing the heart.[98] The Association for the Advancement of Medical Instrumentation recommends a minimum electrode size of 50 cm[2] for individual electrodes. The sum of the electrode areas should be a minimum of 150 cm[2].[99] For adult defibrillation, both handheld paddle electrodes and self-adhesive pad electrodes 8 to 12 cm in diameter perform well, although defibrillation success may be higher with electrodes 12 cm in diameter rather than with those 8 cm in diameter.[100,101] Small (4.3-cm) electrodes may be harmful and may cause myocardial necrosis.[102] Use of pediatric pads in larger children and adults can result in unacceptably high transthoracic impedance.[103] It is best to use the largest pads that can fit on the chest without overlap. This transition occurs at approximately 10 kg, the average weight of a 1-year-old child.[126]

Electrode Placement

Placement of pads or paddles for defibrillation and cardioversion is an important but often neglected topic. One of the most common mistakes is to place the pads too close to each other. In one study doctors placed the electrodes incorrectly (Fig. 13-6) over 90% of the time![104] Pads should be

PART THREE • DEFIBRILLATION

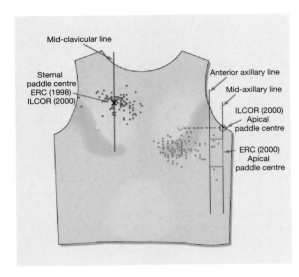

FIGURE 13-6 • Anatomic position of sternal and apical defibril-lation paddles placed by 101 doctors. The apical paddle was placed incorrectly over 90% of the time.

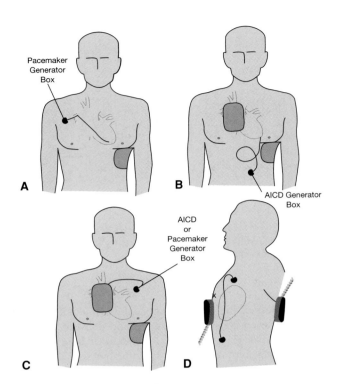

FIGURE 13-8 • Placement of defibrillation pads (or paddles). In a patient in whom a pacemaker or defibrillator generator has been implanted below the right clavicle, one patch should be placed posteriorly over the right scapula, and the second patch over the apex as shown in **A.** In patients who do not have an implanted pacemaker or defibrillator, or in whom the generator lies on the left side or in the abdomen, an anterior-apical position shown in **B** and **C** is acceptable. Alternatively, anterior-posterior patch posi-tions as shown in **D**, are also acceptable, including placement of patches directly opposite each other in an anterior-posterior con-figuration over the mid- or left-chest wall and back; or at the right anterior mid chest wall and the left lower scapular region. Pacemaker and defibrillator manufacturers recommend that defib-rillation patches should be kept at least 6 inches away from an implanted generator (see Chapter 24).

placed in a position that will maximize current flow through the myocardium (Fig. 13-7). This fractional transmyocardial current affects the current density generated in the heart. It has been estimated that even with properly placed paddles, only 4% to 25% of the delivered current actually passes through the heart.[105,106] The recommended placement is termed either "sternal apex" or "anterior apex" (Fig. 13-3). The sternal (or anterior) electrode is placed to the right of the upper part of the sternum below the clavicle. The apex electrode is placed to the left of the nipple with the center of the electrode in the midaxillary line.[107–110] There are several acceptable alternative locations: one paddle anteriorly over the left apex (pre-cordium) and the other posteriorly behind the heart in the left infrascapular location;[100,111,112] placement on the lateral chest wall on the right and left sides (biaxillary); or the left pad in the standard apical position and the other pad on the right or left upper back (Fig. 13-8).[106,113,114]

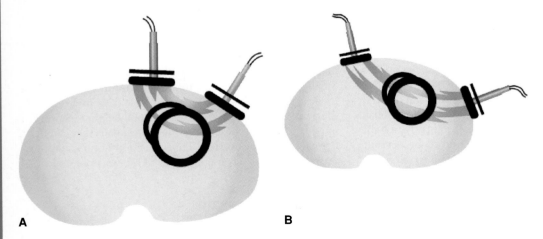

FIGURE 13-7 • Pad or paddle positions showing current pathway for incorrect (**A**) and correct (**B**) place-ment allowing an optimal current pathway. These figures depict how the patient would be viewed from the head of the bed.

Placement should be avoided directly over any implanted pacemaker or defibrillator or other metallic implanted device. (*See* Chapter 24, Electrical Therapies). Also, avoid placing the defibrillation electrode directly on the breast of female patients. This position can significantly increase transthoracic impedance.[115]

Providers also should make sure that the pads are separate and not touching. If electrode paddles are used instead of pads, the paddles should be well separated, and the paste or gel used to create the interface between the paddles and the skin should not be smeared on the chest between the paddles. Smearing of the paste or gel may allow current to follow a superficial pathway (arc) along the chest wall, "missing" the heart.

Paddles Versus Pads

Studies have shown self-adhesive electrode pads to be as effective as rigid metal paddles.[108,111,116] Many clinicians consider them to be safer and more convenient to use. These pads have an adhesive, nonconductive perimeter that reduces the chance of arcing. For many newer models of defibrillators (including all AEDs), pads are set as the "default" method of defibrillation. They can be placed before or at the onset of cardiac arrest to allow for monitoring and then rapid administration of a shock when necessary.[117] Consequently self-adhesive pads are recommended to be used routinely instead of standard paddles by the AHA ECC 2005 guidelines.

Electrode Contact/Impedance

Efforts should be made to avoid excessively high thoracic impedance in delivering shock therapy. Defibrillators are designed to deliver a therapeutic current dose based on a range of impedance around the average human adult impedance of about 70 to 80 ohms.[100,118] When transthoracic impedance is too high, a shock may not generate sufficient current to achieve defibrillation.[101,119,120]

The main modifiable factor that affects thoracic impedance is the interface between the defibrillation electrode and the skin. This interface is optimized by:

1. Use of conductive interface, such as non–alcohol-based gels or pads designed to enhance electrical conduction.[121] Do not use medical gels or pastes with poor electrical conductivity, such as ultrasound gel.[122]
2. Application of firm pressure when using paddles to assure tight contact with skin (25 lb of pressure is recommended).
3. Assurance of firm, circumferential adhesion of self-adhesive pads; this may require wiping off very wet skin or shaving very hairy skin.[123]

The degree of lung inflation can also affect the impedance, with greater lung volumes associated with higher impedance.[124] Most patients in cardiac arrest will default to an end-expiratory position, even after a positive-pressure ventilation. The application of 25 lb of pressure on handheld pads further decreases lung volume and decreases impedance.[125] This is not felt to provide a significant advantage with self-adhesive pads; therefore, applying pressure with them is not recommended.

Another reason to assure tight, full circumferential adhesion of the self-adhesive pads and applying firm pressure with paddles is to avoid arcing. This typically occurs when there is poor contact with even a small portion of both electrodes, and is more likely to occur when electrodes are close together or there is a conducting material between them. This may be conducting gel inadvertently smeared, saline spilled on chest, or very humid air. If manual paddles are used, gel pads are preferable to electrode pastes and gels that can more easily smear. Although extremely rare, arcing has ignited fires in oxygen-rich environments, such as critical care units or the patient compartment of an ambulance.

Energy Level

Defibrillation is achieved by generating adequate current flow through the myocardium and sustaining that flow for an effective time interval. Although the defibrillator operator selects the shock energy (in joules), it is the current flow (in amperes) that actually depolarizes the myocardium. Current depends in part on the selected shock dose and is affected by the thoracic pathway between the defibrillator electrodes, the position of the heart in that pathway, and the impedance to current flow between the electrodes. The complexity of thoracic current flow has been observed experimentally.[126]

At present it is clear that both low- and high-energy biphasic waveform shocks are effective, but definitive recommendations for the first and subsequent energy levels for all devices cannot be made because devices vary in waveform and reported shock success. Although both escalating-energy and nonescalating-energy defibrillators are available, there are insufficient data to recommend one approach over another pending results of ongoing investigation.

As noted, biphasic defibrillators use one of two waveforms, and each waveform has been shown to be effective in terminating VF over a specific dose range. The ideal shock dose with a biphasic device is one that falls within the range that has been documented to be effective using that specific device. Manufacturers should display the device-specific effective waveform dose range on the face of the device, and providers should use that dose range in attempting defibrillation with that device. Providers should be aware of the range of energy levels at which the specific waveform they use has been shown to be effective for terminating VF, and they should use that device-specific dose for attempted defibrillation. As noted above, there is no evidence that one biphasic waveform is more effective than another.

It is reasonable to select energies of 150 J to 200 J with a biphasic truncated exponential waveform or 120 J with a rectilinear biphasic waveform for the initial shock. For second and subsequent shocks, it is acceptable to use the same or higher energy. The selected energy and the delivered energy may differ owing to automated adjustments made by most models to meet certain parameters, such as peak or total current. With the rectilinear biphasic waveform device, delivered energy is typically higher in the usual range of impedance. For example, in a patient with impedance of 80 Ω, a selected energy of 120 J will deliver 150 J.

If a provider is operating a manual biphasic defibrillator and is unaware of the effective dose range for that device to terminate VF, the rescuer may use a selected dose of 200 J (or the highest selectable dose if <200 J) for the first shock and an equal or higher dose for the second and subsequent shocks. Conversely, for a manual monophasic defibrillator, the initial recommended energy level for defibrillation is 360 J.

Some but not all studies have found first-shock efficacy for monophasic shocks to be generally lower than first-shock efficacy for biphasic shocks at comparable energy settings.[127–130] In the past, 200 J was recommended as the energy setting for the first monophasic defibrillation shock. This was based on a study comparing the effectiveness of 175 J versus 320 J monophasic waveform shocks for out-of-hospital VF cardiac arrest. Approximately 61% of patients who received shocks with either 175 J or 320 J monophasic damped sine waveforms were defibrillated with the first shock, which was delivered an average of 10.6 minutes after the call to EMS. There was no significant difference in the percentage of patients who developed advanced atrioventricular (AV) block after one shock. AV block was more likely to develop after two or three shocks of 320 J than after two or three shocks of 175 J, but the block was transient and did not affect survival to hospital discharge.[131]

Although the optimal energy level for defibrillation using any of the monophasic or biphasic waveforms has not been determined, a recommendation for higher initial energy in using a monophasic waveform was weighed by expert consensus with consideration of the potential negative effects of a high first-shock energy versus the negative effects of prolonged VF. The consensus was that rescuers using monophasic AEDs should give an initial shock of 360 J; if VF persists after the first shock, second and subsequent shocks of 360 J should be given. This single dose for monophasic shocks is designed to simplify instructions to rescuers but is not a mandate to recall monophasic AEDs for reprogramming. If the monophasic AED being used is programmed to deliver a different first or subsequent dose, that dose is acceptable.

Special Situations

Water

Defibrillation may be performed safely in light rain, on wet, nonmetallic surfaces and when the patient's skin is wet, but should not be done if the victim is lying in free-standing water or there is pooling of water on the patient's chest. In these instances it is best to move the victim quickly to a drier location or wipe off the patient's chest. AEDs can be used when the victim is lying on snow or ice.

Oxygen

Several case reports have described fires ignited by sparks from poorly applied defibrillator paddles in the presence of an oxygen-enriched atmosphere. Fires have been reported when ventilator tubing is disconnected from the endotracheal tube and then left adjacent to the patient's head, blowing oxygen across the chest during defibrillation. When ventilation is interrupted for shock delivery, rescuers should try

to ensure that oxygen does not flow across the patient's chest during defibrillation attempts. Rescuers should take precautions to minimize sparking during attempted defibrillation. The use of self-adhesive defibrillation pads is probably the best way to minimize the risk of sparks igniting during defibrillation. In general, rescuers should try to avoid defibrillation in an oxygen-enriched atmosphere.[122,132–136]

Medication Patches

Do not place electrode pads directly on top of a transdermal medication patch (e.g., patches containing nitroglycerin, nicotine, analgesics, hormone replacements, antihypertensives) because the patch may block delivery of energy from the electrode pad to the heart and may cause burns to the skin. Explosion of a nitroglycerin patch has been reported.[137] Remove medication patches and wipe the area before attaching the electrode pad.

Defibrillation of Patient with Implanted Device (Implantable Cardioverter-Defibrillators, Pacemakers, Medication Pumps, Electrical Stimulators)

(*See also* Chapter 24)

Never withhold defibrillation or synchronized cardioversion from patients with an implanted pacemaker or defibrillator if either intervention is indicated. In patients with a known implantable cardioverter-defibrillator (ICD), unless the collapse itself has been witnessed by EMS responders, it should be assumed that the ICD has already unsuccessfully administered its therapies and responders should proceed with standard treatment measures, including provision of CPR and external defibrillation. If the collapse is witnessed, however, it is reasonable to wait 15 to 20 seconds to allow the first ICD therapy to be administered before proceeding with standard treatment measures. Occasionally the analysis and shock cycles of automatic ICDs and AEDs will conflict,[138,139] in that a shock may have already been administered by one device as the other is preparing to shock. Use of a manual defibrillator, when available, avoids this conflict by permitting direct vision of the rhythm at the time that administration of external shock is being considered.

Direct defibrillation can cause temporary or permanent pacemaker malfunction. Because some of the defibrillation current flows down the pacemaker leads, permanent pacemakers and ICDs should be reevaluated after the patient receives a shock.[140] Such problems can be minimized by proper placement of defibrillation electrodes (see Fig. 13-8 and preceding discussion).

Defibrillation in Children

Manual

The lowest energy dose for effective defibrillation in infants and children is not known. The upper limit for safe defibrillation is also not known, but doses >4 J/kg (as high as 9 J/kg) have effectively defibrillated children[141,142] and pediatric animal models[143] with no significant adverse effects. Based on adult clinical data[96,144] and pediatric animal models,[145] biphasic shocks appear to be at least as effective as monophasic shocks and less harmful. Recommended manual defibrillation (monophasic or biphasic) doses are 2 J/kg for the first attempt and 4 J/kg for subsequent attempts.[145,146]

Automated External Defibrillators

Many AEDs now have pediatric capability, which means that they can deliver lower-energy shocks for use in children. Different models have different mechanisms to achieve this function—some use special cables with an in-line resistance and others alter the energy output of the device. These AEDs can accurately differentiate shockable from non-shockable rhythms with a high degree of sensitivity and specificity in children.[58,59] The FDA has approved a number of these modified devices or electrodes for use in children 1 to 8 years of age.

For children 1 to 8 years of age the rescuer should use a pediatric device if one is available.[142,147,148] If the provider initiates CPR to a child in cardiac arrest but does not have an AED with a pediatric attenuator system, she or he should use a standard adult AED. There are insufficient data to make a recommendation for or against the use of AEDs for infants <1 year of age.[149]

In-Hospital Use of Automated External Defibrillators

The expectation and perhaps assumption among the medical and lay-communities is that treatment of cardiac arrest is much better inside hospitals than outside.[150] Yet a report from the AHA National Registry of Cardiopulmonary Resuscitation,[151] a voluntary registry and database of in-hospital cardiac arrests from 369 hospitals, raises concerns. This report found an overall survival-to-discharge rate from VF and pulseless VT of 34%. The median time from recognition of arrest to shock delivery was an impressive 1 minute, but it was >2 minutes in 30% of cases. Delay in defibrillation was associated with decreased survival.[152]

Defibrillation is more likely to be delayed when patients develop SCA in unmonitored hospital beds and in outpatient and diagnostic facilities. In such areas, several minutes may elapse before centralized response teams arrive with the defibrillator, attach it, and deliver shocks. This prompted consideration for use of AEDs. In-hospital AED use has been associated with increased survival rates from VF arrest.[153,154] Despite limited evidence, AEDs should be considered for the hospital setting as a way to facilitate early defibrillation (a goal of ≤3 minutes from collapse), especially in areas where staff have no rhythm-recognition skills or defibrillators are used infrequently.

Early defibrillation capability should be available in ambulatory care facilities as well as throughout hospital inpatient areas.

When hospitals deploy AEDs, an effective system for rapid response and training and retraining of initial responders should be in place.[155] Hospitals should monitor collapse-to–first-shock intervals and resuscitation outcomes.

Lay-Responder Public Access Defibrillation Programs

Automated external defibrillators (AEDs) have the capacity to save lives. This has recently been confirmed by a large retrospective review reporting that bystander use of CPR combined with the use of an AED actually more than doubled the chances of survival of out-of-hospital cardiac arrest. When CPR was done and the AED delivered a shock, survival increased to 36%, which was approximately four times greater than with CPR alone.[156] However, the potential benefit of AEDs is fully realized only if they are used and used promptly and effectively by on-site responders. The implementation of a quality public access defibrillation (PAD) program with medical direction oversight is fundamental and will increase the likelihood of bystanders performing CPR and using the AED.

See Web site for AHA Science Advisory Statement—Lay Rescuer (Public Access) Automatic External Defibrillation Programs

A system approach integrating an AED program can have an impact beyond just early defibrillation. Although a critical goal, early defibrillation is integrated in a system that provides committed and increased provider training, early system activation, and advanced life support (Fig. 13-9).

The cost-effectiveness of PAD programs is difficult to evaluate because of the variability in potential costs and the determination of all incremental costs. One study estimated a median incremental cost of $44,000 per additional quality-adjusted life year (QALY) for on-site lay-responders and $27,200 per QALY for police responders.[157] Another analysis reported that the cost per QALY in casinos was $56,700.[158] These studies noted that the primary factors influencing cost were frequency of arrest and the number of defibrillators deployed.

The following section provides an overview of important elements in developing and maintaining an effective PAD program.

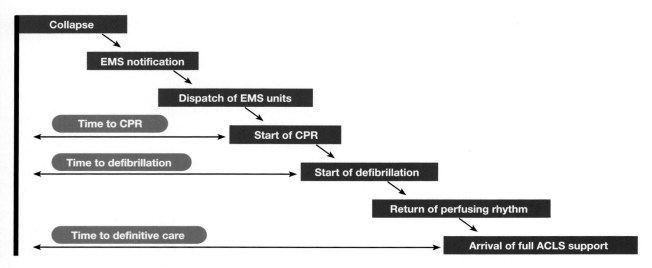

FIGURE 13-9 • An AED program accomplishes very early defibrillation in the setting of trained providers in increased numbers and early activation of additional components of the chain of survival. Preplanning provides a system structure and quality review, and debriefing maintains quality and improve care.

Types of Automated External Defibrillator Programs

There are different types of PAD programs, mainly related to the specific site, population, or purpose, such as those described below.

Community/Neighborhood

These are community-wide programs typically with designated first responders dispatched through the local 911 center. Typical first responders are firefighters (especially in urban areas with fire departments staffed with in-house crews) and police officers (more common in suburban areas). A national survey found that about 80% of local law enforcement agencies responded to medical emergencies, with about 39% of those equipped with AEDs.[35] In many rural areas, volunteers often serve on an on-call basis as part of a quick response service (QRS). All of these prehospital defibrillation programs are usually integrated as part of the local EMS system.

Some neighborhoods and gated communities have developed PAD programs for their well-defined small areas. These have utilized AEDs deployed by on-site security personnel when available or placed in central areas, often with a lock-box type of system. This model shares characteristics of a community and an on-site program.

On-Site for Public and Private Nonresidential Locations

These programs comprise specific buildings or a defined location such as office buildings, industrial plants, schools, churches, and public squares or parks. Such programs are often run by the site owner or management firm and not directly owned and operated by local EMS. However, these programs should be coordinated with local EMS and the 911 call center.

In some communities, the local EMS has provided consultation or program coordination services for these programs.

Home (Residential) and Personal

A newer concept is the deployment of AEDs in private residences and vehicles. This concept has garnered attention because 75% to 80% of all SCAs occur at home. However, many of these are unwitnessed or occur during sleep, hence are unrecognized. Additional concerns regarding the effectiveness of this strategy are whether family members or others would be willing and able to promptly use the AED and that attention to the AED would not lead to delay or failure to call 911. A multicenter trial that studied this concept in 7001 patients with myocardial infarction found that overall mortality (about 6.5%) did not differ between subjects who were provided AEDs and those who were not. Four of 32 patients on whom AED was used survived and no inappropriate shocks were reported.[159]

However, use of a home defibrillator may still be a consideration for the small group of persons with risk factors for SCA but who are not candidates for an implanted defibrillator. Some "worried well" individuals have deployed AEDs not only in their private residences but also their personal vehicles, planes, and vacation homes. Currently there is one AED model (Home Defibrillator, Philips Medical Systems, Andover, MA) with FDA approval for sale without a prescription.

The similar components among these types of programs allow for a general format to set up and maintain any PAD program. The components that are different provide specifics that make a particular PAD program successful.

Liability and Regulatory Issues

All states have some form of "good Samaritan" AED legislation. In general, these laws provide immunity from legal liability for those who use and deploy AEDs without gross negligence or willful and wanton misconduct, but the details vary from state to state. Some states require training by nationally recognized training organizations, coordination with EMS, medical direction, and record keeping.

The National Cardiac Arrest Survival Act provides liability protection for good Samaritans in states without such legislation. Now that all states do have this in place, whether the federal statute provides any additional protections is unclear and likely will depend on court interpretations.

This information can be accessed via the Internet at many different Web sites, such as the AHA, American Red Cross, Sudden Cardiac Arrest Association, as well as state-based legislative Web sites.

Critical Elements of a Quality Public Access Defibrillation Program

Coordination and Leadership

Leadership is critical for the development and maintenance of a quality PAD program. There must be someone passionate and dedicated to making the program work, preferably someone in a leadership position in the organization or empowered by leadership. This person can make sure that the necessary resources are available and can motivate other individuals when necessary.

A key part of leadership is medical direction oversight. This element is like an insurance policy, making sure that all the components are in place and functioning properly. The medical director is ideally a physician with interest and expertise in prehospital care or resuscitation medicine. For the majority of AEDs a prescription is required in order to purchase the device, which is considered a class III medical device by the FDA (http://www.fda.gov/cdrh/devadvice/313.html). A good knowledge base of the different AEDs available in the market is useful, since AEDs have differing options that make some better for PAD programs (such as the need for a basic AED) versus medical or advanced use by professional responders, such as an EMS agency or cardiac testing facility (where the need for visualization of the real-time ECG, manual override of preset energy levels, or pacing capabilities may be required). Medical direction oversight helps to assure protective legal steps are addressed, such as the use of checklists for expiration dates, battery-life status, and equipment requirements. Other components of a medical direction oversight program are listed below.

The medical direction oversight team is composed of the physician and at least one coordinator, such as a nurse, EMT, EMT-P, or anyone knowledgeable about AEDs. Having a medical background is helpful but not necessary in the role of coordinator. This team provides the prescription, standard operating guidelines (SOG), and possibly training; it can also offer consultation on the need for PAD programs. Leadership is important, so that awareness of AEDs can be promoted, proper use of AEDs—in conjunction with CPR—can be recommended, providing a source of support to all involved for consistency and comfort of both the lay-public and the medical personnel.

Another key person is someone at the site who is willing and able to be responsible for the AED and SOG, and serve as liaison between the site and medical direction oversight team. This person is called the on-site coordinator. If there is a safety committee or emergency response team already on-site, this is a good source to use. If there is security on-site, as at the entrance to the site/building, this is not only a good location to place the AED but a good source to use for the daily equipment check, since such security is probably going to be making rounds and will be a consistent presence on-site.

It is important to notify the local EMS agency that an AED is on-site. EMS also provides a source of support, information and possibly training. This also promotes communication and awareness between the general public and the local EMS agency.

Response Planning and Device Deployment

Assessment of the Site and/or Facility   This is an important step in any PAD program so the site can be visually inspected for its size and scope, entrances to buildings, access for EMS, deterrents that may hinder response time (such as automatically locking doors in stairways), location of elevators and stairs, and any other emergency equipment on-site. Two other components to assess would be the form of communication (overhead public access system, pagers, cell phones, walkie-talkies/radios, or nothing) and the current emergency response plan.

An emerging goal, based on published studies and expert opinion, is to deploy devices such that they can be retrieved and brought to the victim within 3 minutes. This step should actually be walked through and timed with a stopwatch from the furthest point from the AED location.

Information collected on the site assessment will help to determine how many AEDs are ideal for the site as well as placement and location for storage and signage to direct the responder to the AED in the timeliest manner. The most central, easily accessed, and visual location is the optimal location for the AED.

Written Standard Operating Guidelines   This is a key element, since it basically ties all the elements of the PAD program together. The chain of survival is a good model for any emergency response plan. The links include calling 911, performing CPR, obtaining and using the AED, and EMS arrival. An emergency response plan should address the following elements:

- Recognition of possible cardiac arrest.
- How to call 911:
  - Is it a direct line or must an outside line be dialed first?
  - How is the public made aware of this information (sign by the phones, stickers on the phone)?
- What is the form of communication on-site to alert others of an emergency?

– How is the public made aware of this information (forms posted at key locations, frequent reminders at staff meetings)?
- What is the location of the AED (or AEDs)?
- Statement that the AED should be brought to all events.
- EMS access (designated entrance, hold the elevator, unlock any doors)

The standard operating guidelines (SOG) serve as the blueprint that will guide and maintain organization of the PAD program for both the medical direction oversight team and the site itself. Components of the SOG include the justification for the AED by using current knowledge and statistics on how CPR and AED use affect the survival of the victim. Other components would be the emergency response plan, a list of the exact location of the AED(s) on-site, AED manufacturer and model number, CPR and AED "how to" steps, listing of ownership, responsibilities of the different entities involved (such as the medical direction oversight team, on-site coordinator, and responders). Contact information for key persons should be included. Information specific to the AED's functioning should be outlined. Helpful hints for troubleshooting are valuable and should be specific to the AED, including technical support contact information and referral to the manufacturer's owner's manual. Checklists for checking the AED's state-of-readiness indicator as well as checking the equipment for expiration dates and lot numbers, battery-life status, and that all required equipment is intact. Event documentation forms are important for event data collection and quality-assurance review. This process must be outlined to detail who will collect data, in what time frame, and what equipment is necessary to obtain event data from the AED device. Quality assurance should include review of the entire event, time sequence and role of responders, AED event review for initial rhythm, rhythm at each analysis, rhythm at each shock or "no shock advised" assessment, and final rhythm. This also presents the opportunity to provide feedback to the program personnel.

Personnel and Training

All responding personnel should be trained in CPR and AED use. It is important to document and maintain this training. Some sites have designated response teams or safety committees of which all of those members should be trained. Another helpful training aspect is an in-service on the site on the specifics of the AED(s) by providing information and a demonstration. It is optimal to do this at time of initial deployment and as review. A mock drill is another way to evaluate the PAD program, providing staff involvement and teaching with the post-mock-drill review. Another option is the AHA's Heartsaver AED Anytime" self-training, which allows for viewing a DVD while practicing on the manikin provided, and then having an AHA instructor evaluate the procedure at a later time to be certified as having passed the AHA Heartsaver course.

Equipment and Supplies

The suggested equipment that should be considered for storage with the AED includes the following:

- Battery (installed)
- Two sets of adult pads
- Carry case to hold the above in an organized and safe manner (recommended is a carry case specifically made for the AED, since it holds the AED firmly and has slots for extra supplies; this is preferable to any other carry bag format)
- "CPR kit," which would include medical scissors, razor, towel, gloves, and barrier device (face shield or face mask)
- Event report form
- All this equipment allows for a grab-and-go concept, since all is encapsulated inside the carry case (AED, battery, pads) and attached to the handle (CPR kit), so that it can easily be carried from storage to the victim for optimal response time.

Other equipment to consider based on specific circumstances would include:

- Pediatric pads
- Spare battery (refer to manufacturer's owner's manual and medical director for recommendation on specifics of spare battery location; generally spare needed only for rechargeable batteries or if under unusual stress)
- Paper pad and pen to make notes of event
- Forms such as the emergency response plan and the CPR and AED "how to" and Event Report form

Storage and Signage There are several options for storage of the AED. Wall-mounted cabinets can be recessed, semirecessed, or in on-the-wall format. There are also stand-alone cabinets. The cabinet can have different alert systems, such as a local alarm system (usually audible and visual) or an autodial phone mechanism to alert the 911 center and/or an on-site call center. The cabinet can house just the AED or also other first aid equipment. The cabinet is usually metal with a clear front so that the AED can easily be seen, including the state-of-readiness indicator. There are also options for temperature-controlled and security cabinets ideal for outdoor settings, such as parks and pools. The cabinet door generally should not be locked, so that anyone can pull the door open to access the AED when needed. A cabinet is best for public locations so that the AED can be visualized but still kept protected.

Another storage mode for AEDs employs a wall bracket or hook. This would be appropriate for a location that is not accessed by the general public, such as a doctor's office.

Signage is very important to make everyone aware that there is an AED on-site and where it is located. It seems redundant, but having a 3D AED sign (one that protrudes from the wall versus being flat on the wall) above the cabinet is useful so that it can be more easily seen. Directional signage with words or arrows to help the responder reach the AED location may be warranted in some settings. Having a sign stating that there is an AED on the premises and where it is located within the site is also useful. Signs can usually be purchased from the manufacturer of the AED, or they can be custom-made or even printed out and laminated (the Sudden Cardiac Arrest Association Web site offers the option of printing out the universal AED symbol).

Maintenance (Equipment and Program)

Most AEDs conduct self-checks, and this generates a readiness indicator on the device. This information can be found in the manufacturer's owner's manual. Most AEDs will make a chirping sound similar to the sound a smoke detector makes when its battery is low. There is also a change with the state-of-readiness indicator. All this is important for the on-site coordinator to know and assess for when checking the state-of-readiness indicator. This should be done daily for most sites or at minimum on a weekly basis, such as at a church. Such a checkup is ideally done in the morning, since most AEDs do the self-check after midnight.

Since the battery is being used every day by the AED so as to be maintained in a state-of-readiness, this will lead to wear on the battery. Hence the state-of-readiness indicator and daily visible check are important for ensuring that the AED is in optimal ready-to-use format at all times. It is important to document in the SOG when the battery was first installed in the AED. It is recommended to place an insertion date on the battery pack, using a permanent marker. This date will help determine when the battery will need to be replaced within a safe time margin. For example, the Philips lithium battery is a 4-year battery, but it will need to be replaced after about 3.5 years. If the AED is used for an event, this also means wear on the battery. Some manufacturers replace the battery pack at the same time as the pads, as with the Medtronic CR Plus and Express. One of the AED self-checks is to check the status of the battery; it will alert if it is low according to the state-of-readiness indicator. The AED is still usable in a limited format even in this low-battery state for a certain number of shocks and certain amount of time. The battery must be replaced with a new battery (or recharged if it is a rechargeable battery) so that the AED is maintained in a state-of-readiness and is not left with a dead battery, in which case the AED is not operational.

The pads also have expiration dates, usually 2 years, but some manufacturers are now providing longer expiration dates. The package in which the pads come is sealed and should remain sealed to maintain the optimal life span of the pads, specifically the conductivity of the gel on the pads. When the seal is broken and the gel is exposed to air, the time during which the pads are usable—with good conductivity and adherence to the skin—is reduced. The pads are designed for one-time use only and will need to be replaced after an event. It is important to have two sets of adult pads, so that if the first set is not placed properly or does not adhere adequately (for example, on a male victim with a hairy chest), the second set can be used.

Pediatric pads are optional; usually just one set of these is needed. They are considered preferable for children 1 to 8 years of age who weigh <55 lb (25 kg). Adult pads can be used in the anteroposterior location if pediatric pads are not available.

Some of the materials from the CPR kit can be cleaned and reused and some, once used, must be discarded and replaced after the event. The medical scissors can be cleaned appropriately and reused. The razor, towel, gloves, and barrier device will have to be replaced. If the barrier device is a face mask, only the valve will need replacement. Some face masks can be cleaned appropriately and reused.

The SOG should include the procedure for restocking the AED after an event or when items expire. The medical direction oversight team may keep supplies in stock for quick turnover postevent. If there is an event, the coordinator goes to the site to retrieve the necessary forms and download the information from the AED. At this time the AED is restocked with supplies. After the event, the site is given an order form to reorder whatever additional supplies may be needed. This allows for quick turnover and consistency of supplies and maintenance.

Incident Follow-up

Post-AED actions should include several important components. Documentation of the event from the responder(s) on a designated form is recommended. Information should include the date and time, location, when CPR was initiated, whether the AED was used, what the AED advised, whether there were any problems with CPR or AED use, whether all necessary emergency equipment was available, EMS notification and response, and any other anecdotal information. The recorded information from the AED is downloaded and made available to the appropriate medical personnel. A designated individual is then responsible for cleaning and restocking the AED.

Postevent response from the medical direction oversight team would be for quality assurance purposes to review the event forms and AED ECG; obtain follow-up, if able, on the victim; and provide a report and feedback to the site. The event ECG should be forwarded to the appropriate medical personnel if that had not already been done, including the victim's medical records. It is obviously very important to do this in a timely fashion, especially if the victim survives, so that the physician can assess the event ECG to possibly help determine what occurred and plan for treatment. The medical direction oversight program should have the means to do this, either by having the necessary equipment (software, infrared cable, laptop, etc.) or having access to such equipment from another source (possibly local EMS agencies or local AED manufacturer sales or technical support representative).

Quality Improvement

The quality-improvement program should comprise both system and individual incident review. The program should be reviewed annually by the medical direction oversight team by actually going to the site again, reviewing the SOG, visually inspecting the AEDs, and discussing the program with the on-site coordinator and then updating the SOG as needed to maintain it at an optimal level. This review should assure that responses are initiated to all potential SCAs.

The medical oversight team should also review the responder actions and AED function for every response. This includes reviewing data collected from the AED.

Summary of PAD

Lay-rescuer PAD programs save lives. An organized and consistent approach to the PAD program fosters success. Success will promote the program and save more lives. Remember that the AED is easy to use and difficult to misuse. The AED has self-checks that provide alerts showing whether it is functioning appropriately, so performing a check is easy and takes little time. A quality medical direction oversight program as the foundation of the PAD program enhances success.

References

1. Larsen MP, Eisenberg MS, Cummins RO, et al. Predicting survival from out-of-hospital cardiac arrest: a graphic model. *Ann Emerg Med* 1993;22(11):1652–1658.
2. Valenzuela TD, Roe DJ, Cretin S, et al. Estimating effectiveness of cardiac arrest interventions: a logistic regression survival model. *Circulation* 1997;96(10):3308–3313.
3. Swor RA, Boji B, Cynar M, et al. Bystander vs EMS first-responder CPR: initial rhythm and outcome in witnessed nonmonitored out-of-hospital cardiac arrest. *Acad Emerg Med* 1995;2(6):494–498.
4. Holmberg M, Holmberg S, Herlitz J. Incidence, duration and survival of ventricular fibrillation in out-of-hospital cardiac arrest patients in Sweden. *Resuscitation* 2000;44(1):7–17.
5. Wik L, Hansen TB, Fylling F, et al. Delaying defibrillation to give basic cardiopulmonary resuscitation to patients with out-of-hospital ventricular fibrillation: a randomized trial. *JAMA* 2003;289(11):1389–1395.
6. Cobb LA, Fahrenbruch CE, Walsh TR, et al. Influence of cardiopulmonary resuscitation prior to defibrillation in patients with out-of-hospital ventricular fibrillation. *JAMA* 1999;281(13):1182–1188.
7. Cummins RO, Eisenberg MS, Hallstrom AP, et al. Survival of out-of-hospital cardiac arrest with early initiation of cardiopulmonary resuscitation. *Am J Emerg Med* 1985;3(2):114–119.
8. Holmberg M, Holmberg S, Herlitz J. Effect of bystander cardiopulmonary resuscitation in out-of-hospital cardiac arrest patients in Sweden. *Resuscitation* 2000;47(1):59–70.
9. Waalewijn RA, Tijssen JG, Koster RW. Bystander initiated actions in out-of-hospital cardiopulmonary resuscitation: results from the Amsterdam Resuscitation Study (ARRESUST). *Resuscitation* 2001;50(3):273–279.
10. Weaver WD, Copass MK, Bufi D, et al. Improved neurologic recovery and survival after early defibrillation. *Circulation* 1984;69(5):943–948.
11. Cobb LA, Werner JA, Trobaugh GB. Sudden cardiac death: II. outcome of resuscitation—management, and future directions. *Mod Concepts Cardiovasc Dis* 1980;49(7):37–42.
12. Cobb LA, Werner JA, Trobaugh GB. Sudden cardiac death: I. A decade's experience with out-of-hospital resuscitation. *Mod Concepts Cardiovasc Dis* 1980;49(6):31–36.
13. Cobb LA, Hallstrom AP. Community-based cardiopulmonary resuscitation: what have we learned? *Ann N Y Acad Sci* 1982;382:330–342.
14. Eisenberg MS, Bergner L, Hallstrom A. Cardiac resuscitation in the community: importance of rapid provision and implications for program planning. *JAMA* 1979;241(18):1905–1907.
15. Eisenberg M, Bergner L, Hallstrom A. Paramedic programs and out-of-hospital cardiac arrest, I: factors associated with successful resuscitation. *Am J Public Health* 1979;69(1):30–38.
16. Bayes de Luna A, Coumel P, Leclercq JF. Ambulatory sudden cardiac death: mechanisms of production of fatal arrhythmia on the basis of data from 157 cases. *Am Heart J* 1989;117(1):151–159.
17. Cummins RO, Ornato JP, Thies WH, et al. Improving survival from sudden cardiac arrest: the "chain of survival" concept. A statement for health professionals from the Advanced Cardiac Life Support Subcommittee and the Emergency Cardiac Care Committee, American Heart Association. *Circulation* 1991;83(5):1832–1847.
18. Van Camp SP, Peterson RA. Cardiovascular complications of outpatient cardiac rehabilitation programs. *JAMA* 1986;256(9):1160–1163.
19. Haskell WL. Cardiovascular complications during exercise training of cardiac patients. *Circulation* 1978;57(5):920–924.
20. Swor RA, Jackson RE, Cynar M, et al. Bystander CPR, ventricular fibrillation, and survival in witnessed, unmonitored out-of-hospital cardiac arrest. *Ann Emerg Med* 1995;25(6):780–784.
21. Cummins RO, Eisenberg MS. Prehospital cardiopulmonary resuscitation. Is it effective? *JAMA* 1985;253(16):2408–2412.
22. Cummins RO. Witnessed collapse and bystander cardiopulmonary resuscitation: what is really going on? *Acad Emerg Med* 1995;2(6):474–477.
23. Eisenberg MS, Cummins RO. Defibrillation performed by the emergency medical technician. *Circulation* 1986;74(pt 2)(6):IV9–IV12.
24. Stults KR, Brown DD, Schug VL, et al. Prehospital defibrillation performed by emergency medical technicians in rural communities. *N Engl J Med* 1984;310(4):219–223.
25. Vukov LF, Johnson DQ. External transcutaneous pacemakers in interhospital transport of cardiac patients. *Ann Emerg Med* 1989;18(7):738–740.
26. Bachman JW, McDonald GS, O'Brien PC. A study of out-of-hospital cardiac arrests in northeastern Minnesota. *JAMA* 1986;256(4):477–483.
27. Olson DW, LaRochelle J, Fark D, et al. EMT-defibrillation: the Wisconsin experience. *Ann Emerg Med* 1989;18(8):806–811.
28. Cummins RO. From concept to standard-of-care? Review of the clinical experience with automated external defibrillators. *Ann Emerg Med* 1989;18(12):1269–1275.
29. Eisenberg MS, Horwood BT, Cummins RO, et al. Cardiac arrest and resuscitation: a tale of 29 cities. *Ann Emerg Med* 1990;19(2):179–186.
30. Eisenberg MS, Cummins RO, Damon S, et al. Survival rates from out-of-hospital cardiac arrest: recommendations for uniform definitions and data to report. *Ann Emerg Med* 1990;19(11):1249–1259.
31. Every NR, Fahrenbruch CE, Hallstrom AP, et al. Influence of coronary bypass surgery on subsequent outcome of patients resuscitated from out of hospital cardiac arrest. *J Am Coll Cardiol* 1992;19(7):1435–1439.
32. White RD, Asplin BR, Bugliosi TF, et al. High discharge survival rate after out-of-hospital ventricular fibrillation with rapid defibrillation by police and paramedics. *Ann Emerg Med* 1996;28(5):480–485.
33. Mosesso VN, Jr, Davis EA, Auble TE, et al. Use of automated external defibrillators by police officers for treatment of out-of-hospital cardiac arrest. *Ann Emerg Med* 1998;32(2):200–207.
34. Davis EA, Mosesso VN Jr. Performance of police first responders in utilizing automated external defibrillation on victims of sudden cardiac arrest. *Prehosp Emerg Care* 1998;2(2):101–107.
35. Hawkins SC, Shapiro AH, Sever AE, et al. The role of law enforcement agencies in out-of-hospital emergency care. *Resuscitation* 2007;72(3):386–393.
36. Alonso-Serra HM, Delbridge TR, Auble TE, et al. Law enforcement agencies and out-of-hospital emergency care. *Ann Emerg Med* 1997;29(4):497–503.
37. Weisfeldt ML, Becker LB. Resuscitation after cardiac arrest: a 3-phase time-sensitive model. *JAMA* 2002;288(23):3035–3038.
38. Valenzuela TD, Roe DJ, Nichol G, et al. Outcomes of rapid defibrillation by security officers after cardiac arrest in casinos. *N Engl J Med* 2000;343(17):1206–1209.
39. O'Rourke MF, Donaldson E, Geddes JS. An airline cardiac arrest program. *Circulation* 1997;96(9):2849–2853.
40. Page RL, Joglar JA, Kowal RC, et al. Use of automated external defibrillators by a U.S. airline. *N Engl J Med* 2000;343(17):1210–1216.
40a. Caffrey SL, Willoughby PJ, Pepe PE, et al. Public use of automated external defibrillators. *N Engl J Med* 2002;347(16):1242–1247.
41. *Automatic External Defibrillators (AEDs) and Public Access Defibrillation (PAD) Programs*. Bethesda, Md: Center for Devices

and Radiological Health, U.S. Food and Drug Administration; 2000. http://www.fda.gov/cdrh/consumer/aed_pad.html.

42. Weisfeldt ML. Bystander administered shock improves survival from out of hospital cardiac arrest in U.S. and Canada. *Circulation.* 2007;116:II-386.

43. Finn JC, Jacobs IG, Holman CD, et al. Outcomes of out-of-hospital cardiac arrest patients in Perth, Western Australia, 1996–1999. *Resuscitation* 2001;51(3):247–255.

44. Sedgwick ML, Watson J, Dalziel K, et al. Efficacy of out of hospital defibrillation by ambulance technicians using automated external defibrillators. The Heartstart Scotland Project. *Resuscitation* 1992;24(1):73–87.

45. Diack AW, Welborn WS, Rullman RG, et al. An automatic cardiac resuscitator for emergency treatment of cardiac arrest. *Med Instrum* 1979;13(2):78–83.

46. Cummins RO, Eisenberg MS, Litwin PE, et al. Automatic external defibrillators used by emergency medical technicians: a controlled clinical trial. *JAMA* 1987;257(12):1605–1610.

47. Jaggarao NS, Heber M, Grainger R, et al. Use of an automated external defibrillator-pacemaker by ambulance staff. *Lancet* 1982;2(8289):73–75.

48. Jakobsson J, Nyquist O, Rehnqvist N. Effects of early defibrillation of out-of-hospital cardiac arrest patients by ambulance personnel. *Eur Heart J* 1987;8(11):1189–1194.

49. Gray AJ, Redmond AD, Martin MA. Use of the automatic external defibrillator-pacemaker by ambulance personnel: the Stockport experience. *BMJ* 1987;294:1133–1135.

50. Eisenberg MS, Moore J, Cummins RO, et al. Use of the automatic external defibrillator in homes of survivors of out-of-hospital ventricular fibrillation. *Am J Cardiol* 1989;63(7):443–446.

51. Weaver WD, Hill D, Fahrenbruch CE, et al. Use of the automatic external defibrillator in the management of out-of-hospital cardiac arrest. *N Engl J Med* 1988;319(11):661–666.

52. White RD, Vukov LF, Bugliosi TF. Early defibrillation by police: initial experience with measurement of critical time intervals and patient outcome. *Ann Emerg Med* 1994;23(5):1009–1013.

53. White RD, Hankins DG, Bugliosi TF. Seven years' experience with early defibrillation by police and paramedics in an emergency medical services system. *Resuscitation* 1998;39(3):145–151.

54. Cummins RO, Eisenberg M, Bergner L, et al. Sensitivity, accuracy, and safety of an automatic external defibrillator. *Lancet* 1984;2(8398):318–320.

55. Dull SM, Graves JR, Larsen MP, et al. Expected death and unwanted resuscitation in the prehospital setting. *Ann Emerg Med* 1994;23(5):997–1002.

56. Kerber RE, Becker LB, Bourland JD, et al. Automatic external defibrillators for public access defibrillation: recommendations for specifying and reporting arrhythmia analysis algorithm performance, incorporating new waveforms, and enhancing safety. A statement for health professionals from the American Heart Association Task Force on Automatic External Defibrillation, Subcommittee on AED Safety and Efficacy. *Circulation* 1997;95(6):1677–1682.

57. Dickey W, Dalzell GW, Anderson JM, et al. The accuracy of decision-making of a semi-automatic defibrillator during cardiac arrest. *Eur Heart J* 1992;13(5):608–615.

58. Atkinson E, Mikysa B, Conway JA, et al. Specificity and sensitivity of automated external defibrillator rhythm analysis in infants and children. *Ann Emerg Med* 2003;42(2):185–196.

59. Cecchin F, Jorgenson DB, Berul CI, et al. Is arrhythmia detection by automatic external defibrillator accurate for children? Sensitivity and specificity of an automatic external defibrillator algorithm in 696 pediatric arrhythmias. *Circulation* 2001;103(20):2483–2488.

60. Atkins DL, Hartley LL, York DK. Accurate recognition and effective treatment of ventricular fibrillation by automated external defibrillators in adolescents. *Pediatrics* 1998;101(pt 1)(3):393–397.

61. Hazinski MF, Walker C, Smith J, et al. Specificity of automatic external defibrillator rhythm analysis in pediatric tachyarrhythmias. *Circulation* 1997;96(suppl I):I-561.

62. Cummins RO, Eisenberg MS, Stults KR. Automatic external defibrillators: clinical issues for cardiology. *Circulation* 1986;73(3):381–385.

63. Stolzenberg BT, Kupas DF, Wieczorek BJ, et al. Automated external defibrillators appropriately recognize ventricular fibrillation in electromagnetic fields. *Prehosp Emerg Care* 2002;6(1):65–66.

64. Ornato JP, Shipley J, Powell RG, et al. Inappropriate electrical countershocks by an automated external defibrillator. *Ann Emerg Med* 1992;21:1278–1282.

65. Macdonald RD, Swanson JM, Mottley JL, et al. Performance and error analysis of automated external defibrillator use in the out-of-hospital setting. *Ann Emerg Med* 2001;38(3):262–267.

66. Wik L, Kramer-Johansen J, Myklebust H, et al. Quality of cardiopulmonary resuscitation during out-of-hospital cardiac arrest. *JAMA* 2005;293(3):299–304.

67. Abella BS, Alvarado JP, Myklebust H, et al. Quality of cardiopulmonary resuscitation during in-hospital cardiac arrest. *JAMA* 2005;293(3):305–310.

68. Lloyd MS, Heeke B, Walter PF, et al. Hands-on defibrillation: an analysis of electrical current flow through rescuers in direct contact with patients during biphasic external defibrillation. *Circulation* 2008;117:2510–2515.

69. Eftestol T, Sunde K, Aase SO, et al. Predicting outcome of defibrillation by spectral characterization and nonparametric classification of ventricular fibrillation in patients with out-of-hospital cardiac arrest. *Circulation* 2000;102(13):1523–1529.

69a. ACC/AHA/ESC 2006 Guidelines for Management of Patients with Ventricular Arrhythmias and the Prevention of Sudden Cardiac Death. *JACC* 2006;48:5.

70. Callaway CW, Sherman LD, Mosesso VN Jr, et al. Scaling exponent predicts defibrillation success for out-of-hospital ventricular fibrillation cardiac arrest. *Circulation* 2001;103(12):1656–1661.

70a. Epstein AE, Dimarco JP, Ellenbogen KA. ACC/AHA/HRS 2008 Guidelines for Device-Based Therapy of Cardiac Rhythm Abnormalities. A Report of the American College of Cardiology/American Heart Association Task Force on Practice Guidelines (Writing Committee to Revise the ACC/AHA/NASPE 2002 Guideline Update for Implantation of Cardiac Pacemakers and Antiarrhythmia Devices). *Circulation.* 2008 May 15. [Epub ahead of print]

71. Weaver WD, Cobb LA, Dennis D, et al. Amplitude of ventricular fibrillation waveform and outcome after cardiac arrest. *Ann Intern Med* 1985;102(1):53–55.

72. Brown CG, Dzwonczyk R. Signal analysis of the human electrocardiogram during ventricular fibrillation: frequency and amplitude parameters as predictors of successful countershock. *Ann Emerg Med* 1996;27(2):184–188.

73. Callaham M, Braun O, Valentine W, et al. Prehospital cardiac arrest treated by urban first-responders: profile of patient response and prediction of outcome by ventricular fibrillation waveform. *Ann Emerg Med* 1993;22(11):1664–1677.

74. Strohmenger HU, Lindner KH, Brown CG. Analysis of the ventricular fibrillation ECG signal amplitude and frequency parameters as predictors of countershock success in humans. *Chest* 1997;111(3):584–589.

75. Strohmenger HU, Eftestol T, Sunde K, et al. The predictive value of ventricular fibrillation electrocardiogram signal frequency and amplitude variables in patients with out-of-hospital cardiac arrest. *Anesth Analg* 2001;93(6):1428–1433.

76. Podbregar M, Kovacic M, Podbregar-Mars A, et al. Predicting defibrillation success by 'genetic' programming in patients with out-of-hospital cardiac arrest. *Resuscitation* 2003;57(2):153–159.

77. Povoas HP, Weil MH, Tang W, et al. Predicting the success of defibrillation by electrocardiographic analysis. *Resuscitation* 2002;53(1):77–82.

78. Noc M, Weil MH, Gazmuri RJ, et al. Ventricular fibrillation voltage as a monitor of the effectiveness of cardiopulmonary resuscitation. *J Lab Clin Med* 1994;124(3):421–426.

79. Lightfoot CB, Nremt P, Callaway CW, et al. Dynamic nature of electrocardiographic waveform predicts rescue shock outcome in porcine ventricular fibrillation. *Ann Emerg Med* 2003;42(2):230–241.

80. Marn-Pernat A, Weil MH, Tang W, et al. Optimizing timing of ventricular defibrillation. *Crit Care Med* 2001;29(12):2360–2365.

81. Hamprecht FA, Achleitner U, Krismer AC, et al. Fibrillation power, an alternative method of ECG spectral analysis for prediction of countershock success in a porcine model of ventricular fibrillation. *Resuscitation* 2001;50(3):287–296.

82. Amann A, Achleitner U, Antretter H, et al. Analysing ventricular fibrillation ECG-signals and predicting defibrillation success during cardiopulmonary resuscitation employing N(alpha)-histograms. *Resuscitation* 2001;50(1):77–85.

83. Amann A, Rheinberger K, Achleitner U, et al. The prediction of defibrillation outcome using a new combination of mean frequency and amplitude in porcine models of cardiac arrest. *Anesth Analg* 2002;95(3):716–722, table of contents.

84. Brown CG, Griffith RF, Van Ligten P, et al. Median frequency— a new parameter for predicting defibrillation success rate. *Ann Emerg Med* 1991;20(7):787–789.

85. Yu T, Weil MH, Tang W, et al. Adverse outcomes of interrupted precordial compression during automated defibrillation. *Circulation* 2002;106(3):368–372.

86. Sato Y, Weil MH, Sun S, et al. Adverse effects of interrupting precordial compression during cardiopulmonary resuscitation. *Crit Care Med* 1997;25(5):733–736.

87. Berg RA, Sanders AB, Kern KB, et al. Adverse hemodynamic effects of interrupting chest compressions for rescue breathing during cardiopulmonary resuscitation for ventricular fibrillation cardiac arrest. *Circulation* 2001;104(20):2465–2470.

88. Kern KB, Hilwig RW, Berg RA, et al. Importance of continuous chest compressions during cardiopulmonary resuscitation: improved outcome during a simulated single lay-rescuer scenario. *Circulation* 2002;105(5):645–649.

89. Eftestol T, Sunde K, Steen PA. Effects of interrupting precordial compressions on the calculated probability of defibrillation success during out-of-hospital cardiac arrest. *Circulation* 2002; 105(19):2270–2273.

90. van Alem AP, Sanou BT, et al. Interruption of cardiopulmonary resuscitation with the use of the automated external defibrillator in out-of-hospital cardiac arrest. *Ann Emerg Med* 2003;42(4): 449–457.

91. Hess EP, White RD. Recurrent ventricular fibrillation in out-of-hospital cardiac arrest after defibrillation by police and firefighters: implications for automated external defibrillator users. *Crit Care Med* 2004;32(9 Suppl):S436–S439.

92. Bain AC, Swerdlow CD, Love CJ, et al. Multicenter study of principles-based waveforms for external defibrillation. *Ann Emerg Med* 2001;37(1):5–12.

93. Poole JE, White RD, Kanz KG, et al. Low-energy impedance-compensating biphasic waveforms terminate ventricular fibrillation at high rates in victims of out-of-hospital cardiac arrest. LIFE Investigators. *J Cardiovasc Electrophysiol* 1997;8(12):1373–1385.

94. White RD, Blackwell TH, Russell JK, et al. Transthoracic impedance does not affect defibrillation, resuscitation or survival in patients with out-of-hospital cardiac arrest treated with a non-escalating biphasic waveform defibrillator. *Resuscitation* 2005;64 (1):63–69.

95. Mittal S, Ayati S, Stein KM, et al. Comparison of a novel rectilinear biphasic waveform with a damped sine wave monophasic waveform for transthoracic ventricular defibrillation. ZOLL Investigators. *J Am Coll Cardiol* 1999;34(5):1595–1601.

96. Schneider T, Martens PR, Paschen H, et al. Multicenter, randomized, controlled trial of 150-J biphasic shocks compared with 200- to 360-J monophasic shocks in the resuscitation of out-of-hospital cardiac arrest victims. Optimized Response to Cardiac Arrest (ORCA) Investigators. *Circulation* 2000;102(15): 1780–1787.

97. Blouin D, Topping C, Moore S, et al. Out-of-hospital defibrillation with automated external defibrillators: postshock analysis should be delayed. *Ann Emerg Med* 2001;38(3):256–261.

98. Hoyt R, Grayzel J, Kerber RE. Determinants of intracardiac current in defibrillation. Experimental studies in dogs. *Circulation* 1981;64(4):818–823.

99. *American National Standard: Automatic External Defibrillators and Remote Controlled Defibrillators (DF39)*. Arlington, VA: Association for the Advancement of Medical Instrumentation, 1993.

100. Kerber RE, Grayzel J, Hoyt R, et al. Transthoracic resistance in human defibrillation. Influence of body weight, chest size, serial shocks, paddle size and paddle contact pressure. *Circulation* 1981;63(3):676–682.

101. Dalzell GW, Cunningham SR, Anderson J, et al. Electrode pad size, transthoracic impedance and success of external ventricular defibrillation. *Am J Cardiol* 1989;64(12):741–744.

102. Dahl CF, Ewy GA, Warner ED, et al. Myocardial necrosis from direct current countershock: effect of paddle electrode size and time interval between discharges. *Circulation* 1974;50(5): 956–961.

103. Samson RA, Atkins DL, Kerber RE. Optimal size of self-adhesive preapplied electrode pads in pediatric defibrillation. *Am J Cardiol* 1995;75(7):544–545.

104. Heames RM, Sado D, Deakin CD. Do doctors position defibrillation paddles correctly? Observational study. *BMJ* 2001;322 (7299):1393–1394.

105. Deale OC, Lerman BB. Intrathoracic current flow during transthoracic defibrillation in dogs. Transcardiac current fraction. *Circ Res* 1990;67(6):1405–1419.

106. Karlon WJ, Eisenberg SR, Lehr JL. Effects of paddle placement and size on defibrillation current distribution: a three-dimensional finite element model. *IEEE Trans Biomed Eng* 1993;40(3): 246–255.

107. Garcia LA, Kerber RE. Transthoracic defibrillation: does electrode adhesive pad position alter transthoracic impedance? *Resuscitation* 1998;37(3):139–143.

108. Kerber RE, Martins JB, Ferguson DW, et al. Experimental evaluation and initial clinical application of new self-adhesive defibrillation electrodes. *Int J Cardiol* 1985;8(1):57–66.

109. Jones FD, Fahy BG. Intraoperative use of automated external defibrillator. *J Clin Anesth* 1999;11(4):336–338.

110. Panescu D, Webster JG, Tompkins WJ, et al A. Optimization of cardiac defibrillation by three-dimensional finite element modeling of the human thorax. *IEEE Trans Biomed Eng* 1995;42(2): 185–192.

111. Kerber RE, Martins JB, Kelly KJ, et al. Self-adhesive preapplied electrode pads for defibrillation and cardioversion. *J Am Coll Cardiol* 1984;3(3):815–820.

112. Lown B. Electrical reversion of cardiac arrhythmias. *Br Heart J* 1967;29(4):469–489.

113. Camacho MA, Lehr JL, Eisenberg SR. A three-dimensional finite element model of human transthoracic defibrillation: paddle placement and size. *IEEE Trans Biomed Eng* 1995;42(6):572–578.

114. Moulton C, Dreyer C, Dodds D, et al. Placement of electrodes for defibrillation—a review of the evidence. *Eur J Emerg Med* 2000;7(2):135–143.

115. Pagan-Carlo LA, Spencer KT, Robertson CE, et al. Transthoracic defibrillation: importance of avoiding electrode placement directly on the female breast. *J Am Coll Cardiol* 1996;27(2):449–452.

116. Stults KR, Brown DD, Cooley F, et al. Self-adhesive monitor/defibrillation pads improve prehospital defibrillation success. *Ann Emerg Med* 1987;16(8):872–877.

117. Perkins GD, Roberts C, Gao F. Delays in defibrillation: influence of different monitoring techniques. *Br J Anaesth* 2002;89(3): 405–408.

118. Lerman BB, DiMarco JP, Haines DE. Current-based versus energy-based ventricular defibrillation: a prospective study. *J Am Coll Cardiol* 1988;12(5):1259–1264.

119. Kerber RE, Kouba C, Martins J, et al. Advance prediction of transthoracic impedance in human defibrillation and cardioversion: importance of impedance in determining the success of low-energy shocks. *Circulation* 1984;70(2):303–308.

120. Kerber RE, Martins JB, Kienzle MG, et al. Energy, current, and success in defibrillation and cardioversion: clinical studies using an automated impedance-based method of energy adjustment. *Circulation* 1988;77(5):1038–1046.

121. Sirna SJ, Ferguson DW, Charbonnier F, et al. Factors affecting transthoracic impedance during electrical cardioversion. *Am J Cardiol* 1988;62(16):1048–1052.

122. Hummel RS III, Ornato JP, Weinberg SM, et al. Spark-generating properties of electrode gels used during defibrillation. A potential fire hazard. *JAMA* 1988;260(20):3021–3024.

123. Bissing JW, Kerber RE. Effect of shaving the chest of hirsute subjects on transthoracic impedance to self-adhesive defibrillation electrode pads. *Am J Cardiol* 2000;86(5):587–589.

124. Sirna SJ, Kieso RA, Fox-Eastham KJ, et al. Mechanisms responsible for decline in transthoracic impedance after DC shocks. *Am J Physiol* 1989;257(pt 2)(4):H1180–H1183.

125. Ewy GA, Hellman DA, McClung S, et al. Influence of ventilation phase on transthoracic impedance and defibrillation effectiveness. *Crit Care Med* 1980;8(3):164–166.

126. Yoon RS, DeMonte TP, Hasanov KF, et al. Measurement of thoracic current flow in pigs for the study of defibrillation and cardioversion. *IEEE Trans Biomed Eng* 2003;50(10):1167–1173.

127. van Alem AP, Vrenken RH, de Vos R, et al. Use of automated external defibrillator by first responders in out of hospital cardiac arrest: prospective controlled trial. *BMJ* 2003;327(7427):1312.

128. Carpenter J, Rea TD, Murray JA, et al. Defibrillation waveform and post-shock rhythm in out-of-hospital ventricular fibrillation cardiac arrest. *Resuscitation* 2003;59(2):189–196.

129. Morrison LJ, Dorian P, Long J, et al. Out-of-hospital cardiac arrest rectilinear biphasic to monophasic damped sine defibrillation waveforms with advanced life support intervention trial (ORBIT). *Resuscitation* 2005;66(2):149–157.

130. Kudenchuk PJ, Cobb LA, Copass MK, et al. Transthoracic incremental monophasic verus biphasic defibrillation by emergency responders (TIMBER). *Circulation* 2006;114:2010–2018.

131. Weaver WD, Cobb LA, Copass MK, et al. Ventricular defibrillation: a comparative trial using 175-J and 320-J shocks. *N Engl J Med* 1982;307(18):1101–1106.

132. Miller PH. Potential fire hazard in defibrillation. *JAMA* 1972;221(2):192.

133. Fires from defibrillation during oxygen administration. *Health Devices* 1994;23(7):307–309.

134. Sparking during discharge testing on Physio-Control Lifepak 9 defibrillator/monitors. *Health Devices* 1994;23(3):98–99.

135. Lefever J, Smith A. Risk of fire when using defibrillation in an oxygen enriched atmosphere. *Medical Devices Agency Safety Notices* 1995;3:1–3.

136. Theodorou AA, Gutierrez JA, Berg RA. Fire attributable to a defibrillation attempt in a neonate. *Pediatrics* 2003;112(3 Pt 1):677–679.

137. Panacek EA, Munger MA, Rutherford WF, et al. Report of nitropatch explosions complicating defibrillation. *Am J Emerg Med* 1992;10(2):128–129.

138. Monsieurs KG, Conraads VM, Goethals MP, et al. Semi-automatic external defibrillation and implanted cardiac pacemakers: understanding the interactions during resuscitation. *Resuscitation* 1995;30(2):127–131.

139. Calle PA, Buylaert W. When an AED meets an ICD . . . Automated external defibrillator. Implantable cardioverter defibrillator. *Resuscitation* 1998;38(3):177–183.

140. Levine PA, Barold SS, Fletcher RD, et al. Adverse acute and chronic effects of electrical defibrillation and cardioversion on implanted unipolar cardiac pacing systems. *J Am Coll Cardiol* 1983;1(6):1413–1422.

141. Gurnett CA, Atkins DL. Successful use of a biphasic waveform automated external defibrillator in a high-risk child. *Am J Cardiol* 2000;86(9):1051–1053.

142. Atkins DL, Jorgenson DB. Attenuated pediatric electrode pads for automated external defibrillator use in children. *Resuscitation* 2005;66(1):31–37.

143. Berg RA, Hilwig RW, Ewy GA, et al. Precountershock cardiopulmonary resuscitation improves initial response to defibrillation from prolonged ventricular fibrillation: a randomized, controlled swine study. *Crit Care Med* 2004;32(6):1352–1357.

144. van Alem AP, Chapman FW, Lank P, et al. A prospective, randomised and blinded comparison of first shock success of monophasic and biphasic waveforms in out-of-hospital cardiac arrest. *Resuscitation* 2003;58(1):17–24.

145. Berg RA, Chapman FW, Berg MD, et al. Attenuated adult biphasic shocks compared with weight-based monophasic shocks in a swine model of prolonged pediatric ventricular fibrillation. *Resuscitation* 2004;61(2):189–197.

146. Gutgesell HP, Tacker WA, Geddes LA, et al. Energy dose for ventricular defibrillation of children. *Pediatrics* 1976;58(6):898–901.

147. Samson RA, Berg RA, Bingham R, et al. Use of automated external defibrillators for children: an update: an advisory statement from the pediatric advanced life support task force, International Liaison Committee on Resuscitation. *Circulation* 2003;107(25):3250–3255.

148. Jorgenson D, Morgan C, Snyder D, et al. Energy attenuator for pediatric application of an automated external defibrillator. *Crit Care Med* 2002;30(4 Suppl):S145–S147.

149. Samson R, Berg R, Bingham R, et al. Use of automated external defibrillators for children: an update. An advisory statement from the Pediatric Advanced Life Support Task Force, International Liaison Committee on Resuscitation. *Resuscitation* 2003;57(3):237–243.

150. Saxon LA. Survival after tachyarrhythmic arrest—what are we waiting for? *N Engl J Med* 2008;358(1):77–79.

151. Peberdy MA, Kaye W, Ornato JP, et al. Cardiopulmonary resuscitation of adults in the hospital: a report of 14720 cardiac arrests from the National Registry of Cardiopulmonary Resuscitation. *Resuscitation* 2003;58(3):297–308.

152. Chan PS, Krumholz HM, Nichol G, et al. American Heart Association National Registry of Cardiopulmonary Resuscitation Investigators. *N Engl J Med* 2008;358(1):9–17.

153. Zafari AM, Zarter SK, Heggen V, et al. A program encouraging early defibrillation results in improved in-hospital resuscitation efficacy. *J Am Coll Cardiol* 2004;44(4):846–852.

154. Destro A, Marzaloni M, Sermasi S, et al. Automatic external defibrillators in the hospital as well? *Resuscitation* 1996;31(1):39–43.

155. Kaye W, Mancini ME, Richards N. Organizing and implementing a hospital-wide first-responder automated external defibrillation program: strengthening the in-hospital chain of survival. *Resuscitation* 1995;30(2):151–156.

156. Weisfeldt ML, Griffith C, Aufderheide TP, et al. for the ROC investigators. Abstract 1810: Bystander Administered AED Shock Improves Survival from Out of Hospital Cardiac Arrest in U.S. and Canada. *Circulation* 2007;116:385–386.

157. Nichol G, Hallstrom AP, Ornato JP, et al. Potential cost-effectiveness of public access defibrillation in the United States. *Circulation* 1998;97(13):1315–1320.

158. Nichol G, Valenzuela T, Roe D, et al. Cost effectiveness of defibrillation by targeted responders in public settings. *Circulation* 2003;108(6):697–703.

159. Bardy GH, Lee KL, Mark DB, et al. HAT Investigators. Home use of automated external defibrillators for sudden cardiac arrest. *N Engl J Med* 2008;358(17):1793–1804.

Chapter 14
Ventricular Fibrillation and Defibrillation: Experimental and Clinical Experience with Waveforms and Energy

Roger D. White and Richard E. Kerber

In human studies increasing evidence supports the observation that ventricular fibrillation (VF) is very organized, consisting of large structured wavefronts with origins in one or only a few reentrant circuits rather than many simultaneously circulating reentrant circuits.[15,23–24] To terminate VF, a defibrillation shock must extinguish these circuits and at the same time not itself induce VF. The transition of biphasic waveforms from implantable cardioverters-defibrillators (ICDs) to external defibrillators constituted a significant technological advance for transthoracic defibrillation.

- Two types of VF have been reported to occur: wandering wavelets and a mother rotor with "spinoff" daughter wavelets.
- Defibrillation is dependent upon creating refractoriness in myocardial cells so that they cannot propagate fibrillation wavefronts.
- Shock efficacy has been defined and accepted as termination of VF during the 5 seconds after shock delivery. Biphasic waveform defibrillation shocks have greater efficacy in the termination of VF than monophasic shocks.
- Currently available research indicates that biphasic shock energies, regardless of waveform, for initial shocks of 120 to 200 J are safe and effective. More limited data are available on 300- to 360-J biphasic shocks because of the very high efficacy (90%) of initial shocks with lower energies.

Ventricular Fibrillation: Electrophysiologic Mechanisms

The mechanisms that initiate and sustain ventricular fibrillation (VF) are still not fully understood.[1–8] A variety of experimental models have helped define mechanisms of VF and have been reviewed in detail.[9–11] New terminology is being used along with traditional terms to describe the activation patterns that launch and sustain VF. Two types of VF have been reported to occur, type I, consisting of wandering wavelets, and type II, consisting of a mother rotor with "spinoff" daughter wavelets.[12–14] Recent observations in human VF indicate that both of these mechanisms may be operative, even in the same patient.[15] The multiple-wavelet mechanism states that VF is maintained by multiple wandering wavelets with constantly changing patterns of activation. Self-sustaining reentrant circuits are formed from these wavelets, resulting in continuing VF. Once initiated, VF can be sustained by the incessant recirculation of re-entrant activation fronts moving along randomly changing pathways at varying conduction velocities. Excitable myocardium in their path assures their survival. The unstable and fragmented activation characteristic of VF can be understood as the result of wavefronts that have been disrupted by interaction with refractory tails of other waves. As these wavefronts fracture, some may propagate unchanged until they are annihilated by random collision with other waves, whereas others can create new wavefronts. The final result would be fragmentation into multiple daughter wavelets. In this manner, the "pernicious stability" of VF can be sustained.

Another mechanism described in human hearts is the mother-rotor hypothesis recently described and illustrated.[16] This description proposes that VF is sustained by a single rapid source of excitation that cannot maintain uniform conduction throughout the myocardium; as a result, the rotor generates fibrillatory conduction with intermittent conduction block, leading to the formation of multiple patterns of irregular activation.

Re-entry can also be understood within the hypothesis of virtual electrode polarization (VEP).[17–23]

This hypothesis has been invoked to explain both successful and failed defibrillation shocks as well as the greater efficacy of biphasic shocks. VEP describes a complex global myocardial polarization characterized by the simultaneous presence of positive and negative areas of polarization adjacent to each other. In virtual electrode terminology, "negative polarization" describes repolarization (hyperpolarization) and "positive polarization" describes depolarization. Shortening of action potential duration by negative polarization is referred to as "de-excitation," which can be understood to be equivalent to repolarization. Thus, in essence, "excitation" refers to shock-induced depolarization of de-excited (repolarized) tissue. VEP is a result of redistribution of charge between neighboring areas of myocardium. Re-entry can develop because of the proximity of areas of shock-induced positive and negative polarization.

In human studies, increasing evidence supports the observation that VF is very organized, consisting of large structured wavefronts with origins in one or only a few reentrant circuits rather than many simultaneously circulating reentrant circuits.[15,24,25] To terminate VF, a defibrillation shock must extinguish these circuits and at the same time not itself induce VF. The mechanisms by which this might be achieved are discussed in the next section.

Defibrillation: Hypotheses and Electrophysiologic Mechanisms

The mechanisms by which an electric shock terminates cardiac tachyarrhythmias have not been conclusively demonstrated. Various hypotheses have been described and include the "critical mass" hypothesis and the "upper limit of vulnerability" hypothesis.[26–28] The hypotheses of "extension of refractoriness" and "virtual electrode polarization" are discussed in more detail because they provide insights into the mechanism of defibrillation with biphasic waveforms. These various hypotheses are not necessarily mutually exclusive. Some or all of them may be applicable at any one time. Also, it should be noted that these hypotheses have been derived specifically from studies of VF; their applicability to the atrial myocardium for cardioversion of atrial fibrillation (AF) is unknown. Kerber et al. have shown that more organized tachyarrhythmias, such as ventricular tachycardia and atrial flutter, require lower energy to terminate than do VF and AF. This may be because only regional depolarization in the pathway of an advancing waveform is required to terminate these arrhythmias.[29]

Defibrillation is dependent upon creating refractoriness in myocardial cells so that they cannot propagate fibrillation wavefronts. This is achieved by depolarizing the cell membrane sufficiently to trigger an action potential, which propagates throughout the membrane and to adjacent cells. Following an action potential, the cell membrane becomes absolutely refractory. As it repolarizes toward its resting potential, it becomes first relatively refractory and then fully excitable. Myofibrils are oriented at a variety of angles with respect to any electrical field (voltage gradient). Thus cell membranes vary in their susceptibility to depolarization by a local voltage gradient, in part due to the variation in the angle they subtend with respect to the electrical field. Also, some portions of the cell membrane will be oriented to the field in such a manner that depolarization will occur while other portions of the cell membrane will be repolarized.[20]

During VF, cells are unsynchronized so that some are in an absolute refractory state, some in various degrees of relative refractoriness, and some in a resting state, readily depolarized by a stimulus. All of these factors combine to create a range of responsiveness of cells to an electrical field. A monophasic shock of a given strength will depolarize some mass of myocardial cells. At sufficient strength, the vast majority of cells will be depolarized and defibrillation will be achieved. Biphasic shocks can defibrillate with local electrical fields of less intensity than can monophasic shocks—for several reasons, which are discussed in the next section. As a result, at any given intensity, a biphasic shock can depolarize a larger portion of the myocardium than can a monophasic shock of the same strength and, therefore, is more likely to defibrillate.

Most of what is known about VF and defibrillation has been derived from a wide variety of animal models. The complexity and duration of commonly present underlying structural heart disease in human VF, the typical substrate for arrhythmogenesis, makes extrapolation from these experimental studies challenging, and it must be done with caution. In long-duration VF degradation of VF amplitude, frequency, and conduction properties progressively impairs the likelihood that a defibrillation shock will restore an organized rhythm. It can be anticipated that advances in waveform design and energy delivery will increase the probability that human VF can be terminated with longer durations and various underlying myocardial substrates. Whether such advances will be translated into improved survival remains to be determined. Given the complexities of cardiac arrest and resuscitation, including multiple interventions in many events, survival as an outcome measure of defibrillation waveform performance will be difficult to confirm.

Mechanisms of Superior Efficacy of Biphasic Shocks

It is well accepted that biphasic waveform defibrillation shocks have greater efficacy in the termination of VF than monophasic shocks. This greater efficacy resides in the ability of the second phase to achieve defibrillation more easily by creating a homogeneous distribution of postshock transmembrane voltage. As pointed out above, myocytes stimulated by an extracellular electrical field are depolarized on one side and hyperpolarized on the other, depending upon

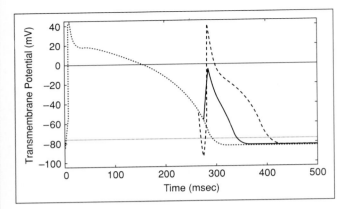

FIGURE 14-1 • Responses of a computer-generated ventricular action potential (*left dotted line*) shocked by monophasic (*solid line*) and biphasic (*dashed line*) waveforms. The hyperpolarizing first phase of the biphasic waveform shock recruits sodium channels from the inactivated state, enabling the second phase to induce an action potential with prolonged refractoriness. The extended refractoriness blocks incoming ventricular fibrillation (VF) wavefronts. (From Jones JL, Jones RE, Milner KB. Refractory period prolongation by biphasic defibrillator waveforms is associated with enhanced sodium current in a computer model of the ventricular action potential. *IEEE Trans Biomed Eng* 1994;41:60–68, with permission.)

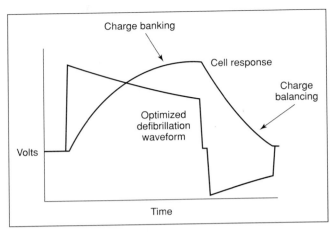

FIGURE 14-2 • Charge balancing. Depiction of a well-designed biphasic truncated exponential waveform. The first-phase duration and leading-edge voltage maximize cell membrane voltage, shown by the charge-banking curve. The second-phase duration and leading-edge voltage remove the charge on myocyte membranes, shown by the charge-balancing curve. This represents the charge-burping mechanism of defibrillation with optimally designed biphasic waveforms. (From Bain AC, Swerdlow CD, Love CJ, et al. Multicenter study of principles-based waveforms for external defibrillation. *Ann Emerg Med* 2001;37:5–12, with permission.)

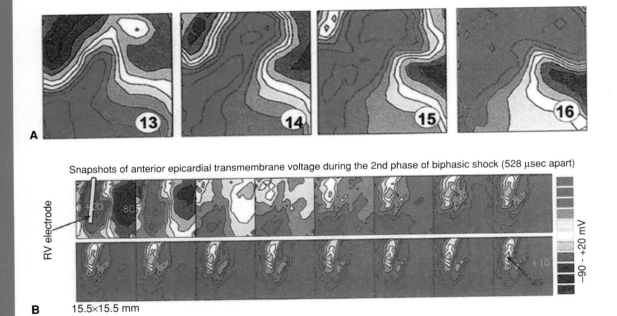

FIGURE 14-3 • Virtual electrode polarization. **A.** Isochrone maps depict transmembrane voltage at the end of a failed monophasic shock.[13–16] **B.** Changes in transmembrane voltage are shown for a successful biphasic shock. At the end of the first phase, changes in voltage are similar to those at the end of the monophasic shock. However, during the second phase, which follows, virtual electrode polarization is eliminated, shown by the progressive transition of the membrane voltage to complete depolarization. The hyperpolarized areas, shown in blue, have been eliminated as the second phase transitions the membrane voltage to depolarization, shown in red. (Adapted from Efimov IR, Cheng Y, Yamanouchi Y, et al. Direct evidence of the role of virtual electrode-induced phase singularity in success and failure of defibrillation. *J Cardiovasc Electrophysiol* 2000;11:861–868, with permission.)

their orientation to the electrical field. A monophasic shock will be successful if it is able to activate sufficient sodium current to cause depolarization of the entire cell. A biphasic shock will succeed at a lower shock strength because the activation threshold is lowered on the side of myocytes hyperpolarized by the first phase.[30] This is because the hyperpolarized side of the cell is more excitable and thus more readily activated when the polarity of the shock is reversed and the hyperpolarized membranes are depolarized (Fig. 14-1). Depolarization-induced refractoriness will abort excitation by fibrillation wavefronts.[31,32] Another benefit of biphasic pulses is removal of excess charge left on myocardial cell membranes at the end of the first phase. This has been described and referred to as charge balancing, or "charge burping"[33,34] (Fig. 14-2). The first phase of a well-designed biphasic waveform shock prepares the cell membrane for uniform depolarization by the second phase.[23,33,35] The charge-burping hypothesis states that the first phase of a biphasic shock depolarizes most of the myocytes and that the second phase removes excess charge from cells that retain such charge. Removal of residual charge on cell membranes by the second phase of a biphasic shock prevents the launch of new wavefronts, which would cause sustained VF or immediate refibrillation after a shock[33,36] (Fig. 14-3).

Introduction and Evolution of Biphasic Waveform Defibrillation Technology

In 1996, the first biphasic waveform approved for external defibrillation was incorporated into an automated external defibrillator (AED). It is an impedance-compensated biphasic truncated exponential (BTE) waveform, which delivers a fixed energy of 150 J.[37–42] Since 1996, other biphasic waveforms have been approved for clinical use, most of them utilizing a BTE design.[42] Compensation for impedance is typically achieved by extending the phasic durations and adjusting the tilt of the first phase and/or by altering the voltage of the phases.[42] Maximum total duration is limited to 20 milliseconds so as to minimize the risk of shock-induced refibrillation. Examples of BTE waveforms are shown in Figures 14-4 and 14-5. Some of these incorporate escalating energy protocols, with energy capability up to 360 J.

Another biphasic waveform is the rectilinear biphasic waveform (RBW)[43] (Fig. 14-6). This waveform maintains a relatively constant current during the first phase, based upon the rationale that it is first-phase current that primarily accounts for defibrillation. Impedance compensation is achieved by increasing the voltage applied in order to maintain delivered first-phase current as constant as possible while the phasic durations remain fixed at 6 milliseconds for the first phase and 4 milliseconds for the second phase. Because of this mechanism to achieve impedance compensa-

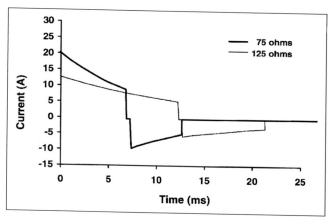

FIGURE 14-4 • Biphasic truncated exponential (BTE) waveform delivering 150 J into 75- and 125-Ω impedances. Compensation for impedance is achieved by extending the duration of the waveform while controlling tilt and limiting total duration to a maximum of 20 milliseconds. (Courtesy of Philips Healthcare, Seattle, WA.)

tion, delivered energy is typically higher than that selected (Fig. 14-7).

Yet another biphasic waveform that has been approved for clinical use in Europe and is awaiting FDA approval for use in the United States is a biphasic pulsed waveform. Chopping the waveform at high frequency is intended to achieve high shock efficacy with 150 J. There are no peer-reviewed published studies defining the performance of this waveform when applied for VF in out-of-hospital cardiac arrest. The pulsed waveform is shown in Figure 14-8.

Experimental Defibrillation Waveforms

A number of new waveforms for defibrillation have been investigated in animal models. Multipulse/multipathway encircling and overlapping shocks have been evaluated. These waveforms have been proposed in the hope of taking advantage of a well-known property of myocytes: they are directionally sensitive to their orientation to current flow. If a single myocyte is suspended in a bath, it takes 10 times as much energy to depolarize the myocyte if the current flow from electrodes placed in the bath traverses the myocyte perpendicular to its long axis compared with parallel to its long axis. Since at any given time millions of myocytes in the heart are oriented in various directions, a monophasic or biphasic shock following a single pathway through the heart will be optimally oriented to some but not all of the myocytes. The assumption underlying the use of multipulse/multipathway shocks is that the rapidly changing shock vectors will, at some point during the shock, be optimally oriented to virtually all of the myocytes, thereby depolarizing a much larger number of them. These shocks have been effective in the laboratory.[44] However, a potential drawback to the clinical use of these waveforms is that they require fairly elaborate circuitry and/or additional capacitors,

PART THREE • DEFIBRILLATION

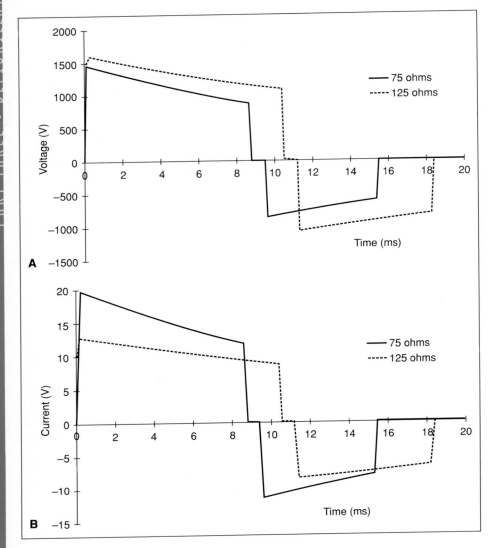

FIGURE 14-5 • Biphasic truncated exponential waveform delivering 200 J. In **(A)** voltage is plotted against time. Impedance compensation is achieved by adjusting the leading-edge voltage and extending the waveform duration. In **(B)** current is plotted against time for the same impedances. (Courtesy of Physio-Control Inc., Redmond, WA.)

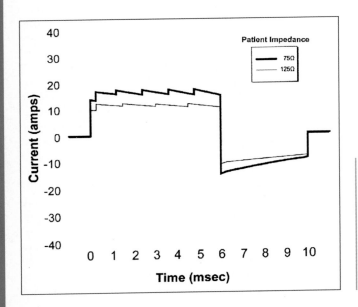

FIGURE 14-6 • The rectilinear biphasic waveform displayed with 120-J selected energy. The durations of the two phases are fixed at 6 and 4 milliseconds, respectively, despite changes in imped-ance. A relatively constant current is maintained during the first phase by means of an internal resistor network that changes the resistance in series with the patient and increases current as capacitor voltage decays. The leading-edge voltage applied to the patient increases with transthoracic impedance because the inter-nal resistance is set lower for high-impedance patients. (Courtesy of Zoll Medical Corp, Chelmsford, MA.)

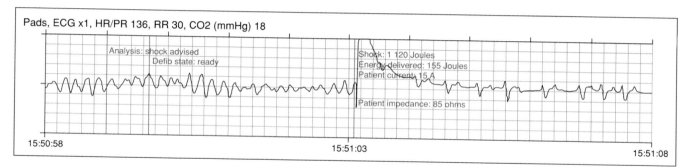

Pads, ECG x1, HR/PR 136, RR 30, CO2 (mmHg) 18

Analysis: shock advised
Defib state: ready

Shock: 1 120 Joules
Energy delivered: 155 Joules
Patient current: 15 A

Patient impedance: 85 ohms

15:50:58   15:51:03   15:51:08

FIGURE 14-7 • Example of the difference between selected and delivered energy with the rectilinear biphasic waveform shown in Figures 14-4 and 14-5. In this case 120 J was selected, and the defibrillator delivered 155 J into an impedance of 85 Ω. This increased energy delivery was derived from an increased leading-edge voltage as described in the legend for Figure 14-3. The average current during the first phase was 15 A.

thus adding weight and complexity to defibrillators, an obviously undesirable attribute. Avoiding this problem are waveforms which simply add one or two additional pulses to biphasic waveforms, resulting in triphasic or quadriphasic waveforms. These may add the advantage of the biphasic waveform already discussed without requiring additional capacitors or other components. Again, laboratory evaluation has been promising.[45] These waveforms may be particularly useful when impedance is high, such as may be encountered in a very large or emphysematous patient.[46]

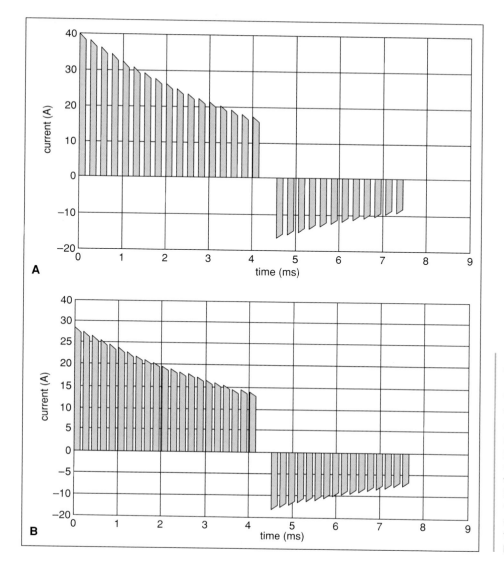

A

B

FIGURE 14-8 • The pulsed biphasic waveform. The waveform in **(A)** shows 150 J delivered into an impedance of 70 Ω. The pulses are depicted as bars with pauses between the bars. The duty cycle (pulse/pause) is 150/100 microseconds. The duration of each phase is fixed as shown, with a total duration <8 milliseconds. In **(B)** the waveform is shown delivering 150 J into a 100-Ω impedance. In this case the duty cycle is 150/50 microseconds and total waveform duration is similar to that for 70 Ω. (Courtesy of Schiller Medical, Wissembourg, France.)

None of these waveforms have yet been evaluated in clinical studies.

Clinical Experience and Recommendations

Biphasic waveforms, regardless of design and delivered energy, have largely replaced non-impedance-compensated monophasic waveforms for external defibrillation; the latter are no longer being manufactured. Despite some variation in study design and interpretation among different studies, clinical experience with several of these waveforms confirms high shock efficacy in terminating VF,[47–56] although a definitive effect from waveform on clinical outcome is still unproven. Shock efficacy has been defined and accepted as termination of VF during the 5 seconds after shock delivery.[57] This definition of shock success is based upon the observation that termination of VF occurs within 400 to 500 ms of shock delivery.[58,59] When this definition has been employed in the clinical studies cited above, termination of VF as the presenting rhythm has been reported to be in the range of 90% to 98% with BTE waveforms.[36–42] Importantly, "termination of VF" in all these studies was defined broadly, to include its conversion to asystole or an organized rhythm regardless of whether there was a return of spontaneous circulation (ROSC). One study evaluated both VF upon initial presentation of cardiac arrest and VF occurring at any time during resuscitation. For all these episodes, VF was terminated with the first rectilinear biphasic waveform shock in 67% of patients at 5 seconds.[55] In a recent randomized trial, 23% of patients presenting in VF were converted to an "organized rhythm" at 5 seconds after the first shock delivered with the rectilinear biphasic waveform.[56] However, extrapolation of the data in that study using the standard definition of shock success (that is, to include asystole or an organized rhythm) revealed that presenting VF was terminated in 73 of 86 patients (85%). Although more successful in terminating VF, no overall benefit on ROSC, survival, or neurologic recovery was observed from biphasic as compared with monophasic shock in this study.

Primary clinical endpoints, in addition to termination of VF at 5 seconds postshock, have also been used to evaluate the effectiveness of biphasic waveform defibrillation.[57,60] Return of an organized rhythm after a shock has been suggested as a more clinically meaningful measure of defibrillation shock performance than removal of VF at 5 seconds postshock.[60] However, it must be understood that postshock rhythms extending beyond the time immediately after a shock can be influenced by postshock interventions not directly related to the shock itself, most importantly resumption of chest compressions. The recommendation in the 2005 guidelines that chest compressions be resumed immediately after a shock and continued without interruption for 2 minutes complicates interpretation of the specific role of the shock per se on the postshock rhythm extending beyond the 5-second postshock period. A literal interpretation of "immediate" resumption of chest compressions after a shock might even obscure determination of the postshock rhythm at this time. Similarly, survival after cardiac arrest may be influenced by many factors other than defibrillation itself.

With these considerations in mind, there is currently no certain clinical evidence of superiority of one type of biphasic waveform over another—or, necessarily, of the superior performance of biphasic over monophasic waveform defibrillation—in altering clinical outcomes after cardiac arrest due to VF. That is, despite the growing use of biphasic waveform defibrillation, its theoretical advantages over monophasic waveform shock, and its greater success in terminating VF, this has not been regularly accompanied by reports of improved clinical outcomes. To the contrary, a recent randomized trial performed in Seattle, Washington, found that termination of VF, ROSC, admission alive to hospital, survival, and neurologic outcome from out-of-hospital cardiac arrest due to VF were not significantly improved with BTE waveforms employing escalating energy to 360 J when compared with monophasic waveforms with similar escalation.[61] Although some trends were observed favoring biphasic defibrillation in this study, relatively large numbers of patients would be required to establish their statistical significance (Fig. 14-9). Such results may reflect the difficulty of discerning a clinical benefit derived from a defibrillation waveform per se, given the complexity and multiple variables that determine patient outcome after a cardiac arrest and resuscitation, or they may suggest that such variables may minimize any theoretical advantage of a biphasic over a monophasic waveform. This issue is now largely moot in that monophasic defibrillators are no longer being manufactured, but it has practical implications in suggesting that continued use of existing monophasic waveform

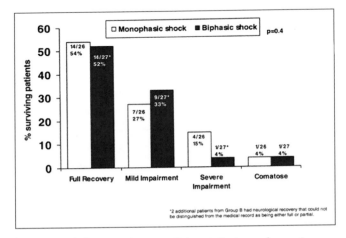

FIGURE 14-9 • Neurologic condition at discharge for survivors of after monophasic or biphasic shocks. Full recovery is CPC 1, mild impairment CPC 2, severe impairment CPC 3, and comatose CPC 4. CPC was not determined in one patient in each group. There are no significant differences between the two groups in any category of recovery. (From Kudenchuk PJ, Cobb LA, Copass MK, et al. Transthoracic incremental monophasic versus biphasic defibrillation by emergency responders [TIMBER]. *Circulation* 2006;114:2010–2018. Used with permission.)

devices is acceptable practice until replacement is required for other reasons.

Currently available research indicates that biphasic shock energies, regardless of waveform, for initial shocks of 120 to 200 J are safe and effective. More limited data are available on 300- to 360-J biphasic shocks because of the very high efficacy (90%) of initial shocks with lower energies. In one study comparing nonescalating energy (150–150–150 J) with escalating energy (200–300–360 J), it was reported that shocking with escalating energy was more effective for "secondary" shocks than shocking with fixed energy.[62] Conversion to organized rhythm and termination of VF at 5 seconds postshock were higher in patients who required additional shocks, mostly for recurrent VF, and in those who received escalating energy. All BTE shocks were delivered from a 200-μF capacitor. A commonly used 150-J BTE waveform delivers charge from a 100-μF capacitor, which results in a higher peak current.[63] Thus the observations in this study are not readily transposed to other 150-J BTE waveforms. Certainly more studies are needed to clarify these observations.

The 2005 American Heart Association Guidelines for Cardiopulmonary Resuscitation and Emergency Cardiovascular Care and the European Resuscitation Council (ILCOR) guidelines state that for the first shock using a BTE waveform of 150 to 200 J is safe and effective and that 120-J selected energy is safe and effective with the RBW, whereas 360 J is the initial recommended energy setting for monophasic defibrillation. As pointed out earlier, delivered energy with the RBW waveform is typically higher than that selected because of the mechanism of impedance compensation. If additional shocks are needed to terminate persistent VF, the same or a higher dose can be used. There is no unequivocal evidence that escalation is needed. The appropriateness of energy escalation may vary among defibrillator waveform designs, in part because of the indirect relationship between energy and defibrillation efficacy. If VF recurs after initial termination, the energy dose that terminated the VF should be used.[64,65]

While there is experimental evidence of at least transient myocardial dysfunction after high-energy shocks, there is no clinical evidence of shock-induced myocardial dysfunction in settings in which higher energies (300–360 J) have been used.[66] Of course it would be difficult to identify such shock-induced myocardial injury in a clinical setting of cardiac arrest without immediate preshock data because of the other variables that influence myocardial function during cardiac arrest and resuscitation. Certainly the trend appears to be a transition toward lower energies for defibrillation, which will render the question of clinically significant myocardial injury a nonissue.

Conclusions

The transition of biphasic waveforms from ICDs to external defibrillators constituted a significant technologic advance for transthoracic defibrillation. Impedance compensation has enabled the delivery of defibrillation current adapted to each patient and to each shock in the same patient. Optimally designed biphasic waveforms have been shown clinically to have greater efficacy than monophasic waveforms in terminating VF, and because peak current delivery is typically lower, these waveforms are less likely to be injurious to myocardial function. Advances in our understanding of the mechanisms of fibrillation and defibrillation have identified the electrophysiologic events that initiate and sustain VF and the effects of defibrillation shocks on those events. The ability of the second phase of well-designed biphasic waveforms to exploit recruited sodium channels in negatively polarized areas and thus induce rapid propagation of postshock excitation assures uniform depolarization and prevention of reentry. This appears to be the major mechanism of greater efficacy of biphasic waveforms. Translation of experimental observations to mechanisms of defibrillation in human hearts with long-standing underlying structural heart disease, which often has a multifactorial etiology, remains a major challenge. Clinical investigations are likely to be the most relevant source of additional understanding of defibrillation in the presence of underlying heart disease.

Although biphasic waveforms have largely replaced monophasic waveforms, some monophasic and various configurations of biphasic waveforms are in clinical use, including biphasic truncated exponential, rectilinear biphasic, and pulsed biphasic waveforms. All biphasic waveform devices are impedance-compensated. At this time both fixed and escalating energy protocols for biphasic shock in VF are used, employing low energy (120–200 J) or higher energy (300–360 J) with or without escalating energy protocols. Current guidelines recommend administration of monophasic shock at maximum energy (360 J) for initial therapy of VF. There is no persuasive clinical evidence indicating that any one type of biphasic waveform is clearly superior to any other; nor is there compelling evidence that currently mandates premature replacement of monophasic defibrillators with biphasic devices until required for other reasons. While there is no definite clinical evidence of shock-induced myocardial dysfunction with higher-energy shocks, there is a trend toward the utilization of lower energies with biphasic waveforms because of the very high success with low-energy defibrillation.

References

1. Ideker RE, Rogers JM. Human ventricular fibrillation: wandering wavelets, mother rotors, or both? *Circulation* 2006;114:530–532.
2. Ideker RE, Chattipakorn TN, Gray RA. Defibrillation mechanisms: the parable of the blind men and the elephant. *J Cardiovasc Electrophysiol* 2000;11:1008–1013.
3. Laurita KR. Has the chaos of ventricular fibrillation become clearer? *J Cardiovasc Electrophysiol* 2002;13:1042–1043.
4. Karagueuzian HS. Ventricular fibrillation: an organized delirium or uncoordinated reason? *Heart Rhythm* 2004;1:24–26.
5. Efimov IR. Fibrillation or neurillation: back to the future in our concepts of sudden cardiac death? *Circ Res* 2003;92:1062–1064.
6. Ideker RE, Rogers J, Huang J. Types of ventricular fibrillation: 1,2,4,5, or 3000,000? *J Cardiovasc Electrophysiol* 2004;15: 1441–1443.
7. Ideker RE, Walcott GP, Epstein AE, et al. Ventricular fibrillation and defibrillation—what are the major unresolved issues? *Heart Rhythm* 2005;2:555–558.

8. Callans DJ. Can we learn about ventricular fibrillation in man by studying animal models of defibrillation? *J Cardiovasc Electrophysiol* 2003;14:70–71.

9. Jalife J. Spatial and temporal organization in ventricular fibrillation. *Trends Cardiovasc Med* 1999;9:119–127.

10. Jalife J. Ventricular fibrillation: mechanisms of initiation and maintenance. *Annu Rev Physiol* 2000;62:25–50.

11. Samie FH, Jalife J. Mechanisms underlying ventricular tachycardia and its transition to ventricular fibrillation in the structurally normal heart. *Cardiovasc Res* 2001;50:242–250.

12. Liu YB, Pak HN, Lamp ST, et al. Coexistence of two types of ventricular fibrillation during acute regional ischemia in rabbit ventricle. *J Cardiovasc Electrophysiol* 2004;15:1433–1440.

13. Wu TJ, Lin SF, Weiss JN, et al. Two types of ventricular fibrillation in isolated rabbit hearts: importance of excitability and action potential duration restitution. *Circulation* 2002;106:1859–1866.

14. Chen PS, Wu TJ, Ting CT, et al. A tale of two fibrillations. *Circulation* 2003;108:2298–2303.

15. Nash MP, Mourad A, Clayton RH, et al. Evidence for multiple mechanisms in human ventricular fibrillation. *Circulation* 2006;114:536–542.

16. Scheinman MM, Keung E. The year in clinical electrophysiology. *J Am Coll Cardiol* 2006;47:1207–1213.

17. Efimov IR, Aguel F, Cheng Y, et al. Virtual electrode polarization in the far field: implications for external defibrillation. *Am J Physiol Heart Circ Physiol* 2000;279:H1055–H1070.

18. Efimov IR, Cheng Y, Van Wagoner DR, et al. Virtual electrode-induced phase singularity: a basic mechanism of defibrillation failure. *Circ Res* 1998;82:918–925.

19. Efimov IR, Cheng Y, Yamanouchi Y, et al. Direct evidence of the role of virtual electrode-induced phase singularity in success and failure of defibrillation. *J Cardiovasc Electrophysiol* 2000;11:861–868.

20. Efimov IR, Gray RA, Roth BJ. Virtual electrodes and deexcitation: new insights into fibrillation induction and defibrillation. *J Cardiovasc Electrophysiol* 2000;11:339–353.

21. Lindblom AE, Aguel F, Trayanova NA. Virtual electrode polarization leads to reentry in the far field. *J Cardiovasc Electrophysiol* 2001;12:946–956.

22. Cheng Y, Mowrey KA, Van Wagoner DR, et al. Virtual electrode-induced reexcitation: A mechanism of defibrillation. *Circ Res* 1999;85:1056–1066.

23. Trayanova N, Skouibine K, Moore P. Virtual electrode effects in defibrillation. *Prog Biophys Mol Biol* 1998;69:387–403.

24. Walcott GP, Kay GN, Plumb VJ, et al. Endocardial wave front organization during ventricular fibrillation in humans. *J Am Coll Cardiol* 2002;39:109–115.

25. Nanthakumar K, Walcott GP, Melnick S, et al. Epicardial organization of human ventricular fibrillation. *Heart Rhythm* 2004;1:14–23.

26. Zipes DP, Fischer J, King RM, et al. Termination of ventricular fibrillation in dogs by depolarizing a critical amount of myocardium. *Am J Cardiol* 1975;36:37–44.

27. Shibata N, Chen PS, Dixon EG, et al. Epicardial activation after unsuccessful defibrillation shocks in dogs. *Am J Physiol* 1988;255:H902–H909.

28. Ideker RE. Ventricular fibrillation: How do we put the genie back in the bottle? *Heart Rhythm* 2007;4:665–674.

29. Kerber RE, Kienzle MG, Olshansky B, et al. Ventricular tachycardia rate and morphology determine energy and current requirements for transthoracic cardioversion. *Circulation* 1992;85: 158–163.

30. Jones JL, Jones RE, Milne KB. Refractory period prolongation by biphasic defibrillator waveforms is associated with enhanced sodium current in a computer model of the ventricular action potential. *IEEE Trans Biomed Eng* 1994;41:60–68.

31. Tovar OH, Jones JL. Relationship between "extension of refractoriness" and probability of successful defibrillation. *Am J Physiol* 1997;272:H1011–H1019.

32. Jones JL, Tovar OH. Threshold reduction with biphasic defibrillator waveforms. Role of charge balance. *J Electrocardiol* 1995;28 (Suppl):25–30.

33. Bain AC, Swerdlow CD, Love CJ, et al. Multicenter study of principles-based waveforms for external defibrillation. *Ann Emerg Med* 2001;37:5–12.

34. Kroll MW. A minimal model of the single capacitor biphasic defibrillation waveform. *Pacing Clin Electrophysiol* 1994;17: 1782–1792.

35. Efimov I, Ripplinger CM. Virtual electrode hypothesis of defibrillation. *Heart Rhythm* 2006;3:1100–1102.

36. Kroll MW, Efimov IR, Tchou PJ. Present understanding of shock polarity for internal defibrillation: the obvious and non-obvious clinical implications. *Pacing Clin Electrophysiol* 2006;29:885–891.

37. White RD. Early out-of-hospital experience with an impedance-compensating low-energy biphasic waveform automatic external defibrillator. *J Intervent Cardiol Electrophysiol* 1997;1:203–208; discussion 9–10.

38. Poole JE, White RD, Kanz KG, et al. Low-energy impedance-compensating biphasic waveforms terminate ventricular fibrillation at high rates in victims of out-of-hospital cardiac arrest. LIFE investigators. *J Cardiovasc Electrophysiol* 1997;8:1373–1385.

39. Gliner BE, Jorgenson DB, Poole JE, et al. Treatment of out-of-hospital cardiac arrest with a low-energy impedance-compensating biphasic waveform automatic external defibrillator. The LIFE Investigators. *Biomed Instrum Technol* 1998;32:631–644.

40. White RD. Technologic advances and program initiatives in public access defibrillation using automated external defibrillators. *Curr Opin Crit Care* 2001;7:145–151.

41. White RD. Waveforms for defibrillation and cardioversion: recent experimental and clinical studies. *Curr Opin Crit Care* 2004;10: 202–207.

42. White RD. New concepts in transthoracic defibrillation. *Emerg Med Clin North Am* 2002;20:785–807.

43. Mittal S, Ayati S, Stein KM, et al. Comparison of a novel rectilinear biphasic waveform with a damped sine wave monophasic waveform for transthoracic ventricular defibrillation. ZOLL Investigators. *J Am Coll Cardiol* 1999;34:1595–1601.

44. Pagan-Carlo LA, Allan JJ, Spencer KT, et al. Encircling overlapping multipulse shock waveforms for transthoracic defibrillation. *J Am Coll Cardiol* 1998;32:2065–2071.

45. Zhang Y, Ramabadran RS, Boddicker KA, et al. Triphasic waveforms are superior to biphasic waveforms for transthoracic defibrillation: experimental studies. *J Am Coll Cardiol* 2003;42: 568–575.

46. Zhang Y, Rhee B, Davies LR, et al. Quadriphasic waveforms are superior to triphasic waveforms for transthoracic defibrillation in a cardiac arrest swine model with high impedance. *Resuscitation* 2006;68:251–258.

47. Higgins SL, Herre JM, Epstein AE, et al. A comparison of biphasic and monophasic shocks for external defibrillation. Physio-Control Biphasic Investigators. *Prehosp Emerg Care* 2000;4:305–313.

48. Schneider T, Martens PR, Paschen H, et al. Multicenter, randomized, controlled trial of 150-J biphasic shocks compared with 200- to 360-J monophasic shocks in the resuscitation of out-of-hospital cardiac arrest victims. Optimized Response to Cardiac Arrest (ORCA) investigators. *Circulation* 2000;102: 1780–1787.

49. Martens PR, Russell JK, Wolcke B, et al. Optimal Response to Cardiac Arrest study: defibrillation waveform effects. *Resuscitation* 2001;49:233–243.

50. White RD, Hankins DG, Atkinson EJ. Patient outcomes following defibrillation with a low energy biphasic truncated exponential waveform in out-of-hospital cardiac arrest. *Resuscitation* 2001;49:9–14.

51. Carpenter J, Rea TD, Murray JA, et al. Defibrillation waveform and post-shock rhythm in out-of-hospital ventricular fibrillation cardiac arrest. *Resuscitation* 2003;59:189–196.

52. Faddy SC, Powell J, Craig JC. Biphasic and monophasic shocks for transthoracic defibrillation: a meta analysis of randomised controlled trials. *Resuscitation* 2003;58:9–16.

53. van Alem AP, Chapman FW, Lank P, et al. A prospective, randomised and blinded comparison of first shock success of monophasic and biphasic waveforms in out-of-hospital cardiac arrest. *Resuscitation* 2003;58:17–24.

54. Walsh SJ, McClelland AJ, Owens CG, et al. Efficacy of distinct energy delivery protocols comparing two biphasic defibrillators for cardiac arrest. *Am J Cardiol* 2004;94:378–380.

55. Stothert JC, Hatcher TS, Gupton CL, et al. Rectilinear biphasic waveform defibrillation of out-of-hospital cardiac arrest. *Prehosp Emerg Care* 2004;8:388–392.

56. Gliner BE, White RD. Electrocardiographic evaluation of defibrillation shocks delivered to out-of-hospital sudden cardiac arrest patients. *Resuscitation* 1999;41:133–144.

57. Morrison LJ, Dorian P, Long J, et al. Out-of-hospital cardiac arrest rectilinear biphasic to monophasic damped sine defibrillation waveforms with advanced life support intervention trial (ORBIT). *Resuscitation* 2005;66:149–157.
58. Chen PS, Shibata N, Dixon EG, et al. Activation during ventricular defibrillation in open-chest dogs. Evidence of complete cessation and regeneration of ventricular fibrillation after unsuccessful shocks. *J Clin Invest* 1986;77:810–823.
59. Usui M, Callihan RL, Walker RG, et al. Epicardial sock mapping following monophasic and biphasic shocks of equal voltage with an endocardial lead system. *J Cardiovasc Electrophysiol* 1996;7:322–334.
60. Koster RW, Walker RG, van Alem AP. Definition of successful defibrillation. *Crit Care Med* 2006;34:S423–S426.
61. Kudenchuk PJ, Cobb LA, Copass MK, et al. Transthoracic incremental monophasic versus biphasic defibrillation by emergency responders (TIMBER): a randomized comparison of monophasic with biphasic waveform ascending energy defibrillation for the resuscitation of out-of-hospital cardiac arrest due to ventricular fibrillation. *Circulation* 2006;114:2010–2018.
62. Stiell IG, Walker RG, Nesbitt LP, et al. BIPHASIC Trial: a randomized comparison of fixed lower versus escalating higher energy levels for defibrillation in out-of-hospital cardiac arrest. *Circulation* 2007;115:1511–1517.
63. Achleitner U, Rheinberger K, Furtner B, et al. Waveform analysis of biphasic external defibrillators. *Resuscitation* 2001;50:61–70.
64. American Heart Association. Guidelines for cardiopulmonary resuscitation and emergency cardiovascular care: Part 2. Ethical issues. *Circulation* 2005;112 (Suppl IV):IV-6–IV-11.
65. European Resuscitation Council. Guidelines for resuscitation 2005. *Resuscitation* 2005;67:157–342.
66. Walcott GP, Killingsworth CR, Ideker RE. Do clinically relevant transthoracic defibrillation energies cause myocardial damage and dysfunction? *Resuscitation* 2003;59:59–70.

Airway Management in Basic and Advanced Life Support

Elizabeth H. Sinz and Kane High

The arrested circulation requires both ventilation and gas transport to sustain vital organ function while attempts are made to establish a perfusing rhythm. Thus, both ventilations and compressions are important for patients in prolonged cardiac arrest, when the oxygen stores are depleted, and for patients in asphyxial arrest, such as children and drowning patients who were hypoxemic at the time of cardiac arrest.

■ Optimizing ventilation during cardiopulmonary resuscitation (CPR)
■ Controversy regarding optimal compression-to-ventilation ratios—the science
■ Airway anatomy and lung–thorax relationships affecting ventilation

Overview

Health care providers learn to use a systematic approach to adult resuscitation based on the Basic Life Support (BLS) Primary Survey and the Advanced Cardiac Life Support (ACLS) Secondary Survey. Many of the topics in this initial assessment are organized around the A (airway) and B (breathing) components of these surveys. An organized approach to airway management is critical and monitoring of ventilation and oxygenation is mandatory.

Respiratory Physiology

Although respiration is commonly perceived as the act of breathing, respiration is more precisely defined as the provision of gas exchange at the tissue and cellular level. There are three other functional components of respiration. *Pulmonary ventilation* is the exchange of gas between the atmosphere and alveoli. The end result of pulmonary ventilation is *diffusion* of oxygen and carbon dioxide between the alveoli and blood. Circulation or *transport* of gases to and from the tissues is dependent on normal cardiovascular function. Four structural components provide the skeleton for respiration and can modify the functional components: *the central nervous system, chest bellows component, airway component, and an alveolar component.*

Acute respiratory failure results from diverse causes affecting these functional or structural components. However, the final end result is an impairment of gas exchange resulting in either low blood oxygen content (hypoxemic respiratory failure), high carbon dioxide content (hypercapnic respiratory failure), or both. Clinical management involves identification of the failure or impending failure of respiration and emergency measures to support ventilation. The cause may be obvious or can require an extensive differential diagnosis if the patient can be resuscitated or stabilized.

Oxygenation and Ventilation During CPR

The arrested circulation requires both ventilation and gas transport to sustain vital organ function while attempts are made to establish a perfusing rhythm. Thus, both ventilations and compressions are important for patients in prolonged cardiac arrest, when the oxygen stores are depleted, and for patients in asphyxial arrest, such as children and drowning patients who were hypoxemic at the time of cardiac arrest.

If the primary event is cardiac arrest, oxygen levels in the blood are normal and remain adequate for the first several minutes after cardiac arrest (Fig. 15.1). During the phase of early cardiac arrest, myocardial and cerebral oxygen

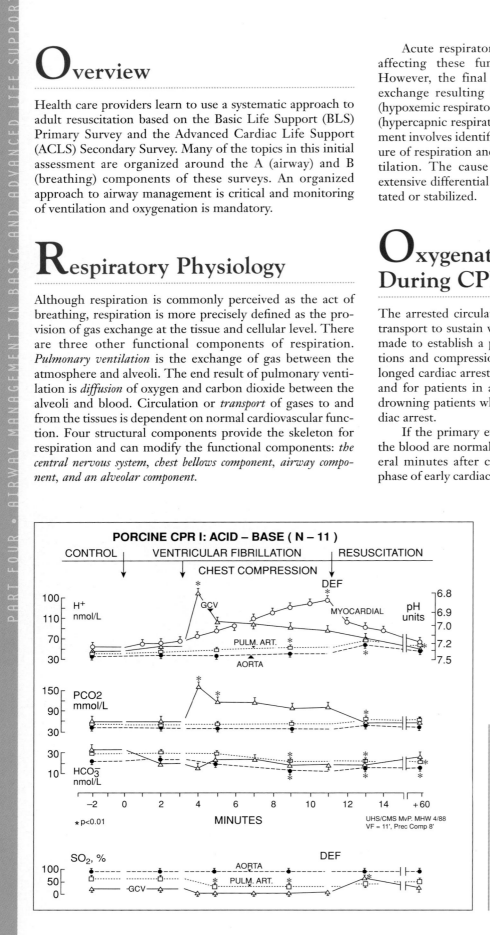

FIGURE 15-1 • Plots of mean ± SEM of intramyocardial [H+] and pH, great cardiac vein (GCV), mixed venous (PULM ART) and aortic [H+], P_{CO_2}, and $SO_2\%$ before, during, and after resuscitation from ventricular fibrillation in pigs. External chest compression was begun after 3 minutes, and spontaneous circulation was restored by defibrillation at 11 minutes. (Modified from von Planta M, Weil MH, Gazmuri RJ, et al. Myocardial acidosis associated with CO_2 production during cardiac arrest and resuscitation. *Circulation* 1989;80[3]: 684–692, with permission.)

delivery is limited more by the diminished blood flow (cardiac output) than a lack of oxygen in the lungs and blood. For these reasons, during the first minutes of ventricular fibrillation (VF) sudden cardiac arrest (SCA), rescue breaths are probably not as important as chest compressions.[1] In either situation the overall goal is return of oxygen to tissues and organs.

Important Lung–Thorax Relationships

During normal ventilation, the mechanics of ventilation are very important. Elastic forces exist in the lung and chest wall that must be overcome by the respiratory muscles. During CPR, this elasticity returns the chest wall and lungs to their resting state and must be overcome by positive-pressure ventilation to deliver oxygen and remove carbon dioxide during mechanical ventilation and CPR. The resulting airway and transpulmonary pressures have a complex relationship, but the resulting net intrathoracic pressure can significantly affect blood flow during low-flow states such as shock and CPR. In one study, incomplete chest recoil preventing return to baseline intrathoracic pressures increased intrathoracic pressure, decreased coronary perfusion pressure, and decreased cerebral perfusion pressure.[3] Increased intrathoracic pressure decreases both venous return and cardiac output. In a clinical study, about 50% of patients had incomplete chest relaxation at some point during CPR.[4] In contrast, in an experimental situation, negative intrathoracic pressure significantly improved hemodynamics, vital organ perfusion pressure, and common carotid organ flow[5] (Fig. 15-2). Whether these beneficial effects can be translated into patient survival is under current investigation.

Basic Principles of Ventilation in CPR

During CPR, blood flow to the lungs is substantially reduced, so an adequate ventilation–perfusion ratio can be maintained with lower tidal volumes and respiratory rates than normal.[6] Excessive ventilation is unnecessary and is harmful because it increases intrathoracic pressure, decreases venous return to the heart, and diminishes cardiac output and survival.[7]

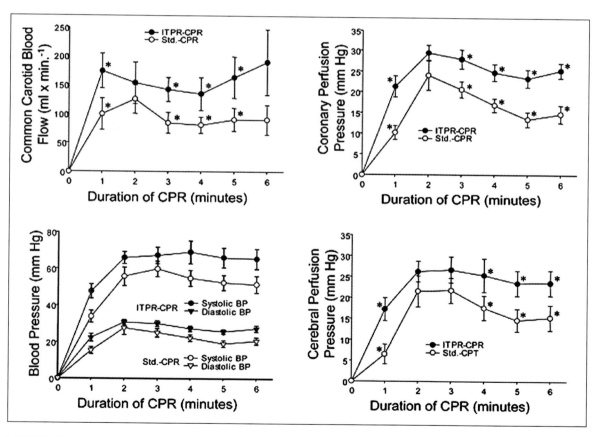

FIGURE 15-2 • Protocol 1: Mean±SEM values of common carotid blood flow coronary and cerebral perfusion pressure, and systolic (SAoP) and diastolic (DAoP) pressures with ITPR and STD-CPR during 6 minutes of CPR. *P < 0.05. C. There was statistically significant difference (0.04>P>0.0001) between 2 groups in every minute, except minute 2, in which P = 0.07. When comparison was performed with Friedman's repeated measures ANOVA of ranks, there was significant difference between ITPR-CPR and STD-CPR in all parameters shown, with P<0.001. (From Yannopoulas D, Nadkarni V, McKnite S, et al. Intrathoracic pressure regulator during continuous-chest-compression advanced cardiac resuscitation improves vital organ perfusion pressures in a porcine model of cardiac arrest. Circulation 2005;112[6]:807, with permission.)

Tidal Volumes

Studies in anesthetized adults (with normal perfusion) suggest that a tidal volume of 8 to 10 mL/kg maintains normal oxygenation and elimination of CO_2. During CPR, cardiac output is approximately 25% to 33% of normal,[8] so oxygen uptake from the lungs and CO_2 delivery to the lungs are also reduced.[9] As a result, low minute ventilation (lower than normal tidal volume and respiratory rate) can maintain effective oxygenation and ventilation during CPR.[10–13] During adult CPR, tidal volumes of approximately 500 to 600 mL (6–7 mL/kg) should be sufficient. Although a provider cannot estimate tidal volume, this guide may be useful for setting automatic transport ventilators and as a reference for manikin manufacturers. If providers generate a tidal volume sufficient to cause visible chest rise in adults, this will approximate the necessary tidal volume.

Optimizing Ventilation During CPR

Current controversy has emerged regarding the need for ventilation early in CPR and the optimal ventilation–perfusion ratio matching tidal volume and rate and cardiac output generated by chest compressions. Importantly, interruption of chest compressions decreased optimal hemodynamic parameters determining cerebral and myocardial blood flow.[1]

Ventilation Rate and Compression–Ventilation Ratio

The ideal compression–ventilation ratio to achieve an optimal ventilation–perfusion ratio during CPR has not been defined. Babbs and Kern evaluated the optimum ratio of compressions to ventilations in CPR using a mathematical model[14] (Fig. 15-3). These investigators found that guidelines overestimate the need for ventilation during standard CPR by two- to fourfold and that blood flow and oxygen delivery to the periphery can be improved by eliminating interruptions. Optimal oxygen delivery to peripheral tissues or a combination of oxygen delivery and waste product removal was determined by equations describing oxygen delivery and blood flow during CPR as functions of the number of compressions and the number of ventilations delivered over time, as developed from principles of classic physiology. For typical standard CPR variables, maximum values occurred at compression–ventilation ratios near 30:2. For variables typical of actual lay-rescuer performance in the field, maximal values occurred at compression/ventilation ratios near 60:2.

A manikin study suggests that rescuers may find a compression–ventilation ratio of 30:2 more tiring than a ratio of 15:2.[15] Further studies are needed to define the best method for coordinating chest compressions and ventilations during CPR as well as the best compression-ventilation ratio in terms of survival and neurologic outcome in patients with or without an advanced airway in place.

The updated 2005 AHA emergency cardiovascular care (ECC) guidelines recommend a compression–ventilation ratio of 30:2 and encourage further validation of this guideline. This recommendation was based on a consensus of

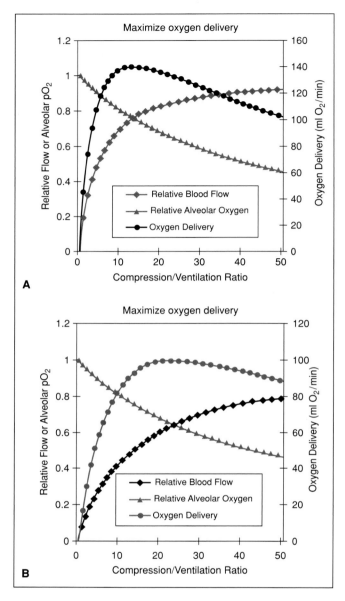

FIGURE 15-3 • Components of oxygen delivery as a function of compression–ventilation ratio in a physiologic model of cardiac arrest and CPR. **A**. Results for professionally trained rescuers, assumed to deliver two rescue breaths in 5 seconds. **B**. Results for lay rescuers, assumed to deliver two rescue breaths in 16 seconds. (From Babbs CF, Kern KB. Optimum compression to ventilation ratios in CPR under realistic, practical conditions: a physiological and mathematical analysis. *Resuscitation* 2002;54 [2]:147–157, with permission.)

experts rather than clear evidence. It is designed to increase the number of compressions, reduce the likelihood of hyperventilation, minimize interruptions in chest compressions for ventilation, and simplify instruction for teaching and skills retention.

In addition, "compression rate" refers to the *speed* of compressions, not the actual *number* of compressions delivered per minute. The actual number of chest compressions delivered per minute is determined by the rate of chest compressions and the number and duration of interruptions to open the airway, deliver rescue breaths, and allow automatic external defibrillator (AED) analysis.[14,16] However, efforts should be made to minimize these interruptions in chest compressions. In one out-of-hospital study, rescuers intermittently achieved compression rates of 100 to 121 compressions per minute, but the mean number of compressions delivered per minute was reduced to 64 compressions per minute by frequent interruptions.[17]

See Web site for AHA guidelines for cardiopulmonary resuscitation and emergency cardiovascular care—adult basic life support.

Compression-Only CPR

One possible reason for lack of bystander CPR is reluctance to perform ventilation during CPR. In surveys, health care providers[18] as well as lay-rescuers[20] were reluctant to perform mouth-to-mouth ventilation for unknown victims of cardiac arrest. The outcome of chest compressions without ventilations is significantly better than the outcome of no CPR for adult cardiac arrest.[21,22] In observational studies of adults with cardiac arrest treated by lay rescuers, survival rates were better with chest compressions only than with no CPR but were best with compressions and ventilation.[23,24] Some animal studies[1,25,26] and extrapolation from clinical evidence[22] suggest that rescue breathing is not essential during the first 5 minutes of adult CPR for VF SCA. If the airway is open, occasional gasps and passive chest recoil may provide some air exchange.[27,28] But a recent study suggests this would be inadequate when initial oxygen levels are depleted.[29] In addition, a low minute ventilation may be all that is necessary to maintain a normal ventilation–perfusion ratio during CPR.[30] As a result, current investigations continue into the optimal compression–ventilation ratio for children and adults.[31] Also, whether an initial period of no-ventilation chest compression improves outcome is the subject of several clinical studies. Laypersons should be encouraged to do compression-only CPR if they are unable or unwilling to provide rescue breaths, although the best method of CPR is compressions coordinated with ventilations.

Current AHA ECC Recommendations for Ventilation in Cardiac Arrest

See Web site for AHA scientific statement on compression only CPR and Guidelines for Ventilation in BLS (See also Chapter 11).

Functional and Clinical Anatomy of the Airway

A basic understanding of important airway structures and relationships is critical to management of related airway emergencies in ECC and SCA. An appreciation of the potential difficulties in obtaining and maintaining a patent airway is essential for optimal outcomes. Anticipation and intervention of difficult airway issues similarly can prevent or lesson complications and comorbidities in the postarrest and critical care recovery of patients.

Upper Respiratory System

The upper airway includes the nose, nasal cavity, the mouth or oral cavity, and the pharynx. The pharynx is subdivided into three regions called the nasopharynx, oropharynx, and hypopharynx (Fig. 15-4).

The nose, a framework of bones and cartilages, is composed of two parts divided by a septum. The anteromedial portion of this septum has a rich vascular supply and can be damaged during insertion of an nasopharyngeal airway or nasotracheal intubation. This blood supply is located in Little's area of the anteromedial aspect of the nasal septum. The arterial supply from several arteries, called Kiesselbach's plexus, originates ultimately from the carotid artery; bleeding from this area can be brisk and become a serious problem.

The nasal cavities open into the nasopharynx. The lower border is the soft palate. This is clinically important during insertion of a nasotracheal tube. The posterior portion of this area contains a depression that may hinder advancement of the tube. If not recognized, the use of force applied at this point causes perforation of the mucosa and submucosal dissection.

The mouth or oral cavity extends from the lips to the oropharynx, comprising the lips, cheeks, and hard and soft palates. There is a potential space in the hollow of the mandible below the floor of the oral cavity. It is into this space that the tongue is largely displaced during laryngoscopy and endotracheal intubation. Variations and distortion of the oral cavity can make visualization of structures and insertion of an endotracheal tube difficult.

The mouth opens into the oropharynx, a muscular tube, comprising skeletal musculature with a basal resting tone. Loss of basal tone or impairment by sedatives can cause obstruction of the upper airway. Obstruction of the oropharynx by posterior displacement of the tongue is the most common cause of upper airway obstruction.

Larynx

Below the oropharynx is the hypopharynx or laryngopharynx. The larynx extends from an opening in the hypopharynx bordered by the aryepiglottic folds, tip of the epiglottis,

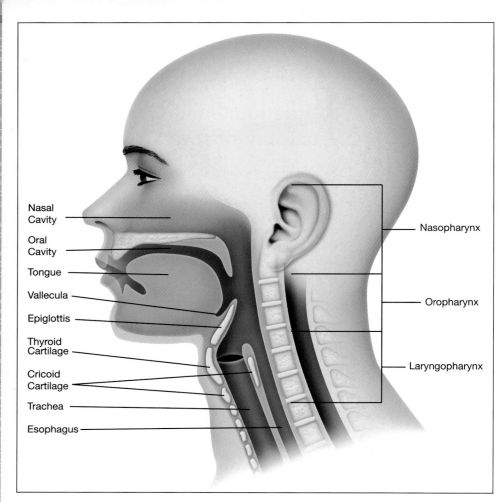

Nasal Cavity

Oral Cavity

Tongue

Vallecula

Epiglottis

Thyroid Cartilage

Cricoid Cartilage

Trachea

Esophagus

Nasopharynx

Oropharynx

Laryngopharynx

FIGURE 15-4 • Clinical and functional structures of the upper airway. These structures include the nose, nasal cavity, mouth or oral cavity, and the pharynx subdivided into the nasopharynx, oropharynx, and hypopharynx (see text).

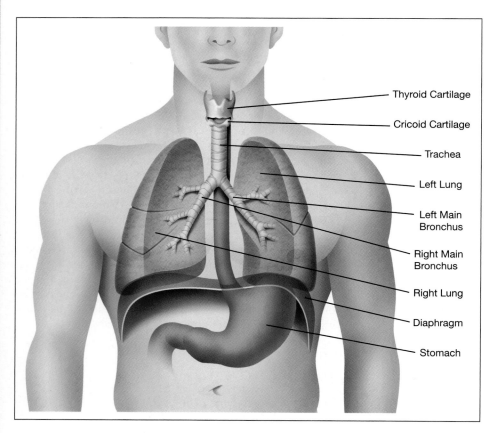

Thyroid Cartilage

Cricoid Cartilage

Trachea

Left Lung

Left Main Bronchus

Right Main Bronchus

Right Lung

Diaphragm

Stomach

FIGURE 15-5 • The respiratory system.

and the posterior commissure between the arytenoid carti-lages. The larynx is in essence a box formed by nine carti-lages (three single and three pairs). The thyroid cartilage is anterior. The arytenoid, corniculate, and cuneiform carti-lages are posterior. The epiglottal cartilage is the top of the box. The cricoid cartilage (Greek *cricos*, meaning "ring") is in the shape of a signet ring with the signet portion poste-rior, forming part of the back and lower bottom of the box. The arytenoid (Greek, meaning "pitcher") cartilages bear a resemblance when they are approximated to the lip of a pitcher. Important structures to recognize include the thy-roid and cricothyroid cartilages, the cricothyroid mem-brane, and the vocal cords (Figs. 15-5 and 15-6). The larynx is the most heavily innervated sensory structure in humans.

Stimulation of the larynx causes significant sympathetic response.

Thyroid and Cricoid Cartilages

The first and second cartilages of the larynx are the thyroid and cricoid cartilage, respectively. Between these two struc-tures anteriorly is the cricothyroid membrane (Fig. 15-6A and B).

The thyroid cartilage is the largest and has a subcuta-neous anterior projection called the *pomum Adami*, or Adam's apple, and is more prominent in men than in women. The cricothyroid membrane extends between from the lower bor-der of the thyroid cartilage to the upper border of the cricoid

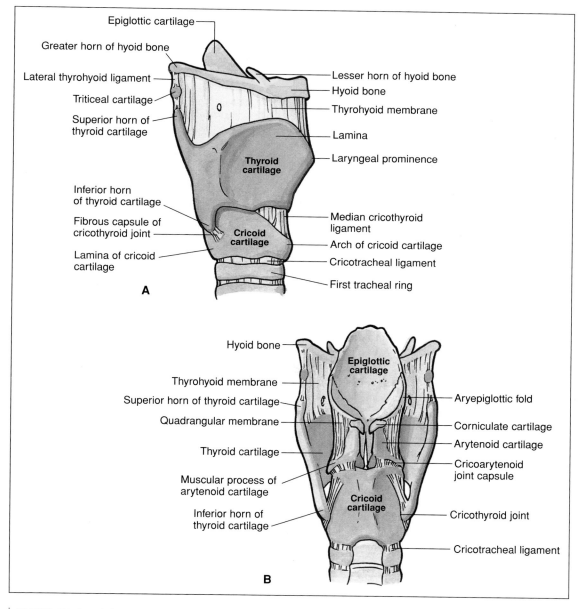

FIGURE 15-6 • Skeleton of the larynx and associated ligaments and membranes. **A.** Right lateral view. **B.** Posterior view. (From Moore K L, Agur AM. *Essential Clinical Anatomy*, 2nd ed. Philadelphia: Lippincott Williams & Wilkins, 2003, with permission.)

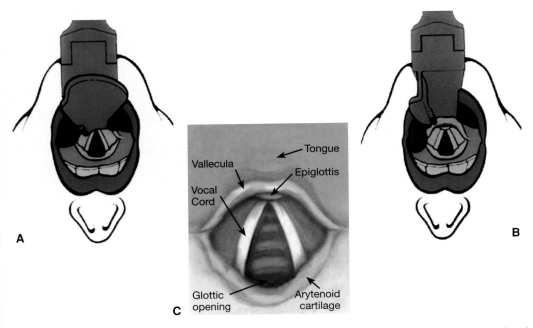

FIGURE 15-7 • Visualization of vocal cords. **A.** View of vocal cords with straight-blade laryngoscope (epiglottis is covered by straight blade and not visible). **B.** View of the vocal cords with curved-blade laryngoscope (epiglottis is visible). **C.** Anatomy.

cartilage. The cricothyroid membrane is also generally located higher in the neck in women than in men. Locating these structures can be critical in an airway emergency.

Glottic Opening and Vocal Cords

The glottic opening and vocal cords are important clinical landmarks to be identified during endotracheal intubation. Figure 15-7 shows the larynx as visualized from the oropharynx. In Figure 15-7A, the straight blade of a laryngoscope has been placed in front of the tip of the epiglottis and displaces it anteriorly so that it is hidden by the blade. In Figure 15-7B, the tip of a curved blade has been placed in the vallecula and pressure on the median glossoepiglottic fold displaces the epiglottis anteriorly, exposing the vocal cords. Depressions between the median and lateral epiglottic folds are called *valleculae*, meaning crevices or depressions.

Lower Respiratory System

The lower respiratory system extends from the larynx to the parenchyma of the lung and is composed of the trachea, bronchi, alveoli, and chest wall (Fig. 15-5).

References

1. Kern KB, Hilwig RW, Berg RA, et al. Importance of continuous chest compressions during cardiopulmonary resuscitation: improved outcome during a simulated single lay-rescuer scenario. *Circulation* 2002;105(5):645–649.
2. von Planta M, Weil MH, Gazmuri RJ, et al. Myocardial acidosis associated with CO_2 production during cardiac arrest and resuscitation. *Circulation* 1989;80(3):684–692.
3. Yannopoulos D, McKnite S, Aufderheide TP, et al. Effects of incomplete chest wall decompression during cardiopulmonary resuscitation on coronary and cerebral perfusion pressures in a porcine model of cardiac arrest. *Resuscitation* 2005;64(3):363–372.
4. Aufderheide TP, Pirrallo RG, Yannopoulos D, et al. Incomplete chest wall decompression: A clinical evaluation of CPR performance by trained laypersons and an assessment of alternative manual chest compression–decompression techniques. *Resuscitation* 2006; 71(3):341–351.
5. Yannopoulos D, Aufderheide TP, McKnite S, et al. Hemodynamic and respiratory effects of negative tracheal pressure during CPR in pigs. *Resuscitation* 2006;69(3):487–494.
6. Baskett P, Nolan J, Parr M. Tidal volumes which are perceived to be adequate for resuscitation. *Resuscitation* 1996;31(3):231–234.
7. Aufderheide TP, Sigurdsson G, Pirrallo RG, et al. Hyperventilation-induced hypotension during cardiopulmonary resuscitation. *Circulation* 2004;109(16):1960–1965.
8. Paradis NA, Martin GB, Goetting MG, et al. Simultaneous aortic, jugular bulb, and right atrial pressures during cardiopulmonary resuscitation in humans. Insights into mechanisms. *Circulation* 1989;80(2):361–368.
9. Idris AH, Staples ED, O'Brien DJ, et al. Effect of ventilation on acid–base balance and oxygenation in low blood-flow states. *Crit Care Med* 1994;22(11):1827–1834.
10. Idris A, Wenzel V, Banner MJ, et al. Smaller tidal volumes minimize gastric inflation during CPR with an unprotected airway. *Circulation* 1995;92(Suppl):I-759.
11. Idris A, Gabrielli A, Caruso L. Smaller tidal volume is safe and effective for bag-valve-ventilation, but not for mouth-to-mouth ventilation: an animal model for basic life support. *Circulation* 1999;100(Suppl I):I-644.
12. Dorph E, Wik L, Steen PA. Arterial blood gases with 700 ml tidal volumes during out-of-hospital CPR. *Resuscitation* 2004;61(1): 23–27.
13. Winkler M, Mauritz W, Hackl W, et al. Effects of half the tidal volume during cardiopulmonary resuscitation on acid–base balance and haemodynamics in pigs. *Eur J Emerg Med* 1998;5(2):201–206.

14. Babbs CF, Kern KB. Optimum compression to ventilation ratios in CPR under realistic, practical conditions: a physiological and mathematical analysis. *Resuscitation* 2002;54(2):147–157.
15. Greingor JL. Quality of cardiac massage with ratio compression–ventilation 5/1 and 15/2. *Resuscitation* 2002;55(3):263–267.
16. Kern KB, Hilwig RW, Berg RA, et al. Efficacy of chest compression-only BLS CPR in the presence of an occluded airway. *Resuscitation* 1998;39(3):179–188.
17. Wik L, Kramer-Johansen J, Myklebust H, et al. Quality of cardiopulmonary resuscitation during out-of-hospital cardiac arrest. *JAMA* 2005;293(3):299–304.
18. Ornato JP, Hallagan LF, McMahan SB, et al. Attitudes of BCLS instructors about mouth-to-mouth resuscitation during the AIDS epidemic. *Ann Emerg Med* 1990;19(2):151–156.
19. Brenner BE, Van DC, Cheng D, et al. Determinants of reluctance to perform CPR among residents and applicants: the impact of experience on helping behavior. *Resuscitation* 1997;35(3):203–211.
20. Hew P, Brenner B, Kaufman J. Reluctance of paramedics and emergency medical technicians to perform mouth-to-mouth resuscitation. *J Emerg Med* 1997;15(3):279–284.
21. Berg RA, Kern KB, Sanders AB, et al. Bystander cardiopulmonary resuscitation. Is ventilation necessary? *Circulation* 1993;88(pt 1)(4):1907–1915.
22. Hallstrom AP. Dispatcher-assisted "phone" cardiopulmonary resuscitation by chest compression alone or with mouth-to-mouth ventilation. *Crit Care Med* 2000;28(11 Suppl):N190–N192.
23. Waalewijn RA, Tijssen JG, Koster RW. Bystander initiated actions in out-of-hospital cardiopulmonary resuscitation: results from the Amsterdam Resuscitation Study (ARRESUST). *Resuscitation* 2001;50(3):273–279.
24. Van Hoeyweghen RJ, Bossaert LL, Mullie A, et al. Quality and efficiency of bystander CPR. Belgian Cerebral Resuscitation Study Group. *Resuscitation* 1993;26(1):47–52.
25. Chandra NC, Gruben KG, Tsitlik JE, et al. Observations of ventilation during resuscitation in a canine model. *Circulation* 1994;90(6):3070–3075.
26. Tang W, Weil MH, Sun S, et al. Cardiopulmonary resuscitation by precordial compression but without mechanical ventilation. *Am J Respir Crit Care Med* 1994;150(6 pt 1):1709–1713.
27. Berg RA, Kern KB, Hilwig RW, et al. Assisted ventilation does not improve outcome in a porcine model of single-rescuer bystander cardiopulmonary resuscitation. *Circulation* 1997;95(6):1635–1641.
28. Berg RA, Kern KB, Hilwig RW, et al. Assisted ventilation during 'bystander' CPR in a swine acute myocardial infarction model does not improve outcome. *Circulation* 1997;96(12):4364–4371.
29. Deakin CD, O'Neill JF, Tabor T. Does compression-only cardiopulmonary resuscitation generate adequate passive ventilation during cardiac arrest? *Resuscitation* 2007;75(1):53–59.
30. Weil MH, Rackow EC, Trevino R, et al. Difference in acid–base state between venous and arterial blood during cardiopulmonary resuscitation. *N Engl J Med* 1986;315(3):153–156.
31. Koster RW, Deakin CD, Bottiger BW, et al. Chest-compression-only or full cardiopulmonary resuscitation? *Lancet* 2007;369(9577):1924; author reply 1925.

Chapter 16
Monitoring and Maintaining a Patent Airway

Elizabeth H. Sinz and Kane High

The major general objectives of respiratory support in emergency cardiovascular care (ECC) are to provide a patent airway and adequate oxygenation and ventilation. These objectives require prioritization according to patient condition and potential precipitating cause.

- Assessing the need for oxygenation and ventilation
- Determinants of adequate respiration at the cellular level
- Pearls and pitfalls of oximetry and capnometry

Principles of Oxygenation and Ventilation

The major general objectives of respiratory support in ECC are to provide a patent airway and adequate oxygenation and ventilation. These objectives require prioritization according to patient condition and potential precipitating cause. The major objectives of respiratory support can be organized into initial primary, or basic life support (BLS), priorities and secondary, or advanced cardiac life support (ACLS), priorities. Methods of maintaining the airway and administering oxygen are predicated upon clinical circumstances and may change with time; therefore, serial repeated evaluation of the airway and patient is critical.

The objectives of airway intervention and assessment are as follows:

BLS Primary A—Airway
- Ensure a patent and protected airway; use manual techniques as needed.
- Ensure a patent and protected airway; use simple, noninvasive airway adjuncts as needed.

BLS Primary B—Breathing
- Provide supplementary oxygen.
- Monitor the quality of oxygenation and ventilation with noninvasive devices.
- Provide positive-pressure oxygenation and ventilation with manual techniques or noninvasive airway devices when spontaneous breathing is inadequate or absent.

ACLS Secondary A—Airway
- Establish a patent and protected airway with invasive advanced airway devices.
- Confirm proper placement of these devices with both clinical and device confirmation techniques.

ACLS Secondary B—Breathing
- Provide effective positive-pressure oxygenation and ventilation through properly inserted advanced airway devices.
- Secure the advanced airway devices to prevent displacement.
- Monitor oxygenation and ventilation and tailor support as needed.

Cardiac or Respiratory Arrest?

Professional as well as lay-rescuers may be unable to accurately determine the presence or absence of adequate or normal breathing in unresponsive patients[32–34] because the airway is not open[35] or the patient has occasional agonal gasps, which can occur in the first minutes after SCA and may be confused with adequate breathing. Agonal gasps are not effective breaths.[29] The patient who has agonal gasps should be treated as if he or she were not breathing by giving rescue breaths. CPR training should emphasize how to recognize agonal gasps and should instruct rescuers to give rescue breaths and proceed with the steps of CPR when the unresponsive patient demonstrates agonal gasps.

Initial Airway Sequence to Determine Adequate Breathing

Health care providers should quickly determine if the patient demonstrates spontaneous breathing efforts.

- Is the patient making spontaneous breathing efforts?
- Do these efforts appear adequate?
- Can you feel the patient exhale into your hand?
- If the efforts are inadequate, are the inadequate efforts caused by fatigue or one of the many causes of respiratory depression?

- If the patient is making spontaneous breathing efforts, is there evidence of partial or complete upper airway obstruction caused by foreign material such as food, vomitus, or blood clots, or posterior displacement of the tongue or epiglottis?
- If spontaneous breathing is absent or inadequate, provide positive-pressure ventilation with one of the following ventilation techniques described in this chapter:
  - –Mouth-to-mouth
  - –Mouth-to-mask
  - –Ventilation with a bag through a face mask, endotracheal tube, esophageal–tracheal Combitube, or laryngeal mask airway (LMA).

Clues to the Presence of Airway Obstruction

Significant partial upper airway obstruction typically causes noisy airflow during inspiration (stridor or "crowing") and cyanosis (late sign). Another sign of airway obstruction is use of accessory muscles, indicated by retractions of the suprasternal, supraclavicular, and intercostal spaces. Complete airway obstruction results in patient efforts at breathing against a closed airway this typically causes a rocking or "see-saw" motion of the chest and abdomen as the diaphragm moves into the abdomen, pushing the abdomen upward and the chest collapses in the absence of airflow to fill the lungs. If the patient is not making spontaneous breathing efforts, airway obstruction becomes more difficult to recognize and must be determined during attempts to provide positive-pressure ventilation. Occasionally, isolated bradycardia, secondary to occult hypoxemia, provides an early sign of airway obstruction. It is important to recognize the presence of airway obstruction caused by the tongue and epiglottis, as this is common in the unconscious patient due to loss of muscle tone.

Assessing the Need for Supplementary Oxygen and Ventilation

Health-care providers must be able to accurately assess *oxygenation* and *ventilation* to detect and treat respiratory distress and failure. Clinical parameters form the cornerstone of initial assessment and intervention. Frequently, pulse oximetry and capnography provide useful supplemental and continuous information. The two major functions of respiration are to achieve and maintain:

- Oxygenation (oxygenate arterial blood)
  - –Evaluate oxygenation with pulse oximetry
- Ventilation (remove carbon dioxide from venous blood)
  - –Evaluate ventilation with capnography

Oximetry: Basic Principles

To understand the clinical utility of oximetry—as well as its limitations and pitfalls—one must understand the physics involved in measurement and the clinical principles of adequate tissue oxygenation. Here too, "treat the patient and not the number" is most important.

Basic Physics of Pulse Oximetry

The concentration of a substance in a fluid can be determined by its ability to transmit light. Oxygenated hemoglobin absorbs and reflects red and infrared light differently than nonoxygenated hemoglobin. Oxygenated hemoglobin primarily absorbs *infrared* light; reduced (nonoxygenated) hemoglobin primarily absorbs *red* light. In pulse oximetry, red and infrared light are passed through a pulsatile tissue bed, and a photodetector captures any nonabsorbed light on the other side of the tissue bed. A microprocessor calculates the relative absorption of red and infrared light that occurred as it passed through the tissue bed and can determine the percentage of oxygenated and nonoxygenated hemoglobin present in that tissue bed. In this way the pulse oximeters calculate the *percent of hemoglobin that is saturated with oxygen (percent saturation, percent SO2; percent SaO2)*. In the absence of abnormal hemoglobins, such as carboxyhemoglobin or methemoglobin, if the arterial oxygen saturation is greater than 70%, there should be no more than 3% variance between pulse oximetry and the arterial oxyhemoglobin saturation measured by co-oximeter used in arterial blood gas determinations. Studies have shown pulse oximetry to be an accurate and useful guide for patient care in the in-hospital setting as well as in the prehospital EMS setting,[36–39] including transport by rotary-wing aircraft.[40]

Hemoglobin and Tissue Oxygen Delivery

Analysis of arterial blood is an invasive procedure, and arterial blood gases are infrequently ordered, available, or clinically useful during cardiac arrest. *Pulse oximetry* was developed to provide a noninvasive, painless approximation of the percent of hemoglobin saturated with oxygen, usually designated as SpO_2 to distinguish it from the value measured by co-oximetry of an arterial blood sample (SaO_2). In cardiac arrest, the pulse oximeter will not function well because there must be pulsatile blood flow through the tissue where the light measurements are being made to obtain an accurate measurement although a reading may appear with adequate chest compressions. But pulse oximetry is commonly used for monitoring patients who are not in arrest, because it provides a simple, continuous method of tracking oxyhemoglobin saturation. There are three major determinants of adequate tissue oxygenation:

1. There must be an adequate amount of oxygen to saturate the hemoglobin molecules.
2. There must be enough hemoglobin to carry adequate oxygen.
3. Cardiac output must be sufficient to deliver the saturated hemoglobin to peripheral tissues.

Arterial oxygen content is determined by the hemoglobin concentration and its saturation with oxygen. Normal pulse oximetry saturation, however, does not ensure adequate systemic *oxygen delivery* because it does not calculate the total oxygen content (O_2 bound to hemoglobin + dissolved O_2) *and* adequacy of blood flow (cardiac output):

Arterial oxygen content (mL of oxygen per dL of blood)
= Hemoglobin concentration (g/dL)
× 1.34 (mL oxygen/g hemoglobin)
× Oxyhemoglobin saturation
+ (PaO_2 × 0.003)

(normal oxygen content = 18-20 ml/dL)

Measurement of the oxygen content is only part of the determination of effective oxygenation. The oxygen present must be delivered to the tissues for use. Peripheral cells must be able to uptake and use oxygen for cellular metabolism. Oxygen delivery is defined by how much oxygen is present and how much of it is delivered to the body. Oxygen delivery is defined by the following equation:

Oxygen delivery (mL of oxygen/min)
= arterial oxygen content (mL oxygen/dL blood)
× cardiac output (L/min)
(× 10 dL/L)

Pulse Oximetry Precautions and Limitations

Pulse oximetry readings, even those that are accurate, do not necessarily correlate with cardiac output and oxygen delivery. In clinically evaluating a patient's cardiac output and oxygen delivery, always assess systemic perfusion and be aware of the hemoglobin concentration. If cardiac output or hemoglobin concentration is low, oxygen delivery can be inadequate even if oxyhemoglobin saturation is normal.

Abnormal Hemoglobins (e.g., Carbon Dioxide Poisoning)

The light absorption of carboxyhemoglobin (carbon monoxide) and of methemoglobin (nitrates or aromatic amines) differs from that of normal hemoglobin, so carboxyhemoglobin and methemoglobin are *not* recognized by pulse oximeters. If these altered forms of hemoglobin are present, the SaO_2 calculated by the pulse oximeters will be falsely high because most pulse oximeters calculate the percent of normal hemoglobin that is saturated with oxygen rather than the percent of *total* hemoglobin that is saturated with oxygen. When you suspect the presence of carbon monoxide poisoning or methemoglobin toxicity, you should measure the oxyhemoglobin saturation with a co-oximeter (this requires arterial blood sampling).

Abnormal Conditions Affecting Pulse Oximetry

In several clinical situations, abnormal or inaccurate oximetry readings may occur. In a large review of pulse oximeter devices, the major sources of error were finger thickness, hemoglobin level, skin color, and peripheral temperature.

- Motion artifact and low perfusion are the most common sources of SpO_2 inaccuracies. Motion artifacts can occur with patient transport, movement, twitching, and agitation.

ACCURACY OF PULSE OXIMETERS IN THE PRESENCE OF CARBOXYHEMOGLOBINEMIA AND METHEMOGLOBINEMIA

Most commercially available pulse oximeters use two light-emitting diodes and a photodetector in a sensor. The two diodes emit a red and an infrared light. Oxygenated hemoglobin in the pulsatile tissue bed primarily absorbs infrared light, but reduced (nonoxygenated) hemoglobin in the pulsatile tissue bed primarily absorbs red light. A microprocessor in the unit determines the relative absorption of red and infrared light to calculate the percentage of oxygenated versus reduced (nonoxygenated) hemoglobin present in the tissue bed.

The light absorption of methemoglobin and carboxyhemoglobin is different from that of normal hemoglobin, so pulse oximeters will not accurately reflect total hemoglobin saturation in the presence of these two products.[41] With significant methemoglobinemia, pulse oximeters display an oxygen saturation of approximately 85%. With significant carboxyhemoglobinemia (as occurs in carbon monoxide poisoning), the pulse oximeter will typically reflect the oxygen saturation of *normal* hemoglobin, not the percentage of hemoglobin bound to carbon monoxide. If these or other conditions affecting oxyhemoglobin saturation are present, arterial hemoglobin oxygen saturation must be determined by using co-oximetry.

- When the systolic blood pressure is low, oximetry becomes inaccurate because of decreased pulsatile flow, response time, or calibration characteristics of the instrument. Oximetry may also read falsely high when the SaO_2 is <70% or may become inaccurate when the hemoglobin level is very low (2–3 g/dL).
- Peripheral hypoperfusion from hypothermia, low cardiac output, or vasoconstrictive drugs may cause or increase inaccuracies.
- Very dark skin, fingernail polish, and fungal infections of the nails (onychomycosis) may cause spurious readings when digital monitors are used.

Safety Considerations

There are some safety precautions regarding use of the pulse oximetry equipment:

- Do not use oximetry probes with broken or cracked casings. Burns have been reported when the lights from the probes come into direct contact with the skin.
- Do not connect the probes from one manufacturer to base units made by another manufacturer.

Capnography and Capnometry

Detection of exhaled CO_2 is one of several independent methods of confirming endotracheal tube position. Given the simplicity of the exhaled CO_2 detector (waveform, colorimetry, or digital), it can be used as the initial method for detecting correct tube placement even in the patient in cardiac arrest. Detection of exhaled CO_2, however, is not infallible as a means of confirming tube placement, particularly during cardiac arrest. Evidence from a meta-analysis in adults[42] indicated a range of results:

- Positive predictive value (probability of endotracheal placement if CO_2 is detected): 100%
- Negative predictive value (probability of esophageal placement if no CO_2 is detected): 20% to 100%

Therefore, exhaled carbon dioxide almost certainly indicates that ventilation of the lungs is occuring; however absence of exhaled carbon dioxide may be due to esophageal intubation or to cardic arrest with no pefusion of the lungs. The use of CO_2 detecting devices to determine the correct placement of other advanced airways (e.g., Combitube, LMA) has not been adequately studied.

Basic Principles

The body eliminates carbon dioxide through *ventilation*. When blood passes through the lungs, carbon dioxide moves from the blood, across the alveolar capillary membrane into the alveoli and then into the airways and is exhaled. Alveolar P_{CO_2} should be approximately equal to pulmonary venous, left atrial and arterial P_{CO_2}. If there is a good match of ventilation and perfusion in the lungs and there is no airway obstruction, exhaled CO_2 should correlate well with arterial P_{CO_2}, and exhaled carbon dioxide can be used to estimate arterial carbon dioxide tension. Carbon dioxide can be detected by either of two techniques:

- *Capnometry* is a *qualitative* method that detects the presence of CO_2 in exhaled air. *Colorimetric* capnometers are semiquantitative devices based on a chemical reaction between exhaled CO_2 and a chemical detector impregnated in a strip of paper. These devices are used to identify the presence or absence of a sufficient quantity of CO_2 to produce a color change at a point in time.
- *Capnography* devices are *quantitative* devices that measure the concentration of CO_2 using infrared absorption detectors. Carbon dioxide concentration is typically displayed by these devices as a continuous exhaled CO_2 concentration waveform with a digital display of end-tidal CO_2. This plot of CO_2 concentration against time is called a capnograph.

Capnometry

A CO_2 concentration of >2% will react with the chemical reagent in a colorimetric CO_2 detector and change the color (Fig. 18-1). If the endotracheal tube is actually in the trachea, the CO_2 detector will turn a color determined by the manufacturer. In the *absence* of expired CO_2, the color of the colorimetric indicator will remain unchanged. Health care providers commonly use this color change with a disposable device as a quick check to provide one method of device confirmation of the success or failure of endotracheal intubation.[43]

COLOR CHANGE WITH COLORIMETRIC DEVICE: KNOW YOUR DEVICE

The 2000 Guidelines for Advanced Cardiovascular Life Support (ACLS) and Pediatric Advanced Life Support (PALS) as well as associated training materials offer examples of how colorimetric CO_2 detection devices work and suggest mnemonic schemes for interpretation. Those details were meant to help providers remember the significance of specific colors indicating the relative concentration of CO_2 present in the expired air. Some of the materials, for example, link the color purple with a sign of low CO_2 and yellow with high CO_2. New devices have been introduced on the market with new indicators and color schemes. The indicators in some commercially available devices respond to detection of increasing CO_2 concentration by transitioning in color using one of the following schemes:

- Purple-to-yellow
- Blue-to-yellow
- White-to-purple

Even more possibilities will likely appear on the market in the coming years. Clearly, any one mnemonic that relies on color will not fit all available devices.

The product inserts for some commercially available semiqualitative colorimetric capnometers recommend that after intubation, six positive-pressure breaths be provided by hand or mechanical ventilation before attempting to identify exhaled CO_2. Six breaths will wash out any CO_2 that is present in the stomach or esophagus from bag-mask ventilation. Any CO_2 detected after six breaths can be presumed to be from the lungs.[44,45] There is no need to continue ventilation attempts if the endotracheal tube is clearly misplaced.

In patients who weigh >2 kg with a perfusing rhythm (not in cardiac arrest), the sensitivity and specificity of colorimetric capnometry methods approaches 100% if six ventilations have been provided following intubation. This means that if the endotracheal tube is in the trachea of a patient with a perfusing rhythm, the colorimetric device will change color with few exceptions (see "False-Positive Results," below). If the tube is in the esophagus, there should be no CO_2 detected after six breaths, so a colorimetric CO_2 detector should remain unchanged.

False-Positive Results   When exhaled CO_2 is detected (positive reading for CO_2) in cardiac arrest, it is usually a reliable indicator of tube position in the trachea. False-positive readings (CO_2 is detected but the tube is located in the esophagus) have been observed in animals that ingested large amounts of carbonated liquids before the arrest.[44]

A color change is generally a reliable indicator of the presence of CO_2 and endotracheal intubation. False-positive color changes are uncommon but can occur when the tip of the tube is in the supraglottic area rather than in the trachea. A false-positive may also be possible following prolonged bag-mask ventilation,[8–10] which is why some manufacturers recommend that six ventilations be provided after intubation and before the check for exhaled CO_2. Finally, if the colorimetric detector is contaminated with acidic gastric contents or acidic drugs, such as endotracheal administration of epinephrine, a colorimetric detector may remain unchanged during the entire respiratory cycle.

False-Negative Results   *False-negative* results occur if the tube is in the trachea but the colorimetric indicator remains unchanged. A false-negative result is most often associated with cardiac arrest (see below). False-negative results may also occur with severe airway obstruction or pulmonary edema, which can impair CO_2 elimination so that inadequate CO_2 is detected in exhaled gas. Administration of an intravenous (IV) bolus of epinephrine in patients with cardiac arrest or very low cardiac output may transiently reduce pulmonary blood flow and reduce exhaled CO_2.[46]

False-negative readings (in this context defined as failure to detect CO_2 despite tube placement in the trachea) may be present during cardiac arrest for several reasons. The most common explanation for false-negative readings during CPR is that blood flow and delivery of CO_2 to the lungs are low. False-negative results have also been reported in association with pulmonary embolus because pulmonary blood flow is reduced. In addition, elimination and detection of CO_2 can be drastically reduced with severe airway obstruction (e.g., status asthmaticus) and pulmonary edema.[47] For these reasons, if CO_2 is not detected, the AHA 2005 guidelines recommend that a second method be used to confirm endotracheal tube placement, such as auscultation of the lungs, direct visualization of the tube passing through the vocal cords with a laryngoscope, or the esophageal detector device.

Capnography

Some *capnography devices* are infrared devices in which a light-emitting diode is used to measure the intensity of light transmitted across a short distance, usually the diameter of an endotracheal tube. The measured light absorption varies inversely with the concentration of CO_2 passing through the endotracheal tube. When attached to the end of an endotracheal tube, these infrared devices are called *mainstream capnometers*. These devices readily reveal low exhaled CO_2 indicative of esophageal intubation, and they can provide estimates of the adequacy of ventilation and the effectiveness of circulation during CPR. Conversely, *sidestream capnometers* draw a small sample of gas from the airway through a small tube to measure the CO_2 concentration in a device detached from the airway and the patient.

Capnography devices provide a continuous readout of the concentration of CO_2. They are used to monitor the quality of ventilation in nonarrest patients. Because of their high degree of sensitivity to expired CO_2, however, capnographs can often detect a sufficient quantity of CO_2 to indicate the presence of an endotracheal tube in the trachea even when cardiac arrest is present. Continuous capnography monitoring devices can identify and signal a fall in exhaled CO_2 consistent with endo-

tracheal tube dislodgment. This may be very helpful when patients are being moved or during emergencies.

Capnometry and Capnography in Cardiac Arrest

End-tidal CO_2 monitoring is a safe and effective noninvasive indicator of cardiac output during CPR capnography may be an early indicator of return of spontaneous circulation (ROSC) in intubated patients because an increase in exhaled CO_2 typically occurs when cardiac output increases and perfusion of the lungs improves. During cardiac arrest, CO_2 continues to be generated throughout the body; however, there is little pulmonary blood flow, and the level of CO_2 in exhaled gas may be too low to produce a color change or a graphic exhaled CO_2 waveform. In such situations, when a colorimetric device is attached to the distal end of a properly placed endotracheal tube, the color remains unchanged or the CO_2 level remains very low. Because the unchanged color and lack of exhaled CO_2 may also indicate that the tube has been placed in the esophagus, the health care provider must decide whether the lack of carbon dioxide indicates esophageal intubation or reflects the absence of blood flow to the lungs. The major determinant of CO_2 excretion is its rate of delivery from the peripheral production sites to the lungs. In the low-flow state during CPR, ventilation is relatively high compared with blood flow, so the end-tidal CO_2 concentration is low. If ventilation is reasonably constant, then changes in end-tidal CO_2 concentration reflect changes in cardiac output. Patients who are successfully resuscitated from cardiac arrest have significantly higher end-tidal CO_2 levels than those who cannot be resuscitated.

References

1. Kern KB, Hilwig RW, Berg RA, et al. Importance of continuous chest compressions during cardiopulmonary resuscitation: improved outcome during a simulated single lay-rescuer scenario. *Circulation* 2002;105(5):645–649.
2. von Planta M, Weil MH, Gazmuri RJ, et al. Myocardial acidosis associated with CO2 production during cardiac arrest and resuscitation. *Circulation* 1989;80(3):684–692.
3. Yannopoulos D, McKnite S, Aufderheide TP, et al. Effects of incomplete chest wall decompression during cardiopulmonary resuscitation on coronary and cerebral perfusion pressures in a porcine model of cardiac arrest. *Resuscitation* 2005;64(3):363–372.
4. Aufderheide TP, Pirrallo RG, Yannopoulos D, et al. Incomplete chest wall decompression: A clinical evaluation of CPR performance by trained laypersons and an assessment of alternative manual chest compression–decompression techniques. *Resuscitation* 2006;71(3):341–351.
5. Yannopoulos D, Aufderheide TP, McKnite S, et al. Hemodynamic and respiratory effects of negative tracheal pressure during CPR in pigs. *Resuscitation* 2006;69(3):487–494.
6. Baskett P, Nolan J, Parr M. Tidal volumes which are perceived to be adequate for resuscitation. *Resuscitation* 1996;31(3):231–234.
7. Aufderheide TP, Sigurdsson G, Pirrallo RG, et al. Hyperventilation-induced hypotension during cardiopulmonary resuscitation. *Circulation* 2004;109(16):1960–1965.
8. Paradis NA, Martin GB, Goetting MG, et al. Simultaneous aortic, jugular bulb, and right atrial pressures during cardiopulmonary resuscitation in humans. Insights into mechanisms. *Circulation* 1989;80(2):361–368.
9. Idris AH, Staples ED, O'Brien DJ, et al. Effect of ventilation on acid-base balance and oxygenation in low blood-flow states. *Crit Care Med* 1994;22(11):1827–1834.

10. Idris A, Wenzel V, Banner MJ, et al. Smaller tidal volumes minimize gastric inflation during CPR with an unprotected airway. *Circulation* 1995;92(suppl):I-759.
11. Idris A, Gabrielli A, Caruso L. Smaller tidal volume is safe and effective for bag-valve-ventilation, but not for mouth-to-mouth ventilation: an animal model for basic life support. *Circulation* 1999;100 (suppl I):I-644.
12. Dorph E, Wik L, Steen PA. Arterial blood gases with 700 ml tidal volumes during out-of-hospital CPR. *Resuscitation* 2004;61(1): 23–27.
13. Winkler M, Mauritz W, Hackl W, et al. Effects of half the tidal volume during cardiopulmonary resuscitation on acid-base balance and haemodynamics in pigs. *Eur J Emerg Med* 1998;5(2): 201–206.
14. Babbs CF, Kern KB. Optimum compression to ventilation ratios in CPR under realistic, practical conditions: a physiological and mathematical analysis. *Resuscitation* 2002;54(2):147–157.
15. Greingor JL. Quality of cardiac massage with ratio compression–ventilation 5/1 and 15/2. *Resuscitation* 2002;55(3):263–267.
16. Kern KB, Hilwig RW, Berg RA, et al. Efficacy of chest compression-only BLS CPR in the presence of an occluded airway. *Resuscitation* 1998;39(3):179–188.
17. Wik L, Kramer-Johansen J, Myklebust H, et al. Quality of cardiopulmonary resuscitation during out-of-hospital cardiac arrest. *JAMA* 2005;293(3):299–304.
18. Ornato JP, Hallagan LF, McMahan SB, et al. Attitudes of BCLS instructors about mouth-to-mouth resuscitation during the AIDS epidemic. *Ann Emerg Med* 1990;19(2):151–156.
19. Brenner BE, Van DC, Cheng D, et al. Determinants of reluctance to perform CPR among residents and applicants: the impact of experience on helping behavior. *Resuscitation* 1997;35(3):203–211.
20. Hew P, Brenner B, Kaufman J. Reluctance of paramedics and emergency medical technicians to perform mouth-to-mouth resuscitation. *J Emerg Med* 1997;15(3):279–284.
21. Berg RA, Kern KB, Sanders AB, et al. Bystander cardiopulmonary resuscitation. Is ventilation necessary? *Circulation* 1993;88(pt 1) (4):1907–1915.
22. Hallstrom AP. Dispatcher-assisted "phone" cardiopulmonary resuscitation by chest compression alone or with mouth-to-mouth ventilation. *Crit Care Med* 2000;28(11 Suppl): N190–N192.
23. Waalewijn RA, Tijssen JG, Koster RW. Bystander initiated actions in out-of-hospital cardiopulmonary resuscitation: results from the Amsterdam Resuscitation Study (ARRESUST). *Resuscitation* 2001; 50(3):273–279.
24. Van Hoeyweghen RJ, Bossaert LL, Mullie A, et al. Quality and efficiency of bystander CPR. Belgian Cerebral Resuscitation Study Group. *Resuscitation* 1993;26(1):47–52.
25. Chandra NC, Gruben KG, Tsitlik JE, et al. Observations of ventilation during resuscitation in a canine model. *Circulation* 1994; 90(6):3070–3075.
26. Tang W, Weil MH, Sun S, et al. Cardiopulmonary resuscitation by precordial compression but without mechanical ventilation. *Am J Respir Crit Care Med* 1994;150(6 pt 1):1709–1713.
27. Berg RA, Kern KB, Hilwig RW, et al. Assisted ventilation does not improve outcome in a porcine model of single-rescuer bystander cardiopulmonary resuscitation. *Circulation* 1997;95(6): 1635–1641.
28. Berg RA, Kern KB, Hilwig RW, et al. Assisted ventilation during "bystander" CPR in a swine acute myocardial infarction model does not improve outcome. *Circulation* 1997;96(12): 4364–4371.
29. Deakin CD, O'Neill JF, Tabor T. Does compression-only cardiopulmonary resuscitation generate adequate passive ventilation during cardiac arrest? *Resuscitation* 2007;75(1):53–59.
30. Weil MH, Rackow EC, Trevino R, et al. Difference in acid-base state between venous and arterial blood during cardiopulmonary resuscitation. *N Engl J Med* 1986;315(3):153–156.
31. Koster RW, Deakin CD, Bottiger BW, et al. Chest-compression-only or full cardiopulmonary resuscitation? *Lancet* 2007;369 (9577):1924; author reply 1925.
32. Eberle B, Dick WF, Schneider T, et al. Checking the carotid pulse check: diagnostic accuracy of first responders in patients with and without a pulse. *Resuscitation* 1996;33(2):107–116.
33. Bahr J, Klingler H, Panzer W, et al. Skills of lay people in checking the carotid pulse. *Resuscitation* 1997;35(1):23–26.
34. Ruppert M, Reith MW, Widmann JH, et al. Checking for breathing: evaluation of the diagnostic capability of emergency medical services personnel, physicians, medical students, and medical laypersons. *Ann Emerg Med* 1999;34(6):720–729.
35. Safar P, Escarraga LA, Chang F. Upper airway obstruction in the unconscious patient. *J Appl Physiol* 1959;14:760–764.
36. Carlson KA, Jahr JS. An update on pulse oximetry. Part II: limitations and future applications. *Anesthesiol Rev* 1994;21(2):41–46.
37. Aughey K, Hess D, Eitel D, et al. An evaluation of pulse oximetry in prehospital care. *Ann Emerg Med* 1991;20(8):887–891.
38. Bota GW, Rowe BH. Continuous monitoring of oxygen saturation in prehospital patients with severe illness: the problem of unrecognized hypoxemia. *J Emerg Med* 1995;13(3):305–311.
39. Brown LH, Manring EA, Kornegay HB, et al. Can prehospital personnel detect hypoxemia without the aid of pulse oximeters? *Am J Emerg Med* 1996;14(1):43–44.
40. Valko PC, Campbell JP, McCarty DL, et al. Prehospital use of pulse oximetry in rotary-wing aircraft. *Prehosp Disast Med* 1991;6(4): 421–428.
41. Wahr JA, Tremper KK. Noninvasive oxygen monitoring techniques. *Crit Care Clin* 1995;11(1):199–217.
42. Li J. Capnography alone is imperfect for endotracheal tube placement confirmation during emergency intubation. *J Emerg Med* 2001;20(3):223–229.
43. Chow LH, Lui PW, Cheung EL, et al. Verification of endotracheal tube misplacement with the colorimetric carbon dioxide detector during anesthesia. *Chung Hua I Hsueh Tsa Chih* 1993;51(6):415–418.
44. Sum Ping ST, Mehta MP, Symreng T. Accuracy of the FEF CO2 detector in the assessment of endotracheal tube placement. *Anesth Analg* 1992;74(3):415–419.
45. Ornato JP, Shipley JB, Racht EM, et al. Multicenter study of a portable, hand-size, colorimetric end-tidal carbon dioxide detection device. *Ann Emerg Med* 1992;21(5):518–523.
46. Cantineau JP, Merckx P, Lambert Y, et al. Effect of epinephrine on end-tidal carbon dioxide pressure during prehospital cardiopulmonary resuscitation. *Am J Emerg Med* 1994;12(3): 267–270.
47. Ward KR, Yealy DM. End-tidal carbon dioxide monitoring in emergency medicine. Part 2: clinical applications. *Acad Emerg Med* 1998;5(6):637–646.
48. Thomas M, Malmcrona R, Shillingford J. Haemodynamic effects of oxygen in patients with acute myocardial infarction. *Br Heart J* 1965;27:401–407.
49. Daly WJ, Cline D, Bondurant S. Effects of breathing oxygen on atrioventricular conduction. *Am Heart J* 1963;66:321–324.
50. Daly WJ, Behnke RH. Hemodynamic consequences of oxygen breathing in left ventricular failure. *Circulation* 1963;27:252–256.
51. Kenmure AC, Murdoch WR, Beattie AD, et al. Circulatory and metabolic effects of oxygen in myocardial infarction. *Br Med J* 1968;4(5627):360–364.
52. Foster GL, Casten GG, Reeves TJ. The effects of oxygen breathing in patients with acute myocardial infarction. *Cardiovasc Res* 1969;3(2):179–189.
53. Bourassa MG, Campeau L, Bois MA, et al. The effects of inhalation of 100 percent oxygen on myocardial lactate metabolism in coronary heart disease. *Am J Cardiol* 1969;24(2):172–177.
54. Sukumalchantra Y, Levy S, Danzig R, et al. Correcting arterial hypoxemia by oxygen therapy in patients with acute myocardial infarction. Effect on ventilation and hemodynamics. *Am J Cardiol* 1969;24(6):838–852.
55. Neill WA. Effects of arterial hypoxemia and hyperoxia on oxygen availability for myocardial metabolism. Patients with and without coronary heart disease. *Am J Cardiol* 1969;24(2):166–171.
56. Madias JE, Hood WB Jr. Reduction of precordial ST-segment elevation in patients with anterior myocardial infarction by oxygen breathing. *Circulation* 1976;53(3 Suppl):I198–I200.
57. Madias JE, Madias NE, Hood WB Jr. Precordial ST-segment mapping. 2. Effects of oxygen inhalation on ischemic injury in patients with acute myocardial infarction. *Circulation* 1976;53(3):411–417.
58. Madias JE, Hood WB Jr. Precordial ST-segment mapping. 4. Experience with mapping of ST-segment depression in anterior transmural myocardial infarction. *J Electrocardiol* 1976;9(4):315–320.
59. Rawles JM, Kenmure AC. Controlled trial of oxygen in uncomplicated myocardial infarction. *Br Med J* 1976;1(6018):1121–1123.
60. Nicholson C. A systematic review of the effectiveness of oxygen in reducing acute myocardial ischaemia. *J Clin Nurs* 2004;13(8): 996–1007.

61. Antman EM, Anbe DT, Armstrong PW, et al. ACC/AHA guidelines for the management of patients with ST-elevation myocardial infarction; A report of the American College of Cardiology/American Heart Association Task Force on Practice Guidelines (Committee to Revise the 1999 Guidelines for the Management of patients with acute myocardial infarction). *J Am Coll Cardiol* 2004;44(3):E1–E211.

62. Anderson JL, Adams CD, Antman EM, et al. ACC/AHA 2007 guidelines for the management of patients with unstable angina/non-ST-Elevation myocardial infarction: a report of the American College of Cardiology/American Heart Association Task Force on Practice Guidelines (Writing Committee to Revise the 2002 Guidelines for the Management of Patients With Unstable Angina/Non-ST-Elevation Myocardial Infarction) developed in collaboration with the American College of Emergency Physicians, the Society for Cardiovascular Angiography and Interventions, and the Society of Thoracic Surgeons endorsed by the American Association of Cardiovascular and Pulmonary Rehabilitation and the Society for Academic Emergency Medicine. *J Am Coll Cardiol* 2007;50(7):e1–e157.

63. Anderson JL, Adams CD, Antman EM, et al. ACC/AHA 2007 guidelines for the management of patients with unstable angina/non ST-elevation myocardial infarction: a report of the American College of Cardiology/American Heart Association Task Force on Practice Guidelines (Writing Committee to Revise the 2002 Guidelines for the Management of Patients With Unstable Angina/Non ST-Elevation Myocardial Infarction): developed in collaboration with the American College of Emergency Physicians, the Society for Cardiovascular Angiography and Interventions, and the Society of Thoracic Surgeons: endorsed by the American Association of Cardiovascular and Pulmonary Rehabilitation and the Society for Academic Emergency Medicine. *Circulation* 2007;116(7):e148–304.

64. Davies AE, Kidd D, Stone SP, et al. Pharyngeal sensation and gag reflex in healthy subjects. *Lancet* 1995;345(8948):487–488.

65. Bleach NR. The gag reflex and aspiration: a retrospective analysis of 120 patients assessed by videofluoroscopy. *Clin Otolaryngol Allied Sci* 1993;18(4):303–307.

66. Gallagher WJ, Pearce AC, Power SJ. Assessment of a new nasopharyngeal airway. *Br J Anaesth* 1988;60(1):112–115.

67. Feldman SA, Fauvel NJ, Ooi R. The cuffed pharyngeal airway. *Eur J Anaesthesiol* 1991;8(4):291–295.

68. Ellis DY, Lambert C, Shirley P. Intracranial placement of nasopharyngeal airways: is it all that rare? *Emerg Med J* 2006;23(8):661.

69. Muzzi DA, Losasso TJ, Cucchiara RF. Complication from a nasopharyngeal airway in a patient with a basilar skull fracture. *Anesthesiology* 1991;74(2):366–368.

70. Schade K, Borzotta A, Michaels A. Intracranial malposition of nasopharyngeal airway. *J Trauma* 2000;49(5):967–968.

71. Martin JE, Mehta R, Aarabi B, et al. Intracranial insertion of a nasopharyngeal airway in a patient with craniofacial trauma. *Mil Med* 2004;169(6):496–497.

72. Simons RW, Rea TD, Becker LJ, et al. The incidence and significance of emesis associated with out-of-hospital cardiac arrest. *Resuscitation* 2007;74(3):427–431.

73. Kozak RJ, Ginther BE, Bean WS. Difficulties with portable suction equipment used for prehospital advanced airway procedures. *Prehosp Emerg Care* 1997;1(2):91–95.

74. Rowe BH, Shuster M, Zambon S, et al. Preparation, attitudes and behaviour in nonhospital cardiac emergencies: evaluating a community's readiness to act. *Can J Cardiol* 1998;14(3):371–377.

75. Locke CJ, Berg RA, Sanders AB, et al. Bystander cardiopulmonary resuscitation concerns about mouth-to-mouth contact. *Arch Intern Med* 1995;155(9):938–943.

76. Brenner BE, Kauffman J. Reluctance of internists and medical nurses to perform mouth-to-mouth resuscitation. *Arch Intern Med* 1993;153(15):1763–1769.

77. Brenner B, Stark B, Kauffman J. The reluctance of house staff to perform mouth-to-mouth resuscitation in the inpatient setting: what are the considerations? *Resuscitation* 1994;28(3):185–193.

78. Mejicano GC, Maki DG. Infections acquired during cardiopulmonary resuscitation: estimating the risk and defining strategies for prevention. *Ann Intern Med* 1998;129(10):813–828.

79. Axelsson A, Thoren A, Holmberg S, et al. Attitudes of trained Swedish lay rescuers toward CPR performance in an emergency: a survey of 1012 recently trained CPR rescuers. *Resuscitation* 2000;44(1):27–36.

80. Melanson SW, O'Gara K. EMS provider reluctance to perform mouth-to-mouth resuscitation. *Prehosp Emerg Care* 2000;4(1):48–52.

81. Rossi R, Lindner KH, Ahnefeld FW. Devices for expired air resuscitation. *Prehosp Disast Med* 1993;8(2):123–126.

82. Cydulka RK, Connor PJ, Myers TF, et al. Prevention of oral bacterial flora transmission by using mouth-to-mask ventilation during CPR. *J Emerg Med* 1991;9(5):317–321.

83. Lawrence PJ, Sivaneswaran N. Ventilation during cardiopulmonary resuscitation: which method? *Med J Aust* 1985;143(10):443–446.

84. Harrison RR, Maull KI, Keenan RL, et al. Mouth-to-mask ventilation: a superior method of rescue breathing. *Ann Emerg Med* 1982;11(2):74–76.

85. Seidelin PH, Stolarek IH, Littlewood DG. Comparison of six methods of emergency ventilation. *Lancet* 1986;2(8518):1274–1275.

86. Thomas AN, O'Sullivan K, Hyatt J, et al. A comparison of bag mask and mouth mask ventilation in anaesthetised patients. *Resuscitation* 1993;26(1):13–21.

87. Paal P, Falk M, Sumann G, et al. Comparison of mouth-to-mouth, mouth-to-mask and mouth-to-face-shield ventilation by lay persons. *Resuscitation* 2006;70(1):117–123.

88. Johannigman JA, Branson RD, Davis K Jr, et al. Techniques of emergency ventilation: a model to evaluate tidal volume, airway pressure, and gastric insufflation. *J Trauma* 1991;31(1):93–98.

89. Elling R, Politis J. An evaluation of emergency medical technicians' ability to use manual ventilation devices. *Ann Emerg Med* 1983;12(12):765–768.

90. Cummins RO, Austin D, Graves JR, et al. Ventilation skills of emergency medical technicians: a teaching challenge for emergency medicine. *Ann Emerg Med* 1986;15(10):1187–1192.

91. Hess D, Baran C. Ventilatory volumes using mouth-to-mouth, mouth-to-mask, and bag-valve-mask techniques. *Am J Emerg Med* 1985;3(4):292–296.

92. De Regge M, Vogels C, Monsieurs KG, et al. Retention of ventilation skills of emergency nurses after training with the SMART BAG compared to a standard bag-valve-mask. *Resuscitation* 2006;68(3):379–384.

93. Walsh K, Loveday K, O'Rathaille M. A comparison of the effectiveness of pre-hospital bag-valve-mask ventilation performed by Irish emergency medical technicians and anaesthetists working in a tertiary referral teaching hospital. *Ir Med J* 2003;96(3):77–79.

94. Osterwalder JJ, Schuhwerk W. Effectiveness of mask ventilation in a training mannikin. A comparison between the Oxylator EM100 and the bag-valve device. *Resuscitation* 1998;36(1):23–27.

95. Martin PD, Cyna AM, Hunter WA, et al. Training nursing staff in airway management for resuscitation: A clinical comparison of the facemask and laryngeal mask. *Anaesthesia* 1993;48(1):33–37.

96. Alexander R, Hodgson P, Lomax D, et al. A comparison of the laryngeal mask airway and Guedel airway, bag and face mask for manual ventilation following formal training. *Anaesthesia* 1993;48(3):231–234.

97. Jesudian MC, Harrison RR, Keenan RL, et al. Bag-valve-mask ventilation; two rescuers are better than one: preliminary report. *Crit Care Med* 1985;13(2):122–123.

98. Davidovic L, LaCovey D, Pitetti RD. Comparison of 1- versus 2-person bag-valve-mask techniques for manikin ventilation of infants and children. *Ann Emerg Med* 2005;46(1):37–42.

99. Dunkley CJ, Thomas AN, Taylor RJ, et al. A comparison of standard and a modified method of two resuscitator adult cardiopulmonary resuscitation: description of a new system for research into advanced life support skills. *Resuscitation* 1998;38(1):7–12.

100. Wheatley S, Thomas AN, Taylor RJ, et al. A comparison of three methods of bag valve mask ventilation. *Resuscitation* 1997;33(3):207–210.

101. Thomas AN, Dang PT, Hyatt J, et al. A new technique for two-hand bag valve mask ventilation. *Br J Anaesth* 1992;69(4):397–398.

102. Wenzel V, Idris AH, Dorges V, et al. The respiratory system during resuscitation: a review of the history, risk of infection during assisted ventilation, respiratory mechanics, and ventilation strategies for patients with an unprotected airway. *Resuscitation* 2001;49(2):123–134.

103. Dorges V, Ocker H, Wenzel V, et al. Emergency airway management by non-anaesthesia house officers—a comparison of three strategies. *Emerg Med J* 2001;18(2):90–94.

104. Wenzel V, Keller C, Idris AH, et al. Effects of smaller tidal volumes during basic life support ventilation in patients with respiratory arrest: good ventilation, less risk? *Resuscitation* 1999;43(1):25–29.

105. Dorges V, Ocker H, Hagelberg S, et al. Smaller tidal volumes with room-air are not sufficient to ensure adequate oxygenation during bag-valve-mask ventilation. *Resuscitation* 2000;44(1):37–41.

106. Tourtier JP, Compain M, Petitjeans F, et al. Acid aspiration prophylaxis in obstetrics in France: a comparative survey of 1998 vs. 1988 French practice. *Eur J Anaesthesiol* 2004;21(2):89–94.

107. Soreide E, Holst-Larsen H, Steen PA. Acid aspiration syndrome prophylaxis in gynaecological and obstetric patients. A Norwegian survey. *Acta Anaesthesiol Scand* 1994;38(8):863–868.

108. Schlesinger S, Blanchfield D. Modified rapid-sequence induction of anesthesia: a survey of current clinical practice. *AANA J* 2001; 69(4):291–298.

109. Morris J, Cook TM. Rapid sequence induction: a national survey of practice. *Anaesthesia* 2001;56(11):1090–1097.

110. Kluger MT, Willemsen G. Anti-aspiration prophylaxis in New Zealand: a national survey. *Anaesth Intens Care* 1998;26(1):70–77.

111. Lawes EG, Campbell I, Mercer D. Inflation pressure, gastric insufflation and rapid sequence induction. *Br J Anaesth* 1987;59 (3):315–318.

112. Lawes EG, Rea TD. The incidence and rapid sequence induction. *Br J Anaesth* 2007;74(3):315–318.

113. Admani M, Yeh TF, Jain R, et al. Prevention of gastric inflation during mask ventilation in newborn infants. *Crit Care Med* 1985; 13(7):592–593.

114. Moynihan RJ, Brock-Utne JG, Archer JH, et al. The effect of cricoid pressure on preventing gastric insufflation in infants and children. *Anesthesiology* 1993;78(4):652–656.

115. Neilipovitz DT, Crosby ET. No evidence for decreased incidence of aspiration after rapid sequence induction. *Can J Anaesth* 2007; 54(9):748–764.

116. Quigley P, Jeffrey P. Cricoid pressure: assessment of performance and effect of training in emergency department staff. *Emerg Med Australas* 2007;19(3):218–222.

117. Howells TH, Chamney AR, Wraight WJ, et al. The application of cricoid pressure. An assessment and a survey of its practice. *Anaesthesia* 1983;38(5):457–460.

118. Lawes EG, Duncan PW, Bland B, et al. The cricoid yoke—a device for providing consistent and reproducible cricoid pressure. *Br J Anaesth* 1986;58(8):925–931.

119. Vanner RG, O'Dwyer JP, Pryle BJ, et al. Upper oesophageal sphincter pressure and the effect of cricoid pressure. *Anaesthesia* 1992; 47(2):95–100.

120. Ellis DY, Harris T, Zideman D. Cricoid Pressure in Emergency Department Rapid Sequence Tracheal Intubations: A risk-benefit analysis. *Ann Emerg Med* 2007.

121. Brimacombe JR, Berry AM. Cricoid pressure. *Can J Anaesth* 1997;44(4):414–425.

122. Levitan RM, Kinkle WC, Levin WJ, et al. Laryngeal view during laryngoscopy: a randomized trial comparing cricoid pressure, backward-upward-rightward pressure, and bimanual laryngoscopy. *Ann Emerg Med* 2006;47(6):548–555.

123. Stone B. The use of the laryngeal mask airway by nurses during cardiopulmonary resuscitation: Results of a multicentre trial. *Anaesthesia* 1994;49(1):3–7.

124. Stone BJ, Chantler PJ, Baskett PJ. The incidence of regurgitation during cardiopulmonary resuscitation: a comparison between the bag valve mask and laryngeal mask airway. *Resuscitation* 1998;38(1): 3–6.

125. Guly UM, Mitchell RG, Cook R, et al. Paramedics and technicians are equally successful at managing cardiac arrest outside hospital. *BMJ* 1995;310(6987):1091–1094.

126. Stiell IG, Wells GA, Field B, et al. Advanced cardiac life support in out-of-hospital cardiac arrest. *N Engl J Med* 2004;351(7): 647–656.

127. Gausche M, Lewis RJ, Stratton SJ, et al. Effect of out-of-hospital pediatric endotracheal intubation on survival and neurological outcome: a controlled clinical trial. *JAMA* 2000;283(6):783–790.

128. Jones JH, Murphy MP, Dickson RL, et al. Emergency physician-verified out-of-hospital intubation: miss rates by paramedics. *Acad Emerg Med* 2004;11(6):707–709.

129. Sayre MR, Sakles JC, Mistler AF, et al. Field trial of endotracheal intubation by basic EMTs. *Ann Emerg Med* 1998;31(2):228–233.

130. Katz SH, Falk JL. Misplaced endotracheal tubes by paramedics in an urban emergency medical services system. *Ann Emerg Med* 2001;37(1):32–37.

131. Dorges V, Wenzel V, Knacke P, et al. Comparison of different airway management strategies to ventilate apneic, nonpreoxygenated patients. *Crit Care Med* 2003;31(3):800–804.

132. Kurola JO, Turunen MJ, Laakso JP, et al. A comparison of the laryngeal tube and bag-valve mask ventilation by emergency medical technicians: a feasibility study in anesthetized patients. *Anesth Analg* 2005;101(5):1477–1481.

133. Kette F, Reffo I, Giordani G, et al. The use of laryngeal tube by nurses in out-of-hospital emergencies: preliminary experience. *Resuscitation* 2005;66(1):21–25.

134. Vertongen VM, Ramsay MP, Herbison P. Skills retention for insertion of the Combitube and laryngeal mask airway. *Emerg Med* 2003;15(5-6):459–464.

135. Brimacombe J. A proposed classification system for extraglottic airway devices. *Anesthesiology* 2004;101(2):559.

136. Jones JH, Murphy MP, Dickson RL, et al. Emergency physician-verified out-of-hospital intubation: miss rates by paramedics. *Acad Emerg Med* 2004;11(6):707–709.

137. Beyer AJ III, Land G, Zaritsky A. Nonphysician transport of intubated pediatric patients: a system evaluation. *Crit Care Med* 1992; 20(7):961–966.

138. Bradley JS, Billows GL, Olinger ML, et al. Prehospital oral endotracheal intubation by rural basic emergency medical technicians. *Ann Emerg Med* 1998;32(1):26–32.

139. Sayre MR, Sakles JC, Mistler AF, et al. Field trial of endotracheal intubation by basic EMTs. *Ann Emerg Med* 1998;31(2):228–233.

140. Miller DM. A proposed classification and scoring system for supraglottic sealing airways: a brief review. *Anesth Analg* 2004;99 (5):1553–1559; table of contents.

141. Soar J. The I-gel supraglottic airway and resuscitation—some initial thoughts. *Resuscitation* 2007;74(1):197.

142. 2005 American Heart Association Guidelines for Cardiopulmonary Resuscitation and Emergency Cardiovascular Care. *Circulation* 2005;112(24 Suppl):IV1-203.

143. Brain AI. The development of the laryngeal mask—a brief history of the invention, early clinical studies and experimental work from which the Laryngeal Mask evolved. *Eur J Anaesthesiol Suppl* 1991; 4:5–17.

144. Brain AI. The laryngeal mask—a new concept in airway management. *Br J Anaesth* 1983;55(8):801–805.

145. Flaishon R, Sotman A, Ben-Abraham R, et al. Antichemical protective gear prolongs time to successful airway management: a randomized, crossover study in humans. *Anesthesiology* 2004;100(2): 260–266.

146. Goldik Z, Bornstein J, Eden A, et al. Airway management by physicians wearing anti-chemical warfare gear: comparison between laryngeal mask airway and endotracheal intubation. *Eur J Anaesthesiol* 2002;19(3):166–169.

147. Pennant JH, Pace NA, Gajraj NM. Role of the laryngeal mask airway in the immobile cervical spine. *J Clin Anesth* 1993;5(3):226–230.

148. Flaishon R, Sotman A, Ben-Abraham R, et al. Antichemical protective gear prolongs time to successful airway management: a randomized, crossover study in humans. *Anesthesiology* 2004;100 (2):260–266.

149. Davies PR, Tighe SQ, Greenslade GL, et al. Laryngeal mask airway and tracheal tube insertion by unskilled personnel. *Lancet* 1990;336(8721):977–979.

150. Pennant JH, Walker MB. Comparison of the endotracheal tube and laryngeal mask in airway management by paramedical personnel. *Anesth Analg* 1992;74(4):531–534.

151. Reinhart DJ, Simmons G. Comparison of placement of the laryngeal mask airway with endotracheal tube by paramedics and respiratory therapists. *Ann Emerg Med* 1994;24(2):260–263.

152. Deakin CD, Peters R, Tomlinson P, et al. Securing the prehospital airway: a comparison of laryngeal mask insertion and endotracheal intubation by UK paramedics. *Emerg Med J* 2005;22(1):64–67.

153. Burgoyne L, Cyna A. Laryngeal mask vs intubating laryngeal mask: insertion and ventilation by inexperienced resuscitators. *Anaesth Intens Care* 2001;29(6):604–608.

154. Coulson A, Brimacombe J, Keller C, et al. A comparison of the ProSeal and classic laryngeal mask airways for airway management

by inexperienced personnel after manikin-only training. *Anaesth Intens Care* 2003;31(3):286–289.

155. Dingley J, Baynham P, Swart M, et al. Ease of insertion of the laryngeal mask airway by inexperienced personnel when using an introducer. *Anaesthesia* 1997;52(8):756–760.

156. Roberts I, Allsop P, Dickinson M, et al. Airway management training using the laryngeal mask airway: a comparison of two different training programmes. *Resuscitation* 1997;33(3):211–214.

157. Yardy N, Hancox D, Strang T. A comparison of two airway aids for emergency use by unskilled personnel: the Combitube and laryngeal mask. *Anaesthesia* 1999;54(2):181–183.

158. Verghese C, Prior-Willeard PF, Baskett PJ. Immediate management of the airway during cardiopulmonary resuscitation in a hospital without a resident anaesthesiologist. *Eur J Emerg Med* 1994; 1(3):123–125.

159. Samarkandi AH, Seraj MA, el Dawlatly A, et al. The role of laryngeal mask airway in cardiopulmonary resuscitation. *Resuscitation* 1994;28(2):103–106.

160. Kokkinis K. The use of the laryngeal mask airway in CPR. *Resuscitation* 1994;27(1):9–12.

161. Leach A, Alexander CA, Stone B. The laryngeal mask in cardiopulmonary resuscitation in a district general hospital: a preliminary communication. *Resuscitation* 1993;25(3):245–248.

162. Carrillo Alvarez A, Lopez-Herce Cid J, Moral Torrero R, et al. [Evaluation of basic and advanced pediatric resuscitation courses]. *An Esp Pediatr* 2000;53(2):125–134.

163. Grantham H, Phillips G, Gilligan JE. The laryngeal mask in prehospital emergency care. 1994;6:193–197.

164. Rumball CJ, MacDonald D. The PTL, Combitube, laryngeal mask, and oral airway: a randomized prehospital comparative study of ventilatory device effectiveness and cost-effectiveness in 470 cases of cardiorespiratory arrest. *Prehosp Emerg Care* 1997;1(1):1–10.

165. Ho BY, Skinner HJ, Mahajan RP. Gastro-oesophageal reflux during day case gynaecological laparoscopy under positive pressure ventilation: laryngeal mask vs. tracheal intubation. *Anaesthesia* 1998;53(9):921–924.

166. Maltby JR, Beriault MT, Watson NC, et al. LMA-Classic and LMA-ProSeal are effective alternatives to endotracheal intubation for gynecologic laparoscopy. *Can J Anaesth* 2003;50(1):71–77.

167. Rewari W, Kaul HL. Regurgitation and aspiration during gynaecological laparoscopy: Comparison between laryngeal mask airway and tracheal intubation. *Journal of Anaesthesiology Clin Pharmacol* 1999;15(1):67–70.

168. Atherton GL, Johnson JC. Ability of paramedics to use the Combitube in prehospital cardiac arrest. *Ann Emerg Med* 1993;22(8):1263–1268.

169. Rabitsch W, Schellongowski P, Staudinger T, et al. Comparison of a conventional tracheal airway with the Combitube in an urban emergency medical services system run by physicians. *Resuscitation* 2003;57(1):27–32.

170. Staudinger T, Brugger S, Roggla M, et al. [Comparison of the Combitube with the endotracheal tube in cardiopulmonary resuscitation in the prehospital phase]. *Wien Klin Wochenschr* 1994;106 (13):412–415.

171. Rumball C, Macdonald D, Barber P, Wong H, Smecher C. Endotracheal intubation and esophageal tracheal Combitube insertion by regular ambulance attendants: a comparative trial. *Prehosp Emerg Care* 2004;8(1):15–22.

172. Davis DP, Valentine C, Ochs M, Vilke GM, Hoyt DB. The Combitube as a salvage airway device for paramedic rapid sequence intubation. *Ann Emerg Med* 2003;42(5):697–704.

173. Ochs M, Davis D, Hoyt D, Bailey D, Marshall L, Rosen P. Paramedic-performed rapid sequence intubation of patients with severe head injuries. *Ann Emerg Med* 2002;40(2):159–167.

174. Frass M, Frenzer R, Zdrahal F, Hoflehner G, Porges P, Lackner F. The esophageal tracheal combitube: preliminary results with a new airway for CPR. *Ann Emerg Med* 1987;16(7):768–772.

175. Frass M, Frenzer R, Ilias W, Lackner F, Hoflehner G, Losert U. [The esophageal tracheal Combitube (ETC): animal experiment results with a new emergency tube]. *Anasth Intensivther Notfallmed* 1987;22(3):142–144.

176. Frass M, Frenzer R, Rauscha F, Schuster E, Glogar D. Ventilation with the esophageal tracheal combitube in cardiopulmonary Resuscitation Promptness and effectiveness. *Chest* 1988;93(4):781–784.

177. Staudinger T, Brugger S, Watschinger B, Roggla M, Dielacher C, Lobl T, Fink D, Klauser R, Frass M. Emergency intubation with the Combitube: comparison with the endotracheal airway. *Ann Emerg Med* 1993;22(10):1573–1575.

178. Lefrancois DP, Dufour DG. Use of the esophageal tracheal combitube by basic emergency medical technicians. *Resuscitation* 2002;52(1):77–83.

179. Tanigawa K, Shigematsu A. Choice of airway devices for 12,020 cases of nontraumatic cardiac arrest in Japan. *Prehosp Emerg Care* 1998;2(2):96–100.

180. Oczenski W, Krenn H, Dahaba AA, Binder M, El-Schahawi-Kienzl I, Kohout S, Schwarz S, Fitzgerald RD. Complications following the use of the Combitube, tracheal tube and laryngeal mask airway. *Anaesthesia* 1999;54(12):1161–1165.

181. Rabitsch W, Krafft P, Lackner FX, Frenzer R, Hofbauer R, Sherif C, Frass M. Evaluation of the oesophageal-tracheal double-lumen tube (Combitube) during general anaesthesia. *Wien Klin Wochenschr* 2004;116(3):90–93.

182. Vezina D, Lessard MR, Bussieres J, Topping C, Trepanier CA. Complications associated with the use of the Esophageal-Tracheal Combitube. *Can J Anaesth* 1998;45(1):76–80.

183. Stoppacher R, Teggatz JR, Jentzen JM. Esophageal and pharyngeal injuries associated with the use of the esophageal-tracheal Combitube. *J Forens Sci* 2004;49(3):586–591.

184. Urtubia RM, Aguila CM, Cumsille MA. Combitube: a study for proper use. *Anesth Analg* 2000;90(4):958–962.

185. Hagberg CA, Vartazarian TN, Chelly JE, Ovassapian A. The incidence of gastroesophageal reflux and tracheal aspiration detected with pH electrodes is similar with the Laryngeal Mask Airway and Esophageal Tracheal Combitube—a pilot study. *Can J Anaesth* 2004;51(3):243–249.

186. Mercer MH. An assessment of protection of the airway from aspiration of oropharyngeal contents using the Combitube airway. *Resuscitation* 2001;51(2):135–138.

187. Petring OU, Adelhoj B, Jensen BN, Pedersen NO, Lomholt N. Prevention of silent aspiration due to leaks around cuffs of endotracheal tubes. *Anesth Analg* 1986;65(7):777–780.

188. Dorges V, Ocker H, Wenzel V, Steinfath M, Gerlach K. The Laryngeal Tube S: a modified simple airway device. *Anesth Analg* 2003;96(2):618–621.

189. Ochs M, Vilke GM, Chan TC, Moats T, Buchanan J. Successful prehospital airway management by EMT-Ds using the combitube. *Prehosp Emerg Care* 2000;4(4):333–337.

190. Genzwuerker HV, Dhonau S, Ellinger K. Use of the laryngeal tube for out-of-hospital resuscitation. *Resuscitation* 2002;52(2):221–224.

191. Asai T, Hidaka I, Kawachi S. Efficacy of the laryngeal tube by inexperienced personnel. *Resuscitation* 2002;55(2):171–175.

192. Cook TM, McCormick B, Asai T. Randomized comparison of laryngeal tube with classic laryngeal mask airway for anaesthesia with controlled ventilation. *Br J Anaesth* 2003;91(3):373–378.

193. Ocker H, Wenzel V, Schmucker P, Steinfath M, Dorges V. A comparison of the laryngeal tube with the laryngeal mask airway during routine surgical procedures. *Anesth Analg* 2002;95(4):1094–1097.

194. Asai T, Moriyama S, Nishita Y, Kawachi S. Use of the laryngeal tube during cardiopulmonary resuscitation by paramedical staff. *Anaesthesia* 2003;58(4):393–394.

195. Genzwurker H, Finteis T, Hinkelbein J, Ellinger K. [First clinical experiences with the new LTS. A laryngeal tube with an oesophageal drain]. *Anaesthesist* 2003;52(8):697–702.

196. Gaitini LA, Vaida SJ, Somri M, Kaplan V, Yanovski B, Markovits R, Hagberg CA. An evaluation of the laryngeal tube during general anesthesia using mechanical ventilation. *Anesth Analg* 2003; 96(6):1750–1755.

197. Asai T, Murao K, Shingu K. Apparatus: efficacy of the laryngeal tube during intermittent positive-pressure ventilation. *Anaesthesia* 2000;55(11):1099–1102.

198. Kurola J, Harve H, Kettunen T, Laakso JP, Gorski J, Paakkonen H, Silfvast T. Airway management in cardiac arrest—comparison of the laryngeal tube, tracheal intubation and bag-valve mask ventilation in emergency medical training. *Resuscitation* 2004;61(2):149–153.

199. Genzwuerker HV, Finteis T, Slabschi D, Groeschel J, Ellinger K. Assessment of the use of the laryngeal tube for cardiopulmonary resuscitation in a manikin. *Resuscitation* 2001;51(3):291–296.

200. Dorges V, Wenzel V, Neubert E, Schmucker P. Emergency airway management by intensive care unit nurses with the intubating

laryngeal mask airway and the laryngeal tube. *Crit Care* 2000;4 (6):369–376.

201. Frass M, Frenzer R, Rauscha F, Weber H, Pacher R, Leithner C. Evaluation of esophageal tracheal Combitube in cardiopulmonary Resuscitation *Crit Care Med* 1987;15(6):609–611.

202. Pepe PE, Copass MK, Joyce TH. Prehospital endotracheal intubation: rationale for training emergency medical personnel. *Ann Emerg Med* 1985;14(11):1085–1092.

203. Bowman FP, Menegazzi JJ, Check BD, Duckett TM. Lower esophageal sphincter pressure during prolonged cardiac arrest and resuscitation. *Ann Emerg Med* 1995;26(2):216–219.

204. Weiler N, Heinrichs W, Dick W. Assessment of pulmonary mechanics and gastric inflation pressure during mask ventilation. *Prehosp Disast Med* 1995;10(2):101–105.

205. Ruben H, Knudsen EJ, Carugati G. Gastric inflation in relation to airway pressure. *Acta Anaesth Scand* 1961;5:107–114.

206. Wenzel V, Idris AH, Banner MJ, Kubilis PS, Band R, Williams JL, Jr., Lindner KH. Respiratory system compliance decreases after cardiopulmonary resuscitation and stomach inflation: impact of large and small tidal volumes on calculated peak airway pressure. *Resuscitation* 1998;38(2):113–118.

207. Stept WJ, Safar P. Rapid induction-intubation for prevention of gastric-content aspiration. *Anesth Analg* 1970;49(4):633–636.

208. Wang HE, Sweeney TA, O'Connor RE, Rubinstein H. Failed prehospital intubations: an analysis of emergency department courses and outcomes. *Prehosp Emerg Care* 2001;5(2):134–141.

209. Wang HE, O'Connor RE, Megargel RE, Bitner M, Stuart R, Bratton-Heck B, Lamborn M, Tan L. The utilization of midazolam as a pharmacologic adjunct to endotracheal intubation by paramedics. *Prehosp Emerg Care* 2000;4(1):14–18.

210. Wayne MA, Slovis CM, Pirrallo RG. Management of difficult airways in the field. *Prehosp Emerg Care* 1999;3(4):290–296.

211. Brownstein D, Shugerman R, Cummings P, Rivara F, Copass M. Prehospital endotracheal intubation of children by paramedics. *Ann Emerg Med* 1996;28(1):34–39.

212. Ma OJ, Atchley RB, Hatley T, Green M, Young J, Brady W. Intubation success rates improve for an air medical program after implementing the use of neuromuscular blocking agents. *Am J Emerg Med* 1998;16(2):125–127.

213. Kociszewski C, Thomas SH, Harrison T, Wedel SK. Etomidate versus succinylcholine for intubation in an air medical setting. *Am J Emerg Med* 2000;18(7):757–763.

214. Syverud SA, Borron SW, Storer DL, Hedges JR, Dronen SC, Braunstein LT, Hubbard BJ. Prehospital use of neuromuscular blocking agents in a helicopter ambulance program. *Ann Emerg Med* 1988;17(3):236–242.

215. Walls R. The emergency airway algorithms. In: RS, ed. *Manual of Emergency Airway Management*. Philadelphia: Lippincott Williams & Wilkins, 2000.

216. Pace SA, Fuller FP. Out-of-hospital succinylcholine-assisted endotracheal intubation by paramedics. *Ann Emerg Med* 2000;35(6):568–572.

217. O'Connor RE, Swor RA. Verification of endotracheal tube placement following intubation. National Association of EMS Physicians Standards and Clinical Practice Committee. *Prehosp Emerg Care* 1999;3(3):248–250.

218. Wang HE, O'Connor RE, Domeier RM. Prehospital rapid-sequence intubation. *Prehosp Emerg Care* 2001;5(1):40–48.

219. Schneider RE WR, Luten RC, Murphy MF. *Manual of Emergency Airway Management*. Philadelphia: Lippincott Williams & Wilkins; 2000.

220. McGowan P, Skinner A. Preoxygenation—the importance of a good face mask seal. *Br J Anaesth* 1995;75(6):777–778.

221. Berthoud M, Read DH, Norman J. Pre-oxygenation: how long? *Anaesthesia* 1983;38(2):96–102.

222. Nocera A. A flexible solution for emergency intubation difficulties. *Ann Emerg Med* 1996;27(5):665–667.

223. Kidd JF, Dyson A, Latto IP. Successful difficult intubation. Use of the gum elastic bougie. *Anaesthesia* 1988;43(6):437–438.

224. Dogra S, Falconer R, Latto IP. Successful difficult intubation. Tracheal tube placement over a gum-elastic bougie. *Anaesthesia* 1990;45(9):774–776.

225. Nolan JP, Wilson ME. An evaluation of the gum elastic bougie. Intubation times and incidence of sore throat. *Anaesthesia* 1992;47(10):878–881.

226. Nolan JP, Wilson ME. Orotracheal intubation in patients with potential cervical spine injuries. An indication for the gum elastic bougie. *Anaesthesia* 1993;48(7):630–633.

227. Viswanathan S, Campbell C, Wood DG, et al. The Eschmann Tracheal Tube Introducer. (Gum elastic bougie). *Anesthesiol Rev* 1992;19(6):29–34.

228. Hopkins PM. Use of suxamethonium in children. *Br J Anaesth* 1995;75(6):675–677.

229. Morell RC, Berman JM, Royster RI, et al. Revised label regarding use of succinylcholine in children and adolescents. *Anesthesiology* 1994;80(1):242–245.

230. Scheiber G, Ribeiro FC, Marichal A, et al. Intubating conditions and onset of action after rocuronium, vecuronium, and atracurium in young children. *Anesth Analg* 1996;83(2):320–324.

231. McDonald PF, Sainsbury DA, Laing RJ. Evaluation of the onset time and intubation conditions of rocuronium bromide in children. *Anaesth Intens Care* 1997;25(3):260–261.

232. Fuchs-Buder T, Tassonyi E. Intubating conditions and time course of rocuronium-induced neuromuscular block in children. *Br J Anaesth* 1996;77(3):335–338.

233. Maddineni VR, McCoy EP, Mirakur RK, McBride RJ. Onset and duration of action and hemodynamic effects of rocuronium bromide in balanced and volatile anesthesia. *Acta Anaesthesiol Belg* 1994;45(2):41–47.

234. Khuenl-Brady KS, Pomaroli A, Puhringer F, Mitterschiffthaler G, Koller J. The use of rocuronium (ORG 9426) in patients with chronic renal failure. *Anaesthesia* 1993;48(10):873–875.

235. Magorian T, Wood P, Caldwell J, Fisher D, Segredo V, Szenohradszky J, Sharma M, Gruenke L, Miller R. The pharmacokinetics and neuromuscular effects of rocuronium bromide in patients with liver disease. *Anesth Analg* 1995;80(4):754–759.

236. Khalil M, D'Honneur G, Duvaldestin P, Slavov V, De Hys C, Gomeni R. Pharmacokinetics and pharmacodynamics of rocuronium in patients with cirrhosis. *Anesthesiology* 1994;80(6):1241–1247.

237. Ferres CJ, Crean PM, Mirakhur RK. An evaluation of Org NC 45 (vecuronium) in paediatric anaesthesia. *Anaesthesia* 1983;38(10):943–947.

238. Mirakhur RK, Ferres CJ, Clarke RS, Bali IM, Dundee JW. Clinical evaluation of Org NC 45. *Br J Anaesth* 1983;55(2):119–124.

239. Lynam DP, Cronnelly R, Castagnoli KP, Canfell PC, Caldwell J, Arden J, Miller RD. The pharmacodynamics and pharmacokinetics of vecuronium in patients anesthetized with isoflurane with normal renal function or with renal failure. *Anesthesiology* 1988;69(2):227–231.

240. Sellick BA. Cricoid pressure to control regurgitation of stomach contents during induction of anaesthesia. *Lancet* 1961;2:404–406.

241. Grmec S. Comparison of three different methods to confirm tracheal tube placement in emergency intubation. *Intens Care Med* 2002;28(6):701–704.

242. Anton WR, Gordon RW, Jordan TM, Posner KL, Cheney FW. A disposable end-tidal CO_2 detector to verify endotracheal intubation. *Ann Emerg Med* 1991;20(3):271–275.

243. Bhende MS, Thompson AE. Evaluation of an end-tidal CO2 detector during pediatric cardiopulmonary resuscitation. *Pediatrics* 1995;95(3):395–399.

244. Bhende MS, Thompson AE, Cook DR, Saville AL. Validity of a disposable end-tidal CO2 detector in verifying endotracheal tube placement in infants and children. *Ann Emerg Med* 1992;21(2):142–145.

245. Hayden SR, Sciammarella J, Viccellio P, Thode H, Delagi R. Colorimetric end-tidal CO_2 detector for verification of endotracheal tube placement in out-of-hospital cardiac arrest. *Acad Emerg Med* 1995;2(6):499–502.

246. MacLeod BA, Heller MB, Gerard J, Yealy DM, Menegazzi JJ. Verification of endotracheal tube placement with colorimetric end-tidal CO2 detection. *Ann Emerg Med* 1991;20(3):267–270.

247. Takeda T, Tanigawa K, Tanaka H, Hayashi Y, Goto E, Tanaka K. The assessment of three methods to verify tracheal tube placement in the emergency setting. *Resuscitation* 2003;56(2):153–157.

248. Tanigawa K, Takeda T, Goto E, Tanaka K. The efficacy of esophageal detector devices in verifying tracheal tube placement: a randomized cross-over study of out-of-hospital cardiac arrest patients. *Anesth Analg* 2001;92(2):375–378.

249. Varon AJ, Morrina J, Civetta JM. Clinical utility of a colorimetric end-tidal CO2 detector in cardiopulmonary resuscitation and emergency intubation. *J Clin Monit* 1991;7(4):289–293.

250. Cantineau JP, Lambert Y, Merckx P, Reynaud P, Porte F, Bertrand C, Duvaldestin P. End-tidal carbon dioxide during cardiopulmonary resuscitation in humans presenting mostly with asystole: a predictor of outcome. *Crit Care Med* 1996;24(5):791–796.
251. Hand IL, Shepard EK, Krauss AN, Auld PA. Discrepancies between transcutaneous and end-tidal carbon dioxide monitoring in the critically ill neonate with respiratory distress syndrome. *Crit Care Med* 1989;17(6):556–559.
252. Tobias JD, Meyer DJ. Noninvasive monitoring of carbon dioxide during respiratory failure in toddlers and infants: end-tidal versus transcutaneous carbon dioxide. *Anesth Analg* 1997;85(1):55–58.
253. Pelucio M, Halligan L, Dhindsa H. Out-of-hospital experience with the syringe esophageal detector device. *Acad Emerg Med* 1997;4(6):563–568.
254. Bozeman WP, Hexter D, Liang HK, Kelen GD. Esophageal detector device versus detection of end-tidal carbon dioxide level in emergency intubation. *Ann Emerg Med* 1996;27(5):595–599.
255. Sharieff GQ, Rodarte A, Wilton N, Silva PD, Bleyle D. The self-inflating bulb as an esophageal detector device in children weighing more than twenty kilograms: A comparison of two techniques. *Ann Emerg Med* 2003;41(5):623–629.
256. Wee MY, Walker AK. The oesophageal detector device: an assessment with uncuffed tubes in children. *Anaesthesia* 1991;46(10):869–871.
257. Williams KN, Nunn JF. The oesophageal detector device: a prospective trial on 100 patients. *Anaesthesia* 1989;44(5):412–424.
258. Zaleski L, Abello D, Gold MI. The esophageal detector device. Does it work? *Anesthesiology* 1993;79(2):244–247.
259. Haynes SR, Morton NS. Use of the oesophageal detector device in children under one year of age. *Anaesthesia* 1990;45(12):1067–1069.
260. Baraka A, Khoury PJ, Siddik SS, Salem MR, Joseph NJ. Efficacy of the self-inflating bulb in differentiating esophageal from tracheal intubation in the parturient undergoing cesarean section. *Anesth Analg* 1997;84(3):533–537.
261. Blanc VF, Tremblay NA. The complications of tracheal intubation: a new classification with a review of the literature. *Anesth Analg* 1974;53(2):202–213.
262. Jones GO, Hale DE, Wasmuth CE, Homi J, Smith ER, Viljoen J. A survey of acute complications associated with endotracheal intubation. *Cleve Clin Q* 1968;35(1):23–31.
263. Taryle DA, Chandler JE, Good JTJ, Potts DE, Sahn SA. Emergency room intubations: complications and survival. *Chest* 1979;75(5):541–543.
264. Thompson DS, Read RC. Rupture of the trachea following endotracheal intubation. *JAMA* 1968;204(11):995–997.
265. Wolff AP, Kuhn FA, Ogura JH. Pharyngeal-esophageal perforations associated with rapid oral endotracheal intubation. *Ann Otol Rhinol Laryngol* 1972;81(2):258–261.
266. Stauffer JL, Petty TL. Accidental intubation of the pyriform sinus: a complication of "roadside" resuscitation. *JAMA* 1977;237(21):2324–2325.
267. Pollard BJ, Junius F. Accidental intubation of the oesophagus. *Anaesth Intens Care* 1980;8(2):183–186.
268. Bernhard WN, Cottrell JE, Sivakumaran C, Patel K, Yost L, Turndorf H. Adjustment of intracuff pressure to prevent aspiration. *Anesthesiology* 1979;50(4):363–366.
269. Nordin U. The trachea and cuff-induced tracheal injury. An experimental study on causative factors and prevention. *Acta Otolaryngol Suppl* 1977;345:1–71.
270. Cheney FW, Posner KL, Caplan RA. Adverse respiratory events infrequently leading to malpractice suits. A closed claims analysis. *Anesthesiology* 1991;75(6):932–939.
271. Cheney FW, Posner K, Caplan RA, Ward RJ. Standard of care and anesthesia liability. *JAMA* 1989;261(11):1599–1603.
272. Caplan RA, Posner KL, Ward RJ, Cheney FW. Adverse respiratory events in anesthesia: a closed claims analysis. *Anesthesiology* 1990;72(5):828–833.
273. Cooper JB, Newbower RS, Kitz RJ. An analysis of major errors and equipment failures in anesthesia management: considerations for prevention and detection. *Anesthesiology* 1984;60(1):34–42.
274. Cooper JB, Newbower RS, Long CD, McPeek B. Preventable anesthesia mishaps: a study of human factors. *Anesthesiology* 1978;49(6):399–406.
275. Cooper JB, Cullen DJ, Nemeskal R, Hoaglin DC, Gevirtz CC, Csete M, Venable C. Effects of information feedback and pulse oximetry on the incidence of anesthesia complications. *Anesthesiology* 1987;67(5):686–694.
276. Cooper JB. Accidents and mishaps in anesthesia: how they occur; how to prevent them. *Minerva Anestesiol* 2001;67(4):310–313.
277. Cooper JB. Towards patient safety in anaesthesia. *Ann Acad Med Singapore* 1994;23(4):552–557.
278. Florete OG. Airway management. In: Civetta JM, Taylor RW, Kirby RR, eds. *Critical Care*. 2nd ed. Philadelphia: Lippincott, 1992:1430–1431.
279. Brantigan CO, Grow JBS. Cricothyroidotomy: elective use in respiratory problems requiring tracheotomy. *J Thorac Cardiovasc Surg* 1976;71(1):72–81.
280. McGill J, Clinton JE, Ruiz E. Cricothyrotomy in the emergency department. *Ann Emerg Med* 1982;11(7):361–364.
281. Simon RR, Brenner BE, Rosen MA. Emergency cricothyroidotomy in the patient with massive neck swelling. Part 2: Clinical aspects. *Crit Care Med* 1983;11(2):119–123.
282. Simon RR, Brenner BE. Emergency cricothyroidotomy in the patient with massive neck swelling: Part 1: Anatomical aspects. *Crit Care Med* 1983;11(2):114–118.

Chapter 17
Oxygen Administration and Supraglottic Airways

Michael Shuster

A first priority in treating any critical patient is assessment of the airway and the establishment of a patent airway if one is not already present. Endotracheal intubation requires skill, competence, and recurrent training. Bag-mask ventilation (BMV) is a fundamental skill of emergency airway management that has been taught to health care providers for more than 40 years, but effective BMV is difficult to perform. Supraglottic airways have been adopted both in and out of hospital because they are associated with ease of training, ease of skill maintenance, effectiveness, and paucity of serious complications.

- Indications and methods of administering supplementary oxygen
- Proper use and technique for supraglottic airways
- Bag-mask versus supraglottic airway versus endotracheal intubation

Supplementary Oxygen

Cardiac Arrest

Ventilation using exhaled air, whether mouth-to-mouth or mouth-to-mask rescue breathing, can deliver only about 16% to 17% inspired oxygen concentration to the patient. Under ideal conditions, this can produce an alveolar oxygen tension of only about 80 mm Hg. In cardiac arrest, metabolic requirements may be reduced, but many factors such as low cardiac output, reduced peripheral oxygen delivery, and a wide arteriovenous oxygen difference or underlying respiratory disease and ventilation–perfusion mismatch can contribute to decreased tissue perfusion. Untreated tissue hypoxia leads to anaerobic metabolism, lactate production, and metabolic acidosis, which will blunt the beneficial effects of chemical and electrical therapy. Continued use of expired air will lead to lower and lower blood oxygen concentrations; therefore health care providers should give supplementary 100% inspired oxygen ($FiO_2 = 1.0$) as soon as it is available.

Myocardial Ischemia

Supplementary oxygen is frequently administered in the care of patients encountered in emergency cardiovascular care. For patients with chest discomfort of possible ischemic origin, the administration of oxygen has become routine practice. There is, however, no evidence that supplemental oxygen has beneficial effect on myocardial ischemia in patients with normal oxygen saturation, and some evidence suggests that supplemental oxygen may potentially cause harm. Hence, administration of oxygen for short periods during assessment of chest discomfort and other life-threatening conditions is prudent, but continuing or long-term administration should be based on clear indications.

A series of studies in the 1960s showed that, in both normal patients and patients with myocardial infarction, high-flow oxygen increased arterial pressure, increased systemic vascular resistance, and when oxygen saturation was >90%, reduced cardiac output.[1–6] In contrast, when arterial oxygen saturations were <90%, oxygen administration increased both oxygen content and cardiac output.[7] In another study, in patients with coronary artery disease, a fall in oxygen saturation to between 70% and 85% produced anaerobic metabolism indicative of myocardial ischemia.[8] In this same study, there was no evidence that hyperoxia relieved myocardial ischemia in patients with coronary artery disease.

FROM THE ACC AHA GUIDELINES

No evidence is available to support the (routine continuing) administration of oxygen to all patients with acute coronary syndromes in the absence of signs of respiratory distress or arterial hypoxemia. Its use based on the evidence base can be limited to those with questionable respiratory status and documented hypoxemia. Nevertheless, it is the opinion of the Writing Committee that a short period of initial routine oxygen supplementation is reasonable during initial stabilization of the patient, given its safety and the potential for underrecognition of hypoxemia.

In 1976, Madias et al. performed precordial ST-segment mapping in a controlled trial of 17 patients and concluded that oxygen administration may reduce ischemic injury; they demonstrated that administration of oxygen to patients experiencing a myocardial infarction may reduce the sum of ST-segment elevations as well as their number.[9–11]

Also in 1976, a randomized, double-blind, controlled trial of oxygen therapy in the first 24 hours of uncomplicated myocardial infarction found that the group of 80 patients receiving 6 L/min of oxygen by mask for the initial 24-hour period had indications of greater myocardial damage than the group of 77 patients receiving room air. There was a greater proportion of deaths in the group receiving oxygen, 9 of 80 (11.3%) versus 3 of 77 (3.9%), but the difference did not reach statistical significance.[12]

A systematic review of the evidence for the use of oxygen to treat acute myocardial ischemia found only nine clinical trials in human subjects (randomized and nonrandomized) and concluded that "any effect of oxygen is likely to be marginal so a suitably powered trial is necessary."[13]

Current guidelines recommend that supplemental oxygen be provided to patients during an initial period of stabilization and evaluation. Oxygen should be continued when oxygen saturation is <90%, but there is little evidence that oxygen is beneficial beyond this period. There is general consensus that, in patients with ongoing myocardial ischemia or signs of respiratory insufficiency or congestive heart failure, oxygen should be continued and oxygen saturation estimated by pulse oximetry or determined by direct arterial measurement.[14,15]

See Web site for AHA guidelines for the management of patients with unstable angina and NSTEMI.

Indications for the method and administration of oxygen are general recommendations and require consideration of patient comfort and ongoing or anticipated patient requirements such as the work of breathing and comorbidity. Pulse oximetry can estimate oxygen saturation and methods of administration can be guided by the degree of hypoxia.

Devices Used to Deliver Supplementary Oxygen

Several devices can be used to deliver supplementary oxygen to patients. Beyond the first minutes of cardiac arrest, tissue hypoxia develops. Additional factors that contribute to hypoxia include intrapulmonary shunting with microcirculatory dysfunction and attendant ventilation–perfusion abnormalities. Some patients may also have underlying respiratory disease. Tissue hypoxia leads to anaerobic metabolism and metabolic acidosis. To improve oxygenation, health care providers should give 100% inspired oxygen (FiO_2 = 1.0) during basic life support and advanced cardiovascular

life support as soon as it becomes available. High inspired oxygen tension will tend to maximize arterial oxygen saturation and, in turn, arterial oxygen content. This will help support oxygen delivery (cardiac output × arterial oxygen content) when cardiac output is limited. This short-term oxygen therapy does not produce oxygen toxicity.

In other patients, supplementary oxygen is given to improve arterial oxygenation and tissue delivery. The amount of oxygen delivered and the method of delivery will depend on several variables. These will include the degree of arterial hypoxemia, underlying condition and airway jeopardy and compromise, respiratory effort, and patient comfort, cooperation, and preference.

Nasal Cannula

The nasal cannula is a simple, comfortable, inexpensive low-flow oxygen administration device which adds oxygen to room air as the patient inspires (Fig. 17-1A). The inspired oxygen concentration will vary widely depending on the oxygen flow rate through the cannula, the patient's tidal volume, and the amount of mouth-breathing. For every 1 L/min increase in the oxygen flow rate, the inspired oxygen concentration increases by approximately 4%, to a maximum flow rate of about 6 L/min. Use of a nasal cannula with rates >4 L/min or for prolonged periods may cause local irritation and drying of mucous membranes.

Face Mask

A simple oxygen face mask delivers oxygen to the patient's nose and mouth. It can deliver a higher concentration of oxygen than is possible with nasal prongs and must be used with a minimum oxygen flow rate of 6 L/min to prevent rebreathing of exhaled carbon dioxide and to maintain increased inspired oxygen concentration. Exhalation ports on either side of the mask allow exhaled air to escape and also allow the patient to entrain room air during inspiration. A flow rate of 6 to 10 L/min is required to deliver an inspired oxygen concentration of 35% to 60%, but the actual concentration delivered is highly dependent on the fit of the mask and the patient's spontaneous rate of breathing and tidal volume.

Face Mask with Oxygen Reservoir

Adding an oxygen reservoir bag (200 mL) to the face mask makes available higher oxygen concentrations at lower flow rates than are possible with a simple face mask (Fig. 17-1B). A mask with an oxygen reservoir can be either a partial rebreathing mask or a nonrebreathing mask. With a partial rebreathing mask, the first 200 mL of exhaled air flows into the reservoir bag and combines with fresh oxygen flowing into the reservoir, while the remainder of the exhaled gas is expelled through the exhalation ports. Since the initial portion of exhaled gas comes from the upper airway and is not involved in gas exchange, the oxygen concentration in the reservoir remains high. During inspiration, the inspired air will initially come from the bag and

PART FOUR • AIRWAY MANAGEMENT IN BASIC AND ADVANCED LIFE SUPPORT

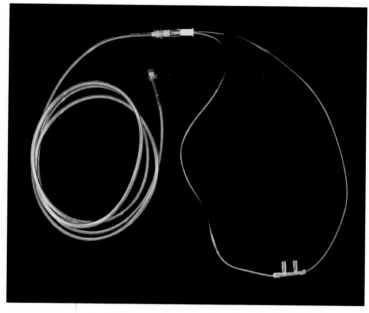

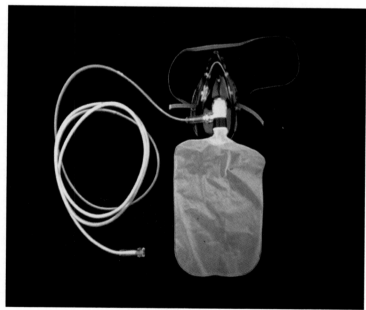

FIGURE 17-1 • Airway adjunct devices. **A.** Nasal cannula. **B.** Face mask.

the fresh oxygen inflow. If the oxygen flow rate is maintained above the patient's minute ventilation and the mask fits securely, an oxygen concentration of 60% to 80% can be achieved. To assess the adequacy of oxygen flow, water mist may be added to the oxygen with a humidifier; thus the mist can be watched to escape from the exhalation ports of the mask during both inspiration and expiration. If mist does not escape during inspiration, room air is being entrained by the patient, effectively reducing the inspired oxygen concentration.

A nonrebreathing mask incorporates a valve into one or both exhalation ports to prevent room air from being entrained during inspiration. In addition, a valve between the reservoir bag and the mask prevents flow of exhaled gas into the reservoir. During inspiration, the patient draws air from the reservoir bag being filled by oxygen inflow. Each 1

L/min of increase in oxygen flow >6 L/min will increase the inspired oxygen concentration by 10%. If oxygen inflow is adjusted to prevent collapse of the reservoir bag (flow rates of 10–15 L/min), inspired oxygen concentrations of 90% to 95% can be achieved provided that the mask is well sealed.

Venturi Mask

The Venturi mask system entrains air into the mask at a specific ratio by passing oxygen through a calibrated opening under pressure. By varying the calibration of the opening, the Venturi mask delivers a reliable oxygen concentration of 24% to 50% as long as the flow rate specified for each caliber of opening is maintained.

Airway Adjuncts

Assessing and Establishing a Patent Airway

The first priority in treating any critical patient is assessment of the airway and the establishment of a patent airway if one is not already present.

The first priority in treating any critically ill patient is assessment of the airway and the establishment of a patent airway if one is not already present. Without adequate ventilation and oxygenation, circulation cannot be sustained. In the conscious patient, upper airway patency can be compromised by obstruction from a swollen tongue or the soft tissues surrounding the airway, from dentures or other foreign body, or by excessive bleeding or secretions (Fig. 17-2). Obtundation, cyanosis, agitation, retractions, and stridorous or snoring respirations may all be signs of airway or ventilatory compromise. In the unconscious patient, upper airway obstruction results from loss of tone in the submandibular muscles which provide direct support to the tongue and indirect support to the epiglottis. Airway patency is often established simply by repositioning the head and neck but the maneuver may also require chin lift or jaw thrust and insertion of an oropharyngeal or nasopharyngeal airway.

Once airway patency and ventilations are established, consideration must be given to the patient's ability to protect against aspiration of gastric contents, which can produce significant morbidity and mortality. There is no evidence that the presence of the gag reflex corresponds to airway protective reflexes.[17] A gag reflex is an unreliable indicator of the ability to protect the airway as it may be absent in as many as 22% to 37% of normal adults.[16,17] The ability of the patient to swallow may be a more reliable indicator, but this is untested. In general, if a maneuver is needed to establish a patent airway, intubation should be considered.

Suspected Cervical Spine or Facial Injury

Airway control and breathing remain top priorities in caring for patients with facial trauma or with suspected cervical spine injury, but the approach to airway management must be altered to minimize the potential for causing inadvertent harm through treatment. Although there is no published case of a spinal cord injury as a result of airway management, the potential for serious cord injury exists. Spine injury should be suspected on the basis of the type and mechanism of injury, and in the presence of any suggestive injury (face, head, neck, multiple trauma) that is apparent. Airway control should be established with in-line stabilization of the neck without a head tilt, using a jaw thrust or chin lift. With the head maintained in the neutral position by one rescuer and protected from excessive flexion, extension, or lateral movement, a second rescuer should perform whatever interventions are required to open the airway and ensure adequate ventilation (Fig. 17-3).

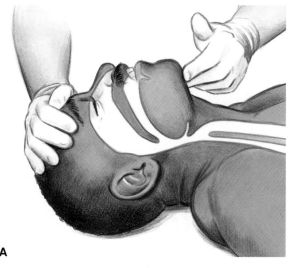

A

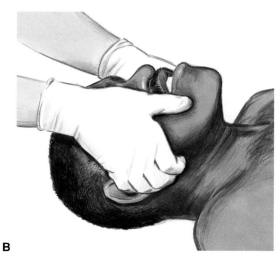

B

FIGURE 17-3 • **A.** Head tilt–chin lift. **B.** Jaw thrust without head tilt.

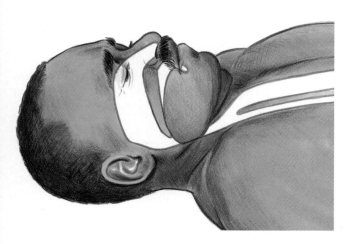

FIGURE 17-2 • Obstruction by the tongue and epiglottis.

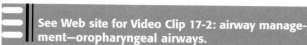

See Web site for Video Clip 17-1: airway management—opening airway C-spine injury suspected

General Considerations

The patient who is immobilized on his or her back, even if airway reflexes are intact, may not be able to cope with excessive salivation or oral bleeding. Suction should be immediately available if required and consideration should be given to how the patient might be safely turned to the side if necessary.

If the patient is breathing spontaneously but unable to protect the airway or if ventilation must be controlled, an advanced airway should be established. Endotracheal or nasotracheal intubation were formerly the only options for advanced airway control short of cricothyrotomy, but excellent options now exist with the availability of supraglottic airways. Endotracheal intubation requires enough space behind the head for the rescuer to work and a sufficient view of the glottis to be able to direct the tube. Endotracheal intubation may be extremely difficult in a patient where limited movement of the head and neck is possible and where bleeding or secretions may obscure the visual field. "Blind" nasotracheal intubation, once recommended only for expert providers, is rarely considered any longer: the failed insertion rate is high and the complications are frequent and significant. Nasotracheal intubation can shear off turbinates, cause major nasal bleeding, or be misdirected into the brain or the retropharyngeal tissues.

Supraglottic airways such as the Combitube or the laryngeal tube are considered to provide excellent protection from aspiration because of the dual cuffs sealing the airway from contamination from above and protecting the airway from regurgitated stomach contents from below. The laryngeal mask airway (LMA), once thought not to provide protection from regurgitation, has not been shown to increase the risk of aspiration compared with face-mask ventilation. The supraglottic airways may be inserted with the rescuer in any position relative to the patient, and insertion requires little or no movement of the head and neck.

Maintaining a Patent Airway with an Airway Adjunct

Oropharyngeal Airway

When submandibular muscles relax while a person is in a recumbent position, the tongue falls against the posterior pharyngeal wall and may obstruct the pharynx. The oropharyngeal airway (OPA) is designed to create a conduit through the oropharynx and posterior pharynx, keeping the airway open. The OPA is a rigid, comma-shaped device that has either a hollow inner channel or a solid core and hollow side channels (Fig. 17-4). Because the placement of the OPA stimulates the posterior pharynx, its use should be reserved for the *unconscious and unresponsive patient with no cough or gag reflex*. There are three methods for placing the OPA: (1) invert the device and rotate it into place when it reaches the posterior pharynx, or (2) turn the device 90 degrees and rotate it into place when it reaches the posterior pharynx, or (3) insert it directly by following the curve of the tongue, with or without the help of a tongue depressor. Whichever technique is chosen, care must be taken not to push the tongue into the posterior pharynx, thus causing airway obstruction. If there are problems ventilating the patient after insertion of the OPA, the device should be removed and reinserted. Although studies have not specifically addressed use of the OPA in cardiac arrest, clinical experience shows that it may aid ventilation with a bag-mask device by preventing the tongue from occluding the airway.

See Web site for Video Clip 17-2: airway management—oropharyngeal airways.

Nasopharyngeal Airway

The nasopharyngeal airway (NPA) is a soft rubber, Silastic, or plastic hollow tube that is inserted through the nose to the posterior pharynx, creating an opening

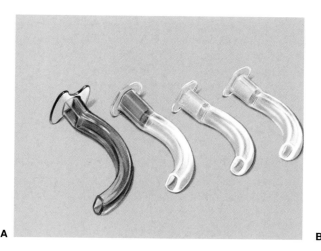

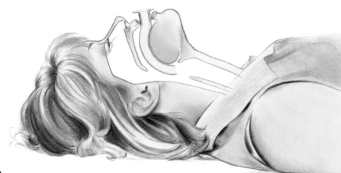

A   B

FIGURE 17-4 • Oropharyngeal airways. **A.** Four oropharyngeal airway devices. **B.** One oropharyngeal airway device inserted.

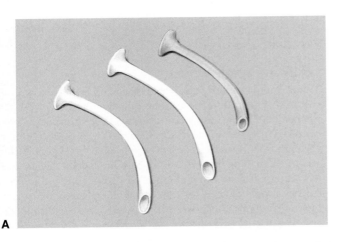

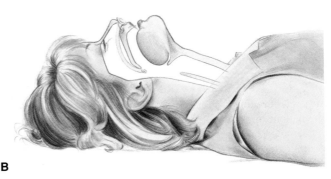

A   **B**

FIGURE 17-5 • Nasopharyngeal airways. **A.** Three nasopharyngeal airway devices. **B.** One nasopharyngeal airway device inserted.

between the tongue and posterior pharyngeal wall (Fig. 17-5). NPAs are particularly useful when conditions such as a clenched jaw prevent placement of an OPA. NPAs are less likely than OPAs to stimulate the gag reflex, so are a better choice in patients who are not deeply unconscious. In studies of anesthetized patients, 5% to 30% have bleeding with insertion of an NPA.[18,19] To minimize or prevent bleeding, care must be taken to first lubricate the NPA well, then insert the airway with the beveled edge facing the septum pushing it into the nares while rotating the airway once it has passed the cartilaginous area of the septum, and directing it along the floor of the nose until the flared end of the NPA is against the nasal orifice. If available, a vasoconstricting nasal spray administered before placement may be helpful. Particular care must be taken when placing the NPA in patients with craniofacial injury: inadvertent intracranial placement of an NPA in patients with basilar skull fracture has been described in four case reports.[20–23]

As with all adjunctive equipment, safe use of the NPA requires adequate training, practice, and retraining. Although studies have not specifically addressed the use of the NPA in cardiac arrest, clinical experience shows that it may aid ventilation with a bag-mask device by preventing the tongue from occluding the airway.

> See Web site for Video Clip 17-3: airway management—nasopharyngeal airway.

Suctioning

Regurgitation is a frequent occurrence in cardiac arrest, and survival to hospital discharge after aspiration of regurgitated materials is very low.[24] Suctioning is thus an essential aspect of airway management. Either a portable or installed suction device should be immediately available for resuscitation emergencies. An installed suction unit should be powerful enough to provide an airflow of >40 L/min at the end of the delivery tube and a vacuum of >300 mm Hg when the tube is clamped. The amount of suction should be adjustable to allow for use in children and intubated patients.

Portable units should provide vacuum pressure and flow that is adequate for pharyngeal suction. The suction device should be fitted with large-bore, nonkinking suction tubing and semirigid pharyngeal tips of sufficient size to suction thick fluids and large particulate matter. Also, suction units must be checked regularly and maintained. When 51 paramedics from nine paramedic units were anonymously surveyed, 26 paramedics (51%) reported difficulties with the portable suction equipment. The difficulty most commonly cited (21 times) was clogging of the tubing as a result of thick emesis. Poor suction power and battery problems were cited 13 times. As a result of frequent problems with portable suction units, some emergency medical services (EMS) systems may choose to carry both a battery-operated device and a manual hand-operated suction pump.[25]

Both soft flexible and rigid suctioning catheters are available. *Rigid catheters* (e.g., Yankauer) are used to suction the oropharynx. These are better for suctioning thick secretions and particulate matter (Fig. 17-6). *Soft, flexible catheters* may be used in the mouth or nose. They can also be used for deep suctioning with an endotracheal (ET) tube. Soft, flexible catheters come in sterile wrappers.

> See Web site for Video Clip 17-4: airway management—suctioning.

Several methods can be used to suction the upper airway and trachea. Central to each of these is the prevention both of hypoxia during the procedure and stimulation of reflexes leading to bradycardia and hypotension. Care must

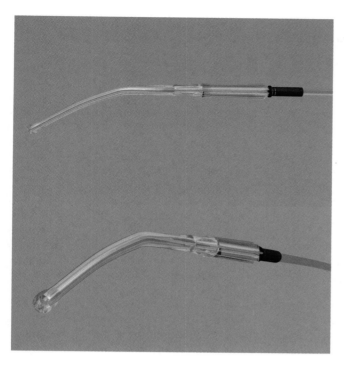

FIGURE 17-6 • Rigid catheter. Rigid catheters (e.g., Yankauer) are used to suction the oropharynx. These are better for suctioning thick secretions and particulate matter.

| TABLE 17-2 • Endotracheal Tube Suctioning Procedure

Step	Action
1	Use sterile technique to reduce the likelihood of airway contamination.
2	Gently insert the catheter into the ET tube. Be sure the side opening is not occluded during insertion. Insertion of the catheter beyond the tip of the ET tube is not recommended because it may injure the endotracheal mucosa or stimulate coughing or bronchospasm.
3	Apply suction by occluding only the side opening while withdrawing the catheter with a rotating or twisting motion. **Suction attempts should not exceed 10 seconds.** To avoid hypoxemia, precede and follow suctioning attempts with a short period of administration of 100% oxygen. To help remove thick mucus or other material from the airway, instill 1 or 2 mL of sterile saline into the airway before suctioning. Provide positive-pressure ventilation to disperse the saline throughout the airways for maximum effect before suctioning.

be taken to prevent damage to the airway structures. During the procedure, the patient's heart rate, pulse, oxygen saturation, and clinical appearance during suctioning should be monitored. If bradycardia develops, oxygen saturation drops, or the patient's clinical appearance deteriorates, suctioning must be interrupted at once. High-flow oxygen is then administered until the heart rate returns to normal and the patient's clinical condition improves. Ventilation is assisted as needed.

One method for suctioning the oropharynx and trachea through an endotracheal tube is given in Tables 17-1 and 17-2.

| TABLE 17-1 • Oropharyngeal Suctioning Procedure

Step	Action
1	Gently insert the suction catheter or device into the oropharynx beyond the tongue. Measure the catheter before suctioning and do not insert it any further than the estimated distance from the tip of the nose to the earlobe.
2	Apply suction by occluding the side opening while withdrawing the catheter with a rotating or twisting motion. **Typically limit suction attempts to 10 seconds or less.** To avoid hypoxemia, precede and follow suctioning attempts with a short period of administration of 100% oxygen.

Mouth-to-Barrier Device (Face Shield, Tube, or Mask)

For many years, mouth-to-mouth ventilation has been taught as the basic rescue ventilation technique. Mouth-to-barrier-device has now superseded mouth-to-mouth as the basic ventilation technique recommended for training and for resuscitation, because the interposition of a protective barrier between rescuer and patient addresses a concern that rescuers may have about disease transmission. Although the risk of contagion is very low—there are only 15 reported cases of possible disease transmission during CPR and none during CPR training—surveys of both health care providers and the lay public have repeatedly cited the concern of contagion as a factor affecting the respondent's expressed willingness to perform mouth-to-mouth ventilation.[26–34] While the interposition of a barrier device is likely to be more aesthetically pleasing to potential rescuers and will perhaps reduce their fears of contagion, whether rescuers actually undertake CPR more often when the device is available is unknown. Clearly, though, a barrier device can increase the likelihood of CPR performance only if health care providers and other potential rescuers carry such a device with them at all times.

The three types of barrier devices are face shields, tubes, and masks (Fig. 17-7). The devices are typically plastic, they may be disposable or reusable, and they often incorporate a unidirectional valve that will direct the victim's expired air away from the rescuer. In addition, a one-way valve is available that fits to the inlet of a regular face mask,

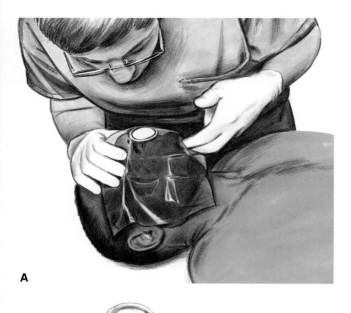

A

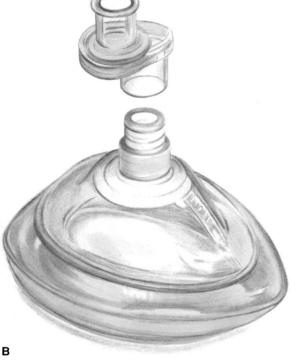

B

FIGURE 17-7 • **A.** Face shield. Place the face shield over the victim's mouth and nose, positioning the opening at the center of the shield over the victim's mouth. The technique of rescue breathing with a barrier device is the same as that for mouth-to-mouth breathing. **B.** Pocket face mask.

so that the mask may be used for mouth-to-mask or bag-mask ventilation. Each of the devices has its own performance characteristics, and effectiveness in protecting against infection transmission varies from device to device. Drawbacks associated with some devices include the creation of inspiratory or expiratory resistance and valve leak-

age. One study that tested a variety of barrier devices found that few of them had low inspiratory and expiratory resistances and that some of the one-way valves failed.[35] In another study, where cultures were performed after mock CPR, none of the masks with one-way valves were culture-positive but one of three face shields that incorporated a one-way valve was culture positive and five of five face shields that did not have a one-way valve were contaminated with the victim's oral aerobic flora.[36] It has not been proven that a barrier device will prevent disease transmission in real-world use, and, given the very low rate of disease transmission that has been reported, it is unlikely that effectiveness will be established.

Mouth-to-barrier ventilation, like mouth-to-mouth ventilation, relies on the rescuer's expired air to ventilate the victim. Most rescuers will have the vital capacity necessary to provide the 5 to 6 L/min of air required for lung inflation but will be able to provide only 17% oxygen, which is the approximate concentration of oxygen in expired air. If an oxygen source is available, the rescuer should wear a nasal cannula or should breathe from the oxygen source between rescue breaths. As soon as possible, the rescuer should switch to a barrier device that has an oxygen inlet, a bag-mask device with attached oxygen, or some other airway adjunct that will allow for the administration supplementary oxygen.

Both tube and face-shield devices fit adults of all sizes, but any given mask fits people only within a particular size range, so the rescuer must have masks of different sizes available. If a mask is too big or too small for the given patient, an air leak will occur, which may reduce the effectiveness of ventilation. A leak can often be tolerated, however, since a full breath often provides more air than is required. The mouth-to-mask technique is easier than bag-mask ventilation, since the rescuer is able to use two hands to correctly elevate the mandible, position the head, and seal the mask to the face. Studies on manikins have found that mouth-to-mask ventilation is capable of delivering significantly larger tidal volumes than bag-mask ventilation, and a similar study on patients after induction of anesthesia endorsed mouth-to-mask ventilation for its ease of use by inexperienced operators.[37–40] No matter which barrier device is used, adequate training is important to ensure effective ventilation.[41]

Pocket face masks can be used effectively by a provider who is trained in their use and effectively maintains an open airway. Most have side ports for the administration of oxygen. (Fig. 17-8).

Bag-Mask Devices

See Web site for **Video Clip 17-5: airway management—details of bag mask.**

Bag-mask ventilation (BMV) is a fundamental skill of emergency airway management that has been taught to health care providers as part of both basic and advanced airway management for more than 40 years. Effective BMV is difficult to perform: in several studies, both inexperienced and experienced providers delivered inadequate tidal volumes

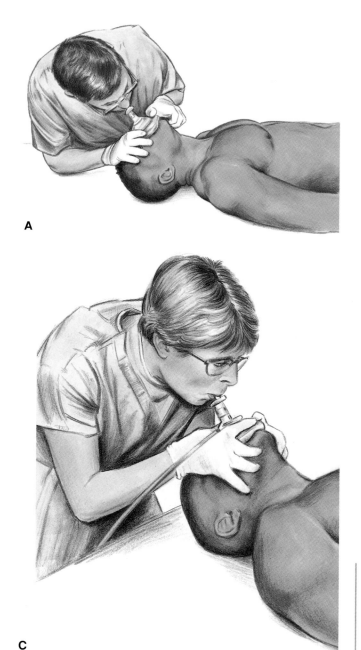

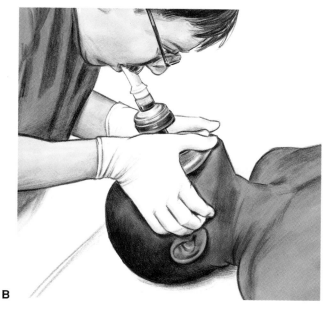

FIGURE 17-8 • **A.** Pocket face mask, lateral technique. **B.** Pocket face mask, cephalic technique. The rescuer places the thumb and thenar eminence on top of the mask. **C.** Pocket face mask, cephalic technique with oxygen tube attached. The rescuer uses the "E-C" technique (the "E" is formed by the three fingers and the "C" is formed by the thumb and first finger curving around the face mask).

when tested on manikins.[42–48] When tested on anesthetized subjects, where the face is more malleable and the lungs are more compliant than in a manikin, ventilation with a bag-mask is still frequently inadequate: in a study of BMV use by 30 inexperienced nurses, the tidal volume averaged only 239 mL.[49] In another study, 10 nurses were able to adequately ventilate 100 patients only 43% of the time.[50] Ventilation is unlikely to be performed any better under resuscitation conditions than it is under the controlled conditions of a study.

In order to provide effective ventilation with a bag-mask, the head, neck, and mandible must be positioned so that the tongue does not obstruct the airway and a correctly sized mask must then be chosen so that a tight seal of the mask to the face can be achieved (Fig. 17-9). Next, the bag

must be squeezed in a deliberate, consistent manner over 1 second so as to avoid high inspiratory pressures and thus prevent gastric inflation. Each of these steps may pose difficulty. The head must be tilted back and maintained in neutral or slightly extended position while pulling the jaw forward and pressing the mask down, all with one hand, while the second hand must hold and squeeze the bag (Fig. 17-9A, Table 17-3A). If the patient is edentulous or bearded, the mask seal will be more difficult to achieve. Maintaining a seal in the back of a moving ambulance can be especially challenging.

To improve the mask seal and ensure that the hand squeezing the bag is large enough to hold and compress a sufficient volume of air from the bag, an effective strategy

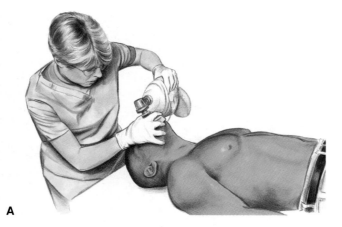

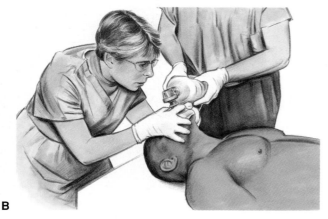

FIGURE 17-9 • **A.** Mouth-to-mask E-C clamp technique of holding mask while lifting the jaw. Position yourself at the victim's head. Circle the thumb and first finger around the top of the mask (forming a "C") while using the third, fourth, and fifth fingers (forming an "E") to lift the jaw. **B.** Two-rescuer use of the bag mask. The rescuer at the victim's head tilts the victim's head and seals the mask against the victim's face with the thumb and first finger of each hand creating a "C" to provide a complete seal around the edges of the mask. The rescuer uses the remaining three fingers (the "E") to lift the jaw (this holds the airway open). The second rescuer slowly squeezes the bag (over 1 second) until the chest rises. Both rescuers should observe chest rise.

is for one rescuer to open the airway and seal the mask using both hands, while a second rescuer uses both hands to squeeze the bag. Two rescuers may provide more effective ventilation than one rescuer. When two rescuers use the bag-mask system, one rescuer opens the airway with a head tilt and jaw lift and holds the mask to the face while the other rescuer squeezes the bag (Fig. 17-9B, Table 17-3B). Squeezing the bag requires minimal explanation and can typically be performed even by untrained assistants.

Techniques for holding the mask are the same as those for the mouth-to-mask devices described above.[51–55]

Peak inspiratory pressure is a key factor causing gastric inflation, which in turn results in increased pulmonary compliance and hypoinflation of the lungs and an

| TABLE 17-3A • One-Hand Mask Hold

Step	Action
1	Position yourself directly above the patient's head.
2	Place the mask on the patient's face, using the bridge of the nose as a guide for correct position.
3	Use the E-C clamp technique to hold the mask in place while you lift the jaw to hold the airway open: • Perform a head tilt. • Use the thumb and index finger of one hand to make a "C," pressing the edges of the mask to the face. • Use the remaining fingers to lift the angles of the jaw (three fingers form an "E") and open the airway.
4	Squeeze the bag to give breaths (1 second each) while watching for chest rise. The delivery of breaths is the same whether you use supplementary oxygen or not.

See Web site for Video Clips 17-6 and 17-7: airway management—ventilation by one provider with bag-mask device and ventilation by two providers with bag-mask device.

| TABLE 17-3B • Two-Hand Mask Hold

Step	Action
1	Position yourself directly above the patient's head.
2	Place the mask on the patient's face, using the bridge of the nose as a guide for correct position.
3	Use either of these techniques: • Lift the patient's head and seal the mask against the patient's face with the thumb and first finger of each hand, creating a "C" to provide a complete seal around the edges of the mask. Use the remaining three fingers of both hands (the "E") to lift the jaw. • Hold the mask in place with the thumb and the thenar prominence of the palm of the hands; use the remaining four fingers of both hands to lift the chin and open the airway.
4	Squeeze the bag to give breaths (1 second each) while watching for chest rise. The delivery of breaths is the same whether you use supplementary oxygen or not.

increased incidence of regurgitation.[56] It is possible to limit peak inspiratory pressure by controlling tidal volume, flow rate, and inflation time and maintaining an unobstructed airway: a bench study comparing a pediatric bag (700 mL) to an adult bag (1,500 mL) showed that the former produced comparable lung tidal volumes (245 ± 19 versus 271 ± 33 mL; P = NS); but a significantly ($P <$ 0.001) lower gastric tidal volume (149 ± 11 versus 272 ± 24 mL).[57]

A study comparing the two bag sizes for ventilating adult patients undergoing anesthesia found that the pediatric bag resulted in less mean exhaled tidal volume (365 ± 55 versus 779 ± 22 mL; $P <$ 0.0001), lower peak airway pressure (20 ± 2 versus 25 ± 5 cm H_2O; $P <$ 0.0001), and comparable oxygen saturation (97% ± 1% versus 98 ± 1%; NS); no patients experienced stomach inflation, whereas 5 of 40 patients ventilated with an adult bag did experience stomach inflation (P = 0.054).[58] It should be noted, however, that when small volumes are used to ventilate, oxygen saturation can be maintained only when supplemental oxygen is provided.[59] An advanced airway should be considered if the device can be inserted without significantly disrupting compressions.

Cricoid Pressure Cricoid pressure is widely used as a technique to reduce gastric inflation and prevent vomiting and regurgitation in patients undergoing rapid sequence induction and for resuscitation when being ventilated with a bag-mask.[60–64]

Cricoid pressure is intended to displace the trachea posteriorly, causing the cricoid cartilage to compress the esophagus against the vertebrae, providing a barrier both to air being pushed down the esophagus into the stomach and stomach contents being pushed up and out of the esophagus (Fig. 17-10). Bag-mask ventilation, which produces only moderate peak inspiratory pressure, can still cause gastric inflation, which then predisposes to vomiting and regurgitation.[65] Vomiting is a negative predictor of survival in cardiac arrest.[66] When cricoid pressure is applied to anesthetized adults or children during bag-mask ventilation, even high peak inspiratory pressures do not cause gastric inflation.[65,67,68] However, a recent review of the literature failed to find confirmation that cricoid pressure is safe or evidence that it is an effective technique to decrease the risk of aspiration in rapid sequence induction.[69] While cricoid pressure sounds easy to apply, studies show that it is difficult to estimate the optimal recommended pressure (30–44 newtons).[70–73] If too little pressure is used, the esophagus is incompletely occluded, while too much pressure can distort the airway and make ventilation more difficult or impossible. In a review of cricoid pressure for emergency department rapid sequence intubation, Ellis notes that in 10 studies, functional occlusion of the airway occurred between 6% and 50% of the time and that two studies of cricoid pressure observed cases of airway obstruction with the application of cricoid pressure.[74] In the absence of evidence, it seems reasonable to apply cricoid pressure in patients requiring manual ventilation whenever there are sufficient rescuers available. However,

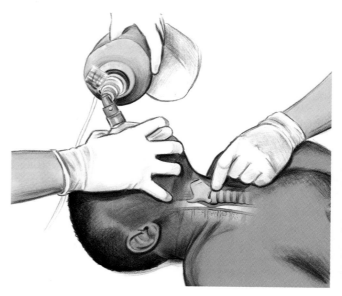

FIGURE 17-10 • Cricoid pressure, or Sellick's technique, is the application of pressure to the *unresponsive* patient's cricoid cartilage. The pressure is intended to push the trachea posteriorly, compressing the esophagus against the cervical vertebra. Cricoid pressure is effective in preventing gastric inflation during positive-pressure ventilation of *unresponsive* patients. Step 1: Locate the thyroid cartilage (Adam's apple) with your index finger. Step 2: Slide your index finger to the base of the thyroid cartilage and palpate the prominent horizontal ring below the thyroid cartilage (this is the cricoid cartilage). Step 3: Using the tips of your thumb and index finger, apply firm backward pressure to the cricoid cartilage.

when performing bag-mask ventilation in conjunction with cricoid pressure, the pressure should be adjusted, relaxed or released if it impedes ventilation. Cricoid pressure in conjuction with laryngoscopy may make visualization of the vocal cords more difficult, and although there is little hard evidence, some studies have attributed failed intubation to cricoid pressure.[75,76] When intubating while applying cricoid pressure, the pressure should be maintained until the endotracheal tube is passed through the cords unless the pressure interferes with intubation, in which case cricoid pressure can be relaxed or released.

See Web site for Video Clip 17-8: airway management—cricoid pressure.

Ventilation with Supraglottic Airways

Use of Bag-Mask versus Advanced Airway

Bag-mask ventilation has long been considered a temporizing maneuver until either the patient was able to protect the airway and to breathe independently or a definitive airway—endotracheal intubation—was employed. Bag-mask ventilation was taught to virtually all health care providers, while only anesthetists at first, and then other physicians, and then specific categories of nonphysicians were permitted to perform endotracheal intubation (ETI). While BMV is certainly easier to perform than endotracheal intubation, it is clearly not without problems: not only do rescuers have difficulty delivering adequate ventilation with a bag-mask, but the bag-mask is difficult to use in certain physical situations (e.g., trapped in a car in a ditch or in a small overcrowded elevator) or with certain body types (edentulous, bearded). Other serious disadvantages of BMV are the need to interrupt chest compressions during CPR and the increased likelihood of regurgitation.

Recent studies suggest that not only advanced providers but also basic providers can safely use supraglottic airways in place of ETI and BMV. In a multicenter prospective observational trial, nurses successfully used the LMA as the primary ventilation method in 56 of 164 (34%) patients and in 144 of 164 (88%) patients overall. The authors note that regurgitation occurred in 20 patients before LMA insertion (BMV had been used in 17 of 20) and in 3 cases during LMA use (BMV had been used in all three cases).[77] In another prospective trial, 797 cardiac arrests occurring over 3.5 years were examined. The regurgitation rate was 12.4% when BMV was the primary method of ventilation followed by endotracheal intubation, 11.8% when BMV was the primary method of ventilation followed by LMA, and 3.5% when LMA was the primary airway adjunct used.[78]

No prospective randomized trials have directly assessed the outcome of adult victims of cardiac arrest after bag-mask ventilation compared to those who had been treated with an advanced airway. Studies comparing outcomes of out-of-hospital cardiac arrest in adults treated by either emergency medical technicians or paramedics failed to show a link between long-term survival rates and various paramedic skills, including intubation.[79,80] One prospective randomized, controlled trial in an EMS system with short out-of-hospital transport intervals showed no survival advantage for endotracheal intubation over bag-mask ventilation in children where providers had limited training and experience in intubation.[81]

Endotracheal intubation, once considered the optimal method of managing an airway in cardiac arrest, is no longer an automatic intervention. The change is due to the increasing recognition that the failure and complication rates of ETI are high, especially when performed by less experienced or less practiced practitioners, that adequate practitioner-training is time- and labor-intensive, and that many trained rescuers get inadequate experience with the device.[82–84] Trials of supraglottic airways have demonstrated that they can be successfully used by all levels of providers.[85–87]

Supraglottic airways are quickly being adopted both in and out of hospital because they are associated with ease of training, ease of skill maintenance, effectiveness, and paucity of serious complications.[88] Despite the positive aspects of these newer advanced airway devices, insertion can be difficult, failure can occur and practitioners must maintain their insertion skills through frequent experience or practice.[88] The optimal method of managing the airway during any particular cardiac arrest will vary according to provider experience, the characteristics of the EMS or health care system, and the patient's condition.

Supraglottic Airways

"Supraglottic airway" is a term used to describe any airway that is "above the glottis"—the glottis, of course, being the space between the vocal cords. Supraglottic airways may also be referred to as "extraglottic" devices[89] and are distinct from the endotracheal tube, which passes through the glottis to lie within the trachea. Although there is a long list of these devices, only a few have been studied in resuscitation.

While the endotracheal tube is an effective airway, significant complications, including death, occur as a result of its use.[90,91] Practitioners require considerable training and experience to become proficient in inserting the endotracheal tube as well as significant ongoing experience and practice to maintain their skills. There is a high failure rate in the hands of those who are less skilled or practiced.[92,93] Supraglottic airways were originally developed to avoid the problems of the endotracheal tube, and new versions continue to be developed in an effort to find the perfect airway.

The perfect airway for use in resuscitation would be easy to insert in all patients and in all situations on the first attempt. The user would require little or no training to be proficient at insertion and would require no practice to maintain insertion skills. The device itself would be an inexpensive, single-use device that could effectively maintain airway patency and provide a conduit for ventilation regardless of the size of the patient, the pressures required to ventilate, or the presence of anatomic anomalies. This ideal airway would be easy to secure so it stayed in place during CPR and patient transport, yet its presence would not damage the tissues, and it would protect against aspiration. The perfect airway does not yet exist. More than 25 supraglottic devices have so far been described and others are no doubt in development.

In an attempt to organize thinking about supraglottic airways, Miller has proposed a classification of these devices according to their sealing mechanism: cuffed perilaryngeal sealers (CPLS), cuffed pharyngeal sealers (CPS), and cuffless anatomically preshaped sealers (CAPS).[94] This classification is especially useful in a discussion about resuscitation, since the sealing mechanism of the supraglottic airway has implications for stability of the device during CPR and for protection from aspiration. The CAPS are the newest of the three classes of devices, and their use has been reported in resuscitation only once.[95] Initial reports of CAPS make them appear promising as airways, but their role in resuscitation has yet to be defined.

Since the AHA's 2000 guidelines regarding emergency cardiovascular care (ECC), both the laryngeal mask airway (LMA) (a cuffed perilaryngeal sealer device) and the Combitube (a cuffed pharyngeal sealer) have been recommended for use in resuscitation, initially as an alternative to bag-valve-mask ventilation and then in the AHA's 2005 Guidelines also as an alternative to the endotracheal tube.[96]

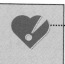
See Web site for AHA guidelines on airway interventions: Supraglottis Airways

Laryngeal Mask Airway

A laryngeal mask airway (LMA) is an advanced airway device that is an acceptable alternative to the endotracheal tube (ETT). The LMA is composed of a tube with a cuffed mask-like projection at the end of the tube (Fig. 17-11).

The LMA was designed by British anesthesiologist Archie Brain (and called the Brain airway); it has been used in general anesthesia since 1988.[97,98] Its chief advantages over bag-mask ventilation are that once it is inserted, it can be left in place and used "hands free" by a minimally trained rescuer to maintain a reliable conduit for ventilation. The LMA is designed to be inserted "blindly," without use of a laryngoscope and without visualization of the vocal cords, so it can be quicker and easier to insert than the endotracheal tube, with less extensive training needed to develop competence. Another major advantage of the LMA is that it can be inserted without interrupting cardiopulmonary resuscitation. The LMA may also have advantages over the endotracheal tube when access to the patient is limited,[99,100] when the patient may have an unstable neck injury,[101] or when some other factor makes it impossible to appropriately position the patient for endotracheal intubation.

See Web site for Video Clips 17-9 and 17-10: airway management—LMA details and LMA insertion technique.

The LMA has been studied extensively in anesthesia as well as in direct comparison to bag-mask ventilation, to endotracheal intubation, and to ventilation with other devices. In randomized controlled trials (RCTs) on anesthetized patients, the LMA is generally as easy or more easy to insert as compared with the endotracheal tube, whether the users are experienced[102–106] physicians, nurses, respiratory therapists, or EMS personnel. Inexperienced personnel were also quickly and easily taught to successfully insert the device into anesthetized patients in RCTs comparing the LMA to bag-mask ventilation or another alternate airway (not compared with the ETT).[50,85,107–111]

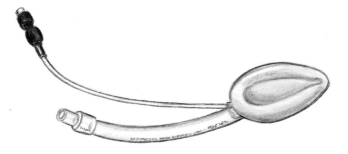

| FIGURE 17-11 • Laryngeal mask airway.

It is important that novice users or users with limited ongoing experience be able to use the airway quickly, reliably, and safely. In nonrandomized studies of patients undergoing resuscitation, novice users successfully performed intubation and ventilation with LMA in a high proportion of adult patients.[112–117] In a pseudorandomized study comparing the LMA to bag-mask ventilation and to the Combitube, successful insertion and ventilation was accomplished in 73% of patients randomized to LMA compared with 86% of patients randomized to Combitube.[118]

The idea of using the LMA in resuscitation was initially treated skeptically because the LMA does not fully seal the airway. However, studies have not shown an increased incidence of aspiration with the LMA. In RCTs with anesthetized patients, there was no reflux on intubation or with intermittent positive pressure ventilation (IPPV) with the LMA as compared with four cases with the ETT ($P = 0.11$).[119] There was no gastric distention[120] and no aspiration when tested with methylene blue.[121]

Resuscitation studies have yielded results similar to those of the anesthesia studies with regard to aspiration. In a multicenter study of cardiac arrest ventilatory management by RNs in 164 patients, regurgitation was observed in 20 patients before the LMA was inserted and in three patients during LMA use. In only one case (not involving LMA use) was there clinical evidence of aspiration. Where the LMA was inserted mainly by junior anesthesia staff with no previous experience in its use in a series of 50 cardiac arrest cases, the LMA was inserted successfully in 98% of the patients and no signs of regurgitation or aspiration were detected.[114] In a study of 797 patients in cardiac arrest, when the LMA was used as the first-line airway management device, the incidence of regurgitation was significantly less than when bag-mask ventilation was used first (3.5% versus 12.3%; $P <0.05$).[78]

All of the resuscitation studies carried out with the LMA have used the LMA Classic (a reusable airway) or the LMA Unique (a single-use airway). In resuscitation, particularly in prehospital resuscitation, a single-use device is preferable to a reusable device because of the difficulty in storing then cleaning a soiled airway and the possibility of transmission of infection. Other LMA models, such as the LMA Fastrach (a reusable LMA designed to allow intubation through the LMA) or the LMA Supreme (a single-use LMA with built-in gastric access) have not been studied in resuscitation. Anyone contemplating using these alternative LMAs should carefully review their characteristics. The ability to perform endotracheal intubation without removing the LMA or the addition of a gastric vent may seem to be desirable, but these features must be weighed against the possibility that such alternative LMAs will be more difficult to insert or will produce more complications than the LMA designs that have already been studied.

While studies show that the LMA can be used reliably and safely by relatively inexperienced personnel with minimal training, experience with the LMA, as with all technical devices, can be expected to increase the user's confidence and ability. Success rates and the occurrence of complications should be monitored closely. Providers who insert the LMA should receive adequate initial training and should regularly practice insertion of the device.

Studies report cases of failure to insert the LMA and a small number of cases where insertion is achieved but ventilation cannot be accomplished through the LMA. With these cases in mind, it is important for providers to have an alternative strategy for management of the airway. The LMA can provide safe, effective ventilation during cardiac arrest and is an acceptable alternative to bag-mask ventilation, ventilation with another supraglottic device, or the endotracheal tube for airway management in cardiac arrest.

Steps used to properly insert an LMA are shown in Table 17-4 and demonstrated in Figure 17-12.

TABLE 17-4 • Steps Used to Insert the Laryngeal Mask Airway (LMA)

Step	Action
1	*Equipment preparation:* Check the integrity of the mask and tube according to the manufacturer's instructions. Lubricate only the posterior surface of the cuff to avoid blocking the airway aperture.
2	*Patient preparation:* Provide oxygenation and ventilation and position the patient. Note that use of the LMA poses risks of regurgitation and aspiration in unresponsive patients, but studies have shown that regurgitation is less likely with the LMA than a bag-mask and that aspiration is uncommon. You must weigh these risks against the benefit of establishing an airway using this specific device.
3	*Insertion technique:* • Introduce the LMA into the pharynx and advance it blindly until you feel resistance. Resistance indicates that the distal end of the tube has reached the hypopharynx. • Inflate the cuff of the mask. Cuff inflation pushes the mask up against the tracheal opening, allowing air to flow through the tube and into the trachea. • Ventilation through the tube is ultimately delivered to the opening in the center of the mask and into the trachea. • To avoid trauma, do not use force at any time during insertion of the LMA. • Never overinflate the cuff after inflation. Excessive intracuff pressure can result in misplacement of the device. It also can cause pharyngolaryngeal injury (e.g., sore throat, dysphagia, or nerve injury).
4	Ensure proper placement of the LMA by auscultation of the neck (should hear clear, smooth gas flow) and chest and check expired CO_2.
5	Insert a bite block, provide ventilation, and continue to monitor the patient's condition and the position of the LMA. A bite block reduces the possibility of airway obstruction and tube damage. Keep the bite block in place until you remove the LMA.

Esophageal–Tracheal Combitube and Laryngeal Tube S

The Esophageal–Tracheal Combitube (ETC) is a double-lumen airway classed as a cuffed pharyngeal sealer because of the large balloon that inflates at the base of the tongue and isolates the upper oropharyngeal airway from the lower. A second balloon inflates in the esophagus to isolate the stomach from the airway (Fig. 17-13). This second feature is an important attribute of the Combitube, since regurgitation is common in cardiac arrest.[24,118] Because of the two-balloon seal, the ETC resists displacement and provides reliable ventilation—qualities that are especially helpful in the out-of-hospital environment, where transporting the patient may displace a less stable airway or make maintaining a seal with a face mask difficult or impossible (Fig. 17-14).

See Web site for Video Clips 17-11, 17-12, and 17-13: airway management—Combitube LTS, Combitube details, and Combitube insertion technique.

Studies have compared the ETC to the endotracheal tube in patients undergoing anesthesia as well as in those suffering cardiac arrest. In three studies of in- and out-of-hospital cardiac arrest, a total of 391 victims were randomized by alternate-day allocation to receive the Combitube or the endotracheal tube. High levels of success were achieved by both methods of airway management regardless of whether the airway was managed by paramedics, nurses, or physicians.[122–125] When placement of the allocated airway device failed, there was moderate to high success in placing the other device.[122,123,126,127] And in studies comparing the effectiveness of ventilation for the ETT and the Combitube, results were similar for both devices.[128–131] A case series of patients with out-of-hospital cardiac arrest reported ventilation by Combitube was successful in 695 of 760 patients (91.4%).[132] When the Combitube was compared with the LMA in an out-of-hospital observational study, successful ventilation was achieved in 1,242 of 1,574 patients (78.9%) with the Combitube and 1,931 of 2,701 patients (71.5%) with the LMA.[133] In a randomized controlled trial, paramedics successfully ventilated 66 of 77 patients (86%) with the Combitube and 79 of 108 patients (73%) with the LMA.[118]

Three problems are common to many of the supraglottic airways as well as to the endotracheal tube: inability to insert the airway, inability to ventilate, and aspiration, with some problems occurring more commonly with one airway than another. A complication reported with the Combitube but not with other airways is a finding of superficial lacerations or hematomas or subcutaneous emphysema in a small proportion of patients following use of the airway.[132,134–137] In one anesthesia study, 7.2% of Combitube patients experienced superficial laceration not requiring intervention.[135]

Three studies examined tracheal soiling while using these devices (in anesthetized patients) and found no soiling in 25 of 27, 24 of 25, and 25 of 25 patients.[138–140] These

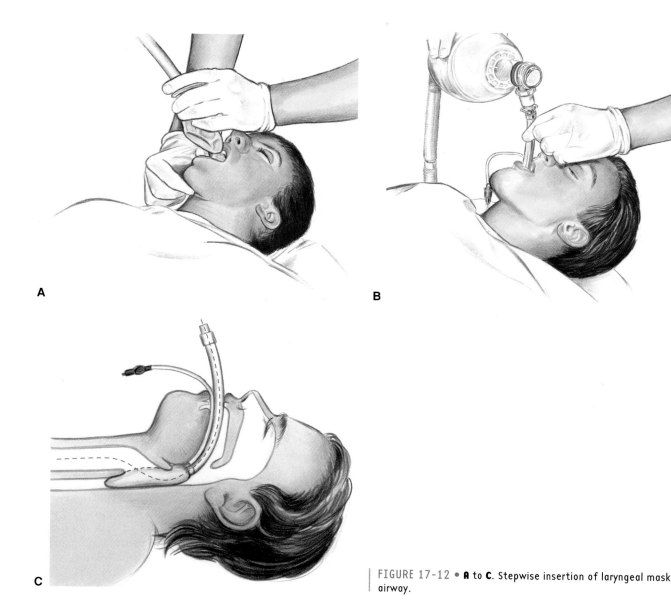

A

B

C

FIGURE 17-12 • **A** to **C**. Stepwise insertion of laryngeal mask airway.

results are similar to those of a like study performed with endotracheal tubes.[141]

Ease of training is an important issue, and maintenance of skills can be especially difficult when use of a procedure is infrequent. When training methods are reported, outcomes suggest that inexperienced personnel require relatively little training to be proficient at Combitube insertion.[88,111,125,131,132,142,143] As with all technical devices, lack of use results in skill decay. In a manikin study, intubation success rates fell from 91% posttraining to 77% at 6 months.[88] No study has examined maintenance of skills when regular use of the Combitube or regular practice, whether supervised or not, has occurred. As with other technical devices, experience with the Combitube can be expected to increase the user's confidence and ability. Success rates and the occurrence of complications should be monitored closely. Providers who insert the Combitube should receive ade-

quate initial training and should regularly practice insertion of the device.

The Combitube will normally be placed in the esophagus because of its shape and rigidity, but in a small number of cases the tube is placed in the trachea (Ochs found the Combitube placed in the trachea in only 9% of cases).[143] Both placements are acceptable, but placement location must be verified so that the correct lumen is ventilated. In one study, paramedics were found to be ventilating the wrong lumen of the Combitube in 16 of 725 cases (2.2%): this error is equivalent to unrecognized esophageal intubation with a standard endotracheal tube and can be fatal. To avoid this error, confirmation of the location of tube placement is essential.

Although there are a number of cuffed pharyngeal sealer airways now being used in anesthesia—notably the PA Express, the Airway Management Device (AMD), and the

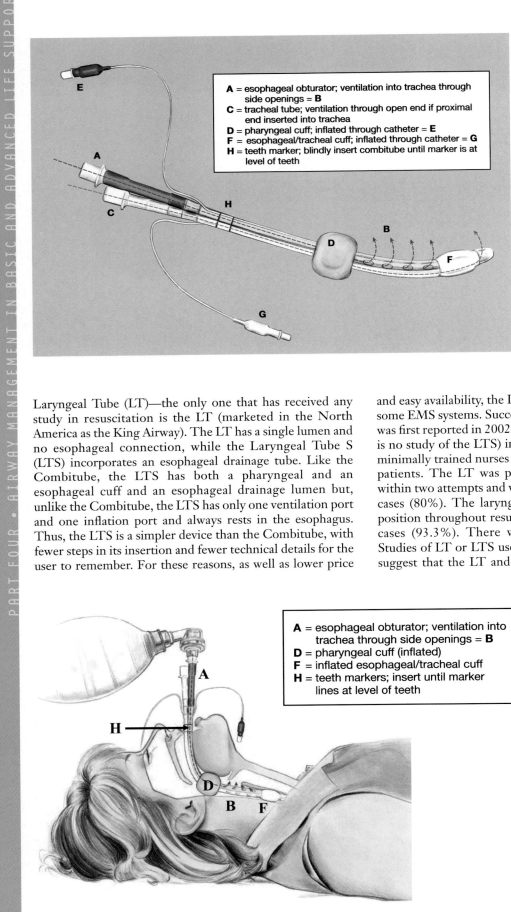

A = esophageal obturator; ventilation into trachea through side openings = **B**
C = tracheal tube; ventilation through open end if proximal end inserted into trachea
D = pharyngeal cuff; inflated through catheter = **E**
F = esophageal/tracheal cuff; inflated through catheter = **G**
H = teeth marker; blindly insert combitube until marker is at level of teeth

FIGURE 17-13 • Esophageal–tracheal Combitube.

Laryngeal Tube (LT)—the only one that has received any study in resuscitation is the LT (marketed in the North America as the King Airway). The LT has a single lumen and no esophageal connection, while the Laryngeal Tube S (LTS) incorporates an esophageal drainage tube. Like the Combitube, the LTS has both a pharyngeal and an esophageal cuff and an esophageal drainage lumen but, unlike the Combitube, the LTS has only one ventilation port and one inflation port and always rests in the esophagus. Thus, the LTS is a simpler device than the Combitube, with fewer steps in its insertion and fewer technical details for the user to remember. For these reasons, as well as lower price

and easy availability, the LTS has replaced the Combitube in some EMS systems. Successful use of the LT in resuscitation was first reported in 2002.[144] The only study of the LT (there is no study of the LTS) in resuscitation was performed with minimally trained nurses in 30 out-of-hospital cardiac arrest patients. The LT was placed in 27 of 30 patients (90%) within two attempts and ventilation was adequate in 24 of 30 cases (80%). The laryngeal tube remained in the correct position throughout resuscitation and transport in 28 of 30 cases (93.3%). There were no cases of regurgitation.[87] Studies of LT or LTS use during anesthesia or on manikins suggest that the LT and LTS require little training, are as

A = esophageal obturator; ventilation into trachea through side openings = **B**
D = pharyngeal cuff (inflated)
F = inflated esophageal/tracheal cuff
H = teeth markers; insert until marker lines at level of teeth

FIGURE 17-14 • Esophageal–tracheal Combitube inserted in esophagus.

| TABLE 17-5 • Method for Insertion of the Combitube

Step	Action
1	*Equipment preparation:* Check the integrity of both cuffs according to the manufacturer's instructions and lubricate the tube.
2	*Patient preparation:* Provide oxygenation and ventilation, and position the patient. Rule out the contraindications to insertion of the Combitube.
3	*Insertion technique:* • Hold the device with cuffs deflated so that the curvature of the tube matches the curvature of the pharynx. • Lift the jaw and insert the tube gently until the black lines on the tube are positioned between the patient's teeth. (Do not force, and do not attempt for more than 30 seconds.) • Inflate the proximal/pharyngeal (blue) cuff with 100 mL of air. (Inflate with 85 mL for the smaller Combitube.) Then inflate the distal (white or clear) cuff with 15 mL of air. (Inflate with 12 mL for the smaller Combitube.)
4	Confirm tube location and select the lumen for ventilation. To select the appropriate lumen to use for ventilation, you must determine where the tip of the tube is located. The tip of the tube can rest in either the esophagus or the trachea. • *Esophageal placement:* Breath sounds should be present bilaterally with no epigastric sounds. Provide ventilation through the blue (proximal/pharyngeal) lumen. This action delivers ventilation through the pharyngeal side holes between the two cuffs, and air will enter the trachea. Because the tip of the tube rests in the esophagus, do not use the distal (white or clear) tube for ventilation. The distal cuff will also lie within the esophagus; inflation of this cuff prevents the ventilations that you deliver through the pharyngeal tube from entering the esophagus. • *Tracheal placement:* Breath sounds are absent and epigastric sounds are present when you attempt to provide ventilation through the blue (proximal/pharyngeal) lumen. Immediately stop providing ventilations through the blue lumen and provide them through the distal (white or clear) lumen that opens at the tip of the tube in the trachea. With endotracheal placement of the tube, the distal cuff performs the same function as a cuff on an ETT. Detection of exhaled CO_2 (through the ventilating white or clear lumen) should be used for confirmation, particularly if the patient has a perfusing rhythm. • *Unknown placement:* Breath sounds and epigastric sounds are absent. Deflate both cuffs and withdraw the tube slightly, reinflate the blue cuff, and then reinflate the white (or clear) cuff (see steps above). If breath sounds and epigastric sounds are still absent, remove the tube.

easy to use as the Combitube or the LMA, and provide reliable ventilation with few complications.[142,145–154] It remains to be seen whether this airway will perform as well as other supraglottic airways in resuscitation.

While there is no evidence that any airway device is effective in improving outcome from cardiac arrest, the Combitube can provide safe, effective ventilation during cardiac arrest and is an acceptable alternative to bag-mask ventilation, ventilation with another supraglottic device, or the endotracheal tube for airway management in cases of cardiac arrest.[118,122–125,130,131,155]

Steps for one method of inserting the Combitube are shown in Table 17-5.

References

1. Thomas M, Malmcrona R, Shillingford J. Haemodynamic effects of oxygen in patients with acute myocardial infarction. *Br Heart J* 1965;27:401–407.
2. Daly WJ, Cline D, Bondurant S. Effects of breathing oxygen on atrioventricular conduction. *Am Heart J* 1963;66:321–324.
3. Daly WJ, Behnke RH. Hemodynamic consequences of oxygen breathing in left ventricular failure. *Circulation* 1963;27:252–256.
4. Kenmure AC, Murdoch WR, Beattie AD, et al. Circulatory and metabolic effects of oxygen in myocardial infarction. *Br Med J* 1968;4(5627):360–364.
5. Foster GL, Casten GG, Reeves TJ. The effects of oxygen breathing in patients with acute myocardial infarction. *Cardiovasc Res* 1969;3(2):179–189.
6. Bourassa MG, Campeau L, Bois MA, et al. The effects of inhalation of 100 percent oxygen on myocardial lactate metabolism in coronary heart disease. *Am J Cardiol* 1969;24(2):172–177.
7. Sukumalchantra Y, Levy S, Danzig R, et al. Correcting arterial hypoxemia by oxygen therapy in patients with acute myocardial infarction. Effect on ventilation and hemodynamics. *Am J Cardiol* 1969;24(6):838–852.
8. Neill WA. Effects of arterial hypoxemia and hyperoxia on oxygen availability for myocardial metabolism. Patients with and without coronary heart disease. *Am J Cardiol* 1969;24(2):166–171.
9. Madias JE, Hood WB Jr. Reduction of precordial ST-segment elevation in patients with anterior myocardial infarction by oxygen breathing. *Circulation* 1976;53(3 Suppl):I198–I200.
10. Madias JE, Madias NE, Hood WB Jr. Precordial ST-segment mapping. 2. Effects of oxygen inhalation on ischemic injury in patients with acute myocardial infarction. *Circulation* 1976;53(3):411–417.
11. Madias JE, Hood WB Jr. Precordial ST-segment mapping. 4. Experience with mapping of ST-segment depression in anterior transmural myocardial infarction. *Journal of Electrocardiology* 1976;9(4):315–320.
12. Rawles JM, Kenmure AC. Controlled trial of oxygen in uncomplicated myocardial infarction. *Br Med J* 1976;1(6018):1121–1123.
13. Nicholson C. A systematic review of the effectiveness of oxygen in reducing acute myocardial ischaemia. *J Clin Nurs* 2004;13(8):996–1007.
14. Antman EM, Anbe DT, Armstrong PW, et al. ACC/AHA guidelines for the management of patients with ST-elevation myocardial infarction: A report of the American College of Cardiology/American Heart Association Task Force on Practice Guidelines (Committee to Revise the 1999 Guidelines for the Management of Patients With Acute Myocardial Infarction). *J Am Coll Cardiol* 2004;44(3):E1–E211.
15. Anderson JL, Adams CD, Antman EM, et al. ACC/AHA 2007 guidelines for the management of patients with unstable angina/non-ST-Elevation myocardial infarction: a report of the American College of Cardiology/American Heart Association Task Force on Practice Guidelines (Writing Committee to Revise the 2002 Guidelines for the Management of Patients With Unstable Angina/Non-ST-Elevation Myocardial Infarction) developed in collaboration with the American College of Emergency

Physicians, the Society for Cardiovascular Angiography and Interventions, and the Society of Thoracic Surgeons endorsed by the American Association of Cardiovascular and Pulmonary Rehabilitation and the Society for Academic Emergency Medicine. *J Am Coll Cardiol* 2007;50(7):e1–e157.

16. Davies AE, Kidd D, Stone SP, et al. Pharyngeal sensation and gag reflex in healthy subjects. *Lancet* 1995;345(8948):487–488.

17. Bleach NR. The gag reflex and aspiration: a retrospective analysis of 120 patients assessed by videofluoroscopy. *Clin Otolaryngol Allied Sci* 1993;18(4):303–307.

18. Gallagher WJ, Pearce AC, Power SJ. Assessment of a new nasopharyngeal airway. *Br J Anaesth* 1988;60(1):112–115.

19. Feldman SA, Fauvel NJ, Ooi R. The cuffed pharyngeal airway. *Eur J Anaesthesiol* 1991;8(4):291–295.

20. Ellis DY, Lambert C, Shirley P. Intracranial placement of nasopharyngeal airways: is it all that rare? *Emerg Med J* 2006;23(8):661.

21. Muzzi DA, Losasso TJ, Cucchiara RF. Complication from a nasopharyngeal airway in a patient with a basilar skull fracture. *Anesthesiology* 1991;74(2):366–368.

22. Schade K, Borzotta A, Michaels A. Intracranial malposition of nasopharyngeal airway. *J Trauma* 2000;49(5):967–968.

23. Martin JE, Mehta R, Aarabi B, et al. Intracranial insertion of a nasopharyngeal airway in a patient with craniofacial trauma. *Mil Med* 2004;169(6):496–497.

24. Simons RW, Rea TD, Becker LJ, et al. The incidence and significance of emesis associated with out-of-hospital cardiac arrest. *Resuscitation* 2007;74(3):427–431.

25. Kozak RJ, Ginther BE, Bean WS. Difficulties with portable suction equipment used for prehospital advanced airway procedures. *Prehosp Emerg Care* 1997;1(2):91–95.

26. Ornato JP, Hallagan LF, McMahan SB, et al. Attitudes of BCLS instructors about mouth-to-mouth resuscitation during the AIDS epidemic. *Ann Emerg Med* 1990;19(2):151–156.

27. Hew P, Brenner B, Kaufman J. Reluctance of paramedics and emergency medical technicians to perform mouth-to-mouth resuscitation. *J Emerg Med* 1997;15(3):279–284.

28. Rowe BH, Shuster M, Zambon S, et al. Preparation, attitudes and behaviour in nonhospital cardiac emergencies: evaluating a community's readiness to act. *Can J Cardiol* 1998;14(3):371–377.

29. Locke CJ, Berg RA, Sanders AB, et al. Bystander cardiopulmonary resuscitation. Concerns about mouth-to-mouth contact. *Arch Intern Med* 1995;155(9):938–943.

30. Brenner BE, Kauffman J. Reluctance of internists and medical nurses to perform mouth-to-mouth resuscitation. *Arch Intern Med* 1993;153(15):1763–1769.

31. Brenner B, Stark B, Kauffman J. The reluctance of house staff to perform mouth-to-mouth resuscitation in the inpatient setting: what are the considerations? *Resuscitation* 1994;28(3):185–193.

32. Mejicano GC, Maki DG. Infections acquired during cardiopulmonary resuscitation: estimating the risk and defining strategies for prevention. *Ann Intern Med* 1998;129(10):813–828.

33. Axelsson A, Thoren A, Holmberg S, et al. Attitudes of trained Swedish lay rescuers toward CPR performance in an emergency: a survey of 1012 recently trained CPR rescuers. *Resuscitation* 2000;44(1):27–36.

34. Melanson SW, O'Gara K. EMS provider reluctance to perform mouth-to-mouth resuscitation. *Prehosp Emerg Care* 2000;4(1):48–52.

35. Rossi R, Lindner KH, Ahnefeld FW. Devices for expired air resuscitation. *Prehospital Disaster Med* 1993;8(2):123–126.

36. Cydulka RK, Connor PJ, Myers TF, et al. Prevention of oral bacterial flora transmission by using mouth-to-mask ventilation during CPR. *J Emerg Med* 1991;9(5):317–321.

37. Lawrence PJ, Sivaneswaran N. Ventilation during cardiopulmonary resuscitation: which method? *Med J Aust* 1985;143(10):443–446.

38. Harrison RR, Maull KI, Keenan RL, et al. Mouth-to-mask ventilation: a superior method of rescue breathing. *Ann Emerg Med* 1982;11(2):74–76.

39. Seidelin PH, Stolarek IH, Littlewood DG. Comparison of six methods of emergency ventilation. *Lancet* 1986;2(8518):1274–1275.

40. Thomas AN, O'Sullivan K, Hyatt J, et al. A comparison of bag mask and mouth mask ventilation in anaesthetised patients. *Resuscitation* 1993;26(1):13–21.

41. Paal P, Falk M, Sumann G, et al. Comparison of mouth-to-mouth, mouth-to-mask and mouth-to-face-shield ventilation by lay persons. *Resuscitation* 2006;70(1):117–123.

42. Johannigman JA, Branson RD, Davis K Jr, et al. Techniques of emergency ventilation: a model to evaluate tidal volume, airway pressure, and gastric insufflation. *J Trauma* 1991;31(1):93–98.

43. Elling R, Politis J. An evaluation of emergency medical technicians' ability to use manual ventilation devices. *Ann Emerg Med* 1983;12(12):765–768.

44. Cummins RO, Austin D, Graves JR, et al. Ventilation skills of emergency medical technicians: a teaching challenge for emergency medicine. *Ann Emerg Med* 1986;15(10):1187–1192.

45. Hess D, Baran C. Ventilatory volumes using mouth-to-mouth, mouth-to-mask, and bag-valve-mask techniques. *Am J Emerg Med* 1985;3(4):292–296.

46. De Regge M, Vogels C, Monsieurs KG, et al. Retention of ventilation skills of emergency nurses after training with the SMART BAG compared to a standard bag-valve-mask. *Resuscitation* 2006;68(3):379–384.

47. Walsh K, Loveday K, O'Rathaille M. A comparison of the effectiveness of pre-hospital bag-valve-mask ventilation performed by Irish emergency medical technicians and anaesthetists working in a tertiary referral teaching hospital. *Ir Med J* 2003;96(3):77–79.

48. Osterwalder JJ, Schuhwerk W. Effectiveness of mask ventilation in a training mannikin. A comparison between the Oxylator EM100 and the bag-valve device. *Resuscitation* 1998;36(1):23–27.

49. Martin PD, Cyna AM, Hunter WA, et al. Training nursing staff in airway management for resuscitation. A clinical comparison of the facemask and laryngeal mask. *Anaesthesia* 1993;48(1):33–37.

50. Alexander R, Hodgson P, Lomax D, et al. A comparison of the laryngeal mask airway and Guedel airway, bag and face mask for manual ventilation following formal training. *Anaesthesia* 1993;48(3):231–234.

51. Jesudian MC, Harrison RR, Keenan RL, et al. Bag-valve-mask ventilation; two rescuers are better than one: preliminary report. *Crit Care Med* 1985;13(2):122–123.

52. Davidovic L, LaCovey D, Pitetti RD. Comparison of 1- versus 2-person bag-valve-mask techniques for manikin ventilation of infants and children. *Ann Emerg Med* 2005;46(1):37–42.

53. Dunkley CJ, Thomas AN, Taylor RJ, et al. A comparison of standard and a modified method of two resuscitator adult cardiopulmonary resuscitation: description of a new system for research into advanced life support skills. *Resuscitation* 1998;38(1):7–12.

54. Wheatley S, Thomas AN, Taylor RJ, et al. A comparison of three methods of bag valve mask ventilation. *Resuscitation* 1997;33(3):207–210.

55. Thomas AN, Dang PT, Hyatt J, et al. A new technique for two-hand bag valve mask ventilation. *Br J Anaesth* 1992;69(4):397–398.

56. Wenzel V, Idris AH, Dorges V, et al. The respiratory system during resuscitation: a review of the history, risk of infection during assisted ventilation, respiratory mechanics, and ventilation strategies for patients with an unprotected airway. *Resuscitation* 2001;49(2):123–134.

57. Dorges V, Ocker H, Wenzel V, et al. Emergency airway management by non-anaesthesia house officers—a comparison of three strategies. *Emerg Med J* 2001;18(2):90–94.

58. Wenzel V, Keller C, Idris AH, et al. Effects of smaller tidal volumes during basic life support ventilation in patients with respiratory arrest: good ventilation, less risk? *Resuscitation* 1999;43(1):25–29.

59. Dorges V, Ocker H, Hagelberg S, et al. Smaller tidal volumes with room-air are not sufficient to ensure adequate oxygenation during bag-valve-mask ventilation. *Resuscitation* 2000;44(1):37–41.

60. Tourtier JP, Compain M, Petitjeans F, et al. Acid aspiration prophylaxis in obstetrics in France: a comparative survey of 1998 vs. 1988 French practice. *Eur J Anaesthesiol* 2004;21(2):89–94.

61. Soreide E, Holst-Larsen H, Steen PA. Acid aspiration syndrome prophylaxis in gynaecological and obstetric patients. A Norwegian survey. *Acta Anaesthesiol Scand* 1994;38(8):863–868.

62. Schlesinger S, Blanchfield D. Modified rapid-sequence induction of anesthesia: a survey of current clinical practice. *AANA J* 2001;69(4):291–298.

63. Morris J, Cook TM. Rapid sequence induction: a national survey of practice. *Anaesthesia* 2001;56(11):1090–1097.

64. Kluger MT, Willemsen G. Anti-aspiration prophylaxis in New Zealand: a national survey. *Anaesth Intens Care* 1998;26(1):70–77.

65. Lawes EG, Campbell I, Mercer D. Inflation pressure, gastric insufflation and rapid sequence induction. *Br J Anaesth* 1987;59(3):315–318.

66. Lawes EG, Rea TD. The incidence and rapid sequence induction. *Br J Anaesth* 2007;74(3):315–318.

67. Admani M, Yeh TF, Jain R, et al. Prevention of gastric inflation during mask ventilation in newborn infants. *Crit Care Med* 1985;13(7):592–593.

68. Moynihan RJ, Brock-Utne JG, Archer JH, et al. The effect of cricoid pressure on preventing gastric insufflation in infants and children. *Anesthesiology* 1993;78(4):652–656.

69. Neilipovitz DT, Crosby ET. No evidence for decreased incidence of aspiration after rapid sequence induction. *Can J Anaesth* 2007;54(9):748–764.

70. Quigley P, Jeffrey P. Cricoid pressure: assessment of performance and effect of training in emergency department staff. *Emerg Med Australas* 2007;19(3):218–222.

71. Howells TH, Chamney AR, Wraight WJ, et al. The application of cricoid pressure. An assessment and a survey of its practice. *Anaesthesia* 1983;38(5):457–460.

72. Lawes EG, Duncan PW, Bland B, et al. The cricoid yoke—a device for providing consistent and reproducible cricoid pressure. *Br J Anaesth* 1986;58(8):925–931.

73. Vanner RG, O'Dwyer JP, Pryle BJ, et al. Upper oesophageal sphincter pressure and the effect of cricoid pressure. *Anaesthesia* 1992;47(2):95–100.

74. Ellis DY, Harris T, Zideman D. Cricoid pressure in emergency department rapid sequence tracheal intubations: a risk-benefit analysis. *Ann Emerg Med* 2007;50(6):653–665.

75. Brimacombe JR, Berry AM. Cricoid pressure. *Can J Anaesth* 1997;44(4):414–425.

76. Levitan RM, Kinkle WC, Levin WJ, et al. Laryngeal view during laryngoscopy: a randomized trial comparing cricoid pressure, backward-upward-rightward pressure, and bimanual laryngoscopy. *Ann Emerg Med* 2006;47(6):548–555.

77. Stone B. The use of the laryngeal mask airway by nurses during cardiopulmonary resuscitation. Results of a multicentre trial. *Anaesthesia* 1994;49(1):3–7.

78. Stone BJ, Chantler PJ, Baskett PJ. The incidence of regurgitation during cardiopulmonary resuscitation: a comparison between the bag valve mask and laryngeal mask airway. *Resuscitation* 1998;38(1):3–6.

79. Guly UM, Mitchell RG, Cook R, et al. Paramedics and technicians are equally successful at managing cardiac arrest outside hospital. *BMJ* 1995;310(6987):1091–1094.

80. Stiell IG, Wells GA, Field B, et al. Advanced cardiac life support in out-of-hospital cardiac arrest. *N Engl J Med* 2004;351(7):647–656.

81. Gausche M, Lewis RJ, Stratton SJ, et al. Effect of out-of-hospital pediatric endotracheal intubation on survival and neurological outcome: a controlled clinical trial. *JAMA* 2000;283(6):783–790.

82. Jones JH, Murphy MP, Dickson RL, et al. Emergency physician-verified out-of-hospital intubation: miss rates by paramedics. *Acad Emerg Med* 2004;11(6):707–709.

83. Sayre MR, Sakles JC, Mistler AF, et al. Field trial of endotracheal intubation by basic EMTs. *Ann Emerg Med* 1998;31(2):228–233.

84. Katz SH, Falk JL. Misplaced endotracheal tubes by paramedics in an urban emergency medical services system. *Ann Emerg Med* 2001;37(1):32–37.

85. Dorges V, Wenzel V, Knacke P, et al. Comparison of different airway management strategies to ventilate apneic, nonpreoxygenated patients. *Crit Care Med* 2003;31(3):800–804.

86. Kurola JO, Turunen MJ, Laakso JP, et al. A comparison of the laryngeal tube and bag-valve mask ventilation by emergency medical technicians: a feasibility study in anesthetized patients. *Anesth Analg* 2005;101(5):1477–1481.

87. Kette F, Reffo I, Giordani G, et al. The use of laryngeal tube by nurses in out-of-hospital emergencies: preliminary experience. *Resuscitation* 2005;66(1):21–25.

88. Vertongen VM, Ramsay MP, Herbison P. Skills retention for insertion of the Combitube and laryngeal mask airway. *Emerg Med* 2003;15(5–6):459–464.

89. Brimacombe J. A proposed classification system for extraglottic airway devices. *Anesthesiology* 2004;101(2):559.

90. Jones JH, Murphy MP, Dickson RL, et al. Emergency physician-verified out-of-hospital intubation: miss rates by paramedics. *Acad Emerg Med* 2004;11(6):707–709.

91. Beyer AJ III, Land G, Zaritsky A. Nonphysician transport of intubated pediatric patients: a system evaluation. *Crit Care Med* 1992;20(7):961–966.

92. Bradley JS, Billows GL, Olinger ML, et al. Prehospital oral endotracheal intubation by rural basic emergency medical technicians. *Ann Emerg Med* 1998;32(1):26–32.

93. Sayre MR, Sakles JC, Mistler AF, et alM. Field trial of endotracheal intubation by basic EMTs. *Ann Emerg Med* 1998;31(2):228–233.

94. Miller DM. A proposed classification and scoring system for supraglottic sealing airways: a brief review. *Anesth Analg* 2004;99(5):1553–1559; table of contents.

95. Soar J. The I-gel supraglottic airway and resuscitation—some initial thoughts. *Resuscitation* 2007;74(1):197.

96. 2005 American Heart Association Guidelines for Cardiopulmonary Resuscitation and Emergency Cardiovascular Care. *Circulation* 2005;112(24 Suppl):IV1–IV203.

97. Brain AI. The development of the Laryngeal Mask—a brief history of the invention, early clinical studies and experimental work from which the Laryngeal Mask evolved. *Eur J Anaesthesiol Suppl* 1991;4:5–17.

98. Brain AI. The laryngeal mask—a new concept in airway management. *Br J Anaesth* 1983;55(8):801–805.

99. Flaishon R, Sotman A, Ben-Abraham R, et al. Antichemical protective gear prolongs time to successful airway management: a randomized, crossover study in humans. *Anesthesiology* 2004;100(2):260–266.

100. Goldik Z, Bornstein J, Eden A, et al. Airway management by physicians wearing anti-chemical warfare gear: comparison between laryngeal mask airway and endotracheal intubation. *Eur J Anaesthesiol* 2002;19(3):166–169.

101. Pennant JH, Pace NA, Gajraj NM. Role of the laryngeal mask airway in the immobile cervical spine. *J Clin Anesth* 1993;5(3):226–230.

102. Flaishon R, Sotman A, Ben-Abraham R, et al. Antichemical protective gear prolongs time to successful airway management: a randomized, crossover study in humans. *Anesthesiology* 2004;100(2):260–266.

103. Davies PR, Tighe SQ, Greenslade GL, et al. Laryngeal mask airway and tracheal tube insertion by unskilled personnel. *Lancet* 1990;336(8721):977–979.

104. Pennant JH, Walker MB. Comparison of the endotracheal tube and laryngeal mask in airway management by paramedical personnel. *Anesth Analg* 1992;74(4):531–534.

105. Reinhart DJ, Simmons G. Comparison of placement of the laryngeal mask airway with endotracheal tube by paramedics and respiratory therapists. *Ann Emerg Med* 1994;24(2):260–263.

106. Deakin CD, Peters R, Tomlinson P, et al. Securing the prehospital airway: a comparison of laryngeal mask insertion and endotracheal intubation by UK paramedics. *Emerg Med J* 2005;22(1):64–67.

107. Burgoyne L, Cyna A. Laryngeal mask vs intubating laryngeal mask: insertion and ventilation by inexperienced resuscitators. *Anaesth Intens Care* 2001;29(6):604–608.

108. Coulson A, Brimacombe J, Keller C, et al. A comparison of the ProSeal and classic laryngeal mask airways for airway management by inexperienced personnel after manikin-only training. *Anaesth Intens Care* 2003;31(3):286–289.

109. Dingley J, Baynham P, Swart M, et al. Ease of insertion of the laryngeal mask airway by inexperienced personnel when using an introducer. *Anaesthesia* 1997;52(8):756–760.

110. Roberts I, Allsop P, Dickinson M, et al. Airway management training using the laryngeal mask airway: a comparison of two different training programmes. *Resuscitation* 1997;33(3):211–214.

111. Yardy N, Hancox D, Strang T. A comparison of two airway aids for emergency use by unskilled personnel: the Combitube and laryngeal mask. *Anaesthesia* 1999;54(2):181–183.

112. Verghese C, Prior-Willeard PF, Baskett PJ. Immediate management of the airway during cardiopulmonary resuscitation in a hospital without a resident anaesthesiologist. *Eur J Emerg Med* 1994;1(3):123–125.

113. Samarkandi AH, Seraj MA, el Dawlatly A, et al. The role of laryngeal mask airway in cardiopulmonary resuscitation. *Resuscitation* 1994;28(2):103–106.

114. Kokkinis K. The use of the laryngeal mask airway in CPR. *Resuscitation* 1994;27(1):9–12.

115. Leach A, Alexander CA, Stone B. The laryngeal mask in cardiopulmonary resuscitation in a district general hospital: a preliminary communication. *Resuscitation* 1993;25(3):245–248.

116. Carrillo Alvarez A, Lopez-Herce Cid J, et al. [Evaluation of basic and advanced pediatric resuscitation courses]. *An Esp Pediatr* 2000;53(2):125–134.

117. Grantham H, Phillips G, Gilligan JE. The laryngeal mask in prehospital emergency care. 1994;6:193–197.

118. Rumball CJ, MacDonald D. The PTL, Combitube, laryngeal mask, and oral airway: a randomized prehospital comparative study of ventilatory device effectiveness and cost-effectiveness in 470 cases of cardiorespiratory arrest. *Prehosp Emerg Care* 1997;1(1):1–10.

119. Ho BY, Skinner HJ, Mahajan RP. Gastro-oesophageal reflux during day case gynaecological laparoscopy under positive pressure ventilation: laryngeal mask vs. tracheal intubation. *Anaesthesia* 1998;53(9):921–924.

120. Maltby JR, Beriault MT, Watson NC, et al. LMA-Classic and LMA-ProSeal are effective alternatives to endotracheal intubation for gynecologic laparoscopy. *Can J Anaesth* 2003;50(1):71–77.

121. Rewari W, Kaul HL. Regurgitation and aspiration during gynaecological laparoscopy: Comparison between laryngeal mask airway and tracheal intubation. *J Anaesthesiol Clin Pharmacol* 1999;15(1):67–70.

122. Atherton GL, Johnson JC. Ability of paramedics to use the Combitube in prehospital cardiac arrest. *Ann Emerg Med* 1993;22(8):1263–1268.

123. Rabitsch W, Schellongowski P, Staudinger T, et al. Comparison of a conventional tracheal airway with the Combitube in an urban emergency medical services system run by physicians. *Resuscitation* 2003;57(1):27–32.

124. Staudinger T, Brugger S, Roggla M, et al. [Comparison of the Combitube with the endotracheal tube in cardiopulmonary resuscitation in the prehospital phase]. *Wien Klin Wochenschr* 1994;106(13):412–415.

125. Rumball C, Macdonald D, Barber P, et al. Endotracheal intubation and esophageal tracheal Combitube insertion by regular ambulance attendants: a comparative trial. *Prehosp Emerg Care* 2004;8(1):15–22.

126. Davis DP, Valentine C, Ochs M, et al. The Combitube as a salvage airway device for paramedic rapid sequence intubation. *Ann Emerg Med* 2003;42(5):697–704.

127. Ochs M, Davis D, Hoyt D, et al. Paramedic-performed rapid sequence intubation of patients with severe head injuries. *Ann Emerg Med* 2002;40(2):159–167.

128. Frass M, Frenzer R, Zdrahal F, et al. The esophageal tracheal combitube: preliminary results with a new airway for CPR. *Ann Emerg Med* 1987;16(7):768–772.

129. Frass M, Frenzer R, Ilias W, et al. [The esophageal tracheal Combitube (ETC): animal experiment results with a new emergency tube]. *Anasth Intensivther NotfallMed* 1987;22(3):142–144.

130. Frass M, Frenzer R, Rauscha F, et al. Ventilation with the esophageal tracheal combitube in cardiopulmonary resuscitation. Promptness and effectiveness. *Chest* 1988;93(4):781–784.

131. Staudinger T, Brugger S, Watschinger B, et al. Emergency intubation with the Combitube: comparison with the endotracheal airway. *Ann Emerg Med* 1993;22(10):1573–1575.

132. Lefrancois DP, Dufour DG. Use of the esophageal tracheal combitube by basic emergency medical technicians. *Resuscitation* 2002;52(1):77–83.

133. Tanigawa K, Shigematsu A. Choice of airway devices for 12,020 cases of nontraumatic cardiac arrest in Japan. *Prehosp Emerg Care* 1998;2(2):96–100.

134. Oczenski W, Krenn H, Dahaba AA, et al. Complications following the use of the Combitube, tracheal tube and laryngeal mask airway. *Anaesthesia* 1999;54(12):1161–1165.

135. Rabitsch W, Krafft P, Lackner FX, et al. Evaluation of the oesophageal-tracheal double-lumen tube (Combitube) during general anaesthesia. *Wien Klin Wochenschr* 2004;116(3):90–93.

136. Vezina D, Lessard MR, Bussieres J, et al. Complications associated with the use of the esophageal-tracheal Combitube. *Can J Anaesth* 1998;45(1):76–80.

137. Stoppacher R, Teggatz JR, Jentzen JM. Esophageal and pharyngeal injuries associated with the use of the esophageal-tracheal Combitube. *J Forens Sci* 2004;49(3):586–591.

138. Urtubia RM, Aguila CM, Cumsille MA. Combitube: a study for proper use. *Anesth Analg* 2000;90(4):958–962.

139. Hagberg CA, Vartazarian TN, Chelly JE, et al. The incidence of gastroesophageal reflux and tracheal aspiration detected with pH electrodes is similar with the Laryngeal Mask Airway and Esophageal Tracheal Combitube—a pilot study. *Can J Anaesth* 2004;51(3):243–249.

140. Mercer MH. An assessment of protection of the airway from aspiration of oropharyngeal contents using the Combitube airway. *Resuscitation* 2001;51(2):135–138.

141. Petring OU, Adelhoj B, Jensen BN, et al. Prevention of silent aspiration due to leaks around cuffs of endotracheal tubes. *Anesth Analg* 1986;65(7):777–780.

142. Dorges V, Ocker H, Wenzel V, et al. The Laryngeal Tube S: a modified simple airway device. *Anesth Analg* 2003;96(2):618–621.

143. Ochs M, Vilke GM, Chan TC, et al. Successful prehospital airway management by EMT-Ds using the combitube. *Prehosp Emerg Care* 2000;4(4):333–337.

144. Genzwuerker HV, Dhonau S, Ellinger K. Use of the laryngeal tube for out-of-hospital resuscitation. *Resuscitation* 2002;52(2):221–224.

145. Asai T, Hidaka I, Kawachi S. Efficacy of the laryngeal tube by inexperienced personnel. *Resuscitation* 2002;55(2):171–175.

146. Cook TM, McCormick B, Asai T. Randomized comparison of laryngeal tube with classic laryngeal mask airway for anaesthesia with controlled ventilation. *Br J Anaesth* 2003;91(3):373–378.

147. Ocker H, Wenzel V, Schmucker P, et al. A comparison of the laryngeal tube with the laryngeal mask airway during routine surgical procedures. *Anesth Analg* 2002;95(4):1094–1097.

148. Asai T, Moriyama S, Nishita Y, et al. Use of the laryngeal tube during cardiopulmonary resuscitation by paramedical staff. *Anaesthesia* 2003;58(4):393–394.

149. Genzwurker H, Finteis T, Hinkelbein J, et al. [First clinical experiences with the new LTS. A laryngeal tube with an oesophageal drain]. *Anaesthesist* 2003;52(8):697–702.

150. Gaitini LA, Vaida SJ, Somri M, et al. An evaluation of the Laryngeal Tube during general anesthesia using mechanical ventilation. *Anesth Analg* 2003;96(6):1750–1755.

151. Asai T, Murao K, Shingu K. Apparatus: efficacy of the laryngeal tube during intermittent positive-pressure ventilation. *Anaesthesia* 2000;55(11):1099–1102.

152. Kurola J, Harve H, Kettunen T, et al. Airway management in cardiac arrest—comparison of the laryngeal tube, tracheal intubation and bag-valve mask ventilation in emergency medical training. *Resuscitation* 2004;61(2):149–153.

153. Genzwuerker HV, Finteis T, Slabschi D, et al. Assessment of the use of the laryngeal tube for cardiopulmonary resuscitation in a manikin. *Resuscitation* 2001;51(3):291–296.

154. Dorges V, Wenzel V, Neubert E, et al. Emergency airway management by intensive care unit nurses with the intubating laryngeal mask airway and the laryngeal tube. *Crit Care* 2000;4(6):369–376.

155. Frass M, Frenzer R, Rauscha F, et al. Evaluation of esophageal tracheal Combitube in cardiopulmonary resuscitation. *Crit Care Med* 1987;15(6):609–611.

Chapter 18
Endotracheal Intubation and Management of the Difficult Airway

Kane High

When emergency health care providers cannot maintain an airway or support ventilation with a bag-mask or other airway devices, insertion of an endotracheal tube by experienced providers is indicated. Importantly, only experienced and continually qualified individuals should perform endotracheal intubation after a careful assessment of the risks and benefits in an emergency setting.

- When and how to intubate during cardiac arrest
- "Crash" endotracheal intubation
- Anticipating complications during emergency airway intubation
- Confirming endotracheal tube placement and displacement

Indications for Endotracheal Intubation

When emergency health care providers cannot maintain an airway or support ventilation with a bag-mask or other airway devices, insertion of an endotracheal tube by experienced providers is indicated. Importantly, only experienced and continually qualified individuals should perform endotracheal intubation after a careful assessment of the risks and benefits in an emergency setting. Urgent or emergent endotracheal intubation will pose additional challenges.

Currently, advanced cardiac life support (ACLS) experts consider the cuffed endotracheal tube the ventilation adjunct of choice for providers who are skilled and experienced in its use. The cuffed endotracheal tube

- Keeps the airway patent
- Allows suctioning of airway secretions
- Ensures delivery of a high concentration of oxygen
- Provides a route for administration of certain drugs
- Facilitates delivery of a specific tidal volume
- Protects the airway from aspiration of gastric contents
- Protects the airway from aspiration of blood and mucus from above the trachea.[1]

Indications

Indications for insertion of an endotracheal tube in an emergency situation include cardiac arrest and acute respiratory insufficiency. General indications in these settings are:

- Inability of the provider to ventilate the unconscious patient with less invasive methods. In general, attempt to provide oxygenation and ventilation of the lungs with exhaled-air methods, simple airway adjuncts, or bag-mask ventilation before attempting endotracheal intubation.
- Inability of the patient to protect the airway (e.g., because of coma, absent reflexes, or cardiac arrest). To provide adequate lung inflation, rescuers often generate airway and esophageal pressures that exceed the closing pressure of the gastroesophageal junction. This can lead rapidly to gastric inflation and subsequent regurgitation. When the airway is unprotected, regurgitated gastric contents can enter the lungs.[2–5]
- Prolonged need for chest compressions during resuscitation. Simple, noninvasive airway adjuncts may be used to maintain oxygenation and ventilation during cardiac arrest of short duration such as ventricular fibrillation (VF) or pulseless ventricular tachycardia (VT) arrest responsive to defibrillation. When resuscitation is prolonged, however, gastric inflation often becomes problematic and airway control is needed. As soon as practical during the resuscitative effort, intubate the trachea or insert one of the two acceptable alternative advanced airways—the laryngeal mask airway (LMA) or Combitube.

Endotracheal Intubation in Cardiac Arrest

The principles of assessment and management of airway emergencies are complex; the specific approach required is influenced by the training, skills, and experience of emergency health care providers, the assistance and resources available in different clinical settings, and local protocols.

Rapid Sequence Intubation Versus "Crash Airway" (Cardiac Arrest) Intubation

"Rapid sequence intubation" (RSI) and "rapid sequence induction" both describe a sequential protocol for the rapid induction of anesthesia and intubation in patients at risk for aspiration of gastric contents. Peter Safar's pioneer description of such a protocol used both terms: "rapid induction/intubation for prevention of gastric-content aspiration."[6] The more inclusive term "rapid sequence intubation" is preferred now because "induction" currently refers only to the step of "inducing" anesthesia via sedative agents.

Crash Airway Intubation for Cardiorespiratory Arrest

Obvious differences exist between a patient who is breathing spontaneously—the usual candidate for RSI—and someone in cardiac (cardiorespiratory) arrest. The term "crash airway" describes patients who are unresponsive (no airway protective reflexes), without effective respirations or circulation.

Assess the Patient: The Primary and Secondary ABCD Surveys
On arriving at the scene of a cardiac arrest or respiratory emergency in any setting, ACLS personnel follow the steps of the primary ABCD survey: assess/ manage airway, breathing, circulation, and ventricular fibrillation—with an automatic external defibrillator (AED) or conventional defibrillator.

The steps of endotracheal intubation are part of the secondary ABCD survey. Correct performance of the primary ABCD survey, however, accomplishes a number of critical steps required for endotracheal intubation:

- Open airway. If patient is unresponsive, insert oropharyngeal airway.
- Administer high-flow (10–15 L/min) 100% oxygen.
- Provide positive-pressure ventilation with bag and mask if spontaneous ventilation is absent or inadequate (see "Preoxygenation," below).

If bag-mask ventilation is provided for the unresponsive patient (with no airway protective reflexes), provide cricoid pressure if personnel are available.

Begin the secondary ABCD survey:

- Designated intubator verifies effectiveness of ventilation and oxygenation and prepares to intubate (secondary A and B).
- Designated IV accessor/medication provider gains peripheral vein access (see Table 18-1) to provide appropriate resuscitation medications and premedications for intubation if needed.

Initial Steps of Crash Airway (Cardiac Arrest) Intubation

The patient with a crash airway requires chest compressions and positive-pressure ventilation before and after endotracheal intubation. In such circumstances several steps in the sequence of RSI—such as preoxygenation, premedication, defasciculation, and sedation—are either unnecessary or have a lower priority. When endotracheal intubation is performed for the crash airway, the intubation steps (see below) are modified according to the following steps:

Step 1. Preparation per routine appropriate for the setting
Step 2. Assessment
Step 3. Preoxygenation, accomplished during resuscitation
Step 4. *Premedication*, omitted because the "LOAD" agents (lidocaine, opioids, atropine, and defasciculating agents) add little if any clinical value to benefit the cardiac arrest patient
Step 5. *Induction of anesthesia and paralysis*, omitted because the patient is already unresponsive and flaccid due to cerebral anoxia from lack of blood flow

Use of Paralytic Agents With the Crash Airway
Although the *paralysis step* is often omitted for patients with crash airway, residual muscle spasm and hypertonicity during the first minutes after cardiac arrest may complicate attempted endotracheal intubation. In one emergency medical services (EMS) system in which paramedics were not allowed to use paralytic agents, 49% of failed intubations were due to "inadequate relaxation."[7] Some EMS systems have initiated programs that train and protocols that authorize advanced life support (ALS) personnel to administer sedative agents,[8] paralytic agents,[9] or both.[10] Many such protocols are based on published experience in air medical transport systems, involving trauma patients[11–13] and others who require a crash airway.[14] Because most experience with RSI protocols using sedatives and paralytic agents in the prehospital setting have actually involved management of the crash airway, the need for—and effects of—RSI medications has not been demonstrated. There have been no reports of outcomes of airway management by systems that have prospectively studied the use of paralytic agents in cardiac arrest.[9] In fact, many published protocols for the use of succinylcholine specifically exclude patients in cardiac arrest.[15] Intubation of some victims of cardiac arrest may be facilitated by the use of neuromuscular blocking agents if protocols and programs are based on the consensus guidelines of organizations such as the National Association of EMS Physicians.[16,17]

The "RAPIDS" Approach to Endotracheal Intubation for Crash Airway Patients[18]

In the crash airway situation usually presented to health care responders, the patient is unresponsive without effective respiration (agonal gasps may be present) and no circulation.[14] No monitoring or treatment action other than basic CPR is ongoing. The following approach is one method to rapidly intubate the trachea and control the airway.

R: Resuscitate Patient—Continue CPR while planning to establish a definitive airway.

- **Personnel.** Two or preferably three persons are assigned to airway management. One person is designated in advance as the intubator; this person must have proper training and experience and documented intubation success.
- **Equipment and medications.** Regular (daily or every shift) review of the checklist is essential (see the pre-event checklist at the end of this chapter).
- **Begin primary ABCD survey: assess and support**

Airway: Insert oropharyngeal airway.
Breathing: Administer supplementary oxygen.
 Provide bag-mask (or mouth-to-mask/shield) ventilation.
 Apply cricoid pressure (see Chapter 17).
Circulation: Ensure that adequate chest compressions are performed. Evaluate rhythm.
Defibrillate: Attempt defibrillation as appropriate.

A: Access—Establish peripheral venous access and start secondary ABCD survey.

- Establish peripheral vein access.
- Designated intubator prepares to intubate.

P: Position Patient—Align the respiratory axes to best facilitate laryngoscopy.

- Flex the neck relative to the thorax.
- Extend the head relative to the neck (see Fig. 18-1).

I: Intubate

- Intubator makes one oral intubation attempt without using pharmacologic agents.
- If successful, see step D—"Determine tube location."
- If unsuccessful on first attempt, resume bag-mask ventilation:

 1. **Bag-mask ventilation:** Consider: do the bag-mask ventilations produce effective chest rise per clinical evaluation? If yes, see step 2; further endotracheal tube attempts are OK. If no, make only one more attempt; then go to step 3.
 2. **Review relaxation/flaccidity:** During the first intubation attempt, was there complete skeletal muscle relaxation? If yes, more intubation attempts are OK. If no, see step 3: succinylcholine 1.5 mg/kg.
 3. **Paralyze the patient:** Administer *succinylcholine* 1.5 mg/kg to ensure complete relaxation of the patient for intubation.

 A. Give one dose only; no sedative or anesthetic.
 B. After 30 to 40 seconds, check jaw and neck muscles for flaccidity.
 C. If flaccid, attempt endotracheal intubation.

D: Determine Tube Location

- Perform confirmation with physical examination and five point auscultation.

- Perform confirmation with a device such as a CO_2 detector or esophageal detector device (EDD).

S: Secure Tube—To prevent dislodgment, use tape or a commercial tube holder. Monitor position of the tube frequently.

Rapid Sequence Intubation

Initial Steps of Rapid Sequence Intubation

RSI is used primarily for patients who need to be intubated but who are usually breathing spontaneously, are variably responsive to stimuli, have intact airway protective reflexes, and—most critically—may have a full stomach. Consequently the recommended RSI steps incorporate actions to prevent pain, anxiety, and distress; to blunt multiple adverse physiologic responses to laryngoscopy and endotracheal intubation; and to reduce the risk of aspiration of gastric contents.

Step 1 is pre-event preparation.
Step 2 is *preoxygenation*. A high concentration of inspired oxygen is administered to the spontaneously-breathing patient to maximize arterial and alveolar oxygen content. To prevent gastric inflation, bag-mask ventilation is not *routinely* provided at this time. If adequate spontaneous ventilation is present.

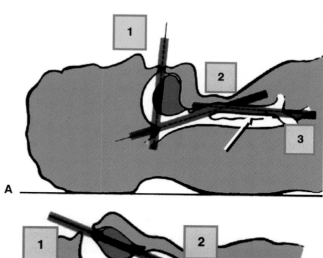

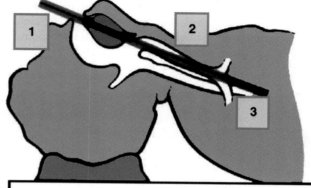

FIGURE 18-1 • Aligning axes of upper airway. 1, oral axis; 2, pharyngeal axis; 3, tracheal axis. **A.** Normal position. **B.** Neck flexed on the shoulders to align axis 2 with axis 3, and head extended on the neck to align axis 1 with axes 2 and 3.

Step 3 is *premedication*. Pharmaceutical agents are administered to blunt specific reflex reactions to airway manipulation. The Airway Course, an advanced emergency airway management course,[19] has developed the mnemonic "LOAD" as a memory aid for the premedication (pretreatment) agents: lidocaine, opioids, atropine, and defasciculating agents. (See the next section for further information about the use of these medications.)

Step 4 is induction of *anesthesia or sedation and paralysis.*

See Web site for ACEP policy statement on rapid sequence intubation.

The Seven "Ps" of Rapid Sequence Intubation

The "Seven P's of Rapid Sequence Intubation" was developed as a memory aid for advanced airway providers.[18] As modified for ACLS use, seven steps or "Ps" are as follows:

1. **Pre-event Preparation.** Prepare personnel, equipment, medications, and monitoring and begin primary ABCD survey. Note any history that will influence intubation procedure or choice of medication. This preparation will be influenced by the setting and acuity of the intubation procedure.
2. **Preoxygenate.**
3. **Pretreatment/Premedication.**
4. **Paralyze** after sedation. Induce anesthesia.
5. **Protection/Positioning.** Cricoid pressure applied: just as airway protective reflexes (cough, gag) are lost and before positive-pressure ventilation.
6. **Placement** of endotracheal tube with both clinical conformation and a device.
7. **Postintubation** management, including securing of tube and radiographic verification of tube placement; continuous monitoring of tube position, oxygenation, and ventilation.

Step 1: Pre-event Preparation Multiple advanced resuscitation interventions must be performed simultaneously during an intubation procedure. This is particularly true when intubation is required during resuscitation. Resuscitation teams should have predesignated responsibilities so that in the event of an emergency, rescuers can act without waiting for instructions.

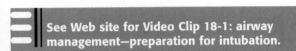

See Web site for Video Clip 18-1: airway management—preparation for intubation.

Personnel Two or preferably three providers should be assigned to airway management, with one of the providers designated to perform intubation. As the designated provider prepares for the intubation attempt, the other "airway" providers perform bag-mask ventilation (see discussion of bag-mask ventilation in preceding pages) and assist with intubation.

One provider is typically assigned to establish vascular access. Vascular access will be needed during resuscitation to provide vasoactive and other medications and will be needed during intubation of the responsive patient if sedatives and paralytic agents are used during RSI.

Inexperienced providers should use only those airway management devices for which they have adequate training. Providers who perform endotracheal intubation require either frequent experience or frequent retraining.[1,20,21]

- Advanced skills are required to place an endotracheal tube and verify correct position.
- Delays in intubation or failure to intubate will adversely affect the outcome of cardiac arrest. Failure-to-intubate rates are as high as 50% in EMS systems with low patient volume and providers who perform intubation infrequently.[22,23]
- Intubation attempts may produce serious complications that are more common when the provider is inexperienced. These potential complications include trauma to the oropharynx, hypoxia and hypercarbia from long interruptions in ventilation, delayed or withheld chest compressions, esophageal intubation, failure to secure the tube, and failure to recognize tube misplacement or displacement.

EMS systems should establish a system of quality improvement monitoring for intubation attempts, documenting for each provider and patient the number of intubations attempted, number of confirmed successful intubations, complications, and outcomes.

One successful model for out-of-hospital response to cardiac arrest is a two-tier response: a two- to three-member BLS-D response team followed by a two-member ALS response team. In this system it is common for BLS responders to perform chest compressions, bag-mask ventilation, and defibrillation. One member of the two-person ALS team gains intravenous access and administers medications, and the other performs endotracheal intubation and airway management. This should be the default response model for emergencies both in and out of hospital. In the absence of procedural delays, one ALS provider should be ready to attempt intubation when the other ALS responder is ready to administer IV medications after ensuring chest.

Equipment

CUFFED ENDOTRACHEAL TUBE   A typical cuffed endotracheal tube

- Is open at both ends
- Is measured in length (cm) from the distal end and marked at several intervals (in adults the tube depth mark visible at the front teeth should be approximately 20–22 cm)
- Has *size markings* indicating the internal diameter of the tube in millimeters. For an average-sized woman, the tube size should be 7 mm; for an average-sized man, 8 mm.
- Has a standard 15-mm/22-mm end connector that will fit positive-pressure ventilation devices.
- Has a high-volume, low-pressure inflatable cuff attached to an inflating tube with a one-way valve for the cuff-inflation syringe.

- Has a pilot balloon between the one-way valve and inflating syringe to indicate cuff inflation.

Always check the inflatable cuff for integrity by testing it just before insertion. Use the same syringe that will be used to inflate the cuff after insertion.

STYLET   A stylet is typically a plastic-coated, malleable metal rod that can be inserted through the endotracheal tube to curve and stiffen the tube to the desired configuration. This procedure will facilitate insertion of the tube into the larynx and trachea by allowing easier manipulation of the direction of the tube. Apply a water-soluble lubricant to the stylet before inserting it to a point 1 to 2 cm from the end of the tube. Do not allow the end of the stylet to extend beyond the end of the tube, because it could injure the vocal cords and laryngeal mucosa. Once the stylet is properly positioned in the tube, bend the stylet over the edge of the connector to prevent inadvertent advance of the stylet during attempted intubation.

GUM ELASTIC BOUGIE   The Eschmann endotracheal tube introducer, more commonly called the *gum elastic bougie*, is another device used to assist with placement of the endotracheal tube[24] (Fig. 18-2). Currently the gum elastic bougie is used by trained providers only for difficult or unsuccessful oral intubations. It is a semirigid, resin-coated device, about 2 feet long (60 cm), made of braided polyester. As seen in Figure 18-2, use of the gum elastic bougie is quite analogous

to the Seldinger wire technique for inserting intravascular catheters. The device is inserted with a laryngoscope, but only partial visualization of laryngeal structures is required. The small-diameter flexible device is inserted in the trachea largely by "feel"; the design allows the provider to feel the bumping of the tracheal rings when the device enters the trachea. Once the bougie has been passed into the trachea, it essentially acts as a "guidewire" over which an endotracheal tube is passed and advanced blindly into position in the trachea. The endotracheal tube is then stabilized and the rescuer slides the bougie back out.[25–30] The tip of the endotracheal tube sometimes gets caught on laryngeal structures and cannot be advanced. In such cases, rotation of the tube with gentle pressure will allow it to advance into the trachea. Some endotracheal tubes (e.g., the Parker endotracheal tube) are designed to reduce this problem by having a curved bevel that causes the tip of the tube to more closely follow the introducer.

LARYNGOSCOPE (HANDLE/BLADE-HOLDER PLUS CURVED AND STRAIGHT BLADE)   The laryngoscope is used to expose the glottis and allow direct visualization of the vocal cords and the tracheal entrance (see Fig. 18-2). The laryngoscope consists of three parts:

- The handle, which holds batteries for the light source
- The blade, which has a bulb in the distal third of the blade
- The fitting, which is the connection point between the blade and the handle where electrical contact is made

Always check that the light is working.

- Attach the indentation of the blade to the bar of the handle.
- Elevate the blade to the point where it makes a right angle to the handle. The light should come on. If it does not, check the bulb or the batteries.

There are two common types of blades:

- Curved (Fig. 18-3A, the MacIntosh design)
- Straight (see Fig. 18-4A, the Miller design). The choice of blade is a matter of personal preference. Variations in design usually alter the technique used by the operator.

Medications   All medications that may be needed during the intubation attempt should be prepared and at hand. These medications may include

- Premedications ("LOAD": lidocaine, opioids, atropine, and defasciculating agents)
- Paralyzing agents, sedatives, and anesthetics

Monitoring   Before any attempted intubation, providers should establish appropriate monitoring based on the setting and the type of intubation to be performed. This monitoring should include

- Continuous electrocardiographic (ECG) rhythm monitoring
- Pulse oximetry
- Intermittent blood pressure measurements

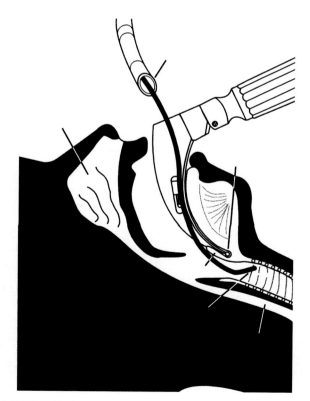

FIGURE 18-2 • The gum elastic bougie is used to assist endotracheal intubation by the oral route. (Figure is reprinted with permission from *Annals of Emergency Medicine.* 1996; 27:665–667. © 1996 *Annals of Emergency Medicine.*)

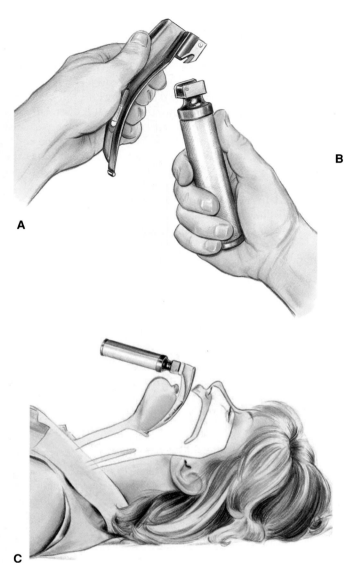

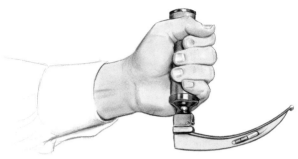

FIGURE 18-3 • **A.** Curved blade attaches to laryngoscope handle. **B.** Attached to laryngoscope handle. **C.** Inserted against epiglottis. During laryngoscopy, the handle is held in the left hand.

Continuous end-tidal CO_2 is valuable but not required. Always designate one provider to monitor the patient throughout the intubation attempt. This monitor should immediately inform the intubator if the patient's heart rate slows or becomes irregular or if there is any fall in the oxyhemoglobin saturation.

Note that emergent monitoring of the cardiac arrest patient cannot include pulse oximetry. There is no pulsatile signal for the pulse oximeter to use to measure oxyhemoglobin saturation. Cardiac monitoring is also distorted by artifact from chest compressions. Base assessment of how the patient is tolerating the intubation attempt on general appearance and on duration.

Step 2: Preoxygenation

- When RSI is performed for a spontaneously breathing, adequately ventilated patient, provide preoxygenation by delivering 100% oxygen through a well-fitted face mask for at least 3 minutes. Preoxygenation maximizes hemoglobin and arterial oxygen saturation and provides an oxygen reservoir in the lungs.
- A typical preoxygenation period is not possible for victims of cardiac arrest who are apneic or lack adequate ventilations or have no airway protective (cough and gag) reflexes. In this situation deliver high-flow 100% oxygen by bag-mask ventilation plus cricoid pressure. See "Protect the Airway With Cricoid Pressure," below.

Step 3: Premedication   Provide premedication to *responsive* patients. Do not provide premedication to an *unresponsive*, or "crash airway" (cardiac arrest) patient. Properly trained providers, in an appropriate setting, should administer the following "LOAD" medications when indications are present:

- **Lidocaine *1.5 mg/kg IV***. Administer to patients with elevated intracranial pressure or reactive airways disease. In

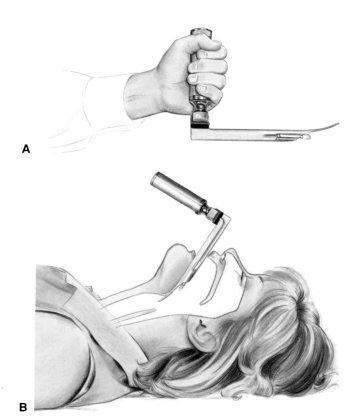

FIGURE 18-4 • **A.** Straight-blade laryngoscope. **B.** Inserted past epiglottis. During laryngoscopy, the handle is held in the left hand.

patients with elevated intracranial pressure (ICP), lidocaine prevents a reflex rise in intracranial pressure stimulated by laryngoscopy and intubation. Lidocaine mitigates bronchospasm induced by laryngoscopy and intubation in reactive airways patients. Administer lidocaine 3 minutes before the paralytic agent.

- **Opioids,** most commonly **fentanyl, 3 μg/kg IV.** Administer to patients who have no contraindications. Opioids blunt the catecholamine discharge that accompanies laryngeal manipulation. Opioids are particularly useful in patients with elevated ICP because any elevations in blood pressure would further elevate ICP. Opioids are also useful in patients for whom an increase in sympathetic activity or in cardiovascular "shear" pressure would pose a risk (i.e., those with ischemic heart disease, aortic dissection, or ruptured intracranial aneurysm). Like lidocaine, opioids should be given 3 minutes before the paralytic agent.

- **Atropine 0.02 mg/kg; given IV.** Administer to patients who are bradycardic immediately before an intubation attempt (first rule out hypoxia); to all infants younger than 1 year of age and in children 1 to 5 years of age who are going to receive succinylcholine; and to all older children or adults who are to receive a *second* dose of succinylcholine. Atropine is also given 3 minutes before the paralytic agent.

- **Defasciculating agents** (most often a nondepolarizing agent) given at **10% of the usual paralytic dose.** Administer to patients who are to receive succinylcholine and to those who could be harmed by the rise in intracranial pressure that can accompany succinylcholine-induced fasciculations.

Step 4: Paralysis After Sedation Approximately 3 minutes after the last premedication (see above), induce deep *sedation* (to the point of *anesthesia*) by rapid IV administration of a benzodiazepine (such as **midazolam**), or **etomidate** or one of several other types of anesthetic agents. Follow immediately with rapid IV administration of a *paralytic agent* (neuromuscular blocking agent) such as **succinylcholine** or **vecuronium.** The sedative agents rapidly induce loss of consciousness, loss of airway protective reflexes, and loss of muscle tone, thereby permitting rapid intubation.

As the patient becomes unconscious, perform *Sellick's maneuver* (firm pressure applied on the cricoid cartilage) to occlude the esophagus and prevent passive regurgitation of gastric contents (see Chapter 17 and Video Clip 17-8).

Cricoid pressure must be timed to occur with the onset of deep sedation (loss of consciousness, loss of cough, gag, and airway protective reflexes). Bag-mask ventilation can begin with the application of cricoid pressure. Maintain steady pressure on the cricoid while the endotracheal tube is inserted, correct tube placement is confirmed, and the cuff is inflated.

The majority of crash airway patients will be unresponsive to such a degree that *step 4: paralysis after sedation*, is unnecessary. Many patients, however, will maintain a degree of postarrest muscle tone and spasm such that bag-mask ventilation and endotracheal intubation are difficult or even impossible. Administer one of the paralyzing agents to these hypertonic patients. Sedatives or the LOAD premedications are unnecessary.

Neuromuscular Blockade to Facilitate Endotracheal Intubation in Cardiac Arrest For patients whose cardiac arrest has been witnessed, the intubation goal is to intubate *every* patient, on the *first* attempt, and *within seconds*.

- The first objective in achieving this goal is to *paralyze* the patient. Numerous studies have confirmed the value of effective paralysis, which facilitates the challenging task of aligning the airway axes in most cases and determines success in others.
- The second objective is to paralyze the patient *early* and *quickly*, before positive-pressure ventilation induces gastric inflation, regurgitation, and the devastating consequences of aspiration.
- The third objective is to paralyze the patient *briefly*, so that, upon return of spontaneous circulation, the patient can resume spontaneous respirations as well.

Clinical indicators of adequate paralysis in the nonarrested patient include lack of spontaneous movements, respiratory effort, and blink reflex and jaw relaxation as manifested by the provider's ability to fully open the patient's mouth without resistance.

WHICH PARALYTIC AGENT TO USE? The ideal paralytic agent to use for endotracheal intubation would have the following characteristics:

- Rapid onset of action
- Short duration of action
- Minimal adverse effects

No paralytic agent possesses all three of these characteristics. Therefore, the final choice of paralytic agent depends on the setting (in hospital versus out of hospital) and the specific protocol (RSI versus cardiac arrest or crash airway). Neuromuscular blocking agents used in endotracheal intubation during cardiac arrest are summarized in Table 18-1.

Many experts consider *succinylcholine* the drug of choice for endotracheal intubation during both RSI and cardiac arrest. It is the only agent that meets two of the three criteria for a paralytic agent: rapid onset of action (30–60 seconds) plus ultrashort duration (3–5 minutes). But succinylcholine does not meet the criterion for minimal adverse effects, because it possesses numerous, sometimes fatal, side effects (see below and Table 18-2).

Two nondepolarizing agents, *rocuronium* and *vecuronium*, also have rapid onset of action but more benign side effects than succinylcholine. Consequently these two drugs may be used in emergency departments and in-hospital settings. Many experts prefer them as paralytic agents over succinylcholine. Rocuronium and vecuronium, however, do not fulfill the criterion of short duration of action. The slower onset and long duration of action of rocuronium and vecuro-

nium render them unacceptable for use in the out-of-hospital setting.

For appropriately trained prehospital personnel responding to out-of-hospital cardiac arrest, the general consensus is that *succinylcholine* remains the paralytic agent of choice. In the National Emergency Airway Registry project, a multicenter study of emergency department intubations, only a few of the more than 7,000 rapid sequence intubations reported were accomplished with any neuromuscular blocking agent.

PHARMACOLOGY OF SUCCINYLCHOLINE In the nonarrest patient, succinylcholine produces onset of paralysis within 30 to 60 seconds and almost universal effective (intubation-level) paralysis within 45 seconds. The effects of sudden complete loss of all tone and the onset of complete flaccidity in all the muscles of the head, neck, and thorax are dramatic and obvious. Onset of action may be delayed in patients in cardiac arrest. The effects of succinylcholine may be difficult to ascertain in the patient in cardiac arrest because the arrest itself produces many of the same effects on muscle tone as succinylcholine-induced paralysis. However, the lack of spontaneous movements, respiratory effort and blink reflex, and jaw relaxation (the provider should be able to completely open the patient's mouth without resistance) indicate onset of action. An appropriate IV dose of succinylcholine is 1.5 mg/kg. Duration of action is normally about 3 to 5 minutes. Effective spontaneous respirations may not be possible for approximately 8 minutes.

The advantage of an agent with an ultrashort duration of action is that if the intubation attempt is unsuccessful, the agent will quickly wear off, and the patient may be able to

TABLE 18-1 • Neuromuscular Blocking Agents Used in Endotracheal Intubation During Cardiac Arrest

Drug	Dose[a]	Route	Duration of Paralysis	Side Effects	Comments
Neuromuscular Blocking Agents					
Succinylchaline (Anectine)	1 to 2 mg/kg IV; 2 to 4 mg/kg IM	IV, IM[b]	3-5 minutes	Muscle fasciculations; Rise in intraocular, intragastric, intracranial pressure; Life-threatening high level of potassium; Hypertension	Depolarizing muscle relaxant; Rapid onset; short duration of action; Renal failure, burns, high potassium level are contraindications; Consider defasciculation with nondepolarizing agent; Do not use for maintenance of paralysis
Vecuronium (Norcuron)	0.1–0.2 mg/kg	IV	30–60 minutes	Minimal cardiovascular side effects	Nondepolarizing agent; Onset of action: 2–3 minutes
Rocuroium (Zemuron)	0.6–1.2 mg/kg	IV	40+ minutes	Minimal cardiovascular side effects	Nondepolarizing agent; Rapid-action onset like succinylcholine

[a]Doses shown are guidelines only.
[b]Actual dosing may vary depending on patient's clinical status.

| TABLE 18-2 • Succinylcholine: Adverse Effects and Relative Contraindications

Adverse Effects	Contraindications
• Muscle fasciculations	• Denervation syndrome (stroke, spinal cord injury) >72 hours earlier
• Muscle pain	• Neuromuscular disorders
• Rhabdomyolysis	• Increased intracranial pressure
• Myoglobinuria	• Open injury of the eye globe
• Hyperkalemia	• Glaucoma
• Hypertension	• History (patient or family) of malignant hyperthermia
• Increased intracranial pressure	• History of plasma cholinesterase deficiency
• Increased intraocular pressure	• Major crush injuries
• Increased intragastric pressure	• Trauma or burns >48 hours after injury
• Malignant hyperthermia	• Hyperkalemia
• Bradycardia, asystole	• Renal failure

resume spontaneous ventilation, minimizing the period of bag-mask ventilation. Many patients, however, may have underlying disease that will prevent effective ventilation. So if intubation is unsuccessful, the provider should be prepared to provide a prolonged period of bag-mask ventilation, thereby negating the advantage of a short-acting agent.

Succinylcholine has numerous contraindications and potential side effects, which may occasionally be fatal (Table 18-2). Providers who use succinylcholine must be completely familiar with its potential dangers and contraindications and must carefully weigh its risk–benefit ratio against those of the nondepolarizing agents available. Because of its potential detrimental effects, succinylcholine should never be used to maintain paralysis after intubation.[31,32]

Alternative Paralytics Rocuronium is an aminosteroid nondepolarizing agent with rapid onset and intermediate duration of action. Acceptable intubation conditions can be achieved within 60 seconds at doses of 0.6 to 1.2 mg/kg IV with a duration of >40 minutes.[33–35] At these doses rocuronium has minimal to no cardiovascular side effects.[36] It is safe to use in patients with renal[37] and hepatic failure, although the duration of neuromuscular blockade may be prolonged with liver disease.[38,39] Another advantage of rocuronium is that it is available as a premixed solution.

Vecuronium is considerably more potent than rocuronium. Because onset is inversely related to potency, vecuronium has a slower onset. Doses of 0.1 to 0.2 mg/kg IV will produce a level of muscle relaxation acceptable for intubation within 90 to 120 seconds and that can last from 30 minutes up to 1 hour.[40,41] Higher doses produce more rapid onset but at the expense of prolonged duration of action.

Vecuronium also has minimal side effects and is safe for patients with renal and hepatic failure.[42] Unlike rocuronium, vecuronium is supplied as a powder that must be reconstituted before it can be administered.

Step 5: Protection of Airway with Cricoid Pressure (Sellick's Maneuver) and Positioning of Patient

Protect Airway With Cricoid Pressure Cricoid pressure occludes the esophagus, minimizing air entry into the stomach. It should be provided *before* initiation of bag-mask ventilation, so it may be necessary early in the preparation for intubation or later for an RSI sequence.

If the victim is in cardiac arrest (crash airway), bag-mask ventilation is initiated as one of the first steps of resuscitation. Sedatives are not administered and paralysis is seldom required before intubation. If adequate personnel are available, one rescuer should apply cricoid pressure *before* positive-pressure ventilation is provided and should maintain it until intubation is complete, the tube cuff is inflated, and correct tube placement is verified. In the prehospital setting, however, a third rescuer is often not available to provide cricoid pressure.

In an RSI sequence, sedative and paralytic drugs are administered to a patient who is breathing spontaneously. Providers should apply cricoid pressure *as soon as* the patient becomes sedated (i.e., loses consciousness with loss of airway protective and gag reflexes) and *before* bag-mask ventilation is initiated. When possible, maintain cricoid pressure continuously until the endotracheal tube is successfully placed.[43] Cricoid pressure during the intubation attempt can improve visualization of the vocal cords because the maneuver displaces the larynx back into visual alignment with the laryngoscope.

The application of cricoid pressure will not prevent all regurgitation or aspiration. A portable suction device (battery powered) or access to a wall-vacuum source and an adequately sized suction catheter must be readily available (see Video Clip 17-8).

Position the Patient: Align the Respiratory Axes to Best Facilitate Laryngoscopy

- Flex the neck relative to the thorax.
- Extend the head relative to the neck.

ALIGNING THE AIRWAY AXES   The most common cause of unsuccessful intubation is the intubator's inability to see the vocal cords through the laryngoscope (see Fig. 18-5C). The laryngoscope (Figs. 18-2 and 18-3) is a rigid metal device that is not well designed for intubation; it allows the intubator to see the vocal cords only along a straight visual axis between the provider's eye and the vocal cords. The difficulties are created by the presence of three separate, angulated lines of sight and by the patient's teeth, tongue, and uvula, which vary in size and consistency.

Visualization is best accomplished by moving the patient's head, neck, and thorax into the "sniffing position" (see Fig 18-4).

- Three axes—the oral, pharyngeal, and tracheal—must be aligned to achieve direct visualization of the larynx.
- To accomplish this, first flex the neck forward relative to the chest; then lift the chin (which extends the head backward relative to the neck). An exaggerated attempt to "sniff" (the sniffing position) duplicates the position needed. One recent study using cervical spine radiography concluded that precise "alignment of the axes" seldom if ever occurs.
- Do not allow the head to hang over the end of a bed or stretcher, because intubation is virtually impossible in that position.

For proper flexion of the neck, it is often helpful to place several towels under the patient's head to elevate it a few centimeters above the level of the bed. The intubator can then extend the head and visualize the vocal cords.

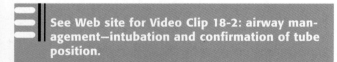

See Web site for Video Clip 18-2: airway management—intubation and confirmation of tube position.

Step 6: Perform Oral Endotracheal Intubation and Confirmation of Endotracheal Placement

- During cardiac arrest, the intubator typically makes one oral intubation attempt without using sedative or paralytic agents.
- If successful, see step 7. If unsuccessful, resume bag-mask ventilation. See Figure 18-8.

Perform Oral Endotracheal Intubation

DIRECTLY VISUALIZE THE VOCAL CORDS WITH THE LARYNGOSCOPE

- Open the patient's mouth with your right hand. If an assistant is applying cricoid pressure, he or she may retract the right corner of the mouth.

- Hold the laryngoscope in your left hand.
- Insert the blade in the right side of the mouth, displacing the tongue to the left.
- Move the blade toward the midline and advance it to the base of the tongue.
- Simultaneously move the lower lip away from the blade with your right index finger. Be gentle and avoid applying pressure on the lips and teeth.

Using a curved blade (Fig. 18-5B), advance its tip into the vallecula (i.e., the space between the base of the tongue and the pharyngeal surface of the epiglottis).

Using a straight blade (Fig. 18-5A), insert its tip under the epiglottis.

Expose the glottic opening by exerting upward traction on the handle. Do not use a prying motion, and *do not* use the upper teeth as a fulcrum. Point and firmly lift the end of the handle at an angle of 30 to 45 degrees above and toward the patient's feet. This helps to create the sniffing position and allows the best view of the vocal cords (Fig. 18-4B).

- Keeping the vocal cords under direct vision, advance the tube from the right side of the mouth through the cords.
- Continue inserting the tube until the cuff appears and completely passes through the cords.
- Then advance the tube 1.25 to 2.5 cm further into the trachea. The tip of the tube should now be about halfway between the vocal cords and the carina. In the average adult, this position will result in the front teeth aligning between the 19- and 23-cm depth markings on the tube. This position allows for some movement of the tip of the tube during neck flexion or extension without extubation or movement of the tip into a main bronchus.
- If you used a stylet, remove it now.
- Inflate the cuff with enough air to occlude the trachea (usually 10–20 mL).
- *Note:* Oxyhemoglobin saturation and oxygen delivery will quickly fall during an intubation attempt. Hypoxia develops rapidly because bag-mask ventilation and oxygen delivery have stopped abruptly and no ventilations or chest compressions can be provided. Intubation attempts should, therefore, be expeditious but gentle, exposing the glottic opening as quickly as possible and placing the tube through the cords under direct vision in a controlled manner. It may be necessary to interrupt the intubation attempt to provide oxygen if the patient's heart rate, oxyhemoglobin saturation, or clinical appearance deteriorates significantly during the attempt.
- As soon as the tube is placed, inflate the cuff. Then:
  - Confirm tube position. Various approaches to confirmation of tube placement are acceptable provided one critical principle is always followed: a *combination* of both clinical (physical examination) and device (e.g., capnometery or EDD) confirmation techniques must be used to confirm tube placement. See "Confirmation of Endotracheal Tube Placement," below.

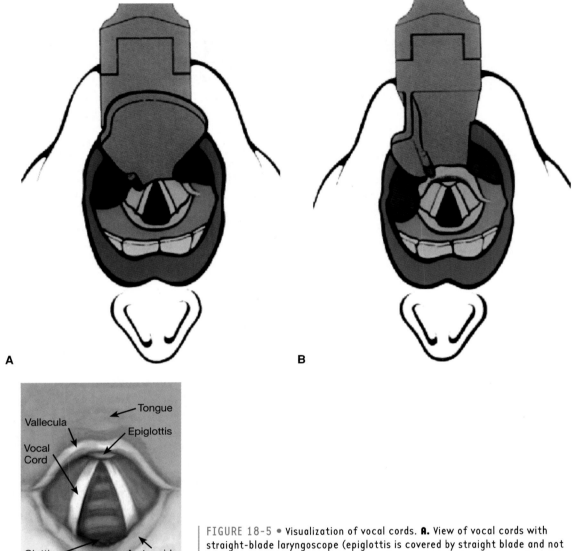

A

B

Tongue
Vallecula
Epiglottis
Vocal
Cord
Glottic
opening
Arytenoid
cartilage

C

FIGURE 18-5 • Visualization of vocal cords. **A.** View of vocal cords with straight-blade laryngoscope (epiglottis is covered by straight blade and not visible). **B.** View of the vocal cords with curved-blade laryngoscope (epiglottis is visible). **C.** Anatomy.

- Confirm effective seal of the trachea by the cuff with these steps: listen over the larynx with a stethoscope, provide a ventilation (normal tidal volume), and if an air leak is heard around the cuff, add more air from the syringe. Repeat this sequence of providing ventilations and adding air to the cuff until the audible air leak disappears.

Confirmation of Endotracheal Tube Placement A thorough assessment of endotracheal tube position should be performed immediately after placement. For patients in cardiac arrest, this assessment should not require interruption of chest compressions. Assessment by physical examination consists of visualizing chest expansion bilaterally and listening over the epigastrium (breath sounds should not be heard) and the lung fields bilaterally (breath sounds should be equal and adequate). A device should also be used to confirm correct placement in the trachea (see below). If there is

doubt about correct tube placement, use the laryngoscope to visualize the tube passing through the vocal cords. If still in doubt, remove the tube and provide bag-mask ventilation until the tube can be replaced.

Use of Devices to Confirm Tube Placement

Providers should always use both clinical assessment and devices to confirm endotracheal tube location immediately after placement and each time the patient is moved. No study, however, has identified a single device as both sensitive and specific for endotracheal tube placement in the trachea or esophagus. All confirmation devices should be considered adjuncts to other confirmation techniques. There are no data to quantify the capability of devices to monitor tube position after initial placement. False-positive and false-negative results can occur for a variety of reasons (Table 18-3).

| TABLE 18-3 • Reasons for Misleading Results Using End-Tidal CO_2 Detector and Esophageal Detector Device

A: Colorimetric End-Tidal CO_2 Detector		
Reading	**Actual Location of ETT: Trachea**	**Actual Location of ETT: Esophagus (or Hypopharynx)**
Carbon Dioxide Detected Color change: positive = CO_2 present (or as specified by manufacturer)	*ETT in trachea* Proceed with ventilations.	*Reasons for apparent CO_2 detection despite tube in esophagus* **Causes:** Distended stomach, recent ingestion of carbonated beverage, non-pulmonary sources of CO_2. **Consequences:** Unrecognized esophageal intubation; can lead to iatrogenic death.
No CO_2 Detected No color change: negative = CO_2 absent (or as specified by manufacturer)	*No CO_2 detection with tube in trachea* **Causes:** Low or no blood flow state (e.g., cardiac arrest); any cardiac arrest with no, prolonged, or poor CPR. **Consequences:** Leads to unnecessary removal of properly placed ETT. Reintubation attempts increase chances of other adverse consequences.	*No CO_2 detection and tube is not in trachea (i.e., tube is in esophagus)* **Causes:** Rescuer has inserted ETT in esophagus/hypopharynx. A life-threatening adverse event has occurred. **Consequences:** Rescuer recognizes ETT is not in trachea; properly and rapidly identified; tube is removed at once; patient is reintubated.
B: Esophageal Detector Device		
Reading	**Actual Location of ETT: Esophagus**	**Actual Location of ETT: Trachea**
Consistent With Tube in Esophagus Bulb does not refill or refills slowly (>5 seconds × 2), or syringe cannot be aspirated, suggesting that tip of ETT is in esophagus	*Device suggests tube in esophagus when it is in esophagus* **Causes:** Rescuer has inserted tube in esophagus/hypopharynx. A life-threatening adverse event has occured. **Consequences:** Rescuer correctly recognizes ETT is in esophagus; ETT is removed at once; patient is reintubated.	*Device suggests tube in esophagus when it is in trachea* **Causes:** Secretions in trachea (mucus, gastric contents, acute pulmonary edema); insertion in right main bronchus; pliable trachea (morbid obesity, late-term pregnancy). **Consequences:** Leads to unnecessary removal of properly placed ETT. Reintubation attempts increase chances of other adverse consequences.
Consistent with Tube in Trachea Bulb fills immediately or syringe can be aspirated, suggesting that ETT is in trachea	*Results suggest that tube is NOT in esophagus (i.e., that it is in trachea) when tube IS in esophagus* **Causes:** • Conditions that cause increased lung expansion (e.g., COPD, status asthmaticus). • Conditions that fill stomach with air (e.g., recent bag-mask ventilation, mouth-to-mask or mouth-to-mouth breathing). • Conditions that cause poor tone in esophageal sphincter or increased gastric pressure (late pregnancy). **Consequences:** Unrecognized esophageal intubation can lead to death.	*Results suggest that tube is NOT in the esophagus (i.e., that it is in the trachea) when it IS in the trachea.* Esophageal detector device indicates ETT is in trachea. Proceed with ventilations.

See Web site for ACEP policy statement on confirmation of endotracheal tube placement.

Exhaled CO_2 Detectors (Fig. 18-6) Detection of exhaled CO_2 is one of several independent methods of confirming endotracheal tube position. Given the simplicity of the exhaled CO_2 detector, it can be used as the initial method for detecting correct tube placement even in the victim of cardiac arrest. Detection of exhaled CO_2, however, is not infallible as a means of confirming tube placement, particularly during cardiac arrest. But evidence from one meta-analysis in adults,[44] one prospective controlled cohort study,[45] and several case series and reports[46–54] indicates that exhaled CO_2 detectors (waveform, colorimetry, or digital) may be useful as adjuncts to confirm endotracheal tube placement during cardiac arrest. The range of results obtained from the reviewed papers is as follows:

- Sensitivity (percentage of correct endotracheal placement detected when CO_2 is detected): 33% to 100%
- Specificity (percentage of incorrect esophageal placements detected when no CO_2 is detected): 97% to 100%
- Positive predictive value (probability of endotracheal placement if CO_2 is detected): 100%

- Negative predictive value (probability of esophageal placement if no CO_2 is detected): 20% to 100%.

When exhaled CO_2 is detected (positive reading for CO_2) in cardiac arrest, it is usually a reliable indicator of tube position in the trachea. False-positive readings (CO_2 is detected but the tube is located in the esophagus) have been observed in animals that ingested large amounts of carbonated liquids before the arrest.[55] False-negative readings (in this context defined as failure to detect CO_2 despite tube placement in the trachea) may be present during cardiac arrest for several reasons. The most common explanation for false-negative readings during CPR is that blood flow and delivery of CO_2 to the lungs is low. False-negative results have also been reported in association with pulmonary embolus because pulmonary blood flow to the lungs is reduced. If the detector is contaminated with gastric contents or acidic drugs (e.g., endotracheally administered epinephrine), a colorimetric device may display a constant color rather than breath-to-breath color change. In addition, elimination and detection of CO_2 can be drastically reduced following an intravenous bolus of epinephrine[56] or with severe airway obstruction (e.g., status asthmaticus) and pulmonary edema.[46,57–59] For these reasons, if CO_2 is not detected, a second method should be used to confirm endotracheal tube placement, such as direct visualization or the esophageal detector device.

Use of CO_2-detecting devices to determine the correct placement of other advanced airways (e.g., Combitube, LMA) has not been adequately studied; however, the

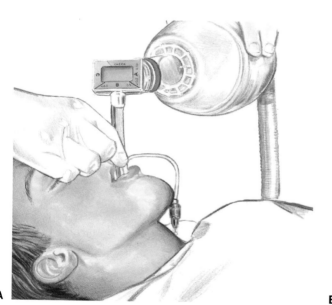

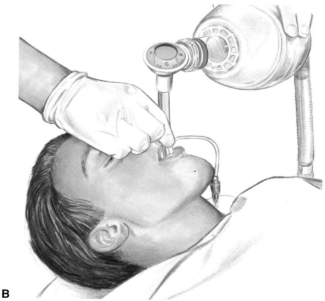

A   B

FIGURE 18-6 • Confirmation of endotracheal tube placement. **A.** End-tidal colorimetric carbon dioxide indicator: purple color indicates lack of carbon dioxide—probably in the esophagus. **B.** End-tidal colorimetric carbon dioxide indicators: yellow indicates the presence of carbon dioxide and tube in the airway. Note that the carbon dioxide detection cannot ensure proper *depth* of tube insertion. Different manufacturers may use different color indicators.

presence of a CO_2 tracing using capnography is the standard of care for LMAs used in anesthesia consistent with lung ventilation.

Esophageal Detector Devices The esophageal detector device (EDD) consists of a bulb that is compressed and attached to the endotracheal tube (Fig. 18-7). If the tube is in the esophagus (positive result for an EDD), the suction created by the EDD will collapse the lumen of the esophagus or pull the esophageal tissue against the tip of the tube and the bulb will not re-expand. The EDD may also consist of a syringe attached to the endotracheal tube; the provider attempts to pull the barrel of the syringe. If the tube is in the esophagus, it will not be possible to pull the barrel (aspirate air) with the syringe.

Eight studies of at least fair quality evaluated the accuracy of the EDD (self-inflating bulb or syringe),[52,53,60–65] but many suffer from small numbers and lack of a control group.

The EDD was highly sensitive for detection of endotracheal tubes that were misplaced in the esophagus (sensitive for esophageal placement) in five case series.[49–53] But in two studies[52,53] involving patients in cardiac arrest, the EDD had poor specificity for indicating endotracheal placement of an endotracheal tube. In these studies up to 30% of correctly placed tubes may have been removed because the EDD suggested esophageal placement.[53] In the operating room, the EDD had poor sensitivity and specificity in 20 children <1 year of age.[66] With these findings in mind, use of the EDD should be considered as just one of several independent methods for confirmation of correct endotracheal tube placement.

The EDD may yield misleading results in patients with morbid obesity, late pregnancy, or status asthmaticus, or when there are copious endotracheal secretions,[67] because

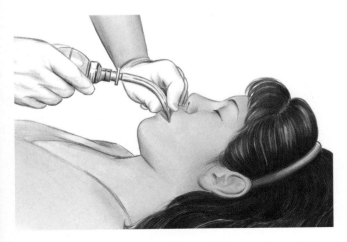

FIGURE 18-7 • Esophageal detector bulb device: the aspiration technique. The tube should be held in place and then secured once correct position is verified.

with these conditions the trachea tends to collapse. There is no evidence that the EDD is accurate for the continued monitoring of endotracheal tube placement.

Confirming Endotracheal Tube Placement When "Confirmation" Results Are Equivocal As a general rule, whenever there is doubt about the results from clinical and device confirmation, the best course of action is to remove the endotracheal tube and provide reoxygenation and ventilation with bag and mask. One or two reattempts at intubation may be appropriate, depending on available resources. The most experienced and highly skilled intubator available should reattempt intubation.

If chest movement or breath sounds are asymmetric, particularly if breath sounds are heard over only one lung, consider whether inadvertent intubation of the right or left main bronchus has occurred. Do not wait for a chest radiograph to determine proper tube position or whether intubation of a main bronchus has occurred. Slowly withdraw the endotracheal tube centimeter by centimeter until equal breath sounds are heard bilaterally and chest expansion is symmetric.

Complications of Endotracheal Intubation The most frequent complications of endotracheal intubation[68–70] are described below.

Trauma Trauma to the lips, mouth, teeth, or oral mucosa can easily occur during intubation. The lips or tongue can be compressed and lacerated between the blade of the laryngoscope and the teeth. The teeth themselves may be chipped. The tip of the tube or stylet may lacerate the pharyngeal or endotracheal mucosa, resulting in bleeding, hematoma, or formation of an abscess. Rupture of the trachea has been reported.[71] Avulsion of an arytenoid cartilage and injury to the vocal cords is also possible. Other complications are pharyngeal–esophageal perforation[72] and intubation of the pyriform sinus.[73]

Vomiting and Aspiration Vomiting can occur and gastric contents may be aspirated into the lower airway. This complication is most likely to occur during emergent intubation of the semiconscious patient who has preserved airway protective reflexes (cough and gag). Vomiting and stimulation of a strong cough or gag reflex can also contribute to increased intracranial pressure.

Reflex Sympathetic and Parasympathetic Stimulation Patients who are not in circulatory arrest receive intense stimulation from laryngoscopy and endotracheal intubation. This adverse stimulation can trigger a complex series of sympathetic and parasympathetic reflexes, including release of high levels of catecholamines from the adrenals. Clinically this can lead to increased intracranial pressure, bronchospasm, hypertension, hypotension, bradycardias, tachycardias, and other arrhythmias.[14] The use of lidocaine, opioids, and atropine at the "premedication step" helps prevent these reactions. These reflexes are much less pronounced in the cardiac arrest patient because the absence of circulation dominates the clinical picture.

Main Bronchus Intubation Insertion of the endotracheal tube into a main bronchus is a relatively common complication. Auscultate the chest to check for bilateral breath sounds and examine it for equal expansion of both sides during ventilation. Intubation of a bronchus can result in hypoxemia and atelectasis caused by underinflation of the other lung.

Esophageal Intubation Unrecognized insertion of the endotracheal tube into the esophagus will result in ineffective ventilation and oxygenation. If this situation remains uncorrected for more than a few minutes, the result can be fatal.[74]

Preventing Complications of Endotracheal Intubation To minimize complications of endotracheal intubation, follow these recommendations:

- Only properly trained personnel should perform endotracheal intubation. This is the key to preventing complications.
- Try to limit intubation attempts to approximately 20 to 30 seconds per attempt. When the time limit is reached or if clinical deterioration occurs (e.g., significant bradycardia, hypoxia, or deterioration in color), provide bag-mask ventilation with 100% oxygen until the clinical appearance improves. Typically another attempt can be made approximately 30 to 60 seconds later.
- If the provider has proper training, experience, and support and the patient is responsive with spontaneous ventilation, consider use of the RSI sequence (with premedication, sedation, and paralysis).
- Use endotracheal tubes with a high-volume, low-pressure cuff, which can be used for prolonged intubation after resuscitation. Measure intracuff pressure and adjust it to 25 to 35 cm H_2O. The minimum intracuff pressure to prevent aspiration in adults appears to be 25 cm H_2O,[75] and the pressure that produces a decrease in mucosal capillary blood flow (ischemia) in adults is >40 cm H_2O.[76]

If Step 6 (First Intubation Attempt) Is Unsuccessful, Resume Bag-Mask Ventilation See Figure 18-8. Numbered boxes below refer to this figure.

"Successful" Bag-Mask Ventilation If the first endotracheal intubation attempt does not succeed, immediately resume bag-mask ventilation (Box 3). If bag-mask ventilation is "successful," with return and maintenance of oxygen saturation at a level ≥90% (or good color for the patient with cardiac arrest), then proceed to clinical and device confirmation (Box 2).

"Unsuccessful" Bag-Mask Ventilation If bag-mask ventilation cannot achieve and maintain an oxygen saturation level ≥90% (or good color for the patient with cardiac arrest), attempt endotracheal intubation once more. But review the level of relaxation and flaccidity in the patient's neck and jaw muscles during the first intubation attempt (Box 4) before making the next attempt. This will determine whether the patient should be paralyzed before the next intubation attempt. If the second attempt is unsuccessful, the clinical situation has now become the dreaded "unable to oxygenate—unable to ventilate" scenario (Box 7).[14] In many settings this is the major indication for initiating a surgical airway protocol (e.g., cricothyrotomy; see "Cricothyrotomy," below).

In other settings, most often in the prehospital setting or emergency department, this scenario represents the major indication for use of a temporizing airway adjunct, such as the Combitube or LMA (Box 8). The value of these two newly recommended devices (see "Alternative Advanced Airways") derives from the requirement for blind insertion only. The provider does not face the challenge of direct visualization of the vocal cords.

Evaluate Relaxation/Flaccidity The *intubator* actually gathers this information during the first endotracheal intubation attempt. It is only upon failure to intubate that the rescuer can determine if there was complete skeletal muscle relaxation. If jaw and neck muscle flaccidity was nearly absolute, then endotracheal intubation can be attempted again. If there was *any* resistance to intubation, paralysis is indicated (Box 6).

Paralyze the Patient When you administer succinylcholine 1.5 mg/kg IV, you should immediately resume the most effective bag-mask ventilations possible with 100% oxygen. In many in-hospital settings, the person who performs emergency intubations has already drawn up a syringe containing 100 mg of succinylcholine, an appropriate dose for a patient weighing 65 to 70 kg. This will ensure complete paralysis of the patient for intubation.

A. If the patient is in cardiac arrest, give one dose (for a patient in cardiac arrest sedation is not necessary).
B. After 30 to 40 seconds, check the jaw and neck muscles for flaccidity.
C. If flaccid, attempt endotracheal intubation again.

Step 7: Postintubation Management—Prevent Endotracheal Tube Dislodgment The endotracheal tube may be displaced if the tube is not secured, particularly in pre-hospital settings or during any transport of the patient. Maintenance of proper tube position requires frequent assessment, not only immediately after intubation, but whenever the patient is moved.

The endotracheal tube is secured with tape or a commercial endotracheal tube holder (Fig. 18-9). It is acceptable to use locally derived, ad hoc tape-and-tie systems if they are supported by formal teaching and demonstrations or protocols.

The tube may still be displaced or dislodged, regardless of how it is secured, particularly during patient transfer. Continuous monitoring of end-tidal CO_2 and oxygen

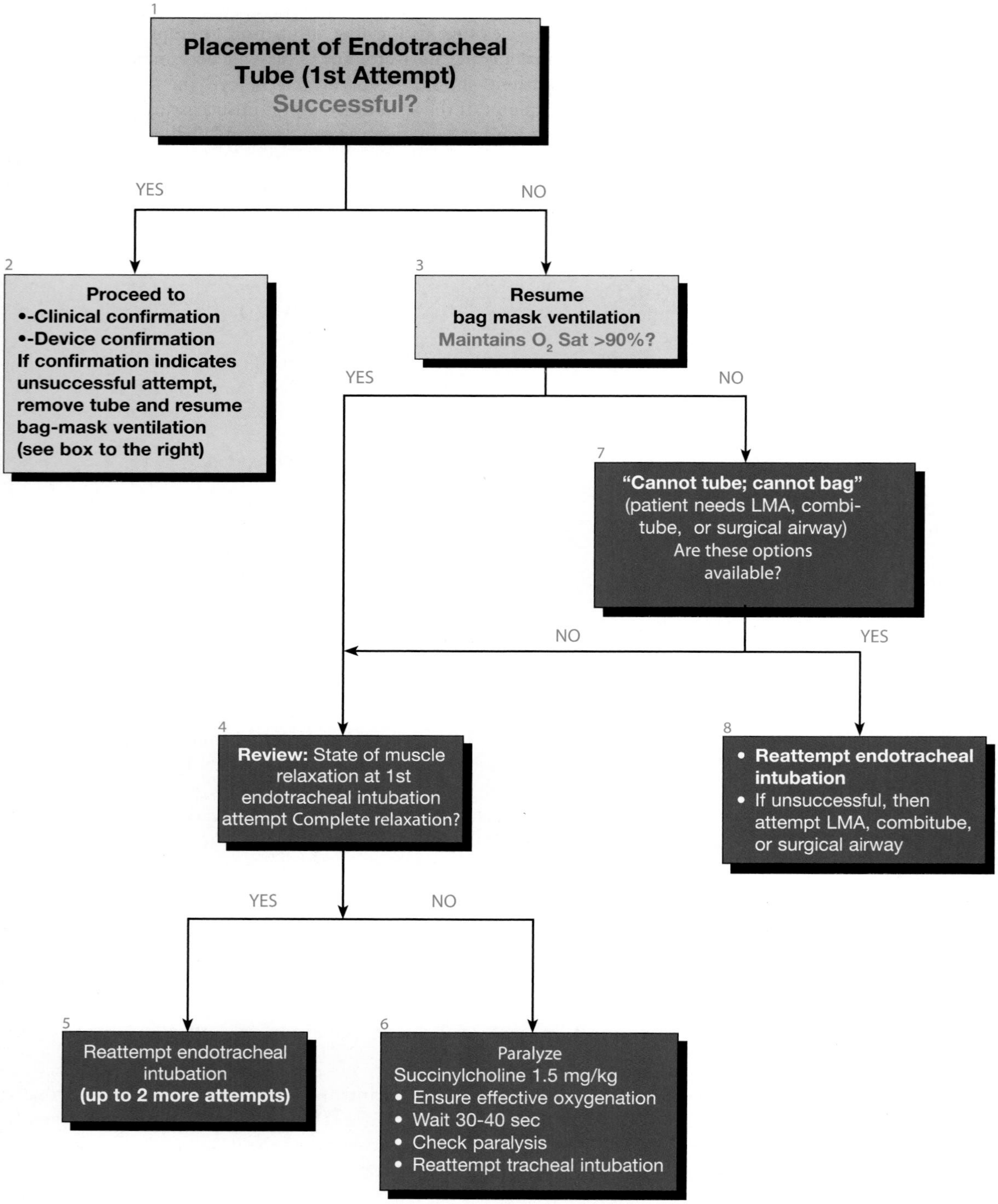

1

Placement of Endotracheal Tube (1st Attempt)
Successful?

YES ← → NO

2

Proceed to
- -Clinical confirmation
- -Device confirmation

If confirmation indicates unsuccessful attempt, remove tube and resume bag-mask ventilation (see box to the right)

3

Resume bag mask ventilation
Maintains O_2 Sat >90%?

YES ← → NO

7

"Cannot tube; cannot bag"
(patient needs LMA, combitube, or surgical airway)
Are these options available?

NO ← → YES

4

Review: State of muscle relaxation at 1st endotracheal intubation attempt Complete relaxation?

8

- **Reattempt endotracheal intubation**
- If unsuccessful, then attempt LMA, combitube, or surgical airway

YES ← → NO

5

Reattempt endotracheal intubation
(up to 2 more attempts)

6

Paralyze
Succinylcholine 1.5 mg/kg
- Ensure effective oxygenation
- Wait 30-40 sec
- Check paralysis
- Reattempt tracheal intubation

FIGURE 18-8 • Actions for provider if first attempted intubation is unsuccessful (see text for full explanation). Major actions are try to place tube with first oral intubation attempt, resume bag-mask ventilations, review relaxation/ flaccidity, and paralyze the patient.

saturation is recommended. In the prehospital setting, immobilization of the cervical spine with a collar, backboard, or both can serve as an additional precaution, although the use and effect of these immobilizers on tube placement has not been reported.

Checklists for Endotracheal Intubation

Checklists provide means to improve the performance of complex, psychomotor skills that are difficult to learn and remember. A variety of helpful checklists have been developed for advanced airway management,[77–79] particularly

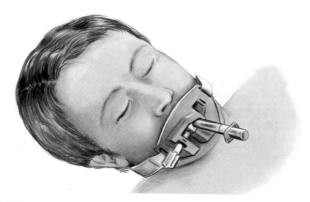

FIGURE 18-9 • Actions for rescuer if first attempted intubation is unsuccessful (see text for full explanation). Major actions are try to place tube with first oral intubation attempt, resume bag-mask ventilations, review relaxation/flaccidity, and paralyze the patient.

endotracheal intubation.[79–84] The purpose of these checklists is to have all equipment and personnel in place and in working order before every intubation attempt. One of many possible Preparation-Action Checklists that lists actions, intubation team members, and designated duties as shown here. This checklist for resuscitation personnel reviews areas and topics to be considered. Different settings, personnel, and resources will require different preparation-action checklists. Some items on this sample checklist must be completed before an actual clinical event occurs. Others are performed urgently, just before an endotracheal intubation attempt in cardiac arrest.

Pre-Event Equipment Checklist for Endotracheal Intubation: Equipment and Drugs Recommended for Endotracheal Intubation

Yes?	No?	Equipment
☐	☐	Cardiac monitor
☐	☐	Automatic blood pressure cuff
☐	☐	Intravenous infusion equipment
☐	☐	Oxygen supply, equipment for connections to airway adjunct device
☐	☐	Esophageal detector device (aspiration technique)
☐	☐	Exhaled CO_2 detector device: capnometry (qualitative) **or** Exhaled CO_2 measuring device: capnography (continuous, quantitative)
☐	☐	Pulse oximeters
☐	☐	Suction device and suction catheter (confirm working; catheter near patient head)
☐	☐	Bag-mask connected to high-flow oxygen source
☐	☐	Endotracheal tubes, proper size (all sizes should be available for emergent use; typically the size above and below anticipated size for the patient should be within reach during the attempt)
☐	☐	Endotracheal tube stylet
☐	☐	Laryngoscope blade (curved and straight available)
☐	☐	Laryngoscope handle with working light
☐	☐	Backup light source (another laryngoscope handle and blade)
☐	☐	5- to 10-mL syringe to test-inflate endotracheal tube balloon (attached to pilot balloon)
☐	☐	**Premedication agents:** lidocaine, opioids (such as fentanyl), atropine, and defasciculating agents
☐	☐	**Analgesic agents:** opioids
☐	☐	**Sedative/anesthetic agents:** etomidate, propofol, methohexital, thiopental, midazolam, ketamine
☐	☐	**Paralytic agents:** succinylcholine, vancuronium, pancuronium
☐	☐	Commercial endotracheal tube holder if used instead of tape
☐	☐	Restraints for patient's hands if awake
☐	☐	Container for patient's dentures if needed
☐	☐	Towel or pad to place under patient's neck (to elevate neck 10 cm)

Modify where appropriate. Modifications will depend on specific settings (e.g., critical care unit versus paramedic-staffed ambulance). For intubation during cardiac arrest, adjunctive and analgesic agents are typically omitted. Paralytic agents, most often succinylcholine, may be the only medications used. This checklist can serve as a pre-event checklist for *endotracheal intubation during cardiac arrest*. In practice, similar checklists must be incorporated into the daily/every shift *supply check* or *stocking rounds* standard in emergency departments, critical care units and EMS.

Sample Checklist for Personnel Preparation and Responsibilities During Endotracheal Intubation

This sample checklist includes actions, intubation team members, and designated duties for intubation of the unresponsive patient with no spontaneous respirations and no spontaneous circulation. Some items on this checklist must be completed before an actual clinical event. Other actions are performed urgently, just before attempting endotracheal intubation in a cardiac arrest. The checklist concept provides a quality-improvement/assurance tool with the purpose of having all equipment and personnel in place and in working order before *every* intubation attempt.

Yes?	No?	Equipment
☐	☐	*Assistant to intubator.* At start of shift (before time of arrest), designate and identify an *assistant to the intubator*. These duties are assumed by intubator if no assistant is available. These duties include responsibility for equipment and devices, including the following: • Attach *cardiac monitor*; maintain continuous surveillance of rhythm before, during, and after intubation; announce any rhythm change • Attach and maintain automatic blood pressure device • Attach and maintain O_2 saturation device; survey readings; announce drops in readings, O_2 saturation; state response to changes in FiO_2 or in response to intubation attempt • Assess for signs of decompensation • Track periods without ventilation; announce any >30 seconds in duration • Remove patient's dentures as needed before intubation attempt • Apply cricoid pressure when bag-mask ventilation begins; maintain throughout laryngoscopy and insertion of endotracheal tube until cuff inflated and primary and secondary confirmations completed • Perform or assist with clinical confirmation of tube placement (five-point auscultation, chest rise and fall, tube condensation) • Perform or assist with device confirmation of tube placement (colorimetric exhaled CO_2 device, esophageal detector device, quantitative exhaled CO_2 device) • For in-hospital intubation: call radiology for postintubation radiograph of chest after confirmation of tube placement
☐	☐	*IV accessor/medications.* At start of shift, designate person responsible for IV access and administration of drugs; review her or his duties: • Establish peripheral vein access • Verify ready availability of drugs most likely to be needed, administer agents when ordered (drugs used will vary by clinical setting and protocols) • Premedications: lidocaine, opioids—such as fentanyl, atropine • Defasciculating/paralytic agents: succinylcholine, vecuronium, rocuronium, etc. • Sedative/hypnotic/anesthetic agents: *fentanyl, etomidate, propofol, methohexital, thiopental, ketamine, midazolam, diazepam*
☐	☐	*Oxygen:* locate oxygen source; make sure connecting tubing is in place; attach to bag mask (start at 15 L/min)
☐	☐	*Endotracheal tube:* select size (7 mm for average-size woman; 8 mm for average-size man); check volume of inflatable cuff; using syringe, inject that volume into balloon; check for leaks, deflate; leave syringe attached • Insert stylet into endotracheal tube (if needed) • Check that additional endotracheal tubes are available
☐	☐	*Laryngoscope:* select blade (straight or curved); check that light is ON; confirm availability of backup light source
☐	☐	*Oral suction:* confirm that wall suction source or battery-powered portable unit is available and in working order and that connecting tube is in place. Use Yankauer-type suction tip. • Start suction, place suction tip near patient's head (in hospital: under pillow)
☐	☐	*Final steps before picking up laryngoscope and endotracheal tube:* 1. Place a towel under patient's head to elevate it 10 cm 2. Check head positioning: neck is slightly flexed, head extended 3. Review latest vital signs 4. Identify rhythm on monitor 5. Obtain oxygen saturation reading 6. Ask if *intubator assistant* and *IV accessor/medications* are ready to start intubation 7. Announce *"I am ready to begin intubation"*

Surgical Airways

Cricothyrotomy

Description

The term "cricothyrotomy" refers to the procedure of creating an opening in the cricothyroid membrane so that an airway tube can be inserted directly into the trachea (Fig. 18-10). There are two acceptable techniques for the ACLS provider:

- *Percutaneous dilational cricothyrotomy.* This is the preferred technique, using one of the prepackaged commercial cricothyrotomy kits to gain access to the trachea via a modified Seldinger technique. After a suitably sized opening is produced with an introducer, guidewire, and dilator, a commercially produced *cricothyrotomy tube* is advanced over the guidewire.[85]
- *Surgical cricothyrotomy.* This technique makes use of a scalpel incision with ad hoc dilation of the opening by rotation of the scalpel handle and insertion of a pediatric-sized endotracheal tube (without an inflatable cuff) or a cuffed tracheostomy tube. This technique is acceptable if a cricothyrotomy kit is unavailable. Use of the scalpel surgical technique is discouraged, especially in emergency settings, where cricothyrotomies are rarely if ever performed.[85–89] The ventilation through small-diameter tubes allows emergency oxygen administration but severely limits ventilation (CO_2 elimination).

Safe performance of a cricothyrotomy requires specialized training. It should be performed by only highly skilled medical providers who encounter complete upper airway obstruction that is unresponsive to standard interventions.

Indications

An invasive procedure, cricothyrotomy is indicated only when airway control is impossible by other available methods. These "difficult airway" situations are caused by upper airway obstruction by trauma, allergic reactions with swelling and angioedema, foreign bodies, anatomic variations, and bleeding.

Insertion Technique: Simple Cricothyrotomy

- Position the patient supine with the neck extended and the larynx as anterior as possible.
- Palpate the prominent thyroid cartilage (Adam's apple) and locate the cricothyroid membrane with your gloved fingernail as the transverse indentation below the thyroid cartilage and above the cricoid cartilage.
- Clean the area with antiseptic solution.
- With the commercial cricothyrotomy kits, the general approach is to make a small horizontal opening in the cricothyroid membrane with a scalpel. This allows easy insertion of the larger introducer needle, through which a Seldinger-like guidewire is introduced.
- The introducer needle is replaced by a dilator to enlarge the opening.
- Next, the kit's cricothyrotomy tube is inserted into the opening over the guidewire.
- The surgical technique requires a larger scalpel incision through the skin, through the cricothyroid membrane, and into the trachea.
- After enlarging the opening by rotation of the scalpel handle, insert the largest pediatric-sized endotracheal tube or tracheostomy tube that will fit through this opening.
- Attach a bag-mask device connected to the highest available oxygen concentration and begin ventilation.

Complications

Possible complications are hemorrhage, false passage of the tube, perforation of the esophagus, and subcutaneous or mediastinal emphysema.

Tracheostomy

Tracheostomy is familiar to most emergency health care providers but is rarely a procedure that even experienced ACLS providers should ever expect to perform.

Description

The term "tracheostomy" refers to the procedure of surgically creating an opening through the cartilage rings of the trachea. This procedure is considerably more involved and complicated than a cricothyrotomy, which requires only a simple incision through the cricothyroid membrane.

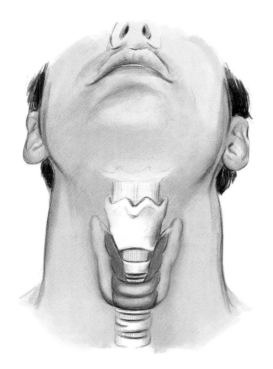

FIGURE 18-10 • Neck with cricoid membrane displayed, with an arrow indicating location for an emergency cricothyrotomy.

Indications and Prevention of Complications

- A patient becomes a candidate for a tracheostomy only after the airway is first secured with one of the following: an endotracheal tube inserted through a cricothyrotomy, an endotracheal tube inserted through the mouth and hypopharynx, or a translaryngeal catheter.
- A tracheostomy is a follow-up or secondary procedure.
- A tracheostomy is not appropriate for urgent situations such as airway obstruction or cardiac arrest.
- Surgical opening of the trachea and insertion of a tracheostomy tube should be performed only under controlled conditions in the operating room or emergency department by a health care professional skilled in the procedure.

References

1. Pepe PE, Copass MK, Joyce TH. Prehospital endotracheal intubation: rationale for training emergency medical personnel. *Ann Emerg Med* 1985;14(11):1085–1092.
2. Bowman FP, Menegazzi JJ, Check BD, et al. Lower esophageal sphincter pressure during prolonged cardiac arrest and resuscitation. *Ann Emerg Med* 1995;26(2):216–219.
3. Weiler N, Heinrichs W, Dick W. Assessment of pulmonary mechanics and gastric inflation pressure during mask ventilation. *Prehosp Disaster Med* 1995;10(2):101–105.
4. Ruben H, Knudsen EJ, Carugati G. Gastric inflation in relation to airway pressure. *Acta Anaesth Scand* 1961;5:107–114.
5. Wenzel V, Idris AH, Banner MJ, et al. Respiratory system compliance decreases after cardiopulmonary resuscitation and stomach inflation: impact of large and small tidal volumes on calculated peak airway pressure. *Resuscitation* 1998;38(2):113–118.
6. Stept WJ, Safar P. Rapid induction-intubation for prevention of gastric-content aspiration. *Anesth Analg* 1970;49(4):633–636.
7. Wang HE, Sweeney TA, O'Connor RE, et al. Failed prehospital intubations: an analysis of emergency department courses and outcomes. *Prehosp Emerg Care* 2001;5(2):134–141.
8. Wang HE, O'Connor RE, Megargel RE, et al. The utilization of midazolam as a pharmacologic adjunct to endotracheal intubation by paramedics. *Prehosp Emerg Care* 2000;4(1):14–18.
9. Wayne MA, Slovis CM, Pirrallo RG. Management of difficult airways in the field. *Prehosp Emerg Care* 1999;3(4):290–296.
10. Brownstein D, Shugerman R, Cummings P, et al. Prehospital endotracheal intubation of children by paramedics. *Ann Emerg Med* 1996;28(1):34–39.
11. Ma OJ, Atchley RB, Hatley T, et al. Intubation success rates improve for an air medical program after implementing the use of neuromuscular blocking agents. *Am J Emerg Med* 1998;16(2):125–127.
12. Kociszewski C, Thomas SH, Harrison T, et al. Etomidate versus succinylcholine for intubation in an air medical setting. *Am J Emerg Med* 2000;18(7):757–763.
13. Syverud SA, Borron SW, Storer DL, et al. Prehospital use of neuromuscular blocking agents in a helicopter ambulance program. *Ann Emerg Med* 1988;17(3):236–242.
14. Walls R. The emergency airway algorithms. In: Walls RN, Luten RC, Murphy MF, et al, eds. *Manual of Emergency Airway Management*. Philadelphia: Lippincott Williams & Wilkins, 2000.
15. Pace SA, Fuller FP. Out-of-hospital succinylcholine-assisted endotracheal intubation by paramedics. *Ann Emerg Med* 2000;35(6):568–572.
16. O'Connor RE, Swor RA. Verification of endotracheal tube placement following intubation. National Association of EMS Physicians Standards and Clinical Practice Committee. *Prehosp Emerg Care* 1999;3(3):248–250.
17. Wang HE, O'Connor RE, Domeier RM. Prehospital rapid-sequence intubation. *Prehosp Emerg Care* 2001;5(1):40–48.
18. Walls RN, Luten RC, Murphy MF, et al, eds. *Manual of Emergency Airway Management*. Philadelphia: Lippincott Williams & Wilkins, 2000.
19. Anderson JL, Adams CD, Antman EM, et al. ACC/AHA 2007 guidelines for the management of patients with unstable angina/non ST-elevation myocardial infarction: a report of the American College of Cardiology/American Heart Association Task Force on Practice Guidelines (Writing Committee to Revise the 2002 Guidelines for the Management of Patients With Unstable Angina/Non ST-Elevation Myocardial Infarction): developed in collaboration with the American College of Emergency Physicians, the Society for Cardiovascular Angiography and Interventions, and the Society of Thoracic Surgeons: endorsed by the American Association of Cardiovascular and Pulmonary Rehabilitation and the Society for Academic Emergency Medicine. *Circulation* 2007;116(7):e148–e304.
20. McGowan P, Skinner A. Preoxygenation—the importance of a good face mask seal. *Br J Anaesth* 1995;75(6):777–778.
21. Berthoud M, Read DH, Norman J. Pre-oxygenation: how long? *Anaesthesia* 1983;38(2):96–102.
22. Mejicano GC, Maki DG. Infections acquired during cardiopulmonary resuscitation: estimating the risk and defining strategies for prevention. *Ann Intern Med* 1998;129(10):813–828.
23. Axelsson A, Thoren A, Holmberg S, et al. Attitudes of trained Swedish lay rescuers toward CPR performance in an emergency: a survey of 1012 recently trained CPR rescuers. *Resuscitation* 2000;44(1):27–36.
24. Melanson SW, O'Gara K. EMS provider reluctance to perform mouth-to-mouth resuscitation. *Prehosp Emerg Care* 2000;4(1):48–52.
25. Nocera A. A flexible solution for emergency intubation difficulties. *Ann Emerg Med* 1996;27(5):665–667.
26. Kidd JF, Dyson A, Latto IP. Successful difficult intubation. Use of the gum elastic bougie. *Anaesthesia* 1988;43(6):437–438.
27. Dogra S, Falconer R, Latto IP. Successful difficult intubation. Tracheal tube placement over a gum-elastic bougie. *Anaesthesia* 1990;45(9):774–776.
28. Nolan JP, Wilson ME. An evaluation of the gum elastic bougie. Intubation times and incidence of sore throat. *Anaesthesia* 1992;47(10):878–881.
29. Nolan JP, Wilson ME. Orotracheal intubation in patients with potential cervical spine injuries. An indication for the gum elastic bougie. *Anaesthesia* 1993;48(7):630–633.
30. Viswanathan S, Campbell C, Wood DG, et al. The Eschmann Tracheal Tube Introducer. (Gum elastic bougie). *Anesthesiol Rev* 1992;19(6):29–34.
31. Hopkins PM. Use of suxamethonium in children. *Br J Anaesth* 1995;75(6):675–677.
32. Morell RC, Berman JM, Royster RI, et al. Revised label regarding use of succinylcholine in children and adolescents. *Anesthesiology* 1994;80(1):242–245.
33. Scheiber G, Ribeiro FC, Marichal A, et al. Intubating conditions and onset of action after rocuronium, vecuronium, and atracurium in young children. *Anesth Analg* 1996;83(2):320–324.
34. McDonald PF, Sainsbury DA, Laing RJ. Evaluation of the onset time and intubation conditions of rocuronium bromide in children. *Anaesth Intens Care* 1997;25(3):260–261.
35. Fuchs-Buder T, Tassonyi E. Intubating conditions and time course of rocuronium-induced neuromuscular block in children. *Br J Anaesth* 1996;77(3):335–338.
36. Maddineni VR, McCoy EP, Mirakur RK, et al. Onset and duration of action and hemodynamic effects of rocuronium bromide under balanced and volatile anesthesia. *Acta Anaesthesiol Belg* 1994;45(2):41–47.
37. Khuenl-Brady KS, Pomaroli A, Puhringer F, et al. The use of rocuronium (ORG 9426) in patients with chronic renal failure. *Anaesthesia* 1993;48(10):873–875.
38. Magorian T, Wood P, Caldwell J, et al. The pharmacokinetics and neuromuscular effects of rocuronium bromide in patients with liver disease. *Anesth Analg* 1995;80(4):754–759.
39. Khalil M, D'Honneur G, Duvaldestin P, et al. Pharmacokinetics and pharmacodynamics of rocuronium in patients with cirrhosis. *Anesthesiology* 1994;80(6):1241–1247.
40. Ferres CJ, Crean PM, Mirakhur RK. An evaluation of Org NC 45 (vecuronium) in paediatric anaesthesia. *Anaesthesia* 1983;38(10):943–947.
41. Mirakhur RK, Ferres CJ, Clarke RS, et al. Clinical evaluation of Org NC 45. *Br J Anaesth* 1983;55(2):119–124.
42. Lynam DP, Cronnelly R, Castagnoli KP, et al. The pharmacodynamics and pharmacokinetics of vecuronium in patients anesthetized with isoflurane with normal renal function or with renal failure. *Anesthesiology* 1988;69(2):227–231.

43. Sellick BA. Cricoid pressure to control regurgitation of stomach contents during induction of anaesthesia. *Lancet* 1961;2:404–406.

44. Li J. Capnography alone is imperfect for endotracheal tube placement confirmation during emergency intubation. *J Emerg Med* 2001;20(3):223–229.

45. Grmec S. Comparison of three different methods to confirm tracheal tube placement in emergency intubation. *Intens Care Med* 2002;28(6):701–704.

46. Ornato JP, Shipley JB, Racht EM, et al. Multicenter study of a portable, hand-size, colorimetric end-tidal carbon dioxide detection device. *Ann Emerg Med* 1992;21(5):518–523.

47. Anton WR, Gordon RW, Jordan TM, et al. A disposable end-tidal CO_2 detector to verify endotracheal intubation. *Ann Emerg Med* 1991;20(3):271–275.

48. Bhende MS, Thompson AE. Evaluation of an end-tidal CO2 detector during pediatric cardiopulmonary resuscitation. *Pediatrics* 1995;95(3):395–399.

49. Bhende MS, Thompson AE, Cook DR, et al. Validity of a disposable end-tidal CO_2 detector in verifying endotracheal tube placement in infants and children. *Ann Emerg Med* 1992;21(2):142–145.

50. Hayden SR, Sciammarella J, Viccellio P, et al. Colorimetric end-tidal CO_2 detector for verification of endotracheal tube placement in out-of-hospital cardiac arrest. *Acad Emerg Med* 1995;2(6):499–502.

51. MacLeod BA, Heller MB, Gerard J, et al. Verification of endotracheal tube placement with colorimetric end-tidal CO_2 detection. *Ann Emerg Med* 1991;20(3):267–270.

52. Takeda T, Tanigawa K, Tanaka H, et al. The assessment of three methods to verify tracheal tube placement in the emergency setting. *Resuscitation* 2003;56(2):153–157.

53. Tanigawa K, Takeda T, Goto E, et al. The efficacy of esophageal detector devices in verifying tracheal tube placement: a randomized cross-over study of out-of-hospital cardiac arrest patients. *Anesth Analg* 2001;92(2):375–378.

54. Varon AJ, Morrina J, Civetta JM. Clinical utility of a colorimetric end-tidal CO2 detector in cardiopulmonary resuscitation and emergency intubation. *J Clin Monit* 1991;7(4):289–293.

55. Sum Ping ST, Mehta MP, Symreng T. Accuracy of the FEF CO2 detector in the assessment of endotracheal tube placement. *Anesth Analg* 1992;74(3):415–419.

56. Cantineau JP, Lambert Y, Merckx P, et al. End-tidal carbon dioxide during cardiopulmonary resuscitation in humans presenting mostly with asystole: a predictor of outcome. *Crit Care Med* 1996;24(5):791–796.

57. Ward KR, Yealy DM. End-tidal carbon dioxide monitoring in emergency medicine. Part 2: clinical applications. *Acad Emerg Med* 1998;5(6):637–646.

58. Hand IL, Shepard EK, Krauss AN, et al. Discrepancies between transcutaneous and end-tidal carbon dioxide monitoring in the critically ill neonate with respiratory distress syndrome. *Crit Care Med* 1989;17(6):556–559.

59. Tobias JD, Meyer DJ. Noninvasive monitoring of carbon dioxide during respiratory failure in toddlers and infants: end-tidal versus transcutaneous carbon dioxide. *Anesth Analg* 1997;85(1):55–58.

60. Pelucio M, Halligan L, Dhindsa H. Out-of-hospital experience with the syringe esophageal detector device. *Acad Emerg Med* 1997;4(6):563–568.

61. Bozeman WP, Hexter D, Liang HK, Kelen GD. Esophageal detector device versus detection of end-tidal carbon dioxide level in emergency intubation. *Ann Emerg Med* 1996;27(5):595–599.

62. Sharieff GQ, Rodarte A, Wilton N, et al. The self-inflating bulb as an esophageal detector device in children weighing more than twenty kilograms: A comparison of two techniques. *Ann Emerg Med* 2003;41(5):623–629.

63. Wee MY, Walker AK. The oesophageal detector device: an assessment with uncuffed tubes in children. *Anaesthesia* 1991;46(10):869–871.

64. Williams KN, Nunn JF. The oesophageal detector device: a prospective trial on 100 patients. *Anaesthesia* 1989;44(5):412–424.

65. Zaleski L, Abello D, Gold MI. The esophageal detector device. Does it work? *Anesthesiology* 1993;79(2):244–247.

66. Haynes SR, Morton NS. Use of the oesophageal detector device in children under one year of age. *Anaesthesia* 1990;45(12):1067–1069.

67. Baraka A, Khoury PJ, Siddik SS, et al. Efficacy of the self-inflating bulb in differentiating esophageal from tracheal intubation in the parturient undergoing cesarean section. *Anesth Analg* 1997;84(3):533–537.

68. Blanc VF, Tremblay NA. The complications of tracheal intubation: a new classification with a review of the literature. *Anesth Analg* 1974;53(2):202–213.

69. Jones GO, Hale DE, Wasmuth CE, et al. A survey of acute complications associated with endotracheal intubation. *Cleve Clin Q* 1968;35(1):23–31.

70. Taryle DA, Chandler JE, Good JTJ, et al. Emergency room intubations: complications and survival. *Chest* 1979;75(5):541–543.

71. Thompson DS, Read RC. Rupture of the trachea following endotracheal intubation. *JAMA* 1968;204(11):995–997.

72. Wolff AP, Kuhn FA, Ogura JH. Pharyngeal-esophageal perforations associated with rapid oral endotracheal intubation. *Ann Otol Rhinol Laryngol* 1972;81(2):258–261.

73. Stauffer JL, Petty TL. Accidental intubation of the pyriform sinus: a complication of "roadside" resuscitation. *JAMA* 1977;237(21): 2324–2325.

74. Pollard BJ, Junius F. Accidental intubation of the oesophagus. *Anaesth Intens Care* 1980;8(2):183–186.

75. Bernhard WN, Cottrell JE, Sivakumaran C, et al. Adjustment of intracuff pressure to prevent aspiration. *Anesthesiology* 1979;50(4): 363–366.

76. Nordin U. The trachea and cuff-induced tracheal injury. An experimental study on causative factors and prevention. *Acta Otolaryngol Suppl* 1977;345:1–71.

77. Cheney FW, Posner KL, Caplan RA. Adverse respiratory events infrequently leading to malpractice suits. A closed claims analysis. *Anesthesiology* 1991;75(6):932–939.

78. Cheney FW, Posner K, Caplan RA, et al. Standard of care and anesthesia liability. *JAMA* 1989;261(11):1599–1603.

79. Caplan RA, Posner KL, Ward RJ, et al. Adverse respiratory events in anesthesia: a closed claims analysis. *Anesthesiology* 1990;72(5): 828–833.

80. Cooper JB, Newbower RS, Kitz RJ. An analysis of major errors and equipment failures in anesthesia management: considerations for prevention and detection. *Anesthesiology* 1984;60(1):34–42.

81. Cooper JB, Newbower RS, Long CD, et al. Preventable anesthesia mishaps: a study of human factors. *Anesthesiology* 1978;49(6): 399–406.

82. Cooper JB, Cullen DJ, Nemeskal R, et al. Effects of information feedback and pulse oximetry on the incidence of anesthesia complications. *Anesthesiology* 1987;67(5):686–694.

83. Cooper JB. Accidents and mishaps in anesthesia: how they occur; how to prevent them. *Minerva Anestesiol* 2001;67(4):310–313.

84. Cooper JB. Towards patient safety in anaesthesia. *Ann Acad Med Singapore* 1994;23(4):552–557.

85. Florete OG. Airway management. In Civetta JM, Taylor RW, Kirby RR, eds. *Critical Care*, 2nd ed. Philadelphia: Lippincott, 1992:1430–1431.

86. Brantigan CO, Grow JBS. Cricothyroidotomy: elective use in respiratory problems requiring tracheotomy. *J Thorac Cardiovasc Surg* 1976;71(1):72–81.

87. McGill J, Clinton JE, Ruiz E. Cricothyrotomy in the emergency department. *Ann Emerg Med* 1982;11(7):361–364.

88. Simon RR, Brenner BE, Rosen MA. Emergency cricothyroidotomy in the patient with massive neck swelling. Part 2: Clinical aspects. *Crit Care Med* 1983;11(2):119–123.

89. Simon RR, Brenner BE. Emergency cricothyroidotomy in the patient with massive neck swelling: Part 1: Anatomical aspects. *Crit Care Med* 1983;11(2):114–118.

Arrhythmias

Chapter 19
Life-Threatening Arrhythmias: Evaluation, Identification, and Assessment

Peter J. Kudenchuk

If a patient is pulseless or in shock, a wide-complex tachycardia is best presumed to be ventricular tachycardia (VT) until proved otherwise. In a study of patients who presented with a wide-QRS-complex tachycardia, if they said yes to two questions ("Have you ever had a heart attack in the past?" and "Did [these kind of symptoms] start after your heart attack?") VT was the culprit arrhythmia in nearly all (28 of 29) cases.

- Evaluation and assessment of patients with life-threatening arrhythmias
- Diagnostic clues in the 12-lead electrocardiogram
- Triggers for actions and interventions
- Knowing when to call expert consultation for complicated rhythm interpretation or pharmacologic or management decisions

Evaluation of the Arrhythmia Patient

Basic Principles

Cardiac arrhythmias present with a wide variety of symptoms, including palpitations, chest discomfort, dyspnea, dizziness, confusion, syncope, as well as unheralded collapse (cardiac arrest). These symptoms may be intermittent when caused by self-terminating (paroxysmal) arrhythmias and can range in severity from bothersome but not necessarily life-threatening to catastrophic, requiring immediate intervention. The initial assessment of an arrhythmia should focus on the patient, her or his clinical status, and whether there is time to establish a rhythm diagnosis before treatment or before moving to immediate lifesaving measures—cardiopulmonary resuscitation (CPR) and electrical cardioversion or defibrillation—in the case of someone who is unconscious, markedly hypotensive, or pulseless.

In presentations with a wide complex tachycardia (WCT), the hemodynamic stability (or instability) of the patient is singularly unhelpful in discriminating whether it represents a supraventricular or a ventricular tachycardia.[1] Typically heart rate, not the supraventricular or ventricular etiology of the arrhythmia, is the single most important determinant of symptoms and their severity. From a hemodynamic standpoint, arrhythmias are also generally better tolerated among patients with better underlying heart function than in those whose ventricular function is significantly impaired.

History

A brief history focused on whether the patient has heart disease can be revealing. Ventricular arrhythmias predominate in patients with known structural heart disease as well in as older adults with other risk factors for heart disease. Supraventricular arrhythmias tend to be more common in younger, healthier patients and in those in whom arrhythmias may have preceded their development of heart disease. In a study of conscious patients who presented with a wide-QRS-complex tachycardia, an affirmative answer to two questions ("Have you ever had a heart attack in the past?" and "Did [these kind of symptoms] start after your heart attack?") correctly identified VT as the culprit arrhythmia in nearly all (28 of 29) cases.[1] Comparison of a prior ECG (if available) with an ECG of the current arrhythmia can also be quite helpful.

In a study of conscious patients who presented with a wide-QRS-complex tachycardia, an affirmative answer to two questions ("Have you ever had a heart attack in the past?" and "Did [these kind of symptoms] start after your heart attack?") correctly identified VT as the culprit arrhythmia in nearly all (28 of 29) cases.

Physical Examination

The physical examination of patients in arrhythmia should initially assess for signs of hemodynamic instability or evidence that the arrhythmia is being poorly tolerated, including level of consciousness, heart rate, and blood pressure, followed by evidence of heightened sympathetic drive, including skin pallor, cool extremities, and diaphoresis. Auscultation of lung fields may reveal diffuse crackles suggestive of pulmonary edema. The pulse may be regular, irregularly irregular, thready, or absent. Variability in the intensity of the first heart sound (S1) and cannon "A" waves in the jugular pulse are highly sensitive and specific indications of atrioventricular dissociation associated VT. Although these signs are helpful when detected, very often the rapid ventricular rate precludes making a rhythm diagnosis on the basis of physical findings alone. Documenting the rhythm through rhythm monitoring or an electrocardiogram (ECG) is required.

Electrocardiogram

ECG monitoring should be instituted as soon as possible, ideally simultaneous with the initial assessment of the patient. In emergent or semiemergent circumstances, this can be done most efficiently by applying defibrillation electrodes (from which the ECG can be monitored) or by use of the "quick-look paddles" feature available on most conventional defibrillators. Early ECG monitoring is also important in high-risk patients, such as those with acute myocardial infarction (AMI) or severe ischemia. Because the greatest risk for serious arrhythmias exists during the first hour after onset of symptoms of infarction or ischemia, health care professionals should start cardiac monitoring as soon as possible.

All ECG and rhythm information should be interpreted in context of other available information about the patient, including ventilation, oxygenation, heart rate, blood pressure, level of consciousness, acid-base status, and medication use. In specific clinical settings, care providers should consider possible aggravation of arrhythmias by antiarrhythmic drugs (proarrhythmia), adverse drug effects from intentional or unintentional overdose, or drug toxicity occurring with normal dosing patterns or as a result of drug-drug interactions.

With these principles in mind, care providers should:

1. Recognize the symptoms and signs requiring immediate treatment of the patient with cardioversion or defibrillation.
2. Understand the initial diagnostic, electrical, and pharmacologic treatment approaches for rhythms that are hemodynamically unstable and those that are not.
3. Know when to call expert consultation for complicated rhythm interpretation or pharmacologic or management decisions.

Providers of acute cardial life support (ACLS) should also participate in training and evaluation sessions that will establish their ability to detect and treat serious arrhythmias, including regular updates to enhance their expertise in rhythm interpretation and in using and troubleshooting ECG monitoring equipment.

Arrhythmia Recognition and Classification

Advanced providers and professionals should be able to distinguish true arrhythmias from normal heart rhythms occurring at other than usual rates and from fictitious arrhythmias. Patients in acute distress are likely to manifest normal rhythms at more rapid rates, which should not be confused with a primary arrhythmia unless the rate is not appropriate for the clinical situation. Confusion can sometimes occur when the heart rate is sufficiently rapid that the P wave blends into the preceding T wave, making it difficult to see and, therefore, difficult to distinguish a supraventricular tachycardia (SVT) from what is simply sinus tachycardia. Obtaining a 12-lead ECG in this instance can be helpful because P waves may be more easily distinguished in some leads than in others, making the rhythm diagnosis more apparent.

Obtaining a 12-lead ECG can be helpful because P waves may be more easily distinguished in some leads than in others, making the rhythm diagnosis more apparent.

The following rhythms should be recognized by experienced health care professionals:

- Fictitious rhythms (artifact)
- Sinus rhythm (including sinus bradycardia and sinus tachycardia)
- Sinus pause and arrest
- Atrioventricular (AV) blocks of all degrees
- Premature atrial complexes (PACs)
- Supraventricular tachycardia (SVT)
- Preexcited arrhythmias (associated with an accessory pathway)
- Premature ventricular complexes (PVCs)
- Ventricular tachycardia (VT)
- Ventricular fibrillation (VF)
- Ventricular asystole
- Accelerated idioventricular rhythm

Fictitious Arrhythmias

Fictitious arrhythmias are those generated by body motion, muscle artifact, electrical interference from nearby equipment, loose electrodes, or loss of the ECG signal.[2] When motion artifact and electrical interference are superimposed upon a normal rhythm, both the appearance of QRS complexes and the normal isoelectric baseline between QRS complexes are typically altered, creating the impression of a rapid tachycardia. Important clues to an apparent arrhythmia being artifactual include the absence of associated symptoms and signs and failure to corroborate the presence of an arrhythmia by physical findings (pulse). Neither VF nor true asystole are associated with a normal level of consciousness, at least not for long! Another important clue as to the fictitious nature of an arrhythmia is the ability to distinguish normal-appearing QRS complexes amid the baseline artifact with a rate and regularity that appear undisturbed (as compared with the preceding normal rhythm) by the apparent arrhythmia (Fig. 19-1).

Another important clue as to the fictitious nature of an arrhythmia is the ability to distinguish normal-appearing QRS complexes amidst the baseline artifact with a rate and regularity that appears undisturbed (as compared with the preceding normal rhythm) by the apparent arrhythmia.

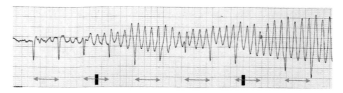

FIGURE 19-1 • Fictitious arrhythmia. The tracing illustrates motion artifact. In this instance the patient is brushing his teeth while being monitored and is in normal sinus rhythm throughout. The first sinus rhythm complex on the left appears to change to an apparent atrial arrhythmia (atrial flutter), then to an apparent wide complex tachycardia (ventricular tachycardia). However, as indicated by the arrows (shown between alternate QRS complexes), one is able to "march out" QRS complexes without a change in their rate or regularity throughout the apparent arrhythmias, a telltale sign that the apparent arrhythmias are artifactual.

Classifying Tachycardias

QRS Appearance

Tachycardias can be classified in a number of ways. One useful system is based on the width (or duration) of the QRS interval. The QRS interval reflects the time required for complete depolarization of the ventricles. This normally occurs within 80 to 100 milliseconds (0.08–0.10 seconds) due to the rapid conduction of impulses through the His–Purkinje system. Depolarization of the ventricles via the specialized conduction tissue comprising the His–Purkinje system is an order of magnitude faster than muscle-to-muscle conduction would be outside this conduction system.[3] Hence, any disruption in conduction in the His–Purkinje system (as, for example, by right or left bundle-branch block), results in the corresponding portion of the ventricles being depolarized by slower muscle-to-muscle conduction. The ventricular depolarization that now transpires over a longer time interval results in widening of the QRS and is referred to as aberrant conduction, or aberrancy. Similarly, ventricular arrhythmias (VF and VT) are associated with a wide QRS because ventricular depolarization in this instance originates from muscle tissue outside the His–Purkinje system and thereafter propagates by muscle-to-muscle conduction throughout the ventricles. Notably, one should not confuse widening of the QRS (which represents the longer time required to depolarize the ventricles with each impulse) with the actual rate of a tachycardia (which represents how rapidly such impulses may come in succession). Wide- or narrow-complex tachycardias can each be quite rapid.

Preexcitation

Preexcited rhythms are also manifested by a wider than normal QRS.[4] "Preexcitation" refers to early ventricular activation as a result of one or more congenitally acquired muscular connections between the atria and ventricles. The atrioventricular node, which is ordinarily the only electrical connection between the atria and ventricles, transiently slows the conduction of impulses between the atria and ventricles, resulting in the typical PR interval of 0.12 to 0.20 seconds between the onset of the P wave and beginning of the QRS complex. In contrast, conduction through an atrioventricular accessory pathway "bypasses" the atrioventricular node and starts to excite the ventricles almost immediately after the P wave [represented by a foreshortened PR interval (<0.12 seconds)]. This earlier than normal activation of ventricular muscle via the accessory pathway is called "preexcitation." The accessory pathway typically inserts directly into ventricular muscle (rather than into the His–Purkinje system, although it can occasionally be found to insert directly into this conduction system as well). Accordingly, although the ventricles are electrically activated earlier via the accessory pathway than they would been via the AV node and His–Purkinje system (that is, are "preexcited"), the subsequent spread of conduction occurs outside the His–Purkinje system via muscle-to-muscle conduction, resulting in a wider than normal QRS. Hence preexcited rhythms are manifested by a wide QRS complex. During normal sinus rhythm, the QRS complex is the result of fusion of two processes: muscle-to-muscle conduction initiated from the site where the accessory pathway inserts in the ventricle and depolarization of the ventricle via the His–Purkinje system. In effect, the sinus P wave (atrial impulse) follows two paths to the ventricle, one via the atrioventricular node and the other via the atrioventricular accessory pathway. Conduction via the atrioventricular accessory pathway reaches the ventricle first, whereas the corresponding atrial impulse is delayed in the atrioventricular node. Ventricular excitation begins early as a result of early activation of the ventricle from the accessory pathway and spreads by muscle-to-muscle conduction. However, once the corresponding impulse emerges from the atrioventricular node, activation of the ventricle through the His–Purkinje system proceeds at an order of magnitude faster than muscle-to-muscle spread of activation from the accessory pathway. The appearance of the resulting QRS is a melding of initial muscle-to-muscle conduction and later more rapid His–Purkinje conduction, resulting in the typical appearance of preexcitation: a foreshortened PR interval (due to early activation of the ventricle by the accessory pathway) and an initial slurred QRS or delta wave (representing early muscle-to-muscle depolarization of ventricular muscle from the accessory pathway) followed by the remaining QRS, which rapidly normalizes in its appearance (due to His–Purkinje depolarization of the remaining portions of the ventricles) (Fig. 19-2).

The sinus P wave (atrial impulse) follows two paths to the ventricle, one via the atrioventricular node and the other via the atrioventricular accessory pathway resulting in the typical appearance of preexcitation: a foreshortened PR interval, an initially slurred QRS complex (delta wave), with the remaining portion of the QRS having a more normal appearance.

Patients with an accessory pathway are predisposed to reentry arrhythmias [paroxysmal supraventricular tachycardias (PSVT)] that involve the atrioventricular node as one limb and the atrioventricular accessory pathway as the other limb of a spinning circuit between the atria and ventricles. This can result in a regular narrow-complex tachycardia when forward (antegrade) conduction to the ventricles occurs via the atrioventricular node and His–Purkinje system (referred to as orthodromic tachycardia), or it can lead to a wide complex tachycardia when forward conduction to the ventricles occurs via the accessory pathway that inserts directly into ventricular muscle (antidromic tachycardia). Patients with an accessory pathway may also experience other atrial arrhythmias, during which conduction to the ventricles occurs via the atrioventricular node and accessory pathway, often resulting in a mixture of wide, intermediate, and narrow QRS complexes. To complicate things further, some patients may have multiple accessory pathways.

QRS Uniformity

Another useful criterion to apply to wide-complex tachycardia is whether the QRS complexes are uniform from beat to

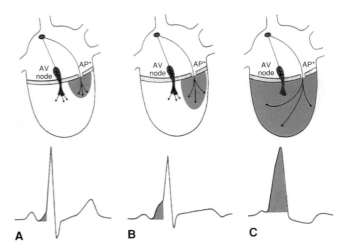

FIGURE 19-2 • Preexcitation. The preexcited QRS: Conduction of a sinus node impulse is shown via the atrioventricular node (AV node) and an accessory pathway (AP). The red areas in the upper portion of the figure demarcate excitation of the ventricle via the accessory pathway and, in the lower figure (A, B, and C), the portion of the QRS that corresponds to such early muscle-to-muscle conduction. The white areas in the upper portion of the figure demarcate excitation of the ventricle via the atrioventricular node and His-Purkinje system, and, in the lower figure (A, B, and C), the portion of the QRS that corresponds to this later but much more rapid activation of the ventricle. In **(A)**, conduction through the AV node is relatively brisk, with only a small portion of the ventricle being preexcited by the accessory pathway before being rapidly depolarized via the His-Purkinje system. In **(B)**, a longer delay of the atrial impulse in the AV node allows for a greater degree of the ventricle to be depolarized by the accessory pathway. Part **(C)** illustrates complete depolarization of the ventricle via the accessory pathway, where conduction through the AV node is completely blocked. The "delta wave" (initial red portion of the ECG) represents early activation of the ventricle by the accessory pathway (reflected in the shorter than normal PR interval) and thereafter slower muscle-to-muscle spread of conduction, creating a widening of the QRS. The later, more normal-(narrow) appearing portion of the QRS represents the more rapid depolarization of the ventricle by the His-Purkinje system once the atrial impulse has conducted through the AV node. Patients with accessory pathways may show a smaller or larger degree of ventricular preexcitation (*red areas*), depending on the degree of conduction slowing in the AV node (and is not present when the QRS complex is completely preexcited). This may be dependent on autonomic tone or medications being administered. (Modified from Sandoe E, Sigurd B. Arrhythmia: A Guide to Clinical Electrocardiology. 1991, page 192. Publishing Partners Verlags GmbH, Bingen.)

beat (are monomorphic) or vary greatly in configuration (are polymorphic). The extreme case is represented by VF, defined as a completely disorganized tachycardia for which individual QRS complexes are not even distinguishable. Polymorphic tachycardias manifest some organization in that distinct QRS complexes are identifiable but vary in rate and appearance from beat to beat; whereas monomorphic tachycardias are typically uniform in both their rate and the appearance of QRS complexes (Fig. 19-3).

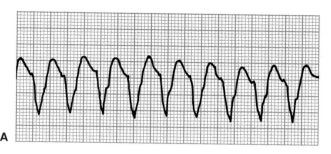

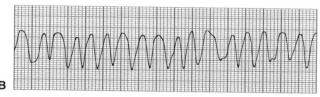

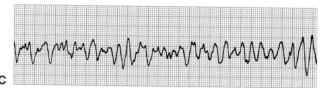

FIGURE 19-3 • Various morphologies of ventricular tachy-arrhythmia. Monomorphic VT **(A)**, polymorphic ventricular tachy-cardia **(B)**, and VF **(C)** are depicted. **A.** Monomorphic VT is charac-terized by QRS complexes that are uniform in appearance from one complex to the next. **B.** Distinct QRS complexes are identifi-able in polymorphic VT but are less organized than in monomor-phic VT, varying in rate and appearance. **C.** In VF, individual QRS complexes are completely disorganized and not individually dis-tinguishable. Distinguishing rapid polymorphic VT from VF is aca-demic because, in practice, both are hemodynamically unstable and treated similarly with electrical defibrillation.

Discriminating SVT from VT

Experienced health care professionals must be able to dis-tinguish between supraventricular and ventricular rhythms, recognizing that organized wide-complex (broad-complex) tachycardias may be either supraventricular or ventricular in origin. If a patient is pulseless or in shock, a wide-complex tachycardia is best presumed to be VT until proved other-wise. Initial management should proceed under this pre-sumption. In patients who are sufficiently stable to afford a few minutes delay in treatment, a 12-lead ECG of the tachy-cardia should be obtained as soon as practicable. A 12-lead ECG can provide a number of important clues about the origin of a wide-complex tachycardia, including whether the QRS configuration matches that from a previous ECG obtained during sinus rhythm (suggesting the arrhythmia is likely of supraventricular origin) and the presence of atri-oventricular dissociation.

Atrioventricular dissociation, the hallmark of ventricular tachycardia, is characterized by the presence of a greater num-ber of ventricular (QRS) than atrial (P) complexes. An esophageal lead tracing (see Chapter 22) obtained during tachycardia will amplify P waves and may be helpful in estab-lishing atrioventricular dissociation if the origin of the arrhyth-mia remains in doubt.[5] Even if such documentation is not found useful at the time of treatment, it may provide impor-tant clues as to rhythm diagnosis for an expert consultant "after the fact" and assist in the patient's future management.

If a patient is pulseless or in shock, a wide-complex tachycardia is best presumed to be VT until proved otherwise.

With these principles in mind, the various tachycardias can be categorized in the following manner:

Narrow-QRS-complex (supraventricular) tachycardias
- Sinus tachycardia
- Sinus node reentry tachycardia
- Paroxysmal supraventricular tachycardia (PSVT)
- Atrioventricular nodal reentry tachycardia (AVNRT)
- Atrioventricular reentry tachycardia (AVRT) with forward conduction to the ventricles via the atrioventricular node
- Ectopic (focal) atrial tachycardia (EAT)
- Multifocal atrial tachycardia (MAT)
- Junctional tachycardia (rare in adults)
- Intra-atrial reentry tachycardia
- Atrial fibrillation (AF)
- Atrial flutter

Wide-QRS-complex tachycardias
- Ventricular tachycardia (monomorphic and polymorphic)
- Ventricular fibrillation
- Accelerated idioventricular rhythm
- Supraventricular tachycardia (SVT) with aberrancy
- Preexcited tachycardias
- Atrial tachycardia with accessory pathway conduction
- Atrial flutter (AF) with accessory pathway conduction
- Atrioventricular reentry tachycardia (AVRT) with forward conduction to the ventricles via the accessory pathway

Approaches to the management of these tachycardias depends upon the clinical setting in which they occur: pulse-less cardiac arrest (which can also be caused by asystole and pulseless electrical activity, in subsequent chapters) and hemodynamically stable tachycardia. Each is addressed by a specific algorithm.

References

1. Tchou P, Young P, Mahmud R, et al. Useful clinical criteria for the diagnosis of ventricular tachycardia. *Am J Med* 1988;84:53–56.
2. Goldman MJ. *Principles of Clinical Electrocardiography*, 11th ed. Los Altos, CA: Lange, 1982.
3. Marriott H. *Practical Electrocardiography*, 8th ed. Baltimore: Williams & Wilkins, 1988.
4. Rowlands DJ. Miscellaneous abnormalities: ventricular pre-excitation. *Clinical Electrocardiography*. New York: Gower, 1991: 212–220.
5. Shaw M, Niemann JT, Haskell RJ, et al. Esophageal electrocardio-graphy in acute cardiac care: efficacy and diagnostic value of a new technique. *Am J Med* 1987;82:689–696.

Chapter 20
The Electrophysiology of Arrhythmias

Peter J. Kudenchuk

Patient management suffers when health care providers base clinical decisions solely on ECG findings and neglect to evaluate the patient's clinical condition or correlate symptoms and findings with rhythm disturbances. Similarly, rhythm management suffers when arrhythmias are treated without some understanding of their electrophysiologic mechanisms.

- Review of basic electrophysiology to clarify clinical arrhythmias
- Mechanisms of arrhythmia generation and propagation
- Anatomy and physiology of the conduction system
- Relationship of electrophysiology to the surface electrocardiogram (ECG)

Introduction

This chapter presents the basic mechanisms and clinical significance of commonly encountered cardiac rhythm disturbances. To support this understanding, it offers an overview of the cardiac cellular environment and the mechanisms governing the heart's "electrical cells" and "muscle cells."

Cell Types

Two groups of cells in the myocardium, muscle (or contractile) and electrical cells, determine the heart's function as a pump. *Muscle cells* produce the cardiac contractions by means of elaborate protein-contractile structures within them. They are activated by *electrical cells, composed of pacemaker cells* and *electrical conducting cells*, from which electrical activity originates and is then transmitted via specialized conducting pathways in the heart. Muscle (contractile) and electrical cells are intricately interwoven in a manner that facilitates rapid and efficient propagation of electrical impulses from their site of origin in *pacemaker cells* (such as the sinus node) and their spread via *electrical conducting cells* (such as the His–Purkinje network) to their final muscle cell destinations throughout the heart. Muscle cells are also electrically active and can conduct electrical impulses from cell to cell, but not as rapidly or efficiently as electrical conducting cells. Proper interactions between the *electrical conducting cells* and the *muscle cells* produce repetitive, coordinated contraction/relaxation cycles. These cycles produce an effective cardiac output over a wide range of physiologic conditions and stress.

Charged ions, predominantly calcium, potassium, and sodium, cross myocardial (muscle and electrical) cell membranes back and forth. These ion movements mediate electrical excitation and muscle contraction. Many conditions can alter ionic movement across cell membranes or charged cell components and thereby interfere with coordinated electrical and mechanical function. This interference can produce symptomatic arrhythmias or even sudden cardiac death.

Basic Cardiac Electrophysiology: Cellular Level

Ion Gradients

For a cell to do work or conduct an impulse, the cell's membrane must be electrically charged. This charge arises from concentrations of potassium, sodium, and calcium inside the cell that vary from those outside the cell. Normally the concentration gradient of ions produces a negative electrical charge across the membrane. When the cell is activated, or *depolarized*, this negative charge moves rapidly towards a positive membrane charge. This change in membrane charge initiates depolarization (or activation). A similar process results in cell-to-cell spread of this activation, referred to as *conduction*, which is ultimately electromechanically linked to mechanical contraction.

Depolarization: The Process

With *depolarization*, there is a momentary change in the physical properties of the cell membrane. Positively charged ions begin to enter the cell through one of two channels, causing the inside to become less negative and ultimately positive:

- The *fast* channel permits rapid entry of sodium ions and is responsible for depolarizing myocardial muscle (contractile) cells.

- The *slow channel* permits entry of calcium ions and possibly sodium ions. Slow channel depolarization produces the spontaneous pacemaker activity of the sinus node, the atrioventricular (AV) junction, and other pacemaker cells of the heart.

Action Potential of a Myocardial Muscle Cell

In a typical ventricular myocardial muscle (contractile) cell, the resting membrane potential is electrically negative compared with the outside of the cell membrane. Sodium exists in high concentration outside the cell and in low concentration inside the cell. Figure 20-1A depicts the change in movement of ions across a myocardial muscle cell membrane as it propagates an action potential. The concentration gradient of the sodium ions and the electrical charge across the membrane provide the driving force for the sodium during the action potential. The cell membrane expends considerable energy to pump sodium ions out of the cell to maintain the concentration gradient.

Phases of the Action Potential

Preparing for Phase 0: Between contractions, the cell membrane is relatively impermeable to sodium. Potassium, high in concentration inside the cell and low in concentration outside the cell, is able to cross the cell membrane. During phase 3 and to some extent during phase 2 of the action potential, potassium moves across the cell membrane from inside to outside. This outward flow of positive ions causes the interior of the cell to become electrically negative and the exterior of the cell to become positive. The resting membrane potential, therefore, depends primarily on the potassium gradient across the cell membrane. This is also why the transmembrane potential just prior to phase 0 is depicted in Figure 20-1A in the negative millivolt range.

Phase 0: Depolarization When depolarization starts, the cell membrane's *fast channel* opens briefly, for about 1 millisecond. This permits very rapid sodium entry into the cell, as shown by the long Na^+ arrow at the cell membrane in Figure 20-1A. The inward flow of positively charged sodium ions across the cell membrane makes the inside of the cell electrically positive relative to the outside of the cell membrane. The transmembrane potential moves rapidly past 0 mV into the positive range. Phase 0 in the atrial muscle mass generates the P wave and in ventricular muscle the QRS complex. This depolarization (phase 0) propagates through the atrial muscle mass, generating the atrial P wave and, in the ventricular muscle mass, the ventricular QRS complex. (Note the parallel ECG tracing at the top of Fig. 20-1A.)

Phase 1: Start of Repolarization As the *fast channel* closes, sodium entry slows down (note the smaller Na^+ arrows in Fig. 20-1A). Potassium begins its exit from cells, making the electrical charge inside the cell less positive and starting the repolarization process (*phase 1*).

Phase 2: Isoelectric or Plateau Phase During *phase 2*, the action potential is approximately isoelectric (horizontal line in Fig. 20-1A), but the cell remains depolarized. Significant amounts of sodium are no longer entering the cell through the fast channel, whereas calcium (depicted by the Ca^{2+} arrows in Fig. 20-1A) begins to enter the cell through the slow channel. Phase 2 of the ventricular muscle action potential is reflected by the ST segment of the ECG. When calcium enters the cell, it activates an interaction between *actin* and *myosin* filaments in the muscle cells' *sarcomeres*. This interaction results in a contraction. The *sarcomere* functions as the basic contractile unit of the myocardial fiber.

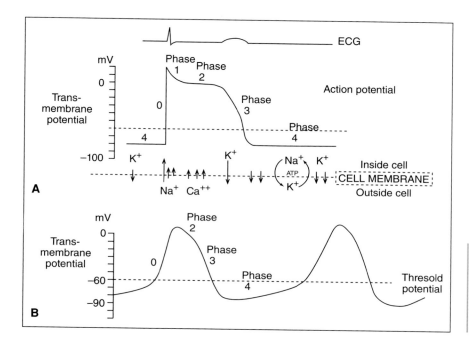

FIGURE 20-1 • **A.** Schematic representation of the action potential of a ventricular myocardial muscle cell. Arrows indicate times of major ionic movement across the cell membrane. **B.** Schematic representation of the action potential of a pacemaker cell.

Phase 3: Rapid Repolarization

Phase 3 represents rapid repolarization, during which the inside of the cell returns to negative (note the transmembrane potential drop in Fig. 20-1A). This return to negative is caused by an increased movement of potassium ions (see long K$^+$ arrow in the figure) from inside to outside the cell. Phase 3 in the ventricular muscle action potential is reflected by the T wave. Repolarization is completed at the end of phase 3. The interior of the cell is again approximately –90 mV.

Phase 4: Sodium/Potassium Pump Activation

Now, immediately after the action potential, the distribution of ions across the cell membrane is different from what it was immediately before depolarization started. Because of sodium entry into the cell and potassium loss from the cell during depolarization, a higher concentration of intracellular sodium and a lower concentration of intracellular potassium now exists. Repeated depolarizations without a redistribution of sodium and potassium ions would soon lead to serious impairment of cell function.

Therefore a special pumping mechanism in the cell membrane is activated during phase 4. (Fig. 20-1A represents this sodium/potassium pump with the curved arrows connecting Na$^+$ and K$^+$ at the cell membrane.) This pumping mechanism, which transports sodium ions from inside to outside the cell and brings potassium ions from outside to inside the cell, depends on adenosine triphosphate (see ATP in Fig. 20-1A) as its energy source. Of note, during phase 4 of the *muscle cell* as described here, the membrane potential remains at a constant level. This differs from phase 4 of specialized *pacemaker cells*, described in the following section, during which there is a gradual lessening of membrane potential.

The Action Potential of a Pacemaker Cell and Its Phases

Phase 4: Automaticity: Spontaneous Diastolic Depolarization

Whereas a description of the electrical activity of a muscle (contractile) myocardial cell begins with phase 0, a description of the activity of the electrical pacemaker cell best begins with phase 4. The action potential of a pacemaker cell differs significantly from that of a working myocardial cell. Pacemaker cells possess the property of *automaticity*, meaning that the cells are able to depolarize spontaneously. The most important feature of the pacemaker cell's action potential is that the membrane potential during *phase 4* does not remain at a constant level, as it does in working myocardial cells (see previous section). During phase 4 in pacemaker cells, as depicted in Figure 20-1B, there is a gradual lessening of the resting membrane potential. This occurs because small amounts of calcium and sodium enter the cell during phase 4, while the outward flow of potassium decreases. The resting membrane potential, therefore, becomes less negative—a process called *spontaneous diastolic depolarization*.

The slope of phase 4 is important in the rate of impulse formation and ultimately heart rate. The steeper the slope, the faster the rate of the pacemaker cell; the more gradual the slope, the slower the rate. Activation of the sympathetic nervous system (or administration of a catecholamine) makes the slope steeper and thereby enhances automaticity. Stimulation of the parasympathetic nervous system (i.e., vagal stimulation) produces the opposite effect. Drugs such as beta-blockers also decrease the rate of spontaneous depolarization, thus diminishing automaticity.

Phase 0: Threshold Potential

Phase 0 begins when the resting membrane potential reaches a critical voltage (the *threshold potential*) (see Fig. 20-1B). The rate of rise of phase 0 is slower (less steep) than that of a normal myocardial working cell. The rate of action potential rise (*slope*) in cells of the sinus node and AV junction depends on the rate of calcium ion entry through the slow channel.

Phases 1 to 3

Phases 1 to 3 of the action potential in pacemaker cells proceed similarly to those described above in myocardial muscle cells.

Groups of Pacemaker Cells Clinically, the most important groups of *pacemaker cells* are located in

- The sinus node
- The AV junction
- The bundle of His
- The bundle branches
- The ventricular Purkinje system

The rate of spontaneous depolarization (the "firing rate") differs in these different locations:

- The firing rate of the sinus node, the primary pacemaker of the heart is 60 to 100 bpm
- The firing rate of the AV junction and bundle of His is 40 to 60 bpm
- The firing rate of the ventricle (Purkinje fibers) is <40 bpm

Escape Pacemakers This decrement in the firing rate as one descends from the sinus node to the AV junction and to the ventricles has important physiologic implications. The lower and slower pacemakers at the AV junction and ventricle are depolarized by a sinus node impulse while still in their phase 4. This depolarization occurs before they can reach their phase 0 threshold potential. Thus, they are prevented from spontaneously depolarizing.

The pacemakers in the AV junction and ventricle can, therefore, become *"escape pacemakers."* This means that they do not spontaneously produce an electrical impulse unless there is failure of a faster pacemaker, such as the sinus node. If the sinus rate falls significantly below 60 bpm, a junctional escape beat should occur. Likewise, if a supraventricular impulse does not reach the ventricles within approximately 1.5 seconds (equivalent to a rate of 40 bpm), a ventricular escape beat should occur. The rates of these escape pacemakers can be increased or decreased by various disease states, drugs, or sympathetic or parasympathetic stimulation.

Refractory Periods: Absolute and Relative

Both muscle and electrical cells have a refractory period (look ahead to Fig. 20-3B) during which they recover their ability to be electrically excited again. The refractory period of the ventricle starts immediately after the completion of phase 0 (corresponding to QRS complex) and ends with phase 3 (the end of the T wave). The refractory period can be divided into two portions:

- The *absolute refractory period*, during which the cell cannot be immediately electrically reexcited. The absolute refractory period begins immediately after phase 0 and ends midway through phase 3 (at about the apex of the T wave).
- *The relative refractory period*, during which a strong stimulus can electrically reexcite the cell but which usually results in an abnormal action potential because the cell is still in an incomplete state of recovery. The relative refractory period extends through the remainder of phase 3 (from the apex to the end of the T wave).

Normal and Abnormal Rhythm Mechanisms

Electrical impulses can produce normal and abnormal heart rhythms through two basic mechanisms: *automaticity (normal and triggered)* and *reentry*.

Mechansim 1: Automaticity

Normal Automaticity An impulse may start through the normal mechanism of automaticity (phase 4 depolarization of pacemaker cells) described above. Depending upon the location of the pacemaker cell affected, sinus tachycardia, junctional tachycardia, and accelerated idioventricular rhythms result from such an increase in phase 4 depolarization. For example, sinus tachycardia generated by such a mechanism during periods of stress (such as exercise) would be regarded as a normal rhythm resulting from increased automaticity.

"Triggered" Automaticity Other forms of automaticity occur that are related to abnormalities in slow-channel activity and can be a cause of arrhythmias. *Triggered automaticity* is the induction of an arrhythmia by *after-potentials*. *After-potentials* are transient inflections in resting membrane potential resulting from abnormal ion fluxes that occur during or immediately after repolarization (during phase 3 or 4 of the action potential). If *after-potentials* reach the threshold potential, spontaneous depolarization will occur, a so-called "triggered" action potential. Successive triggered action potentials can result in a series of premature beats or promote reentry rhythms (by the mechanism below) in susceptible tissues. Atrial or ventricular arrhythmias may result, depending upon the location of the cells that are "triggered" to depolarize by this mechanism.

Mechansim 2: Reentry

A second mechanism for creating arrhythmias is *reentry*, which may occur in the sinus node, the atrium, the AV junction, or the ventricle. *Reentry* occurs in tissues that have altered electrical properties that can facilitate a "circulating" flow of electrical impulses. This can result in isolated beats, such as PVCs, or sustained abnormal rhythms, such as ventricular tachycardia. Figure 20-2 provides an example of this mechanism:

A—An electrical impulse (A) traveling in ventricular muscle may encounter two branches (or pathways), each of which has differing electrical properties. The manner in which this impulse is conducted through these branches sets up the series of events described below, called reentry.

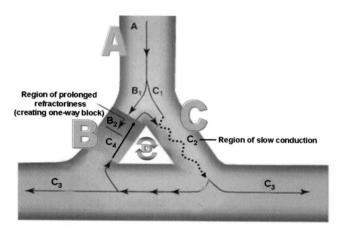

Ventricular muscle fiber

FIGURE 20-2 • Diagrammatic representation of the mechanism of reentry. **A.** An electrical impulse (A) travelling in ventricular muscle encounters 2 branches (or pathways), each of which has differing electrical properties, and into which the impulse is directed as (B₁) and (C₁). The manner in which this impulse is conducted through these branches sets up a series of events, called reentry. **B.** One of the branches that the impulse (B₁) encounters has a long refractory period, which does not permit passage of the impules, particularly if it is premature, creating what is called one-way or unidirectional block. This impulse is blocked in this pathway (B₂). **C.** The alternate branch (entered by impulse (C₁) has slow conduction properties. It allows passage of the impulse, but at a slower than normal speed (C₂). This slower conduction results in a transit time that is just long enough to allow the pathway with the longer refractory period described in B to recover. When the impulse reaches the vicinity of this recovered branch it conducts through it, but in the opposite direction (retrograde) from what it would have originally taken (C₄). Upon reaching the top of the branching circuit, the impulse reenters the slow conducting branch (C₂) and may repeat the same cycle of events. Each "spin" of the impulse in this circuit results in an ectopic impulse (C₃). The process described in C above may repeat itself over and over again. Each "spin" in the circuit "kicks out" an ectopic impulse (C₃) to the surrounding tissue. Successive spins in the circuit generate repetitive impulses, resulting in a tachycardia. Depending upon the anatomic location of the reentry circuit, generated tachycardias can include atrial fibrillation and flutter, AV nodal reentry, atrioventricular reentry, ventricular tachycardia, and ventricular fibrillation.

B—One of these branches has a long refractory period, which does not permit passage of the impulse (B_1), particularly if it is premature, creating what is called one-way or unidirectional block (B_2).

C—The alternate branch has slow conduction properties. It allows passage of the impulse, but at a slower than normal speed (C_2). This slower conduction results in a transit time that is just long enough to allow the pathway with the longer refractory period (described in **B**) to recover. When the impulse reaches the vicinity of this recovered branch it conducts through it, but in the opposite direction (retrograde) from what it would have originally taken (C_4). Upon reaching the top of the branching circuit, the impulse reenters the slow conducting branch (C_2) and may repeat the same cycle of events. Each "spin" of the impulse in this circuit results in an ectopic impulse (C_3).

D—The process described in C above may repeat itself over and over again. Each "spin" in the circuit "kicks out" an ectopic impulse (C_3) to the surrounding tissue. Successive spins in the circuit (depicted by the semicircular arrows in Figure 20-2) generate repetitive impulses, resulting in a tachycardia. Depending upon the anatomic location of the reentry circuit, generated tachycardias can include atrial fibrillation and flutter, AV nodal reentry, atrioventricular reentry, ventricular tachycardia, and ventricular fibrillation.

BASIC COMPONENTS OF THE REENTRY MECHANISM

- There are at least two conducting pathways between the site of origin of an impulse and its destination.
- Each pathway has differing electrical properties. Typically, one pathway has a longer refractory period than the other and one pathway has slower conduction properties than the other.
- An electrical impulse (often premature) that reaches the two pathways initiates the reentry process.
- The pathway with a longer refractory (recovery) period is initially unable to conduct the premature impulse in one direction (sometimes called one-way or unidirectional block) because it has not as yet completely recovered from having conducted the previous impulse.
- The slow-conducting pathway permits passage of this impulse. This transit time through this slow conducting pathway is just long enough to allow the alternate pathway with the longer refractory period to recover by the time the electrical impulse again reaches its vicinity.
- This combination of two pathways, one with a longer refractory period and one with slow conduction, allows just the right timing for the impulse to perpetually "spin" in the circuit without encountering refractory tissue. Each spin creates an impulse, and repetitive spins create a tachycardia.

Diseases such as coronary artery disease and cardiomyopathy cause many of these changes in tissue that promote reentry arrhythmias.

From Cells to Tissue: Conduction through the Heart

Anatomy of the Cardiac Conduction System (Fig. 20-3a)

Sinus Node and Internodal Pathways   The normal cardiac impulse originates in the electrical (pacemaker) cells comprised by the sinus node, a structure located in the superior portion of the right atrium at its junction with the superior vena cava. Historically, conduction from the sinus node was thought to occur over electrical conducting cells that make up the internodal pathways. These "internodal pathways" continue to be depicted in figures and diagrams of the cardiac conduction system and are described here. However, their existence is controversial and many experts now believe that the atria may not have specialized conduction pathways analogous to the His-Purkinje system in the ventricles. Rather, how conduction spreads through the atria is believed to be primarily related to the orientation of the muscle fibers and their electrical properties, which typically conduct impulses at speeds of about 1,000 millimeters per second.

- The *anterior internodal pathway* arises at the cranial end of the sinus node. It divides into branches, one to the left atrium (Bachman's bundle) and the other along the right side of the interatrial septum to the AV node.
- The *middle internodal pathway* arises along the endocardial surface of the sinus node and descends through the interatrial septum to the AV node.
- The *posterior internodal pathway* arises from the caudal end of the sinus node and approaches the AV node at its posterior aspect.

Atrioventricular Node   The AV node (comprising both pacemaker and electrical conducting cells) is located inferiorly in the right atrium, anterior to the ostium of the coronary sinus and above the tricuspid valve. The speed of conduction is slowed (to about 200 millimeters per second) through the AV node. The AV node is anatomically a complicated network of fibers made up of electrically conducting cells. These fibers converge at its lower margin to form a discrete bundle of fibers, the *bundle of His*. This structure penetrates the annulus fibrosis and arrives at the upper margin of the muscular intraventricular septum. There, the bundle of His gives origin to the bundle branches.

Bundle Branches   The *left bundle branch* arises as a series of radiations, or *fascicles*, at right angles to the bundle of His. A superior, anterior fascicle courses down the anterior aspect of the interventricular septum to the anterolateral papillary muscle, where it breaks up into a Purkinje network. The shorter and thicker inferoposterior fascicle passes posterior to the base of the posteromedial papillary muscle, where it branches into the Purkinje network. Purkinje fibers to the interventricular septum may arise as a separate radiation or as fibers from either the anterior or posterior fascicles.

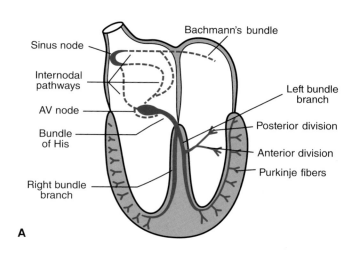

A

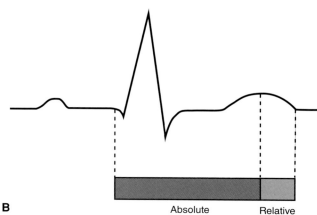

B

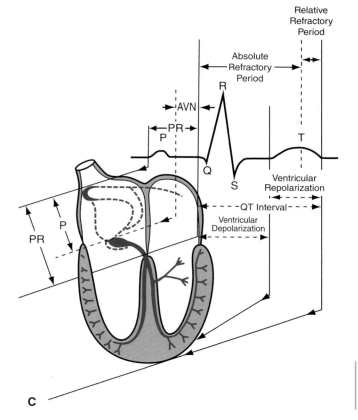

C

FIGURE 20-3 • **A.** Anatomy of the cardiac conduction system. **B.** Absolute and relative refractory periods depicted on the ECG. **C.** Relation of cardiac conduction system and events to the surface ECG, depicting nomenclature for complexes and intervals.

The *right bundle branch* courses down the interventricular septum on the right side. It contributes Purkinje fibers to the septum only near the apex of the right ventricle. At the lower end of the septum, it passes into the right ventricular wall, where it branches into a Purkinje network. Conduction through the bundle branches and His–Purkinje system are rapid, on the order of 10 times faster than spread of electrical activity from muscle to muscle.

Ventricles As the electrical impulse leaves the AV node, it passes into the bundle of His and then down the bundle branches simultaneously. The first section of the ventricle to begin depolarization is the midportion of the interventricular septum from the left side. The walls of the left and right ventricles are depolarized simultaneously. The speed of conduction through the ventricular Purkinje network is rapid, about 4,000 millimeters per second. Conduction in ventricular muscle itself is considerably slower (about 400 millimeters per second).

The Electrocardiogram: Waves, Intervals, and Segments

The ECG can be considered the sum of the multitude of action potentials from electrically excited muscle cells that make up the myocardial tissue. The ECG records these small electrical forces produced by the heart from the body

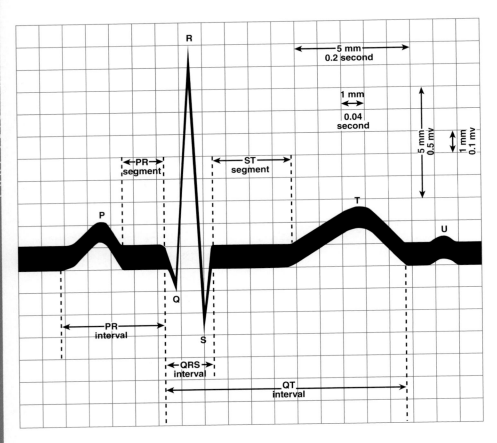

FIGURE 20-4 • Surface ECG depicting nomenclature for complexes and intervals.

surface.[1,2] Because the body acts as a giant conductor of electrical currents, any two points on the body can be connected by electrical "leads" to register the heart's electrical activity. This electrical activity forms a series of waves and complexes that have been arbitrarily labeled (in alphabetical order) the P wave, the QRS complex, the T wave, and the U wave (Fig. 20-4). The waves or deflections are separated in most patients by regularly occurring intervals.[3] From the perspective of the *ventricular* action potential, the QRS can be thought of as corresponding to phases 0 to 1 of the action potential; the ST segment to phase 2, and the T–U wave to phase 3. From the perspective of the *atrial* action potential, the P wave can be thought of as corresponding to phases 0 to 1, the PR segment to phase 2, and the atrial "T wave" (which is hidden within the QRS complex) as phase 3.

The Electrocardiogram and Anatomy of the Cardiac Conduction System

Depolarization of different parts of the heart and its conduction system produces different waves and complexes:

- The atria, which produce the P wave
- The ventricles, which produce the QRS complex during depolarization
- The ventricles, which produce the T wave during repolarization
- The repolarization of the Purkinje system, which is believed to produce the U wave

These relationships between the waves, segments, and intervals of the ECG and the anatomy of the cardiac conduction system are depicted in Fig. 20-3C.

Summary: Causes of Cardiac Arrhythmias

Cardiac arrhythmias (both tachycardias and bradycardias) can result from the following mechanisms:[4]

1. **Disturbed automaticity.** This may involve a speeding up or slowing down of areas of automaticity such as in the sinus node (resulting in sinus tachycardia or sinus bradycardia), the atrioventricular (AV) node (resulting in accelerated junctional rhythm), or at other atrial or ventricular sites. Triggered automaticity in these tissues can result in tachycardias such as atrial or ventricular tachycardia.

2. **Disturbed conduction.** Conduction may be either too slow (as in AV block)[5] or altered in tissue in such a manner as to create reentry circuits and resulting tachycardias.

3. **Combinations of disturbed automaticity and disturbed conduction.** Two examples are
   - A premature atrial impulse (due to disturbed automaticity) in combination with first-degree AV block (disturbed conduction). The resulting ECG would show a premature atrial complex conducted to the ventricle with a prolonged PR interval of first-degree AV block.
   - A premature atrial impulse (due to disturbed automaticity) may encounter tissue that is susceptible to reentry (altered conduction) resulting in a supraventricular tachycardia.

The Basics of Rhythm Recognition

Inaccurate diagnoses and inappropriate therapy occur when health care providers base clinical decisions solely on cardiac rhythm and neglect to evaluate the patient's clinical condition.

Clinical Correlation

ECG and rhythm information should be interpreted within the context of total patient assessment. Inaccurate diagnoses and inappropriate therapy occur when health care providers base clinical decisions solely on cardiac rhythm and neglect to evaluate the patient's clinical condition. Definitive rhythm evaluation must include clinical parameters such as ventilation, oxygenation, heart rate, blood pressure, level of consciousness, signs of inadequate organ perfusion, and metabolic and acid-base status. Many clinical scenarios require consideration of possible proarrhythmic drug effects, adverse drug reactions from intentional or unintentional overdose, and the possibility of drug toxicity following normal dosing patterns.

Skill Development and Maintenance

Many health care providers derive value from participation in regular training and evaluation sessions that increase their ability to recognize and treat serious arrhythmias. Experienced providers must also know how to use ECG monitoring equipment and be able to troubleshoot the most common technical problems.[1] Quality improvement can take the form of regular periodic reviews of difficult, missed, and misdiagnosed tracings from clinical cases. An expert provider in electrocardiography or electrophysiology can provide insightful guidance and education.

A Systematic Approach to Rhythm Analysis

Every rhythm interpretation must be correlated with other signs of the patient's condition to properly assess and manage indicated interventions. A consistent approach to rhythm analysis is helpful and, when applied to every rhythm, is key to consistent and accurate interpretation.

Cardiac Monitoring: Monitoring Systems

Cardiac monitoring systems generally consist of a monitor screen that displays the ECG and a recording system that transcribes the rhythm onto paper. Lights and tones may provide visual and audible signals of the heart rate. Monitor leads or electrodes may be attached to the patient's chest or

KEY QUESTION AREAS FOR SYSTEMATIC EVALUATION OF THE RHYTHM

One method of rhythm interpretation on the ECG is based on a series of questions which, taken in sequence, can help differentiate many arrhythmias.

1. Is the QRS complex narrow or wide (> 0.12 seconds)?
2. Is the ventricular rate regular or irregularly irregular?
3. Are the QRS complexes preceded by P waves in a 1:1 fashion?
4. Are PR intervals (when seen) constant or variable?

These questions, the rationale for which is further developed in subsequent chapters, allow the health care provider to break down the parts of the ECG and better separate rhythms into descriptive categories. Even if a rhythm diagnosis is not readily apparent from the answers, describing an arrhythmia in this fashion may better communicate its attributes to an expert who could assist with the diagnosis. For example, using this series of questions, were one to describe a narrow complex tachycardia (question 1) that was regular at a rate of 150 bpm (question 2), with two P waves for each QRS (question 3) and unchanging PR intervals (question 4), an expert might suggest a likely diagnosis of atrial flutter with 2:1 AV block. Alternatively, if one were to describe a wide-complex rhythm (question 1) that was regular at a rate of 40 bpm (question 2), with more Ps than QRS complexes such that there was not a 1:1 correspondence between each P and each QRS (question 3) and widely variable PR intervals from beat-to-beat (question 4), a possible diagnosis might be third-degree heart block.

extremities. A 3-lead ECG continues to be commonly used for monitoring, but 5-lead ECG monitoring is a growing norm. The chest leads must be placed to show clearly the waves and complexes of the ECG strip and to leave the chest clear for defibrillation if necessary. The most common lead used to evaluate and monitor the cardiac rhythm is a modified lead II (Fig. 20-5). This lead parallels the direction (vector) of the P wave during normal activation of the atria from the sinus node and, therefore, provides the best display of atrial activity.

Monitoring electrodes are color-coded for ease of application and location. In the United States (a different color system is used in Europe), for a 3-lead ECG the convention is for the right arm electrode to be colored white, the left arm electrode black and the left leg electrode red. For the 5-lead ECG, to additional electrodes are provided, green for the right leg (ground), and brown for chest. These electrodes can all be placed on the torso (they do not necessarily have to be placed on the arms and legs), so long as they are oriented in such a manner that what is left is placed on the left side of the torso, what is right is placed on the right, and that an arm lead is placed above a leg lead (and vice versa). Typically, the white electrode is placed below the clavicle on the right side, the black electrode below the clavicle on the left, and the red electrode on the left lower chest wall often adjacent to the cardiac apex. If a green electrode is provided, it can be placed on the right side of the lower chest opposite the red electrode; a brown or chest electrode

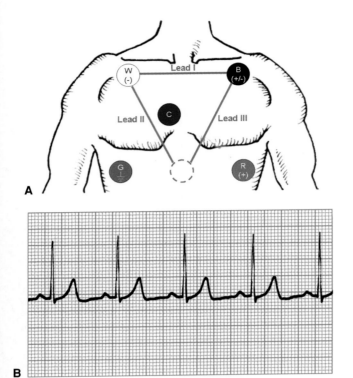

A

B

FIGURE 20-5 • Placement of ECG electrodes for best recording of lead II. When using a 3-lead ECG system to monitor lead II, only the white, black and red electrodes are required; white in this instance is the negative electrode, red is positive, whereas the black electrode switches polarity depending on whether lead II or another lead is selected for monitoring. The green (right leg or ground as denoted by its symbol) and brown (chest) electrodes represent those applied to the chest when a 5-lead ECG is used for monitoring. The red triangle in the center of the chest represents "Einthoven's triangle" which depicts how the electrical signal from the heart is monitered by the white(-), black (-) and red (+) electrodes to create the ECG shown in lead II. In Einthoven's triangle, the dotted the red electrode represents the "electrical location" of the red electrode even though it is physically located on the left chest wall. Lead 2 usually displays upright complexes for P wave, QRS complex, and T wave.

can be placed anywhere a typical "V_{1-6}" ECG lead might be located. See figure 20-5A. The popular mnemonics **"white-to-right, red-to-ribs, and black-on-top"** and **"white-to-right, smoke [black]-over-the-fire [red]"** are aids to remembering where to place the monitor electrodes for lead II when using a 3 or 5 lead ECG for monitoring.

Cardiac Monitoring: Key Points

1. A prominent P wave should be displayed if organized atrial activity is present. Use lead II, which in most patients provides the clearest display of the P wave.
2. The QRS amplitude should be sufficient to properly trigger the rate meter.
3. The patient's precordium must be kept exposed so that defibrillation paddles can be readily used if necessary.
4. Monitoring is for rhythm interpretation only. One should not try to read ST abnormalities or attempt more elaborate interpretation without obtaining a 12-lead ECG. If such changes are observed on the monitored rhythm, a 12-lead ECG should be obtained.
5. Artifacts should be recognized and eliminated as much as possible. Loose electrodes, for example, may produce a perfectly straight line or a bizarre, wavy baseline that resembles ventricular fibrillation. The appearance of patient movement and 60-cycle electrical interference on the monitor should be immediately recognizable and corrected.

References

1. Marriott H. *Practical Electrocardiography*, 8th ed. Baltimore: Williams & Wilkins, 1988.
2. Marriott H. Recognition of cardiac arrhythmias and conduction disturbances. In Hurst JW, ed. *The Heart, Arteries, and Veins*, 7th ed. New York: McGraw-Hill, 1990:489–534.
3. Smith W. Mechanisms of cardiac arrhythmias and conduction disturbances. In Hurst JW, ed. *The Heart, Arteries and Veins*, 7th ed. New York: McGraw-Hill, 1990:473–488.
4. Zipes D. Genesis of cardiac arrhythmias: electrophysiological considerations. In Braunwald E, ed. *Heart Disease: A Textbook of Cardiovascular Medicine*, 4th ed. Philadelphia: Saunders, 1992: 588–627.
5. Task Force of the Working Group on Arrhythmias of the European Society of Cardiology. The Sicilian gambit. A new approach to the classification of antiarrhythmic drugs based on their actions on arrhythmogenic mechanisms. *Circulation* 1991;84:1831–1851.

Chapter 21
Pulseless Cardiac Arrest

Peter J. Kudenchuk

The most critical interventions during the first minutes of a cardiac arrest are immediate bystander cardiopulmonary resuscitation (CPR) providing high-quality chest compressions with minimal interruption.

- Primary emphasis on high quality uninterrupted chest compressions and CPR
- Immediate defibrillation for ventricular fibrillation (VF)/pulseless ventricular tachycardia (VT)
- Secondary emphasis on vasoactive agents and endotracheal intubation
- Coordinated team approach with defined team leader

 See Web site for AHA ECC guidelines on management of pulseless cardiac arrest.

Pulseless Arrest Due to Ventricular Fibrillation or Pulseless VT

Pulseless cardiac arrest is caused by four rhythms: VF, pulseless VT, asystole, or pulseless electrical activity (Fig. 21-1). The basic life support (BLS) algorithm is followed (see Chapter 11, Fig. 11-2); an automatic electrical defibrillator (AED) or manual defibrillator is placed as soon as possible and the rhythm determined (Fig. 21-1, Box 2). Based upon rhythm analysis, a shockable or nonshockable rhythm is determined to be present and further interventions are based on the type of rhythm (Boxes 3 and 9).

The 2005 AHA ECC guidelines gave renewed emphasis to the importance of high-quality, minimally interrupted CPR during the course of resuscitation. A single-shock strategy with subsequent shocks separated by 2 minutes (five cycles) of CPR also displaced the former algorithm of three serial "stacked" shocks. This was recommended in part because it was recognized that serial AED analyses and repeated shocks have limited yield and can deprive patients in cardiac arrest of needed CPR for protracted periods of time.[1,2] For similar reasons, it is now recommended that 2 minutes (five cycles) of CPR be interposed before rhythm and pulse checks following all interventions, including shock. In the current AHA ECC guidelines, pharmacologic therapies (epinephrine or vasopressin) to bolster coronary perfusion pressure are recom-

mended after failure of one or more shocks, and antiarrhythmic therapies for recurrent or resistant VF/VT are recommended after failure of two or more shocks to restore an organized perfusing rhythm. In particular, patients in whom a perfusing rhythm can be transiently restored but not successfully maintained between repeated shocks (recurrent VF/VT) are appropriate candidates for early treatment with antiarrhythmic medications. In such patients the antiarrhythmics may facilitate and stabilize the return of circulation that shock alone has failed to accomplish. As is true for virtually all interventions, the likelihood of benefit from antiarrhythmic drug therapies declines rapidly with the lengthening duration of cardiac arrest.

Defibrillation

The optimal number of attempted defibrillatory shocks that should be administered for refractory VF/VT before initiating pharmacologic therapy is unknown. Traditionally, given the established efficacy of early defibrillation, pharmacologic therapy was recommended after at least three precordial shocks failed to restore a stable perfusing rhythm.

If VF/pulseless VT is present (Fig. 21-1, Box 3), providers should deliver one shock (Box 4) and then resume CPR immediately, beginning with chest compressions. If a biphasic defibrillator is available, providers should use the dose at which that defibrillator has been shown to be effective for terminating VF (typically a selected energy of 120–200 J). If the provider is unaware of the effective dose range of the device, a dose of 200 J for the first shock may be used and an equal or higher shock dose for the second and subsequent shocks. If a monophasic defibrillator is used, providers should deliver an initial shock of 360 J and use that dose for subsequent shocks. If VF is initially terminated by a shock but then recurs later in the arrest, subsequent shocks may be delivered at the previously successful energy level.

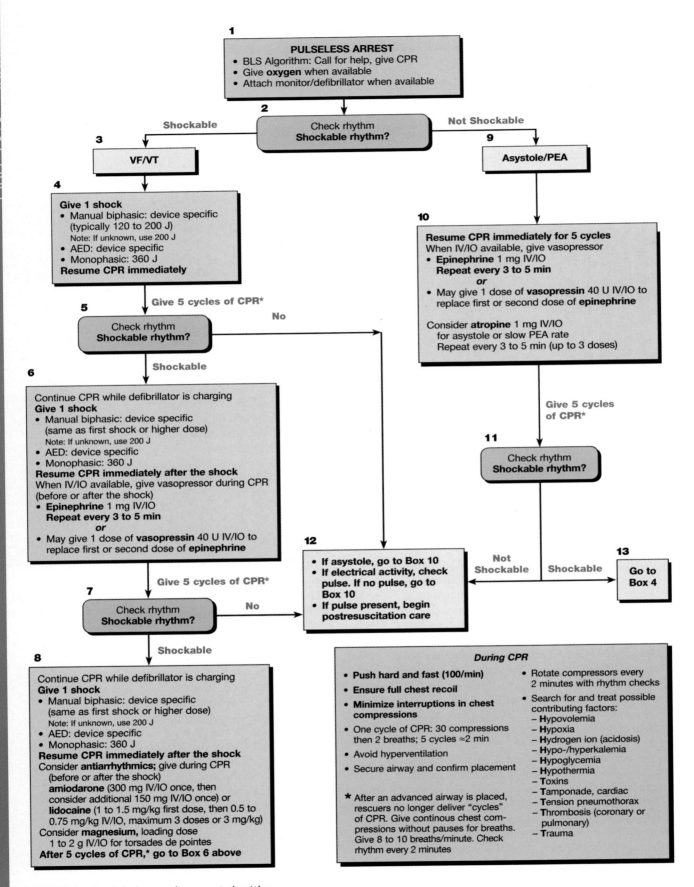

| FIGURE 21-1 • Pulseless cardiac arrest algorithm.

Intravenous Access, Pharmacologic Therapy, and Endotracheal Intubation

Establishing IV access is important (see below), but it should not interfere with CPR and the delivery of shocks. The pulseless arrest algorithm (Fig. 21-1) does not specify precisely when providers should accomplish endotracheal intubation and gain access to the circulation except that these should be accomplished as soon as feasible in unconscious patients who are not responsive to shock and that these activities do not or only minimally interfere with CPR and defibrillation. Since administration of drugs requires intravenous or intraosseous access or endotracheal intubation (see Chapter 18), these interventions should ideally be performed during the CPR interludes between shocks once skilled providers who are trained in such tasks are on scene.

Importantly, efficacy studies of vasoactive agents and antiarrhythmic drugs in VF/VT arrest have addressed only short-term outcomes. Thus recommendations for their use are based on surrogate or immediate or intermediate outcome measures (such as admission alive to hospital) that may not correlate with the preferred outcome of neurologically intact survival to hospital discharge after the cardiac arrest. This is detailed in the subsequent sections with respect to antiarrhythmic agents.

Rhythm, Pulse Checks, and Team Coordination

Rhythm checks should be brief, and pulse checks should generally be performed only if an organized rhythm is observed. If there is any doubt about the presence of a pulse, resume CPR. During treatment of VF/pulseless VT, health care providers must practice efficient coordination between CPR and shock delivery. When VF is present for more than a few minutes, the myocardium is depleted of oxygen and metabolic substrates. A brief period of chest compressions can deliver oxygen and energy substrates, increasing the likelihood that a perfusing rhythm will return after shock delivery.[3] Analyses of VF waveform characteristics predictive of shock success have documented that the shorter the time between chest compression and shock delivery, the more likely it is that the shock will be successful.[3,4] Reduction in the interval from compression to shock delivery by even a few seconds can increase the probability of shock success[4] (Fig. 21-2).

Pulseless Arrest due to Asystole or Pulseless Electrical Activity (PEA)

Definitions

Asystole is defined as the absence of any electrical cardiac activity (either atrial or ventricular) for seconds to minutes or electrical activity that is so profoundly slow (perhaps seen as only a single QRS complex) that for all practical purposes it is a "straight line" rhythm (Fig. 21-3). It should be distinguished from bradycardia (in which successive QRS complexes at a definable albeit slow rate are seen), complete atrioventricular block with ventricular asystole (in which there is evidence of atrial electrical activity without either ventricular conduction or a ventricular escape rhythm), and pulseless electrical activity (an organized rhythm without a corresponding detectable pulse).

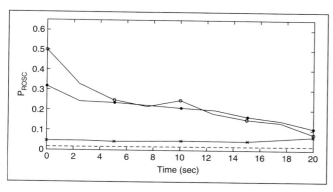

FIGURE 21-2 • This graph illustrates the change in probability for successful defibrillation with return of spontaneous circulation (P$_{ROSC}$) based on the number of seconds without CPR ("hands off" period) between when ECG analysis was initiated and a shock was actually administered (a median of 20 seconds later) to patients in cardiac arrest. It uses a surrogate measure for ROSC, P$_{ROSC}$(v), which is derived based on a variety of factors that can affect the ECG signal (centroid frequency, peak power frequency, spectral flatness and energy features of the signal) and has been used to predict the likelihood of ROSC after shock. The graph illustrates the effect of the pause in CPR upon the ECG signal for 3 groups of patients, those whose analyzed ECG before shock (time 0 on the graph) would have predicted a high likelihood of ROSC (40 to 100%; "[black dot]"), those in whom their ECG predicted a moderate likelihood of ROSC (25 to 40%: "★") and those with a low likelihood (0 to 25% "x"). Among patients in cardiac arrest in whom their ECG would have predicted a high or moderate likelihood of ROSC (top most lines in the graph), saw that probability steadily decline during the 20 second time period before shock was actually administered. In patients in whom P$_{ROSC}$(v) was already low (bottom most line in the graph) when their ECG was first analyzed, the effect of time without CPR on predicted outcome was less apparent, probably because their predicted outcome was already so poor at the outset. (Adapted from Eftestol T, Sunde K, Steen PA. Effects of interrupting precordial compressions on the calculated probability of defibrillation success during out-of-hospital cardiac arrest. *Circulation* 2002;105[19]:2270–2273, revised with permission.)

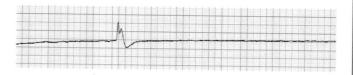

FIGURE 21-3 • Asystole. Although asystole is commonly regarded as the complete absence of any electrical activity on the ECG, it can also present in the manner shown here, with a rare QRS complex. In fact the isolated QRS complex confirms that the baseline is indeed "flat" and does not represent "fine" ventricular fibrillation. Because only a single QRS complex is evident in this instance, no rate can be assigned to this rhythm. The protracted "straight line" appearance of the rhythm following the QRS best characterizes it as asystole.

Pulseless electrical activity (PEA) (terminology that has displaced "electromechanical dissociation," or EMD) is defined as the presence of an organized ventricular rhythm for which a corresponding pulse would ordinarily be expected but is noticeably absent. It does not refer to ventricular fibrillation or pulseless ventricular tachycardia, for which the rapid rate and character of the arrhythmia explain the absence of a pulse. PEA can represent the complete absence of mechanical cardiac contraction in association with each QRS complex. It can also refer to poor mechanical contraction that is insufficient to create a discernible pulse but for which more sensitive methods demonstrate a blood pressure (so-called pseudo-PEA), mechanical contraction that would be adequate were it not compromised by inadequate cardiac filling (such as that caused by pericardial tamponade, tension pneumothorax, or exsanguination), or obstruction to outflow from the heart (such as a large pulmonary embolus).[6]

If rhythm analysis confirms asystole or PEA, resume CPR immediately. A vasopressor (epinephrine or vasopressin) may be administered at this time. Epinephrine can be administered approximately every 3 to 5 minutes during cardiac arrest; one dose of vasopressin may be substituted for either the first or second epinephrine dose (Fig. 21-1, Box 10). For a patient in asystole or slow PEA, consider atropine. Do not interrupt CPR to deliver these medications.

After drug delivery and approximately 5 cycles (or about 2 minutes) of CPR, recheck the rhythm (Fig. 21-1, Box 11). If a shockable rhythm is present, deliver a shock (Box 4). If no rhythm is present or if there is no change in the appearance of the electrocardiogram, immediately resume CPR (Box 10). If an organized rhythm is present (Box 12), try to palpate a pulse. If no pulse is present (or if there is any doubt about the presence of a pulse), continue CPR (Box 10). If a pulse is present, the provider should identify the rhythm and treat appropriately.

Treatment and Prognosis

Prognosis for cardiac arrest due to asystole or PEA is poor. Asystolic cardiac arrest is rarely salvaged unless found in association with a readily reversible problem, such as severe hyperkalemia. Cardiac arrest associated with PEA carries a better prognosis than asystole if its wider range of causes (see below) can be readily identified and corrected.[7] From a practical standpoint, both rhythms are treated empirically with CPR, epinephrine, or vasopressin and/or atropine. Notably, transcutaneous pacing (which is recommended for symptomatic bradycardia when a pulse is present) is not recommended for either PEA or asystole because of poor efficacy and resulting distraction from performing CPR. Antiarrhythmic drugs have no benefit and in theory may be harmful because of their rhythm-suppression and hypotensive effects. Asystole and particularly PEA have a "differential diagnosis" in terms of what entities can produce these heterogenous rhythms (Table 21-1). Accordingly, particularly victims of PEA should be thoughtfully evaluated to discover a potential reversible cause.

Reversible Causes

Underlying and potentially reversible causes of cardiac arrest should be considered regardless of the rhythm presentation.

TABLE 21-1 • The Most Common Causes of Pulseless Electrical Activity Presented as Hs and Ts

Hs	Ts
Hypovolemia	**T**oxins
Hypoxia	**T**amponade (cardiac)
Hydrogen ion (acidosis)	**T**ension pneumothorax
Hyper-/hypokalemia	**T**hrombosis (coronary and pulmonary)
Hypoglycemia	**T**rauma
Hypothermia	

VF/VT may be precipitated by acute myocardial ischemia or infarction, electrolyte abnormalities, hypoxia, or drug toxicity, recognition and correction of which may facilitate the success of defibrillation. Effective therapeutic options are far more limited when cardiac arrest stems from asystole or PEA, for which the successful restoration of circulation depends almost entirely on recognizing and treating a potentially reversible cause. As a memory aid, such causes can be classified as "the Hs and Ts." The "Hs" are:

- Hypovolemia
- Hypoxia
- Hydrogen ion (acidosis)
- Hyperkalemia/hypokalemia and metabolic disorders
- Hypothermia
- Hypoglycemia

The "Ts" are:

- Toxins/tablets (drug overdose, illicit drugs)
- Tamponade, cardiac
- Tension pneumothorax
- Thrombosis, coronary
- Thrombosis, pulmonary

References

1. Yu T, Weil MH, Tang W, et al. Adverse outcomes of interrupted precordial compression during automated defibrillation. *Circulation* 2002;106(3):368–372.
2. Rea TD, Shah S, Kudenchuk PJ, et al. Automated external defibrillators: to what extent does the algorithm delay CPR? *Ann Emerg Med* 2005;46(2):132–141.
3. Eftestol T, Wik L, Sunde K, et al. Effects of cardiopulmonary resuscitation on predictors of ventricular fibrillation defibrillation success during out-of-hospital cardiac arrest. *Circulation* 2004;110(1):10–15.
4. Eftestol T, Sunde K, Aase SO, et al. Predicting outcome of defibrillation by spectral characterization and nonparametric classification of ventricular fibrillation in patients with out-of-hospital cardiac arrest. *Circulation* 2000;102(13):1523–1529.
5. Eftestol T, Sunde K, Steen PA. Effects of interrupting precordial compressions on the calculated probability of defibrillation success during out-of-hospital cardiac arrest. *Circulation* 2002;105(19):2270–2273.
6. Breitkreutz R, Walcher F, Seeger FH. Focused echocardiographic evaluation in resuscitation management: concept of an advanced life support-conformed algorithm. *Crit Care Med* 2007;35(5 Suppl): S150–S161.
7. Cobb LA, Fahrenbruch CE, Olsufka M, et al. Changing incidence of out-of-hospital ventricular fibrillation, 1980–2000. *JAMA* 2002; 288(23):3008–3013.

Chapter 22
Tachycardia with Pulses: Narrow and Wide

Peter J. Kudenchuk

Guesses as to whether a wide-complex tachycardia is ventricular or supraventricular in origin are wrong as often they are right. Differentiating a wide-complex tachycardia that is supraventricular from one of ventricular origin is important because of the differing treatment and prognostic implications for the patient. The most common presumption is that a hemodynamically stable wide-complex tachycardia must be supraventricular (with aberrancy) in origin, whereas the hemodynamic characteristics of an arrhythmia have little to do with its site or origin. Accordingly, the clinician then proceeds to inappropriately treat a true VT with agents meant for SVT, which are not only ineffective but also expose the patient to adverse effects.

- Definition and approach to the patient with a tachycardia
- Differential diagnosis of narrow-complex tachycardias
- Emergency differential diagnosis of wide-complex tachycardias
- Initial treatment, including "expert consultation advised"

See Web site for AHA/ECC guidelines for cardiopulmonary resuscitation and management of tachycardia with pulses.

Overview

Although, convention tachycardia is defined as a heart rate ≥100 bpm, abnormal tachycardias are somewhat arbitrarily defined by a resting rate of >120 bpm. It should be recognized, however, that a normal rhythm (sinus tachycardia) may reach or exceed this resting rate under some conditions.

Therefore, in light of the appearance and clinical circumstances surrounding the rhythm and rate, the provider must initially ascertain whether an abnormal tachycardia is actually present. Is it a real tachyarrhythmia? (Fig. 22-1, Box 1.) If the rate and appearance of the tachycardia suggest that it truly represents an arrhythmia (rather than a normal rhythm at a faster rate, or an artifactual arrhythmia), the initial approach to its characterization is to assess the patient and determine if serious symptoms are present and due to the tachycardia (Fig. 22-1, Box 2). If serious or significant symptoms are present, then is the patient hemodynamically stable (Fig. 22-1, Box 3)? Unstable signs include altered mental status, ongoing chest pain, hypotension, or other signs of tissue hypoperfusion. A hemodynamically unstable tachycardia prompts the

need for rapid intervention with electrical cardioversion, whereas a hemodynamically stable tachycardia can be approached more deliberately with attention to the most probable rhythm diagnosis and treatment, targeted at its likely origin and mechanism. Or such a patient can potentially be transported to a facility more capable of diagnosing the rhythm.

INITIAL STEPS IN ASSESSING THE 12-LEAD ELECTROCARDIOGRAM

1. Is the QRS complex narrow or wide (≥0.12 seconds)?
2. Is the ventricular rate regular or irregularly irregular?
3. Are the QRS complexes preceded by P waves in a 1:1 fashion?
4. Are PR intervals (when seen) constant or variable?

The next steps in the evaluation of the patient with arrhythmia are to characterize the tachycardia as being wide (QRS ≥0.12 seconds) or narrow in appearance (Fig. 22-1, Boxes 6 and 12); whether it is regular or irregularly irregular in rate (Fig. 22-1 stratification of rhythms shown below Boxes 6 and 12); and whether there is a 1:1 correspondence between each P wave and QRS complex. Finally, determining whether the PR intervals (when seen) are constant or variable can be helpful in determining whether P waves are being conducted to QRS complexes or are more randomly associated with them.

Obtaining a 12-lead ECG of the tachycardia is crucial. A rhythm obtained from a single lead (in which a portion of the QRS complex may be isoelectric and

313

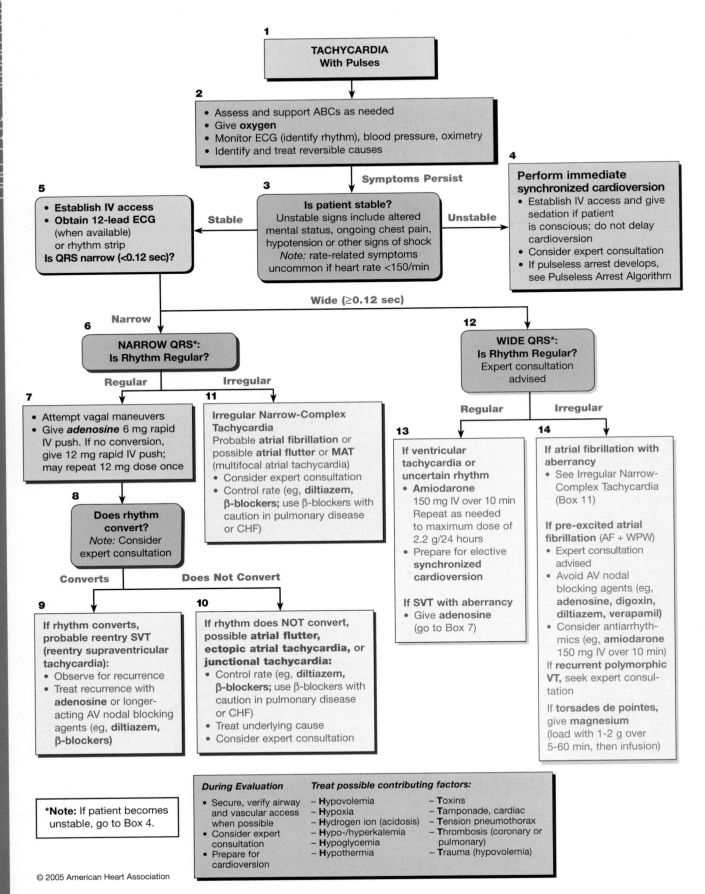

| FIGURE 22-1 • Tachycardia with pulses algorithm.

appear flat on the baseline) can mislead providers into thinking a tachycardia is narrow and presumably of supraventricular origin, when seeing the same rhythm in other leads indicates QRS complexes are actually wide.

If the patient is stable, obtaining a 12-lead ECG of the tachycardia is crucial. A rhythm obtained from a single lead (in which a portion of the QRS complex may be isoelectric and appear flat on the baseline) can mislead providers into thinking a tachycardia is narrow and presumably of supraventricular origin, when seeing the same rhythm in other leads indicates QRS complexes are actually wide.

Narrow-Complex Tachycardias

A narrow-complex tachycardia (<120 milliseconds and especially if <110 milliseconds in duration) can almost always be considered to be of supraventricular origin. The rare exception is a form of ventricular tachycardia (called fascicular tachycardia), which involves one of the fascicles of the His-Purkinje system of the ventricle, and appears relatively narrow (110–120 milliseconds) because it utilizes a portion of the His-Purkinje system for conduction, even though it actually originates in the ventricle. Narrow-complex (supraventricular) tachycardias can be subdivided by whether they are regular or irregular and by their mechanism (whether due to increased automaticity or reentry) (Fig. 22- 2); see below. The differential diagnosis of the supraventricular tachycardia (SVT) includes sinus tachycardia; sinus node reentry tachycardia; paroxysmal supraventricular tachycardia (PSVT) due to atrioventricular nodal reentry (AVNRT) or atrioventricular reentry utilizing an accessory pathway as the retrograde limb of the reentry circuit (AVRT); ectopic (focal) atrial tachycardia; multifocal atrial tachycardia; intra-atrial reentry tachycardia, atrial fibrillation, and atrial flutter. The features and treatment approaches to these arrhythmias are discussed for each specific entity in the section below. In general, treatment of these arrhythmias, if the patient is hemodynamically stable, is approached by use of drugs that block the AV node and result in slower ventricular rates or result in termination of the arrhythmia by creating AV nodal block. The exception to this generality is when one is dealing with an arrhythmia

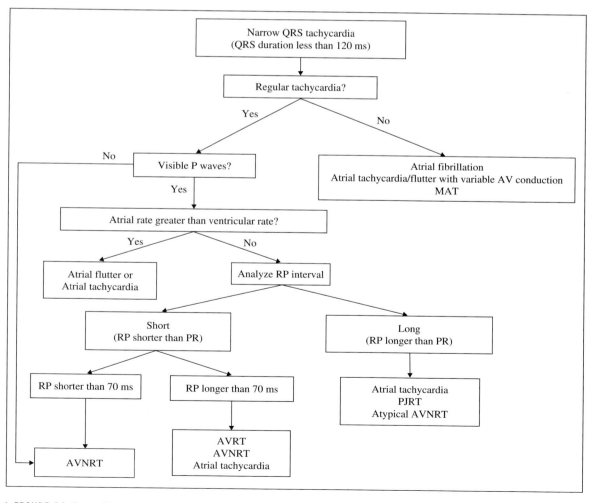

| FIGURE 22-2 • Differential diagnosis for narrow QRS tachycardia. See text for details.

DIFFERENTIAL DIAGNOSIS OF NARROW-COMPLEX (SUPRAVENTRICULAR) TACHYCARDIAS (SVT)

Rhythm	Mechanism
Sinus tachycardia	Increased sinus node automaticity
Sinus node reentry tachycardia	Reentry within the sinus node
Paroxysmal supraventricular tachycardia (PSVT)	
– Atrioventricular nodal reentry tachycardia (AVNRT)	Reentry within or surrounding the AV node
– Atrioventricular reentry tachycardia (AVRT)	Reentry involving an accessory pathway
Ectopic (focal) atrial tachycardia (EAT)	Increased automaticity of an atrial focus
Multifocal atrial tachycardia (MAT)	Increased automaticity of many atrial foci
Junctional tachycardia	Increased automaticity of the AV node
Intra-atrial reentry tachycardia	Reentry within the atria
Atrial fibrillation (AF)	Multiple reentry circuits within the atria
Atrial flutter	Reentry circuit typically within the right atrium

such as atrial tachycardia, atrial flutter, or atrial fibrillation that conducts to the ventricles via an accessory pathway (the clue to whose presence is the appearance of a wide QRS complex when conduction to the ventricle occurs over the accessory pathway). In this instance, slowing the ventricular rate requires treatment that is directed at the accessory pathway itself.

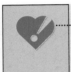 See Web site for ACC/AHA 2007 guidelines for the management of supraventricular tachycardia.

Irregular Narrow-Complex Tachycardias

Narrow-complex tachycardias that are irregularly irregular most commonly represent atrial fibrillation. Atrial fibrillation is defined as an irregularly irregular rhythm without definite P waves. Instead there is a continuous undulation of the baseline between QRS complexes of variable amplitude and contour representing atrial fibrillation waves (Fig. 22-3). The exception to this rule is multifocal atrial tachycardia. Multifocal atrial tachycardia (MAT) is defined as an irregularly irregular tachycardia with distinct P waves of at least three differing morphologies preceding each QRS. The atrial rate may range from 100 to 250 beats/minute. Conduction to the ventricle may be 1:1 as in Fig. 22-4, or variable, in which case each blocked P wave is separated by an isoelectric interval from the next (distinguishing it from atrial fibrillation or flutter where there is no isoelectric interval between successive fibrillation or flutter waves).

In multifocal atrial tachycardia, each blocked P wave is separated by an isoelectric interval from the next. This differential point distinguishes MAT from atrial fibrillation or flutter where there is no isoelectric interval between successive fibrillation or flutter waves.

Regular Narrow-Complex Tachycardias

Regular narrow-complex tachycardias include automatic rhythms, such as sinus tachycardia, junctional tachycardia, and ectopic atrial tachycardia, and reentry rhythms, such as reentrant PSVTs, sinus node reentry tachycardia, intra-atrial reentry tachycardia, and atrial flutter (when conducted with a fixed degree of block). Reentry arrhythmias are distinguished from automatic rhythms by their abrupt onset and termination and their relatively fixed rate, whereas automatic rhythms are characterized by a more gradual "warm up" in rate at their onset.

Reentry Arrhythmias

Reentry arrhythmias (see Chapter 20 for description of mechanisms) typically have an abrupt onset, because once a reentry circuit is activated by a premature complex, the rate of the tachycardia is determined by the conduction properties of the

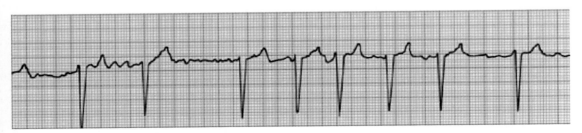

FIGURE 22-3 ● Atrial fibrillation. Arrhythmia characterized by an irregularly irregular rate and undulating baseline between QRS complexes without any regularity or uniformity in the appearance of P (fibrillation) waves.

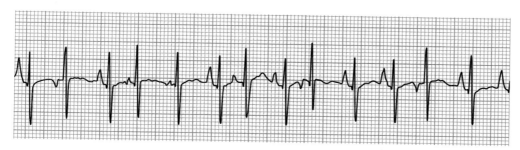

FIGURE 22-4 • Multifocal atrial tachycardia. Irregularly irregular arrhythmia that is distinguished from atrial fibrillation by the presence of clearly discernible P waves preceding each QRS complex. P waves are of differing morphologies, representing their origin from multiple different locations in the atria.

circuit itself, which are relatively constant. Hence the heart rate rapidly increases, becoming steady within a few beats of onset. The term "paroxysmal supraventricular tachycardia" (PSVT), as commonly used, implies a rapid onset of a supraventricular arrhythmia at a regular rate, suggesting a reentry mechanism, usually without easily discernible P waves (although they may be identifiable when not completely hidden within QRS complexes upon closer inspection). The various PSVTs include atrioventricular nodal reentry (AVNRT) and atrioventricular reentry using an accessory pathway (AVRT). These arrhythmias are typically triggered by a premature atrial complex, followed by a rapid, regular tachycardia often without discernible P waves (Fig. 22-5).

Other regular narrow-complex tachycardias caused by reentry include atrial flutter (due to a reentry circuit in the right atrium), intra-atrial reentry tachycardia (analogous to atrial flutter, but using a different reentry circuit within the atria and often presenting at a different rate than typical

atrial flutter), and sinus node reentry tachycardia (where the reentry circuit occurs within the sinus node). Atrial flutter is defined as an atrial arrhythmia with a "sawtooth" appearance (without an isoelectric period between successive flutter waves) (Fig. 22-6). Typically, the atrial rate in flutter is 300 per minute, with a 2:1 AV block, resulting in a regular ventricular rate of 150 per minute. However, both the atrial rate and degree of AV block can vary and atrial flutter can present with varying ventricular rates (an irregular tachycardia).

Automatic Rhythms

In contrast, automatic rhythms (that is, those due to enhanced automaticity, not reentry) typically begin with a more gradual warm-up or gradual acceleration of rate and may terminate the same way, similar to the behavior of sinus rhythm (an automatic rhythm) before, during, and upon completion of exercise. Automatic rhythms include sinus

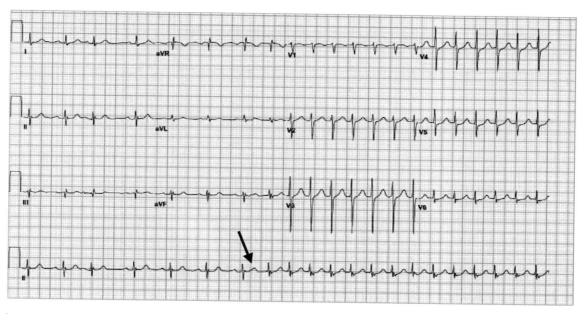

FIGURE 22-5 • PSVT. Sinus rhythm is followed by a premature atrial impulse (arrow) that is hidden in the T wave, followed by a longer than usual PR interval, representing conduction down a more slowly conducting pathway to the ventricle (see Chapter 20). This is immediately followed by a regular narrow-complex tachycardia at a fixed rate without discernible P waves.

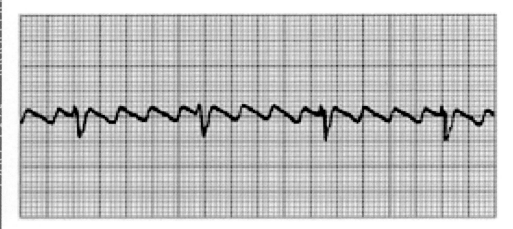

FIGURE 22-6 • Atrial flutter. A typical sawtooth appearance without an isoelectric period between successive flutter waves is seen between QRS complexes. In this case, the atrial rate is 260 per minute with 4:1 AV block, resulting in a ventricular rate of 65 per minute.

tachycardia, ectopic atrial tachycardia (Fig. 22-7), and junctional tachycardia (Fig. 22-8). Junctional tachycardia is a rare arrhythmia in adults and is most commonly confused with PSVT or sinus tachycardia with first-degree AV block (in which the P wave is not discernible because of its fusion with the preceding T wave). Retrograde (inverted) P waves may be visible in junctional tachycardia just preceding or following each QRS, but they may also be hidden from view within the QRS. When seen in adults, junctional tachycardia may be associated with the administration of catecholamine drugs (such as dopamine), which excite a junctional pacemaker focus and result in its more rapid firing.

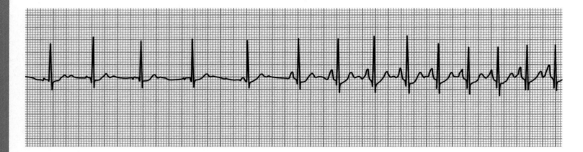

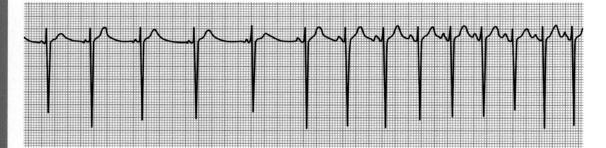

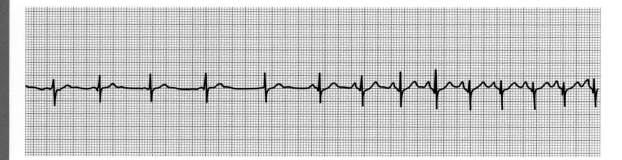

FIGURE 22-7 • Ectopic atrial tachycardia. Three simultaneous ECG leads are shown. Sinus rhythm is followed by a change in P wave morphology followed by a "warmup" acceleration of heart rate. This gradual (as opposed to abrupt) change in heart rate is suggestive of an automatic rather than reentry mechanism for the tachycardia.

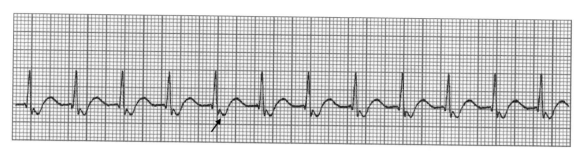

FIGURE 22-8 • Junctional tachycardia. A regular narrow-complex tachycardia is seen. Apparent retrograde (inverted) P waves are seen after each QRS complex (arrow).

Clues to the Diagnosis of Narrow-Complex Tachycardias

Figure 22-2 provides a useful approach to the diagnosis of supraventricular tachycardias, which can be based on a number of serially asked questions:

1. How does the tachycardia begin? Capture of the actual onset of the tachycardia can provide a particularly valuable clue as to its mechanism. Reentry tachycardias typically begin abruptly (with a premature complex), whereas automatic tachycardias more commonly accelerate to their peak rate gradually.
2. Is the tachycardia irregularly irregular? Irregularly irregular supraventricular tachycardias include (most commonly) atrial fibrillation, atrial flutter (when there is variable atrioventricular block), and multifocal atrial tachycardia.
3. If the tachycardia is regular, are P waves visible? In AVNRT, where the reentry circuit "spins" within the AV node, retrograde P waves that are "spun off" to the atrium during the tachycardia are typically hidden within the QRS complex and not discernible on the surface ECG.
4. If P waves are visible, is their rate faster than the ventricular rate? If so, the likely diagnosis is atrial flutter or an atrial tachycardia.
5. What is the character of the RP interval? The R-to-P (or RP) interval is defined as the time between the QRS complex and the next visible P wave (or the converse of the PR interval) and usually refers to the timing of the retrograde P wave resulting from a reentry tachycardia (but it can also refer to atrial or junctional rhythms, as discussed below).

A "short-RP tachycardia" refers to a state in which the RP interval is less than half of the interval between successive QRS complexes (RR interval). That is, the P wave falls closer to the preceding QRS than to the QRS trailing it. Conversely, a "long-RP tachycardia" refers to a state in which the RP interval exceeds half of the interval between successive QRS complexes. That is, the P wave falls closer to the trailing QRS than to the preceding one.

A short RP tachycardia with an extremely short RP interval (<70 milliseconds) means the retrograde P wave is either buried within the QRS complex (and not seen) or might be seen to just coincide with the onset or offset of the QRS. If due to reentry, this is diagnostic of AVNRT. When the RP interval is somewhat longer but still relatively short

(>70 milliseconds), this implies that the reentry circuit takes longer to spin off P waves back to the atrium. This could implicate retrograde P waves generated from AVNRT (with slower than normal conduction of the retrograde P wave back to the atrium) or from AVRT (which typically takes longer to generate a retrograde P wave because the reentry circuit requires that the impulse traverse the ventricles and accessory pathway before being spun back to the atrium).

Conversely, long-RP tachycardias can represent an atypical form of reentry (either the uncommon form of AVNRT or a slowly conducting accessory pathway, including an unusual accessory pathway–mediated arrhythmia called PJRT (permanent form of junctional reciprocating tachycardia). The longer R-to-P interval in these instances results from slower retrograde conduction back to the atrium.

Short- and long-RP tachycardia can also result from automatic (rather than reentrant) arrhythmias, such as atrial tachycardia. For example, an atrial tachycardia with relatively brisk AV conduction might have the appearance of a long-RP tachycardia; whereas an atrial tachycardia with a rate-related first-degree AV block might have the appearance of a short-RP tachycardia.

Finally, in the case of automatic junctional rhythms, retrograde P waves may just slightly precede, be hidden within, or immediately follow the QRS complex, depending upon the speed of retrograde conduction from the AV node back to the atria. When retrograde conduction is more rapid than antegrade conduction, the retrograde P wave may just slightly precede the QRS; when retrograde conduction occurs as rapidly as antegrade conduction to the ventricle, the retrograde P wave will be nearly simultaneous with and hidden within the QRS; whereas when retrograde conduction is slower than antegrade conduction, the retrograde P wave will trail the QRS.

In summary, the relationship of the P wave to the preceding and trailing QRS complex can provide a differential diagnosis for the arrhythmia; in concert with the behavior and other characteristics of the arrhythmia, this may help to establish its diagnosis. The differential diagnosis of a short-RP tachycardia includes reentry arrhythmias (AVNRT or AVRT), atrial tachycardia with first-degree AV block, or junctional rhythms. The differential diagnosis of a long-RP tachycardia includes the uncommon form of AVNRT, or AVRT with a slowly conducting accessory pathway (PJRT), atrial tachycardia, or junctional rhythms.

An additional question to ask that is not addressed in the algorithm shown in Figure 22-2 is: What is the configuration (appearance) of the P wave? A P wave that appears identical to a sinus P wave suggests that the rhythm is sinus tachycardia or possibly sinus node reentry tachycardia. A retrograde P wave may be inverted in leads that would normally see an upright sinus P wave. And the P wave from an ectopic atrial focus will have a different configuration than a sinus P wave. Although a P wave that is clearly different in appearance from a sinus P wave implies that the rhythm is not of sinus origin, the converse is not true. P waves may appear sinus-like but still originate from an ectopic arrhythmia focus lying near the sinus node or even posterior to it (in the left atrium).

As evidenced by the growing complexity of possibilities from these series of questions, rhythm diagnosis is likely to require expert consultation if such a diagnosis has not been made by the time the care providers arrives at question 5.

Wide-Complex Tachycardias

In describing tachycardias with a prolonged QRS duration, "wide" is the common term in the United States, whereas in the United Kingdom "broad" is frequently used. Such rhythms are formally defined by a QRS >120 milliseconds, although many experts would also regard a QRS of 120 milliseconds as wide. Wide- or broad-complex tachycardias present a diagnostic challenge because, in addition to being possibly due to ventricular tachycardia, they can be caused by any supraventricular arrhythmia with aberrant conduction. Aberrant conduction means that one or more of the His–Purkinje pathways normally responsible for depolarizing the ventricles failed to conduct the impulse, resulting in depolarization of that region of the ventricle by slower muscle-to-muscle conduction. Such a failure of conduction may be transient (due to the rapid rate of the tachycardia), or permanent (due to a preexisting conduction abnormality). The longer time required to depolarize the ventricle as a result of this interruption in the His–Purkinje system is expressed by a QRS complex of longer (wider) duration. In addition, conduction to the ventricle via an accessory pathway (see discussion of preexcitation in Chapter 19) will result in a wide QRS because of the direct insertion of the pathway into ventricular muscle outside the His–Purkinje system. A narrow-complex tachycardia can be said in most instances to be of supraventricular origin; virtually any arrhythmia can present as a wide-complex tachycardia.

Aberrant conduction means that one or more of the His–Purkinje pathways normally responsible for depolarizing the ventricles fails to conduct the impulse, resulting in depolarization of that region of the ventricle by slower muscle-to-muscle conduction. A narrow-complex tachycardia can be said, in most instances, to be of supraventricular origin, but virtually any arrhythmia can present as a wide-complex tachycardia.

Differentiating a wide-complex tachycardia (Fig. 22-9) that is supraventricular from one of ventricular origin is important because of the differing treatment and prognostic implications for the patient. Guesses as to whether a wide-complex tachycardia is ventricular or supraventricular in origin are wrong as often they are right. The most common presump-

tion is that a hemodynamically stable wide-complex tachycardia must be supraventricular (with aberrancy) in origin, whereas the hemodynamic characteristics of an arrhythmia have little to do with its site or origin. Accordingly, the clinician then proceeds to treat a true VT inappropriately with agents meant for SVT, which are not only ineffective but also expose the patient to adverse effects.[2,3]

Clinical Clues

Clues about the origin of the arrhythmia may be provided with some knowledge of the patient. Older patients with known structural heart disease are at higher risk for ventricular arrhythmias than younger patients without known heart disease, although both groups can have supraventricular arrhythmias. Thus a wide-complex tachycardia is more likely to represent ventricular tachycardia in an older patient with known heart disease than in a younger, healthy patient. A history of previous supraventricular tachycardia, known accessory pathway, preexisting bundle-branch block, or known rate-dependent bundle-branch blocks also suggests that a wide-complex tachycardia is more likely to be of supraventricular origin (with aberrancy) than of ventricular origin. When the QRS during a wide-complex tachycardia matches the QRS observed on a prior ECG obtained during sinus rhythm, this is further support to the arrhythmia being of supraventricular origin.

CLINICAL CLUES—DIFFERENTIAL DIAGNOSIS OF WIDE-COMPLEX TACHYCARDIA (WCT)

Supports Diagnosis of WCT

1. Older patient with known structural heart disease.
2. Symptoms of acute ischemia/infarction.

Supports Diagnosis of SVT with Aberrancy

1. Young patient without structural heart disease.
2. Prior existing bundle-branch block and the appearance of QRS complex matches previous ECG.
3. History of SVT with aberrancy or known accessory pathway.

ECG Clues and Exceptions

The opportunity to establish a rhythm diagnosis is optimal when the patient is hemodynamically stable and the arrhythmia is ongoing. If possible, a 12-lead ECG should be obtained. Either the ECG or, if unavailable, the rhythm strip tracing should be carefully scrutinized for P waves that are slower in rate and dissociated (fewer in number) from the wide QRS complexes (Fig. 22-10) as this is arguably the most reliable evidence that an arrhythmia represents ventricular tachycardia. This is referred to as atrioventricular (AV) dissociation. Unfortunately, P waves can be challenging to identify amid a tachycardia because of their low amplitude relative to the size of QRS complexes, in which they can easily be hidden from view. Other ECG clues suggesting that a wide-complex tachycardia is due to VT include the presence of fusion and/or capture QRS complexes amid the wide-complex tachycardia. These result when an occasional sinus impulse is successfully

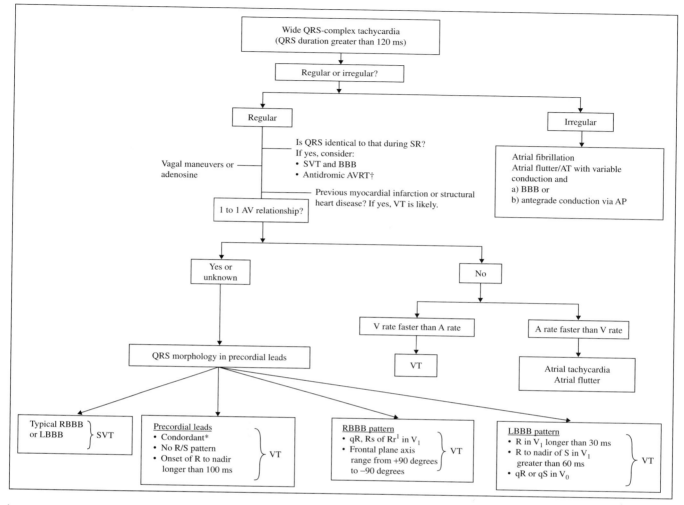

FIGURE 22-9 • Differential diagnosis for wide-QRS-complex tachycardia (QRS >120 milliseconds although many experts would also include QRS of 120 milliseconds in this category). A QRS conduction delay during sinus rhythm, when available for comparison, reduces the value of QRS morphology analysis. *"Concordant" indicates that all precordial leads show either positive or negative deflections. The presence of an occasional narrow QRS "capture" or QRS "fusion" complex of intermediate width amidst a wide QRS arrhythmia suggests a diagnosis of VT. †In preexcited tachycardias, the QRS is wide (i.e., preexcited) compared with sinus rhythm. A, atrial; AF, atrial fibrillation; AP, accessory pathway; AT, atrial tachycardia; AV, atrioventricular; AVRT, atrioventricular reciprocating tachycardia; BBB, bundle-branch block; LBBB, left bundle-branch block; ms, milliseconds; QRS, ventricular activation on ECG; RBBB, right bundle-branch block; SR, sinus rhythm; SVT, supraventricular tachycardias; V, ventricular; VF, ventricular fibrillation; VT, ventricular tachycardia.

conducted across the AV node simultaneously with the tachycardia, resulting in "capture" of the ventricle by the supraventricular impulse. Were this event to occur between successive beats of the tachycardia, a narrow-complex (supraventricular) QRS may be seen amid the otherwise wide-complex tachycardia. Were this event to instead be superimposed on a VT complex, the resulting morphology would be intermediate between a narrow supraventricular and wide-complex VT beat, of a "fusion" of the two complexes (sometimes called a "Dressler" complex). While the occasional presence of either such fusion or capture complexes suggests that the underlying wide-complex rhythm is VT (see Fig. 22-13), unfortunately, this rule is not foolproof. Its notable exception occurs in patients with an accessory pathway (see discussion in Chapter 19). When such patients develop an atrial arrhythmia (such as atrial fibrillation),

conduction to the ventricle may occur variably down the accessory pathway (resulting in a wide QRS), down the AV node (resulting in a narrow QRS), or both (resulting in complexes that combine some of both appearances). This can result in a mixture of wide, narrow and intermediate duration QRS complexes on the ECG due to a supraventricular arrhythmia, not ventricular tachycardia. This principle is illustrated in Figure 19-2 and exemplified in Figure 22-15.

If available, the detailed characterization of QRS configuration on the 12-lead ECG may be helpful in differentiating SVT from VT, but accuracy requires experience.[4–8] Complex rules exist for making the correct rhythm diagnosis by QRS morphology *alone*, as depicted in Figure 22-9. These morphology rules, however, are difficult to teach, learn, remember, and reproducibly apply; they are applicable only when a

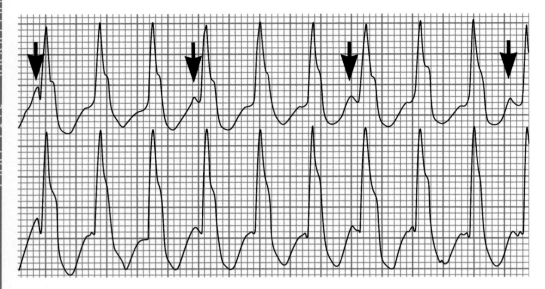

FIGURE 22-10 • Ventricular tachycardia with AV dissociation. A regular wide-complex tachycardia at a rate of 180 per minute is depicted. Occasional deflections are seen preceding some of the QRS complexes that represent dissociated P waves at a rate of 57 per minute. The presence of such AV dissociation (fewer P waves than can account for the number of QRS complexes) confirms a diagnosis of ventricular tachycardia. In addition, the uniform appearance of all QRS complexes would allow for describing this rhythm as monomorphic ventricular tachycardia.

ECG CLUES—DIFFERENTIAL DIAGNOSIS OF WIDE-COMPLEX TACHYCARDIA (WCT)*

Supports Diagnosis of VT

1. P waves present in fewer number than QRS complexes (AV dissociation).
2. Fusion (Dressler) or "capture" beats consistent with occasional AV nodal conduction amid the WCT.

Supports Diagnosis SVT with Aberrancy

1. P waves present in equal or greater number than QRS complexes.
2. Prior ECG with bundle-branch block and similar QRS morphology.
3. Known accessory pathway conduction with similar QRS morphology.

---

*In addition to those listed below, complex rules exist for making the correct rhythm diagnosis by QRS morphology *alone*. These rules, however, are difficult to teach, learn, remember, and reproducibly apply; they can be applied only when a 12-lead ECG has been obtained.[9–13]

12-lead ECG has been obtained.[9–13] Moreover, morphologic QRS criteria are less accurate in patients who have a preexisting QRS conduction abnormality, particularly if they are taking antiarrhythmic medications, and (as with capture and fusion complexes) may also be confounded in patients with preexcitation (an accessory pathway). The challenges associated with these other approaches to rhythm diagnosis, underscores the importance of AV dissociation as arguably the simplest if not most reliable criterion for distinguishing supraventricular tachycardia with aberrancy from VT and why obtaining, either a rhythm strip or a 12-lead ECG is such a useful effort for looking for AV dissociation. If a 12-lead ECG is not available—as, for example, in the prehospital setting—an attempt to document the arrhythmia in at least two or more limb leads before proceeding to transport or with treatment can still serve to provide useful diagnostic information, even if only after the fact.

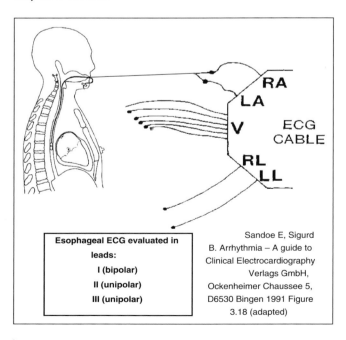

Esophageal ECG evaluated in leads:

I (bipolar)
II (unipolar)
III (unipolar)

Sandoe E, Sigurd B. Arrhythmia – A guide to Clinical Electrocardiography Verlags GmbH, Ockenheimer Chaussee 5, D6530 Bingen 1991 Figure 3.18 (adapted)

FIGURE 22-11 • Typical manner of obtaining and recording an esophageal ECG. The two electrodes from the bipolar esophageal lead are attached to the right and left arm leads of the ECG. Right and left leg leads are placed in their usual locations. Precordial (chest) leads may be attached but are not necessary because a rhythm tracing in leads I, II, and III is used to identify P waves recorded by the esophageal ECG.

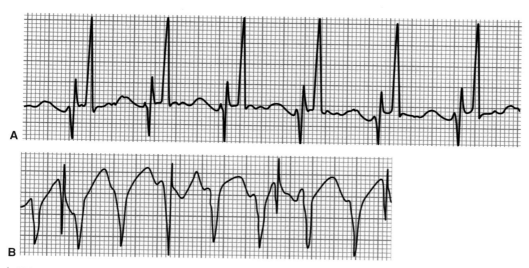

A

B

FIGURE 22-12 • Typical esophageal lead recording obtained in the manner depicted in Figure 22-11. Figure 22-12A depicts the appearance of normal sinus rhythm recorded from an esophageal lead. P waves appear larger in amplitude and more "spike-like" when recorded from a location that is closer to their site of origin compared to their smaller more rounded appearance on the ordinary surface ECG. In Figure 22-12B these higher amplitude, "spike-like" P waves can be more easily distinguished from the underlying wide complex tachycardia. In this instance, the atrial rate is much slower than the ventricular rate (AV dissociation) indicating that the rhythm is ventricular tachycardia.

Esophageal Lead

If P waves are *not* seen on the 12-lead ECG, use of an esophageal lead may be helpful. The esophageal electrogram is a means of amplifying P waves to better evaluate a wide-complex tachycardia for atrioventricular dissociation. A standard transvenous pacing electrode can be used as an esophageal lead, although special esophageal electrodes are also commercially available. This electrode is placed in the esophagus, in similar fashion as a nasogastric tube, with the inserted length estimated to place the distal electrodes at center chest, or approximately behind the heart. In this location, the esophagus lies in close vicinity of and immediately posterior to the left atrium. Attaching the two pacing electrodes from the esophageal lead to the right and left arm electrodes of the ECG (with right and left leg leads in their usual positions) allows for recording amplified P waves in leads I, II, and III during the tachycardia (Fig. 22-11).[14–17] A carefully evaluated 12-lead ECG, monitor tracing, or esophageal lead often permits identification of AV dissociation (Fig. 22-12). This is defined as the loss of a 1-to-1 relationship between atrial electrical activity (P waves) and ventricular response (QRS complexes), with more QRS complexes than can be accounted for by the number of P waves. AV dissociation is a highly specific criterion for VT.

Recently, the American Heart Association, American College of Cardiology, and European Heart Association updated standard definitions for the diagnosis and categorization of arrhythmias.[4,5] These categories (which are modified for presentation here) help to characterize arrhythmias according to the patient's symptoms (Table 22-1), ECG characteristics (Table 22-2), and associated heart disease (Table 22-3).

Regular Wide-Complex Tachycardias

General principles behind the creation of wide complex tachycardias were discussed previously (see page 320 of this chapter). In this section, we will discuss the specific rhythms that can present themselves as regular or irregular wide QRS tachycardias. Whereas regular narrow-complex tachycardias are virtually always of supraventricular origin, regular wide-complex tachycardias are more challenging to diagnose because they can be due to the same supraventricular causes as a regular narrow-complex tachycardia (see Fig. 22-2) but conduct aberrantly or via an accessory pathway to the ventricle; or they may be attributable to ventricular tachycardia. As previously discussed an occasional narrow QRS complex amidst a regular wide-complex tachycardia may represent an interposed sinus beat that happened to conduct to the ventricle between beats (called a capture or fusion beat) and suggests ventricular tachycardia (Fig. 22-13) in patients who are not known to have an accessory pathway (which can occasionally mimic the same finding during an atrial arrhythmia).[18]

Irregular Wide-Complex Tachycardias

In general, an irregularly irregular tachycardia with a uniform beat-to-beat QRS morphology most likely represents atrial fibrillation (Fig. 22-14). The QRS may be narrow or wide if there is aberrant conduction. The differential diagnosis of irregularly irregular tachycardias with QRS complexes that are not uniform across beats (QRS complexes vary in their appearance and in width) suggests the presence of atrial fibrillation with conduction to the ventricle variably

| TABLE 22-1 • Classification of Arrhythmias by Clinical Presentation

Hemodynamically stable	Asymptomatic	The absence of symptoms that could result from an arrhythmia.
	Minimal symptoms, e.g., palpitations	Patient reports palpitations felt in either the chest, throat, or neck as described by the following: • Heartbeat sensations that feel like pounding or racing • An unpleasant awareness of heartbeat • Feeling skipped beats or a pause
Hemodynamically unstable	Presyncope	Patient reports presyncope as described by the following: • Dizziness • Light-headedness • Feeling faint • "Graying out"
	Syncope	Sudden loss of consciousness with loss of postural tone, not related to anesthesia, with spontaneous recovery as reported by the patient or observer. Patient may experience syncope when supine.
	Sudden cardiac death	Death from an unexpected circulatory arrest, usually due to a cardiac arrhythmia occurring within an hour of the onset of symptoms.
	Sudden cardiac arrest	Death from an unexpected circulatory arrest, usually due to a cardiac arrhythmia occurring within an hour of the onset of symptoms, in whom medical intervention (e.g., defibrillation) reverses the event.

| TABLE 22-2 • Classification of Ventricular Arrhythmias by ECG Characteristics

Nonsustained VT		Three or more beats in duration, terminating spontaneously in less than 30 s. VT is a cardiac arrhythmia of three or more consecutive complexes in duration emanating from the ventricles at a rate of greater than 100 bpm (cycle length less than 600 ms.)
	Monomorphic	Nonsustained VT with a single QRS morphology.
	Polymorphic	Nonsustained VT with a changing QRS morphology at cycle length between 600 and 180 ms.
Sustained VT		VT greater than 30 s in duration and/or requiring termination due to hemodynamic compromise in less than 30 s.
	Monomorphic	Sustained VT with a stable single QRS morphology.
	Polymorphic	Sustained VT with a changing or multiform QRS morphology at cycle length between 600 and 180 ms.
Bundle-branch re-entrant tachycardia		VT due to re-entry involving the His-Purkinje system, usually with LBBB morphology; this usually occurs in the setting of cardiomyopathy.
Bidirectional VT		VT with a beat-to-beat alternans in the QRS frontal plane axis, often associated with digitalis toxicity.
Torsades de pointes		Characterized by VT associated with a long QT or QTc when in normal rhythm, and electrocardiographically characterized by twisting of the peaks of the QRS complexes around the isoelectric line during the arrhythmia: • "Typical," initiated following "short-long-short" coupling intervals. • Short coupled variant initiated by normal-short coupling.
Ventricular flutter		A regular (cycle length variability 30 ms or less) ventricular arrhythmia approximately 300 bpm (cycle length—200 ms) with a monomorphic appearance; no isoelectric interval between successive QRS complexes.
Ventricular fibrillation		Rapid, usually more than 300 bpm/200 ms (cycle length 180 ms or less), grossly irregular ventricular rhythm with marked variability in QRS cycle length, morphology, and amplitude.

LBBB, left bundle-branch block; VT, ventricular tachycardia.

| TABLE 22-3 • Heart Diseases Associated with Arrhythmias

Ischemic heart disease

Heart failure (of any cause)

Congenital heart disease

Neurological disorders involving the heart

Valvular heart disease

Primary electrical disease

Sudden infant death syndrome

Cardiomyopathies

  Dilated cardiomyopathy

  Hypertrophic cardiomyopathy

  Arrhythmogenic right ventricular cardiomyopathy

  Infiltrative cardiomyopathies (sarcoid, etc.)

across one or more accessory pathways and the AV node, accounting for the variable appearance of QRS complexes (Fig. 22-15). This is referred to as preexcited atrial fibrillation. Alternatively, such an arrhythmia could represent polymorphic ventricular tachycardia, including torsades de pointes (Fig. 22-17). In this instance the varying QRS appearance is due to the unstable circuits and mechanisms causing the arrhythmia. Because both preexcited atrial fibrillation and polymorphic ventricular tachycardias are often quite rapid in rate and are hemodynamically unstable, they

usually require immediate cardioversion. In addition, when polymorphic VT is sustained, it usually rapidly deteriorates to ventricular fibrillation.

The differential diagnosis of an irregularly irregular wide-complex tachycardia with nonuniform QRS complexes includes atrial fibrillation with preexcitation and polymorphic ventricular tachycardia. Because both preexcited atrial fibrillation and polymorphic ventricular tachycardias are often quite rapid in rate and are hemodynamically unstable, they usually require immediate cardioversion.

Treatment of Hemodynamically Stable Tachycardias

General Considerations

When circumstances and expertise allow, experienced health care providers should make a reasonable attempt to distinguish hemodynamically stable VT from SVT with or without aberrancy based on the QRS duration (width), regularity of the tachycardia, presence of P waves, and direct treatment of the most probable diagnosis. In general, vagal maneuvers or adenosine are recommended in the AHA ECC guidelines and the AHA/ECC guidelines for regular narrow-complex tachycardias. The response to adenosine

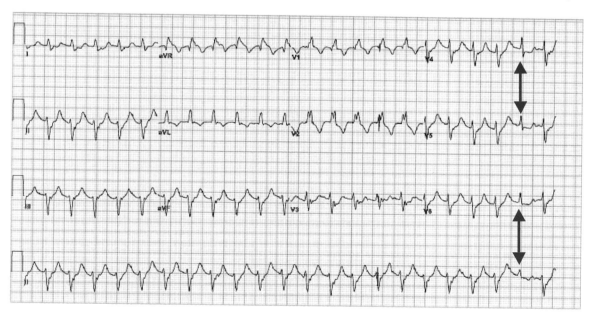

FIGURE 22-13 • Wide-complex tachycardia with a capture complex. A regular wide-complex tachycardia is depicted. The arrows depict a narrow QRS complex in the wide-complex tachycardia, which represents a capture beat. In this case, this complex represents a sinus impulse that happened to be conducted to the ventricle during the tachycardia. This finding suggests that the wide-complex rhythm is most likely ventricular tachycardia. Note that the 12-lead ECG is helpful in defining this single complex as truly narrow and therefore of supraventricular origin.

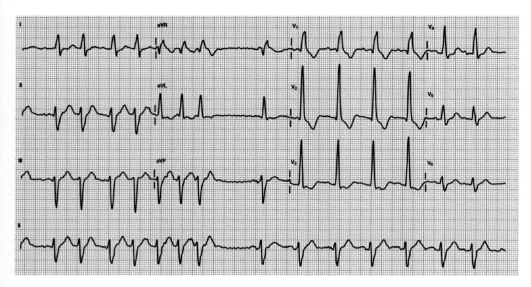

FIGURE 22-14 • Paroxysmal atrial fibrillation with wide-complex conduction. This 12-lead ECG shows an irregularly irregular monomorphic wide-complex tachycardia that spontaneously converts back to sinus rhythm. Both sinus rhythm and the wide-complex tachycardia manifest identical right bundle-branch block morphology. The arrhythmia represents paroxysmal atrial fibrillation with aberrancy.

can help in the diagnosis and treatment of the patient with a regular narrow-complex SVT (Fig. 22-16). The key to understanding the response of a supraventricular tachycardia to adenosine is appreciating the differing effects of the drug on nodal tissue (sinus and AV nodes) as compared with muscle tissue. Adenosine slows sinus node impulse formation and slows (or transiently blocks) conduction in the AV node. Thus, given to a patient in normal sinus rhythm, adenosine would result in sinus bradycardia (or sinus arrest) with transient AV block, after which sinus node and AV node function would recover. Given for reentry arrhythmias that traverse the AV node (such as AVNRT or AVRT) or whose origin is in the sinus node (sinus node reentry tachycardia), adenosine would result in immediate termination of the arrhythmia. However, when given for atrial arrhythmias such as atrial fibrillation, atrial flutter, or an atrial tachycardia (either automatic or due to intra-atrial reentry) whose origin is in atrial muscle, the typical response to adenosine is continuation of the atrial arrhythmia with transient slowing of the ventricular response due the drug's effects on the AV node, followed by resumption of the arrhythmia at its usual ventricular rate. Occasionally, however, adenosine may terminate a focal (automatic) atrial tachycardia.

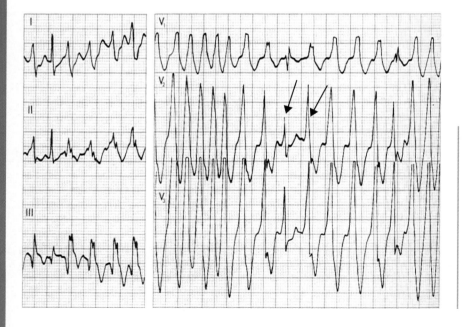

FIGURE 22-15 • Preexcited atrial fibrillation. Preexcited atrial fibrillation is shown with rapid irregularly irregular wide-complex tachycardia due to a rapidly conducting accessory pathway. QRS complexes vary in their morphology, including the occasional appearance of narrow QRS complexes and QRS complexes that have an intermediate morphology between wide and narrow (see arrows in figure). This is due to variable conduction to the ventricle along the accessory pathway (resulting in wide QRS complexes), the AV node (resulting in narrow QRS complexes), or both (resulting in fusion complexes).

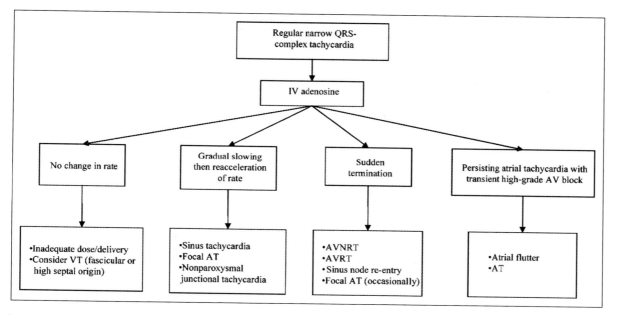

FIGURE 22-16 • Responses of narrow-complex tachycardias to adenosine. AT, atrial tachycardia; AV, atrioventricular; AVNRT, atrioventricular nodal reciprocating tachycardia; AVRT, atrioventricular reciprocating tachycardia; IV, intravenous; QRS, ventricular activation on electrocardiogram; VT, ventricular tachycardia.

IV calcium or beta-blockers are recommended for irregular narrow-complex tachycardias or for regular narrow-complex tachycardias that recur or are resistant to adenosine. Wide-complex tachycardias *known* to be of supraventricular or ventricular origin should be treated in the same way as the suspected supraventricular arrhythmia. An exception is a wide-complex supraventricular tachycardia that is felt to be associated with an accessory pathway (such as preexcited atrial fibrillation or flutter). In this case, expert consultation is recommended before proceeding with treatment. Specifically, preexcited atrial arrhythmias (such as atrial fibrillation or flutter) should *not* be treated with AV-nodal blocking drugs such as adenosine, digoxin, calcium channel blockers, or beta-blockers.

Preexcited atrial arrhythmias (such as atrial fibrillation or flutter) should not be treated with AV nodal blocking drugs such as adenosine, digoxin, calcium channel blockers, or beta-blockers. Seek expert consultation. If a rhythm diagnosis is not possible, expert consultation is not readily available, and treatment is required, a wide-complex tachycardia may be empirically treated with IV amiodarone.

If a rhythm diagnosis is not possible, expert consultation is not readily available, and treatment is required, a wide-complex tachycardia may be empirically treated with IV amiodarone. The broad-range electrophysiologic properties of amiodarone make the drug effective for both ventricular and supraventricular tachycardias, including those involving an accessory pathway.[19] However, if possible, expert consultation should be sought before such empiric treatment is initiated or if there is suspicion for preexcited arrhythmias or polymorphic ventricular tachycardia. If torsades de pointes is suspected, magnesium is the preferred treatment.[20]

MONITOR HEMODYNAMICS CAREFULLY DURING DRUG ADMINISTRATION

Because most drugs used for most tachycardias lower blood pressure, pretreatment blood pressures should be sufficiently high to permit use of such drugs. Typically the hypotensive effect of drugs is more than compensated for by the restoration of sinus rhythm. However, a precipitous drug-induced fall in blood pressure without termination of the arrhythmia should prompt immediate electrical cardioversion. Most but not all arrhythmias ([the notable exceptions being automatic (focal) atrial tachycardia and multifocal atrial tachycardia]) are shock-responsive.

Obtain Pre- and Postconversion 12-Lead Electrocardiograms

If possible, a 12-lead ECG or a continuous rhythm strip should be obtained immediately before and during pharmacologic interventions and after conversion to a regular rhythm.

Treatment of Specific Arrhythmias Ventricular Tachycardia (VT)

Hemodynamically Stable VT

The initial step in the management of any arrhythmia is to determine if the patient is stable or unstable. An unstable patient with a wide-complex tachycardia is presumed to have VT until proven otherwise. If the patient is hemodynamically unstable, immediate cardioversion is performed (see Fig. 22-1, Box 4). If the VT is hemodynamically stable, further evaluation and treatment options can be considered with expert consultation.

VT is considered "hemodynamically stable" if there are no symptoms or clinical evidence of tissue hypoperfusion or shock. Hemodynamically unstable VT requires immediate termination with synchronized cardioversion. Even among patients who appear clinically stable, it is necessary to judge whether there is sufficient time and blood pressure margin for pharmacologic interventions, because success is uncertain, the onset of action often delayed, and side effects, which include hypotension, occur frequently. Electrical cardioversion is, therefore, a preferred treatment strategy for clinically stable ventricular tachycardia, given its high efficacy and ability to rapidly restore sinus rhythm without the uncertainties and potential side effects of antiarrhythmic drugs. However, in instances where cardioversion is not possible (if, for example, the patient is regarded as being at high risk from the required level of sedation for shock), cardioversion has already proven to be unsuccessful, or VT has recurred after successful cardioversion, pharmacologic therapy is reasonable and appropriate.

Even if patients appear clinically stable, it is necessary to judge whether there is sufficient time and blood pressure margin for pharmacologic interventions, because success is uncertain, onset of action often delayed, and side effects, which include hypotension, occur frequently.

Monomorphic VT Monomorphic VT is defined as ventricular tachycardia with a regular rate and with QRS complexes that appear uniform (Fig. 22-10). It likely originates from a single reentry circuit in the ventricle. Although automatic ventricular tachycardias (emerging from an automatic rather than reentrant ventricular focus) can occur, most monomorphic ventricular tachycardias can be presumed to be caused by reentry and approached accordingly. The most typical setting for development of an automatic ventricular rhythm (accelerated idioventricular rhythm) can be during the reperfusion phase of acute myocardial infarction. An accelerated idioventricular rhythm (typically due to an excited automatic focus in the Purkinje system) is usually 120 bpm or slower, as compared with the more rapid rates of reentry VT. It frequently abates spontaneously and may not require specific treatment.

Most monomorphic ventricular tachycardias can be presumed to be caused by reentry and approached accordingly. The principal electrophysiologic effects of drugs used to treat ventricular arrhythmias are to slow conduction and/or increase tissue refractoriness, compromising the ability of a reentry circuit to sustain itself.

The principal electrophysiologic effects of drugs used to treat ventricular arrhythmias are to slow conduction and/or increase tissue refractoriness, thereby compromising the ability of a reentry circuit to sustain itself. However, such electrophysiologic properties can also contribute to worsen-

ing ventricular arrhythmias or create a greater risk for even more malignant forms of ventricular tachycardia, referred to as "proarrhythmia."[21] Patients with impaired heart function are at greater risk for proarrhythmia than those with normal hearts.[22] Among antiarrhythmic drugs, amiodarone appears the least associated with proarrhythmic effects, making it the preferred agent in patients with significantly impaired left ventricular function.[23]

A number of studies have evaluated amiodarone for the treatment of hemodynamically *unstable* VT and VF.[24–35] Although amiodarone has not been specifically evaluated for the pharmacologic termination of hemodynamically stable VT, by extrapolation from these studies its use is reasonable in this setting. For monomorphic VT associated with impaired cardiac function, amiodarone is the agent of first choice because of a lower incidence of proarrhythmia and lesser degree of negative inotropic effects than other drugs.

For monomorphic VT associated with impaired cardiac function, amiodarone is the agent of first choice because of a lower incidence of proarrhythmia and lesser degree of negative inotropic effects than other drugs.

In patients with preserved ventricular function, alternatives to IV amiodarone include IV procainamide,[36] IV quinidine gluconate (which acts similarly to procainamide but has fallen into disuse because of its higher incidence of adverse effects),[37–39] or IV sotalol (not available for use in the United States).[40] There are insufficient data on IV flecainide, IV propafenone, and IV disopyramide (none of these agents are available in the United States) to recommend their use in VT. Although lidocaine can be administered rapidly with minimal effect on blood pressure, studies suggest that it is relatively ineffective for termination of VT[41,42] and less effective against VT than IV procainamide or IV sotalol.[36,40] In treating VT, it is recommended that a single agent be used to maximum doses if necessary. The use of multiple drugs in combination is discouraged because of their potentially additive effects on conduction, which could result in bradycardia or proarrhythmia.

Polymorphic VT VT with varying QRS morphologies is called polymorphic VT (Fig. 22-17). Polymorphic VT is usually irregular in rate, hemodynamically unstable, and likely to quickly degenerate to VF. It often presents as spontaneously terminating paroxysms of tachycardia between interludes of perfusing sinus rhythm.[43] The provider is thus confronted with patients who are hemodynamically unstable when having paroxysms of tachycardia, and relatively stable when these paroxysms spontaneously terminate to sinus rhythm. Defibrillation effectively terminates polymorphic VT but does not prevent its recurrence. Thus the goals of treatment must be to abate and prevent return of the arrhythmia.

Polymorphic VT is often associated with ischemic heart events or electrolyte or toxic conditions.[43] There are also unique forms of polymorphic VT. One form, called torsades de pointes, is often heralded by a preceding sinus bradycardia with a prolonged QT interval.[44] The rhythm's name is derived from its continuously changing VT morphology, often described as appearing to rotate or turn around the ECG

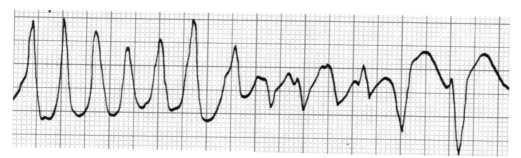

FIGURE 22-17 • A VT with varying QRS morphologies is called polymorphic.

baseline. However, during tachycardia, morphology does not distinguish torsades from polymorphic tachycardia attributable to other causes. Rather, torsades is suspected based on knowledge of the preceding ECG (with QT prolongation) or circumstances that may have predisposed the patient to such an arrhythmia. These include a preceding bradycardia with QT prolongation, particularly in the context of prior treatment with an antiarrhythmic drug, and/or an electrolyte abnormality. Sometimes, if the onset of torsade is captured, the sequence of intervals preceding its onset (such as a transient pause in the rhythm) can provide some clue as to its diagnosis. Making the correct diagnosis is important because the approach to treatment differs in that torsades is an arrhythmia that may be provoked or worsened by antiarrhythmic drugs, which, therefore, should be avoided in its management, whereas polymorphic VT (caused by other mechanisms) may be more responsive to such treatment. Torsades de pointes may be responsive to magnesium and to the combination of pacing and beta-blockers, whereas polymorphic VT of other causes generally is not. Torsades de pointes may be caused by congenital long-QT syndrome or precipitated by drugs that prolong the QT interval.[20] Other unique presentations of polymorphic VT include catecholaminergic polymorphic VT, which is an inherited disorder precipitated by adrenergic stress,[45] and Brugada syndrome, an inherited cardiac disorder associated with ST-segment elevation in the right precordial leads of the ECG.[46] Neither of these disorders is typically associated with structural heart disease.

There are limited data from which to recommend treatment of polymorphic VT. The algorithm for stable ventricular tachycardia, whether monomorphic or polymorphic, is supported largely by extrapolation from studies addressing hemodynamically unstable VT and case series of torsades de pointes. If it is hemodynamically unstable, which more often is the case, polymorphic VT (regardless of cause) is reported to respond similarly as other ventricular arrhythmias to standard advanced cardiac life support measures (VF/pulseless VT algorithm).[47] Recognizing that a polymorphic VT may be due to torsades de pointes invites preferential treatment with magnesium over other antiarrhythmic agents, although amiodarone has been reported to successfully treat torsades de pointes in case reports and is rarely a cause of torsades.[23] It is advisable to seek an expert opinion.

Torsades de Pointes Polymorphic VT of the torsades de pointes type should be treated immediately because of the frequent transition to unstable VT. The first step is to stop medications known to prolong the QT interval. Correct electrolyte imbalance and any other acute precipitants.

Other interventions that may be helpful (based on anecdotal reports that have not been adequately evaluated in controlled trials) include administration of IV magnesium and temporary atrial or ventricular pacing ("overdrive pacing").[48] If patients are free of coronary artery disease, ischemic syndromes, or other contraindications, then isoproterenol may be administered as an interim measure to accelerate heart rate while temporary pacing is initiated.[49] The intent of pacing (or isoproterenol) is to accelerate heart rate to shorten the QT interval by this mechanism. After pacing has been initiated, beta-blockers may be used as adjunctive therapy. Limited studies of lidocaine have shown uncertain efficacy.[50] It is advisable to seek expert opinion.

During tachycardia, morphology does not distinguish torsades from polymorphic tachycardia attributable to other causes. Knowledge of the preceding ECG or circumstances that may have predisposed the patient to such an arrhythmia is helpful. These include a preceding bradycardia with QT prolongation, particularly in the context of prior treatment with an antiarrhythmic drug and/or an electrolyte abnormality.

Other Forms of Polymorphic VT (Ischemia, Catecholaminergic, Brugada Syndrome) Other forms of polymorphic VT, besides torsades de pointes, are not known to be magnesium-responsive[51] and can be treated with conventional antiarrhythmic agents based on extrapolation of data from studies evaluating hemodynamically unstable VT.[47] For patients in whom polymorphic VT may be precipitated by acute coronary syndromes, the use of beta-blockers and anti-ischemic agents is sensible but without tested efficacy. Catecholaminergic polymorphic ventricular tachycardia is an inherited and highly lethal subtype of polymorphic VT that is typically precipitated by adrenergic stress (exercise or emotions), is not associated with structural heart disease or QT prolongation, and is responsive to beta-blockers.[52] Brugada syndrome frequently presents as cardiac arrest due to polymorphic ventricular tachycardia and is treated in accordance with the VF/pulseless VT algorithm.

However, most sodium-channel-blocking antiarrhythmic agents (such as procainamide) should be avoided in patients with known or suspected Brugada syndrome, as these can worsen arrhythmias.[56a]

When polymorphic VT is precipitated by acute myocardial ischemia, lidocaine may be a useful antiarrhythmic agent given its apparent greater efficacy in an acute ischemic event than nonischemic setting.[53–56] Other antiarrhythmic drug options for polymorphic VT not associated with QT prolongation include IV amiodarone, IV procainamide, IV sotalol, or IV phenytoin, based on extrapolation of their use for hemodynamically stable and unstable ventricular tachycardia. It is advisable to seek expert opinion.

Supraventricular Tachycardia (SVT)

Paroxysmal Supraventricular Tachycardia (PSVT)

The term "paroxysmal SVT" (PSVT), as commonly used, refers to a regular tachycardia of supraventricular origin that exceeds the expected limits of sinus tachycardia at rest (>120 bpm), at first glance appears "P-less" (without easily discernible P waves), and is of abrupt onset and abrupt termination. By definition this arrhythmia, whether presenting with a broad or narrow QRS, is of *known* supraventricular origin. Although "PSVT" could technically apply to any supraventricular arrhythmia of sudden onset, the term is conventionally used in specific reference to atrioventricular nodal reentry tachycardia (AVNRT) and atrioventricular reentry tachycardia mediated by an accessory pathway (AVRT). Other supraventricular reentry tachycardias—such as sinus node reentry tachycardia, intra-atrial reentry tachycardia, AF, and atrial flutter—are usually individually characterized and not labeled as PSVT. PSVT is distinguished from junctional tachycardia (which can also appear "P-less" but is very rare in adults) or ectopic (focal) atrial tachycardia (where P waves can be hidden within T waves) by the often gradual onset ("warm up") and termination of automatic tachyarrhythmias (versus the abrupt onset and termination of reentrant PSVT).

Vagal Maneuvers and IV Adenosine   Initial use of vagal maneuvers and IV adenosine in all patients (without contraindications) with PSVT is recommended by the AHA ECC guidelines. This is true even for patients in whom one limb of the reentry pathway contributing to PSVT is mediated by an accessory pathway. Interruption of an arrhythmia whose existence depends upon its "spin" within a reentry circuit only requires block in one or the other of these reentrant limbs in order to be stopped. In the case of atrioventricular reentry due to an accessory pathway, blocking the atrioventricular node with vagal maneuvers or adenosine will terminate the arrhythmia (as will drugs that specifically block conduction in the accessory pathway such as procainamide or amiodarone). The precaution in using atrioventricular blocking drugs for preexcited arrhythmias (see discussion of arrhythmia in Chapter 19) pertains more specifically to arrhythmias such as atrial tachycardia, atrial flutter or atrial fibrillation. The circuits responsible for sustaining these atrial arrhythmias lie outside the atrioventricular node. Thus an AV nodal blocking drug will not terminate these rhythms. Instead, such a drug will only slow conduction of the atrial impulses to the ventricle via the atrioventricular node, while potentially speeding their conduction to the ventricle via the accessory pathway (the latter provoking a potentially dangerous increase in the heart rate).

Other Drugs (Calcium Channel Blockers, Beta-Blockers, Digitalis)   Recurrences of PSVT after vagal maneuvers or adenosine can be treated with calcium channel blockers (verapamil, diltiazem) and beta-blockers. Digitalis (digoxin) is a time-honored drug for treatment of PSVT, but indirect evidence from treatment of AF and atrial flutter suggests that digitalis has a slower onset of action and lower potency relative to other treatment agents.[57] When digitalis is given in combination with other agents, however, its initial use may allow for lower doses of subsequently administered agents for rhythm termination or may blunt their potentially negative inotropic properties by its positive inotropic effects.

PSVT Refractory to Standard Therapy   Treatment of PSVT refractory to vagal maneuvers, adenosine, and AV nodal blocking agents (whether mediated by an accessory pathway or not) includes IV procainamide,[58] IV amiodarone,[59–63] IV flecainide (not available in the United States),[64] IV propafenone (not available in the United States),[65] and IV sotalol (not available in the United States).[66,67] However, these primary antiarrhythmic agents are rarely necessary for treatment of PSVT, require slow administration, and can destabilize marginally compensated patients by virtue of their hypotensive effects. They also have the potential for proarrhythmic effects, including the provocation of life-threatening ventricular arrhythmias. Antiarrhythmic agents should be considered only when AV nodal blocking agents and electrical cardioversion are not feasible, desirable, or successful. *Serial* or combined use of calcium channel blockers, beta-blockers, and primary antiarrhythmic agents is discouraged because of the potential additive hypotensive, bradycardic, and proarrhythmic effects of these drugs.

In the setting of significantly impaired LV function (clinical evidence of congestive heart failure or moderately to severely reduced LV ejection fraction), caution should be exercised in administering drugs with negative inotropic effects to patients with PSVT. These include verapamil, beta-blockers, IV procainamide, IV flecainide, and IV sotalol. Digitalis, amiodarone,[30,34] and perhaps diltiazem[68] are better alternatives in such circumstances. Life-threatening ventricular proarrhythmias may be provoked by primary antiarrhythmic medications in patients with congestive heart failure. In addition, some antiarrhythmic agents, such as flecainide, have been shown to increase mortality in patients with ischemic heart disease[69] and should be avoided in such patients.

In the setting of significantly impaired LV function (clinical evidence of congestive heart failure or moderately to severely reduced LV ejection fraction), caution should be exercised in administering drugs with negative inotropic effects to patients with PSVT. These include verapamil, beta-blockers, IV procainamide, IV flecainide, and IV sotalol.

In summary, in the absence of contraindications, vagal maneuvers or adenosine should be used in an effort to initially terminate PSVT. Treatment of recurrent or resistant PSVT may include calcium channel blockers (verapamil or diltiazem) or beta-blockers. Strong consideration should be given to electrical cardioversion when AV nodal agents are unsuccessful in terminating PSVT. When electrical cardioversion is not feasible, desirable, or successful, patients who "fail" AV nodal blocking agents with either persistent or recurrent PSVT may be treated with antiarrhythmic agents, including IV procainamide, IV amiodarone, IV flecainide (not available in the United States), IV propafenone (not available in the United States), and IV sotalol (not available in the United States). The proarrhythmic potential of this group of medications makes them less desirable options, however, than AV nodal blocking drugs. The serial or combined use of parenteral calcium channel blockers, beta-blockers, and primary antiarrhythmic agents is discouraged.

Automatic Atrial Tachycardias (Ectopic Atrial Tachycardia, Multifocal Atrial Tachycardia)

Ectopic (or focal) atrial tachycardia (EAT) and multifocal atrial tachycardia (MAT) are the result of increased automaticity of a single or multiple (MAT) atrial foci. The term "focal" is intended to imply that these arrhythmias originate from a discrete site, rather than from a relatively larger reentry circut, and are caused by increased automaticity at this focus, no reentry. EAT can be distinguished from sinus tachycardia on the 12-lead ECG by the presence of an abnormal P-wave configuration and P-wave axis that deviates from that seen with normal sinus rhythm. It is important to distinguish MAT from AF, because both can result in an irregularly irregular rhythm but are treated differently. MAT is distinguished from AF by having more organized atrial activity, specifically distinct P waves with three or more different morphologies preceding QRS complexes. By contrast, atrial activity in AF continuously undulates or is incessant between QRS complexes without any organized P wave activity. Automatic arrhythmias such as EAT can be distinguished from reentry–caused PSVT (such as AVNRT or AVRT mediated by an accessory pathway) by their often gradual onset (warm-up) and termination (versus the abrupt onset and termination of reentrant PSVT) and by their continuation even when their conduction is blocked through the AV node by adenosine, vagal maneuvers, or other AV-nodal blocking drugs.

Diagnosis of an atrial tachycardia is made by identifying a P-wave morphology and axis on the 12-lead ECG that differs from that of sinus rhythm. P waves of sinus node origin are typically upright in leads I, II, and aVF, whereas an ectopic atrial tachycardia, by virtue of originating in a different location than the sinus node, will depolarize the atria from a different direction, resulting in P waves that differ in their configuration and P-wave axis from sinus rhythm. In addition, an automatic atrial tachycardia will typically have a more gradual acceleration ("warm up") in rate at its onest, compared to one caused by reentry for which rate acceleration at the onset of the arrhythmia is more sudden and abrupt. Vagal maneuvers or adenosine may be used to demonstrate AV block with persistence of the atrial arrhythmia confirming the rhythm diagnosis of atrial tachycardia. Because automatic atrial tachycardias are due to increased automaticity, they require a different treatment strategy from the reentrant supraventricular arrhythmias (PSVT, AF, atrial flutter, and intra-atrial reentry tachycardia). In particular, automatic rhythms are not treatable by electrical cardioversion; instead, treatment must be directed at the underlying cause and rate control must be achieved through AV-nodal blockade. Many of these automatic arrhythmias are associated with other medical conditions, and require supportive measures and treatment of precipitating causes. MAT, for example, typically is seen in patients with decompensated chronic obstructive pulmonary disease. In patients with preserved LV function, beta-blockers or calcium channel blockers (verapamil or diltiazem) may provide improved rate control by enhancing AV block or conversion of the arrhythmia to normal sinus rhythm. Digitalis is relatively ineffective for slowing heart rate, completely ineffective for terminating ectopic atrial arrhythmias[70] and has actually been associated with provoking EAT.[70] Other useful drugs for EAT or MAT include amiodarone,[61,71] IV flecainide (not available in the United States),[71–73] and IV propafenone (not available in the United States).[74,75] IV quinidine, IV procainamide, and IV phenytoin are not generally effective.[70] In patients with impaired LV function, drugs with significant negative inotropic properties (verapamil, beta-blockers, IV flecainide, and IV propafenone) may provoke heart failure and should be avoided. In the presence of LV impairment, preferred agents include amiodarone and digitalis and perhaps diltiazem.[68]

Masquerading Arrhythmias (Intra-atrial Reentry Tachycardia and Sinus Node Reentry Tachycardia)

Intra-atrial tachycardia is reentry arrhythmia that may be difficult to distinguish from ectopic (focal) atrial tachycardia. Both arrhythmias will typically manifest P waves that differ in their appearance from sinus rhythm. Importantly, intra-atrial reentry, like other reentry-based arrhythmias, is shock-responsive, whereas EAT, like other arrhythmias due to increased automaticity, is not. The most helpful clinical clue in distinguishing the two arrhythmias is found at their onset. The onset of EAT, like that of other automatic rhythms, usually displays a more gradual acceleration (warm-up) to its peak rate; whereas the onset of intra-atrial reentry tachycardia, like other reentry arrhythmias, is usually sudden and reaches its peak heart rate more abruptly. Intra-atrial reentry tachycardia is distinguished from atrial flutter by its slower rate and presence of an isoelectric period (flat segment) between successive P waves. Like atrial flutter and other arrhythmias caused by reentry, it can be acutely treated with electrical cardioversion or similar drug therapies (see next section on atrial flutter).[1]

Sinus node reentry tachycardia, due to reentry in the sinus node, is another arrhythmia masquerader which may be difficult to distinguish from sinus tachycardia.[75a] Both arrhythmias manifest identical-appearing sinus-like P waves. The most useful clinical clue in distinguishing the two arrhythmias is their pattern of onset. The onset of sinus tachycardia (an automatic rhythm) is usually manifested as a warm-up (gradual acceleration) of heart rate, whereas sinus node reentry (a reentry rhythm) begins more abruptly. Because of their differing mechanisms, the two arrhythmias require a different approach to their acute management. Like other reentry tachycardias, sinus node reentry may abruptly terminate with vagal maneuvers, adenosine, beta or calcium channel blockers, antiarrhythmic agents, and cardioversion. Conversely, sinus tachycardia due to enhanced automaticity may gradually slow with administration of beta or calcium channel blockers (which are treatments of choice because of their negative chronotropic effects on pacemaker tissue), but such a tachycardia is not shock-responsive.

Atrial Fibrillation/Flutter

Considerations in the treatment of AF and flutter include pharmacologic control of the rate, restoration of sinus rhythm (rhythm control), indications for anticoagulation, and different treatment approaches for patients without and with significantly impaired LV function (Table 22-4) and those with preexcitation (Table 22-5). Impaired ventricular function is defined as a history of clinical congestive heart failure or a depressed LV ejection fraction (moderate impairment 0.30–0.40; severe impairment <0.30). Because LV ejection fraction is usually not known to care providers, a history of congestive heart failure or its acute presentation is the more pragmatic marker of poor heart function.

Reversible and underlying causes of AF should be investigated and corrected, if possible, including hypoxemia, anemia, hypertension, congestive heart failure, mitral regurgitation, thyrotoxicosis, hypokalemia, hypomagnesemia, and other toxic and metabolic causes. Myocardial ischemia may result from AF with rapid rates, but acute myocardial infarction is an uncommon cause of AF. Most patients with AF have underlying structural heart disease, although a significant minority manifest "lone AF" without evidence of other heart problems.

 See Web site for ACC/AHA 2007 guidelines for the management of atrial fibrillation.

Rate Control IV verapamil,[76–84] beta-blockers,[85–91] and diltiazem[68,92–97] are recommended for rate control in patients with AF or atrial flutter, preserved LV function, and a heart rate ≥120 bpm.[77] Available evidence suggests that digitalis,[98] though effective, is the least potent and has the slowest onset of action of the available pharmacologic options for ventricular rate control. In patients with clinical evidence of congestive heart failure, greater caution should be exercised in use of calcium channel and beta-blocking agents because of their recognized negative inotropic properties and because, in trials of efficacy, patients with congestive heart failure were usually excluded. This risk may be less with diltiazem than with verapamil or beta-blockers.[99] Digoxin remains the only parenteral AV nodal blocking drug with positive inotropic properties, but its usefulness is limited by its relative impotence and slow onset of action, particularly in high-adrenergic states such as congestive heart failure. Sometimes, rate controlling drugs are used in combination when either one,

alone, is unable to achieve satisfactory rate control. Such treatment should be undertaken cautiously, since such combinations (particularly between an IV beta blocker and an IV calcium channel blocker) can provoke a profound bradycardia.

The antiarrhythmic drugs, including procainamide, quinidine, flecainide, propafenone, amioderone and sotalol have conduction slowing properties that can result in a slowing of ventricular rate during atrial fibrillation. However, they should not be regarded as primary rate controlling drugs nor used for this purpose unless there are extenuating circumstances, and the possible risk of their converting atrial fibrillation to sinus rhythm is considered. Their use in atrial flutter is relatively contraindicated unless patients have been treated with a primary rate-slowing drug because they may otherwise paradoxically accelerate ventricular rate. The possible exception is amiodarone, whose combination of beta and calcium channel blocking properties and tolerability in patients with reduced ejection fraction has prompted its use for rate control when other AV nodal blocking drugs are ineffective or contraindicated because of heart failure. IV amiodarone has been used for AF rate control[100] in patients resistant to conventional heart rate control measures[101] or in combination with digitalis.[102] Because conversion to normal sinus rhythm may occur with amiodarone. It is recommended only when other medications for rate control have proved ineffective or are contraindicated and the risk of possible pharmacologic cardioversion is felt to be justified. The highest-risk group for thromboembolic complications from cardioversion are unanticoagulated patients who have been in AF for >48 hours. Because of this concern, amiodarone is ideally reserved for use in patients who have been anticoagulated and/or treated within the first 48 hours of arrhythmia onset or in the setting of other mitigating circumstances,[24,101] recognizing that cardioversion could unpredictably occur within or beyond this 48 hour time window. Some studies have found that although amiodarone was effective for rate control, conversion to sinus rhythm was no greater with conventional doses of IV amiodarone than with placebo or digitalis[60–62,65,70,101–108] unless considerably higher doses were employed.[100] Use of magnesium in the treatment of atrial fibrillation is controversial. Some studies have shown it to be effective, both with respect to control of rate and rhythm, whereas others have not found it to be as effective as more conventional agents such as calcium channel blockers and amiodarone. As yet, magnesium is not generally used or regarded as first-line therapy for atrial arrhythmias.[109,110]

Particular attention should be paid to patients who present with atrial fibrillation or flutter and already have a spontaneously controlled ventricular rate or bradycardia. Efforts to further slow the ventricular rate response or to convert AF to sinus rhythm in such patients can lead to profound bradycardia and even asystole. Consequently, it is advisable to avoid pharmacologic rate control in such patients, be vigilant to the development of bradyarrhythmias during use of drugs to restore sinus rhythm, and have temporary pacing capability (transcutaneous or transvenous) or pharmacologic support (atropine, dopamine, or isoproterenol) available during cardioversion procedures.

TABLE 22-4 • Treatment of Atrial Fibrillation or Flutter Based on Duration (≤48 Hours *or* >48 Hours) and Ventricular Function (Preserved or Impaired)

Duration 48 Hours or Less

1. Control the Rate		2. Convert the Rhythm	
Ventricular Function Preserved	**Ventricular Function Impaired**		
CLASS I • **Diltiazem** (or another calcium channel blocker) *or* • **Metoprolol** (or another beta-blocker) *or*	**CLASS IIb** • **Diltiazem** (only recommended calcium channel blocker) *or* • **Digoxin** *or* • **Amiodarone**	**DC Cardioversion** (recommended)	
		Ventricular Function Preserved	**Ventricular Function Impaired**
CLASS IIb • Flecainide* • Propafenone* • Procainamide* • Amiodarone* • Quinidine** • Sotalol*** • Digoxin		**CLASS IIb** • Ibutilide • Flecainide★ • Propafenone★ • Procainamide★ • Quinidine★ • Amiodarone*	**CLASS IIa** • No antiarrhythmic other than amiodarone is recommended

Duration Greater Than 48 Hours

1. Control the Rate		2. Convert the Rhythm
Ventricular Function Preserved	**Ventricular Function Impaired**	*Urgent Cardioversion*
CLASS I • **Diltiazem** (or another calcium channel blocker) *or* • **Metoprolol** (or another beta-blocker) Class IIb Digoxin	**CLASS IIb** • **Diltiazem** (only recommended calcium channel blocker) *or* • **Digoxin** *or* • **Amiodarone** (if perceived benefit exceeds risk from potential cardioversion by the drug)	• Begin IV heparin at once • Transesophageal echocardiography to exclude atrial clot *then* • Cardioversion within 24 hours *then* • Anticoagulation for 4 more weeks *Delayed Cardioversion* • Anticoagulation (INR = 2 to 3) for at least 3 weeks *then* • Cardioversion *then* • Anticoagulation for 4 more weeks
CLASS III • Flecainide • Quinidine • Sotalol • Propafenone • Procainamide • Amiodarone (may be administered if rate control remains unsatisfactory, and if the perceived benefit exceeds the risk from potential cardioversion by the drug)		

*These drugs can be used for rate control and/or pharmacologic cardioversion in preexcited atrial fribrillation or flutter. IV sotalol has been shown be effective for rate control in preexcited and non-preexcited atrial fibrillation, but not necessarily for pharmacologic cardioversion (Sung RJ, Tan, HL, Karagounis L, Hanyok JJ, Falk R, Platia E, Das G, Hardy SA. Intravenous sotalol for the termination of supraventricular tachycardia and atrial fibrillation and flutter: a multicenter, randomized, double-blind, placebo-controlled study. Sotalol Multicenter Study Group. Am Heart J, 1995 Apr;129(4):739-48).
Note that flecainide, propafenone, and sotalol are not available in IV form in the United States.
Source: Adapted from Cummins RO, Field JM, Hazinski MF eds. ACLS: Principles and Practice. Dallas: American Heart Association 2003, p. 329.

| TABLE 22-5 • Treatment of Atrial Fibrillation or Flutter Associated With Preexcitation Syndrome

1. Control the Rate
and
2. Convert the Rhythm

Note: Do not use the following drugs to treat AF associated with WPW (can be harmful):

CLASS III
- **Adenosine**
- **Beta-Blockers**
- **Calcium channel blockers**
- **Digoxin**

Duration 48 Hours or Less

DC Cardioversion (Recommended) or

Ventricular Function Preserved	Ventricular Function Impaired
CLASS IIb • Amiodarone* • Procainamide* • Flecainide* • Propafenone* • Sotalol* • Quinidine*	**CLASS IIb** • Amiodarone • No antiarrhythmic other than amiodarone is recommended

Duration Greater Than 48 Hours

Urgent Cardioversion (<24 Hours)	**Delayed Cardioversion (>3 weeks)**

• Begin IV heparin at once
 • Transesophageal echocardiography to exclude atrial thrombus
     then
 • Cardioversion within 24 hours
     then
 • Anticoagulation for 4 more weeks
	• Anticoagulation (INR = 2 to 3) for at least 3 weeks
	     then
	 • Cardioversion
	     then
	 • Anticoagulation for 4 more weeks

*These antiarrhythmic drugs should be avoided in patients with atrial flutter, unless first treated with rate controlling drugs, as they may otherwise result in a paradoxical increase in ventricular rate.
**IV sotalol has been shown be effective for rate control in atrial fibrillation, but not necessarily for pharmacologic cardioversion (Sung RJ, Tan HL, Karagounis L, Hanyok JJ, Falk R, Platia E, Das G, Hardy SA. Intravenous sotalol for the termination of supraventricular tachycardia and atrial fibrillation and flutter: a multicenter, randomized, double-blind, placebo-controlled study. Sotalol Multicenter Study Group. Am Heart J, 1995 Apr 129(4):739-48).
Note that flecainide, propafenone, and sotalol are not available in IV form in the United States.

Preexcited Atrial Fibrillation In patients who have conduction between atria and ventricles through an accessory pathway, there is the potential for extremely rapid ventricular responses during AF with degeneration to VF. Preexcited atrial fibrillation and flutter are recognizable by a bizarre wide-complex QRS and, not infrequently, a variable appearance in QRS morphology from beat to beat representing conduction to the ventricles via one or more accessory pathways, the atrioventricular node, or both (fusion complexes) (see Fig. 22-15). If such patients are clinically unstable, synchronized electrical cardioversion is indicated. Otherwise, when a preexcitation syndrome is known or suspected, cardiology consultation is indicated for the selection of the most appropriate management strategy.

Pharmacologic management of preexcited AF or flutter differs markedly from ordinary (nonpreexcited) AF or flutter.

AV nodal blocking agents ordinarily used to control ventricular rate, including verapamil, diltiazem, beta-blockers, and digoxin (as well as the ultrashort AV-nodal blocking agent adenosine) are contraindicated in preexcited AF or flutter (Table 22-5).[111] These may enhance accessory pathway conduction resulting in a paradoxical increase in ventricular rate response. This acceleration is attributable to a number of factors. The direct electrophysiologic effects of these drugs on the accessory pathway or the reflex increase in sympathetic tone resulting from any hypotension provoked by their use may accelerate accessory pathway conduction. In addition, by hindering depolarization of the ventricles via the AV node, these drugs may indirectly facilitate accessory pathway conduction. This is because retrograde activation of the accessory pathway resulting from depolarization of the ventricles via the AV node and His–Purkinje system, may transiently impair the pathway's ability to conduct impulses in a forward direction.[112] By hindering such activation, AV-nodal blockade may paradoxically promote more frequent stimulation of the ventricles by the accessory pathway.

Conversely, antiarrhythmic agents that have direct effects on accessory pathway conduction and refractoriness [such as IV procainamide,[113] IV propafenone,[64] IV flecainide, and IV sotalol[114] (the latter 3 drugs not available in U.S.)] are more likely to slow ventricular response during preexcited AF or atrial flutter. These agents are also likely to convert the arrhythmia to sinus rhythm, and their use requires consideration of thromboembolic risk if the arrhythmia has been present for >48 hours. Oral amiodarone has rate slowing effects in preexcited atrial fibrillation.[115–117] IV amiodarone also increases the refractoriness and slows the conducting properties of accessory pathways.[63] However, there have been case reports of accelerated heart rates when IV amiodarone was administered more rapidly and at higher than recommended initial loading doses to patients with preexcited atrial fibrillation.[118,119] This illustrates how the beneficial electrophysiologic properties of an antiarrhythmic drug may be mitigated by its acute hypotensive effects and result in destabilizing a marginally compensated patient. Such experience underscores the importance of viewing preexcited atrial fibrillation as an inherently unstable arrhythmia for which electrical cardioversion is likely the fastest and safest treatment.

Anticoagulation   Unless required for other reasons, patients who are cardioverted from atrial fibrillation or flutter within 48 hours of the arrhythmias' onset do not need to be anticoagulated before or following the conversion. Conversely, if AF has been present for >48 hours, a risk of systemic embolization exists with conversion to sinus rhythm unless patients are adequately anticoagulated for at least 3 weeks beforehand (followed by a minimum of 4 weeks afterward).[120,121] Electrical cardioversion and the use of antiarrhythmic agents should be avoided unless the patient is unstable or hemodynamically compromised. In patients who are intolerant of atrial fibrillation or flutter and unable to wait for a 3-week course of therapeutic anticoagulation before cardioversion, acute heparinization and cardiology consultation with the use of transesophageal echocardiography to exclude atrial thrombi is indicated to assess the risk and benefits of acute conversion strategies. Such patients, however, still require ongoing and uninterrupted anticoagulation for a minimum of 4 weeks after cardioversion. Some experts initiate anticoagulation with hepain within the first 48 hours of onset of atrial fibrillation or flutter, in hope of extending the time window during which a patient can be safely cardioverted (from a thromboembolic standpoint). If such a patient is successfully cardioverted within 48 hours of rhythm onset, continued anticoagulation is not required; however if cardioverted >48 hours after onset of AF or flutter, anticoagulation should be continued for a minimum of an additional 4 weeks.

Restoring Sinus Rhythm   Electrical cardioversion is the technique of choice, with relatively low risk, for cardioversion of patients with AF or atrial flutter to sinus rhythm.[122] The recommended initial energy settings are discussed in Chapter 24. The efficacy of biphasic shock waveforms for cardioversion of AF and atrial flutter is greater and may allow for lower energy settings than for monophasic waveform shock.[123,124]

If electrical cardioversion is not feasible, desirable, or successful, a number of pharmacologic alternatives are available for cardioversion of patients, including IV ibutilide,[125–128] IV procainamide,[113,125,129–138] IV amiodarone,[24,25,58–61,65,101–108,139–147] IV quinidine,[148] IV flecainide (not available in the United States),[149] IV propafenone (not available in the United States),[150] IV sotalol (not available in the United States),[67] and IV disopyramide (not available in the United States).[151,152] In patients with impaired LV function, the negative inotropic effects of flecainide, propafenone, sotalol, and procainamide as well as the potential proarrhythmic potential of ibutilide make these agents less desirable. IV amiodarone is a preferable agent in such circumstances. It should also be remembered that the likelihood of successful pharmacologic conversion of atrial fibrillation or flutter with any antiarrythmic agent is variable and the precise timing of its occurrence is unpredictable, such that conversion may not necessarily be achieved within 48 hours of the arrhythmias' onset. Beyond 48 hours, anticoagulation issues as discussed in the immediate preceding section must be adequately addressed before cardioversion (electrical or pharmacologic) is performed. Finally, with respect to pharmacologic cardioversion of atrial flutter, an AV-nodal blocking drug (such as diltiazem or a beta-blocker) should be administered before antiarrhythmic agents, which may otherwise paradoxically accelerate ventricular rates. The mechanism for such acceleration is primarily due to a slowing of the atrial flutter rate (for example from 300–200 per minute) by antiarrhythmic drugs. A slower atrial rate may afford a higher proportion of atrial impulses being conducted 1:1 rather than 2:1 across the atrioventricular node, paradoxically increasing the ventricular response (in the example cited, from 150–200 per minute). Pretreatment with a calcium channel or beta-blocker reduces such risk by increasing the degree of AV block.

Accessory Pathway–Mediated Tachycardias

The presence of one or more accessory pathways, linking the atria and ventricles via a muscular bridge, predisposes patients to arrhythmias that fall within the broad category of Wolff-Parkinson-White syndrome. Among these arrhythmias is paroxysmal supraventricular tachycardia (PSVT) due to atrioventricular reentry.

A reentry circuit that involves the atrioventricular node as one limb and the atrioventricular accessory pathway as the other limb can result in PSVT. Most commonly, this reentry circuit "spins" in such a manner that antegrade (forward) conduction to the ventricles occurs via the atrioventricular node, and retrograde (backward) conduction from ventricle to atrium occurs via the accessory pathway. This results in a regular narrow-complex tachycardia of abrupt onset that may be indistinguishable from atrioventricular nodal tachycardia (AVNRT), called orthodromic reciprocating tachycardia, and is treated in the same fashion. Rarely the reentry circuit "spins" in the opposite direction, such that antegrade (forward) conduction to the ventricles occurs via the accessory pathway and retrograde (backward) conduction from the ventricle to atrium occurs via the atrioventricular node. In this instance, a wide-complex tachycardia results, called antidromic reciprocating tachycardia, which, apart from prior knowledge of the existence of an accessory pathway, may not be easily distinguishable from ventricular tachycardia. Both forms of AVRT, orthodromic and antidromic reciprocating tachycardia, are dependent upon conduction through the AV node as one limb of the circuit and will terminate with maneuvers or agents that block the atrioventricular node. This is the single scenario in Wolff-Parkinson-White syndrome where AV-nodal blocking agents (adenosine, calcium channel blockers, beta-blockers, and digoxin) are recommended.

| TABLE 22-6 • Updated Recommendations for the Acute Management of Hemodynamically Stable Regular Tachycardia

ECG	Recommendation[a]	Classification	Level of Evidence
Narrow QRS-complex tachycardia (SVT)	Vagal maneuvers	I	B
	Adenosine	I	A
	Verapamil, diltiazem	I	A
	Beta-blockers	IIb	C
	Amiodarone	IIb	C
	Digoxin	IIb	C
Wide QRS-complex tachycardia			
• SVT and BBB	See above		
• Preexcited SVT/AF[a]	Flecainide[b]	I	B
	Ibutilide[b]	I	B
	Procainamide[b]	I	B
	DC cardioversion	I	C
• Wide QRS-complex tachycardia of unknown origin	Procainamide[b]	I	B
	Sotalol[b]	I	B
	Amiodarone	I	B
	DC cardioversion	I	B
	Lidocaine	IIb	B
	Adenosine[c]	IIb	C
	Beta-blockers[d]	III	C
	Verapamil[e]	III	B
Wide QRS-complex tachycardia of unknown origin in patients with poor LV function	Amiodarone	I	B
	DC cardioversion	I	B
	Lidocaine	I	B

LEVEL OF EVIDENCE: Level A (highest): derived from multiple randomized clinical trials; Level B (intermediate): data are on the basis of a limited number of randomized trials, nonrandomized studies, or observational registries; Level C (lowest): primary basis for the recommendation was expert consensus.

CLASSIFICATION Class I: Conditions for which there is evidence for and/or general agreement that the procedure or treatment is useful and effective; Class II: Conditions for which there is conflicting evidence and/or a divergence of opinion about the usefulness/efficacy of a procedure or treatment; Class IIa: The weight of evidence or opinion is in favor of the procedure or treatment; Class IIb: Usefulness/efficacy is less well established by evidence or opinion; Class III: Conditions for which there is evidence and/or general agreement that the procedure or treatment is not useful/effective and in some cases may be harmful.

AF, atrial fibrillation; BBB, bundle-branch block; DC, direct current; ECG, electrocardiogram; LV, left ventricular; QRS, ventricular activation on ECG; SVT, supraventricular.

The order in which treatment recommendations appear in this table within each class of recommendation does not necessarily reflect a preferred sequence of administration. For pertinent dosing information, please refer to the AHA/ACC/ESC guidelines on the management of patients with atrial fibrillation.

[a]All listed drugs are administered intravenously

[b]Should not be taken by patients with reduced LV function.

[c]Adenosine should be used with caution in patients with severe coronary artery disease because vasodilation of normal coronary vessels may produce ischemia in vulnerable territory. It should be used only with full resuscitative equipment available.

[d]Beta blockers may be used as first-line therapy for those with catecholamine-sensitive tachycardias such as right ventricular outflow techycardia

[e]Verapamil may be used as first-line therapy for those with LV fascicular VT.

Adapted from Blomstrom-Lundqvist C, Scheinman MM, Aliot EM, Alpert JS, Calkins H, Camm AJ, Campbell WB, Haines DE, Kuck KH, Lerman BB, Miller DD, Shaeffer CW, Stevenson WG, Tomaselli GF. ACC/AHA/ESC guidelines for the management of patients with supraventricular arrhythmias. A report of the American College of Cardiology/American Heart Association Task Force on Practice Guidelines and the European Society of Cardiology Committee for Practice Guidelines. (Writing Committee to Develop Guidelines for the Management of Patients With Supraventricular Arrhythmias). J Am Call Cardiol 2003:42:1463-631.

Conversely, patients with an accessory pathway may also experience other atrial arrhythmias, including ectopic atrial tachycardia, multifocal atrial tachycardia, atrial fibrillation and atrial flutter. In such instances, conduction from the atria to the ventricles will likely occur over both the atrioventricular node and the accessory pathway, with a mixture of wide, narrow, and fused QRS complexes. Ventricular rates are likely to be rapid, and in some cases life-threatening, because the accessory pathway will conduct atrial impulses rapidly to the ventricles without the slowing that is usually afforded by conduction that is restricted to the atrioventricular node. Such arrhythmias cannot and should not be treated with atrioventricular nodal blocking agents (such as digoxin, beta-blockers, or calcium channel blockers and also not with adenosine), which will not slow and may accelerate ventricular rates. Instead, if electrical cardioversion is not an immediate option, pharmacologic agents that have the ability to slow conduction in the muscular accessory pathway should be employed, as discussed in the preceding section; these include IV procainamide, IV amiodarone, IV flecainide, IV propafenone, and IV sotalol (the latter drugs are not available in the United States).

Junctional Tachycardia

In adults, true junctional tachycardia is rare. Apparent junctional tachycardia is most commonly due to misdiagnosed PSVT and should be treated accordingly. True junctional tachycardia in adults is often a manifestation of digitalis toxicity (best treated by withdrawal of digitalis) or of exogenous catecholamines or theophylline (best treated with reduction or withdrawal of such infusions). If no apparent cause is found, symptomatic junctional tachycardia may respond to IV amiodarone or to beta-blockers or calcium channel blockers. This recommendation, however, has no specific human evidence to provide support. Instead the recommendation is based on rational extrapolations from the known antisympathetic and nodal effects of beta-blockers and calcium channel blockers or experience with IV amiodarone for such arrhythmias in children.[153]

Summary

In summary, the diagnosis and management of narrow- and wide-complex tachycardias can be difficult and complex. Emergency cardiac care treatment is focused on the principle of identifying the symptomatic patient and immediately treating those who are hemodynamically unstable or imminently so. Treatment of the stable symptomatic patient is also challenging. When the diagnosis is certain and the treatment specific, therapy can be initiated by providers familiar with initial agents used routinely to treat and terminate the arrhythmia. When it is uncertain, treatment of stable patients is best left to experts familiar with the differential diagnosis and alternate therapies available to these patients (Table 22-6). Shotgun therapy runs the risk of bad treatment, induction of unintended arrhythmias (proarrhythmia), and unanticipated side effects of drug–drug interactions.

References

1. Blomstrom-Lundqvist C, Scheinman MM, et al. ACC/AHA/ESC guidelines for the management of patients with supraventricular arrhythmias—executive summary. A report of the American College of Cardiology/American Heart Association task force on practice guidelines and the European Society of Cardiology committee for practice guidelines (writing committee to develop guidelines for the management of patients with supraventricular arrhythmias) developed in collaboration with NASPE–Heart Rhythm Society. *J Am Coll Cardiol* 2003;42(8): 1493–1531.
2. Akhtar M, Shenasa M, Jazayeri M, et al. Wide QRS complex tachycardia. Reappraisal of a common clinical problem. *Ann Intern Med* 1988;109(11):905–912.
3. Stewart RB, Bardy GH, Greene HL. Wide complex tachycardia: misdiagnosis and outcome after emergent therapy. *Ann Intern Med* 1986;104(6):766–771.
4. Brugada P, Brugada J, Mont L, et al. A new approach to the differential diagnosis of a regular tachycardia with a wide QRS complex. *Circulation* 1991;83(5):1649–1659.
5. Antunes E, Brugada J, Steurer G, et al. The differential diagnosis of a regular tachycardia with a wide QRS complex on the 12-lead ECG: ventricular tachycardia, supraventricular tachycardia with aberrant intraventricular conduction, and supraventricular tachycardia with anterograde conduction over an accessory pathway. *Pacing Clin Electrophysiol* 1994;17(9):1515–1524.
6. Steurer G, Gursoy S, Frey B, et al. The differential diagnosis on the electrocardiogram between ventricular tachycardia and preexcited tachycardia. *Clin Cardiol* 1994;17(6):306–308.
7. Wellens HJ, Bar FW, Lie KI. The value of the electrocardiogram in the differential diagnosis of a tachycardia with a widened QRS complex. *Am J Med* 1978;64(1):27–33.
8. Kindwall KE, Brown J, Josephson ME. Electrocardiographic criteria for ventricular tachycardia in wide complex left bundle branch block morphology tachycardias. *Am J Cardiol* 1988;61(15):1279–1283.
9. Halperin BD, Kron J, Cutler JE, et al. Misdiagnosing ventricular tachycardia in patients with underlying conduction disease and similar sinus and tachycardia morphologies. *West J Med* 1990;152(6): 677–682.
10. Littmann L, McCall MM. Ventricular tachycardia may masquerade as supraventricular tachycardia in patients with preexisting bundle-branch block. *Ann Emerg Med* 1995;26(1):98–101.
11. Alberca T, Almendral J, Sanz P, et al. Evaluation of the specificity of morphological electrocardiographic criteria for the differential diagnosis of wide QRS complex tachycardia in patients with intraventricular conduction defects. *Circulation* 1997;96(10): 3527–3533.
12. Herbert ME, Votey SR, Morgan MT, et al. Failure to agree on the electrocardiographic diagnosis of ventricular tachycardia. *Ann Emerg Med* 1996;27(1):35–38.
13. Andrade FR, Eslami M, Elias J, et al. Diagnostic clues from the surface ECG to identify idiopathic (fascicular) ventricular tachycardia: correlation with electrophysiologic findings. *J Cardiovasc Electrophysiol* 1996;7(1):2–8.
14. Schnittger I, Rodriguez IM, Winkle RA. Esophageal electrocardiography: a new technology revives an old technique. *Am J Cardiol* 1986;57(8):604–607.
15. Shaw M, Niemann JT, Haskell RJ, et al. Esophageal electrocardiography in acute cardiac care: efficacy and diagnostic value of a new technique. *Am J Med* 1987;82(4):689–696.
16. Katz A, Guetta V, Ovsyshcher IA. Transesophageal electrocardiography using a temporary pacing balloon-tipped electrode in acute cardiac care. *Ann Emerg Med* 1991;20(9):961–963.
17. Lopez JA, Lufschanowski R, Massumi A. Transesophageal electrocardiography and adenosine in the diagnosis of wide complex tachycardia. *Texas Heart Inst J* 1994;21(2):130–133.
18. Constant JB. *Learning Electrocardiography: A Complete Course*, 3rd ed. Boston: Little, Brown, 1987.
19. Testa A, Ojetti V, Migneco A, Serra M, et al. Use of amiodarone in emergency. *Eur Rev Med Pharmacol Sci* 2005;9(3):183–190.
20. Gupta A, Lawrence AT, Krishnan K, et al. Current concepts in the mechanisms and management of drug-induced QT prolongation and torsade de pointes. *Am Heart J* 2007;153(6):891–899.
21. Friedman PL, Stevenson WG, Ferrick K, et al. Proarrhythmia. *Am J Cardiol* 1998;82(8 A):50N–58N.
22. Naccarelli GV, Wolbrette DL, Luck JC. Proarrhythmia. *Med Clin North Am* 2001;85(2):503–526, xii.

23. Hohnloser SH, Klingenheben T, Singh BN. Amiodarone-associated proarrhythmic effects. A review with special reference to torsade de pointes tachycardia. *Ann Intern Med* 1994;121(7): 529–535.

24. Leak D. Intravenous amiodarone in the treatment of refractory life-threatening cardiac arrhythmias in the critically ill patient. *Am Heart J* 1986;111(3):456–462.

25. Figa FH, Gow RM, Hamilton RM, et al. Clinical efficacy and safety of intravenous Amiodarone in infants and children. *Am J Cardiol* 1994;74(6):573–577.

26. Mooss AN, Mohiuddin SM, Hee TT, et al. Efficacy and tolerance of high-dose intravenous amiodarone for recurrent, refractory ventricular tachycardia. *Am J Cardiol* 1990;65(9):609–614.

27. Schutzenberger W, Leisch F, Kerschner K, et al. Clinical efficacy of intravenous amiodarone in the short term treatment of recurrent sustained ventricular tachycardia and ventricular fibrillation. *Br Heart J* 1989;62(5):367–371.

28. Helmy I, Herre JM, Gee G, et al. Use of intravenous amiodarone for emergency treatment of life-threatening ventricular arrhythmias. *J Am Coll Cardiol* 1988;12(4):1015–1022.

29. Saksena S, Rothbart ST, Shah Y, et al. Clinical efficacy and electropharmacology of continuous intravenous amiodarone infusion and chronic oral amiodarone in refractory ventricular tachycardia. *Am J Cardiol* 1984;54(3):347–352.

30. Remme WJ, Van Hoogenhuyze DC, Krauss XH, et al. Acute hemodynamic and antiischemic effects of intravenous amiodarone. *Am J Cardiol* 1985;55(6):639–644.

31. Kowey PR, Levine JH, Herre JM, et al. Randomized, double-blind comparison of intravenous amiodarone and bretylium in the treatment of patients with recurrent, hemodynamically destabilizing ventricular tachycardia or fibrillation. The Intravenous Amiodarone Multicenter Investigators Group. *Circulation* 1995; 92(11):3255–3263.

32. Levine JH, Massumi A, Scheinman MM, et al. Intravenous amiodarone for recurrent sustained hypotensive ventricular tachyarrhythmias. Intravenous Amiodarone Multicenter Trial Group. *J Am Coll Cardiol* 1996;27(1):67–75.

33. Scheinman MM, Levine JH, Cannom DS, et al. Dose-ranging study of intravenous amiodarone in patients with life-threatening ventricular tachyarrhythmias. The Intravenous Amiodarone Multicenter Investigators Group. *Circulation* 1995;92(11):3264–3272.

34. Remme WJ, Kruyssen HA, Look MP, et al. Hemodynamic effects and tolerability of intravenous amiodarone in patients with impaired left ventricular function. *Am Heart J* 1991;122(pt 1)(1): 96–103.

35. Anastasiou-Nana MI, Nanas JN, Nanas SN, et al. Effects of amiodarone on refractory ventricular fibrillation in acute myocardial infarction: experimental study. *J Am Coll Cardiol* 1994;23(1): 253–258.

36. Gorgels AP, van den Dool A, Hofs A, et al. Comparison of procainamide and lidocaine in terminating sustained monomorphic ventricular tachycardia. *Am J Cardiol* 1996;78(1):43–46.

37. Holzberger PT, Greenberg ML, Paicopolis MC, et al. Prospective comparison of intravenous quinidine and intravenous procainamide in patients undergoing electrophysiologic testing. *Am Heart J* 1998;136(1):49–56.

38. Torres V, Flowers D, Miura D, et al. Intravenous quinidine by intermittent bolus for electrophysiologic studies in patients with ventricular tachycardia. *Am Heart J* 1984;108(6):1437–1442.

39. Hirschfeld DS, Ueda CT, Rowland M, et al. Clinical and electrophysiological effects of intravenous quinidine in man. *Br Heart J* 1977;39(3):309–316.

40. Ho DS, Zecchin RP, Richards DA, et al. Double-blind trial of lignocaine versus sotalol for acute termination of spontaneous sustained ventricular tachycardia. *Lancet* 1994;344(8914):18–23.

41. Armengol RE, Graff J, Baerman JM, et al. Lack of effectiveness of lidocaine for sustained, wide QRS complex tachycardia. *Ann Emerg Med* 1989;18(3):254–257.

42. Nasir N, Jr., Taylor A, Doyle TK, et al. Evaluation of intravenous lidocaine for the termination of sustained monomorphic ventricular tachycardia in patients with coronary artery disease with or without healed myocardial infarction. *Am J Cardiol* 1994;74(12): 1183–1186.

43. Mechleb BK, Haddadin TZ, Iskandar SB, et al. Idiopathic polymorphic ventricular tachycardia with normal QT interval in a structurally normal heart. *Pacing Clin Electrophysiol* 2006;29(7):791–796.

44. Kay GN, Plumb VJ, Arciniegas JG, Henthorn RW, Waldo AL. Torsade de pointes: the long-short initiating sequence and other clinical features: observations in 32 patients. *J Am Coll Cardiol* 1983;2(5):806–817.

45. Mohamed U, Napolitano C, Priori SG. Molecular and electrophysiological bases of catecholaminergic polymorphic ventricular tachycardia. *J Cardiovasc Electrophysiol* 2007;18(7):791–797.

46. Herbert E, Chahine M. Clinical aspects and physiopathology of Brugada syndrome: review of current concepts. *Can J Physiol Pharmacol* 2006;84(8–9):795–802.

47. Brady WJ, DeBehnke DJ, Laundrie D. Prevalence, therapeutic response, and outcome of ventricular tachycardia in the out-of-hospital setting: a comparison of monomorphic ventricular tachycardia, polymorphic ventricular tachycardia, and torsades de pointes. *Acad Emerg Med* 1999;6(6):609–617.

48. Totterman KJ, Turto H, Pellinen T. Overdrive pacing as treatment of sotalol-induced ventricular tachyarrhythmias (torsade de pointes). *Acta Med Scand Suppl* 1982;668:28–33.

49. Inoue H, Matsuo H, Mashima S, et al. Effects of atrial pacing, isoprenaline and lignocaine on experimental polymorphous ventricular tachycardia. *Cardiovasc Res* 1984;18(9):538–547.

50. Assimes TL, Malcolm I. Torsade de pointes with sotalol overdose treated successfully with lidocaine. *Can J Cardiol* 1998;14(5):753–756.

51. Tzivoni D, Banai S, Schuger C, et al. Treatment of torsade de pointes with magnesium sulfate. *Circulation* 1988;77(2):392–397.

52. Liu N, Colombi B, Raytcheva-Buono EV, et al. Catecholaminergic polymorphic ventricular tachycardia. *Herz* 2007;32(3):212–217.

53. Lie KI, Wellens HJ, van Capelle FJ, et al. Lidocaine in the prevention of primary ventricular fibrillation. A double-blind, randomized study of 212 consecutive patients. *N Engl J Med* 1974; 291(25):1324–1326.

54. Hondeghem LM. Selective depression of the ischemic and hypoxic myocardium by lidocaine. *Proc West Pharmacol Soc* 1975;18:27–30.

55. Borer JS, Harrison LA, Kent KM, et al. Beneficial effect of lidocaine on ventricular electrical stability and spontaneous ventricular fibrillation during experimental myocardial infarction. *Am J Cardiol* 1976;37(6):860–863.

56. Spear JF, Moore EN, Gerstenblith G. Effect of lidocaine on the ventricular fibrillation threshold in the dog during acute ischemia and premature ventricular contractions. *Circulation* 1972;46(1): 65–73.

56a. Brugada R, Brugada J, Antzelevitch C, et al. Sodium channel blockers identify risk for sudden death in patients with ST-segment elevation and right bundle branch block but structurally normal hearts. *Circulation* 2000;101:510–515.

57. Tamargo J, Delpon E, Caballero R. The safety of digoxin as a pharmacological treatment of atrial fibrillation. *Exp Opin Drug Saf* 2006;5(3):453–467.

58. Chapman MJ, Moran JL, O'Fathartaigh MS, et al. Management of atrial tachyarrhythmias in the critically ill: a comparison of intravenous procainamide and amiodarone. *Intens Care Med* 1993;19(1):48–52.

59. Gomes JA, Kang PS, Hariman RJ, et al. Electrophysiologic effects and mechanisms of termination of supraventricular tachycardia by intravenous amiodarone. *Am Heart J* 1984;107(2):214–221.

60. Vietti-Ramus G, Veglio F, Marchisio U, et al. Efficacy and safety of short intravenous amiodarone in supraventricular tachyarrhythmias. *Int J Cardiol* 1992;35(1):77–85.

61. Holt P, Crick JC, Davies DW, et al. Intravenous amiodarone in the acute termination of supraventricular arrhythmias. *Int J Cardiol* 1985;8(1):67–79.

62. Cybulski J, Kulakowski P, Makowska E, et al. Intravenous amiodarone is safe and seems to be effective in termination of paroxysmal supraventricular tachyarrhythmias. *Clin Cardiol* 1996;19(7):563–566.

63. Kuga K, Yamaguchi I, Sugishita Y. Effect of intravenous amiodarone on electrophysiologic variables and on the modes of termination of atrioventricular reciprocating tachycardia in Wolff-Parkinson-White syndrome. *Jpn Circ J* 1999;63(3):189–195.

64. O'Nunain S, Garratt CJ, Linker NJ, et al. A comparison of intravenous propafenone and flecainide in the treatment of tachycardias associated with the Wolff-Parkinson-White syndrome. *Pacing Clin Electrophysiol* 1991;14(pt 2)(11):2028–2034.

65. Bertini G, Conti A, Fradella G, et al. Propafenone versus amiodarone in field treatment of primary atrial tachydysrhythmias. *J Emerg Med* 1990;8(1):15–20.

66. Jordaens L, Gorgels A, Stroobandt R, et al. Efficacy and safety of intravenous sotalol for termination of paroxysmal supraventricular tachycardia. The Sotalol Versus Placebo Multicenter Study Group. *Am J Cardiol* 1991;68(1):35–40.

67. Sung RJ, Tan HL, Karagounis L, et al. Intravenous sotalol for the termination of supraventricular tachycardia and atrial fibrillation and flutter: a multicenter, randomized, double-blind, placebo-controlled study. Sotalol Multicenter Study Group. *Am Heart J* 1995;129(4):739–748.

68. Goldenberg IF, Lewis WR, Dias VC, et al. Intravenous diltiazem for the treatment of patients with atrial fibrillation or flutter and moderate to severe congestive heart failure. *Am J Cardiol* 1994;74(9):884–889.

69. Echt DS, Liebson PR, Mitchell LB, et al. Mortality and morbidity in patients receiving encainide, flecainide, or placebo. The Cardiac Arrhythmia Suppression Trial. *N Engl J Med* 1991;324(12):781–788.

70. Mehta AV, Sanchez GR, Sacks EJ, et al. Ectopic automatic atrial tachycardia in children: clinical characteristics, management and follow-up. *J Am Coll Cardiol* 1988;11(2):379–385.

71. Kouvaras G, Cokkinos DV, Halal G, et al. The effective treatment of multifocal atrial tachycardia with amiodarone. *Jpn Heart J* 1989;30(3):301–312.

72. Hellestrand KJ. Intravenous flecainide acetate for supraventricular tachycardias. *Am J Cardiol* 1988;62(6):16D–22D.

73. Kuck KH, Kunze KP, Schluter M, et al. Encainide versus flecainide for chronic atrial and junctional ectopic tachycardia. *Am J Cardiol* 1988;62(19):37L–44L.

74. Reimer A, Paul T, Kallfelz HC. Efficacy and safety of intravenous and oral propafenone in pediatric cardiac dysrhythmias. *Am J Cardiol* 1991;68(8):741–744.

75. Bauersfeld U, Gow RM, Hamilton RM, et al. Treatment of atrial ectopic tachycardia in infants <6 months old. *Am Heart J* 1995;129(6):1145–1148.

75a. Narula OS. Sinus node re-entry: a mechanism for supraventricular tachycardia. *Circulation* 1974;50:1114–1128.

76. Tommaso C, McDonough T, Parker M, et al. Atrial fibrillation and flutter: immediate control and conversion with intravenously administered verapamil. *Arch Intern Med* 1983;143(5):877–881.

77. Phillips BG, Gandhi AJ, Sanoski CA, et al. Comparison of intravenous diltiazem and verapamil for the acute treatment of atrial fibrillation and atrial flutter. *Pharmacotherapy* 1997;17(6):1238–1245.

78. Hwang MH, Danoviz J, Pacold I, et al. Double-blind crossover randomized trial of intravenously administered verapamil. Its use for atrial fibrillation and flutter following open heart surgery. *Arch Intern Med* 1984;144(3):491–494.

79. Gray RJ, Conklin CM, Sethna DH, et al. Role of intravenous verapamil in supraventricular tachyarrhythmias after open-heart surgery. *Am Heart J* 1982;104(Pt 1)(4):799–802.

80. Gonzalez R, Scheinman MM. Treatment of supraventricular arrhythmias with intravenous and oral verapamil. *Chest* 1981;80(4):465–470.

81. Aronow WS, Landa D, Plasencia G, Wong R, Karlsberg RP, Ferlinz J. Verapamil in atrial fibrillation and atrial flutter. *Clin Pharmacol Ther* 1979;26(5):578–583.

82. Haynes BE, Niemann JT, Haynes KS. Supraventricular tachyarrhythmias and rate-related hypotension: cardiovascular effects and efficacy of intravenous verapamil. *Ann Emerg Med* 1990;19(8):861–864.

83. Barnett JC, Touchon RC. Short-term control of supraventricular tachycardia with verapamil infusion and calcium pretreatment. *Chest* 1990;97(5):1106–1109.

84. Heng MK, Singh BN, Roche AH, et al. Effects of intravenous verapamil on cardiac arrhythmias and on the electrocardiogram. *Am Heart J* 1975;90(4):487–498.

85. Schwartz M, Michelson EL, Sawin HS, et al. Esmolol: safety and efficacy in postoperative cardiothoracic patients with supraventricular tachyarrhythmias. *Chest* 1988;93(4):705–711.

86. Shettigar UR, Toole JG, Appunn DO. Combined use of esmolol and digoxin in the acute treatment of atrial fibrillation or flutter. *Am Heart J* 1993;126(2):368–374.

87. Gray RJ, Bateman TM, Czer LS, et al. Esmolol: a new ultrashort-acting β-adrenergic blocking agent for rapid control of heart rate in postoperative supraventricular tachyarrhythmias. *J Am Coll Cardiol* 1985;5(6):1451–1456.

88. Byrd RC, Sung RJ, Marks J, et al. Safety and efficacy of esmolol (ASL-8052: an ultrashort-acting beta-adrenergic blocking agent) for control of ventricular rate in supraventricular tachycardias. *J Am Coll Cardiol* 1984;3(pt 1)(2):394–399.

89. Amsterdam EA, Kulcyski J, Ridgeway MG. Efficacy of cardioselective beta-adrenergic blockade with intravenously administered metoprolol in the treatment of supraventricular tachyarrhythmias. *J Clin Pharmacol* 1991;31(8):714–718.

90. Rehnqvist N. Clinical experience with intravenous metoprolol in supraventricular tachyarrhythmias: a multicentre study. *Ann Clin Res* 1981;13(suppl 30):68–72.

91. Platia EV, Michelson EL, Porterfield JK, et al. Esmolol versus verapamil in the acute treatment of atrial fibrillation or atrial flutter. *Am J Cardiol* 1989;63(13):925–929.

92. Tisdale JE, Padhi ID, Goldberg AD, et al. A randomized, double-blind comparison of intravenous diltiazem and digoxin for atrial fibrillation after coronary artery bypass surgery. *Am Heart J* 1998;135(pt 1)(5):739–747.

93. Schreck DM, Rivera AR, Tricarico VJ. Emergency management of atrial fibrillation and flutter: intravenous diltiazem versus intravenous digoxin. *Ann Emerg Med* 1997;29(1):135–140.

94. Boudonas G, Lefkos N, Efthymiadis AP, et al. Intravenous administration of diltiazem in the treatment of supraventricular tachyarrhythmias. *Acta Cardiol* 1995;50(2):125–134.

95. Salerno DM, Dias VC, Kleiger RE, et al. Efficacy and safety of intravenous diltiazem for treatment of atrial fibrillation and atrial flutter: the Diltiazem–Atrial Fibrillation/Flutter Study Group. *Am J Cardiol* 1989;63(15):1046–1051.

96. Millaire A, Leroy O, de Groote P, et al. Usefulness of diltiazem in the acute management of supraventricular tachyarrhythmias in the elderly. *Cardiovasc Drugs Ther* 1996;10(1):11–16.

97. Ellenbogen KA, Dias VC, Cardello FP, et al. Safety and efficacy of intravenous diltiazem in atrial fibrillation or atrial flutter. *Am J Cardiol* 1995;75(1):45–49.

98. Jordaens L, Trouerbach J, Calle P, et al. Conversion of atrial fibrillation to sinus rhythm and rate control by digoxin in comparison to placebo. *Eur Heart J* 1997;18(4):643–648.

99. Heywood JT, Graham B, Marais GE, et al. Effects of intravenous diltiazem on rapid atrial fibrillation accompanied by congestive heart failure. *Am J Cardiol* 1991;67(13):1150–1152.

100. Cotter G, Blatt A, Kaluski E, et al. Conversion of recent onset paroxysmal atrial fibrillation to normal sinus rhythm: the effect of no treatment and high-dose amiodarone: a randomized, placebo-controlled study. *Eur Heart J* 1999;20(24):1833–1842.

101. Clemo HF, Wood MA, Gilligan DM, et al. Intravenous amiodarone for acute heart rate control in the critically ill patient with atrial tachyarrhythmias. *Am J Cardiol* 1998;81(5):594–598.

102. Galve E, Rius T, Ballester R, et al. Intravenous amiodarone in treatment of recent-onset atrial fibrillation: results of a randomized, controlled study. *J Am Coll Cardiol* 1996;27(5):1079–1082.

103. Cochrane AD, Siddins M, Rosenfeldt FL, et al. A comparison of amiodarone and digoxin for treatment of supraventricular arrhythmias after cardiac surgery. *Eur J Cardiothorac Surg* 1994;8(4):194–198.

104. Kochiadakis GE, Igoumenidis NE, Simantirakis EN, et al. Intravenous propafenone versus intravenous amiodarone in the management of atrial fibrillation of recent onset: a placebo-controlled study. *Pacing Clin Electrophysiol* 1998;21(11 Pt 2):2475–2479.

105. Larbuisson R, Venneman I, Stiels B. The efficacy and safety of intravenous propafenone versus intravenous amiodarone in the conversion of atrial fibrillation or flutter after cardiac surgery. *J Cardiothorac Vasc Anesth* 1996;10(2):229–234.

106. Kerin NZ, Faitel K, Naini M. The efficacy of intravenous amiodarone for the conversion of chronic atrial fibrillation. Amiodarone vs quinidine for conversion of atrial fibrillation. *Arch Intern Med* 1996;156(1):49–53.

107. Donovan KD, Power BM, Hockings BE, et al. Intravenous flecainide versus amiodarone for recent-onset atrial fibrillation. *Am J Cardio.* 1995;75(10):693–697.

108. Hou ZY, Chang MS, Chen CY, et al. Acute treatment of recent-onset atrial fibrillation and flutter with a tailored dosing regimen of intravenous amiodarone. A randomized, digoxin-controlled study. *Eur Heart J* 1995;16(4):521–528.

109. Onalan O, Crystal E, Daoulah A, et al. Meta-analysis of magnesium therapy for the acute management of rapid atrial fibrillation. *Am J Cardiol* 2007;99(12):1726–1732.

110. Ho KM, Sheridan DJ, Paterson T. Use of intravenous magnesium to treat acute onset atrial fibrillation: a meta-analysis. *Heart (British Cardiac Society)* 2007;93(11):1433–1440.

111. Goy JJ, Fromer M. Antiarrhythmic treatment of atrioventricular tachycardias. *J Cardiovasc Pharmacol* 1991;17(Suppl 6):S36–S40.

112. Chen PS, Prystowsky EN. Role of concealed and supernormal conductions during atrial fibrillation in the preexcitation syndrome. *Am J Cardiol* 1991;68(13):1329–1334.

113. Leitch JW, Klein GJ, Yee R, et al. Differential effect of intravenous procainamide on anterograde and retrograde accessory pathway refractoriness. *J Am Coll Cardiol* 1992;19(1):118–124.

114. Touboul P, Atallah G, Kirkorian G, et al. Effects of intravenous sotalol in patients with atrioventricular accessory pathways. *Am Heart J* 1987;114(3):545–550.

115. Wellens HJ, Lie KI, Bar FW, et al. Effect of amiodarone in the Wolff-Parkinson-White syndrome. *Am J Cardiol* 1976;38(2):189–194.

116. Kappenberger LJ, Fromer MA, Steinbrunn W, et al. Efficacy of amiodarone in the Wolff-Parkinson-White syndrome with rapid ventricular response via accessory pathway during atrial fibrillation. *Am J Cardiol* 1984;54(3):330–335.

117. Feld GK, Nademanee K, Stevenson W, et al. Clinical and electrophysiologic effects of amiodarone in patients with atrial fibrillation complicating the Wolff-Parkinson-White syndrome. *Am Heart J* 1988;115(1 Pt 1):102–107.

118. Tijunelis MA, Herbert ME. Myth: Intravenous amiodarone is safe in patients with atrial fibrillation and Wolff-Parkinson-White syndrome in the emergency department. *CJEM* 2005;7(4):262–265.

119. Schutzenberger W, Leisch F, Gmeiner R. Enhanced accessory pathway conduction following intravenous amiodarone in atrial fibrillation. A case report. *Int J Cardiol* 1987;16(1):93–95.

120. Proceedings of the Seventh ACCP Conference on Antithrombotic and Thrombolytic Therapy: evidence-based guidelines. *Chest* 2004;126(3 Suppl):172S–696S.

121. Sachdev GP, Ohlrogge KD, Johnson CL. Review of the Fifth American College of Chest Physicians Consensus Conference on Antithrombotic Therapy: outpatient management for adults. *Am J Health Syst Pharm* 1999;56(15):1505–1514.

122. Guedon-Moreau L, Gayet JL, Galinier M, et al. Incidence of early adverse events surrounding direct current cardioversion of persistent atrial fibrillation. A cohort study of practices. *Therapie* 2007;62(1):45–48.

123. Gurevitz OT, Ammash NM, Malouf JF, et al. Comparative efficacy of monophasic and biphasic waveforms for transthoracic cardioversion of atrial fibrillation and atrial flutter. *Am Heart J* 2005;149(2):316–321.

124. Koster RW, Dorian P, Chapman FW, et al. A randomized trial comparing monophasic and biphasic waveform shocks for external cardioversion of atrial fibrillation. *Am Heart J* 2004;147(5):e20.

125. Stambler BS, Wood MA, Ellenbogen KA. Comparative efficacy of intravenous ibutilide versus procainamide for enhancing termination of atrial flutter by atrial overdrive pacing. *Am J Cardiol* 1996;77(11):960–966.

126. Kafkas NV, Patsilinakos SP, Mertzanos GA, et al. Conversion efficacy of intravenous ibutilide compared with intravenous amiodarone in patients with recent-onset atrial fibrillation and atrial flutter. *Int J Cardiol* 2007;118(3):321–325.

127. Mountantonakis SE, Moutzouris DA, Tiu RV, et al. Ibutilide to expedite ED therapy for recent-onset atrial fibrillation flutter. *Am J Emerg Med* 2006;24(4):407–412.

128. Lombardi F, Terranova P. Pharmacological treatment of atrial fibrillation: mechanisms of action and efficacy of class III drugs. *Curr Med Chem* 2006;13(14):1635–1653.

129. Mattioli AV, Lucchi GR, Vivoli D, et al. Propafenone versus procainamide for conversion of atrial fibrillation to sinus rhythm. *Clin Cardiol* 1998;21(10):763–766.

130. Kochiadakis GE, Igoumenidis NE, Solomou MC, et al. Conversion of atrial fibrillation to sinus rhythm using acute intravenous procainamide infusion. *Cardiovasc Drugs Ther* 1998;12(1):75–81.

131. Heisel A, Jung J, Stopp M, et al. Facilitating influence of procainamide on conversion of atrial flutter by rapid atrial pacing. *Eur Heart J* 1997;18(5):866–869.

132. Hjelms E. Procainamide conversion of acute atrial fibrillation after open-heart surgery compared with digoxin treatment. *Scand J Thorac Cardiovasc Surg* 1992;26(3):193–196.

133. Fulham MJ, Cookson WO, et al. Procainamide infusion and acute atrial fibrillation. *Anaesth Intens Care* 1984;12(2):121–124.

134. Fenster PE, Comess KA, Marsh R, et al. Conversion of atrial fibrillation to sinus rhythm by acute intravenous procainamide infusion. *Am Heart J* 1983;106(3):501–504.

135. Mandel WJ, Laks MM, Obayashi K, et al. The Wolff-Parkinson-White syndrome: pharmacologic effects of procaine amide. *Am Heart J* 1975;90(6):744–754.

136. Boahene KA, Klein GJ, Yee R, et al. Termination of acute atrial fibrillation in the Wolff-Parkinson-White syndrome by procainamide and propafenone: importance of atrial fibrillatory cycle length. *J Am Coll Cardiol* 1990;16(6):1408–1414.

137. Wellens HJ, Braat S, Brugada P, et al. Use of procainamide in patients with the Wolff-Parkinson-White syndrome to disclose a short refractory period of the accessory pathway. *Am J Cardiol* 1982;50(5):1087–1089.

138. Sellers TDJ, Campbell RW, Bashore TM, et al. Effects of procainamide and quinidine sulfate in the Wolff-Parkinson-White syndrome. *Circulation* 1977;55(1):15–22.

139. Noc M, Stajer D, Horvat M. Intravenous amiodarone versus verapamil for acute conversion of paroxysmal atrial fibrillation to sinus rhythm. *Am J Cardiol* 1990;65(9):679–680.

140. Di Biasi P, Scrofani R, Paje A, et al. Intravenous amiodarone vs propafenone for atrial fibrillation and flutter after cardiac operation. *Eur J Cardiothorac Surg* 1995;9(10):587–591.

141. Horner SM. A comparison of cardioversion of atrial fibrillation using oral amiodarone, intravenous amiodarone and DC cardioversion. *Acta Cardiol* 1992;47(5):473–480.

142. Cowan JC, Gardiner P, Reid DS, et al. A comparison of amiodarone and digoxin in the treatment of atrial fibrillation complicating suspected acute myocardial infarction. *J Cardiovasc Pharmacol* 1986;8(2):252–256.

143. Strasberg B, Arditti A, Sclarovsky S, et al. Efficacy of intravenous amiodarone in the management of paroxysmal or new atrial fibrillation with fast ventricular response. *Int J Cardiol* 1985;7(1):47–58.

144. Faniel R, Schoenfeld P. Efficacy of I.V. amiodarone in converting rapid atrial fibrillation and flutter to sinus rhythm in intensive care patients. *Eur Heart J* 1983;4(3):180–185.

145. Sagrista-Sauleda J, Permanyer-Miralda G, Soler-Soler J. Electrical cardioversion after amiodarone administration. *Am Heart J* 1992;123(6):1536–1542.

146. Butler J, Harriss DR, Sinclair M, et al. Amiodarone prophylaxis for tachycardias after coronary artery surgery: a randomised, double blind, placebo controlled trial. *Br Heart J* 1993;70(1):56–60.

147. Holt AW. Hemodynamic responses to amiodarone in critically ill patients receiving catecholamine infusions. *Crit Care Med* 1989;17(12):1270–1276.

148. Allen LaPointe NM, Li P. Continuous intravenous quinidine infusion for the treatment of atrial fibrillation or flutter: a case series. *Am Heart J* 2000;139(1 Pt 1):114–121.

149. Martinez-Marcos FJ, Garcia-Garmendia JL, Ortega-Carpio A, et al. Comparison of intravenous flecainide, propafenone, and amiodarone for conversion of acute atrial fibrillation to sinus rhythm. *Am J Cardiol* 2000;86(9):950–953.

150. Fak AS, Tezcan H, Caymaz O, et al. Intravenous propafenone for conversion of atrial fibrillation or flutter to sinus rhythm: a randomized, placebo-controlled, crossover study. *J Cardiovasc Pharmacol Ther* 1997;2(4):251–258.

151. Fujimura O, Klein GJ, Sharma AD, et al. Acute effect of disopyramide on atrial fibrillation in the Wolff-Parkinson-White syndrome. *J Am Coll Cardiol* 1989;13(5):1133–1137.

152. Stewart DE, Ikram H. The use of intravenous disopyramide for the conversion of supraventricular tachyarrhythmias. *N Z Med J* 1984;97(751):148–150.

153. Saul JP, Scott WA, Brown S, et al. Intravenous amiodarone for incessant tachyarrhythmias in children: a randomized, double-blind, antiarrhythmic drug trial. *Circulation* 2005;112(22): 3470–3477.

Chapter 23
Bradycardia

Peter J. Kudenchuk

In managing patients with a bradycardia, the critical first action is to evaluate whether the heart rate is hemodynamically significant and sufficiently slow to account for serious and related symptoms.

- Definition and approach to the patient with a bradycardia
- Differential diagnosis of bradycardia
- Emergency treatment considerations for patients with symptomatic bradycardias
- Initial treatment, including "expert consultation advised"
- Considerations for treatment in special circumstances: acute coronary syndrome (ACS), cardiac transplantation

 See Web site for AHA ECC guidelines on cardiopulmonary resuscitation and management of bradycardia.

Cardiac Rhythm and Escape Rhyhms

It is the character of the escape rhythm and hemodynamic impact of the resulting heart rate that determines the emergent or nonemergent consequences of an abnormality in impulse formation or conduction.

The normal cardiac rhythm comprises of two electrical processes, impulse formation and impulse conduction. If either of these fails, an escape rhythm (originating from a subsidiary site of impulse formation) can serve as a backup pacemaker. Impulse formation originates in specialized tissue in the sinus node and is dependent on phase 4 (spontaneous depolarization) of the action potential. Phase 4 of the action potential is heavily dependent on autonomic tone, with parasympathetic (vagal) tone typically slowing impulse formation and sympathetic tone accelerating it. In addition to the sinus node, automatic tissues in other portions of the heart serve as subsidiary pacemakers, which can take control of impulse formation should the sinus node fail, but at a slower rate. Impulse formation in junctional automatic tissue, for example, typically occurs at a rate of 40 to 60 beat per minute (bpm); His automaticity at a rate of

40 bpm; and ventricular automaticity at 30 to 40 bpm. Should impulse formation fail at higher levels, the activity of these otherwise suppressed automatic sites may become manifest.

Impulse conduction is the transmission of an impulse, formed in the atria through the atrioventricular (AV) node and specialized His–Purkinje system, to depolarize the ventricles. Impulse conduction may be slowed or blocked completely at any of these levels, resulting in a spectrum of abnormalities ranging from first-degree AV block and bundle-branch block to complete AV block.

Should either impulse formation or impulse conduction fail completely, the consequences of such failure are dependent upon whether an escape rhythm is robust. Complete AV block, for example, may be associated with a junctional escape rate of 40 to 60 bpm with minimum symptoms or with a slow ventricular escape rate of 30 to 40 bpm and hemodynamic compromise. Importantly, it is the character of the escape rhythm and hemodynamic impact of the resulting heart rate that determines the emergent or nonemergent consequences of an abnormality in impulse formation or conduction.

Disorders of Impulse Formation

Disorders of impulse formation include sinus bradycardia, sinus pause (Fig. 23-1A), and sinus arrest (Fig. 23-1B); they represent impaired automaticity.[1] Such disorders are evidenced by failure to generate P waves at an appropriate rate, abrupt pauses between successive P waves, or complete absence of P waves for a protracted period of time. Criteria that define these disorders are somewhat arbitrary. For

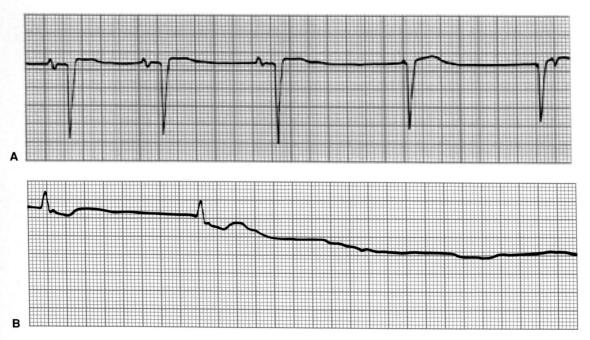

FIGURE 23-1 • Disorders of impulse formation. **A.** Progressive sinus bradycardia is depicted, followed by a sinus pause with junctional escape complexes. **B.** Sinus arrest is shown with junctional escape complexes, followed by asystole (absent atrial and ventricular electrical activity).

example, sinus bradycardia is defined as a heart rate <60 bpm, yet many persons, particularly trained athletes, may be completely asymptomatic with resting heart rates that may average in the range of 40 bpm. Similarly, brief pauses in sinus rhythm of up to 3 seconds may be seen during sleeping periods without adverse consequences. Therefore, bradycardia should become a concern when patients develop symptoms as a result of inappropriately slow heart rates or experience symptomatic pauses in rhythm, provoking significant activity limitations, dizziness, or syncope.

In some cases, inappropriately slow generation of P waves may combine with atrial tachyarrhythmias (such as paroxysmal atrial fibrillation) to create brady-tachy syndrome, also known as sick sinus syndrome. In such patients paroxysms of rapid supraventricular tachycardia may be separated by interludes of excessively slow atrial rates or pauses in sinus rhythm. Permanent pacing is frequently required to allow for pharmacologic control of rapid supraventricular rhythms. Pacing provides a suitable lower heart rate that might otherwise be dangerously suppressed by such rate- or rhythm-controlling agents.

In the acute setting, treatment can include atropine, dopamine, epinephrine and/or temporary pacing for an inappropriately slow heart rate due to impaired automaticity in any of its forms. Attention should be directed to potential causes, such as use of drugs with sinus-slowing properties (e.g., calcium channel blockers, beta-blockers, digoxin, antiarrhythmic agents) or metabolic conditions such as hypothyroidism. Acute hypoxia can also provoke slowing or pauses in heart rate.

Disorders of Impulse Conduction

Disorders of impulse conduction are defined as the failure of a generated impulse to reach its ventricular destination successfully or in timely fashion.[1] Typically, these are broken down into disorders that result in slowing of conduction between the atria and ventricles or within the ventricles (first-degree AV block and intraventricular delay or block, respectively); disorders in which most but not all atrial impulses are conducted to the ventricles (second-degree AV block at the nodal level, and second-degree AV block at the infranodal level); and disorders in which only occasional atrial impulses are conducted to the ventricles (advanced AV block) and in which no impulses are conducted to the ventricles (third-degree or complete AV block).

First-Degree AV Block and Intraventricular Conduction Block

First-degree AV block is defined as prolongation of the PR interval (the onset of the surface P wave to the onset of the QRS complex) to >0.20 second (Fig. 23-2A). The most common location of such slowing is in the AV node. The less common cause is due to slowing of conduction in the bundle of His. Similarly, a slowing or partial block of conduction in the His–Purkinje system (as exemplified by bundle-branch

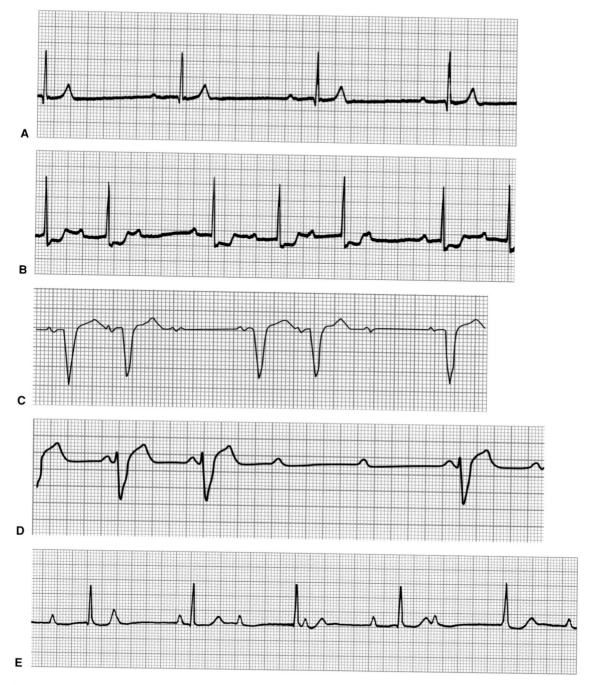

FIGURE 23-2 • Types of AV block. **A.** First-degree AV block, manifested by a prolonged PR interval (>0.20 second). **B.** Mobitz type I (Wenckebach) second-degree AV block, characterized by occasional blocked P waves preceded by successive prolongation of the PR interval. **C.** Mobitz II type second-degree AV block, characterized by occasionally blocked P waves without changes in the PR interval preceding or following block. **D.** Advanced AV block in which two or more P waves fail to conduct to the ventricle. **E.** Third-degree (complete) AV block with complete failure of atrial impulses to conduct to the ventricles. In this instance a subsidiary junctional escape rhythm maintains the ventricular rhythm.

block) results in a lengthening of the time required to completely depolarize the ventricles. This is because conduction via the His–Purkinje system is much faster than conduction of an electrical impulse from muscle to muscle. When a portion of the His–Purkinje system fails to conduct (as in bundle-branch block) or conducts too slowly, the portion of the heart to which it extends is excited instead by muscle-to-muscle conduction. This results in longer time required to completely depolarize the ventricles and is expressed in a prolonged (wider) QRS. This is sometimes called aberrant conduction or intraventricular conduction delay, or it may be described by the characteristic appearance of a right or left bundle-branch block. First degree AV block and intraventricular conduction block can occur independently of one another, or together. Each represents conduction that though slowed, is still ongoing through the AV node, and His-Purkinje system, respectively.

First-degree AV block and intraventricular conduction block do not require treatment. However, their presence can confound rhythm diagnosis, as, for example, when supraventricular tachycardia occurs along with a bundle-branch block, resulting in wide-complex tachycardia, or when the P wave blends into the preceding T wave of a sinus tachycardia, resulting in what appears to be a supraventricular tachycardia without apparent P waves.

Second- and Third-Degree AV Block

Second-degree AV block is divided into two forms, depending upon where the block occurs, either in the AV node or in the bundle of His (infranodal). Intermittent block in the AV node is referred to as Mobitz type I (or Wenckebach-type) second-degree AV block. It is characterized by successive prolongation of the PR interval prior to a P wave that fails to conduct to the ventricle, which results in a pause. This is followed by a shorter PR interval associated with the next conducted P wave, after which the process repeats itself (Fig. 23-2B).

In contrast, Mobitz type II (or infranodal) second-degree AV block is not heralded by PR prolongation before a P wave fails to conduct to the ventricle. This form of block is characteristic of the "all or nothing" conduction properties of the His–Purkinje system, suggesting the block's anatomic location in the conduction system distal (ventricular) side of the AV node (Fig. 23-2C). Whereas Mobitz type I (Wenckebach-type) AV block is frequently benign and often attributable to transient effects of increased parasympathetic tone upon the AV node, Mobitz type II block is always regarded as pathologic and indicative of the need for a permanent pacemaker.

Advanced AV block is a more serious form of second-degree AV block in which multiple (two or more) successive P waves fail to conduct to the ventricle, although occasional P waves may still conduct (Fig. 23-2D). It indicates a more advanced stage of deranged conduction that is leading to complete AV block. Advanced AV block can occur at the level of the AV node, or be infranodal.

Third-degree (or complete) AV block is the complete failure of atrial impulses to conduct to the ventricles (Fig. 23-2E). Such block can occur in the AV node and in or distal to the bundle of His infranodal. Subsidiary pacemaker activity is what maintains a cardiac rhythm in such circumstances, the absence of which would be lethal.

In general, unless they are attributable to an identifiable and reversible cause—such as excessive effects from calcium channel blockers, beta-blockers, antiarrhythmic drugs, or severe hyperkalemia—acquired Mobitz type II

second-degree AV block advanced AV block, and complete AV block (with or without symptoms) usually require permanent pacing. In contrast, Mobitz type 1 second-degree AV block does not usually require pacing, unless it provokes serious symptoms in the absence of a readily reversible cause. The need for temporary pacing in all such patients is determined by their hemodynamic stability and the effectiveness of their escape rhythm.

Evaluation and Treatment of Bradycardia

The bradycardia algorithm (Fig. 23-3) provides an overview of the evaluation and treatment of a bradycardia. Box numbers in the text refer to the numbered boxes in the algorithm.

Evaluation

Bradycardia is conventionally defined as a heart rate of <60 bpm (Fig. 23-3, Box 1). A slow heart rate may be physiologically normal for some patients and not require treatment. Conversely, while it is highly unlikely that a heart rate in the normal range would itself cause hemodynamic compromise, a normal resting heart rate might be inadequate for some clinical situations (such as sepsis or with significant volume depletion), and heart rates >60 bpm may be inadequate for others. The bradycardia algorithm focuses on the management of clinically significant bradycardia (that is, a heart rate that is inadequate under the clinical circumstances).

Initial Patient Stabilization

As with all potential life-threatening arrhythmias, initial management of any patient with bradycardia should focus on the support of airway and breathing in addition to their circulatory status, as necessary given the frequent association of bradycardia with hypoxia (Fig. 23-3). This includes provision of supplementary oxygen, initiation of cardiac rhythm monitoring, measurement of blood pressure and oxyhemoglobin saturation, and initiation of intravenous (IV) access for pharmacologic support of heart rate and blood pressure, if required. If the patient is stable, a 12-lead ECG should be performed to document and better define the cardiac rhythm. The ECG may also identify a potential cause for the arrhythmia, such as acute ischemia or signs suggestive of an electrolyte derangement.

Assessment of Serious Signs and Symptoms

Signs and symptoms of poor perfusion are assessed for whether they are causally related to the bradycardia (Fig. 23-3, Box 3). Signs and symptoms of bradycardia may be

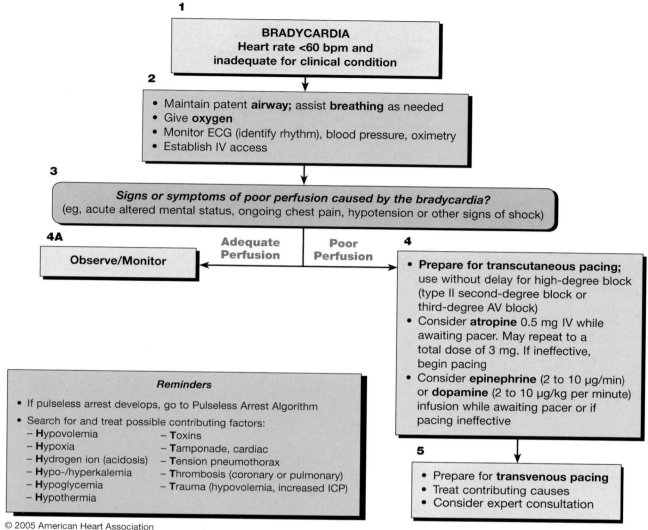

1

BRADYCARDIA
Heart rate <60 bpm and
inadequate for clinical condition

2

- Maintain patent **airway**; assist **breathing** as needed
- Give **oxygen**
- Monitor ECG (identify rhythm), blood pressure, oximetry
- Establish IV access

3

Signs or symptoms of poor perfusion caused by the bradycardia?
(eg, acute altered mental status, ongoing chest pain, hypotension or other signs of shock)

4A

Observe/Monitor

Adequate Perfusion   **Poor Perfusion**

4

- **Prepare for transcutaneous pacing;** use without delay for high-degree block (type II second-degree block or third-degree AV block)
- Consider **atropine** 0.5 mg IV while awaiting pacer. May repeat to a total dose of 3 mg. If ineffective, begin pacing
- Consider **epinephrine** (2 to 10 µg/min) or **dopamine** (2 to 10 µg/kg per minute) infusion while awaiting pacer or if pacing ineffective

Reminders

- If pulseless arrest develops, go to Pulseless Arrest Algorithm
- Search for and treat possible contributing factors:
  - **H**ypovolemia
  - **H**ypoxia
  - **H**ydrogen ion (acidosis)
  - **H**ypo-/hyperkalemia
  - **H**ypoglycemia
  - **H**ypothermia
  - **T**oxins
  - **T**amponade, cardiac
  - **T**ension pneumothorax
  - **T**hrombosis (coronary or pulmonary)
  - **T**rauma (hypovolemia, increased ICP)

5

- Prepare for **transvenous pacing**
- Treat contributing causes
- Consider expert consultation

© 2005 American Heart Association

| FIGURE 23-3 • The bradycardia algorithm.

mild; asymptomatic patients should be monitored expectantly for signs of deterioration (Box 4A) even if they do not require immediate treatment. Provide immediate therapy for patients with hypotension, acute altered mental status, chest pain, congestive heart failure, syncope, or other signs of shock related to the bradycardia (Box 4).

Classification of AV Block and Possible Cause

In appropriate evaluation of the patient with bradycardia includes a general focused assessment of their vital status and the identification of any comorbidities or potential reversible causes (e.g., ischemia, electrolyte abnormalities, or drugs). AV blocks are classified as first-, second-, and third-degree, as described in detail in the preceding section. They may be caused by medications or electrolyte disturbances as well as by structural problems resulting from acute myocardial infarction or ischemia.

Therapy

Once a symptomatic bradycardia is identified, preparations are made for transcutaneous pacing and/or for pharmacologic interventions, whichever is most expedient and appropriate for the circumstances (Fig. 23-3, Box 4). For severely symptomatic patients, especially when the block is at or below the His-Purkinje level or when an escape rhythm is inadequate, these measures should be seen as temporizing. Expert consultation should be quickly sought for placement of a temporary transvenous pacemaker (see Chapter 24 for further discussion of pacing therapies).

Atropine

In the absence of reversible causes, atropine remains the first-line drug for acute symptomatic bradycardia.[2] Atropine works by reversing cholinergic-mediated decreases in heart rate and thereby blocks the effects of vagal nerve discharges on the sinus and AV nodes. It is useful in treating symptomatic sinus bradycardia and AV block at the nodal level.[4] In one randomized clinical trial in adults[2] and additional lower-level studies,[3,4] IV atropine improved heart rate and signs and symptoms associated with bradycardia. If the bradycardic event was acutely mediated by enhanced vagal tone, treatment with atropine may be sufficient to reverse the condition. Transcutaneous pacing is usually indicated if the patient fails to respond to atropine, although second-line drug therapy with drugs such as dopamine or epinephrine may be successful (see below).

Atropine is not indicated in the treatment of bradycardia from infranodal AV block (Morbitz type II second-degree AV block and advanced or third-degree block with wide QRS ventricular escape complexes). Theoretically, atropine may increase the rate of sinus node discharge and accelerate AV conduction, thus worsening the degree of AV block in such circumstances.

Atropine Dosing The recommended atropine dose for asystole and slow pulseless electrical activity is 1 mg IV, repeated in 3 to 5 minutes if the arrhythmias persist. For bradycardia, the dose is 0.5 mg IV every 3 to 5 minutes to a total dose of 3 mg (0.04 mg/kg). A total dose of 3 mg (0.04 mg/kg) results in full vagal blockade in humans and is the maximal total dose recommended by current ACLS guidelines. Doses of atropine sulfate of <0.5 mg may be parasympathomimetic and paradoxically result in further slowing of the heart rate.[6,9] Atropine can be administered intravenously or by intraosseous means and is also well absorbed through the tracheal route of administration. Its administration should not delay implementation of external pacing for patients with poor perfusion.

Atropine Use in Acute Coronary Syndromes Atropine should be used cautiously in the presence of ACS or infarction because excessive increases in heart rate may worsen ischemia or increase the zone of infarction. In rare cases, ventricular fibrillation (VF) and ventricular tachycardia (VT) have followed IV administration of atropine.

Atropine Use Following Cardiac Transplantation The use of atropine in the cardiac transplant patient should be avoided. It will likely be ineffective because the transplanted heart lacks vagal innervation. Paradoxical responses to atropine have also been reported after heart transplantation, including paradoxical slowing of heart rate and development of high-degree AV block, the mechanism of which is unclear.[7,11] Notably, transplanted hearts have increased sensitivity to sympathetic stimulation; therefore, sympathomimetic drugs, as an alternative to atropine, should be used cautiously in such patients.[10]

Pacing

Use of atropine is discouraged in type II second- or third-degree AV block or in patients with third-degree AV block with a new wide-QRS complex (which implies that the location of the block lies in or below the bundle of His in the distal conduction system). These patients require immediate pacing if serious symptoms or hemodynamic instability is present. Even if such patients are hemodynamically stable, one should prepare them for pacing, as clinical deterioration can occur suddenly and unexpectedly.

Transcutaneous pacing is a class I intervention for life-threatening bradycardias. It should be started immediately for patients who are hemodynamically unstable, particularly those with high-degree (second-degree Mobitz type II, advanced, or third-degree infranodal) block.

Transcutaneous pacing is noninvasive and can be performed by ECC providers at the bedside. Initiate transcutaneous pacing immediately if there is no response to atropine, if atropine is unlikely to be effective, or if the patient is severely symptomatic. Verify mechanical capture by pulse or arterial pressure waveform (if such monitoring has been established). Some limitations apply. Transcutaneous pacing is painful, and it may be challenging to confirm effective mechanical capture (see Chapter 24). It is important to verify mechanical capture and reasses the patient's condition after transcutaneous pacing has been established. Use analgesia and sedation for pain control, and continue efforts to identify the cause of the bradyarrhythmia.

If transcutaneous pacing is ineffective (e.g., inconsistent capture), prepare for emergent transvenous pacing and consider obtaining expert consultation. Even if effective, transcutaneous pacing should be regarded as only a temporizing measure, and expert consultation should be expeditiously obtained regarding placement of a transvenous pacemaker.

Alternative Drugs to Consider

Other drugs may be considered when the bradycardia is unresponsive to atropine or for which atropine may be contraindicated and as temporizing measures while awaiting the availability of a pacemaker or if transcutaneous pacing is ineffective. Epinephrine and dopamine are alternative drugs to consider. They are widely available and familiar to clinicians (Fig. 23-3, Box 4).

Epinephrine (2–10 μg/min) If the patient has severe symptoms (e.g., severe bradycardia with hypotension), the drug of choice is a catecholamine infusion (either epinephrine or dopamine). An epinephrine infusion of 2 to 10 μg/min is titrated on the basis of heart rate, blood pressure, and systemic perfusion. Epinephrine infusion is also appropriate if the patient has symptomatic bradycardia unresponsive to dopamine.

Dopamine (2–10 μg/kg/min) Although dopamine can be administered at doses of 2 to 20 μg/kg/min or higher, the vasoconstrictive effects of the drug tend to predominate over its chronotropic properties when doses exceed 10 μg/kg/min. Dopamine may be administered in doses of 2 to 10 μg/kg/min and titrated to desired hemodynamic targets. Conversely, this agent may cause splanchnic vasodilation and relative hypovolemia owing to intravascular volume shifts when given in low doses. For this reason it is necessary to assess intravascular volume and provide fluid support, if necessary, whenever you give dopamine in low doses.

Glucagon   One case series[12] documented improvement in heart rate as well as symptoms and signs associated with bradycardia when IV glucagon (3 mg initially, followed by infusion at 3 mg/hr if necessary) was given to in-hospital patients with drug-induced (e.g., beta-blocker or calcium channel blocker overdose) symptomatic bradycardia not responding to atropine.

Isoproterenol No Longer Recommended   Isoproterenol can increase infarct size and cause life-threatening ventricular arrhythmias, so it requires careful titration. It is no longer included or recommended in the bradycardia algorithm. Isoproterenol is contraindicated in acetylcholinesterase-induced bradycardias, although it may be useful at high doses in refractory bradycardia induced by beta-antagonist receptor blockade.

Aminophylline Not Recommended   Aminophylline, used commonly in patients with bronchospastic disorders, is a competitive antagonist of adenosine. Its use for bradycardia and heart block has been described in several anecdotal reports and small series.[13–15] However, in a recent prospective randomized trial, it demonstrated no evidence of improved return of spontaneous circulation (ROSC) after bradyasystolic cardiac arrest in patients who were unresponsive to epinephrine and atropine.[16]

Bradycardias—Refining the Diagnosis and Treatment

Sinus Bradycardia

Sinus bradycardia (Figs. 23-4 and 23-5) is a slow heart rate with regular P waves, each followed at a consistent interval by a QRS complex. The rhythm is defined by the sinus node being the site of origin for this rhythm, and the heart rate being <60 bpm. Sinus bradycardia is often a symptom of other conditions (e.g., good physical conditioning, vagal tone, or drug effects) rather than a primary arrhythmia that requires treatment. In ACS, it commonly is seen in inferior myocardial infarction (MI).

Pathophysiology

- Sinus bradycardia is caused by a slow rate of spontaneous impulses originating at the sinoatrial node.
- Sinus bradycardia is typically a physical sign of other problems rather than a primary arrhythmia.

Defining ECG Criteria

The key defining criteria of sinus bradycardia on the ECG are regular P waves followed by regular QRS complexes at a rate <60 bpm (Fig. 23-4).

- **Rate:** <60 bpm.
- **Rhythm:** Regular sinus.
- **PR interval:** Regular; may be normal (0.12–0.20 seconds) or prolonged depending upon the concomitant presence of first degree block.
- **P waves:** Configuration (positive and negative deflections) on 12-lead ECG (or in multiple leads) of P waves is consistent with sinus node origin (that is, P wave deflections are positive in leads I, II and a VF); every P wave is followed by a QRS complex; every QRS complex is preceded by a P wave.
- **QRS complex:** Normal or wide (if there is an intraventricular conduction defect).

Clinical Manifestations

- Most people with sinus bradycardia are asymptomatic at rest.
- With increased activity, if the heart rate remains slow or does not rise sufficiently with exertion, a patient may become symptomatic. This is referred to as chronotropic incompetence.
- Common symptoms include fatigue, shortness of breath, dizziness or light-headedness, and frank syncope. Common physical signs include hypotension, diaphoresis, pulmonary congestion, and frank pulmonary edema.
- Apart from its rate, the ECG may otherwise be normal or may independently display acute ST-segment or T-wave deviations or ventricular arrhythmias if there are other underlying conditions. The QT interval normally lengthens as heart rate decreases.

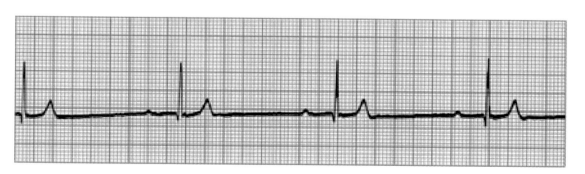

FIGURE 23-4 • Sinus bradycardia with first-degree AV block. Sinus rate is approximately 30 bpm and rhythm is regular. No escape rhythm has emerged.

Common Etiologies

- Sinus bradycardia is often appropriate ("normal") for well-conditioned people. With age, resting heart rate also declines. It is not uncommon to observe significant sinus bradycardia during nighttime telemetry monitoring of patients.
- Sinus bradycardia can occur after an event that stimulates the vasovagal reflex or increases vagal tone, such as vomiting, a Valsalva maneuver, rectal stimuli, or inadvertent pressure on the carotid sinus in the elderly ("shaver's syncope").
- In most patients the blood supply of the sinoatrial node comes from the right coronary artery. For this reason ACS related to the right coronary artery can produce sinus node ischemia and sinus bradycardia.
- Sinus bradycardia can occur as a pharmacologic or adverse clinical drug effect of a number of agents, including beta-blockers, calcium channel blockers, digoxin, quinidine, amiodarone, and other agents that prolong the refractory period of the sinus node.
- Hypoxia can provoke sinus bradycardia. This may be mediated by adenosine, an endogenous metabolite, which is released in increased amounts in response to imbalances in oxygen supply and demand.

Recommended Therapy

- Sinus bradycardia rarely produces rate-related, serious signs and symptoms that merit emergent treatment unless associated with significant comorbidity (e.g., inferior ST-segment elevation myocardial infarction [STEMI]) or ischemia.
- When hemodynamically significant sinus bradycardia does occur, follow the intervention sequence listed in the bradycardia algorithm.
- Try to determine the cause and treat it. Also treat any significant complicating factors (e.g., hypoxia).

Atrioventricular Block

AV block is a delay or interruption in conduction between the atria and ventricles. Such a delay can occur at many levels in the conduction system and may occur insidiously or abruptly. To effectively anticipate progression in AV block, providers need to understand the conduction system, external influences on conduction tissue, and comorbidities that may precipitate high-degree AV block.

Common Etiologies

AV block may be caused by

- Pathological lesions along the conduction pathway (e.g., calcium, fibrosis, necrosis).
- Enhanced vagal stimulation (inferior MI, carotid sinus sensitivity or massage).
- Increases in the refractory period of the conduction pathway (drugs).

- Extrinsic factors, such as hypoxia. This may be mediated by adenosine, an endogenous metabolite, which is released in increased amounts in response to imbalances in oxygen supply and demand.
- Physiologic block due to rapid atrial rates. This is a "protective" rather than pathologic mechanism that prevents the achievement of rapid ventricular rates during arrhythmias such as atrial flutter or fibrillation. The mechanism for this effect is as follows. As the atrial rate becomes more rapid (as with rapid atrial flutter), it encroaches on the refractory period of the AV node. As a result, some impulses will conduct through the AV node more slowly and others not at all. In this manner, electrical impulses are "blocked" from progressing to the ventricle. The AV node may, for example, allow conduction at 150 bpm but not at 300 bpm. This is why the typical conduction pattern for atrial flutter (at an atrial rate of 300 bpm) becomes a 2:1 AV block (with a resulting ventricular rate of 150 bpm). This "protects" the ventricle from excessive rates during supraventricular tachycardias. As compared with this type of physiologic AV block, pathologic heart block occurs when impulses at a normal physiologic rate fail to be appropriately conducted to the ventricle.

Classification of AV Block

AV block may be classified according to the *site* or *degree* of block. The AV node is anatomically a complicated network of fibers—not a discrete structure—located inferiorly in the right atrium, anterior to the ostium of the coronary sinus and above the tricuspid valve. The speed of conduction is normally slowed through the AV node, and the upper limit of normal of the PR interval is 0.20 second. These fibers converge at their lower margin to form a discrete bundle of fibers, the *bundle of His* (or *AV bundle*). This structure penetrates the annulus fibrosus and arrives at the upper margin of the muscular intraventricular septum. Here the infranodal structure of the conduction system gives origin to the bundle branches (Fig. 23-6).

Site of Block

- AV node (sometimes also called "Supra-Hisian" indicating block above the level of the His bundle)
- Infranodal (below the AV node), occurring anatomically at or below the bundle of His (sometimes also called "infraHisian")

Degree of Block

- First-degree AV block
- Second-degree AV block (either type I or type II) including advanced block
- Third-degree or complete AV block

The three degrees of block, along with the character of the QRS complex (wide or narrow), can generally be used to infer the sites of block: within the AV node, or below the AV node (infranodal). The site of block is important because the pathogenesis, treatment, escape rate, and prognosis vary with each site. There are exceptions to this classification, but the

Sinus Bradycardia	
Pathophysiology	• Impulses originate at SA node at a slow rate • Not necessarily pathological or abnormal unless symptomatic
Defining Criteria per ECG **Key:** Regular P waves followed by regular QRS complexes at rate <60 beats/min **Note:** Often a physical sign rather than an abnormal rhythm	• **Rate:** <60 bpm • **Rhythm:** regular sinus • **PR:** regular; may be normal (0.12–0.20 seconds) or prolonged depending upon the concomitant presence of first degree block • **P waves:** configuration (size and shape) on 12-lead ECG (or in multiple leads) is consistent with sinus node origin; every P wave is followed by a QRS complex; every QRS complex is preceded by a P wave. • **QRS complex:** may be narrow or wide
Clinical Manifestations	• At rest, usually asymptomatic • With increased activity, persistent slow rate will lead to symptoms of easy fatigue, SOB, dizziness or lightheadedness, syncope, hypotension
Common Etiologies	• Normal for well-conditioned people • A vasovagal event such as vomiting, Valsalva, rectal stimuli, inadvertent pressure on carotid sinus ("shaver's syncope") • Acute MIs that affect circulation to SA node (right coronary artery); most often inferior MI • Adverse drug effects, e.g., blocking agents (beta or calcium channel), digoxin, quinidine
Recommended Therapy	• Treatment rarely indicated • Treat only if patient has significant signs or symptoms due to the bradycardia • Oxygen (if symptomatic) **Intervention sequence for bradycardia** • Atropine 0.5 mg IV if vagal mechanism • Transcutaneous pacing in readiness for hemodynamic instability **If signs and symptoms are severe, consider catecholamine infusions:** • Dopamine 2 to 10 µg/kg per min • Epinephrine 2 to 10 µg/min

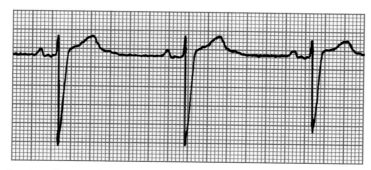

Sinus bradycardia: rate of 45 bpm; with borderline first-degree AV block (PR ≈ 0.20 sec)

| FIGURE 23-5 • Sinus bradycardia.

PART FIVE • ARRHYTHMIAS

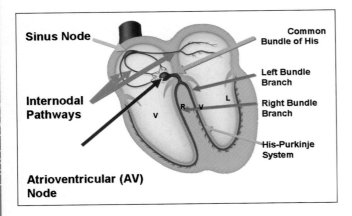

FIGURE 23-6 • Relationship of the AV node to the anatomy of the conduction system. Although often portrayed as a "discrete structure," the AV node is a complicated network of fibers with different electrophysiologic properties.

details involve complicated electrophysiology. Table 23-1 presents the major general ECG features of first-, second-, and third-degree AV block.

First-Degree AV Block

First-degree AV block (Figs. 23-7 and 23-8) is a *delay* in passage of the depolarization impulse from atria to ventri-

cles. This delay manifests as prolongation of the PR interval. The specific site of block can be anywhere from the AV node to at or below the bundle of His, although typically it occurs in the AV node (Fig. 23-6).

Pathophysiology
- In first-degree AV block, conduction of the sinus impulse is slowed at the AV node resulting in a delay between the onset of the atrial P wave and the onset of the ventricular QRS.
- First-degree AV block can be a normal physiologic variant without a specific pathophysiology.
- In some clinical circumstances, first-degree AV block is caused by an extracardiac condition (e.g., excess vagal tone, drug toxicity).

Defining ECG Criteria (Fig. 23-7)
The key defining criterion on the ECG is a PR interval >0.20 second.

- **Rate:** First-degree AV block can be seen with both sinus bradycardia and sinus tachycardia.
- **Rhythm:** Sinus, regular; both atria and ventricles.
- **PR interval:** Prolonged (>0.20 second) but typically does not vary (is relatively *fixed* from beat-to-beat).
- **P waves:** Configuration (size and shape) on 12-lead ECG (or in multiple leads) consistent with sinus node origin; every P wave is followed by a QRS complex; every QRS complex is preceded by a P wave.

| TABLE 23-1 • Major ECG Features of First-, Second-, and Third-Degree AV Block

EGC Feature	First-Degree	Second-Degree	Third-Degree
Rate Atrial Ventricular	Unaffected Same as atrial rate	Unaffected Slower than atrial rate	Unaffected Slower than atrial rate
Ventricular Rhythm	Same as atrial rhythm or regular	Type I: Irregular (may be regularly irregular in a repetitive pattern) Type II: Regular or irregular	Ventricular escape beats are usually regular
P-QRS Relationship	Consistent: 1:1	Type I: Variable PR intervals before the dropped QRS complex Type II: Fixed PR intervals before the dropped QRS complex	Absent (AV dissociation)
QRS Duration	Unaffected	Type I: Narrow Type II: Most often wide; rarely narrow	Wide or narrow, depending on site of escape rhythm
Site of Block	Anywhere from AV node to the Bundle of His, though typically in AV node	Type I: Typically in the node Type II: Typically in or below the bundle of His	Anywhere from AV node to the Bundle of His; or bilateral bundle branch block

Source: Cummins RO. *ACLS: Principles and Practice.* Dallas: American Heart Association, 2003, with permission.

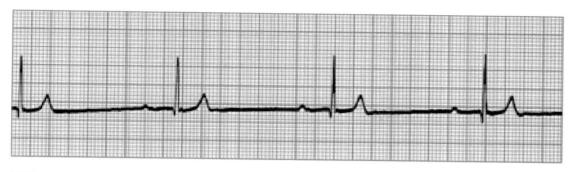

FIGURE 23-7 • First-degree AV block. The PR interval is prolonged to about 0.34 second. Also present is sinus bradycardia.

- **QRS complex:** Normal or wide (if there is an intraventricular conduction defect).

Clinical Manifestations
- The patient with first-degree AV block is usually asymptomatic.

Common Etiologies
- Many first-degree AV blocks are due to the adverse effects of drugs, most commonly drugs known to block conduction through the AV node: beta-blockers, calcium channel blockers, and digoxin. It can also be a manifestation of pathology in the conduction system associated with aging and other disease states.
- First-degree AV block can occur after an event that stimulates vagal activity, such as vomiting, a Valsalva maneuver, rectal stimuli, or inadvertent pressure on the carotid sinus (shaver's syncope).
- Acute coronary syndromes involving the right coronary artery will often affect circulation to the AV node, creating AV nodal ischemia and slowing AV nodal conduction.

Recommended Therapy
- Treatment of first-degree AV block is almost never necessary or indicated because few patients have significant signs or symptoms related to the first-degree AV block. If symptoms or signs are present always search for and consider an alternate cause.
- When a patient develops new-onset first-degree AV block, be alert for progression of the block to second-degree AV block, either type I or type II, and consider an aggravating cause (Fig. 23-8).

Second-Degree AV Block (Mobitz 1 or Wenckebach)

In second-degree AV block, some atrial impulses are conducted through the AV node and others are blocked—that is, "not every P wave is followed by a QRS complex."[17–19] Second-degree AV block is divided into two types:

- *Type I second-degree AV block* (also referred to as AV nodal, *Mobitz I* or *Wenckebach*)
- *Type II second-degree AV block* (also referred to as *infranodal, Mobitz II,* or *non-Wenckebach*)

Type I second-degree AV block almost always occurs at the level of the AV node and is characterized by a progressive prolongation of the PR interval. Conduction velocity slows through the AV node until an impulse is completely blocked. Usually only a single impulse is blocked, and the pattern is then repeated. The sequence of the block can be described by the ratio of the P waves to the QRS complexes (e.g., 2:1 means every other P wave is not followed by a QRS complex; 3:2 means that every third P wave is not followed by a QRS complex). Notably, distinguishing the pattern of type I second-degree block from type II on the ECG is not possible when only alternate P waves conduct to the ventricle (2:1 AV block). Identifying the typical Wenckebach pattern of type I AV block requires at least two consecutively conducted P waves.

Pathophysiology
- Type I second-degree AV block (Mobitz I or Wenckebach) almost always occurs at the level of the AV node). The AV-node cells demonstrate a characteristic gradual and progressive conduction delay in response to a depolarization stimulus, the hallmark of which is a lengthening PR interval before a blocked P wave, followed by a shorter PR interval after the subsequently conducted P wave.
- Type I second-degree AV block is more often caused by increased parasympathetic tone than by ischemia. Because type I block occurs in the AV node, with a reasonable junctional escape rhythm, this form of second-degree block is not as ominous clinically as type II second-degree block (see below). It uncommonly progresses to a high-degree AV block with slow escape rhythm. However, if symptomatic, type I second-degree AV block requires treatment regardless of whether it represents a more "benign" form of AV block by its mechanism and location.
- An increase in parasympathetic tone can cause impulse conduction through the AV node to become slower. This

First-Degree AV Block	
Pathophysiology	• Impulse conduction is slowed at the AV node resulting in a delay between the onset of the atrial P wave and the onset of the ventricular QRS. • Does not in itself usually affect heart rate, but may be precipitated by some of the same causes as bradycardia, and thus the two can appear together.
Defining Criteria per ECG **Key:** PR interval >0.20 sec	• **Rate:** First-degree AV block can be seen with both sinus bradycardia and sinus tachycardia • **Rhythm:** sinus, regular, both atria and ventricles • **PR:** prolonged, >0.20 sec, but does not vary (is relatively fixed from beat-to-beat) • **P waves:** size and shape normal; every P wave is followed by a QRS complex; every QRS complex is preceded by a P wave • **QRS complex:** may be narrow or wide
Clinical Manifestations	• Usually asymptomatic at rest
Common Etiologies	• Large majority of first-degree AV blocks are due to drugs, usually the AV nodal blockers: beta-blockers, calcium channel blockers, and digoxin • Any condition that stimulates the parasympathetic nervous system (e.g., vasovagal reflex) • Acute MIs that affect circulation to AV node (right coronary artery); most often inferior MIs
Recommended Therapy	• Treat only when patient has significant signs or symptoms that are due to an associated bradycardia • Be alert to advancement to second-degree, type I or type II block

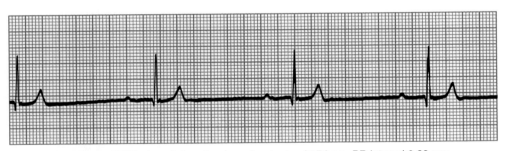

First-degree AV block and sinus bradycardia at rate of 37 bpm; PR interval 0.28 sec

| FIGURE 23-8 • First-degree AV block (in this instance accompanied by sinus bradycardia).

slowed conduction causes the PR interval to increase until one depolarization impulse from the atria is completely blocked before it can depolarize the ventricle ("dropped" QRS complex or "dropped beat").
• This pattern is repeated, resulting in "group beating" (e.g., a few conducted sinus depolarizations with progressive lengthening in their PR intervals followed by a sinus depolarization that is not followed by a QRS complex). Such a "group" is referred to as *4:3 conduction*.
• The conduction ratio (number of Ps to number of QRSs) can change (e.g., 4:3, 3:2, 2:1), or remain constant.

• Type I second-degree AV block is usually transient. The prognosis is generally good and does not usually require pacing, unlike some other forms of AV block.

Defining ECG Criteria (Figs. 23-9 and 23-10) The key defining criterion on the ECG is progressive lengthening of the PR interval until one P wave is not followed by a QRS complex. This represents the nonconducted or "dropped" depolarization impulse or "dropped beat (QRS complex)."

• **Rate:** The atrial rate is unaffected. But the overall atrial rate averaged over a number of complexes is usually faster than the average ventricular rate because some atrial depolarization impulses are not conducted to the ventricles ["blocked complexes" or "dropped beats (QRS complex)"].

- **Rhythm:** The atrial rhythm is usually regular. The ventricular rhythm is usually regularly irregular except in the presence of 2:1 AV block or a changing conduction sequence.
- **PR interval:** The PR interval progressively lengthens from cycle to cycle; then one P wave is not followed by a QRS complex (the blocked P wave or "dropped" QRS complex). The longer PR interval of the conducted beat before a blocked P wave is followed by a shorter PR interval on the subsequently conducted beat. There is also a characteristic progressive shortening of the RR interval before the blocked impulse. The RR interval that brackets the nonconducted P wave is usually less than twice the normal cycle length.
- **P waves:** Configuration (size and shape) on 12-lead ECG (or in multiple leads) of P waves is consistent with sinus node origin; occasionally a P wave is not followed by a QRS complex (the blocked impulse or "dropped" QRS complex).
- **QRS complex:** The QRS complex is usually *narrow*, but a QRS "drops out" periodically (i.e., a QRS complex does not follow every P wave). When the block occurs at the level of the AV node, the QRS complex is typically narrow because distal conduction is unaffected. This is in contrast to Mobitz II AV block, where the distal conduction block creating the Mobitz II pattern is accompanied by other evidence of a distal conduction abnormality, reflected in a wider QRS complex (Fig. 23-9).

Clinical Manifestations In type I second-degree AV block, the symptoms and signs are related to the severity of the bradycardia.

- **Symptoms:** With exertion patients may experience chest discomfort, shortness of breath, and decreased level of consciousness.
- **Signs:** Occasionally the bradycardia is slow enough to produce hypotension, shock, pulmonary congestion, congestive heart failure, and angina.

Common Etiologies

- The most frequent causes of type I second-degree AV block are drugs that slow conduction through the AV node: beta-blockers, calcium channel blockers, and digoxin.
- The second most common cause of type I second-degree AV block is any condition that stimulates the parasympathetic system, increasing parasympathetic tone. Such conditions include any event that stimulates the vasovagal reflex, such as vomiting, a Valsalva maneuver, or rectal stimuli.
- Circulation to the AV node comes from the right coronary artery in most patients. For this reason acute coronary syndromes that affect the *right* coronary artery (or a dominant left circumflex coronary artery) can produce type I second-degree AV nodal block.

Recommended Therapy Specific treatment is rarely needed unless severe signs and symptoms are present. Clinicians should remain comfortable with *watchful waiting* and avoid unnecessary administration of atropine simply to treat the observed block.

- Place a high priority on identifying the underlying cause.
- If the bradycardia resulting from the nonconducted P wave leads to serious signs and symptoms, initiate the bradycardia algorithm intervention sequence.
- If a vagal mechanism appears to be the cause of the type I block, administer a atropine 0.5 mg IV. Further treatment is rarely necessary (see the bradycardia algorithm for additional therapies).

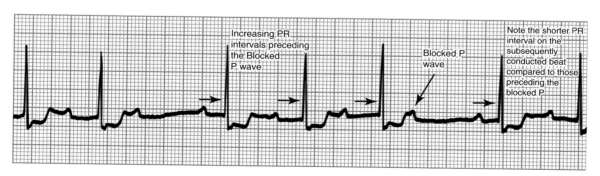

FIGURE 23-9 • Type I second-degree AV block. Atrial rhythm is nearly regular, but there are pauses in ventricular rhythm because the depolarization impulse associated with every fourth P wave does not conduct into the ventricles. Note progressive prolongation of the PR interval, indicating increasing conduction delay in the AV node before the nonconducted impulse (blocked P wave or "dropped" QRS complex) and the shorter PR interval on the subsequently conducted beat. In the center of the strip there are four P waves and three QRS complexes, representing a 4:3 cycle. Note the slight shortening of the RR intervals before the blocked P wave in the middle of the tracing. Note also that the subsequent RR interval that brackets the nonconducted and subsequently conducted P waves is less than twice the cycle length of the conducted QRS complexes. The QRS complexes are normal (narrow) and as such do not indicate the presence of distal conduction system disease, supporting the likely location of block in this instance at the AV node.

Second-Degree AV Block Type I (Mobitz I–Wenckebach)

Pathophysiology	• Site of pathology: AV node • AV node blood supply comes from branches of the right coronary artery • Impulse conduction is increasingly slowed at the AV node (causing a progressive increase in the PR interval before a P wave is blocked ("dropped" QRS)). • The PR interval shortens on the subsequent conducted beat that follows a blocked P wave (or dropped QRS).
Defining Criteria per ECG **Key:** There is progressive lengthening of the PR interval until one P wave is not followed by a QRS complex (the dropped beat)	• **Rate:** atrial rate just slightly faster than ventricular (because of dropped beats); usually normal range • **Rhythm:** regular for atrial beats; irregular for ventricular (because of dropped beats); can show regular P waves marching through irregular QRS • **PR:** progressive lengthening of the PR interval occurs from cycle to cycle; then one P wave is not followed by a QRS complex (blocked P wave or "dropped" QRS) • **P waves:** size and shape remain normal; occasional P wave not followed by a QRS complex (the "dropped beat") • **QRS complex:** ≤0.10 sec most often, but a QRS "drops out" periodically
Clinical Manifestations— Rate-Related	**Due to bradycardia:** • **Symptoms:** chest pain, shortness of breath, decreased level of consciousness • **Signs:** hypotension, shock, pulmonary congestion, CHF, angina
Common Etiologies	• AV nodal blocking agents: beta-blockers, calcium channel blockers, digoxin • Conditions that stimulate the parasympathetic system • An acute coronary syndrome that involves the right coronary artery
Recommended Therapy **Key:** Treat only when patient has significant signs or symptoms that are due to the bradycardia	**Intervention sequence for symptomatic bradycardia:** • Atropine 0.5 mg IV • Transcutaneous pacing in readiness for hydrodynamic instability • Oxygen **If signs and symptoms are severe, consider catecholamine infusions:** • Dopamine 2 to 10 µg/kg per min • Epinephrine 2 to 10 µg/min

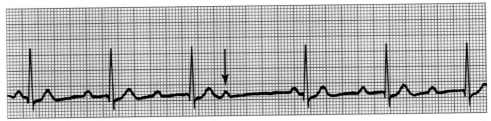

Second-degree AV block type I. Note progressive lengthening of PR interval until one P wave (arrow) is not followed by a QRS.

FIGURE 23-10 • Second-degree AV block type 1: (Mobitz 1 or Wenckebach). The arrow points to a blocked P wave ("dropped" QRS).

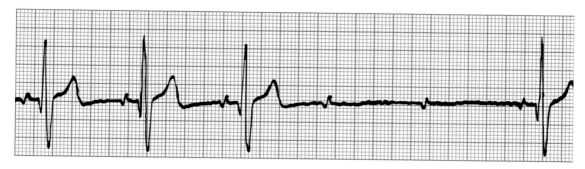

FIGURE 23-11 • Type II second-degree AV block. In this example, three conducted sinus impulses are followed by two nonconducted P waves. The PR interval of the conducted P waves remains constant, and the QRS complex is wide, indicative of distal conduction disease.

Second-Degree AV Block (Mobitz 2 or Infranodal)

Type II second-degree AV block (Figs. 23-11 and 23-12) occurs below the level of the AV node (infranodal), that is, at or below the bundle of His. A hallmark of this type of second-degree AV block is that the PR interval does not lengthen before a blocked impulse; the blocking of the impulse is an abrupt event. More than one nonconducted impulse may occur in succession.

Pathophysiology

- In the type II form of second-degree AV block the conduction pathology occurs *below* the level of the AV node (infranodal) that is at or below the bundle of His.
- Conduction of impulses through the AV node is normal with type II second-degree AV block. For this reason the PR interval does not lengthen before the nonconducted impulse (i.e., no type I second-degree AV block pattern).
- The bundle of His and Purkinje fibers are fast-response cells that tend to be depolarized as an "all or none" phenomenon. This explains why there is no progressive lengthening of the PR interval but instead either a conduction or abrupt nonconduction of the impulse from the atria to the ventricles.
- Type II second-degree AV block is associated with a poorer prognosis. Often it progresses to complete AV block.

Defining ECG Criteria

- The hallmark of type II second-degree AV block is that the PR interval remains constant before an atrial impulse is blocked (not conducted to the ventricles), resulting in "a P wave not followed by a QRS complex." Unlike type I block (Fig. 23-7), in type II block the PR interval does not lengthen before a nonconducted impulse ("dropped beat [QRS complex]" or "blocked impulse").
- **Atrial rate:** The atrial rate is normal (usually between 60 and 100 bpm).
- **Ventricular rate:** By definition the overall ventricular rate (averaged over a number of beats) is slower than the atrial rate because some impulses are blocked between the

atria and the ventricles so that ventricular depolarization does not follow some P waves.

- **Rhythm:** The atrial rhythm is regular; the nonconducted impulses may render the ventricular rhythm irregular. The ventricular rhythm is usually regularly irregular except in the presence of 2:1 AV block or a changing conduction sequence.
- **PR interval:** The PR interval may be normal or prolonged, but it will remain constant. There is no progressive prolongation of the PR interval as is observed with type I second-degree block before a P wave fails to conduct to the ventricle.
- **P waves:** Configuration (size and shape) on 12-lead ECG (or in multiple leads) of P waves is consistent with sinus node origin; by definition the P wave impulses that are blocked will not be followed by a QRS complex.
- **QRS complex:** The QRS complexes are usually abnormal and range from slightly to significantly wider than normal (≥0.11 second). This is because the distal conduction block creating the Mobitz II pattern is accompanied by other evidence of a distal conduction abnormality, reflected in a wider QRS complex.

Clinical Manifestations   In type II second-degree AV block the following symptoms can result from the bradycardia:

- **Symptoms:** Chest discomfort, shortness of breath, and decreased level of consciousness
- **Signs:** Hypotension, shock, pulmonary congestion, congestive heart failure, angina, or acute ST deviation

Common Etiologies

- Unlike type I second-degree AV block, type II second-degree AV block does not result from increased parasympathetic tone, and more commonly implicates pathology of the distal conduction system. It can be exacerbated by some medications that slow cardiac conduction, such as antiarrhythmic agents.
- New-onset type II second-degree block may be caused by an ACS that involves the *left* coronary artery. More specifically type II block develops with occlusion of one of the septal branches of the left anterior descending coronary artery. This occlusion also frequently produces bundle-branch block.

Recommended Therapy New-onset type II second-degree AV block is an indication for consideration for insertion of a transvenous pacemaker. Particularly when associated with a wide QRS, type II second-degree AV block indicates a need for a pacemaker regardless of symptoms. The bradycardia algorithm provides specific instructions for the management of symptomatic bradycardia associated with type II second-degree AV block:

- Prepare for a transvenous pacer.
- If symptoms develop, use a transcutaneous pacemaker until a transvenous pacer is placed.

The intervention sequence for new-onset type II second-degree AV block with serious signs and symptoms is as follows:

- Use transcutaneous pacing (TCP), if available, as a bridge to transvenous pacing. Verify patient tolerance and electrical capture with effective systemic perfusion; use sedation and analgesia as needed and tolerated.
- If severe signs and symptoms are unresponsive to TCP and there are delays to placement of a transvenous pacer, initiate a catecholamine infusion:
  - Epinephrine 2 to 10 μg/min
  - Dopamine 2 to 10 μg/kg/min
- Immediately consult cardiology and begin preparations for a transvenous pacemaker (Fig. 23-12).

Third-Degree AV Block

Third-degree AV block results from injury or damage to the cardiac conduction system so that no impulses are conducted from the atria to the ventricles (Figs. 23-13 and 23-14).

Pathophysiology

- Third-degree AV block (complete AV block) is caused by injury or damage to the cardiac conduction system such that no impulses (*complete*) can pass (*blocked*) between atria and ventricles. The more rapid atrial impulses are not conducted to the ventricles and ventricular, and atrial complexes occur independent of one another.
- This complete block can occur at several different anatomic areas, and each anatomic level of block may be associated with a different pathogenesis, treatment, and prognosis:
  - Block in the AV node. At this anatomic site a junctional or His bundle escape pacemaker frequently will initiate ventricular depolarization. This is usually a stable subsidiary pacemaker with a rate of 40 to 60 per min.
    - When the anatomic site of third-degree AV block is located in the AV node, the resulting escape rhythm also arises high in the conduction system (typically in the lower portion of the AV node or in the bundle of His) resulting in a normal QRS complex (<0.12 second) (Fig. 23-13A).
    - This type of third-degree AV block can result from increased parasympathetic tone associated with inferior infarction, from toxic drug effects (e.g., digitalis, propranolol), or from damage to the AV node.
    - Third-degree AV block with a junctional escape rhythm may be transient and associated with a favorable prognosis.

- Block in or below the bundle of His ("low" or "infranodal" block)
  - Third-degree block at or below the bundle of His indicates the presence of infranodal conduction system disease.
  - When this type of third-degree block is new in onset, it may be associated with extensive anterior MI.
  - The escape pacemaker mechanism originates distal to the site of the heart block. Such a ventricular escape pacemaker has an intrinsic rate that is likely to be slow (<40 per minute), with a wide QRS complex (indicative of distal conduction disease or the origin of the escape pacemaker in ventricular muscle itself), is not usually stable and can result in episodes of ventricular asystole (Fig. 23-13B).

Defining ECG Criteria There are three key defining criteria for third-degree block (Fig. 23-13): (1) the atrial rate exceeds the ventricular rate, (2) the ventricular escape rate is regular, and (3) PR intervals are widely variable indicating that P waves and QRS complexes are dissociated from one another. The latter two criteria provide firm evidence of complete AV block in that no P waves are ever conducted to the ventrical to disrupt the regularity of the slower escape rhythm, nor is there an apparent relationship between any P wave and the subsequent QRS, for which the association (as evidenced by the variable PR interval) is entirely random.

- **Atrial rate:** The atrial rate is faster than the ventricular (escape) rate. The atrial complexes have no relationship with ventricular complexes.
- **Ventricular rate:** The ventricular rate is determined by the rate of the ventricular escape pacemaker.
- **Rhythm:** The ventrcular (escape) rhythm is regular, and completely independent of any atrial activity, nor is its regularity disrupted by any atrial impulses that might traverse to the ventricle.
- **PR interval:** PR intervals are widely variable, indicating the absence of any relationship between the P wave and QRS complex.
- **P waves:** Configuration (size and shape) on a 12-lead ECG (or in multiple leads) of P waves is consistent with sinus node origin.
- **QRS complex:** A normal (narrow) QRS complex implies block in the AV node. A wide (≥0.12 second) QRS complex implies the anatomic level of block is at or below the bundle of His.

Clinical Manifestations

- **Symptoms:** Chest pain, shortness of breath, decreased level of consciousness, and syncope
- **Signs:** Hypotension, shock, pulmonary congestion, signs of congestive heart failure, angina, or AMI

Common Etiologies

- Acute third-degree AV block may occur in the setting of an ACS that involves the *left* coronary artery. In particular the involvement is with the left anterior descending artery, the branches to the interventricular septum, and the corresponding bundle branches. In such instances, the

Second-Degree AV Block Type II (Infranodal) (Mobitz II–Non-Wenckebach)	
Pathophysiology	• The pathology, ie, the site of the block, is most often below the AV node (infranodal); at or below the bundle of His
Defining Criteria per ECG	• **Atrial Rate:** usually 60-100 beats/min • **Ventricular rate:** by definition (due to the blocked impulses) slower than atrial rate • **Rhythm:** atrial = regular; ventricular = irregular (because of blocked impulses) • **PR:** may be normal or prolonged, but without progressive prolongation before a blocked P wave ("dropped" QRS). • **P waves:** typical in size and shape; by definition some P waves will not be followed by a QRS complex • **QRS complex:** typically wider than normal, implying the presence of distal conduction system disease
Clinical Manifestations— Rate-Related	**Due to bradycardia:** • **Symptoms:** chest pain, shortness of breath, decreased level of consciousness • **Signs:** hypotension, shock, pulmonary congestions, CHF, acute MI
Common Etiologies	• An acute coronary syndrome that involves branches of the left coronary artery
Recommended Therapy **Pearl:** New onset type II second-degree AV block in clinical context of acute coronary syndrome is indication for transvenous pacemaker insertion	**Intervention sequence for bradycardia due to type II second-degree or third-degree AV block:** • Prepare for transvenous pacer • Atropine is seldom effective for infranodal block and may paradoxically worsen bradycardia • Use transcutaneous pacing if available as a bridge to transvenous pacing (verify patient tolerance and mechanical capture. Use sedation and analgesia as needed). • Oxygen **If signs/symptoms are severe and unresponsive to TCP, and transvenous pacing is delayed, consider catecholamine infusions:** • Dopamine 2 to 10 μg/kg per min • Epinephrine 2 to 10 μg/min

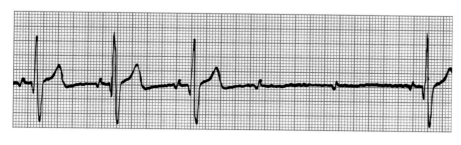
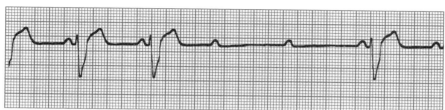

Mobitz type II AV Block: regular PR-QRS intervals until dropped beats; wide QRS complexes suggest the presence of distal conduction system disease and support the infranodal location of the AV block.

| FIGURE 23-12 • Second-degree AV block type 2 (infranodal) (Mobitz 2).

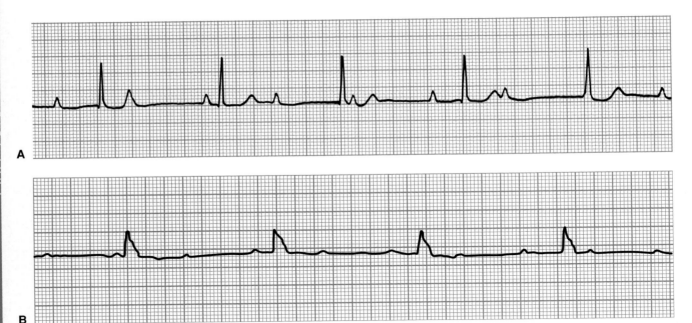

FIGURE 23-13 • **A.** Third-degree AV block occurring at the level of the AV node. The atrial rhythm is slightly irregular owing to the unrelated presence of sinus arrhythmia. The ventricular rhythm is regular at a slower rate (44 bpm). The PR interval is variable; QRS complexes are narrow, indicating that distal conduction is normal. **B.** Third-degree AV block is likely occurring at or below the bundle of His. The atrial rate is faster than the ventricular rate, which is regular at a slow rate of 38 bpm. The QRS is wide, suggesting that the escape pacemaker arises below the bundle of His, indicative of distal conduction block.

level of block is likely to be at or below the bundle of His, with a slow, wide QRS escape rhythm. This is an ominous form of third-degree AV block that requires temporary pacing because of its high likelihood of bradycardia symptoms and/or progression to asystole.

- Third-degree AV block can occur at the AV node, with a resultant junctional or His bundle (narrow QRS) escape rhythm. This type of AV block can result from increased parasympathetic tone, may be associated with inferior ischemia or infarction or toxic drug effects (e.g., digitalis, propranolol) or from injury to the AV node and surrounding tissue. It may resolve spontaneously, and unless symptomatic or persistent, may not necessarily require pacing.

Recommended Therapy New-onset symptomatic third-degree AV block is an indication for insertion of a transvenous pacemaker. The Bradycardia Algorithm indicates the following treatment for symptomatic third-degree AV block:

- Prepare for a transvenous pacer.
- If symptoms develop, use a transcutaneous pacemaker until a transvenous pacer is placed.

The intervention sequence for new-onset third-degree AV block with serious signs and symptoms is as follows (some may be initiated concurrently):

- Begin TCP immediately when available if the patient is unstable due to AV block. Use sedation and analgesia as needed.

- If TCP is not immediately available, consider atropine 0.5 mg; use atropine only if the QRS complex is narrow; atropine is not effective and may be detrimental in infranodal (wide QRS) block.
- If severe signs and symptoms are unresponsive to atropine (if used) and TCP and there are delays to placement of a transvenous pacer, then initiate a catecholamine infusion:
  - Epinephrine 2 to 10 µg/min
  - Dopamine 2 to 10 µg/kg/min
- Consult cardiology and begin preparations for a transvenous pacer. Use TCP if available as a bridge to transvenous pacing. Verify patient tolerance and mechanical capture.

Note: If the patient has third-degree AV block and a ventricular escape rhythm, the ventricular escape rhythm is the only source of ventricular depolarization. ***Do not administer calcium channel or beta-blockers, lidocaine, or amiodarone to these patients.*** These drugs may suppress the ventricular escape rhythm and cause cardiac standstill (Fig. 23-14).

Other Terminology

The classification of AV blocks is simplified to allow providers to initiate emergency therapy for a large number of patients in circumstances where detailed consideration and differential rhythm diagnosis may not be possible. In

Third -degree AV block	
Pathophysiology	• The pathology, ie, the site of the block, may occur at the AV node (nodal), or at or below the bundle of His (infranodal).
Defining Criteria per ECG	• **Atrial Rate:** usually 60-100 bpm and faster than the ventricular (escape) rate. • **Ventricular rate:** escape rhythm is regular, and slower than the atrial rate. The ventricular escape rate is typically faster with nodal than with infranodal AV block. • **Rhythm:** atrial = regular; ventricular = regular escape • **PR:** highly variable, indicating that any apparent relationship between P and QRS complexes is random. • **P waves:** Configuration (size and shape) on 12-lead ECG (or in multiple leads) is consistent with sinus node origin. There is no association of P waves with QRS complexes as evidenced by the regularity of the ventricular escape rate and the wide variation in PR intervals. • **QRS:** QRS may be narrow (implying nodal block) or wide (implying infranodal block).
Clinical Manifestations—Rate-Related	**Due to bradycardia:** • **Symptoms:** chest pain, shortness of breath, decreased level of consciousness • **Signs:** hypotension, shock, pulmonary congestions, CHF, acute MI
Common Etiologies	• An acute coronary syndrome that involves branches of the left coronary artery
Recommended Therapy **Pearl:** New onset type II second-degree AV block in clinical context of acute coronary syndrome is indication for transvenous pacemaker insertion	**Intervention sequence for bradycardia due to type II third-degree AV block:** • Prepare for transvenous pacer • Atropine is seldom effective for infranodal block and may paradoxically worsen bradycardia • Use transcutaneous pacing if available as a bridge to transvenous pacing (verify patient tolerance and mechanical capture. Use sedation and analgesia as needed.) • Oxygen **If signs/symptoms are severe and unresponsive to TCP, and transvenous pacing is delayed, consider catecholamine infusions:** • Dopamine 2 to 10 µg/kg per min • Epinephrine 2 to 10 µg/min

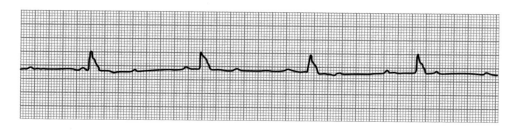

| FIGURE 23-14 • Third-degree AV block and AV classification.

some instances questions of a more advanced context may arise. Although such questions are beyond the scope of this chapter, a brief summary of the more common terminology is provided here to facilitate understanding.

2:1 AV Block

A 2:1 AV conduction ratio is often mistakenly classified as type II AV block when it can be either type I or type II second-degree AV block. Because two consecutive PR intervals are not recorded, an assessment of the PR interval for progressive prolongation or a fixed interval cannot aid in the differential diagnosis. But certain "clues" can be used. For example, if the PR interval of the conducted beat is prolonged and the QRS complex is narrow, the block is more likely type I second-degree AV block. If there is a preexisting bundle branch block or if the QRS complexes are wide, it may not be possible to differentiate between type I and type II second-degree AV block. If the patient has responded favorably to atropine—given for an indicated reason—the block is likely in the AV-nodal portion under vagal influence. But the opposite may not be true. For example, if atropine increases sinus node discharge but minimally increases AV conduction, AV block may paradoxically increase. Importantly, atropine has no known conduction-enhancing effects in the distal conduction system or ventricles. Hence its administration to patients with AV block at or below the bundle of His will accelerate the sinus rate (but do nothing to enhance distal conduction), resulting in further bombardment of the already failing distal conduction system by even more electrical impulses, which may lead to worsening block. Thus atropine is best used therapeutically for AV block only when there is high suspicion for its occurrence at the level of the AV node. Atropine (and other maneuvers such as carotid sinus massage) should not be used for "diagnostic" purposes in this setting.

AV Dissociation

The term "AV dissociation" denotes independent electrical activity of the atria and ventricles. Although this is frequently used in reference to third-degree AV block, such usage can be misleading and should be avoided. "AV dissociation" is a broad term that refers to a variety of rhythms for which there is no association between atrial and ventricular complexes. This can occur for reasons other than AV block. For example, when AV dissociation occurs because the *ventricular* rate is *faster* than the atrial rate (as in ventricular tachycardia), this dissociation is not due to AV block but rather to the ventricular rate simply exceeding the sinus rate. This is not AV block. To qualify as AV block, the *atrial* rate should be *faster* than the ventricular rate, in addition to the other characteristic features of AV block described in previous sections. Because AV dissociation can occur in a variety of circumstances other than AV block, the term is best used to describe arrhythmias where the ventricular rate exceeds the atrial rate, reserving the term "heart (or AV) block" specifically for the opposite (when the atrial rate exceeds the ventricular rate). There are two common scenarios during which AV dissociation may be observed.

- The sinus rhythm may slow (or a bradycardia already present), with the emergence of a subsidiary pacemaker whose rate is somewhat faster than that of the sinus node. For example, a junctional escape rhythm may emerge in patients with significant sinus bradycardia or sinus node dysfunction. Or, in an acute MI with sinus bradycardia, an idioventricular rhythm can emerge. When the rate of this rhythm is increased but <100/min, it is sometimes referred to as an accelerated idioventricular rhythm, or AIVR. These are examples of AV dissociation, not AV block, because the ventricular rate in each of these instance is faster than the atrial rate.
- A reentry or automatic ventricular arrhythmia, such as ventricular tachycardia (VT) may occur and "take over" control of the heart rhythm. During such arrhythmias, the sinus node will typically continue to independently generate P waves but at a slower rate than the VT. This is one of the "footprints" of VT, denoting independent atrial and ventricular activity. This is AV dissociation, not AV block, because in this instance the ventricular rate (VT) is faster than the atrial rate.

High-Degree and Advanced AV Block

High-grade or advanced AV block is a form of second-degree AV block, defined as existing when two or more consecutive P waves fail to conduct to the ventricle regardless of the anatomic level of block (AV nodal or in the distal conduction system). It implies a greater risk for a resulting bradycardia and invites a heightened state of vigilance over a failing conduction system.

References

1. Olgin JE, Zipes DP. Specific arrhythmias: diagnosis and treatment. In Braunwald E, Zipes DP, Libby P, eds. *Heart Disease: A Textbook of Cardiovascular Medicine*, 7th ed. Philadelphia: Saunders; 2005: 803–810.
2. Smith I, Monk TG, White PF. Comparison of transesophageal atrial pacing with anticholinergic drugs for the treatment of intraoperative bradycardia. *Anesth Analg* 1994;78(2):245–252.
3. Brady WJ, Swart G, DeBehnke DJ, et al. The efficacy of atropine in the treatment of hemodynamically unstable bradycardia and atrioventricular block: prehospital and emergency department considerations. *Resuscitation* 1999;41(1):47–55.
4. Chadda KD, Lichstein E, Gupta PK, et al. Effects of atropine in patients with bradyarrhythmia complicating myocardial infarction: usefulness of an optimum dose for overdrive. *Am J Med* 1977;63(4): 503–510.
5. Errando CL, Peiro CM. An additional explanation for atrioventricular block after the administration of atropine. *Can J Anaesth* 2004;51(1):88; author reply 88–89.
6. Maruyama K, Mochizuki N, Hara K. High-degree atrioventricular block after the administration of atropine for sinus arrest during anesthesia. *Can J Anaesth* 2003;50(5):528–529.
7. Brunner-La Rocca HP, Kiowski W, Bracht C, et al. Atrioventricular block after administration of atropine in patients following cardiac transplantation. *Transplantation* 1997;63(12):1838–1839.
8. Bernheim A, Fatio R, Kiowski W, et al. Atropine often results in complete atrioventricular block or sinus arrest after cardiac transplantation: an unpredictable and dose-independent phenomenon. *Transplantation* 2004;77(8):1181–1185.

9. Dauchot P, Gravenstein JS. Effects of atropine on the electrocardiogram in different age groups. *Clin Pharmacol Ther* 1971;12(2):274–280.

10. Ellenbogen KA, Thames MD, DiMarco JP, et al. Electrophysiological effects of adenosine in the transplanted human heart: evidence of supersensitivity. *Circulation* 1990;81(3):821–828.

11. Bernheim A, Fatio R, Kiowski W, et al. Atropine often results in complete atrioventricular block or sinus arrest after cardiac transplantation: an unpredictable and dose-independent phenomenon. *Transplantation* 2004;77(8):1181–1185.

12. Love JN, Sachdeva DK, Bessman ES, et al. A potential role for glucagon in the treatment of drug-induced symptomatic bradycardia. *Chest* 1998;114(1):323–326.

13. Viskin S, Belhassen B, Roth A, et al. Aminophylline for bradyasystolic cardiac arrest refractory to atropine and epinephrine. *Ann Intern Med* 1993;118:279–281.

14. Burton JH, Mass M, Menegazzi JJ, et al. Aminophylline as an adjunct to standard advanced cardiac life support in prolonged cardiac arrest. *Ann Emerg Med* 1997;30:154–158.

15. Mader TJ, Gibson P. Adenosine receptor antagonism in refractory asystolic cardiac arrest: results of a human pilot study. *Resuscitation* 1997;25:3–7.

16. Abu-Laban RB, McIntyre CM, vanBeek CA, et al. Aminophylline in bradyasystolic cardiac arrest: a randomized placebo-controlled trial. *Lancet* 2006;367:1577–1584.

17. Mangrum JM, DiMarco JP. The evaluation and management of bradycardia. *N Engl J Med* 2000;342(10):703–709.

18. Barold SS, Hayes DL. Second-degree atrioventricular block: a reappraisal. *Mayo Clin Proc* 2001;76(1):44–57.

19. Barold SS. Lingering misconceptions about type I second-degree atrioventricular block. *Am J Cardiol* 2001;88(9):1018–1020.

Chapter 24
Electrical Therapies

Peter J. Kudenchuk

A good rule of thumb for determining when to use synchronized versus unsynchronized shock is that if the provider cannot identify each QRS complex with the eye, then the defibrillator will likely not be able to identify them either. In these instances, unsynchronized shock at defibrillation energy settings should be administered.

- Synchronized and unsynchronized shocks
- Indications for treating emergency pacing in emergency cardiovascular care (ECC)
- Special considerations for treating patients with pacemakers and implantable cardioverter defibrillators (ICDs)
- Management of bradyarrhythmia and conduction disturbances in acute myocardial infarction (AMI)
- Safety considerations using electrical therapy

Cardioversion and Defibrillation[1]

Shock therapy (cardioversion or defibrillation) is recommended for any arrhythmia caused by reentry that requires termination. This includes atrioventricular nodal reentry tachycardia, atrioventricular reentry tachycardia, intra-atrial reentry tachycardia, sinus node reentry tachycardia, atrial fibrillation, atrial flutter, ventricular tachycardia, and ventricular fibrillation (see also Chapter 22). These arrhythmias are caused by reentry (an abnormal rhythm circuit that is sustained by circulating upon itself again and again), which can be interrupted by a shock that breaks the circulating pattern (Fig. 24-1).

Shock therapy will not be effective for treatment of automatic tachycardias such as ectopic atrial tachycardia, multifocal atrial tachycardia or junctional tachycardia. Such automatic rhythms are created when local cells become more excited and spontaneously depolarize (fire) more rapidly. Sinus tachycardia is a good example of an automatic rhythm. It results when cells in the sinus node are excited to fire more rapidly. Junctional tachycardia, or ectopic or multifocal atrial tachycardia, is created by the same mechanism but at a different location. An understanding of this mechanism will help to clarify why automatic rhythms are not responsive to shock. Shock stops reentry rhythms by breaking their circulating pattern. Shock cannot stop a rhythm that originates from locally excited cells. In fact, shocking any automatic rhythm is no different than shocking sinus tachycardia—it only results in more of the same. In fact, shock delivery to tachyarrhythmias caused by a rapid automatic focus may actually increase the rate of the tachyarrhythmia because of the enhanced sympathetic tone resulting from shock.

Synchronized Electrical Shock (Cardioversion)

Synchronized cardioversion is recommended for any arrhythmia that is caused by reentry, has distinguishable QRS complexes to which a shock could be synchronized, and that needs to be terminated because of the patient's clinical condition. Synchronized electrical shock (cardioversion) refers to the administration of an electrical shock that is timed to occur simultaneously with the QRS complex. Synchronized cardioversion permits the use of lower-energy settings to convert an organized rhythm, and synchronizing the shock during the QRS complex minimizes the risk of delivering the shock on the T wave, which could induce ventricular fibrillation (VF).

Synchronization is an automated feature of defibrillators that senses QRS complexes based on their electrical characteristics in the lead under evaluation. While mostly reliable, it is not foolproof and on occasion may inappropriately synchronize to another portion of the ECG, such as the T wave, with disastrous consequences. Thus, it is critical for the responder to confirm that synchronization is appropriately timed before shock delivery. This is done by seeing whether the synchronization markers on the defibrillator's ECG screen appropriately correspond to where QRS complexes occur (Fig. 24-2). If the timing is incorrect in the lead, a different ECG lead should be selected where synchronization is reliably timed to the QRS. Done properly, the risk of cardioversion is relatively small.[2]

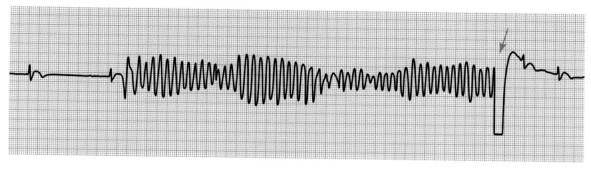

FIGURE 24-1 • This malignant-appearing ventricular arrhythmia, which could be described as course ventricular fibrillation or rapid polymorphic ventricular tachycardia, is terminated by shock (*arrow*).

Unsynchronized Shock (Defibrillation)

For some arrhythmias, synchronization is not possible or recommended (Fig. 24-1). Synchronization requires that the defibrillator be able to reliably recognize a consistent QRS to which a shock can be precisely timed. If the defibrillator is unable to synchronize, it will withhold delivery of any shock. The many QRS configurations and irregular rates comprised by polymorphic ventricular tachycardia and VF may make it difficult or impossible for the defibrillator to reliably synchronize to a QRS complex. Likewise, it may not be possible for a defibrillator to synchronize to a monomorphic ventricular tachycardia that is extremely rapid in rate. This can result in delay of an emergently needed shock. For this reason unsynchronized shock (defibrillation) is recommended in all pulseless states, as for VF and pulseless ventricular tachycardia (VT), where any delay in shock treatment cannot be afforded.

A good rule of thumb for determining when to use synchronized versus unsynchronized shock is that if the provider cannot identify each QRS complex with the eye, then the defibrillator will likely not be able to identify them either. In these instances, unsynchronized shock at defibrillation energy settings should be administered.

A second important rule is that maximum energy settings should be used for any unsynchronized shock. Lower energy settings should not be used for unsynchronized shocks because they have a higher likelihood of provoking VF when given in an unsynchronized fashion.

So-called precordial thump cardioversion, in which the midchest is struck by the fist, should be considered equivalent to unsynchronized, very low energy cardioversion and has been proven ineffective; therefore, it is not a recommended intervention for ventricular tacharrhythmias.[3]

Defibrillation Electrode Position

For ventricular defibrillation, conventional right anterior (infraclavicular) and left lateral (apical) defibrillation electrode locations continue to be recommended because of the ease of placement and the efficacy. The anterior electrode should be placed just below the right clavicle, with the center of its electrode at the midclavicular line; the apical electrode should be placed at the inferolateral left chest, left of and just below the nipple (lateral to the left breast in women), with the center of its electrode in the midaxillary line (Fig. 24-3).

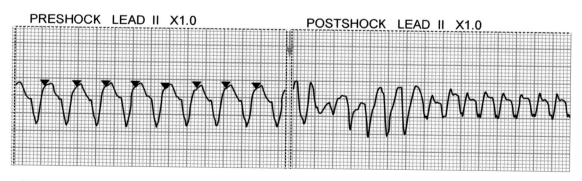

FIGURE 24-2 • Inappropriately synchronized shock. A wide-complex tachycardia is shown, synchronized for anticipated low-energy cardioversion (50 J). However, the synchronization markers (inverted triangles) are falling on the T wave rather than on the QRS complex. The resulting shock (*arrow*) was inappropriately administered on the T wave, resulting in rapid polymorphic VT (shown) which quickly degenerated into VF (not shown).

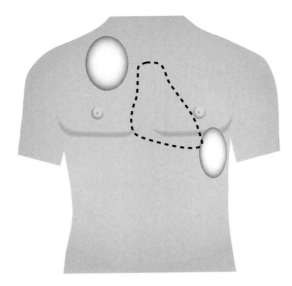

FIGURE 24-3 • Recommended anterior-apex positions for placement of defibrillation paddles or adhesive defibrillation pads. Place the anterior electrode to the right of the upper sternum below the clavicle. Place the apex electrode along the left inferolateral chest wall, to the left of and just below the nipple with the center of the electrode in the midaxillary line.

Mistakes in Pad Position or Size One of the most common errors in pad placement is to place the pads too close together. Figure 24-4A displays a cross section of the heart and thorax showing how most of the current bypasses the heart when the paddles are placed too close together. Notice also that the sternal paddle is indeed over the sternum, which blocks much of the current flow. In Figure 24-4B, the apex paddle is in the proper position in the midaxillary line, which allows all the current to flow through the myocardium, achieving defibrillation.

An interesting manikin study from England supports the idea that improper placement of the apex pad or paddle is the most common positional error.[5] During a course on resuscitation techniques, doctors were asked to place the two defibrillator paddles in the "proper" locations on the breast plate of a resuscitation training manikin. Figure 24-5 presents a composite "map" of all the locations selected by the 101 subjects. This map unequivocally shows how the doctors erred in paddle placement more than 90% of the time, placing the apex paddle too far anterior, well away from the recommended location near the axillary line. Look again at Figure 24-4B to see how, somewhat counterintuitively, moving the apex paddle *away* from the heart and toward the axillary line will lead to more effective defibrillatory shocks.

For cardioversion, particularly of atrial fibrillation, other electrode positions have been suggested, including placement directly opposite each other in an anteroposterior configuration over the mid- or left-chest wall and back or at the right anterior mid-chest wall and the left lower scapular region.[6,7] However, direct comparison of these configurations has not demonstrated a significant difference in shock success.[8] On occasion, electrode positions need to be modified because of patient anatomy, location of an implanted pacemaker or defibrillator (see below), or other extenuating circumstances. Alternate positions may include placement of electrodes on the right and left lateral chest wall (biaxillary) or the left electrode in the standard apical position and the other electrode on the right or left upper back. Whatever defibrillation electrode positions are ultimately selected, conceptually the idea is to "sandwich" the heart between the electrodes to ensure maximum coverage by the shock.

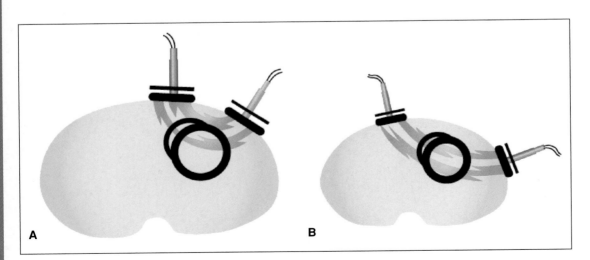

A   B

FIGURE 24-4 • Pad positions. In these figures, the feet of the imaginary supine patient lie towards the viewer, whereas the head faces away. Thus, the chest is viewed from the vantage point of the patient's feet, looking toward the torso. **A.** Pathway of current when the paddles are placed too closely together. **B.** A more optimal current pathway, achieved when the paddles are placed in the standard position. (Reproduced with permission from Ewy GA, Bressler R, eds. *Cardiovascular Drugs and the Management of Heart Disease.* New York: Raven Press, 1982.)

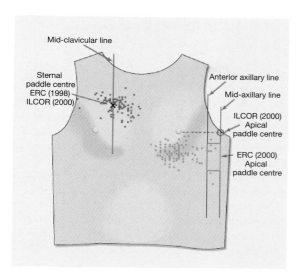

FIGURE 24-5 • Anatomic position of center of sternal and apical defibrillation paddles placed by 101 doctors. [Reproduced from Heames RM, Sado D, Deakin CD. Do doctors position defibrillation paddles correctly? Observational study. *BMJ.* 2001;322(7299):1393–1394. With permission from the BMJ Publishing Group.]

Shock Waveform

Shock waveforms for external cardioversion and defibrillation vary by device manufacturer. The shock waveforms traditionally used, consisted of a single-phase shock (either a damped sinusoidal monophasic or truncated exponential monophasic waveform). These have been largely replaced by biphasic waveform defibrillators, which administer a two-phase shock with each phase being of opposite polarity. Biphasic defibrillators administer differing forms of biphasic waveform shock (such as biphasic truncated exponential and rectilinear biphasic) and have different energy setting options depending upon the manufacturer. Evidence suggests that biphasic waveform shock is more effective than monophasic shock for cardioversion of atrial fibrillation[10,11] and may be as good or better for defibrillation of VF and pulseless VT.[12,13]

Energy Settings: Supraventricular Tachycardia

The recommended initial shock energy setting for cardioversion of atrial fibrillation with a monophasic waveform should be no less than 100 J. Typically a 200-J energy setting is used. Cardioversion of atrial flutter and paroxysmal supraventricular tachycardia (PSVT) may require less energy (25–50 J).[14] Current AHA ECC guidelines recommend starting with a dose of 50 to 100 J and proceeding in a stepwise fashion if the initial shock does not convert the rhythm.[15] However, factors such as patient's clinical condition, use of medications, and transthoracic resistance are important determinants of the energy required for successful cardioversion. From the standpoint of patient comfort, there is little advantage to using lower energy settings. Lower energy settings also risk the need for repeated shock if not initially successful and can precipitate VF if not appropriately timed for delivery precisely on the QRS. For these reasons some experts begin with energy settings of 200 J for virtually all supraventricular arrhythmias, and, if unsuccessful, increasing the setting in a stepwise fashion up to the maximum of 360 J.[16]

Cardioversion with biphasic waveforms is now available,[17] but more data are needed before specific comparative dosing recommendations can be made. In general, for a given shock energy setting, biphasic waveform shock is more likely to terminate atrial arrhythmias than monophasic waveform shock, and biphasic waveform shock can be deployed at a lower energy setting than monophasic shock, with comparable success.[18,19] For example, an initial biphasic shock setting as low as 70 J successfully terminated atrial fibrillation more effectively than a 100-J monophasic waveform shock.[18]

Energy Settings: Ventricular Arrhythmias

Monomorphic VT, defined as having QRS complexes of uniform appearance and occurring at a regular rate, responds to monophasic or biphasic synchronized cardioversion at relatively low energy settings of 25 to 50 J; if there is great urgency to terminate VT, one can begin with energy settings of 100 J or higher.[20] Less organized ventricular arrhythmias, such as polymorphic VT and VF, typically require higher energy settings, which should be administered in unsynchronized fashion. If a monophasic defibrillator is used, 200 to 360 J has generally been used, but current AHA guidelines recommend that 360 J be used for all shocks.

The recommended initial shock energy setting with a biphasic defibrillator is 150 to 200 J; an equal or higher dose is recommended for second and subsequent shocks. Whether the success of defibrillation in out-of-hospital cardiac arrest is improved by using monophasic or biphasic waveform shock is controversial,[12,21] as is whether higher biphasic waveform shock settings (360 J) are more beneficial than lower settings (200 J) during resuscitation of a cardiac arrest patient.[22] After shock delivery, the health care provider should be prepared to provide immediate cardiopulmonary resuscitation (CPR) and other needed support.

Pacing

Emergency pacing of the heart has been greatly simplified by the development of devices able to apply a pacing stimulus through the chest wall. The technique of using these devices is called transcutaneous pacing (TCP). In an emergency setting, TCP can be initiated rapidly and noninvasively, obviating the time to prepare for transvenous pacing and the complications associated with emergency access of the central circulation. Historically, emergency pacing has been employed both in and out of hospital during cardiac arrest and for patients with serious symptoms or hemodynamic instability due to bradycardia.

Other forms of pacing include standby (or "backup") pacing, provided primarily when clinical or electrocardiographic findings indicate the likelihood of progression to high-degree block but pacing is not immediately required. Temporary pacing is often used as a bridge to permanent pacing when a correctable condition cannot be reversed or cardiac pathology causing block is anticipated to be fixed or to transiently compromise function. Emergency health care providers are not usually involved in decisions for permanent pacemaker implantation but should be aware of conditions likely to necessitate continued need for pacemaker therapy. Early involvement of a cardiology or electrophysiology expert is often important in staging devices and procedures.

Emergency Pacing

TCP is an indicated intervention for symptomatic bradycardias. It should be started immediately for patients who are unstable, particularly those with high-degree (Mobitz type II second-degree or third-degree) block. TCP can be painful, and some limitations apply. Pacing spikes may be present, but electrical stimulation may fail to produce effective mechanical capture. After starting pacing, carefully assess the patient for clinical response. Because heart rate is a major determinant of myocardial oxygen consumption, set the pacing rate to the lowest effective rate based on clinical assessment and symptom resolution. If cardiovascular symptoms are not caused by the bradycardia, the patient may not improve despite effective pacing.

Standby Pacing

The indications for *standby pacing* are multiple and most often occur in the setting of an acute coronary syndrome (ACS). These patients typically are clinically stable yet at risk for decompensation in the near future. Often it is the location and size of MI that is ominous in these patients. The development of the rhythm disorder is a secondary event, and pacing has not altered outcome in the past. Priority is given to reperfusion of patients with STEMI, and treatment of symptomatic AV block is supportive in the vast majority of patients.

Because TCP is widely available and inexpensive, when advanced cardiac life support (ACLS) providers are concerned about the possibility of the development of high-degree symptomatic AV block, preparations for TCP should be initiated. Standby TCP has also been used successfully during surgery for high-risk patients who have bifascicular or left bundle-branch block with additional first-degree block.[23,24] If it is then needed to treat hemodynamically significant bradycardia, the device provides a therapeutic bridge until a transvenous pacemaker can be placed under more controlled circumstances. Although it is more invasive, a transcutaneous pacemaker can also be initially placed in standby mode for these and other at-risk patients.

Pacing for Pulseless Bradyasystolic Cardiac Arrest

Pacing has been studied extensively in the treatment of pulseless patients with bradycardia or asystole. Some studies had shown encouraging results in such patients when pacing was initiated within 10 minutes of cardiac arrest, but recent studies have documented no improvement in either short-term outcomes (admission to hospital) or intermediate-term outcomes (survival to hospital discharge).[25-27]

Prehospital studies of TCP for asystolic arrest or post-shock asystole have also shown no benefit of pacing.[28] In a level 1, prospective, controlled trial of TCP for cardiac arrest, investigators observed no benefit even when CPR was combined with pacing, nor did they observe any benefit when the asystole was of only brief duration after a defibrillatory shock.[27]

Pacing for Drug-Induced Cardiac Arrest

An exception to the negative results of pacing for cardiac arrest involves patients in cardiac arrest provoked by overdose of cardiac medications such as calcium channel blockers or antiarrhythmic agents. In such cases, pacing may be successful for the treatment of profound bradycardia or pulseless electrical activity.[29-33] Emergency pacing may also benefit patients with pulseless electrical activity due to acidosis or electrolyte abnormalities. Such patients often possess a normal myocardium with only temporary impairment of the conduction system.

While attempts are made to correct electrolyte abnormalities or profound acidosis, pacing can stimulate effective myocardial contractions. Similarly, pacing can be life-sustaining as the conduction system recovers from the cardiotoxic effects of a drug overdose or poisoning with other substances.[32]

Temporary Pacing

Although TCP is a recommended intervention for symptomatic bradycardia, it can be painful, without complete assurance of capture, and should serve only as an interim measure until more reliable transvenous pacing can be accomplished. TCP is generally ineffective in patients with cardiac arrest due to asystole or pulseless electrical activity,[27,34] perhaps with the exception of where associated with drug overdose.[29-33]

TCP is performed from the same defibrillator electrodes used for cardioversion and defibrillation. However, anteroposterior positioning of the electrodes between the chest and back is recommended in order to capture ventricular muscle. Typically, a left anterior parasternal and left posterior paraspinal (directly opposite the anterior electrode) or left anterior parsternal and right posterior paraspinal position is deployed. If one electrode configuration does not result in ventricular capture, other configurations can be attempted. However, not all patients can be successfully paced with TCP. Such pacing results also in local muscle stimulation and will be painful to the awake patient. It should only serve as a bridge to transvenous temporary pacing if required. Notably, the same electrodes used for pacing may be required for defibrillation (and vice versa). Fortunately, the positions used for TCP usually accommodate their use for defibrillation. However, the care provider may need to prioritize the immediate need of the patient (pacing versus defibrillation) in selecting the location where electrodes are initially placed and be prepared to relocate them if necessary. Output from the pacemaker should be increased from the minimal setting until a pacing artifact appears on the monitor screen, followed by a widened QRS complex and T wave, which indicates ventricular capture. Ventricular capture is not completely reliable, and it can be challenging to determine such capture from the rhythm monitor because of the degree of electrical artifact created by TCP. One should specifically evaluate for the presence of a pacer spike, followed by a QRS complex, followed by a repolarization (T) wave, and confirmed by the presence of a palpable pulse, aterial pressure tracing, or measured blood pressure (Fig. 24-6).[35]

In contrast to TCP, transvenous pacemakers require special expertise for placement, and expert consultation should be sought for patients requiring such treatment.

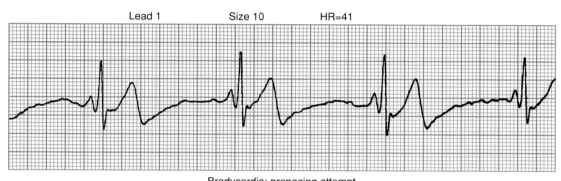

Lead 1   Size 10   HR=41

A   Bradycardia: prepacing attempt

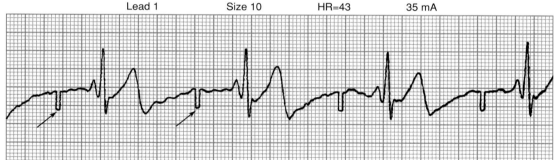

Lead 1   Size 10   HR=43   35 mA

B   Pacing attempted: note pacing stimulus indicator (arrow) which is below threshold; no capture

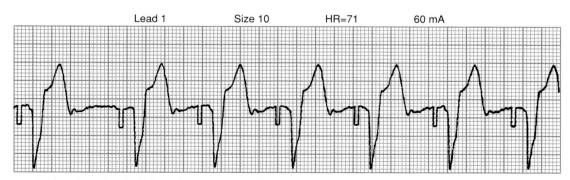

Lead 1   Size 10   HR=71   60 mA

C   Pacing above threshold (60 mA): with capture (QRS complex broad and ventricular; T wave opposite QRS)

FIGURE 24-6 • Transcutaneous pacing. **A.** Sinus bradycardia is shown without evidence of pacing stimulation. **B.** Transcutaneous pacing is activated, evidenced by the presence of pacemaker artifact (*arrow*) but without capture of the ventricle. **C.** At higher pacing output, transcutaneous pacing spikes are each followed by a QRS complex and a repolarization (T) wave, indicative of appropriate ventricular capture.

HISTORY OF CARDIAC PACING

Origins

The modern age of cardiac pacing in humans began in 1952, with the first successful resuscitation using the transcutaneous technique, later reported by Paul Zoll and colleagues.[36] This technique was largely abandoned by the 1960s because it was extremely painful and produced marked muscle contraction and cutaneous burns, especially with prolonged use. In addition, work by Lillehei, Bakken, and Furman led to successful transvenous pacing in the late 1950s and early 1960s.[37-39]

Modern Refinements

Refinements in electrode size and pulse characteristics led to the reintroduction of transcutaneous pacing into clinical practice in the 1980s.[40,41] Increasing the pulse duration from 2 to 20 milliseconds or longer was found to decrease the current output required for cardiac capture.[42] Longer impulse durations also make induction of VF less likely than when shorter impulse durations are used. The pacing stimulus is safe. In animal studies[43] the "safety factor" for VF induction (ratio of fibrillation current to pacing current) of transcutaneous pacing is 12 to 15. This means that 12 to 15 times the pacing current would be required to fibrillate the heart. Electrodes with a larger surface area (8 centimeters in diameter) decrease the current density at the skin, thereby decreasing pain and tissue burns.

Trials of transcutaneous pacemakers using the newer impulse and electrode characteristics have demonstrated the success of these modifications in overcoming the limitations of earlier transcutaneous pacemakers.[44] The mean current required for electrical capture is usually 50 to 100 milliamperes. Although some patients can tolerate pacing at their capture threshold, IV analgesia and sedation should generally be provided when pacing with currents of approximately 50 milliamperes or more because of pain from skeletal muscle stimulation.

Indications for Pacing in Acute Coronary Syndromes

Approximately 20% of patients with acute myocardial infarction (AMI) will develop second- or third-degree AV block. AV block is related to the infarct-related coronary artery, coronary distribution, and site of infarction (Table 24-1). Of those who develop AV block, 42% demonstrate the block on admission, and 66% demonstrate the block within the first 24 hours of presentation. In the majority of cases, these abnormalities are the result of myocardial ischemia or infarction with necrosis of the cardiac pacemaker sites or the conduction system. Other factors responsible for the development of heart block include altered autonomic influence, systemic hypoxia, electrolyte disturbances, acid–base disorders, and complications of various medical therapies.

In general, emergency management of bradycardia and pacing in the setting of acute coronary ischemia and infarction are similar to those implemented with other bradycardias. Caution is advised in the use of atropine and adrener-

gic agents, as noted in Chapter 23. AV block per se is rarely fatal; if death occurs, it is usually caused by an extensive MI with cardiac dysfunction. Heart block is not an independent predictor of mortality, and it is a poor predictor of mortality in patients who survive to discharge. The prognosis for patients with heart block is related most consistently to the size and site of infarction (anterior or inferior). Treatment is influenced by the level of block in the conduction system, the presence and rate of escape rhythms, and the degree of hemodynamic compromise.

In the setting of an ACS, any of the following abnormalities place the patient at risk for complete AV block or another hemodynamically significant deterioration for which placement of transcutaneous pacing electrodes for standby purposes is often advisable, and immediate expert consultation obtained regarding the possible need for a temporary transvenous pacemaker.

- Hemodynamically unstable bradycardia (rate <50 per minute) unresponsive to atropine
- Type II second-degree AV block
- Third-degree AV heart block
- Newly acquired left, right, or alternating bundle-branch block (BBB) or bifascicular block

Management of conduction defects during AMI and convalescence can be complicated, and early involvement of appropriate expert consultants is advised. Management of transient and persistent conduction abnormalities in AMI is complicated and requires expert consultation. For more on this topic see the American College of Cardiology/American Heart Association Guidelines for the Management of ST-Elevation Myocardial Infarction[45] (Table 24-2).

See Web site for ACC/AHA guidelines for management of patients with STEMI and AV block or conduction system abnormalities

Permanent Pacemakers

In general, resuscitation of patients who have a permanent pacemaker should be conducted in similar fashion to those who do not. However, use of external cardioversion or defibrillation calls for special precautions.

Modern pacemakers have protective circuits (an arrangement of Zener diodes) to shield their electronic components from external shock.[46] When exposed to high voltage (as from a defibrillation shock), the Zener diodes divert the energy away from the electronic components in the generator to the electrodes on the pacemaker lead. This can result in concentration of energy at the interface between the electrode tip and the myocardium, causing local trauma and potentially permanent damage reflected in transient or permanently higher pacing thresholds or complete loss of ventricular capture[46-48] and leading to the need for lead replacement.

Occasionally, a patient may be encountered with abandoned pacemaker or defibrillator leads that are not connected to a generator. Typically a plastic cap is placed over the

| TABLE 24-1 • Features of Atrioventricular Conduction in Acute Myocardial Infarction

Feature	Location of AV Conduction Disturbance	
	Proximal	Distal
Site of block	Intranodal	Infranodal
Site of infarction	Inferoposterior	Anteroseptal
Compromised arterial supply	RCA (90%), LCx (10%)	Septal perforators of LAD
Pathogenesis	Ischemia, necrosis, hydropic cell swelling, excess parasympathetic activity	Ischemia, necrosis, hydropic cell swelling
Predominant type of AV nodal block	First degree (PR greater than 200 msec) Mobitz type I second degree	Mobitz type II second degree Third degree
Common promontory features of third-degree AV block	(a) First-second-degree AV block (b) Mobitz type I pattern	
Features of escape following third-degree block (a) Location (b) QRS width (c) Rate (d) Stability of escape rhythm	(a) Proximal conduction system (His bundle) (b) Less than 0.12 sec[a] (c) 45–60 per min but may be as low as 30 per min (d) Rate usually stable; asystole uncommon	(a) Distal conduction system (bundle branches) (b) Greater than 0.12 sec[a] (c) Often less than 30 per min (d) Rate often unstable with moderate to high risk of ventricular asystole
Duration of high-grade AV block	Usually transient (2–3 days)	Usually transient, but some form of AV conduction disturbances and/or intraventricular defect may persist
Associated mortality rate	Low unless associated with hypotension and/or congestive heart failure	High because of extensive infarction associated with power failure or ventricular arrhythmias
Pacemaker therapy (a) Temporary (b) Permanent	(a) Rarely required; may be considered for bradycardia associated with left ventricular power failure, syncope, or angina (b) Almost never indicated; because conduction defect is usually transient	(a) Indicated in patients with anteroseptal infarction and acute bifascicular block (b) Indicated for patients with high-grade AV block with block in His-Purkinje systems and those with transient advanced AV block and associated bundle branch block

AV, atrioventricular; RCA, right coronary artery; LCx, left circumflex artery; LAD, left anterior descending artery.
[a]Some studies suggest that a wide QRS escape rhythm (greater than 0.12 sec) after high-grade AV block in inferior infarction is associated with a worse prognosis.
Modified from Antman EM. *Cardiovascular Therapeutics: A Companion Guide to Braunwald's Heart Disease*, 2nd ed. Philadelphia: Saunders, 2001:273.

portion of the unused lead that would ordinarily fit into the pacemaker or defibrillator generator in order to insulate it from the surrounding soft tissue. Such patients often have a new generator and lead system implanted on the contralateral side of the body. Although the risk of conveying current via the abandoned lead to the heart in such instances is small, one should still avoid placing defibrillation patches directly over pacemaker hardware, whether abandoned or still in use.

In the event that the energy administered to the pacemaker generator itself is greater than can be accommodated by the Zener diodes, the electronic components of the device can also be damaged.[49] Even if not damaged by the

| TABLE 24-2 • Recommendations for Treatment of Atrioventricular and Intraventricular Conduction Disturbances During STEMI

Intraventricular Conduction	Atrioventricular Conduction						
	Normal	First degree AV block		Mobitz I second degree AV block		Mobitz II second degree AV block	
		Anterior MI	Non-Anterior MI	Anterior MI	Non-Anterior MI	Anterior MI	Non-Anterior MI
	Action / Class	Action / Class	Action / Class	Action / Class	Action / Class	Action / Class	Action / Class
Normal	Observe I A III TC III TV III	Observe I A III TC IIb TV III	Observe I A III TC IIb TV III	Observe IIb A * TC I TV III	Observe IIa A * TC I TV III	Observe III A III TC I TV IIa	Observe III A III TC I TV IIa
Old or New Fascicular Block (LAFB or LPFB)	Observe I A III TC IIb TV III	Observe IIb A III TC I TV III	Observe IIb A III TC IIa TV III	Observe IIb A * TC I TV III	Observe IIb A * TC I TV III	Observe III A III TC I TV IIa	Observe III A III TC I TV IIb
Old Bundle Branch Block	Observe I A III TC IIb TV III	Observe III A III TC I TV IIb	Observe III A III TC I TV IIb	Observe III A * TC I TV IIb	Observe III A * TC I TV IIb	Observe III A III TC I TV IIa	Observe III A III TC I TV IIa
New Bundle Branch Block	Observe III A III TC I TV IIb	Observe III A III TC I TV IIa	Observe III A III TC I TV IIa	Observe III A * TC I TV IIa	Observe III A * TC I TV IIa	Observe III A III TC IIb TV I	Observe III A III TC IIb TV I
Fascicular Block + RBBB	Observe III A III TC I TV IIb	Observe III A III TC I TV IIa	Observe III A III TC I TV IIa	Observe III A * TC I TV IIa	Observe III A * TC I TV IIa	Observe III A III TC IIb TV I	Observe III A III TC IIb TV I
Alternating Left and Right Bundle Branch Block	Observe III A III TC IIb TV I	Observe III A III TC IIb TV I	Observe III A III TC IIb TV I	Observe III A * TC IIb TV I	Observe III A * TC IIb TV I	Observe III A III TC IIb TV I	Observe III A III TC IIb TV I

EXPLANATION OF TABLE:

This table is designed to summarize the atrioventricular (column headings) and intraventricular (row headings) conduction disturbances that may occur during acute anterior or nonanterior STEMI, the possible treatment options, and the indications for each possible therapeutic option.

Action

There are four possible actions, or therapeutic options, listed and classified for each bradyarrhythmia or conduction problem:

1. Observe: continued electrocardiographic monitoring, no further action planned.
2. A: atropine administered at 0.6 to 1.0 mg intravenously every 5 minutes to up to 0.04 mg/kg.
3. TC: application of transcutaneous pads and standby transcutaneous pacing with no further progression to transvenous pacing imminently planned.
4. TV: temporary transvenous pacing. It is assumed, but not specified in the table, at the discretion of the clinician, transcutaneous pads will be applied and standby transcutaneous pacing will be in effect as the patient is transferred to the fluoroscopy unit for temporary transvenous pacing.

Class

Each possible therapeutic option is further classified according to ACC/AHA criteria as I, IIa, IIb, and III. The level of evidence for all cells and all treatments is B or C. There are no randomized trials available that address or compare specific treatment options. Moreover, the data for this table and recommendations are largely derived from observational data of prethrombolytic era databases. Thus, the recommendations above must be taken as recommendations and tempered by the clinical circumstances.

Level of Evidence

This table was developed from: (1) published observational case reports and case series; (2) published summaries, not meta-analyses, of these data; and (3) expert opinion, largely from the prereperfusion era. There are no published randomized trials comparing different strategies of managing conduction disturbances post STEMI. Thus, the level of evidence for the recommendations in the table is C.

How to Use the Table

Example: 54-year-old man is admitted with an anterior STEMI and a narrow QRS on admission. On day 1 he develops a right bundle branch block (RBBB), with a PR interval of 0.28 seconds.

1. RBBB is an intraventricular conduction disturbance, so look at row "New BBB."
2. Find the column for "First Degree AV Block."
3. Find the "Action" and "Class" cells at the convergence.
4. Note that Observe and Atropine are class III, not indicated; transcutaneous pacing (TC) is class I. Temporary transvenous pacing (TV) is class IIb.

*In general, because the increase in heart rate with atropine is unpredictable, and may result in worsening ischemia, its administration should be avoided unless there is symptomatic bradycardia (such as sinus bradycardia or Mobitz I heart block) that will likely respond to its vagolytic effects. Administration of atropine should also be avoided when Mobitz I block occurs in the setting of an anterior MI and/or when there is QRS prolongation. This is because Mobitz I block is unusual during anterior MI (which more typically affects the distal conduction system rather than the AV node) and normally occurs in the absence of distal conduction disease (i.e. with a narrow QRS). When either an anterior MI or a widened QRS is present, suspicion should be raised that the level of Mobitz I block may actually be at or below the bundle of His rather than in the AV node, and potentially worsened by receipt of atropine.

Adapted from American College of Cardiology/American Heart Association Guidelines for the Management of ST Elevation Myocardial Infarction 45.

cardioversion shock, the pacemaker generator may be spontaneously reprogrammed to "default" pacing parameters (for example, from dual-chamber to ventricular pacing only) or may falsely indicate its having reached an elective replacement time due to low battery voltage.[50,51]

Avoiding such complications requires taking important precautions in treating patients with permanent pacemakers using cardioversion.[52] First, defibrillation electrodes should be placed as distant as possible from the pacemaker generator (manufacturers recommend 6 or more inches away) to protect the generator itself from exposure to higher shock energies and prevent current from being delivered to the lead via the Zener diode circuitry. Second, shocks should be administered perpendicular rather than parallel to the orientation of the pacemaker lead system. In particular avoiding the administration of shock in an anterolateral direction that parallels the typical anatomical course of transvenous pacemaker leads will minimize the risk of transmitting current along the same path as the pacemaker electrode to the heart. This prevents shock energy from potentially being carried from the proximal portion of the lead (in or near the pacemaker pocket) to its distal tip in the heart, resulting in potential damage to the heart at the lead tip. Figure 24-7 illustrates such positioning in a patient with an implanted pacemaker-defibrillator; the same principles apply to patients with implanted pacemakers.

Third, hospital providers should anticipate the possibility of pacer failure after shock delivery and have a pacemaker programmer (to reprogram a higher pacing output if required) and other bradycardia interventions in readiness. Fourth, all pacemakers should be formally interrogated after cardioversion or defibrillation procedures to evaluate for any changes in their programmed parameters or function. Finally, if possible, expert consultation should be sought in advance for all pacer patients who undergo cardioversion procedures.

Placement of Shock Electrodes

A recent study evaluated the safety of external electrical cardioversion of atrial fibrillation (taking the precautions listed earlier in this section) in patients having a variety of permanent pacemakers and ICDs that had been implanted in either the right or left infraclavicular regions. Cardioversion electrodes were uniformly placed strictly in the anterior-posterior position (to the right of the sternum with the upper edge of the electrode at the fourth anterior intercostal space; and to the left of the patient's spine at the midscapular level posteriorly). In addition, the anterior electrode was kept a minimum of 8 centimeters (approximately 3 inches) away from the implanted device. These precautions assured both a safe distance of shock electrodes away from the

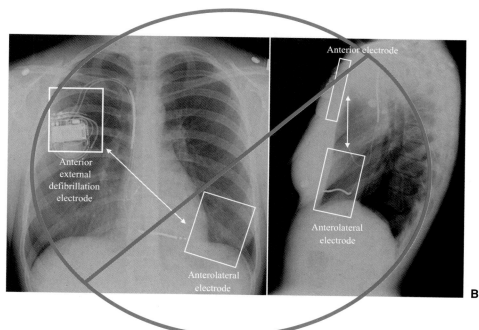

A

B

FIGURE 24-7 • A right pectoral ICD is shown, with overlying external defibrillator electrodes in the traditional right anterior and left anterolateral positions. The location of the defibrillator electrodes is shown in the anterior (**A**) and lateral (**B**) views of the chest x-ray. In this instance, the right anterior electrode directly overlies the ICD, whereas the anterolateral electrode lies at the apex of the heart. While appropriate for cardioversion or defibrillation of patients not having an implanted device, such an external shock configuration is likely to damage the generator (lying directly below one of the defibrillator pads), and the anterior to anterolateral direction of external shock mimics the path of the implanted leads and is likely to be transmitted along their course. This can result in damage at the interface of the lead tip and the heart. The red circle overlay emphasizes the point that placement of defibrillator pads in these locations is contraindicated in patients with an implanted pacemaker or defibrillator. Although exemplified for an ICD in this illustration, the same principles apply to implanted pacemakers.

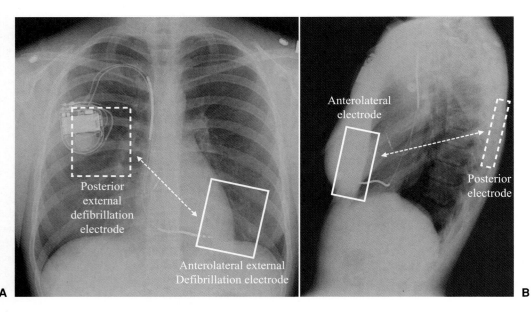

FIGURE 24-8 • Chest x-rays in the anterior (**A**) and lateral (**B**) views depicting the recommended location of external defibrillation electrodes in a patient with a right sided ICD. In this figure, the ICD generator is located on the patient's right side. One external defibrillator pad is placed posteriorly, to the right of the patient's spine at or slightly superior to the midscapular level (dotted rectangle indicates its posterior location) and the other pad is placed in its traditional anterolateral position (overlying the apex of the heart) (solid rectangle). The dotted arrow indicates the direction of the externally administered shock based on the pad locations. This external defibrillation electrode configuration (1) provides a safe distance from the generator (the posterior pad is separated from the generator by the thickness of the chest including soft tissue, ribs, lungs and scapula); (2) delivers a shock in a direction that is perpendicular to the orientation of the implanted leads, thereby minimizing the risk of electrical current passing along their course into the heart, and (3) encompasses the entire heart in the path of the externally administered shock. Although this figure illustrates defibrillation electrode positioning in a patient with an ICD, the same principles apply to patients with implanted pacemakers.

pacemaker or implanted cardioverter-defibrillator (ICD), and a shock direction that was perpendicular to the orientation of the implanted lead systems. Both biphasic and monophasic waveform escalating synchronized shocks were deployed ranging from 100 to 200 J and 200 to 360 J, respectively, including multiple shocks, if required, each separated by a 5-minute interval. No device or lead dysfunction resulting from cardioversion was observed in any patient.[53]

Of note, this external shock configuration may not necessarily be ideal for ventricular defibrillation. And, in cases where the implanted generator lies on the right side, it may be difficult for an anterior external defibrillator pad to avoid being placed too proximal to the generator. Therefore, an alternate, more "universal" location of external defibrillator pads may be preferable in patients with implanted pacemakers or defibrillators. As shown in Figures 24-8 and 24-9, this entails maintaining the left anterolateral defibrillation pad in its traditional left anterolateral position (near the apex of the heart). However the position of the right anterior pad is relocated posteriorly, to the right of the patient's spine at or slightly superior to the midscapular level (that is, directly posterior to the pad's customary right infraclavicular location). This configuration affords a safe distance from the generator (whatever its location), delivers shock in a direction that is always perpendicular to the orientation of the implanted leads, and encompasses the entire heart in the path of the externally administered shock. Its main disadvantage is the need to place one of the defibrillator pads on the patient's

back, which is problematic if defibrillation or cardioversion is being performed with paddles rather than pad electrodes.

Pacemaker Interference with Automatic External Defibrillators

In theory, a problem may be encountered when an automatic external defibrillator (AED) is used in patients with an implanted pacemaker who sustain a cardiac arrest. Should pacemaker activity be ongoing despite the presence of an underlying shockable rhythm, pacemaker spike artifact may mislead the AED arrhythmia detection algorithm to inappropriately withhold shock, mistaking the pacemaker spikes for an organized rhythm.[54] In such instances, use of a manual defibrillator that permits direct observation of the arrhythmia and manually administered defibrillation circumvents the problem.

Implanted Automatic Cardioverter-Defibrillators

The automatic implanted cardioverter-defibrillator (ICD) is increasingly used in patients who have a history of life-threatening ventricular arrhythmias or who are at high risk for developing such arrhythmias. In principle, the ICD detects an arrhythmia by counting its rate. A heart rate that exceeds a

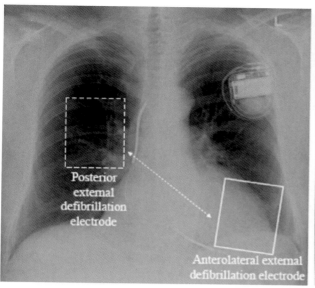
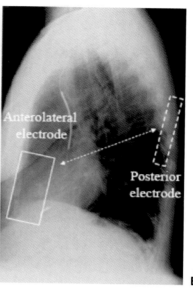

FIGURE 24-9 • Chest x-rays in the anterior (**A**) and lateral (**B**) views depicting the recommended location of external defibrillation electrodes in a patient with a left sided ICD. In this figure, the ICD generator is located on the patient's left side. One external defibrillator pad is placed posteriorly, to the right of the patient's spine at or slightly superior to the midscapular level (dotted rectangle indicates its posterior location) and the other pad is placed in its traditional anterolateral position (overlying the apex of the heart) (solid rectangle). The dotted arrow indicates the direction of the externally administered shock based on the pad locations. This external defibrillation electrode configuration (1) provides a safe distance from the generator (the pad is located contralateral to the generator); (2) delivers a shock in a direction that is perpendicular to the orientation of the implanted leads, thereby minimizing the risk of electrical current passing along their course into the heart; and (3) encompasses the entire heart in the path of the externally administered shock. Although this figures illustrates defibrillation electrode positioning in a patient with an ICD, the same principles apply to patients with implanted pacemakers.

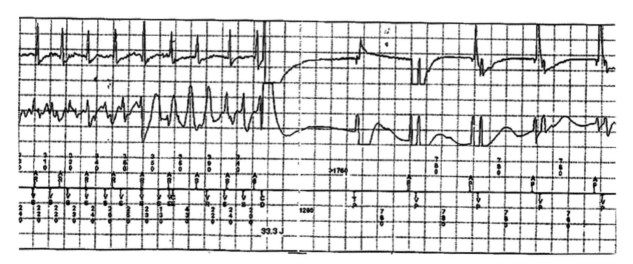

FIGURE 24-10 • Interrogation printout from an implanted dual-chamber ICD. The top tracing is a recording of the atrial electrogram from the right atrial lead of the device. The tracing immediately below this is a recording of the ventricular electrogram from the defibrillator lead. The lettering and numbers on the bottom of the tracing represent the device's interpretation of the events and their cycle length (the time interval between beats, measured in milliseconds) seen in the atrial and ventricular recordings. In this instance, the patient has polymorphic VT at a cycle length of about 220 to 240 milliseconds (rate of about 260 bpm), and a slower atrial cycle length of 360 milliseconds (about 170 bpm). Based on the ventricular rate and the presence of AV dissociation, the device appropriately detects the ventricular arrhythmia, charges, and delivers shock. Successful termination of the arrhythmia is followed by AV pacing (AP, VP) at a cycle length of 780 milliseconds (about 75 per minute).

programmed rate and duration prompts a response from the device, which can be in the form of rapid ventricular pacing and/or defibrillation shock (Fig. 24-10). Following treatment administration, the ICD reevaluates the rhythm to determine if repeated interventions are necessary. Depending upon the device's programming, the ICD can deliver multiple rapid pacing therapies and/or shocks. Once all therapies against an arrhythmia have been exhausted, without success, the ICD goes into a standby mode, without further delivery of therapies. If, however, the arrhythmia were to terminate or its rate falls below the programmed detection of the ICD, the device resets and thereafter approaches any detected arrhythmia as though it were of new onset. The main implication this has for care providers is the possibility that the ICD may be initiating antiarrhythmic therapies at the same time that CPR and other interventions are being administered. Conversely, it is unlikely that CPR itself (chest compressions) would result in false detection of a rhythm by the ICD (John Buysman, personal communication, Medtronic CRM Technical Support, June 7, 2007).

It is, therefore, advised by manufacturers, as with pacemakers, that defibrillator electrodes should be placed at least 6 inches away from the ICD, and shocks should be administered perpendicular to the orientation of the ICD leads and the heart.

In general, an ICD will likely have delivered its full complement of therapies within a few minutes of the patient's collapse. Thus, in encountering an unconscious, pulseless patient with an ICD, the most likely scenario is that the device has exhausted all of its therapies and failed to terminate the arrhythmia. All standard treatment measures should be initiated by providers, as though an implanted device were not present, including external defibrillation. However, ICDs require taking the same precautions as required for patients with pacemakers when external shocks are administered. In particular, providers should note where the ICD generator and leads are located and place external defibrillation electrodes accordingly. Although ICD generators, unlike pacemakers, are better protected from high-energy shock by specialized high-voltage circuitry rather than by Zener diodes, they are nonetheless susceptible to the same spectrum of damage. It is, therefore, advised by manufacturers, as with pacemakers, that defibrillator electrodes should be placed at least 6 inches away from the ICD and that shocks should be administered perpendicular to the orientation of the ICD leads and the heart.

Placement of Shock Electrodes

Placement of external shock electrodes in patients with ICDs is identical to that in those having permanent pacemakers, described and illustrated in the figures above.

Some patients with older ICD systems may have epicardial defibrillation electrodes and an ICD generator implanted in the abdomen rather than a pectoral location. In this instance external defibrillation electrodes may be placed in their traditional positions (right anterior infraclavicular and left antero-

lateral) without the need for other special precautions so long as each is a safe distance from the ICD generator. A theoretical concern in this instance is whether the epicardial defibrillator electrodes may insulate the heart from external shock and require higher energy settings in order to defibrillate successfully. In such instances, external cardioversion or defibrillation be attempted at high-energy settings.[55]

Intentional Suspension of ICD Tachycardia Functions

Malfunction of an ICD generator may result in multiple inappropriate shocks and require inactivation of the device.[56] In other instances, providers may want to prevent an ICD from providing competing treatments during resuscitation. In general, placing and maintaining the position of a donut magnet directly over the generator will usually inhibit its ability to detect tachycardias, resulting in withholding of tachycardia therapies.

Bradycardia pacing, if required, will not be affected by placement of the magnet. This is in contrast to the usual effect of a magnet on a permanent pacemaker, which typically forces asynchronous pacing regardless of the underlying rhythm.

Notably, depending upon the manufacturer, subsequent removal of the magnet may result in the ICD having been permanently inactivated and require reprogramming for reactivation. Thus, anytime a magnet is used in conjunction with an ICD, it should not be presumed that the ICD is necessarily operational upon the magnet's removal. Another caveat is that the ICD or pacemaker's response to magnet application can be device-specific; some manufacturers permit its inactivation by physicians, in which case the function of the implanted device will not be affected at all by magnet placement. Thus, expert consultation should be sought whenever possible in patients with implanted devices.

Interactions between ICDs and Automated External Defibrillators (AEDs)

ICDs and AEDs both deploy automated arrhythmia-detection algorithms. This can lead to "back-to-back" shocks should the ICD and AED simultaneously detect a shockable arrhythmia. In such instances, providers should recognize the sudden muscular contraction that identifies receipt of an ICD shock and, if possible, be prepared to inhibit AED shock delivery. In addition, ICDs deploy both bradycardia pacing and antitachycardia pacing, which can, in theory, mislead the AED detection algorithm as to the nature of the patient's rhythm.[57] Switching to a manual external defibrillator mode can circumvent such issues once providers with rhythm-recognition skills are on scene.

Risk of Shock to Providers

Unlike external defibrillation, which typically deploys 150 to 360 J, the maximum shock output from an ICD is only a fraction of this level and ranges between 30 to 40 J, depending on the manufacturer. However, approximately 20% of an ICD's shock voltage may reach the surface of the patient's skin.[62] Such voltage is not sufficient to cause harm to providers or others who are in contact with the patient at the time of ICD shock but may nonetheless be felt by them. Awareness of this possibility should prevent this from becoming a startling event. The voltage is sufficiently small that the provider is more likely to feel the effect of abrupt muscle contraction when the patient is shocked than the electrical impulse itself. However, the degree of discomfort felt depends on where and how the provider may be in contact with the patient at the time of shock. Transmission of shock from the patient to the provider requires a two-point contact in order to complete the electrical circuit and a conductor (such as sweat or defibrillator paddle gel) that facilitates transmission of current between the patient and care provider. Contact at only one location is unlikely to transmit shock to the provider unless the provider and patient are grounded to one another (for example, both on a wet surface). For the typical "heel of hand" on the chest, with the second hand overlying the first during CPR chest compressions, a relatively small single area is in contact with the patient and shock risk is minimal. In addition, providers who use protective gloves during resuscitation are insulated from the patient and are unlikely to experience shock unless the integrity of the glove has been compromised.[63] As a general rule, other than considering the location where defibrillation electrodes are placed, the presence of an ICD should not alter management of the patient in cardiac arrest.

As a general rule, other than considering the location where defibrillation electrodes are placed, the presence of an ICD should not alter management of the patient in cardiac arrest.

Managing Implanted Devices under Emergent Conditions

Prehospital providers invariably encounter patients in life-threatening emergencies about whom little or nothing is known and in whom searching for an implanted pacemaker or defibrillator may not be feasible before treatments must be initiated. In addition, clothing and other physical restrictions in the out-of-hospital environment may make placing defibrillation electrodes in nontraditional locations either infeasible or too time-consuming. Not all patients with pacemakers or pacemaker-defibrillators are dependent upon their devices for pacing. Hence even if such devices are damaged, the immediate effects may be inconsequential. For these reasons and because, in the final analysis, patient survival is more important than the survival of a pacemaker or pacemaker-defibrillator, it is acceptable, when required, to give implanted devices secondary consideration over the more urgent measures needed to save a life. In contrast, particularly in the hospital setting—where more about the patient is known, device programmers and temporary pacemakers are readily available, and there may be more time and opportunity to properly place defibrillation electrodes—treating patients in context of their implanted device is advisable.

Patient Safety during Operation of an External Defibrillator

Providers should make sure that the pads are separate and not touching. Providers should also ensure that paste or gel has not smeared along the skin between the paddles. Smearing of the paste or gel may allow current to follow a superficial pathway (arc) along the chest wall, "missing" the heart. Self-adhesive monitor/defibrillator electrode pads are as effective as gel pads or paste (level of evidence, 3[58–60]), and they can be placed before cardiac arrest to allow for monitoring and then rapid administration of an initial shock when necessary.[61] As a result, self-adhesive pads should be used routinely instead of standard paddles. Remember that the principles discussed above for correct placement also apply to pads as well. An improperly placed pad can decrease chances of successful defibrillation.

Do not place electrodes directly on top of a transdermal medication patch (e.g., patches containing nitroglycerin, nicotine, analgesics, hormone replacements, or antihypertensives), because the patch may block delivery of energy from the electrode pad to the heart and may cause small burns to the skin. Remove medication patches and wipe the area before attaching the electrode pad.

If an unresponsive patient is lying in water or the chest is covered with water, remove the patient from the water and briskly wipe the chest dry before attaching electrode pads and attempting defibrillation. Defibrillation can be accomplished when a patient is lying on snow or ice.

Fire Hazard and Prevention   Several case reports have described fires ignited by sparks from poorly applied defibrillator paddles in the presence of an oxygen-enriched atmosphere. Severe fires have been reported when ventilator tubing is disconnected from the endotracheal tube and then left adjacent to the patient's head, blowing oxygen across the chest during attempted defibrillation.

The use of self-adhesive defibrillation pads is probably the best way to minimize the risk of sparks igniting during defibrillation. If manual paddles are used, gel pads are preferable to electrode pastes and gels because the pastes and gels can spread between the two paddles, creating the potential for a spark. Do not use medical gels or pastes with poor electrical conductivity, such as ultrasound gel.

Providers should take precautions to minimize sparking during attempted defibrillation; try to ensure that defibrillation is not attempted in an oxygen-enriched atmosphere. When ventilation is interrupted for shock delivery, providers should try to ensure that oxygen does not flow across the patient's chest during defibrillation attempts.

Recommendations for Fire Prevention Defibrillator fires in oxygen-enriched environments, although rare, are an unacceptable danger to patients and health care providers. A defibrillator fire requires three fire-critical ingredients: an electrical arc, atmosphere enriched with oxygen, and an agent for flame propagation. If any one is lacking, a fire cannot occur. Prevention of defibrillator fires is relatively simple: prevent a defibrillation error *or* prevent an oxygen supply error.[64,65]

Proposals to routinely turn off or disconnect the oxygen supply immediately before defibrillation[65] have generated controversy,[66] primarily because supplying oxygen is considered a higher priority than instituting time-consuming steps simply to prevent fires.[67] Much of this controversy loses clinical relevancy when providers focus on proper defibrillation techniques to prevent an electrical arc from ever occurring. Oxygen flow should be turned off and airway adjuncts disconnected for patients at higher risk for electrical arc formation. All ACLS providers and instructors can help generate greater awareness of this danger. Most important, though, is the lesson that simply by performing resuscitation procedures properly and effectively, defibrillator-associated fires will remain a rare problem.

Provider Safety During Operation of an External Defibrillator

It is recommended that no one should be touching the patient during the delivery of external shock. However, recent evidence suggests that there is minimal risk of shock to a gloved rescuer should there be inadvertent contact with the patient while performing CPR.[68] This should not be taken as an "excuse" for unnecessary contact with the patient during administration of shock, but rather reassurance that with proper precautions, the risk of injury from shock to the care provider is minimal even if such contact were to occur.

References

1. Miller JM, Zipes DP. Therapy for cardiac arrhythmias. In Braunwald E, Zipes DP, Libby P, eds. *Heart Disease: A Textbook of Cardiovascular Medicine*, 7th ed. Philadelphia: Saunders, 2005: 736–739.
2. Guedon-Moreau L, Gayet JL, Galinier M, et al. Incidence of early adverse events surrounding direct current cardioversion of persistent atrial fibrillation. A cohort study of practices. *Therapie* 2007; 62(1):45–48.
3. Amir O, Schliamser JE, Nemer S, et al. Ineffectiveness of precordial thump for cardioversion of malignant ventricular tachyarrhythmias. *Pacing Clin Electrophysiol* 2007;30(2):153–156.
4. Ewy GA. Ventricular fibrillation and defibrillation. In: Ewy GA, Bressler R, eds. *Cardiovascular Drugs and the Management of Heart Disease*. New York: Raven Press, 1982:331–340.
5. Heames RM, Sado D, Deakin CD. Do doctors position defibrillation paddles correctly? Observational study. *BMJ* 2001;322(7299): 1393–1394.
6. Botto GL, Politi A, Bonini W, et al. External cardioversion of atrial fibrillation: role of paddle position on technical efficacy and energy requirements. *Heart* 1999;82(6):726–730.
7. Kirchhof P, Monnig G, Wasmer K, et al. A trial of self-adhesive patch electrodes and hand-held paddle electrodes for external cardioversion of atrial fibrillation (MOBIPAPA). *Eur Heart J* 2005;26 (13):1292–1297.
8. Walsh SJ, McCarty D, McClelland AJ, et al. Impedance compensated biphasic waveforms for transthoracic cardioversion of atrial fibrillation: a multi-centre comparison of antero-apical and antero-posterior pad positions. *Eur Heart J* 2005;26(13):1298–1302.
9. Bossaert L. Electrical defibrillation: new technologies. *Curr Opin Anaesthesiol* 1999;12(2):183–193.
10. Gurevitz OT, Ammash NM, Malouf JF, et al. Comparative efficacy of monophasic and biphasic waveforms for transthoracic cardioversion of atrial fibrillation and atrial flutter. *Am Heart J* 2005; 149(2):316–321.
11. Koster RW, Dorian P, Chapman FW, et al. A randomized trial comparing monophasic and biphasic waveform shocks for external cardioversion of atrial fibrillation. *Am Heart J* 2004;147(5):e20.
12. Kudenchuk PJ, Cobb LA, Copass MK, et al. Transthoracic incremental monophasic versus biphasic defibrillation by emergency responders (TIMBER): a randomized comparison of monophasic with biphasic waveform ascending energy defibrillation for the resuscitation of out-of-hospital cardiac arrest due to ventricular fibrillation. *Circulation* 2006;114(19):2010–2018.
13. Morrison LJ, Dorian P, Long J, et al. Out-of-hospital cardiac arrest rectilinear biphasic to monophasic damped sine defibrillation waveforms with advanced life support intervention trial (ORBIT). *Resuscitation* 2005;66(2):149–157.
14. Miller JM, Zipes DP. Specific arrhythmias: diagnosis and treatment. In: Braunwald E, Zipes DP, Libby P, eds. *Heart Disease: A Textbook of Cardiovascular Medicine*, 7th ed. Philadelphia: Saunders, 2005.
15. Kerber RE, Martins JB, Kienzle MG, et al. Energy, current, and success in defibrillation and cardioversion: clinical studies using an automated impedance-based method of energy adjustment. *Circulation* 1988;77(5):1038–1046.
16. Gallagher MM, Yap YG, Padula M, et al. Arrhythmic complications of electrical cardioversion: relationship to shock energy. *Int J Cardiol* 2008;123(3):307–312.
17. Page RL, Kerber RE, Russell JK, et al. Biphasic versus monophasic shock waveform for conversion of atrial fibrillation: the results of an international randomized, double-blind multicenter trial. *J Am Coll Cardiol* 2002;39(12):1956–1963.
18. Mittal S, Ayati S, Stein KM, et al. Transthoracic cardioversion of atrial fibrillation: comparison of rectilinear biphasic versus damped sine wave monophasic shocks. *Circulation* 2000;101(11): 1282–1287.
19. Alatawi F, Gurevitz O, White R. Prospective, randomized comparison of two biphasic waveforms for the efficacy and safety of transthoracic biphasic cardioversion of atrial fibrillation. *Heart Rhythm* 2005;2:382–387.
20. Miller JM. Specific arrhythmias: diagnosis and treatment. In: Braunwald E, Libby P, ed. *Heart Disease: A Textbook of Cardiovascular Medicine*, 7th ed. Philadelphia: Saunders, 2005.
21. Morrison LJ, Dorian P, Long J, et al. Out-of-hospital cardiac arrest rectilinear biphasic to monophasic damped sine defibrillation waveforms with advanced life support intervention trial (ORBIT). *Resuscitation* 2005;66(2):149–157.
22. Stiell IG, Walker RG, Nesbitt LP, et al. BIPHASIC Trial: a randomized comparison of fixed lower versus escalating higher energy levels for defibrillation in out-of-hospital cardiac arrest. *Circulation* 2007;115(12):1511–1517.
23. Gauss A, Hubner C, Radermacher P, et al. Perioperative risk of bradyarrhythmias in patients with asymptomatic chronic bifascicular block or left bundle branch block. *Anesthesiology* 1998;88(3): 679–687.
24. Gauss A, Hubner C, Meierhenrich R, et al. Perioperative transcutaneous pacemaker in patients with chronic bifascicular block or left bundle branch block and additional first-degree atrioventricular block. *Acta Anaesthesiol Scand* 1999;43(7):731–736.
25. Dalsey WC, Syverud SA, Hedges JR. Emergency department use of transcutaneous pacing for cardiac arrests. *Crit Care Med* 1985;13(5):399–401.
26. Eitel DR, Guzzardi LJ, Stein SE, et al. Noninvasive transcutaneous cardiac pacing in prehospital cardiac arrest. *Ann Emerg Med* 1987; 16(5):531–534.
27. Cummins RO, Graves JR, Larsen MP, et al. Out-of-hospital transcutaneous pacing by emergency medical technicians in patients with asystolic cardiac arrest. *N Engl J Med* 1993;328(19): 1377–1382.
28. Paris PM, Stewart RD, Kaplan RM, et al. Transcutaneous pacing for bradyasystolic cardiac arrests in prehospital care. *Ann Emerg Med* 1985;14(4):320–323.

29. Proano L, Chiang WK, Wang RY. Calcium channel blocker overdose. *Am J Emerg Med* 1995;13(4):444–450.

30. Watson NA, FitzGerald CP. Management of massive verapamil overdose. *Med J Aust* 1991;155(2):124–125.

31. Gotz D, Pohle S, Barckow D. Primary and secondary detoxification in severe flecainide intoxication. *Intens Care Med* 1991;17(3):181–184.

32. Cummins R, Graves J, Haulman J, et al. Near-fatal yew berry intoxication treated with external cardiac pacing and digoxin-specific FAB antibody fragments. *Ann Emerg Med* 1991;19:38–43.

33. Quan L, Graves JR, Kinder DR, et al. Transcutaneous cardiac pacing in the treatment of out-of-hospital pediatric cardiac arrests. *Ann Emerg Med* 1992;21(8):905–909.

34. Sherbino J, Verbeek PR, MacDonald RD, et al. Prehospital transcutaneous cardiac pacing for symptomatic bradycardia or bradyasystolic cardiac arrest: a systematic review. *Resuscitation* 2006;70(2):193–200.

35. Craig K. How to provide transcutaneous pacing. *Nursing* 2005;35(10):52–53.

36. Zoll PM. Development of electric control of cardiac rhythm. *JAMA* 1973;226(8):881–886.

37. Zoll PM, Belgard AH, Weintraub MJ, et al. External mechanical cardiac stimulation. *N Engl J Med* 1976;294(23):1274–1276.

38. Schechter DC. *Exploring the Origins of Electrical Cardiac Stimulation.* Minneapolis, MN: Medtronic, 1983.

39. Sutton R, Bourgeois I. *The Foundations of Cardiac Pacing: An Illustrated Practical Guide to Basic Pacing,* vol 1. Mount Kisco, NY: Futura, 1991.

40. Syverud SA, Hedges JR, Dalsey WC, et al. Hemodynamics of transcutaneous cardiac pacing. *Am J Emerg Med* 1986;4(1):17–20.

41. Dalsey WC, Syverud SA, Ross DS, et al. Transcutaneous cardiac pacing. *Ann Emerg Med* 1984;13(5):410–411.

42. Jones M, Geddes LA. Strength-duration curves for cardiac pacemaking and ventricular fibrillation. *Cardiovasc Res Cent Bull* 1977;15(4):101–112.

43. Voorhees WD III, Foster KS, Geddes LA, et al. Safety factor for precordial pacing: minimum current thresholds for pacing and for ventricular fibrillation by vulnerable-period stimulation. *Pacing Clin Electrophysiol* 1984;7(3 Pt 1):356–360.

44. Falk RH, Zoll PM, Zoll RH. Safety and efficacy of noninvasive cardiac pacing. A preliminary report. *N Engl J Med* 1983;309(19):1166–1168.

45. Antman EM, Anbe DT, Armstrong PW, et al. ACC/AHA guidelines for the management of patients with ST-elevation myocardial infarction: a report of the American College of Cardiology/American Heart Association Task Force on Practice Guidelines (Committee to Revise the 1999 Guidelines for the Management of Patients with Acute Myocardial Infarction). *Circulation* 2004;110 (9):e82–e292.

46. Waller C, Callies F, Langenfeld H. Adverse effects of direct current cardioversion on cardiac pacemakers and electrodes: is external cardioversion contraindicated in patients with permanent pacing systems? *Europace* 2004;6(2):165–168.

47. Altamura G, Bianconi L, Lo Bianco F, et al. Transthoracic DC shock may represent a serious hazard in pacemaker dependent patients. *Pacing Clin Electrophysiol* 1995;18(1 Pt 2):194–198.

48. Das G, Staffanson DB. Selective dysfunction of ventricular electrode-endocardial junction following DC cardioversion in a patient with a dual chamber pacemaker. *Pacing Clin Electrophysiol* 1997;20 (2 Pt 1):364–365.

49. Alferness CA. Pacemaker damage due to external countershock in patients with implanted cardiac pacemakers. *Pacing Clin Electrophysiol* 1982;5(3):457–458.

50. Aylward P, Blood R, Tonkin A. Complications of defibrillation with permanent pacemaker in situ. *Pacing Clin Electrophysiol* 1979;2(4):462–464.

51. Das G, Eaton J. Pacemaker malfunction following transthoracic countershock. *Pacing Clin Electrophysiol* 1981;4(5):487–490.

52. External defibrillation or direct current cardioversion (revision B). Minneapolis, MN: CRM Technical Services, Medtronic, 2007.

53. Manegold JC, Israel CW, Ehrlich JR, et al. External cardioversion of atrial fibrillation in patients with implanted pacemaker or cardioverter-defibrillator systems: a randomized comparison of monophasic and biphasic shock energy application. *Eur Heart J* 2007;28(14):1731–1738.

54. Monsieurs KG, Conraads VM, Goethals MP, et al. Semi-automatic external defibrillation and implanted cardiac pacemakers: understanding the interactions during resuscitation. *Resuscitation* 1995;30(2):127–131.

55. Walls JT, Schuder JC, Curtis JJ, et al. Adverse effects of permanent cardiac internal defibrillator patches on external defibrillation. *Am J Cardiol* 1989;64(18):1144–1147.

56. Pinski SL. Emergencies related to implantable cardioverter-defibrillators. *Crit Care Med* 2000;28(10 Suppl):N174–N180.

57. Calle PA, Buylaert W. When an AED meets an ICD. . . automated external defibrillator. Implantable cardioverter defibrillator. *Resuscitation* 1998;38(3):177–183.

58. Stults KR, Brown DD, Cooley F, et al. Self-adhesive monitor/defibrillation pads improve prehospital defibrillation success. *Ann Emerg Med* 1987;16(8):872–877.

59. Kerber RE, Martins JB, Kelly KJ, et al. Self-adhesive preapplied electrode pads for defibrillation and cardioversion. *J Am Coll Cardiol* 1984;3(3):815–820.

60. Kerber RE, Martins JB, Ferguson DW, et al. Experimental evaluation and initial clinical application of new self-adhesive defibrillation electrodes. *Int J Cardiol* 1985;8(1):57–66.

61. Perkins GD, Roberts C, Gao F. Delays in defibrillation: influence of different monitoring techniques. *Br J Anaesth* 2002;89(3):405–408.

62. Peters W, Kowallik P, Reisberg M, et al. Body surface potentials during discharge of the implantable cardioverter defibrillator. *J Cardiovasc Electrophysiol* 1998;9(5):491–497.

63. Lechleuthner A. Electric shock to paramedic during cardiopulmonary resuscitation of patient with implanted cardiodefibrillator. *Lancet* 1995;345(8944):253.

64. ECRI. Defibrillation in oxygen-enriched environments. *Health Dev* 1987;16:113–114.

65. ECRI. Fires from defibrillation during oxygen administration. *Health Dev* 1994;23:307–309.

66. Lefever J, Smith A. Risk of fire when using defibrillation in an oxygen enriched atmosphere. *Med Dev Agency Safety Notices* 1995;03:1–3.

67. McAnulty GR, Robertshaw H. Risk of fire outweighed by need for oxygen and defibrillation. *J Accid Emerg Med* 1999;16(1):77.

68. Lloyd MS, Heeke B, Walter PF, et al. Hand-on defibrillation: An analysis of electrical current flow through rescuers in direct contact with patients during biphasic external defibrillation. *Circulation* 2008;117:2510–2515.

Pharmacology in Emergency Cardiovascular Care

Chapter 25
Drugs for Control of Rhythm

Peter J. Kudenchuk

Antiarrhythmic agents have the potential for benefit as well as harm. Their benefit is maximized when rhythm diagnosis is accurate and when thought is given to targeted treatment.

- Classification of antiarrhythmia drugs
- Risk–benefit for administration: proarrhythmia consideration
- Use of individual antiarrhythmia agents

Using Antiarrhythmics

Antiarrhythmic agents have the potential for benefit as well as harm. Their benefit is maximized when rhythm diagnosis is accurate and when thought is given to targeted treatment. In patients who are hemodynamically compromised by an acute arrhythmia, the approach of choice is to treat first with immediate cardioversion. Conversely, the approach of choice in patients who are hemodynamically stable in the face of an acute arrhythmia is to think first and then treat accordingly. Algorithms are intended to promote such thoughtful approaches to management. Because of the focus on emergency care, only agents that are available in parenteral form are presented in this discussion, not all of which are available in such a formulation within the United States. Recommended dosing guidelines for the drugs discussed, if approved for use in the United States, are taken from published prescribing sources. For drugs not approved for use in the United States, doses are derived from the published studies that evaluated these medications. It is advisable for the reader to refer to these sources for confirmaton of these doses or any change that might have transpired since publication of this text.

Preferred Routes of Drug Administration

Peripheral or Central IV

A peripheral vein is the first choice for intravenous (IV) access in patients, particularly during cardiac arrest. Central line access (internal jugular or subclavian) requires interruption of chest compressions. Peak drug concentrations, however, are lower and circulation times are longer when drugs are administered via peripheral sites compared with central sites.[1–3] When given via a peripheral vein, drugs require 1 to 2 minutes to reach the central circulation; this delay is appreciably shorter with a central venous route. Peripheral venous cannulation, however, is easier to learn, results in fewer complications, and does not require interruption of cardiopulmonary resuscitation (CPR).

If peripheral venous access is used during resuscitative efforts, IV drugs should be administered by bolus injection; follow with a 20-mL bolus of IV fluid and elevation of the extremity to facilitate transport into the central circulation.[4] Unless there are contraindications, if peripheral veins are inaccessible and experienced providers are available, placement of a central line should be considered. Placement of central lines can cause a pneumothorax and potentially increase the risk of bleeding complications for patients who subsequently receive fibrinolytic therapy.

Endotracheal Drug Administration

If an endotracheal tube has been placed before venous access is achieved, lipid-soluble drugs such as epinephrine,[5,6] lidocaine, and atropine[7,8] can be administered via the tube; absorption occurs in the lungs. Much of the evidence for the efficacy of endotracheal administration of drugs stems from studies under normal or near normal circulatory conditions.[9] Notably, there is no clinical evidence that endotracheal administration of drugs at recommended doses is necessarily effective under cardiac arrest conditions. Because pulmonary blood flow is compromised during cardiac arrest and CPR, transalveolar drug absorption is minimal. Therefore, even higher doses of medications may be needed to achieve the same serum levels as when such agents are administered intravenously.[10]

Because administration of resuscitation drugs via the trachea results in lower blood concentrations than when they are given intravenously, it has traditionally been taught to give all endotracheal medications at 2 to 2.5 times the recommended IV dose, diluted in 10 mL of normal saline or distilled water. Lung absorption is greater with distilled water as the diluent than with normal saline, but distilled water has a greater adverse effect on PaO_2. The technique for administration is to pass a catheter beyond the tip of the endotracheal tube, stop chest compressions, inject the drug solution quickly down the catheter, follow immediately with several quick lung insufflations to create a rapidly absorbed aerosol, and then resume chest compressions.[5]

The endotracheal administration of drugs that are not lipid-soluble, such as calcium and sodium bicarbonate, may result in airway injury; therefore, they should not be administered in this manner. While endotracheal use of other drugs such as naloxone and vasopressin is permissible, dosing is uncertain.

Intraosseous Drug Administration

Intraosseous access uses the marrow (medullary) cavity of bones such as the tibia or sternum as a "noncollapsible vein" for parenteral access in both children and adults. This is regarded as a viable alternative to conventional IV line placement under emergency conditions where vascular access is not otherwise possible. The technique requires special training and is described in detail elsewhere.[11] Virtually all fluids and medications that can be administered intravenously can be given by intraosseous means without dose modification and can achieve as rapid an entry into the central circulation, with concentrations and peak effects comparable to those of IV administration.[12] If properly performed, complications from intraosseous access are uncommon; however, they can include extravasation of fluid, fractures at the insertion site, compartment syndrome, fat emboli, cellulitis, and local infection.

Basic Principles of Antiarrhythmic Therapy

No antiarrhythmic agent has yet been proven to improve survival after cardiac arrest. Nonetheless, such drugs are useful for the control of shock-refractory arrhythmias and to restore and maintain sinus rhythm. Their benefits must be balanced against their potential risks. Proarrhythmias are serious tachyarrhythmias or bradyarrhythmias generated by antiarrhythmic agents. All antiarrhythmic agents have some degree of proarrhythmic risk, and sicker hearts appear more susceptible to such effects. Tachyarrhythmias, such as torsade de pointes, account for most proarrhythmia events. Other manifestations of proarrhythmia can include frequent premature ventricular contractions (PVCs) and incessant ventricular tachycardia (VT).

The interactions between antiarrhythmic agents are also complex because of their differing effects on a variety of ionic channels in the heart. Sequential use of two or more antiarrhythmic drugs compounds the adverse effects, particularly for bradycardia, hypotension, and torsades de pointes. Therefore, it is best to avoid use of more than one agent unless absolutely necessary. In most patients, when an appropriate dose of a single antiarrhythmic medication fails to terminate an arrhythmia, it is wiser to turn to electrical cardioversion rather than a second antiarrhythmic medication.

Patients with clinical congestive heart failure or depressed left ventricular (LV) function should also be treated cautiously with antiarrhythmic therapy. In these patients, many antiarrhythmic agents depress LV function further, often precipitating or worsening congestive heart failure. In addition, the risk of proarrhythmia is higher.

Because of its broad antiarrhythmic spectrum, lesser negative inotropic effect, and low incidence of proarrhythmia, amiodarone continues to dominate the management of tachycardias. If amiodarone fails to produce the desired response, the preferred next intervention is to attempt early electrical cardioversion.

Classification of Antiarrhythmic Drugs

Vaughan Williams Classification

Traditionally antiarrhythmic drugs are classified according to site of action or electrophysiologic effects. The Vaughan Williams classification is the most widely used of these classification schemes.[13] The system is practical, although it oversimplifies the complex cellular-level, ionic-channel processes involved in rhythm genesis. The Vaughan Williams system labels antiarrhythmics based on the ion channels or receptors that they block. It classifies a drug according to (1) whether the blocked ionic channel is sodium, potassium, or calcium; (2) whether the drug blocks beta-adrenergic receptors; and (3) the effect of the drug on conduction and repolarization (Table 25-1). Most advanced cardiac life support (ACLS) drugs for rhythm and rate reviewed below are classified according to the Vaughan Williams system (Table 25-2). The following information about scientific evidence, drug indications, and drug doses refers to the parenteral forms of all drugs. During emergencies, antiarrhythmics should be administered by the parenteral route.

Sicilian Gambit

The Sicilian Gambit is a classification of antiarrhythmic agents by the European Society of Cardiology. It is more accurate but more cumbersome[14,15] than the Vaughan Williams system. In the Sicilian Gambit, antiarrhythmic drugs are grouped according to their multiple channel-blocking effects (Fig. 25-1).

The Sicilian Gambit reports the work of a group of basic and clinical investigators who met in Taormina, Sicily, to consider the classification of antiarrhythmic drugs. Paramount to their considerations were

- Their dissatisfaction with the options offered by existing classification systems for inspiring and directing research, development, and therapy
- The disarray in the field of antiarrhythmic drug development and testing following the Cardiac Arrhythmia Suppression Trial (CAST)
- The desire to provide a framework for consideration of antiarrhythmic drugs that will encourage scientific advances and possess the flexibility to grow as advances are made

For more information, the interested reader is encouraged to read the full report,[3] which contains

- A discussion of the shortcomings of the current system for antiarrhythmic classification
- A review of the molecular targets of antiarrhythmic effects (including channels and receptors)
- A consideration of the mechanisms responsible for arrhythmias, including identification of "vulnerable parameters" that might be most accessible to drug effect
- Clinical considerations when deploying antiarrhythmic drugs

Amiodarone

IV amiodarone is a complex drug with effects on sodium, potassium, and calcium channels as well as alpha- and beta-adrenergic blocking properties. The drug is useful for treatment of atrial and ventricular arrhythmias. In patients with severely impaired heart function, IV amiodarone is preferable to other antiarrhythmic agents because of its greater efficacy and lower incidence of proarrhythmic effects. Uses and indications include:

- Cardiac arrest due to persistent VT or ventricular fibrillation (VF)
- Hemodynamically stable VT, polymorphic VT (where torsades de pointes is not suspected), and wide-complex tachycardia of uncertain origin
- Ventricular rate control of rapid atrial arrhythmias in patients with severely impaired LV function when digitalis has proved ineffective
- Pharmacologic conversion of supraventricular arrhythmias that are refractory to other agents
- Control of rapid ventricular rate due to accessory pathway conduction in preexcited atrial arrhythmias

Cardiac Arrest

Amiodarone is a potent and effective antiarrhythmic agent for the termination of hemodynamically unstable ventricular arrhythmias, including treatment of cardiac arrest due to VF and pulseless VT.[16–18] The major drawbacks to its use are a somewhat cumbersome manner of administration in an emergency setting (it is packaged in 150-mg [3-cc] glass ampules, is not available in prefilled syringes, requires dilution prior to administration, and calls for care to prevent foaming of its diluent in this process), and the incidence of hypotension and bradycardia.

Two high-quality randomized trials of shock-resistant out-of-hospital cardiac arrest—one of which compared amiodarone against placebo and another against lidocaine—demonstrated that it improved the likelihood of successful resuscitation and admission alive to hospital but did not have a significant effect on survival to hospital discharge.[18,19] In both of these trials, amiodarone, by design, was administered relatively late in resuscitation. Its potential to improve long-term survival if given earlier in the course of resuscitation is untested.

TABLE 25-1 • Classification of Antiarrhythmic Drugs Modified from the Vaughan Williams System

Vaughan Williams Classification[a]	Channel Effects (Strength)	Effects on Action Potential, Automaticity, and Conduction	ACLS Drugs	Conditions Treated
Class I Ia_{vw}	Sodium channel blockers (moderate)	Phase 0: rapid depolarization phase caused by sodium influx. These drugs produce *moderate slowing* of sodium influx.	Procainamide Disopyramide Quinidine	• Recurrent VF/VT • Stable monomorphic/polymorphic VT • AF/atrial flutter with and without WPW
Ib_{vw}	Sodium channel blockers (weak)	Phase 0: rapid depolarization phase caused by sodium influx. These drugs produce *slight slowing* of sodium influx.	Lidocaine	• Persistent VF/VT • Stable monomorphic/polymorphic VT
Ic_{vw}	Sodium channel blockers (strong)	Phase 0: rapid depolarization phase caused by sodium influx. These drugs produce *marked slowing* of sodium influx.	Propafenone Flecainide	• AF/atrial flutter with and without WPW
Class II_{vw}	Beta-adrenergic blockers	Beta-adrenergic receptor sites → blocked by drugs: • Decreased SA node automaticity • Slowed AV node conduction	Atenolol Metoprolol Propranolol Esmolol Labetalol	• Narrow-complex tachycardias; stable; preserved ventricular function • Stable polymorphic VT; normal QT interval
Class III_{vw}	Potassium channel blockers	Phase 3: rapid repolarization phase; caused by potassium efflux. Phase prolonged by drugs that block potassium efflux: • Prolonged action potential • Prolonged relative refractory period	Amiodarone Bretylium Dofetilide Ibutilide Sotalol	• Persistent VF/VT • Stable monomorphic/polymorphic VT • Narrow-complex tachycardias; stable; preserved/impaired ventricular function
Class IV_{vw}	Calcium channel blockers	Phase 4: spontaneous depolarization; caused by calcium and sodium influx. This phase may be modulated by these drugs. • Decreased SA node automaticity • Slowed AV node conduction	Diltiazem Verapamil	• Control rate in AF/atrial flutter • Narrow-complex tachycardias; stable; preserved ventricular function

[a]The word *Class* with subscript VW (e.g., Class II_{vw}) is used to indicate the Vaughan Williams classification of antiarrhythmics. This use of the word *Class* should not be confused with the AHA Class of Recommendations used in the *ECG Guidelines 2000*.
WPW, Wolff-Parkinson-White syndrome; SA, sinoatrial.
Unclassified: Digoxin (sodium-potassium ATPase inhibitor, vagomimetic) and adenosine (adenosine receptor agonist).

Other Arrhythmias

IV amiodarone is an effective antiarrhythmic agent for virtually any tachyarrhythmia, but it is most commonly used for ventricular arrhythmias and atrial fibrillation or flutter with and without preexcitation.[19–47] It has not been studied specifically for the pharmacologic termination of hemodynamically stable VT, but it is likely to be effective based on experience of its success in treating hemodynamically unstable VT and VF.[16,17,44,47–55]

Dosing and Administration

IV amiodarone is administered as 150 mg over 10 minutes, followed by an infusion of 1 mg/min for 6 hours and then 0.5 mg/min. Supplementary infusions of 150 mg can be repeated as necessary for recurrent or resistant arrhythmias to a maximum manufacturer-recommended total daily dose of 2 g. One study found amiodarone to be effective in the pharmacologic conversion of atrial fibrillation when it is administered at relatively high doses of 125 mg/hr for 24

TABLE 25-2 • Major Pharmacologic Effects of ACLS Medications Arranged According to the Vaughan Williams Classification

Major Pharmacologic Effect	Vaughan Williams Classification of ACLS Medications
Sodium channel blockers	Class Ia: Moderate • Procainamide • Disopyramide • Quinidine Class Ib: Weak • Lidocaine Class Ic: Strong • Propafenone • Flecainide
Beta-adrenergic blockers	Class II • Atenolol • Metoprolol • Propranolol • Esmolol • Labetalol
Potassium channel blockers	Class III • Amiodarone • Bretylium • Dofetilide • Ibutilide • Sotalol
Calcium channel blockers	Class IV • Diltiazem • Verapamil
Other agents that affect rhythm and rate	Miscellaneous • Adenosine • Atropine • Magnesium • Digoxin • Dopamine • Isoproterenol

hours (total dose 3 g).[56] In cardiac arrest due to pulseless VT or VF, IV amiodarone is initially administered as a 300-mg rapid infusion diluted in a volume of 20 to 30 mL of saline or dextrose in water. Based on extrapolation from studies in patients with hemodynamically unstable VT, supplementary doses of 150 mg by rapid infusion may be administered for recurrent or refractory VT/VF, followed by an infusion of 1 mg/min for 6 hours and then 0.5 mg/min, to a maximum daily dose of 2 g.

IV amiodarone has bradycardic and vasodilatory (hypotensive) effects, which can destabilize patients who may already have a tenuous hemodynamic status.[16,57,58] The hypotensive effect is felt to be related to its diluent rather than to amiodarone itself and perhaps to histamine release. Hypotension is most commonly seen during the initial rather than repeat dosing of IV amiodarone. The major adverse effects from amiodarone can be prevented by slowing the rate of drug infusion, or they can be treated as necessary with fluids, pressors, chronotropic agents, or temporary pacing.

Adenosine

Adenosine is an endogenous purine nucleoside that depresses the activity of the atrioventricular (AV) and sinus nodes. Adenosine produces a short-lived pharmacologic response because it is rapidly metabolized by enzymatic degradation in blood and peripheral tissue. The half-life of adenosine is <5 seconds.

Indications

Adenosine is indicated for paroxysmal supraventricular tachycardia (PSVT) whether it is due to AV-nodal reentry or AV reentry mediated by an accessory pathway.[59] These forms of PSVT involve a reentry pathway including the AV node as at least one limb of the circuit. Adenosine is effective in terminating these arrhythmias. If the arrhythmias are not due to reentry involving the AV node (such as atrial flutter, atrial fibrillation, or other atrial arrhythmias), adenosine will not terminate the arrhythmia but may produce transient AV block, which may clarify the diagnosis. However, because of its ultrashort half-life, adenosine is not appropriate for ventricular rate control of AF or atrial flutter.

Adenosine is also not an effective agent for common forms of ventricular arrhythmias and is contraindicated in preexcited atrial arrhythmias such as AF or atrial flutter.[60-64] In the past, use of adenosine was advocated to discriminate VT from supraventricular tachycardia (SVT) with aberrancy in hemodynamically stable wide-complex tachycardia of uncertain origin. This led to instances of worsened hypotension after inappropriate treatment with adenosine for VT.[62] Such practice is discouraged, and adenosine is recommended for use only when a supraventricular origin is strongly suspected.

Dosing

The recommended initial dose of adenosine is a 6-mg rapid bolus over 1 to 3 seconds.[65] The dose should be followed by a 20-mL saline flush. Rapid (bolus) administration is required because the effect of adenosine on nodal tissue is concentration-dependent; slower infusion is more likely to result only in hypotension due to its systemic vasodilatory effects. If no response is observed within 1 to 2 minutes, a 12-mg repeated dose should be administered in the same manner. Experience with larger doses is limited, but patients taking theophylline are less sensitive to adenosine and may require such larger doses.

Side effects with adenosine are common but transient; flushing, dyspnea, and chest pain are the most frequently observed.[66] Adenosine carries the risk of causing angina, bronchospasm, proarrhythmia, and acceleration of accessory pathway conduction.[62] Because of the short half-life of

Drug	Channels					Receptors				Vaughan Wiliams Class
	Na			Ca	K	α	β	M₂	P	
	Fast	Med	Slow							
Lidocaine	●									Ib
Procainamide		Ⓐ			●					Ia
Disopyramide		Ⓐ			●			●		Ia
Quinidine		Ⓐ			●	●		●		Ia
Propafenone		Ⓐ					●			Ic
Flecainide			Ⓐ		●					Ic
Verapamil	●			●		●				IV
Diltiazem				●						IV
Bretylium					●	●	●			III
Sotalol					●		●			III
Amiodarone		●		●	●	●	●			III
Propranolol	●						●			II
Atropine								●		
Adenosine									●	
Digoxin*								●		

Relative blocking potency:

● Low ● Agonist

● Moderate ● Agonist/Antagonist

● High A=Activated state blocker
*Digoxin is also a Na/K ATPase pump blocker (high relative potency)

| FIGURE 25-1 • The Sicilian gambit.

adenosine, PSVT may recur once its effects have abated. Recurrent PSVT may be treated with additional doses of adenosine or with a longer-acting AV-nodal blocking agent (calcium channel blocker or beta-blocker). The systemic hypotensive effects of adenosine are mitigated by successful conversion of PSVT. In the event that the arrhythmia is not terminated, drug-induced hypotension, though transient, may require treatment.

Adenosine has several important drug interactions. Therapeutic concentrations of theophylline or related methylxanthines (caffeine and theobromine) block the receptor responsible for the electrophysiologic and hemodynamic effects of adenosine. Dipyridamole blocks adenosine uptake and potentiates its effects. The effects of adenosine are also prolonged in patients on carbamazepine and those with denervated transplanted hearts. Dose adjustment or alternative therapy should be selected in such patients.

Atropine

Atropine sulfate reverses cholinergic-mediated decreases in heart rate, systemic vascular resistance, and blood pressure.[67] Atropine is useful in treating symptomatic sinus bradycardia. It may be beneficial in the presence of AV block at the nodal level (Mobitz I second-degree AV block) or ventricular asystole but should not be used when infranodal (Mobitz type II) block is suspected. Its use in the latter setting may worsen rather than enhance AV conduction.

Dosing

The recommended dose of atropine sulfate for asystole and slow pulseless electrical activity is 1 mg IV, repeated in 3 to 5 minutes if asystole persists. For bradycardia, the dose is 0.5 mg every 3 to 5 minutes to a total dose of 0.04 mg/kg. A total dose of 3 mg (0.04 mg/kg) results in full vagal blockade in humans. Because atropine increases myocardial oxygen demand and can initiate tachyarrhythmias, the administration of a total vagolytic dose of atropine should be reserved for asystolic cardiac arrest. Doses of atropine sulfate <0.5 mg may be parasympathomimetic and further slow the cardiac rate. Atropine can be administered intravenously or by intraosseous means, and it is also well absorbed via the endotracheal route of administration.

Atropine should be used cautiously in the presence of acute coronary ischemia or myocardial infarction (MI), because excessive increases in rate may worsen ischemia or increase the zone of infarction. VF and VT rarely follow IV administration of atropine. Atropine is not indicated in bradycardia from AV block at the His–Purkinje level (second-degree AV block type II and third-degree AV block with new wide-QRS complexes). In such instances atropine can accelerate sinus rate and worsen AV conduction.

Beta-Adrenergic Blockers

Beta-adrenergic blockers inhibit sympathetic tone on the sinus node and AV node, resulting in sinus bradycardia and slowing of AV-nodal conduction.[68] This makes the drugs useful for termination of PSVT due to AV-nodal reentry or AV reentry mediated by an accessory pathway as well as for rate control of atrial arrhythmias (such as AF, atrial flutter, ectopic atrial tachycardia, and multifocal atrial tachycardia) without preexcitation. Inhibition of sympathetic tone may also have a beneficial effect on recurrent ventricular arrhythmias.[69] Beta-adrenergic blockers also have potential benefits outside the scope of this discussion, as in patients with acute coronary syndromes.

Dosing

The effect of an intravenously administered beta-blocker is transient. In studies where beta-blockers were deployed for acute MI, IV doses were followed by oral regimens soon after the last IV dose. For example, the recommended dose of atenolol in this setting is 5 mg *slow* IV (over 5 minutes); wait 10 minutes; then, if the first dose was well tolerated, give a second dose of 5 mg slow IV (over 5 minutes). An oral regimen is then initiated at 50 mg every 12 hours. Metoprolol is given in doses of 5 mg by slow IV push at 5-minute intervals to a total of 15 mg. An oral regimen is then initiated 15 minutes after the last IV dose at 50 mg twice daily for 24 hours and increased to 100 mg twice a day as tolerated.

IV esmolol is a short-acting (half-life of 2–9 minutes) beta₁-selective beta-blocker that is recommended for the acute treatment of supraventricular tachyarrhythmias, including PSVT, rate control in non-preexcited AF or atrial flutter, ectopic atrial tachycardia, multifocal atrial tachycardia, and polymorphic VT due to torsades de pointes (as adjunctive therapy to cardiac pacing) or myocardial ischemia. It is metabolized by erythrocyte esterases and requires no dose adjustment in patients with renal or hepatic impairment. Continuous IV infusion permits a sustained beta-blocker effect. Esmolol has a complicated dosing regimen and requires an IV infusion pump. It is administered as an IV loading dose of 0.5 mg/kg over 1 minute, followed by a maintenance infusion of 50 µg/kg/min for 4 minutes. If the response is inadequate, a second bolus of 0.5 mg/kg is infused over 1 minute, with an increase of the maintenance infusion to 100 µg/kg. The bolus dose (0.5 mg/kg) and titration of the infusion dose (addition of 50 µg/kg/min) can be repeated every 4 minutes to a maximum infusion of 300 µg/kg/min. Infusions can be maintained for up to 48 hours if necessary. Esmolol 50 to 200 µg/kg/min IV has an effect equivalent to that of 3 to 6 mg IV propranolol.

Side effects related to beta blockade include bradycardias, AV conduction delays, and hypotension. Cardiovascular decompensation and cardiogenic shock after beta-adrenergic blocker therapy are infrequent provided that administration to patients with severe congestive heart failure is avoided and patients with mild and moderate congestive heart failure are monitored closely. Beta-blocker therapy should be withheld from patients with absolute contraindications to these agents.

Contraindications to the use of beta-adrenergic blocking agents include second- or third-degree heart block, hypotension, severe congestive heart failure, and lung disease associated with bronchospasm. Beta-adrenergic blocking agents should be used cautiously in patients with preexisting sinus bradycardia and sick sinus syndrome.

Calcium Channel Blockers: Verapamil and Diltiazem

Verapamil and diltiazem are calcium channel blocking agents that slow sinus node automaticity; they also slow conduction and increase refractoriness in the AV node.[70] These actions may terminate reentrant arrhythmias that require AV nodal conduction for their continuation. Verapamil and diltiazem may also control ventricular response rate in patients with AF, atrial flutter, or multifocal atrial tachycardia. Verapamil, and to a lesser extent diltiazem, may decrease myocardial contractility and exacerbate congestive heart failure in patients with severe LV dysfunction.

Dosing

IV verapamil is effective for terminating narrow-complex PSVT that recurs or is unresponsive to treatment with adenosine. It may also be used for rate control in AF. The initial dose of verapamil is 2.5 to 5 mg IV given over 2 minutes. In the absence of a therapeutic response or drug-induced adverse event, repeated doses of 5 to 10 mg may be administered every 15 to 30 minutes to a maximum of

20 mg. Verapamil should be given *only* to patients with narrow-complex PSVT or arrhythmias known with certainty to be of supraventricular origin. Verapamil should not be given to patients with impaired ventricular function or heart failure.

Diltiazem at a dose of 0.25 mg/kg, followed by a second dose of 0.35 mg/kg, seems to be equivalent in efficacy to verapamil. Diltiazem offers the advantage of producing less myocardial depression than verapamil. Diltiazem may also be used as a maintenance infusion of 5 to 15 mg/hr to control the ventricular rate in AF and atrial flutter.

Digoxin

Digoxin is a time-honored drug for treating supraventricular arrhythmias as well as congestive heart failure. It is unique in being one of the few rhythm agents with a positive (rather than negative) inotropic effect, and it is not a vasodilator. To the contrary, rapid administration of IV digoxin can transiently increase blood pressure. Digoxin is a complicated agent whose AV-nodal blocking properties are indirectly mediated (unlike its direct inotropic and toxic effects) by enhancement of parasympathetic (vagal) tone, which may account in part for the drug's slow onset of action and modest potency compared to other AV-nodal blocking agents.[71] By this mechanism, digoxin acts to terminate PSVT and slow AV-nodal conduction of atrial arrhythmias such as AF and flutter. Vagally denervated hearts (posttransplant) are not responsive, whereas patients with high sympathetic tone are resistant to digoxin's AV-nodal blocking effects.

Dosing

Loading doses of IV digoxin (8–12 μg/kg in adults) are administered in divided fashion with half of the total dose given initially and the remaining portion given as 25% fractions at 4- to 8-hour intervals. Each dose should be given over at least 5 minutes.[72]

IV Disopyramide

Disopyramide is a Vaughn Williams classification I_A antiarrhythmic agent that acts both to slow conduction velocity and prolong the effective refractory period, similar to procainamide. It has potent anticholinergic, negative inotropic, and hypotensive effects that limit its use. It is available in the United States in an oral but not a parenteral formulation.

Dosing

IV disopyramide is given 2 mg/kg over 10 minutes, followed by a continuous infusion of 0.4 mg/kg/hr.[73] The usefulness of IV disopyramide is limited by the need for a relatively slow infusion, which may be impractical and of uncertain efficacy in emergent circumstances, particularly under compromised circulatory conditions.

Dopamine

Dopamine hydrochloride is an endogenous catecholamine agent with dose-related dopaminergic and beta- and alpha-adrenergic agonist activity.[74] At doses between 3 and 7.5 μg/kg/min, dopamine acts as a beta agonist, increasing cardiac output and heart rate. The beta-agonist effects of dopamine are less pronounced than those of isoproterenol, and titration is easier. The inotropic effects of dopamine are modest compared with those of dobutamine. Dopamine is regarded as a safer agent and has displaced isoproterenol as the preferred catecholamine for bradycardias in which atropine is either ineffective or contraindicated.

Dosing

Dopamine is typically initiated at low doses of 3 to 5 μg/kg/min and titrated upward to 6 to 10 μg/kg/min as needed for heart rate and blood pressure support. As doses exceed this amount, the alpha-adrenergic agonist effects of dopamine become more dominant, resulting in vasoconstriction. In the past, dopamine has been used in low doses (2 μg/kg/min) as a renal vasodilator. Dopamine, however, has shown no benefit when used in acute oliguric renal failure[75–77] and is no longer recommended for its management.[77,78]

Flecainide

Flecainide hydrochloride is approved in oral form in the United States (and in IV form outside the United States) for ventricular arrhythmias and for supraventricular arrhythmias in patients without structural heart disease. Flecainide is a potent sodium channel blocker with significant conduction-slowing effects (antiarrhythmic Vaughn Williams classification I_C agent). IV flecainide (not approved for use in the United States) has been effective for the termination of atrial flutter and AF, ectopic atrial tachycardia, AV-nodal reentrant tachycardia, and SVTs associated with an accessory pathway (Wolff-Parkinson-White syndrome), including preexcited atrial fibrillation.[79] Because of its significant negative inotropic effects, flecainide should be avoided in patients with impaired LV function. It has also been observed to increase mortality in patients who have had an MI, and its use should be avoided when coronary artery disease is suspected.

Dosing

Flecainide is usually administered as 2 mg/kg body weight at 10 mg/min.[32] Reported adverse side effects include bradycardia, hypotension, and neurologic symptoms, such as oral paresthesias and visual blurring. Flecainide is limited by the need for a relatively slow infusion, which may be impractical and of uncertain efficacy in emergent circumstances, particularly under compromised circulatory conditions.

Ibutilide

Ibutilide is a short-acting antiarrhythmic available only in parenteral form. It acts by prolonging the duration of the action potential and increasing the refractory period of cardiac tissue (antiarrhythmic Vaughn Williams classification III effect). Ibutilide is recommended for *acute* pharmacologic conversion of atrial flutter or AF or as an adjunct to electrical cardioversion in patients in whom electrical cardioversion alone has been ineffective.[80] Ibutilide has a relatively short duration of action, making it less effective than other antiarrhythmic agents for maintaining sinus rhythm once restored. Ibutilide seems most effective for the pharmacologic conversion of AF or atrial flutter of relatively brief duration.

Dosing

For adults weighing ≥60 kg, ibutilide is administered intravenously, diluted or undiluted, as 1 mg (10 mL) over 10 minutes.[80] If that is unsuccessful in terminating the arrhythmia, a second 1-mg dose can be administered at the same rate 10 minutes after the first. In patients weighing <60 kg, an initial dose of 0.01 mg/kg is recommended. Ibutilide has minimal effects on blood pressure and heart rate. Its major limitation is a relatively high incidence of ventricular proarrhythmia (polymorphic VT), including torsades de pointes. Patients receiving ibutilide should be *continuously monitored* for arrhythmias at the time of its administration and for *at least 4 to 6 hours* after drug administration (longer in patients with hepatic dysfunction in whom the clearance of ibutilide may be prolonged). Patients with significantly impaired LV function may be at higher risk of ibutilide-induced proarrhythmia.

Isoproterenol

Isoproterenol hydrochloride is a pure beta-adrenergic agonist with potent inotropic and chronotropic effects. It increases myocardial oxygen consumption, cardiac output, and myocardial work and can exacerbate ischemia and arrhythmias in patients with ischemic heart disease, congestive heart failure, or impaired ventricular function.[82] At low doses the chronotropic effect (increase in heart rate) of isoproterenol raises blood pressure and compensates for its vasodilatory effects. On the basis of limited evidence, isoproterenol may be considered as a temporizing measure while pacing is being initiated for torsade de pointes. In the past it was recommended for immediate temporary control of hemodynamically significant bradycardia when other alternatives such as temporary pacing were not available. Isoproterenol is not presently regarded as the treatment of choice for this condition and is no longer included or recommended in the bradycardia algorithm, where it has been displaced by epinephrine and dopamine.

Dosing

The recommended infusion rate for isoproterenol is 2 to 10 μg/min titrated according to the heart rate and rhythm response. An isoproterenol infusion is prepared by adding 1 mg of isoproterenol hydrochloride to 500 mL of D_5W; this produces a concentration of 2 μg/mL. Isoproterenol should be used, *if at all*, with extreme caution and at the lowest possible dose. Higher doses are associated with increased myocardial oxygen consumption, increased infarct size, and malignant ventricular arrhythmias. Isoproterenol is not indicated in patients with cardiac arrest or hypotension. For symptomatic bradycardia, epinephrine, dopamine, and temporary pacing are preferred alternatives.

Lidocaine

Lidocaine is one of a number of antiarrhythmic drugs available for the treatment of ventricular ectopy, VT, and VF. It has no efficacy for SVT. Its routine prophylactic use in patients suspected of having AMI is no longer recommended. In fact, lidocaine's effectiveness for any ventricular arrhythmia has been challenged. It is less effective than procainamide or sotalol for treating hemodynamically stable VT and less effective than amiodarone for treating persistent VF or pulseless VT. However, on the basis of established use and historical precedent, lidocaine is an acceptable alternative to amiodarone for persistent VF/pulseless VT when amiodarone is not available and is a second choice behind other alternative agents, such as IV amiodarone, IV procainamide, or IV sotalol (not available in the United States) for hemodynamically stable VT.

Cardiac Arrest

The use of lidocaine for ventricular arrhythmias was supported by initial studies in animals[83–88] and extrapolation from the historical use of the drug to suppress PVCs and prevent VF (but not improve mortality) after acute MI.[89] Lidocaine improved resuscitation rate and the rate for admission alive to the hospital in one retrospective prehospital study,[90] although arguably such improvement may have been attributable to other factors and only incidental to use of lidocaine. Other trials comparing lidocaine and bretylium found no statistically significant differences in outcome.[91–93] Two randomized comparisons between amiodarone and lidocaine found a greater likelihood of successful resuscitation with amiodarone.[18,94] Other studies have suggested that the use of lidocaine for cardiac arrest may be detrimental. A randomized comparison between lidocaine and epinephrine showed a higher incidence of asystole with lidocaine use and no difference in return of spontaneous circulation.[95] Numerous animal studies as well as a retrospective uncontrolled trial suggest that lidocaine may even reduce short-term resuscitation success.[96] Some studies have observed an elevated defibrillation threshold after treatment.[97–103] No benefit and increased morbidity (serious arrhythmias) have been associated with prophylactic administration of lidocaine to patients with acute MI.[104–107]

Thus, although lidocaine is an antiarrhythmic agent of long standing and widespread familiarity, lower in cost and convenient for use in prefilled syringes, it has no proven short- or long-term efficacy in cardiac arrest. Lidocaine should be considered an alternative treatment on the basis of less supportive evidence for its efficacy.

Other Arrhythmias

In the past, lidocaine was frequently used as a first-line agent to treat wide-complex tachycardias. There was a widely held, albeit incorrect belief that lidocaine, like adenosine, had diagnostic utility for discriminating VT (for which it was presumably effective) from aberrantly conducted SVT (for which it was not). In fact, lidocaine is not an effective or appropriate treatment for SVT or a particularly effective treatment for VT. Two studies suggest that lidocaine is ineffective for the termination of hemodynamically stable sustained VT[108,109] and two have found lidocaine to be significantly less effective against VT than IV procainamide[110] or IV sotalol.[111] Thus evidence does not support the use of lidocaine to discriminate the etiology of a wide-complex tachycardia of uncertain origin.

Lidocaine will effectively suppress spontaneous ventricular arrhythmias associated with acute myocardial ischemia and infarction.[89] But the prophylactic use of lidocaine to prevent the arrhythmias in the first place following acute MI does not lower mortality, is associated with a higher frequency of adverse effects (particularly bradycardia), and has been abandoned.[104–107] It is also neither indicated nor useful for SVT.

Dosing

In cardiac arrest, an initial bolus of 1 to 1.5 mg/kg IV is necessary to rapidly achieve and maintain therapeutic lidocaine levels. For refractory VF/VT, an additional bolus of 0.5 to 0.75 mg/kg can be given; repeat in 5 to 10 minutes.[112] Total dose should not exceed 3 mg/kg (or >200–300 mg during a 1-hour period). The more aggressive dosing approach (1.5 mg/kg) is recommended in cardiac arrest due to VF or pulseless VT after failure of defibrillation and epinephrine. Only bolus therapy should be used in cardiac arrest. Administering a continuous infusion of (prophylactic) antiarrhythmic agents to maintain circulation *after* it has been successfully restored is controversial. However, until data are available supporting the prophylactic administration of antiarrhythmic agents after return of circulation, it is reasonable to continue an infusion of the drug associated with the restoration of a stable rhythm. A continuous infusion of lidocaine should be initiated at 1 to 4 mg/min. Reappearance of arrhythmias

during a constant infusion of lidocaine should be treated with a small bolus dose (0.5 mg/kg) and an increase in the infusion rate in incremental doses (maximal infusion rate of 4 mg/min).

The half-life of lidocaine increases after 24 to 48 hours as the drug, in effect, inhibits its own hepatic metabolism. With prolonged infusions, the dosage should be reduced after 24 hours or blood levels should be monitored. The dose should be reduced in the presence of decreased cardiac output (e.g., in acute MI with hypotension or shock, congestive heart failure, or poor peripheral perfusion states), in patients older than 70 years, and in those with hepatic dysfunction. These patients should receive the usual bolus dose first, followed by half the normal maintenance infusion. Lidocaine reaches the central circulation after bolus peripheral administration in approximately 2 minutes. Patients should be observed closely for signs of drug efficacy and toxicity. Toxic reactions and side effects include slurred speech, altered consciousness, muscle twitching, seizures, and bradycardia. Lidocaine blood levels may assist in guiding therapy.

Magnesium

Magnesium exerts a variety of electrophysiologic effects, including calcium antagonism and membrane stabilization,[113] reduced automaticity,[114] and AV-nodal conduction.[115] Severe magnesium deficiency is associated with cardiac arrhythmias, symptoms of cardiac insufficiency, and sudden cardiac death. Anecdotal experience suggests that magnesium may also be an effective treatment for antiarrhythmic drug-induced torsades de pointes even in the absence of magnesium deficiency. Conversely, the routine prophylactic administration of magnesium in patients with acute MI is no longer recommended, nor has it been shown to be beneficial in cardiac arrest except when arrhythmias are suspected to be caused by magnesium deficiency or when torsades de pointes is suspected.

Cardiac Arrest

Use of magnesium for cardiac arrest due to torsades de pointes may be beneficial.[116,117] However, its routine administration during resuscitation is not beneficial.[118,119]

Other Arrhythmias

Use of magnesium in the treatment of atrial fibrillation is controversial. Some studies have shown it to be effective with respect to both control of rate and rhythm, whereas others have not found it to be as effective as more conventional agents such as calcium channel blockers and amiodarone. As yet, magnesium is not generally used or regarded as first-line therapy for atrial arrhythmias.[120,121]

Dosing

A variety of dosing regimens for magnesium sulfate have been described.[122] Magnesium may be administered as a loading dose of 1 to 2 g (8–16 mEq), mixed in 50 to 100 mL D_5W, given over 5 to 60 minutes, followed by an infusion of 0.5 to 1 g (4–8 mEq) per hour. In emergent circumstances, magnesium sulfate 1 to 2 g is diluted in 10 mL D_5W and administered over 1 to 2 minutes. Rapid administration of magnesium may cause clinically significant hypotension or asystole and should be avoided. Therefore, the rate and duration of the infusion should be determined by the clinical situation.

Phenytoin

Phenytoin is commonly used as an anticonvulsant agent but has antiarrhythmic properties similar to those of lidocaine (Vaughn Williams class I_B), making it, in theory, potentially useful for the treatment of ventricular arrhythmias. Experience with phenytoin as an antiarrhythmic agent is mainly found in anecdotal reports in the older literature[123,124] and based on its use for arrhythmias provoked by digitalis intoxication.[125,126] There are limited recent data supporting its benefit for treating ventricular arrhythmias,[127,128] for which a higher failure rate has been found with phenytoin than with other antiarrhythmic agents.[129] Accordingly, IV phenytoin is now rarely used for arrhythmias and does not have an approved label indication for arrhythmias by the U.S. Food and Drug Administration.

Dosing

Phenytoin has been administered as 100 mg IV at 5-minute intervals until the arrhythmia under treatment is abolished or until a total of 1 g is given. The drug may also be infused as 10 to 15 mg/kg at a rate of 50 mg over 1 to 3 minutes.[130] Administration of the drug requires a large vein, with attention to possible precipitation when given as an IV infusion.

Procainamide

Procainamide hydrochloride is a Vaughn Williams class I_A antiarrhythmic agent that slows conduction and increases tissue refractoriness. It is effective for treating both atrial and ventricular arrhythmias. Procainamide is acceptable for the pharmacologic conversion of supraventricular arrhythmias (particularly AF and atrial flutter) to sinus rhythm, for control of rapid ventricular rate due to accessory pathway conduction in preexcited atrial arrhythmias, and for hemodynamically stable VT.[131–142]

Cardiac Arrest

Use of procainamide in cardiac arrest is supported only by a retrospective comparison study involving only 20 patients.[143] In patients with a perfusing rhythm, procainamide must be administered relatively slowly because of its hypotensive effects. Because the way in which it is best administered during pulseless cardiac arrest is not known and its efficacy under such emergent circumstances is uncertain, it has been largely displaced by other agents (lidocaine and amiodarone) for this indication.

Other Arrhythmias

Antiarrhythmic agents such as procainamide have shown efficacy in treating a broad variety of arrhythmias, including supraventricular arrhythmias with and without aberrancy and VT.[110,144,145] Procainamide is effective for treating SVT, including PSVT, AF, and atrial flutter as well as accessory pathway–mediated arrhythmias.[134,136,137,139,146–153] When it is administered for atrial flutter, procainamide should be preceded by an AV-nodal blocking drug in order to prevent potential acceleration of ventricular rates.

Dosing

Procainamide hydrochloride may be given in an infusion of 20 mg/min until the arrhythmia is suppressed, hypotension ensues, the QRS complex is prolonged by 50% from its original duration, or a total of 17 mg/kg (1.2 g for a 70-kg patient) of the drug has been given.[154] Bolus administration of the drug can result in toxic concentrations and significant hypotension. Delay resulting from the need to infuse procainamide slowly presents the major barrier to its use in life-threatening situations, such as persistent or recurrent VF/pulseless VT. In urgent situations, up to 50 mg/min may be administered to a total dose of 17 mg/kg. The maintenance infusion rate of procainamide hydrochloride is 1 to 4 mg/min. The maintenance dosage should be reduced in the presence of renal failure. Blood levels should be monitored in patients with renal failure and in those receiving a constant infusion of more than 3 mg/min for more than 24 hours.

Procainamide should be avoided in patients with preexisting QT prolongation and suspected torsades de pointes. The electrocardiogram and blood pressure must be monitored continuously during procainamide administration. Precipitous hypotension may occur if the drug is injected too rapidly.

Propafenone

Propafenone hydrochloride, like flecainide, is a Vaughn Williams classification I_C antiarrhythmic agent with significant conduction-slowing and negative inotropic effects. In addition, propafenone has nonselective beta-blocking properties. Oral propafenone is approved for use in the United States against ventricular arrhythmias and supraventricular arrhythmias in patients without structural heart disease. IV propafenone (not approved for use in the United States) is used abroad for the same indications as flecainide. Because of its significant negative inotropic effects, propafenone, like flecainide, should be avoided in patients with impaired LV function. Propafenone also falls into the same Vaughn

Williams classification as flecainide, which has been observed to increase mortality in patients who have had an MI. By extrapolation of these data, its use should also probably be avoided when coronary artery disease is suspected.

Dosing

IV propafenone is customarily administered as 1 to 2 mg/kg body weight at 10 mg/min.[155] Reported side effects include bradycardia, hypotension, and gastrointestinal upset. Propafenone is limited by its need to be infused relatively slowly, which may be impractical and of uncertain efficacy in emergent circumstances, particularly under compromised circulatory conditions.

Quinidine

Quinidine, like procainamide, is a Vaughn Williams class I$_A$ antiarrhythmic agent that slows conduction and increases tissue refractoriness. It has been used to treat both atrial and ventricular arrhythmias.[156,157] Like procainamide, it may depress myocardial contractility and is associated with hypotension. IV quinidine gluconate has been used for over half a century for the treatment of atrial and ventricular arrhythmias[158] but has been largely displaced by other agents because of its high incidence of adverse effects, particularly hypotension and concern over ventricular proarrhythmias. It has now fallen into disuse, given the variety of alternative agents available.

Dosing

For atrial arrhythmias, quinidine gluconate is infused at an initial rate of up to 0.25 mg/kg/min. It should be discontinued if the QRS complex or the rate-corrected QT (QT$_c$) interval lengthens to 130% of its pretreatment duration, or if the QT$_c$ exceeds 500 milliseconds. Similar doses have been used for VT.[159]

Alternatively, intermittent regimens of quinidine gluconate have been used in the treatment of severe *Plasmodium falciparum* malaria, consisting of an initial loading dose of 24 mg/kg of quinidine gluconate infused over 4 hours, followed 4 hours later by maintenance doses of 12 mg/kg infused over 4 hours and administered at 8-hour intervals.[160] It has also been administered in this manner for the treatment of VT.[161]

Sotalol

Sotalol hydrochloride is a Vaughn Williams classification III antiarrhythmic agent that, like amiodarone, prolongs action potential duration and increases cardiac tissue refractoriness. In addition, it has nonselective beta-blocking properties. Sotalol is approved in oral form in the United States for atrial and ventricular arrhythmias. Sotalol is administered intravenously for both ventricular and supraventricular arrhythmias outside of the United States but is not available in this form within the United States.

Dosing

IV sotalol is usually administered as 1 to 1.5 mg/kg body weight at a rate of 10 mg/min.[111] Side effects include bradycardia, hypotension, and proarrhythmia (torsades de pointes). IV sotalol is limited by its need to be infused relatively slowly. This may be impractical and has uncertain efficacy in emergent circumstances, particularly under compromised circulatory conditions.

References

1. Kuhn GJ, White BC, Swetnam RE, et al. Peripheral vs central circulation times during CPR: a pilot study. *Ann Emerg Med* 1981;10(8):417–419.
2. Hedges JR, Barsan WB, Doan LA, et al. Central versus peripheral intravenous routes in cardiopulmonary resuscitation. *Am J Emerg Med* 1984;2(5):385–390.
3. Barsan WG, Levy RC, Weir H. Lidocaine levels during CPR: differences after peripheral venous, central venous, and intracardiac injections. *Ann Emerg Med* 1981;10(2):73–78.
4. Emerman CL, Pinchak AC, Hancock D, et al. Effect of injection site on circulation times during cardiac arrest. *Crit Care Med* 1988;16(11):1138–1141.
5. Jasani MS, Nadkarni VM, Finkelstein MS, et al. Effects of different techniques of endotracheal epinephrine administration in pediatric porcine hypoxic–hypercarbic cardiopulmonary arrest. *Crit Care Med* 1994;22(7):1174–1180.
6. Mazkereth R, Paret G, Ezra D, et al. Epinephrine blood concentrations after peripheral bronchial versus endotracheal administration of epinephrine in dogs. *Crit Care Med* 1992;20(11):1582–1587.
7. Johnston C. Endotracheal drug delivery. *Pediatr Emerg Care* 1992;8(2):94–97.
8. Ward JTJ. Endotracheal drug therapy. *Am J Emerg Med* 1983;1(1):71–82.
9. Mielke LL, Frank C, Lanzinger MJ, et al. Plasma catecholamine levels following tracheal and intravenous epinephrine administration in swine. *Resuscitation* 1998;36(3):187–192.
10. Niemann JT, Stratton SJ, Cruz B, et al. Endotracheal drug administration during out-of-hospital resuscitation: where are the survivors? *Resuscitation* 2002;53(2):153–157.
11. LaRocco BG, Wang HE. Intraosseous infusion. *Prehosp Emerg Care* 2003;7(2):280–285.
12. Dubick MA, Holcomb JB. A review of intraosseous vascular access: current status and military application. *Mil Med* 2000;165(7):552–559.
13. Vaughan EM, Williams DM. Classification of antidysrhythmic drugs. *Pharmacol Ther [B]*. 1975;1(1):115–138.
14. The Sicilian gambit. A new approach to the classification of antirhythmic drugs based on their actions on arrhythmogenic mechanisms. Task Force of the Working Group on Arrhythmias of the European Society of Cardiology. *Circulation* 1991; 84(4):1831–1851.
15. Gunnar RM, Lambrew CT, Abrams W, et al. Task force IV: pharmacologic interventions. Emergency cardiac care. *Am J Cardiol* 1982;50(2):393–408.
16. Kowey PR, Levine JH, Herre JM, et al. Randomized, double-blind comparison of intravenous amiodarone and bretylium in the treatment of patients with recurrent, hemodynamically destabilizing ventricular tachycardia or fibrillation. The Intravenous Amiodarone Multicenter Investigators Group. *Circulation* 1995;92(11):3255–3263.
17. Kudenchuk PJ, Cobb LA, Copass MK, et al. Amiodarone for resuscitation after out-of-hospital cardiac arrest due to ventricular fibrillation. *N Engl J Med* 1999;341(12):871–878.
18. Dorian P, Cass D, Schwartz B, et al. Amiodarone as compared with lidocaine for shock-resistant ventricular fibrillation. *N Engl J Med* 2002;346(12):884–890.
19. Gomes JA, Kang PS, Hariman RJ, et al. Electrophysiologic effects and mechanisms of termination of supraventricular tachycardia by intravenous amiodarone. *Am Heart J* 1984;107(2):214–221.

20. Noc M, Stajer D, Horvat M. Intravenous amiodarone versus verapamil for acute conversion of paroxysmal atrial fibrillation to sinus rhythm. *Am J Cardiol* 1990;65(9):679–680.
21. Galve E, Rius T, Ballester R, et al. Intravenous amiodarone in treatment of recent-onset atrial fibrillation: results of a randomized, controlled study. *J Am Coll Cardiol* 1996;27(5):1079–1082.
22. Cochrane AD, Siddins M, Rosenfeldt FL, et al. A comparison of amiodarone and digoxin for treatment of supraventricular arrhythmias after cardiac surgery. *Eur J Cardiothorac Surg* 1994;8(4):194–198.
23. Vietti-Ramus G, Veglio F, Marchisio U, et al. Efficacy and safety of short intravenous amiodarone in supraventricular tachyarrhythmias. *Int J Cardiol* 1992;35(1):77–85.
24. Bertini G, Conti A, Fradella G, et al. Propafenone versus amiodarone in field treatment of primary atrial tachydysrhythmias. *J Emerg Med* 1990;8(1):15–20.
25. Mehta AV, Sanchez GR, Sacks EJ, et al. Ectopic automatic atrial tachycardia in children: clinical characteristics, management and follow-up. *J Am Coll Cardiol* 1988;11(2):379–385.
26. Holt P, Crick JC, Davies DW, et al. Intravenous amiodarone in the acute termination of supraventricular arrhythmias. *Int J Cardiol* 1985;8(1):67–79.
27. Kochiadakis GE, Igoumenidis NE, Simantirakis EN, et al. Intravenous propafenone versus intravenous amiodarone in the management of atrial fibrillation of recent onset: a placebo-controlled study. *Pacing Clin Electrophysiol* 1998;21(11 Pt 2):2475–2479.
28. Clemo HF, Wood MA, Gilligan DM, et al. Intravenous amiodarone for acute heart rate control in the critically ill patient with atrial tachyarrhythmias. *Am J Cardiol* 1998;81(5):594–598.
29. Cybulski J, Kulakowski P, Makowska E, et al. Intravenous amiodarone is safe and seems to be effective in termination of paroxysmal supraventricular tachyarrhythmias. *Clin Cardiol* 1996;19(7):563–566.
30. Larbuisson R, Venneman I, Stiels B. The efficacy and safety of intravenous propafenone versus intravenous amiodarone in conversion of atrial fibrillation or flutter after cardiac surgery. *J Cardiothorac Vasc Anesth* 1996;10(2):229–234.
31. Kerin NZ, Faitel K, Naini M. The efficacy of intravenous amiodarone for the conversion of chronic atrial fibrillation. Amiodarone vs quinidine for conversion of atrial fibrillation. *Arch Intern Med* 1996;156(1):49–53.
32. Donovan KD, Power BM, Hockings BE, et al. Intravenous flecainide versus amiodarone for recent-onset atrial fibrillation. *Am J Cardiol* 1995;75(10):693–697.
33. Hou ZY, Chang MS, Chen CY, et al. Acute treatment of recent-onset atrial fibrillation and flutter with a tailored dosing regimen of intravenous amiodarone. A randomized, digoxin-controlled study. *Eur Heart J* 1995;16(4):521–528.
34. Di Biasi P, Scrofani R, Paje A, et al. Intravenous amiodarone vs propafenone for atrial fibrillation and flutter after cardiac operation. *Eur J Cardiothorac Surg* 1995;9(10):587–591.
35. Chapman MJ, Moran JL, O'Fathartaigh MS, et al. Management of atrial tachyarrhythmias in the critically ill: a comparison of intravenous procainamide and amiodarone. *Intens Care Med* 1993;19(1):48–52.
36. Horner SM. A comparison of cardioversion of atrial fibrillation using oral amiodarone, intravenous amiodarone and DC cardioversion. *Acta Cardiol* 1992;47(5):473–480.
37. Cowan JC, Gardiner P, Reid DS, et al. A comparison of amiodarone and digoxin in the treatment of atrial fibrillation complicating suspected acute myocardial infarction. *J Cardiovasc Pharmacol* 1986;8(2):252–256.
38. Strasberg B, Arditti A, Sclarovsky S, et al. Efficacy of intravenous amiodarone in the management of paroxysmal or new atrial fibrillation with fast ventricular response. *Int J Cardiol* 1985;7(1):47–58.
39. Faniel R, Schoenfeld P. Efficacy of I.V. amiodarone in converting rapid atrial fibrillation and flutter to sinus rhythm in intensive care patients. *Eur Heart J* 1983;4(3):180–185.
40. Soult JA, Munoz M, Lopez JD, et al. Efficacy and safety of intravenous amiodarone for short-term treatment of paroxysmal supraventricular tachycardia in children. *Pediatr Cardiol* 1995;16(1):16–19.
41. Sagrista-Sauleda J, Permanyer-Miralda G, Soler-Soler J. Electrical cardioversion after amiodarone administration. *Am Heart J* 1992;123(6):1536–1542.
42. Butler J, Harriss DR, Sinclair M, et al. Amiodarone prophylaxis for tachycardias after coronary artery surgery: a randomised, double blind, placebo controlled trial. *Br Heart J* 1993;70(1):56–60.
43. Holt AW. Hemodynamic responses to amiodarone in critically ill patients receiving catecholamine infusions. *Crit Care Med* 1989;17(12):1270–1276.
44. Leak D. Intravenous amiodarone in the treatment of refractory life-threatening cardiac arrhythmias in the critically ill patient. *Am Heart J* 1986;111(3):456–462.
45. Kuga K, Yamaguchi I, Sugishita Y. Effect of intravenous amiodarone on electrophysiologic variables and on the modes of termination of atrioventricular reciprocating tachycardia in Wolff-Parkinson-White syndrome. *Jpn Circ J* 1999;63(3):189–195.
46. Kouvaras G, Cokkinos DV, Halal G, et al. The effective treatment of multifocal atrial tachycardia with amiodarone. *Jpn Heart J* 1989;30(3):301–312.
47. Figa FH, Gow RM, Hamilton RM, et al. Clinical efficacy and safety of intravenous Amiodarone in infants and children. *Am J Cardiol* 1994;74(6):573–577.
48. Mooss AN, Mohiuddin SM, Hee TT, et al. Efficacy and tolerance of high-dose intravenous amiodarone for recurrent, refractory ventricular tachycardia. *Am J Cardiol* 1990;65(9):609–614.
49. Schutzenberger W, Leisch F, Kerschner K, et al. Clinical efficacy of intravenous amiodarone in the short term treatment of recurrent sustained ventricular tachycardia and ventricular fibrillation. *Br Heart J* 1989;62(5):367–371.
50. Helmy I, Herre JM, Gee G, et al. Use of intravenous amiodarone for emergency treatment of life-threatening ventricular arrhythmias. *J Am Coll Cardiol* 1988;12(4):1015–1022.
51. Saksena S, Rothbart ST, Shah Y, et al. Clinical efficacy and electropharmacology of continuous intravenous amiodarone infusion and chronic oral amiodarone in refractory ventricular tachycardia. *Am J Cardiol* 1984;54(3):347–352.
52. Remme WJ, Van Hoogenhuyze DC, Krauss XH, et al. Acute hemodynamic and antiischemic effects of intravenous amiodarone. *Am J Cardiol* 1985;55(6):639–644.
53. Levine JH, Massumi A, Scheinman MM, et al. Intravenous amiodarone for recurrent sustained hypotensive ventricular tachyarrhythmias. Intravenous Amiodarone Multicenter Trial Group. *J Am Coll Cardiol* 1996;27(1):67–75.
54. Scheinman MM, Levine JH, Cannom DS, et al. Dose-ranging study of intravenous amiodarone in patients with life-threatening ventricular tachyarrhythmias. The Intravenous Amiodarone Multicenter Investigators Group. *Circulation* 1995;92(11):3264–3272.
55. Remme WJ, Kruyssen HA, Look MP, et al. Hemodynamic effects and tolerability of intravenous amiodarone in patients with impaired left ventricular function. *Am Heart J* 1991;122(pt 1)(1):96–103.
56. Cotter G, Blatt A, Kaluski E, et al. Conversion of recent onset paroxysmal atrial fibrillation to normal sinus rhythm: the effect of no treatment and high-dose amiodarone: a randomized, placebo-controlled study. *Eur Heart J* 1999;20(24):1833–1842.
57. Jawad-Kanber G, Sherrod TR. Effect of loading dose of procaine amide on left ventricular performance in man. *Chest* 1974;66(3):269–272.
58. Harrison DC, Sprouse JH, Morrow AG. The antiarrhythmic properties of lidocaine and procaine amide: clinical and physiologic studies of their cardiovascular effects in man. *Circulation* 1963;28:486–491.
59. Holdgate A, Foo A. Adenosine versus intravenous calcium channel antagonists for the treatment of supraventricular tachycardia in adults. *Cochrane Database Syst Rev* 2006(4):CD005154.
60. Griffith MJ, Linker NJ, Ward DE, et al. Adenosine in the diagnosis of broad complex tachycardia. *Lancet* 1988;1(8587):672–675.
61. Griffith MJ, Linker NJ, Garratt CJ, et al. Relative efficacy and safety of intravenous drugs for termination of sustained ventricular tachycardia. *Lancet* 1990;336(8716):670–673.

62. Sharma AD, Klein GJ, Yee R. Intravenous adenosine triphosphate during wide QRS complex tachycardia: safety, therapeutic efficacy, and diagnostic utility. *Am J Med* 1990;88(4): 337–343.

63. Garratt CJ, Griffith MJ, O'Nunain S, et al. Effects of intravenous adenosine on antegrade refractoriness of accessory atrioventricular connections. *Circulation* 1991;84(5):1962–1968.

64. Brodsky MA, Hwang C, Hunter D, et al. Life-threatening alterations in heart rate after the use of adenosine in atrial flutter. *Am Heart J* 1995;130(pt 1)(3):564–571.

65. American Society of Health-System Pharmacists. *AHFS Drug Information*. Bethesda, MD: American Society of Health-System Pharmacists, 2001:3540.

66. Camm AJ, Garratt CJ. Adenosine and supraventricular tachycardia. *N Engl J Med* 1991;325(23):1621–1629.

67. American Society of Health-System Pharmacists. *AHFS Drug Information*. Bethesda, MD: American Society of Health-System Pharmacists, 2001:1188–1191.

68. American Society of Health-System Pharmacists. *AHFS Drug Information*. Bethesda, MD: American Society of Health-System Pharmacists, 2001:1532–1538, 1591–1597, 1622–1629.

69. Nademanee K, Taylor R, Bailey WE, et al. Treating electrical storm: sympathetic blockade versus advanced cardiac life support–guided therapy. *Circulation* 2000;102(7):742–747.

70. American Society of Health-System Pharmacists. *AHFS Drug Information*. Bethesda, MD: American Society of Health-System Pharmacists, 2001:1557–1565, 1695–1604.

71. American Society of Health-System Pharmacists. *AHFS Drug Information*. Bethesda, MD: American Society of Health-System Pharmacists, 2001:1500–1510.

72. American Society of Health-System Pharmacists. ASoH-S. *AHFS Drug Information*. Bethesda, MD: American Society of Health-System Pharmacists, 2001.

73. Fujimura O, Klein GJ, Sharma AD, et al. Acute effect of disopyramide on atrial fibrillation in the Wolff-Parkinson-White syndrome. *J Am Coll Cardiol* 1989;13(5):1133–1137.

74. American Society of Health-System Pharmacists. *AHFS Drug Information*. Bethesda, MD: American Society of Health-System Pharmacists, 2001:1227–1231.

75. Bersten AD, Holt AW. Vasoactive drugs and the importance of renal perfusion pressure. *New Horiz* 1995;3(4):650–661.

76. Marik PE. Low-dose dopamine in critically ill oliguric patients: the influence of the renin-angiotensin system. *Heart Lung* 1993; 22(2):171–175.

77. Chertow GM, Sayegh MH, Allgren RL, et al. Is the administration of dopamine associated with adverse or favorable outcomes in acute renal failure? Auriculin Anaritide Acute Renal Failure Study Group. *Am J Med* 1996;101(1):49–53.

78. Thadhani R, Pascual M, Bonventre JV. Acute renal failure. *N Engl J Med* 1996;334(22):1448–1460.

79. Hellestrand KJ. Intravenous flecainide acetate for supraventricular tachycardias. *Am J Cardiol* 1988;62(6):16D–22D.

80. Ellenbogen KA, Stambler BS, Wood MA, et al. Efficacy of intravenous ibutilide for rapid termination of atrial fibrillation and atrial flutter: a dose-response study [published correction appears in *J Am Coll Cardiol* 1996;28:1082]. *J Am Coll Cardiol* 1996;28(1): 130–136.

81. American Society of Health-System Pharmacists. *AHFS Drug Information*. Bethesda, MD: American Society of Health-System Pharmacists, 2001:1607–1608.

82. American Society of Health-System Pharmacists. *AHFS Drug Information*. Bethesda, MD: American Society of Health-System Pharmacists, 2001:1244–1249.

83. Borer JS, Harrison LA, Kent KM, et al. Beneficial effect of lidocaine on ventricular electrical stability and spontaneous ventricular fibrillation during experimental myocardial infarction. *Am J Cardiol* 1976;37(6):860–863.

84. Spear JF, Moore EN, Gerstenblith G. Effect of lidocaine on the ventricular fibrillation threshold in the dog during acute ischemia and premature ventricular contractions. *Circulation* 1972;46(1): 65–73.

85. Carden NL, Steinhaus JE. Lidocaine in cardiac resuscitation from ventricular fibrillation. *Circ Res* 1956;4(6):680–683.

86. Lazzara R, el-Sherif N, Scherlag BJ. Electrophysiological properties of canine Purkinje cells in one-day-old myocardial infarction. *Circ Res* 1973;33(6):722–734.

87. Lazzara R, Hope RR, El-Sherif N, et al. Effects of lidocaine on hypoxic and ischemic cardiac cells. *Am J Cardiol* 1978;41(5): 872–879.

88. Hanyok JJ, Chow MS, Kluger J, et al. Antifibrillatory effects of high dose bretylium and a lidocaine-bretylium combination during cardiopulmonary resuscitation. *Crit Care Med* 1988;16(7): 691–694.

89. Lie KI, Wellens HJ, van Capelle FJ, et al. Lidocaine in the prevention of primary ventricular fibrillation. A double-blind, randomized study of 212 consecutive patients. *N Engl J Med* 1974; 291(25):1324–1326.

90. Herlitz J, Ekstrom L, Wennerblom B, et al. Lidocaine in out-of-hospital ventricular fibrillation. Does it improve survival? *Resuscitation* 1997;33(3):199–205.

91. Harrison EE. Lidocaine in prehospital countershock refractory ventricular fibrillation. *Ann Emerg Med* 1981;10(8):420–423.

92. Haynes RE, Chinn TL, Copass MK, et al. Comparison of bretylium tosylate and lidocaine in management of out of hospital ventricular fibrillation: a randomized clinical trial. *Am J Cardiol* 1981;48(2):353–356.

93. Olson DW, Thompson BM, Darin JC, et al. A randomized comparison study of bretylium tosylate and lidocaine in resuscitation of patients from out-of-hospital ventricular fibrillation in a paramedic system. *Ann Emerg Med* 1984;13(Pt 2)(9):807–810.

94. Kentsch M, Berkel H, et al. Intravenous amiodarone application for refractory ventricular fibrillation. *Intensivmedizin* 1988;25:70–74.

95. Weaver WD, Fahrenbruch CE, Johnson DD, et al. Effect of epinephrine and lidocaine therapy on outcome after cardiac arrest due to ventricular fibrillation. *Circulation* 1990;82(6):2027–2034.

96. van Walraven C, Stiell IG, Wells GA, et al. Do advanced cardiac life support drugs increase resuscitation rates from in-hospital cardiac arrest? The OTAC Study Group. *Ann Emerg Med* 1998;32(5): 544–553.

97. Redding JS, Pearson JW. Resuscitation from ventricular fibrillation: drug therapy. *JAMA* 1968;203(4):255–260.

98. Chow MS, Kluger J, Lawrence R, et al. The effect of lidocaine and bretylium on the defibrillation threshold during cardiac arrest and cardiopulmonary resuscitation. *Proc Soc Exp Biol Med* 1986;182(1): 63–67.

99. Babbs CF, Yim GK, Whistler SJ, et al. Elevation of ventricular defibrillation threshold in dogs by antiarrhythmic drugs. *Am Heart J* 1979;98(3):345–350.

100. Echt DS, Black JN, Barbey JT, et al. Evaluation of antiarrhythmic drugs on defibrillation energy requirements in dogs: sodium channel block and action potential prolongation. *Circulation* 1989;79(5):1106–1117.

101. Dorian P, Fain ES, Davy JM, et al. Lidocaine causes a reversible, concentration-dependent increase in defibrillation energy requirements. *J Am Coll Cardiol* 1986;8(2):327–332.

102. Kerber RE, Pandian NG, Jensen SR, et al. Effect of lidocaine and bretylium on energy requirements for transthoracic defibrillation: experimental studies. *J Am Coll Cardiol* 1986;7(2):397–405.

103. Vachiery JL, Reuse C, Blecic S, et al. Bretylium tosylate versus lidocaine in experimental cardiac arrest. *Am J Emerg Med* 1990; 8(6):492–495.

104. MacMahon S, Collins R, Peto R, et al. Effects of prophylactic lidocaine in suspected acute myocardial infarction: an overview of results from the randomized, controlled trials. *JAMA* 1988; 260(13):1910–1916.

105. Hine LK, Laird N, Hewitt P, et al. Meta-analytic evidence against prophylactic use of lidocaine in acute myocardial infarction. *Arch Intern Med* 1989;149(12):2694–2698.

106. Sadowski ZP, Alexander JH, Skrabucha B, et al. Multicenter randomized trial and a systematic overview of lidocaine in acute myocardial infarction. *Am Heart J* 1999;137(5):792–798.

107. Alexander JH, Granger CB, Sadowski Z, et al. Prophylactic lidocaine use in acute myocardial infarction: incidence and outcomes from two international trials. The GUSTO-I and GUSTO-IIb Investigators. *Am Heart J* 1999;137(5):799–805.

108. Armengol RE, Graff J, Baerman JM, et al. Lack of effectiveness of lidocaine for sustained, wide QRS complex tachycardia. *Ann Emerg Med* 1989;18(3):254–257.

109. Nasir N Jr, Taylor A, Doyle TK, et al. Evaluation of intravenous lidocaine for the termination of sustained monomorphic ventric-

ular tachycardia in patients with coronary artery disease with or without healed myocardial infarction. *Am J Cardiol* 1994;74(12): 1183–1186.

110. Gorgels AP, van den Dool A, Hofs A, et al. Comparison of procainamide and lidocaine in terminating sustained monomorphic ventricular tachycardia. *Am J Cardiol* 1996;78(1):43–46.

111. Ho DS, Zecchin RP, Richards DA, et al. Double-blind trial of lignocaine versus sotalol for acute termination of spontaneous sustained ventricular tachycardia. *Lancet* 1994;344(8914):18–23.

112. American Society of Health-System Pharmacists. *AHFS Drug Information.* Bethesda, MD: American Society of Health-System Pharmacists, 2001:1614–1618.

113. Fawcett WJ, Haxby EJ, Male DA. Magnesium: physiology and pharmacology. *Br J Anaesth* 1999;83(2):302–320.

114. Iseri LT, Allen BJ, Ginkel ML, et al. Ionic biology and ionic medicine in cardiac arrhythmias with particular reference to magnesium. *Am Heart J* 1992;123(5):1404–1409.

115. Christiansen EH, Frost L, Andreasen F, et al. Dose-related cardiac electrophysiological effects of intravenous magnesium. A double-blind placebo-controlled dose-response study in patients with paroxysmal supraventricular tachycardia. *Europace* 2000;2(4):320–326.

116. Tzivoni D, Keren A, Cohen AM, et al. Magnesium therapy for torsades de pointes. *Am J Cardiol* 1984;53(4):528–530.

117. Tzivoni D, Banai S, Schuger C, et al. Treatment of torsade de pointes with magnesium sulfate. *Circulation* 1988;77(2):392–397.

118. Miller B, Craddock L, Hoffenberg S, et al. Pilot study of intravenous magnesium sulfate in refractory cardiac arrest: safety data and recommendations for future studies. *Resuscitation* 1995;30(1): 3–14.

119. Thel MC, Armstrong AL, McNulty SE, et al. Randomised trial of magnesium in in-hospital cardiac arrest. Duke Internal Medicine Housestaff. *Lancet* 1997;350(9087):1272–1276.

120. Onalan O, Crystal E, Daoulah A, et al. Meta-analysis of magnesium therapy for the acute management of rapid atrial fibrillation. *Am J Cardiol* 2007;99(12):1726–1732.

121. Ho KM, Sheridan DJ, Paterson T. Use of intravenous magnesium to treat acute onset atrial fibrillation: a meta-analysis. *Heart* 2007;93(11):1433–1440.

122. American Society of Health-System Pharmacists. *AHFS Drug Information.* Bethesda, MD: American Society of Health-System Pharmacists, 2001:2104–2108.

123. Wit AL, Rosen MR, Hoffman BF. Electrophysiology and pharmacology of cardiac arrhythmias. VIII. Cardiac effects of diphenylhydantoin. B. *Am Heart J* 1975;90(3):397–404.

124. Bernstein H, Gold H, Lang TW, et al. Sodium diphenylhydantoin in the treatment of recurrent cardiac arrhythmias. *JAMA* 1965;191:695–697.

125. Ewy GA, Marcus FI, Fillmore SJ, et al. Digitalis intoxication—diagnosis, management and prevention. *Cardiovasc Clin* 1974; 6(2):153–174.

126. Bashour FA, Edmonson RE, Gupta DN, et al. Treatment of digitalis toxicity by diphenylhydantoin (Dilantin). *Dis Chest* 1968;53 (3):263–270.

127. Kavey RE, Blackman MS, Sondheimer HM. Phenytoin therapy for ventricular arrhythmias occurring late after surgery for congenital heart disease. *Am Heart J* 1982;104(4 Pt 1):794–798.

128. Fogoros RN, Fiedler SB, Elson JJ. Efficacy of phenytoin in suppressing inducible ventricular tachyarrhythmias. *Cardiovasc Drugs Ther* 1988;2(2):171–176.

129. Karlsson E. Procainamide and phenytoin. Comparative study of their antiarrhythmic effects at apparent therapeutic plasma levels. *Br Heart J* 1975;37(7):731–740.

130. American Society of Health-System Pharmacists. *AHFS Drug Information.* Bethesda, MD: American Society of Health-System Pharmacists, 2001:2080–2083.

131. Boahene KA, Klein GJ, Yee R, et al. Termination of acute atrial fibrillation in the Wolff-Parkinson-White syndrome by procainamide and propafenone: importance of atrial fibrillatory cycle length. *J Am Coll Cardiol* 1990;16(6):1408–1414.

132. Fenster PE, Comess KA, Marsh R, et al. Conversion of atrial fibrillation to sinus rhythm by acute intravenous procainamide infusion. *Am Heart J* 1983;106(3):501–504.

133. Fulham MJ, Cookson WO, Sher M. Procainamide infusion and acute atrial fibrillation. *Anaesth Intens Care* 1984;12(2): 121–124.

134. Heisel A, Jung J, Stopp M, et al. Facilitating influence of procainamide on conversion of atrial flutter by rapid atrial pacing. *Eur Heart J* 1997;18(5):866–869.

135. Hjelms E. Procainamide conversion of acute atrial fibrillation after open-heart surgery compared with digoxin treatment. *Scand J Thorac Cardiovasc Surg* 1992;26(3):193–196.

136. Kochiadakis GE, Igoumenidis NE, Solomou MC, et al. Conversion of atrial fibrillation to sinus rhythm using acute intravenous procainamide infusion. *Cardiovasc Drugs Ther* 1998; 12(1):75–81.

137. Leitch JW, Klein GJ, Yee R, et al. Differential effect of intravenous procainamide on anterograde and retrograde accessory pathway refractoriness. *J Am Coll Cardiol* 1992;19(1):118–124.

138. Mandel WJ, Laks MM, Obayashi K, et al. The Wolff-Parkinson-White syndrome: pharmacologic effects of procaine amide. *Am Heart J* 1975;90(6):744–754.

139. Mattioli AV, Lucchi GR, Vivoli D, et al. Propafenone versus procainamide for conversion of atrial fibrillation to sinus rhythm. *Clin Cardiol* 1998;21(10):763–766.

140. Stambler BS, Wood MA, Ellenbogen KA. Comparative efficacy of intravenous ibutilide versus procainamide for enhancing termination of atrial flutter by atrial overdrive pacing. *Am J Cardiol* 1996;77(11):960–966.

141. Wellens HJ, Braat S, Brugada P, et al. Use of procainamide in patients with the Wolff-Parkinson-White syndrome to disclose a short refractory period of the accessory pathway. *Am J Cardiol* 1982;50(5):1087–1089.

142. Wellens HJ, Bar FW, Lie KI, et al. Effect of procainamide, propranolol and verapamil on mechanism of tachycardia in patients with chronic recurrent ventricular tachycardia. *Am J Cardiol* 1977;40(4):579–585.

143. Stiell IG, Wells GA, Hebert PC, et al. Association of drug therapy with survival in cardiac arrest: limited role of advanced cardiac life support drugs. *Acad Emerg Med* 1995;2(4):264–273.

144. Callans DJ, Marchlinski FE. Dissociation of termination and prevention of inducibility of sustained ventricular tachycardia with infusion of procainamide: evidence for distinct mechanisms. *J Am Coll Cardiol* 1992;19(1):111–117.

145. Giardina EG, Heissenbuttel RH, Bigger JT Jr. Intermittent intravenous procaine amide to treat ventricular arrhythmias: correlation of plasma concentration with effect on arrhythmia, electrocardiogram, and blood pressure. *Ann Intern Med* 1973;78(2): 183–193.

146. Stambler BS, Wood MA, Ellenbogen KA. Comparative efficacy of intravenous ibutilide versus procainamide for enhancing termination of atrial flutter by atrial overdrive pacing. *Am J Cardiol* 1996;77(11):960–966.

147. Hjelms E. Procainamide conversion of acute atrial fibrillation after open-heart surgery compared with digoxin treatment. *Scand J Thorac Cardiovasc Surg* 1992;26(3):193–196.

148. Fulham MJ, Cookson WO, Sher M. Procainamide infusion and acute atrial fibrillation. *Anaesth Intens Care* 1984;12(2):121–124.

149. Fenster PE, Comess KA, Marsh R, et al. Conversion of atrial fibrillation to sinus rhythm by acute intravenous procainamide infusion. *Am Heart J* 1983;106(3):501–504.

150. Mandel WJ, Laks MM, Obayashi K, et al. The Wolff-Parkinson-White syndrome: pharmacologic effects of procaineamide. *Am Heart J* 1975;90(6):744–754.

151. Boahene KA, Klein GJ, Yee R, et al. Termination of acute atrial fibrillation in the Wolff-Parkinson-White syndrome by procainamide and propafenone: importance of atrial fibrillatory cycle length. *J Am Coll Cardiol* 1990;16(6):1408–1414.

152. Wellens HJ, Braat S, Brugada P, et al. Use of procainamide in patients with the Wolff-Parkinson-White syndrome to disclose a short refractory period of the accessory pathway. *Am J Cardiol* 1982;50(5):1087–1089.

153. Sellers TDJ, Campbell RW, Bashore TM, et al. Effects of procainamide and quinidine sulfate in the Wolff-Parkinson-White syndrome. *Circulation* 1977;55(1):15–22.

154. American Society of Health-System Pharmacists. *AHFS Drug Information.* Bethesda, MD: American Society of Health-System Pharmacists, 2001:1643–1649.

155. Fresco C, Proclemer A, Pavan A, et al. Intravenous propafenone in paroxysmal atrial fibrillation: a randomized, placebo-controlled, double-blind, multicenter clinical trial. Paroxysmal Atrial

Fibrillation Italian Trial (PAFIT)-2 Investigators. *Clin Cardiol* 1996;19(5):409–412.

156. Swerdlow CD, Yu JO, Jacobson E, et al. Safety and efficacy of intravenous quinidine. *Am J Med* 1983;75(1):36–42.

157. Allen LaPointe NM, Li P. Continuous intravenous quinidine infusion for the treatment of atrial fibrillation or flutter: a case series. *Am Heart J* 2000;139(1 Pt 1):114–121.

158. Clagett AH Jr. Intravenous use of quinidine, with particular reference to ventricular tachycardia. *Am J Med Sci* 1950;220(4): 381–388.

159. Hirschfeld DS, Ueda CT, Rowland M, et al. Clinical and electro-physiological effects of intravenous quinidine in man. *Br Heart J* 1977;39(3):309–316.

160. American Society of Health-System Pharmacists. *AHFS Drug Information*. Bethesda, MD: American Society of Health-System Pharmacists, 2001:1669–1675.

161. Torres V, Flowers D, Miura D, et al. Intravenous quinidine by intermittent bolus for electrophysiologic studies in patients with ventricular tachycardia. *Am Heart J* 1984;108(6):1437–1442.

Chapter 26
Cardiovascular Function and Vascular Tone: Physiology for ECC

Raúl J. Gazmuri and Beatrice M. Correa

When using potent vasoactive drugs in emergency cardiovascular care (ECC), specific hemodynamic goals should be established. These goals are aimed at preventing or reversing life-threatening conditions pending the reestablishment of effective hemodynamic function through spontaneous recovery or therapeutic intervention. Likewise, ECC providers should avoid prolonged use of these drugs without establishing the underlying hemodynamic diagnosis and instituting specific etiologic interventions.

- During the treatment of cardiac arrest, pharmacologic support should be initiated as soon as possible after the rhythm is checked.
- The required drugs should be anticipated and the agents prepared before a rhythm check so that they can be administered as soon as possible after the rhythm check.
- Epinephrine 1 mg remains the initial recommended intravenous (IV) dose for shock-refractory ventricular fibrillation (VF). Higher additional doses may be harmful because of its beta-adrenergic effects.
- Vasopressin has not been shown to elicit effects substantially different from those of epinephrine for the purpose of cardiac resuscitation. One dose of vasopressin 40 U may replace either the first or second dose of epinephrine in the treatment of cardiac arrest.

Overview: Pharmacology of Cardiac Function and Vascular Tone

In this chapter, drugs that can alter cardiac function and vascular tone are discussed in relation to their role in the management of cardiovascular emergencies, with primary focus on (1) hemodynamic stabilization to avert cardiac arrest, (2) resuscitation if cardiac arrest has occurred, and (3) management of postresuscitation hemodynamic dysfunction and related acute cardiovascular crises. From a didactic perspective, these drugs can be grouped into those that alter cardiac function and those that alter vascular tone. However, most of them affect cardiac function and vascular tone simultaneously in a dose-dependent manner, yielding complex physiologic effects compounded by potential side effects. An understanding of the cardiovascular effects of these drugs is of paramount importance for their proper use by ECC providers and in the proper clinical context.

Specific hemodynamic goals should be established in using these drugs, which are aimed at averting or reversing life-threatening conditions pending the reestablishment of competent hemodynamic function through spontaneous recovery or therapeutic intervention. Likewise, ECC providers should avoid prolonged use of these drugs without establishing the underlying hemodynamic diagnosis and instituting specific etiologic interventions. For example, use of vasopressor agents to reverse life-threatening hypotension associated with cardiac tamponade, massive pulmonary embolism, exsanguinating hemorrhage, or severe sepsis is appropriate, but only as a temporary measure pending definitive treatment.

Drugs targeting the cardiovascular system are used to (1) enhance myocardial contractility, (2) secure a physiologically appropriate rate and rhythm, and (3) increase or decrease vascular tone. This array of effects permits ECC providers to manipulate cardiac output and peripheral vascular resistance. However, these effects may come at the expense of unwanted side effects. Increasing contractility and heart rate will increase myocardial energy requirements, which could be detrimental, predisposing to myocardial ischemia when there is limited coronary blood supply (i.e., acute or chronic coronary artery obstruction compounded by hypotension). Inotropic agents also predispose to supraventricular and ventricular arrhythmias. Use of vasopressor agents will redistribute blood flow away from tissue beds that are not immediately vital (e.g., splanchnic territory, kidneys, skeletal muscle, skin), potentially leading to subsequent organ dysfunction.

Among the various drugs that affect the cardiovascular system, those that act through modulation of adrenergic receptors occupy a central role in the management of acute cardiovascular emergencies. A synopsis of adrenergic receptors and their physiology is, therefore, useful.

Adrenergic Receptors

Adrenergic receptors (adrenoceptors) are molecular structures present in plasma membranes. They all have seven transmembrane-spanning domains and are coupled to guanosine triphosphate–binding proteins (G proteins). After binding by specific extracellular ligands, they signal their biological effects through various cellular effector systems (Fig. 26-1). In the heart, adrenoceptors mediate changes in contractile function, pacemaker activity, and conduction velocity, leading to increases in cardiac output. In veins and arteries, adrenoceptors mediate changes in the tone of smooth muscle cells, prompting adaptive redistribution of blood flow through vasoconstriction or vasodilation of specific vascular beds. Adrenoceptors also mediate metabolic, endocrine, respiratory, gastrointestinal, urinary, and central

nervous system function, but discussion of these effects exceeds the scope of this chapter. Adrenergic agonists include the endogenous catecholamines epinephrine and norepinephrine and sympathomimetic drugs such as isoproterenol, dobutamine, phenylephrine, and methoxamine (Table 26-1).

Two main adrenoceptors were originally described by Ahlquist[1] based on the vascular response to endogenous agonists. Adrenoceptors that mediated vasoconstriction were designated as alpha adrenoceptors and those that mediated vasodilation as beta adrenoceptors. Subsequently it was discovered that these primary adrenoceptors included multiple subtypes, totaling, at the time of this writing, nine distinctive adrenoceptors (Fig. 26-2).[2]

Alpha Adrenoceptors

The main cardiovascular effect mediated by alpha adrenoceptor is vasoconstriction. This effect leads to redistribution of blood flow away from nonvital territories, favoring myocardial and cerebral perfusion under low-flow conditions. Alpha$_1$ adrenoceptors also mediate inotropic effects, but with less potency than beta adrenoceptors. Two types

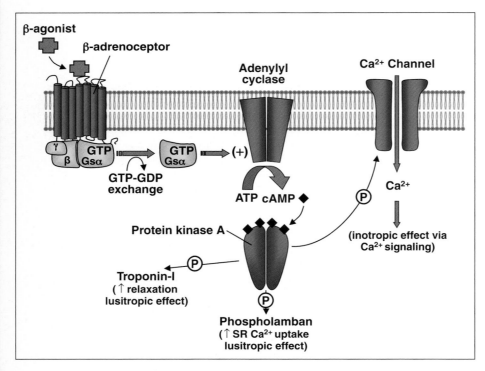

FIGURE 26-1 • Schematic representation of signal transduction through adrenergic receptors. Shown is a beta$_1$ adrenoceptor with its seven transmembrane-spanning domains. The receptor is coupled to a heterotrimeric G protein signaling activation of adenylyl cyclase upon binding by its specific beta agonist (e.g., norepinephrine, epinephrine, isoproterenol, dobutamine). Adenylyl cyclase is activated by the stimulatory subunit Gsα and catalyzes the formation of cAMP from ATP. cAMP signals downstream activation of protein kinase A, which in turn phosphorylates Ca^{2+} channels, phospholamban, and troponin I, among other targets, enhancing contractile activity. GTP, guanosine triphosphate; GDT, guanosine triphosphate; alpha, beta, and gamma refer to subunits of the heterotrimeric GTP-binding protein; ATP, adenosine triphosphate; P, phosphate group; SR, sarcoplasmic reticulum.

| TABLE 26-1 • Drugs for Cardiovascular Support

Drugs	Receptor or Target	Cardiovascular Effects					Dosing	
		Heart			Blood Vessels			
		Inotropy	Rate	Arrhythmias	Arteries	Veins	Bolus	Continuous
Adrenergic Agonists *Natural catecholamines*								
Epinephrine	α_1, α_2, β_1, β_2	+++	+++	++	vd/vc	vd/vc	1 mg[a]	1–10 μg/min
Norepinephrine	α_1, α_2, β_1	+++	++	++	vc	vc		0.5–30 μg/min[b]
Dopamine	D_1, D_2	++	++	+	vd/vc	vd/vc		2–20 μg/kg/min[c]
Sympathomimetic drugs								
Dobutamine	α_1, β_1, β_2	+++	+	+	vd	vd		2–20 μg/kg/min
Isoproterenol	β_1, β_2	+++	+++	++	vd	vd		2–10 μg/min
Phenylephrine	α_1	+	−	+	vc	vc	0.1–0.5 mg/10–15 min	0.4–9.0 μg/kg/min
Nonadrenergic Agonists								
Vasopressin	V_1, V_2	ne	ne	ne	vc	vc	40 U[d]	0.01–0.04 U/min[e]
Milrinone	Phosphodiesterase	+++	+	+	vd	vd	50 μg/kg	0.375–0.75 μg/kg/min
Inamrinone	Phosphodiesterase	+++	+	+	vd	vd	0.75 mg/kg	5–15 μg/kg/min
Nitroglycerin	NO production	ne	ne	ne	vd	vd	12.5–25 μg	10–500 μg/min[f]
Nitroprusside	NO production	ne	ne	ne	vd	vd		0.1–10 μg/kg/min[g]

vc, vasoconstriction; vd, vasodilation; vd/vc, vasodilation at low and vasoconstriction at high doses; *ne*, no effect.
[a]For cardiac arrest, repeated every 3 to 5 minutes.
[b]Delivered through a central venous catheter; titrated to maintain a target systolic blood pressure (e.g., 90 mm Hg).
[c]Effect is dose-dependent, causing a predominant dopaminergic effect at 2 to 4 μg/kg/min, leading to vasodilation and mild inotropic effects; beta1 and beta2 effect at 5 to 10 μg/kg/min, increasing contractility; and alpha-adrenoceptor effect at 11 to 20 μg/kg/min, causing predominantly vasoconstriction.
[d]For cardiac arrest, substituting for one epinephrine dose.
[e]For vasodilation refractory to adrenergic vasopressor agents in patients with septic shock.
[f]Low doses of 10 to 40 μg/min produce predominantly venodilation, whereas high doses of 150 to 500 μg/min produce arteriolar dilation.
[g]Under continuous blood pressure monitoring for optimal safety.

of alpha adrenoceptors have been identified: alpha$_1$ and alpha$_2$.

Alpha$_1$ Adrenoceptors These adrenoceptors are located postsynaptically in the immediate vicinity of sympathetic nerve terminals and in peripherally targeted organs.[3] Alpha$_1$ adrenoceptors signal their effects through $G_{q/11}$ and are coupled to several effector mechanisms, with the main mechanism linked to activation of phospholipase C_B and inositol trisphosphate (IP3), causing increases in cytosolic Ca^{2+}.[4] In smooth muscle cells, Ca^{2+} activates Ca^{2+}-sensitive kinases such as calmodulin-dependent myosin light-chain kinase, promoting contraction of smooth muscle cells (i.e., vasoconstriction). Three subtypes of alpha$_1$ adrenoceptors have been

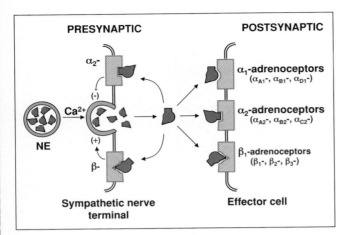

FIGURE 26-2 • Schematic representation of the various adreno-ceptors, illustrating their presynaptic and postsynaptic loca-tions. Note that agonists such as norepinephrine (NE) can acti-vate alpha and beta adrenoceptors with different affinities, as illustrated in the figure by different "lock–key" configurations. In total there are three alpha$_1$-adrenoceptors subtypes (alpha$_{1A}$, alpha$_{1B}$, and alpha$_{1D}$), three alpha$_2$-adrenoceptors subtypes (alpha$_{2A}$, alpha$_{2B}$, and alpha$_{2C}$), and three beta-adrenoceptors types (beta$_1$, beta$_2$, and beta$_3$). Alpha$_2$ and beta adrenoceptors are also located presynaptically and modulate norepinephrine release. (Adapted from Tsuru H, Tanimitsu N, Hirai T. Role of perivascular sympathetic nerves and regional differences in the features of sympathetic innervation of the vascular system. *Jpn J Pharmacol* 2002;88:9–13, with permission.)

identified: alpha$_{1A}$, alpha$_{1B}$, and alpha$_{1D}$. They have different localizations and activation patterns. Subtype alpha$_{1A}$ medi-ates vasoconstriction of specific arteries, including mammary, mesenteric, splenic, hepatic, omental, renal, pulmonary, and epicardial coronary, as well as specific veins, including the vena cava, saphenous, and pulmonary veins. Subtype alpha$_{1D}$ mediates contraction of the aorta and vena cava. In coronary arteries,[5] alpha$_1$-adrenoceptor stimulation may cause vaso-constriction if unopposed by beta$_2$-adrenergic stimulation. In the myocardium, alpha$_1$-adrenoceptors mediate a modest inotropic effect by increases in cytosolic Ca^{2+}.[6]

Alpha$_2$ Adrenoceptors These adrenoceptors are located in the central nervous system, peripheral sympathetic nerve endings, and target organs. They are found presynaptically and postsynaptically.[7] Three subtypes have been identified; alpha$_{2A}$, alpha$_{2B}$, and alpha$_{2C}$. Presynaptic alpha$_2$-adrenocep-tors are predominantly alpha$_{2A}$ and alpha$_{2C}$ in the heart and all three in the adrenal gland.[8,9] Their activation inhibits nor-epinephrine release (Fig. 26-2). Postsynaptic alpha$_2$ adreno-ceptors, centrally located, also reduce sympathetic flow such that central activation of presynaptic and postsynaptic alpha$_2$ adrenoceptors causes a prominent and diffuse sympathoin-hibitory response (i.e., explaining the antihypertensive effects of clonidine). Postsynaptic alpha$_2$ adrenoceptors, located peripherally, are predominantly alpha$_{2B}$ and mediate contrac-tion of smooth muscle cells, leading to vasoconstriction.

These adrenoceptors (alpha$_{2A}$) are also located distant from nerve endings in endothelial and smooth muscle cells and mediate vasoconstriction in response to circulating cate-cholamines.[10] Experimentally, use of the alpha$_2$-adrenoceptor agonist alpha methylnorepinephrine, which does not cross the blood–brain barrier, elicits a prominent vasoconstrictive response and attenuates cardiac sympathetic outflow. Both effects are desirable for resuscitation from cardiac arrest and in animal models improves resuscitation outcomes.[11] This agent, however, is not available for clinical use.

Beta Adrenoceptors

The main cardiovascular effect of beta adrenoceptors is stim-ulation of cardiac activity and relaxation of vascular smooth muscle cells. Beta adrenoceptors mediate their effects through Gs, which activates adenylyl cyclase, enhancing the generation of cAMP, and in turn, signaling downstream through protein kinase A the phosphorylation of several kinases that regulate contractile activity.[12] The same signal-ing mechanism enhances voltage-dependent Ca^{2+} channel activity (Fig. 26-1). Three types of beta adrenoceptors have been identified; beta$_1$, beta$_2$, and beta$_3$. Beta$_1$ and beta$_2$ medi-ate cardiovascular responses. Beta$_3$ has a lesser role in car-diovascular physiology but a prominent one in metabolism-mediating activity in white and brown adipose tissue.

Beta$_1$ Adrenoceptors

These adrenoceptors are expressed predominantly in the heart, attaining high density in the sinus node and ventricular tissue. Their stimulation leads to increased myocardial con-tractility and relaxation, enhanced pacemaker activity, and increased conduction velocity, thus increasing overall cardiac activity as part of the stress response that follows sympathetic activation. Beta$_1$ adrenoceptors are located postsynaptically, mostly in the immediate vicinity of sympathetic nerve termi-nals, but some are distributed more peripherally in target organs, to be stimulated by circulating catecholamines.

Beta$_2$ Adrenoceptors

These adrenoceptors are present in smooth muscle cells of blood vessels. Their stimulation induces vasorelaxation also through signaling cAMP increase. They oppose the vaso-constrictive effects of alpha-adrenoceptor stimulation. Beta$_2$ adrenoceptors are also present in the heart but with a dif-ferent distribution than beta$_1$ adrenoceptors, corresponding to approximately 20% of all beta adrenoceptors in left ven-tricular tissue but close to 50% in the sinus node, explaining the more prominent chronotropic effect of epinephrine and isoproterenol compared to norepinephrine, which lacks sig-nificant beta$_2$-adrenergic agonist activity.[3]

Adrenergic Agonists

Adrenergic agonists include the endogenous catecholamines epinephrine and norepinephrine (Fig. 26-3). Epinephrine is

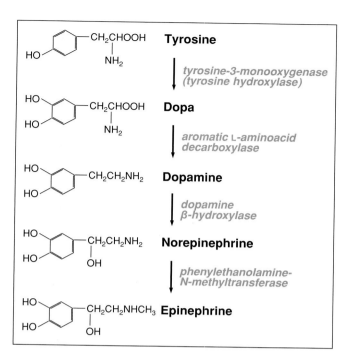

FIGURE 26-3 • Metabolic steps in the synthesis of dopamine, norepinephrine, and epinephrine, with the involved enzymes shown in red. Note that dopamine is the immediate precursor of norepinephrine and epinephrine. Synthesis of norepinephrine is the final step in adrenergic sympathetic neurons. The subsequent step leading to epinephrine occurs in the adrenal medulla and in a few epinephrine-containing neuronal pathways in the brainstem. (Adapted from Nagatsu T. Genes for human catecholamine-synthesizing enzymes. *Neurosci Res* 1991;12:315–345, with permission.)

released from the adrenal glands, whereas norepinephrine is released from sympathetic postganglionic fibers. Epinephrine activates alpha$_1$ and alpha$_2$ and beta$_1$ and beta$_2$ adrenoceptors. Norepinephrine also activates alpha$_1$, alpha$_2$, and beta$_1$ adrenoceptors but exerts minimal effects on beta$_2$ adrenoceptors. Synthetic amines known as sympathomimetic drugs stimulate adrenoceptors, albeit with different adrenoceptor affinities and specificities, as shown in Table 26-1.

Dopamine Receptors

Dopamine (D) receptors are also G protein–coupled receptors. To date, five types have been identified and grouped into two main types based on whether they are coupled to stimulatory (Gsα) or inhibitory (Giα) G-proteins. Thus, D1 receptors (including D1 and D5) are coupled to Gsα and stimulate formation of cAMP by increasing adenylyl cyclase activity. D2 receptors (including D2, D3, and D4) are coupled to Giα and have the opposite effect reducing the formation of cAMP by inhibiting adenylyl cyclase. D receptors play an important role in neurologic processes such as the control of motivation, learning, and fine motor movement.[13] They also mediate neuroendocrine signaling by modulating

the release of prolactin and thyroid hormone from the pituitary gland. Abnormalities in D receptors and dopaminergic nerve function have been implicated in several neuropsychiatric disorders, such as Parkinson's disease, drug addiction, compulsive behavior, attention-deficit/hyperactivity disorder, and schizophrenia.[13]

In the cardiovascular system, D receptors mediate selected vasodilatory responses along with inotropic and chronotropic cardiac responses. In the kidneys, D receptors mediate increased glomerular filtration, diuresis, and natriuresis.[14] These cardiovascular and renal effects are mediated through D1 receptors located postsynaptically in vascular smooth muscle cells and kidney. D2 receptors are located presynaptically at various sites within the sympathetic nervous system. Their activation leads to inhibition of sympathetic nervous system activity.

Dopamine

Dopamine is the naturally occurring agonist of D receptors. Given exogenously at low doses, it promotes vasodilation and increased renal function with minimal central effect because it does not readily cross the blood–brain barrier. Main target vascular beds include cerebral, renal, splanchnic, and coronary arteries. At somewhat higher doses, dopamine exerts inotropic effect by stimulating beta$_1$ adrenoceptors; at even higher doses, it enhances norepinephrine synthesis and release from sympathetic nerve terminals, leading to vasoconstriction, because it is the immediate metabolic precursor in the synthesis of norepinephrine (Fig. 26-3).[15]

Integrated Adrenergic Response

The broad diversity of adrenoceptors presented above permits, at the cellular level, signaling of distinct responses contingent on cell type, effector systems, and target mechanisms. At the organ level, receptor density, specific subtypes, and relative ligand potency allow for specific responses to sympathetic stimulation, circulating catecholamines, and sympathomimetic agents. For example, beta$_1$ adrenoceptors—as discussed above—are distributed predominantly in cardiac tissue, mediating inotropic and chronotropic responses. Blood vessels express alpha and beta adrenoceptors in varying proportions and densities, leading to vasoconstrictive or vasodilatory responses after stimulation by endogenous catecholamines or sympathomimetic drugs contingent on the vascular bed and local concentration of the agonists. For example, cutaneous vessels express almost exclusively alpha adrenoceptors, such that stimulation by epinephrine or norepinephrine leads to vasoconstriction; whereas stimulation by isoproterenol has virtually no effects. Blood vessels that supply skeletal muscles express beta$_2$ and alpha adrenoceptors, such that the predominant effect becomes contingent on the dose of the adrenergic agent. Epinephrine at low doses causes vasodilation, reflecting the predominance of beta$_2$-agonist effect, given a higher receptor affinity, whereas at higher doses, the same epinephrine causes vasoconstriction as the alpha-adrenoceptor effect predominates. This pharmacologic effect is useful during cardiac resuscitation when exogenous epinephrine is given to redistribute blood toward the heart and brain. Dopamine, the natural agonist of dopamine receptor and precursor of norepinephrine and epinephrine, mediates inotropic and vasodilatory responses at relatively low doses. However, as the dopamine dose increases, vasoconstrictive responses occur, related to increased production of norepinephrine in sympathetic nerve terminals.

Besides the primary effect of adrenergic stimulation, many additional factors influence the clinical response to adrenergic agonists, including the baroreflex response slowing the heart rate, activity of the parasympathetic nervous system, release of cotransmitters including ATP and neuropeptide Y from sympathetic nerve terminals, the effects of vasoactive platelet–mediated products such as thromboxane A_2 and prostacyclin, endothelial injury causing paradoxical responses to vasodilating stimuli, and interactions with other drugs.

Accordingly, the clinical effects of adrenergic agonists may vary widely from patient to patient and is further influenced by disease states, including whether the patient is in cardiac arrest. Because of this variability, these drugs may need to be titrated and the patient response closely monitored. In Table 26-1, a simplified selection of vasoactive drugs is summarized, identifying their major receptor sites and their effects on arterial vascular tone, heart rate, myocardial contractility, and the risk for inducing arrhythmias. Their usual clinical doses are also given.

Vasopressor Agents Used for Cardiac Resuscitation

See Web site for AHA ECC 2005 guidelines for CPR—medications for cardiovascular support: usage and dosage of epinephrine, vasopressin, norepinephrine, dopamine, dobutamine, milrinone, inamrinone, calcium chloride, digoxin, nitroglycerin, nitroprusside, furosemide.

Cessation of coronary blood flow after cardiac arrest leads to rapid development of intense global myocardial ischemia, especially when VF is the precipitating mechanism.[16] Unless spontaneous cardiac activity is promptly restored, as when VF is terminated by immediate delivery of electrical shocks (i.e., within a few minutes),[17] successful resuscitation relies on providers' capability for generating coronary blood flow above critical threshold levels.[18] Such blood flow is proportional to the pressure gradient established between the aorta and the right atrium during the relaxation phase of chest compression (i.e., coronary perfusion pressure).[19,20] Critical threshold levels predictive of resuscitation have been identified in various animal models and in human victims of

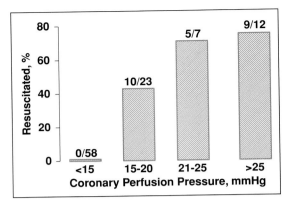

FIGURE 26-4 • Relationship between coronary perfusion pressure and initial resuscitation rates (%) in 100 victims of out-of-hospital cardiac arrest. Victims who failed initial resuscitation attempts at the scene were brought the emergency department and instrumented to measure coronary perfusion pressure during ongoing chest compression. A minimum coronary perfusion pressure of 15 mm Hg was noted before return of spontaneous circulation could be reestablished. Resuscitation rates increased proportional to coronary perfusion pressure after such threshold was exceeded. (Adapted from Paradis NA, Martin GB, Rivers EP, et al. Coronary perfusion pressure and the return of spontaneous circulation in human cardiopulmonary resuscitation. *JAMA* 1990;263:1106–1113, with permission.)

cardiac arrest, corresponding to 20 mm Hg in rats[21] and dogs,[22] 10 mm Hg in pigs,[23] and 15 mm Hg in humans. Once the resuscitability threshold is exceeded, proportionally greater resuscitability rates are expected[18] (Fig. 26-4).

To increase the coronary perfusion pressure, providers must pay close attention to the technique for generating forward blood flow. Current guidelines emphasize the importance of ensuring optimal depth and rate of compression, full chest recoil between compressions, avoiding hyperventilation, and minimizing interruptions of chest compression.[24] However, the forward blood flow generated by chest compression rarely exceeds 20% of the normal cardiac output[20,25] and typically deteriorates over time.[26] Therefore, increases in systemic vascular resistance are required to increase the coronary perfusion pressure above resuscitability thresholds. Although a prominent neuroendocrine stress response, triggered by cardiac arrest, prompts peripheral vasoconstriction, its magnitude is limited and exogenous administration of vasoconstrictive agents is often necessary.

The 2005 guidelines recognized epinephrine and vasopressin as the preferred vasopressor agents for cardiac resuscitation.[24] Yet to date, no placebo-controlled trial has been conducted in humans to determine whether vasopressor agents ultimately increase the rate of neurologically intact survival to hospital discharge.

Epinephrine

Epinephrine is hemodynamically beneficial during cardiac resuscitation because of its alpha-adrenoceptor vasoconstrictive effect.[27] In animal models, alpha-adrenergic stimulation during cardiac resuscitation increases coronary and cerebral blood flow and favors return of spontaneous circulation.[28] Experimentally, differences in the effects mediated through alpha$_1$ and alpha$_2$ adrenoceptors appear relevant. Alpha$_1$ adrenoceptors desensitize faster than alpha$_2$ adrenoceptors during ischemia and acidosis, such that there is a better alpha$_2$-mediated vasoconstrictive response after prolonged cardiac arrest. Alpha$_1$ adrenoceptors signal a modest inotropic effect through increases in cytosolic Ca^{2+}, which can be detrimental by increasing myocardial energy requirements and inducing arrhythmias. In contrast, presynaptic alpha$_2$ adrenoceptors in the heart limit the release of norepinephrine, exerting a favorable antiadrenergic effect.[8] Concomitant beta-adrenergic stimulation by epinephrine may be detrimental by increasing myocardial energy demands. Animal studies have shown that marked increases in myocardial blood flow by epinephrine during chest compression fail to attenuate ischemia, such that intramyocardial lactate and ATP depletion remain unchanged (Fig. 26-5).[29] In other studies, epinephrine has been shown to worsen postresuscitation myocardial function. Such detrimental effects can be reduced by concomitant use of beta-blockers or by use of selective alpha agonists instead of epinephrine.[30]

Despite these considerations, epinephrine is the most used vasopressor agent for resuscitation from cardiac arrest. Previous investigators had suggested that higher initial doses or escalating doses could improve survival rates. However, eight randomized clinical studies—involving more than 9,000 cardiac arrest victims—failed to demonstrate that higher doses of epinephrine improve survival to hospital discharge or neurologic outcomes when compared with standard doses.[31–38]

The 2005 guidelines recommend administration of 1 mg of epinephrine IV or intraosseous (IO) every 3 to 5 minutes during the resuscitation of adult victims in cardiac arrest (class IIb). Higher doses may be used in instances of beta-blocker or calcium channel blocker overdose. If IV or IO access is not available or is being delayed, epinephrine can be given by the endotracheal route at a dose of 2 to 2.5 mg.

Vasopressin (see also Chapter 27)

Arginine vasopressin (also known as antidiuretic hormone) is a neuropeptide hormone synthesized in the supraoptic and paraventricular nuclei of the hypothalamus and stored in the posterior pituitary gland. It is released into the circulation in response to increased plasma osmolality and decreases in blood volume or blood pressure as part of the baroreflex response. Vasopressin signals its effect through distinct types of receptors. V$_2$ receptors present in renal collecting tubules prompt water resorption. V$_{1A}$ receptors present in vascular smooth muscle prompt vasoconstriction, with a potency that exceeds that of angiotensin II and norepinephrine, affecting coronary, renal, and splanchnic beds. V$_{1B}$ (and also V$_2$) receptors promote platelet aggregation, potentially increasing the risk of thromboembolic events.[39,40]

Considerable work has been done in animal models of cardiac arrest examining the potential role of vasopressin for cardiac resuscitation. In VF models, IV vasopressin in doses of 0.4 or 0.8 U/kg promoted higher myocardial blood flows than epinephrine at doses of 0.045 mg/kg (standard dose) or 0.2 mg/kg (high dose).[41,42] Vasopressin had a more gradual onset of action than epinephrine, but the effect was more sustained.[43] Vasopressin also appeared to be more effective after prolonged intervals of cardiac arrest[44] without losing its vasopressor effects after repeated doses.[45]

The 2005 guidelines recommend administration of one dose of vasopressin 40 U IV or IO as replacement for the first or second dose of epinephrine in the treatment of cardiac arrest.

Epinephrine Versus Vasopressin

Several studies have compared epinephrine with vasopressin. Despite one promising randomized study,[46] additional small series of nonrandomized studies[47–49] and multiple well-performed animal studies, two large randomized controlled human trials[50,51] failed to show an increase in rates of return of spontaneous circulation or survival when vasopressin was compared with epinephrine. In one of the studies,[51] a *post hoc* analysis showed higher survival to hospital discharge in patients with asystole who received vasopressin instead of epinephrine. A meta-analysis of five randomized trials[52] showed no statistically significant differences between vasopressin and epinephrine for return of spontaneous circulation or survival at 24 hours or at hospital discharge. Subgroup analysis based on initial cardiac rhythm did not show statistically significant differences in survival to hospital discharge.[52]

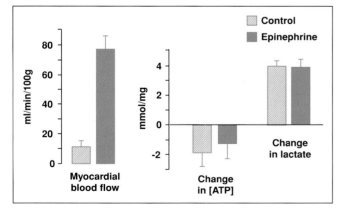

FIGURE 26-5 • Coronary blood flow along with changes in myocardial ATP and lactate during chest compression in dogs. Note that epinephrine failed to improve myocardial ATP and lactate contents despite prominently increasing coronary blood flow. (Adapted from Ditchey RV, Lindenfeld J. Failure of epinephrine to improve the balance between myocardial oxygen supply and demand during closed-chest resuscitation in dogs. *Circulation* 1988;78:382–389, with permission.)

Postresuscitation Hemodynamic Dysfunction

Emergency Medical Services systems are able to initially restore cardiac activity in approximately 30% of victims.[32,53,54] However, more than 30% of these patients die before hospital admission, presumably from recurrent episodes of cardiac arrest.[55] Of those admitted to a hospital, nearly 75% die before hospital discharge. Among the leading causes of postresuscitation deaths are myocardial dysfunction, neurologic dysfunction, and systemic inflammation ushering into a sepsis-like state.[55–57] The discussion below focuses on postresuscitation myocardial dysfunction and the associated hemodynamic abnormalities, which are in part related to a systemic inflammatory state that develops during the postresuscitation phase (see also Chapters 9 and 28).[55,58]

When coronary blood flow ceases after cardiac arrest, an energy imbalance develops, the severity of which is proportional to the myocardial energy requirements. These energy requirements are particularly high when VF is the precipitating cause of arrest[16,59] but less when the precipitating cause is asystole or pulseless electrical activity.[60] The immediate consequence is disruption of mitochondrial oxidative phosphorylation, prompting very limited amounts of ATP generation at the substrate level from breakdown of creatine phosphate and glycolysis.[61–64] A rapid energy deficit develops, accompanied by profound myocardial acidosis.[65,66] Resuscitation interventions play an essential role in ameliorating—at least partially—these metabolic abnormalities through the generation of coronary blood flow. However, reintroduction of oxygen and blood flow to ischemic tissue activates multiple mechanisms of injury, known as "reperfusion injury." This includes the generation of reactive oxygen species and Ca^{2+} overload and is in part responsible for postresuscitation myocardial dysfunction. Additional myocardial injury stems from repetitive electrical shocks[67] and the administration of adrenergic agents.[30] Myocardial injury is further compounded by underlying cardiac abnormalities (mainly coronary artery disease, with its acute and chronic ischemic manifestations).[55] As a result, various myocardial abnormalities develop during cardiac resuscitation, including (1) decreases in myocardial compliance, which may compromise the hemodynamic efficacy of chest compression[68,69]; (2) arrhythmias upon return of spontaneous circulation, accompanied by episodes of VF[70–72]; and (3) left ventricular systolic and diastolic dysfunction of varying severity, which can compromise hemodynamic function and accounts for a significant proportion of in-hospital deaths.[55,73–75] These abnormalities reverse to baseline within days or weeks in survivors (Fig. 26-6), consistent with myocardial stunning (postischemic dysfunction) as the predominant pathogenic mechanism.[73–77]

Laurent et al. reported on 165 patients successfully resuscitated after out-of-hospital cardiac arrest.[55] Hemodynamic instability—defined as hypotension requiring vasoactive drugs after fluid resuscitation—occurred in 55%

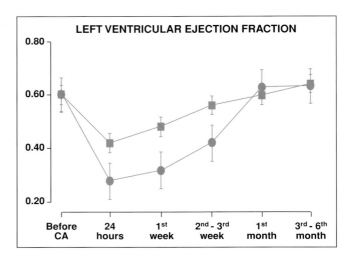

FIGURE 26-6 • Left ventricular ejection fraction estimated by echocardiography in 29 patients successfully resuscitated from cardiac arrest. Patient had no known cardiovascular disease (except for hypertension) and survived a minimum of 72 hours after return of spontaneous circulation. Prearrest echocardiograms were available in 16 patients demonstrating a mean left ventricular ejection fraction of 0.60. Squares represent the entire cohort of 29 patients; circles represent a subset of 20 patients who had myocardial dysfunction. (Adapted from Ruiz-Bailen M, Aguayo dH, Ruiz-Navarro S, et al. Reversible myocardial dysfunction after cardiopulmonary resuscitation. *Resuscitation* 2005;66:175–181, with permission.)

and was associated with longer resuscitation times, a greater number of electrical shocks, and larger amounts of epinephrine. These patients had myocardial dysfunction with a low cardiac index (2.05 L/min/m²) and a high systemic vascular resistance (2,908 dynes·sec/cm⁵·m²) consistent with a pattern of cardiogenic shock. However, within the subsequent 72 hours, a hyperdynamic state developed characterized by a high cardiac index, low peripheral vascular resistance, and large amounts of fluids required to maintain adequate filling pressures (Fig. 26-7). This late hyperdynamic state was consistent with development of a systemic inflammatory response akin to that observed in sepsis.[58,78,79] Adrie et al. measured circulating cytokines in 61 victims of out-of-hospital cardiac arrest; they demonstrated a prominent increase in circulating levels of inflammatory cytokines, including tumor necrosis factor (TNF) alpha and several interleukins as early as 3 hours postresuscitation.[58]

Inotropic Agents

The stunned myocardium is responsive to inotropic stimulation (Fig. 26-8). Conventional inotropic agents signal through increases in cytosolic cAMP or increases in cytosolic Ca^{2+}. The increases in cAMP can be attained by beta₁-adrenoceptor stimulation of adenylyl cyclase and/or by limiting cAMP metabolism, thus inhibiting phosphodiesterase activity. cAMP

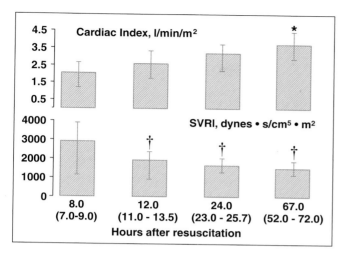

FIGURE 26-7 • Serial measurements of cardiac index and systemic vascular resistance index (SVRI) in a subset of 73 patients who had hemodynamic instability after resuscitation from out-of-hospital cardiac arrest. A cumulative amount of 8,000 mL was required to maintain a pulmonary artery occlusive pressure >12 mm Hg. The mortality rate was 19%. Shown are the median and interquartile range. *P <0.05; † P <0.001 versus baseline. (Adapted from Laurent I, Monchi M, Chiche JD, et al. Reversible myocardial dysfunction in survivors of out-of-hospital cardiac arrest. *J Am Coll Cardiol* 2002;40:2110–2116, with permission.)

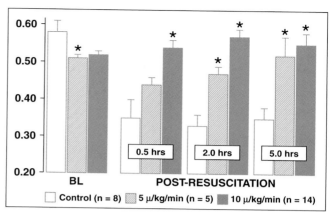

FIGURE 26-8 • Effects of dobutamine infusion on postresuscitation myocardial dysfunction in pigs. VF was induced and left untreated for 15 minutes before attempting resuscitation by conventional closed-chest resuscitation techniques including advanced life support and administration of epinephrine. Dobutamine was started at 15 minutes postresuscitation at either 5 or 10 μ/kg/min and the effects on left ventricular ejection fraction measured. Mean ± SEM. *P <0.05 control. (Adapted from Kern KB, Hilwig RW, Berg RA, et al. Postresuscitation left ventricular systolic and diastolic dysfunction. Treatment with dobutamine. *Circulation* 1997;95: 2610–2613, with permission.)

prompts the phosphorylation of Ca^{2+} regulatory proteins, such as L-type Ca^{2+} channels, phospholamban, the ryanodine receptor, troponin I, and the myosin-binding protein. This mechanism of increases in contractility is associated with increased cytosolic Ca^{2+} cycling, elevated energy consumption, and increased susceptibility to arrhythmias. An alternative approach is to mediate inotropic responses by augmenting the sensitivity of the contractile apparatus to Ca^{2+} acting on troponin C and downstream regulatory proteins but without increasing cAMP or cytosolic Ca^{2+}.[80] Several agents promote inotropy through these mechanisms and are known as Ca^{2+} sensitizers.[81,82] In addition to these newer inotropic agents, contractility can be increased by inhibiting the sarcolemmal Na^+, K^+-ATPase (i.e., digitalis). The inhibition of this pump causes cytosolic Na^+ increases prompting subsequent cytosolic Ca^{2+} increases through the sarcolemmal Na^+–Ca^{2+} exchanger.

Inotropic and Vasoactive Agents to Support Circulation

This section covers the use of inotropic and vasoactive agents for the treatment of hemodynamic dysfunction after cardiac resuscitation and other cardiovascular emergencies. It is important to realize that there is a paucity of clinical studies that specifically address the management of postresuscitation hemodynamic dysfunction. The information presented here has been extrapolated from other cardiovascular emergencies or obtained from work in animal models of cardiac arrest and should be applied with caution, considering that postresuscitation patients may be undergoing primary percutaneous coronary intervention[83,84] or having therapeutic hypothermia induced if they remain unresponsive after the return of cardiac activity.[85,86] A simplified summary of common agents used for cardiovascular support is presented in Table 26-1, listing the receptor or mechanisms of action targeted, the specific cardiac and vascular effects, and the usual clinical doses.

Epinephrine

Indication

The use of epinephrine for resuscitation from cardiac arrest is discussed above. However, epinephrine can also be used in prearrest and postarrest conditions in patients requiring inotropic, chronotropic, or vasopressor support. For example, epinephrine is considered class IIb for symptomatic bradycardia if atropine and transcutaneous pacing fail or pacing is not available. It may also be used for the management of anaphylaxis associated with hemodynamic instability or respiratory distress.[87]

Usage and Dosing

To create a continuous infusion of epinephrine hydrochloride, 1 mg of epinephrine (1 mL of a 1:1,000 solution) is added to 500 mL of normal saline or 5% dextrose in water. The initial dose for adults is 1 μg/min titrated to the desired hemodynamic response, which is typically achieved in doses of 2 to 10 μg/min.

Vasopressin

Indication

The use of arginine vasopressin for resuscitation from cardiac arrest is discussed above and in Chapter 28. Vasopressin in lower doses can be used to treat hypotension associated with septic shock and vasodilation refractory to adrenergic vasopressor agent. It has been shown that circulating levels of vasopressin are elevated during hypovolemic, cardiogenic, and obstructive shock. However, for reasons that are not entirely clear, vasopressin levels remain close to baseline during septic shock despite prominent reductions in blood pressure.[88] Yet the vascular response to vasopressin is not impaired, and prominent vasopressor effects can be elicited even at doses much lower than those typically used to control variceal bleeding.[88–92] The mechanisms of action seem to involve direct stimulation of V_1 receptors and enhanced alpha$_1$-adrenoceptor response to catecholamines. The response is sustained, typically lacks baroreflex reductions in heart rate, and occurs despite unresponsiveness to catecholamines.

Usage and Dosing

The recommended infusion rate for treatment of vasodilation in septic shock in adults is 0.01 to 0.04 U/min. This dosage has been reported to be effective in approximately 85% of patients with hypotension resistant to norepinephrine.[93] Doses >0.04 U/min should be avoided to prevent potential side effects related to vasoconstriction, such as skin, splanchnic, and coronary ischemia.[94]

Norepinephrine

Indication

Norepinephrine exerts a predominant vasoconstrictive effect through alpha-adrenoceptor stimulation and inotropic and chronotropic effects through alpha$_1$ and beta$_1$ adrenoceptors. The effects on cardiac output, however, depend on the magnitude of the afterload increase, the functional state of the left ventricle, and reflex responses. Although norepinephrine—in a dose-dependent manner—can induce renal and mesenteric vasoconstriction, in sepsis, it may improve renal blood flow and urine output.[95,96] Norepinephrine may be effective in the management of severe hypotension (i.e., systolic blood pressure <70 mm Hg), especially in patients with vasodilation associated with sepsis who fail to respond to adequate intravascular volume expansion. Norepinephrine should be avoided in the presence of hypovolemia, in which intravascular volume expan-

sion is the primary intervention. Norepinephrine increases myocardial oxygen requirements and may induce myocardial ischemia in patients with underlying coronary artery disease.

Usage and Dosing

Norepinephrine is administered by adding 4 mg of norepinephrine or 8 mg of norepinephrine bitartrate to 250 mL of 5% dextrose in water or normal saline (but not in normal saline alone), resulting in a concentration of 16 μg/mL of norepinephrine or 32 μg/mL of norepinephrine bitartrate (1 mg of norepinephrine is equivalent to 2 mg of norepinephrine bitartrate). The starting dose is 0.5 to 1 μg/min and is usually titrated up to 30 μg/min in an attempt to maintain a systolic blood pressure of at least 90 mm Hg. To avoid inactivation, norepinephrine should not be administered in the same IV line as alkaline solutions. Norepinephrine should preferably be administered through a central venous catheter, not through a peripheral catheter, in order to avoid the risk of skin extravasation, which can lead to ischemic necrosis and sloughing of superficial tissues.

Dopamine

Indication

Physiologically, dopamine stimulates the heart, presumably through D1 receptors expressed in the heart and through the increased production and release of norepinephrine from sympathetic nerve terminals activating both alpha and beta adrenoceptors. Pharmacologically, the effects of dopamine are dose-dependent, yielding predominantly vasodilation at low doses and vasoconstriction with inotropic effects at higher doses (see below). Dopamine can be used to treat hypotension after resuscitation from cardiac arrest, especially if it is associated with symptomatic bradycardia. If hypotension persists after filling pressure (i.e., intravascular volume) is optimized, drugs with combined inotropic and vasopressor actions, such as epinephrine or norepinephrine, may be used. Positive effects may follow increases in both cardiac output and arterial perfusion pressure. Although low-dose dopamine infusion has been frequently recommended to maintain renal blood flow or improve renal function, more recent data have failed to show a beneficial effect from such therapy, and it is no longer recommended.[97,98]

Usage and Dosing

The usual dose ranges from 2 to 20 μg/kg/min. At a low dose (2–4 μg/kg/min), a dopaminergic effect predominates, leading to vasodilation and mild inotropic and chronotropic effects. At an intermediate dose (5–10 μg/kg/min), a beta$_1$ and beta$_2$ effect is recruited, leading to more prominent increases in contractility and heart rate. At a high dose (11–20 μg/kg/min), the alpha-adrenoceptor effect is incorporated, leading to prominent vasoconstriction. However, this dose can be associated with a significant reduction in splanchnic perfusion.

Dobutamine

Indication

Dobutamine is a sympathomimetic agent designed by Eli Lilly & Company for the management of patients with severe heart failure. The drug is a racemic mixture consisting of both the dextrorotatory (D) and levorotatory (L) isomers of dobutamine. D-dobutamine is a potent beta$_1$ agonist, while L-dobutamine is an alpha$_1$ agonist.[99] Dobutamine also has mild beta$_2$-agonist activity. Dobutamine exerts inotropic and chronotropic effects, leading to increases in cardiac output. Dobutamine can be used to treat acute but potentially reversible heart failure, such as that involving cardiac surgery, septic or cardiogenic shock, and acutely decompensated heart failure. The vasodilating beta$_2$-adrenergic effects counterbalance the vasoconstricting alpha$_1$-adrenergic effects, often leading to little change or a reduction in systemic vascular resistance. The beneficial effects of dobutamine may be associated with decreased left ventricular filling pressure. In addition to its direct inotropic effects, dobutamine may further increase stroke volume through (baroreceptor-mediated) reflex peripheral vasodilation, thus reducing ventricular afterload, so that arterial pressure is unchanged or may even fall despite increases in cardiac output.

Studies in animal models of cardiac arrest have demonstrated substantial reversal of postresuscitation systolic and diastolic dysfunction using doses ranging between 5 and 10 μg/kg/min (Fig. 26-8).[100–102] However, a dose of 5 μg/kg/min was found to provide the best balance by restoring postresuscitation systolic and diastolic function without adverse effects on myocardial oxygen consumption.[101]

Usage and Dosing

The dose of dobutamine ranges from 2 to 20 μg/kg/min, given a wide variation in individual responses. Elderly patients may have a significantly decreased response to dobutamine. At doses >20 μg/kg/min, increases in heart rate of >10% may induce or exacerbate myocardial ischemia. Doses of dobutamine as high as 40 μg/kg/min have been used, but such doses may greatly increase its adverse effects, such as tachycardia and hypotension.

Phosphodiesterase Inhibitors (Inamrinone and Milrinone)

Indication

Inamrinone (formerly amrinone) and milrinone are phosphodiesterase III inhibitors that elicit inotropic and vasodilatory responses. Phosphodiesterase inhibitors are often used in conjunction with catecholamines for severe heart failure, cardiogenic shock, and other forms of shock unresponsive to catecholamine therapy alone. Optimal use requires hemody-namic monitoring. These drugs are contraindicated in patients with heart valve stenosis that limits cardiac output.

Usage and Dosing

Inamrinone is administered as a loading dose of 0.75 mg/kg over 10 to 15 minutes (it may be given over 2–3 minutes in the absence of left ventricular dysfunction), followed by an infusion of 5 to 15 μg/kg/min titrated to clinical effect. An additional bolus may be given in 30 minutes. Milrinone is more often used today because it has a shorter half-life than inamrinone and is less likely to cause thrombocytopenia.[103,104] Milrinone is renally excreted, with a half-life of around 1.5 to 2 hours, so it requires 4.5 to 6 hours to achieve near–steady state concentrations if given without a loading dose. A slow IV loading dose of milrinone (50 μg/kg over 10 minutes) is followed by an IV infusion at a rate of 0.375 to 0.75 μg/kg/min for 2 to 3 days. In renal failure, the dose should be reduced. Adverse effects include nausea, vomiting, and hypotension.

Calcium Salts

Indication

Although Ca^{2+} plays a critical role in myocardial contractility and vascular tone, studies in the cardiac arrest setting have failed to show any benefit associated with administration of calcium salts.[105,106] Instead, there is concern that high serum Ca^{2+} may be toxic. Calcium salts, however, may be used when hyperkalemia, ionized hypocalcemia (e.g., after multiple blood transfusions) or calcium channel blocker toxicity is present.[107] It is important to recognize that it is the ionized form of circulating Ca^{2+} that is physiologically relevant to cardiovascular function. Thus, efforts should be made to measure ionized Ca^{2+} instead of total Ca^{2+}, which correlates poorly with its ionized form in critically ill patients.[108,109]

Usage and Dosing

When necessary, a 10% solution (100 mg/mL) of calcium chloride can be given in a dose of 8 to 16 mg/kg of the salt (usually 5–10 mL) and repeated as necessary.

Digitalis

Indication

Digitalis preparations have limited use as inotropic agents in emergency cardiovascular care. Digitalis decreases the ventricular rate in some patients with atrial flutter or fibrillation by slowing atrioventricular nodal conduction. Digitalis has a narrow therapeutic ratio, especially when potassium depletion is present. Digitalis toxicity may cause serious ventricular arrhythmias and precipitate cardiac arrest. Digoxin-specific antibody is available for the treatment of serious toxicity (Digibind, Digitalis Antidote BM).

Nitroglycerin

Indication

Nitrates are used for their ability to relax vascular smooth muscle of systemic veins and arteries, including the coronary arteries. Nitroglycerin can be helpful in the initial management of acute coronary syndromes, congestive heart failure,[110] and hypertensive emergencies (see also Chapters 4, 5 and 7). Nitroglycerin mediates its effect through local endothelial production of nitric oxide, particularly in venous capacitance vessels. Nitroglycerin is most effective in patients with increased intravascular volume. Hypovolemia blunts the beneficial hemodynamic effects of nitroglycerin and increases the risk of hypotension. Nitrate-induced hypotension typically responds well to intravascular volume expansion. Other potential complications of the use of intravenous nitroglycerin are tachycardia, paradoxical bradycardia, and hypoxemia caused by increased pulmonary ventilation/perfusion mismatch. Headache is a common side effect. Nitroglycerin should be avoided in the presence of bradycardia and extreme tachycardia or within 24 to 48 hours of the use of phosphodiesterase inhibitors for erectile dysfunction.

Usage and Dosing

Nitroglycerin can be administered sublingually, transdermally, or IV as a continuous infusion. This last delivery mechanism is particularly useful in the acute setting, when precise dose titration is desirable. Nitroglycerin (50 or 100 mg) is prepared in 250 mL of 5% dextrose in water or 0.9% sodium chloride and administered at 10 to 20 µg/min. When required, the dose can be increased by 5 to 10 µg/min every 5 to 10 minutes until the desired hemodynamic or clinical response occurs. Low doses (30–40 µg/min) predominantly produce venodilatation; high doses (150–500 µg/min) provide arteriolar dilatation. Uninterrupted administration of nitroglycerin (>24 hours) produces tolerance.[111]

Sodium Nitroprusside

Indication

Sodium nitroprusside is a potent, rapid-acting, direct peripheral vasodilator useful in the treatment of severe heart failure and hypertensive emergencies.[112] It dilates veins and arteries. Venodilation reduces preload, thus helping to alleviate pulmonary and systemic congestion. Arteriolar relaxation causes decreases in peripheral arterial resistance (afterload), resulting in enhanced systolic emptying with reduced left ventricular volume and wall stress. These effects reduce myocardial oxygen consumption. Afterload reduction, especially in patients with left ventricular dysfunction, results in increased cardiac output. These hemodynamic effects are influenced by intravascular volume. In the presence of hypovolemia, nitroprusside can cause hypotension with reflex tachycardia. Continuous blood pressure monitoring is highly desirable during nitroprusside therapy.

Nitroprusside is rapidly metabolized by nonenzymatic means to cyanide, which is then detoxified in the liver and kidney to thiocyanate. Cyanide is also metabolized by forming a complex with vitamin B_{12}.[113] Thiocyanate undergoes renal elimination. Patients with hepatic or renal insufficiency and those requiring >3 µg/kg/min for more than 72 hours may accumulate cyanide or thiocyanate; they should be monitored for signs of cyanide or thiocyanate intoxication, such as metabolic acidosis.[114] When the thiocyanate concentration exceeds 12 mg/dL, toxicity may occur and becomes manifest as confusion, hyperreflexia, and ultimately convulsions. Treatment of elevated cyanide or thiocyanate levels includes immediate discontinuation of the infusion. If the patient is experiencing signs and symptoms of cyanide toxicity, sodium nitrite and sodium thiosulfate should be administered.

Usage and Dosing

Sodium nitroprusside is prepared by adding 50 or 100 mg to 250 mL of 5% dextrose in water. The solution and tubing should be wrapped in opaque material, because nitroprusside deteriorates when exposed to light. The recommended dose is 0.1 to 5 µg/kg/min, but higher doses (up to 10 µg/kg/min) may be needed.

Diuretics

Indication

Furosemide is a potent diuretic agent that inhibits reabsorption of sodium in the proximal and distal renal tubule and the loop of Henle. Furosemide has little or no direct vascular effect, but it reduces venous and pulmonary vascular resistance through stimulation of local prostaglandin production[115] and, therefore, may be useful in the treatment of pulmonary edema. The vascular effects occur within 5 minutes, whereas diuresis is delayed. Although often used in acute renal failure to stimulate increased urine output, there are no data to support this indication, and some data suggests an association with increased mortality.[116]

Usage and Dosing

The initial dose of furosemide is 0.5 to 1 mg/kg IV injected slowly. Newer "loop" diuretics that have an action similar to that of furosemide and a similar profile of side effects include torsemide and bumetanide. In patients who do not respond to high doses of loop diuretics alone, a combination of such agents together with the administration of "proximal tubule"–acting thiazide diuretics (such as chlorothiazide or metolazone) may be effective. Such combinations require close observation with serial measurement of serum electrolytes to avoid profound potassium depletion from their use.

IV Fluid Administration

There is limited evidence available to guide fluid administration during cardiac resuscitation. Early animal studies showed that volume loading during chest compression had a disproportionate effect on right atrial pressure relative to aortic pressure,[117] causing the coronary perfusion pressure to decrease. Even when epinephrine is administered, volume administration given either intravenously or directly into the aorta fails to further increase the coronary perfusion pressure.[118] If cardiac arrest occurs associated with extreme volume losses, however, increasing intravascular volume could be beneficial. More recent studies in animal model suggests that hypertonic saline may improve survival from VF as compared with normal saline.[119,120] However, human studies are needed before the use of hypertonic saline can be recommended. If fluids are administered during cardiac resuscitation, solutions containing dextrose should be avoided unless there is evidence of hypoglycemia.

Administration of fluids, however, is essential in other cardiovascular emergencies in which an absolute or relative intravascular volume deficit is suspected to contribute to hemodynamic instability. That is typically the case in hypovolemic shock and in distributive shock, where blood pooling in venous capacitance vessels and increased capillary permeability contribute to decreased effective intravascular volume. Yet even in instances of cardiogenic and obstructive shock, intravascular volume expansion may be useful to support left or right ventricular function by augmenting preload.

References

1. Ahlquist RP. Development of the concept of alpha and beta adrenotropic receptors. *Ann N Y Acad Sci* 1967;139:549–552.
2. Tsuru H, Tanimitsu N, Hirai T. Role of perivascular sympathetic nerves and regional differences in the features of sympathetic innervation of the vascular system. *Jpn J Pharmacol* 2002;88:9–13.
3. Westfall TC, Westfall DP. Adrenergic agonists and antagonists. In: Brunton LL, Lazo JS, Parker KL, eds. *Goodman and Gilman's the Pharmacological Basis of Therapeutics.* New York: McGraw-Hill, 2006: 237–295.
4. Graham RM, Perez DM, Hwa J, et al. Alpha 1-adrenergic receptor subtypes. Molecular structure, function, and signaling. *Circ Res* 1996;78:737–749.
5. Woodman OL, Vatner SF. Coronary vasoconstriction mediated by alpha 1- and alpha 2-adrenoceptors in conscious dogs. *Am J Physiol* 1987;253:H388–H393.
6. Otani H, Otani H, Das DK. Alpha 1-adrenoceptor-mediated phosphoinositide breakdown and inotropic response in rat left ventricular papillary muscles. *Circ Res* 1988;62:8–17.
7. Tavares A, Handy DE, Bogdanova NN, et al. Localization of alpha 2A- and alpha 2B-adrenergic receptor subtypes in brain. *Hypertension* 1996;27:449–455.
8. Brede M, Wiesmann F, Jahns R, et al. Feedback inhibition of catecholamine release by two different alpha2-adrenoceptor subtypes prevents progression of heart failure. *Circulation* 2002; 106:2491–2496.
9. Brede M, Philipp M, Knaus A, et al. Alpha2-adrenergic receptor subtypes: novel functions uncovered in gene-targeted mouse models. *Biol Cell* 2004;96:343–348.
10. Handy DE, Johns C, Bresnahan MR, et al. Expression of alpha2-adrenergic receptors in normal and atherosclerotic rabbit aorta. *Hypertension* 1998;32:311–317.
11. Klouche K, Weil MH, Tang W, et al. A selective alpha(2)-adrenergic agonist for cardiac resuscitation. *J Lab Clin Med* 2002;140: 27–34.
12. Opie LH. *The Heart: Physiology, from Cell to Circulation*, 3rd ed. Philadelphia: Lippincott-Raven, 1998.
13. Girault JA, Greengard P. The neurobiology of dopamine signaling. *Arch Neurol* 2004;61:641–644.
14. Lokhandwala MF, Barret RJ. Dopamine receptor agonists in cardiovascular therapy. *Drug Dev Res* 1983;3:299–310.
15. Nagatsu T. Genes for human catecholamine-synthesizing enzymes. *Neurosci Res* 1991;12:315–345.
16. Gazmuri RJ, Berkowitz M, Cajigas H. Myocardial effects of ventricular fibrillation in the isolated rat heart. *Crit Care Med* 1999;27:1542–1550.
17. Valenzuela TD, Roe DJ, Nichol G, et al. Outcomes of rapid defibrillation by security officers after cardiac arrest in casinos. *N Engl J Med* 2000;343:1206–1209.
18. Paradis NA, Martin GB, Rivers EP, et al. Coronary perfusion pressure and the return of spontaneous circulation in human cardiopulmonary resuscitation. *JAMA* 1990;263:1106–1113.
19. Maier GW, Tyson GS Jr, Olsen CO, et al. The physiology of external cardiac massage: high impulse cardiopulmonary resuscitation. *Circulation* 1984;70:86–101.
20. Ralston SH, Voorhees WD, Babbs CF. Intrapulmonary epinephrine during prolonged cardiopulmonary resuscitation: improved regional blood flow and resuscitation in dogs. *Ann Emerg Med* 1984;13:79–86.
21. von Planta I, Weil MH, von Planta M, et al. Cardiopulmonary resuscitation in the rat. *J Appl Physiol* 1988;65:2641–2647.
22. Niemann JT, Criley JM, Rosborough JP, et al. Predictive indices of successful cardiac resuscitation after prolonged arrest and experimental cardiopulmonary resuscitation. *Ann Emerg Med* 1985;14:521–528.
23. Gazmuri RJ, von Planta M, Weil MH, et al. Cardiac effects of carbon dioxide–consuming and carbon dioxide–generating buffers during cardiopulmonary resuscitation. *J Am Coll Cardiol* 1990;15: 482–490.
24. American Heart Association. 2005 American Heart Association guidelines for cardiopulmonary resuscitation and emergency cardiovascular care. *Circulation* 2005;112(suppl IV):IV-1–IV-211.
25. Kolarova JD, Ayoub IM, Gazmuri RJ. Cariporide enables hemodynamically more effective chest compression by leftward shift of its flow-depth relationship. *Am J Physiol Heart Circ Physiol* 2005;288:H2904–H2911.
26. Sharff JA, Pantley G, Noel E. Effect of time on regional organ perfusion during two methods of cardiopulmonary resuscitation. *Ann Emerg Med* 1984;13:649–656.
27. Yakaitis RW, Otto CW, Blitt CD. Relative importance of a and b-adrenergic receptors during resuscitation. *Crit Care Med* 1979;7: 293–296.
28. Michael JR, Guerci AD, Koehler RC, et al. Mechanisms by which epinephrine augments cerebral and myocardial perfusion during cardiopulmonary resuscitation in dogs. *Circulation* 1984;69: 822–835.
29. Ditchey RV, Lindenfeld J. Failure of epinephrine to improve the balance between myocardial oxygen supply and demand during closed-chest resuscitation in dogs. *Circulation* 1988;78:382–389.
30. Tang W, Weil MH, Sun S, et al. Epinephrine increases the severity of postresuscitation myocardial dysfunction. *Circulation* 1995;92:3089–3093.
31. Lindner KH, Ahnefeld FW, Prengel AW. Comparison of standard and high-dose adrenaline in the resuscitation of asystole and electromechanical dissociation. *Acta Anaesthesiol Scand* 1991;35: 253–256.
32. Brown CG, Martin DR, Pepe PE, et al. A comparison of standard-dose and high-dose epinephrine in cardiac arrest outside the hospital. *N Engl J Med* 1992;327:1051–1055.
33. Stiell IG, Herbert PC, Weitzman BN, et al. High-dose epinephrine in adult cardiac arrest. *N Engl J Med* 1992;327:1045–1050.
34. Callaham M, Madsen CD, Barton CW, et al. A randomized clinical trial of high-dose epinephrine and norepinephrine vs standard-dose epinephrine in prehospital cardiac arrest [see comments]. *JAMA* 1992;268:2667–2672.
35. Lipman J, Wilson W, Kobilski S, et al. High-dose adrenaline in adult in-hospital asystolic cardiopulmonary resuscitation: a double-blind randomised trial. *Anaesth Intens Care* 1993;21:192–196.
36. Choux C, Gueugniaud PY, Barbieux A, et al. Standard doses versus repeated high doses of epinephrine in cardiac arrest outside the hospital. *Resuscitation* 1995;29:3–9.
37. Sherman BW, Munger MA, Foulke GE, et al. High-dose versus standard-dose epinephrine treatment of cardiac arrest after failure of standard therapy. *Pharmacotherapy* 1997;17:242–247.

38. Gueugniaud PY, Mols P, Goldstein P, et al. A comparison of repeated high doses and repeated standard doses of epinephrine for cardiac arrest outside the hospital. European Epinephrine Study Group. *N Engl J Med* 1998;339:1595–1601.

39. Grant PJ, Tate GM, Davies JA, et al. Intra-operative activation of coagulation—a stimulus to thrombosis mediated by vasopressin? *Thromb Haemost* 1986;55:104–107.

40. Wun T, Paglieroni T, Lachant NA. Physiologic concentrations of arginine vasopressin activate human platelets in vitro. *Br J Haematol* 1996;92:968–972.

41. Lindner KH, Brinkmann A, Pfenninger EG, et al. Effect of vasopressin on hemodynamic variables, organ blood flow, and acid-base status in a pig model of cardiopulmonary resuscitation. *Anesth Analg* 1993;77:427–435.

42. Lindner KH, Prengel AW, Pfenninger EG, et al. Vasopressin improves vital organ blood flow during closed-chest cardiopulmonary resuscitation in pigs. *Circulation* 1995;91:215–221.

43. Mulligan KA, McKnite SH, Lindner KH, et al. Synergistic effects of vasopressin plus epinephrine during cardiopulmonary resuscitation. *Resuscitation* 1997;35:265–271.

44. Wenzel V, Lindner KH, Prengel AW, et al. Vasopressin improves vital organ blood flow after prolonged cardiac arrest with post-countershock pulseless electrical activity in pigs. *Crit Care Med* 1999;27:486–492.

45. Wenzel V, Lindner KH, Krismer AC, et al. Repeated administration of vasopressin but not epinephrine maintains coronary perfusion pressure after early and late administration during prolonged cardiopulmonary resuscitation in pigs. *Circulation* 1999;99:1379–1384.

46. Lindner KH, Dirks B, Strohmenger HU, et al. Randomised comparison of epinephrine and vasopressin in patients with out-of-hospital ventricular fibrillation. *Lancet* 1997;349:535–537.

47. Lindner KH, Prengel AW, Brinkmann A, et al. Vasopressin administration in refractory cardiac arrest. *Ann Intern Med* 1996;124:1061–1064.

48. Mann K, Berg RA, Nadkarni V. Beneficial effects of vasopressin in prolonged pediatric cardiac arrest: a case series. *Resuscitation* 2002;52:149–156.

49. Morris DC, Dereczyk BE, Grzybowski M, et al. Vasopressin can increase coronary perfusion pressure during human cardiopulmonary resuscitation. *Acad Emerg Med* 1997;4:878–883.

50. Stiell IG, Hebert PC, Wells GA, et al. Vasopressin versus epinephrine for inhospital cardiac arrest: a randomised controlled trial. *Lancet* 2001;358:105–109.

51. Wenzel V, Krismer AC, Arntz HR, et al. A comparison of vasopressin and epinephrine for out-of-hospital cardiopulmonary resuscitation. *N Engl J Med* 2004;350:105–113.

52. Aung K, Htay T. Vasopressin for cardiac arrest: a systematic review and meta-analysis. *Arch Intern Med* 2005;165:17–24.

53. Kellermann AL, Hackman BB, Somes G. Predicting the outcome of unsuccessful prehospital advanced cardiac life support. *JAMA* 1993;270:1433–1436.

54. Lombardi G, Gallagher J, Gennis P. Outcome of out-of-hospital cardiac arrest in New York City. The pre-hospital arrest survival evaluation (PHASE) study. *JAMA* 1994;271:678–683.

55. Laurent I, Monchi M, Chiche JD, et al. Reversible myocardial dysfunction in survivors of out-of-hospital cardiac arrest. *J Am Coll Cardiol* 2002;40:2110–2116.

56. Checchia PA, Sehra R, Moynihan J, et al. Myocardial injury in children following resuscitation after cardiac arrest. *Resuscitation* 2003;57:131–137.

57. Laver S, Farrow C, Turner D, et al. Mode of death after admission to an intensive care unit following cardiac arrest. *Intens Care Med* 2004;30:2126–2128.

58. Adrie C, Adib-Conquy M, Laurent I, et al. Successful cardiopulmonary resuscitation after cardiac arrest as a "sepsis-like" syndrome. *Circulation* 2002;106:562–568.

59. Yaku H, Goto Y, Ohgoshi Y, et al. Determinant of myocardial oxygen consumption in fibrillating dog hearts: comparison between normothermia and hypothermia. *J Thorac Cardiovasc Surg* 1993;105:679–688.

60. Kamohara T, Weil MH, Tang W, et al. A comparison of myocardial function after primary cardiac and primary asphyxial cardiac arrest. *Am J Respir Crit Care Med* 2001;164:1221–1224.

61. Neumar RW, Brown CG, Van Ligten P, et al. Estimation of myocardial ischemic injury during ventricular fibrillation with total circulatory arrest using high-energy phosphates and lactate as metabolic markers. *Ann Emerg Med* 1991;20:222–229.

62. Kern KB, Garewal HS, Sanders AB, et al. Depletion of myocardial adenosine triphosphate during prolonged untreated ventricular fibrillation: effect on defibrillation success. *Resuscitation* 1990;20:221–229.

63. Noc M, Weil MH, Gazmuri RJ, et al. Ventricular fibrillation voltage as a monitor of the effectiveness of cardiopulmonary resuscitation. *J Lab Clin Med* 1994;124:421–426.

64. Ayoub IM, Kolarova J, Kantola R, et al. Zoniporide preserves left ventricular compliance during ventricular fibrillation and minimizes post-resuscitation myocardial dysfunction through benefits on energy metabolism. *Crit Care Med* 2007;35:2329–2336.

65. Kette F, Weil MH, Gazmuri RJ, et al. Intramyocardial hypercarbic acidosis during cardiac arrest and resuscitation. *Crit Care Med* 1993;21:901–906.

66. Johnson BA, Weil MH, Tang W, et al. Mechanisms of myocardial hypercarbic acidosis during cardiac arrest. *J Appl Physiol* 1995;78:1579–1584.

67. Gazmuri RJ. Effects of repetitive electrical shocks on postresuscitation myocardial function. *Crit Care Med* 2000;28:N228–N232.

68. Klouche K, Weil MH, Sun S, et al. Echo-Doppler observations during cardiac arrest and cardiopulmonary resuscitation. *Crit Care Med* 2000;28:N212–N213.

69. Ayoub IM, Kolarova JD, Yi Z, et al. Sodium-hydrogen exchange inhibition during ventricular fibrillation: Beneficial effects on ischemic contracture, action potential duration, reperfusion arrhythmias, myocardial function, and resuscitability. *Circulation* 2003;107:1804–1809.

70. White RD, Russell JK. Refibrillation, resuscitation and survival in out-of-hospital sudden cardiac arrest victims treated with biphasic automated external defibrillators. *Resuscitation* 2002;55:17–23.

71. van Alem AP, Post J, Koster RW. VF recurrence: characteristics and patient outcome in out-of-hospital cardiac arrest. *Resuscitation* 2003;59:181–188.

72. Hess EP, White RD. Recurrent ventricular fibrillation in out-of-hospital cardiac arrest after defibrillation by police and firefighters: implications for automated external defibrillator users. *Crit Care Med* 2004;32:S436–S439.

73. Gazmuri RJ, Weil MH, Bisera J, et al. Myocardial dysfunction after successful resuscitation from cardiac arrest. *Crit Care Med* 1996;24:992–1000.

74. Kern KB, Hilwig RW, Rhee KH, et al. Myocardial dysfunction after resuscitation from cardiac arrest: An example of global myocardial stunning. *J Am Coll Cardiol* 1996;28:232–240.

75. Ruiz-Bailen M, Aguayo dH, Ruiz-Navarro S, et al. Reversible myocardial dysfunction after cardiopulmonary resuscitation. *Resuscitation* 2005;66:175–181.

76. Deantonio HJ, Kaul S, Lerman BB. Reversible myocardial depression in survivors of cardiac arrest. *PACE* 1990;13:982–985.

77. Kern KB. Postresuscitation myocardial dysfunction. *Cardiol Clin* 2002;20:89–101.

78. Shyu KG, Chang H, Lin CC, et al. Concentrations of serum interleukin-8 after successful cardiopulmonary resuscitation in patients with cardiopulmonary arrest. *Am Heart J* 1997;134:551–556.

79. Ito T, Saitoh D, Fukuzuka K, et al. Significance of elevated serum interleukin-8 in patients resuscitated after cardiopulmonary arrest. *Resuscitation* 2001;51:47–53.

80. Endoh M. Mechanism of action of Ca^{2+} sensitizers—update 2001. *Cardiovasc Drugs Ther* 2001;15:397–403.

81. Kaheinen P, Pollesello P, Levijoki J, et al. Effects of levosimendan and milrinone on oxygen consumption in isolated guinea-pig heart. *J Cardiovasc Pharmacol* 2004;43:555–561.

82. Lilleberg J, Ylonen V, Lehtonen L, et al. The calcium sensitizer levosimendan and cardiac arrhythmias: an analysis of the safety database of heart failure treatment studies. *Scand Cardiovasc J* 2004;38:80–84.

83. Garot P, Lefevre T, Eltchaninoff H, et al. Six-month outcome of emergency percutaneous coronary intervention in resuscitated patients after cardiac arrest complicating ST-elevation myocardial infarction. *Circulation* 2007;115:1354–1362.

84. Knafelj R, Radsel P, Ploj T, et al. Primary percutaneous coronary intervention and mild induced hypothermia in comatose survivors of ventricular fibrillation with ST-elevation acute myocardial infarction. *Resuscitation* 2007;74:227–234.

85. Bernard SA, Gray TW, Buist MD, et al. Treatment of comatose survivors of out-of-hospital cardiac arrest with induced hypothermia. *N Engl J Med* 2002;346:557–563.
86. Mild therapeutic hypothermia to improve the neurologic outcome after cardiac arrest. *N Engl J Med* 2002;346:549–556.
87. Ellis AK, Day JH. Diagnosis and management of anaphylaxis. *CMAJ* 2003;169:307–311.
88. Landry DW, Levin HR, Gallant EM, et al. Vasopressin deficiency contributes to the vasodilation of septic shock. *Circulation* 1997;95:1122–1125.
89. Malay MB, Ashton RCJ, Landry DW, et al. Low-dose vasopressin in the treatment of vasodilatory septic shock. *J Trauma* 1999;47:699–703.
90. Dunser MW, Mayr AJ, Ulmer H, et al. Arginine vasopressin in advanced vasodilatory shock: a prospective, randomized, controlled study. *Circulation* 2003;107:2313–2319.
91. Mutlu GM, Factor P. Role of vasopressin in the management of septic shock. *Intensive Care Med* 2004;30:1276–1291.
92. Delmas A, Leone M, Rousseau S, et al. Clinical review: Vasopressin and terlipressin in septic shock patients. *Crit Care* 2005;9:212–222.
93. Dellinger RP, Carlet JM, Masur H, et al. Surviving Sepsis Campaign guidelines for management of severe sepsis and septic shock. *Crit Care Med* 2004;32:858–873.
94. den Ouden DT, Meinders AE. Vasopressin: physiology and clinical use in patients with vasodilatory shock: a review. *Neth J Med* 2005;63:4–13.
95. Marin C, Eon B, Saux P, et al. Renal effects of norepinephrine used to treat septic shock patients. *Crit Care Med* 1990;18:282–285.
96. Bellomo R, Giantomasso DD. Noradrenaline and the kidney: friends or foes? *Crit Care* 2001;5:294–298.
97. Bellomo R, Chapman M, Finfer S, et al. Low-dose dopamine in patients with early renal dysfunction: a placebo-controlled randomised trial. Australian and New Zealand Intensive Care Society (ANZICS) Clinical Trials Group. *Lancet* 2000;356:2139–2143.
98. Holmes CL, Walley KR. Bad medicine: low-dose dopamine in the ICU. *Chest* 2003;123:1266–1275.
99. Ruffolo RR Jr. The pharmacology of dobutamine. *Am J Med Sci* 1987;294:244–248.
100. Kern KB, Hilwig RW, Berg RA, et al. Postresuscitation left ventricular systolic and diastolic dysfunction. Treatment with dobutamine. *Circulation* 1997;95:2610–2613.
101. Vasquez A, Kern KB, Hilwig RW, et al. Optimal dosing of dobutamine for treating post-resuscitation left ventricular dysfunction. *Resuscitation* 2004;61:199–207.
102. Studer W, Wu X, Siegemund M, et al. Influence of dobutamine on the variables of systemic haemodynamics, metabolism, and intestinal perfusion after cardiopulmonary resuscitation in the rat. *Resuscitation* 2005;64:227–232.
103. Alousi AA, Johnson DC. Pharmacology of the bipyridines: amrinone and milrinone. *Circulation* 1986;73:III10–III24.
104. Edelson J, Stroshane R, Benziger DP, et al. Pharmacokinetics of the bipyridines amrinone and milrinone. *Circulation* 1986;73:III145–III152.
105. Stueven HA, Thompson B, Aprahamian C, et al. The effectiveness of calcium chloride in refractory electromechanical dissociation. *Ann Emerg Med* 1985;14:626–629.
106. Stueven H, Thompson BM, Aprahamian C, et al. Use of calcium in prehospital cardiac arrest. *Ann Emerg Med* 1983;12:136–139.
107. Ramoska EA, Spiller HA, Winter M, et al. A one-year evaluation of calcium channel blocker overdoses: toxicity and treatment. *Ann Emerg Med* 1993;22:196–200.
108. Urban P, Scheidegger D, Buchmann B, et al. Cardiac arrest and blood ionized calcium levels. *Ann Intern Med* 1988;109:110–113.
109. Cardenas-Rivero N, Chernow B, Stoiko MA, et al. Hypocalcemia in critically ill children. *J Pediatr* 1989;114:946–951.
110. DiDomenico RJ, Park HY, Southworth MR, et al. Guidelines for acute decompensated heart failure treatment. *Ann Pharmacother* 2004;38:649–660.
111. Kirsten R, Nelson K, Kirsten D, et al. Clinical pharmacokinetics of vasodilators. Part II. *Clin Pharmacokinet* 1998;35:9–36.
112. Vaughan CJ, Delanty N. Hypertensive emergencies. *Lancet* 2000;356:411–417.
113. Zerbe NF, Wagner BK. Use of vitamin B12 in the treatment and prevention of nitroprusside-induced cyanide toxicity. *Crit Care Med* 1993;21:465–467.
114. Rindone JP, Sloane EP. Cyanide toxicity from sodium nitroprusside: risks and management. *Ann Pharmacother* 1992;26:515–519.
115. Pickkers P, Dormans TP, Russel FG, et al. Direct vascular effects of furosemide in humans. *Circulation* 1997;96:1847–1852.
116. Mehta RL, Pascual MT, Soroko S, et al. Diuretics, mortality, and nonrecovery of renal function in acute renal failure. *JAMA* 2002;288:2547–2553.
117. Ditchey RV, Lindenfeld J. Potential adverse effects of volume loading on perfusion of vital organs during closed-chest resuscitation. *Circulation* 1984;69:181–189.
118. Gentile NT, Martin GB, Appleton TJ, et al. Effects of arterial and venous volume infusion on coronary perfusion pressures during canine CPR. *Resuscitation* 1991;22:55–63.
119. Fischer M, Dahmen A, Standop J, et al. Effects of hypertonic saline on myocardial blood flow in a porcine model of prolonged cardiac arrest. *Resuscitation* 2002;54:269–280.
120. Breil M, Krep H, Sinn D, et al. Hypertonic saline improves myocardial blood flow during CPR, but is not enhanced further by the addition of hydroxy ethyl starch. *Resuscitation* 2003;56:307–317.

Chapter 27
Nonadrenergic Vasopressors in ECC

Helmut Raab, Martin Dünser, and Volker Wenzel

It had been axiomatic that increased vasoconstriction during CPR improves coronary perfusion pressure and thereby immediate resuscitation success; however, data indicates that vasoconstriction can be excessive. Postresuscitation left ventricular dysfunction is well documented and is a difficult-to-manage problem in the intensive care unit. Accordingly, the stunned left ventricle may be unable to tolerate the increased systemic vascular resistance immediately after resuscitation; therefore, heart failure and malignant ventricular arrhythmias may occur.

- There is long-standing concern that administration of epinephrine during resuscitation may result in detrimental effects during the postresuscitation period.
- Nonadrenergic vasoactive peptides such as arginine vasopressin hold promise, since they may raise perfusion pressure without the beta-receptor–mediated side effects of adrenergic vasopressors.
- A better knowledge of nonadrenergic vasopressors, their underlying mechanisms of action, and their usage in critically ill patients has the potential to save many lives.

Nonadrenergic Pressors

There is a long-standing concern that administration of epinephrine during resuscitation may result in detrimental effects during the postresuscitation period. For example, laboratory studies employing epinephrine during cardiopulmonary resuscitation (CPR) showed increased myocardial oxygen consumption,[1] ventricular arrhythmias,[2] ventilation–perfusion defects,[3] and postresuscitation myocardial dysfunction.[4] Therefore, nonadrenergic vasoactive peptides such as arginine vasopressin hold considerable promise, since they may raise perfusion pressure without the beta-receptor–mediated side effects of adrenergic vasopressors. Another intriguing possibility is that they may act synergistically when administered together with catecholamines, and that concomitant use of adrenergic drugs and nonadrenergic vasoactive peptides may allow lowering of the dosage of each agent.

Arginine Vasopressin as an Endogenous Stress Hormone

A number of fundamental endocrine responses of the human body to cardiac arrest and CPR have been investigated[5–8] and are summarized by Gazmuri (see Chapter 26). Circulating endogenous arginine vasopressin concentrations were found to be high in patients undergoing CPR. In addition, vasopressin levels in successfully resuscitated patients have been shown to be significantly higher than in patients who died.[5] This may indicate that the human body discharges arginine vasopressin as an adjunct endogenous vasopressor to epinephrine in life-threatening situations such as cardiac arrest in order to preserve homeostasis. In a clinical study of 60 out-of-hospital cardiac arrest patients, parallel increases in plasma arginine vasopressin and endothelin during CPR were found only in surviving patients.[6] Thus, plasma concentrations of arginine vasopressin may have a more important effect on CPR outcome than previously thought. These observations prompted several investigations to assess the role of arginine vasopressin in the management of CPR in order to improve patient outcome.

The Physiology of Arginine Vasopressin

Arginine vasopressin is a nonapeptide, an endogenous hormone with osmoregulatory, vasopressor, hemostatic, endocrinologic, thermoregulatory, and central nervous effects (Fig. 27-1). The hormone is produced in the magnocellular and parvocellular nuclei of the hypothalamus and stored in neurosecretory vesicles of the neurohypophysis.[9] It is secreted upon osmotic, hemodynamic, and

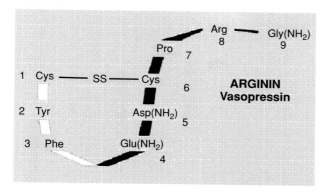

FIGURE 27-1 • Amino acid sequence of arginine–arginine vasopressin. (From Schmittinger CA, Wenzel V, Herff H, et al. [Drug therapy during CPR]. *Anasthesiol Intensivmed Notfallmed Schmerzther* 2003;38:651–672, with permission.)

endocrinologic stimuli. While only 10% to 20% of the total hormonal pool of arginine vasopressin in the neuro-hypophysis can be readily released, the time from synthesis to secretion into the circulation is ~1.5 hours.[10] Once released, the plasma half-life of arginine vasopressin is 4 to 20 minutes. Dose-dependent clearance occurs through arginine vasopressinases in the liver and the kidneys.[11–13]

The most important signals for the secretion of arginine vasopressin are increased plasma osmolality, decreased arterial pressure, and reduced cardiac filling.

The most important signals for the secretion of arginine vasopressin are increased plasma osmolality, decreased arterial pressure, and reduced cardiac filling.[14] Any reduction in blood volume or venous return stimulates the secretion of arginine vasopressin via activation of stretch receptors located in the left atrium and pulmonary arteries (Gauer–Henry reflex). Activation of baroreceptors in the aortic arch and carotid sinus further augments such secretion via the glossopharyngeal and vagal nerves. Baroreceptor stimulation is the primary and most important mechanism for arginine vasopressin release in hypotensive states and cardiac arrest.[15] In acute hypotension, there is an exponential relationship between plasma levels of arginine vasopressin and the decrease in arterial blood pressure. Whereas small reductions in blood pressure (~5%–10% from baseline) usually have only minor or no effect on plasma levels of arginine vasopressin, a 20% to 30% decline in arterial pressure results in concentrations of arginine vasopressin that are severalfold higher.[16] Similarly, unless blood volume decreases by >10% and results in diminished arterial blood pressure, volume depletion produces little elevation in plasma levels of arginine vasopressin.[17] However, the secretion of arginine vasopressin can also be directly stimulated by hypoxia, endotoxin, low concentrations of norepinephrine and angiotensin, or hypoglycemia.[18]

Arginine Vasopressin and its Pharmacologic Effects

Peripheral effects of arginine vasopressin are mediated by different arginine vasopressin receptors; namely V_{1a}, V_{1b}, and V_2 arginine vasopressin receptors. V_{1a} receptors are located on smooth muscle cells in arterial blood vessels and induce vasoconstriction by an increase in cytoplasmic ionized calcium via the phosphatidyl-inositol-bisphosphonate cascade.[19] On a molar basis, arginine vasopressin was shown to be a severalfold more potent vasoconstrictor than norepinephrine and angiotensin II.[20] In contrast to those of catecholamine-mediated vasoconstriction, the effects of arginine vasopressin are preserved during hypoxia and severe acidosis.[21]

Arginine vasopressin–mediated vascular effects differ substantially within particular vascular beds.

However, arginine vasopressin–mediated vascular effects differ substantially within particular vascular beds. Physiologically, most arterial beds exhibit vasoconstriction in response to arginine vasopressin.[22,23] Vasopressor effects are strongest in the muscular, adipose, cutaneous, and probably also the splanchnic vasculature. In a porcine CPR model, Voelckel et al.[24] found a significantly lower blood flow in the superior mesenteric artery in pigs resuscitated with arginine vasopressin when compared to epinephrine; there were no differences in hepatic or renal blood flow. Like oxytocin-mediated paradoxical vasodilatation of vascular smooth muscle, vasodilatation after arginine vasopressin has been described not only in the pulmonary, coronary, and vertebrobasilar circulation but, interestingly, also in the mesenteric vascular bed, suggesting a dose-dependent response.[25–28] The underlying mechanisms for such an arginine vasopressin–mediated vasodilatation seem to be nitric oxide–dependent.[26] Russ and Walker reported that stimulation of V_1 receptors can release nitric oxide, presumably from the endothelium of some vascular regions.[29] Recently, there is increasing evidence of hemodynamically relevant V_1 receptors on cardiomyocytes. *In vitro* and animal experiments have demonstrated an increase of intracellular calcium concentration and inotropy after stimulation of myocardial V_1 receptors.[30,31]

In the kidney, V_2 receptors are located on distal tubules and collecting ducts. Upon stimulation, they facilitate integration of aquaporines into the luminal cell membrane of the collecting ducts, leading to increased resorption of free water via an adenylate cyclase–dependent mechanism.[32] Despite the antidiuretic effect of a continuous infusion of arginine vasopressin, a paradoxical increase of urine output has been reported in patients with advanced vasodilatory shock.[33–35] It is hypothesized that together with increased renal perfusion pressure, arginine vasopressin selectively constricts efferent glomerular arterioles whereas it dilates afferent vessels, thus increasing effective filtration pressure in the glomerulus.[33]

V_{1b} receptors are located on the anterior hypophysis; stimulation induces liberation of ACTH and prolactin.[36] Accordingly, Kornberger et al.[37] reported significantly higher serum ACTH and cortisol concentrations in animals resuscitated from cardiac arrest with arginine vasopressin as compared with epinephrine. However, in patients with advanced vasodilatory shock, a continuous arginine vasopressin infusion at dosages of 4 IU/hr affected neither serum ACTH nor cortisol concentrations.[38] A complex dysfunction of the hypophyseal–adrenal axis in critical illness may explain the lack of effects of the potent stimulator arginine vasopressin on ACTH-producing cells. Nonetheless, arginine vasopressin seems to be able to promote prolactin excretion by stimulating V_{1b} receptors. Additional V_{1b} receptors are expressed on pancreatic islet cells, where they enhance insulin secretion in the presence of high glycemic levels.[39]

Arginine Vasopressin During CPR

In a porcine model simulating ventricular fibrillation, a dose–response investigation of three arginine vasopressin dosages (0.2, 0.4, and 0.8 U/kg) compared with the maximum effective dose of 200 µg/kg of epinephrine showed that 0.8 U/kg of arginine vasopressin was most effective at increasing blood flow to vital organs[40] (Figs. 27-2 and 27-3).

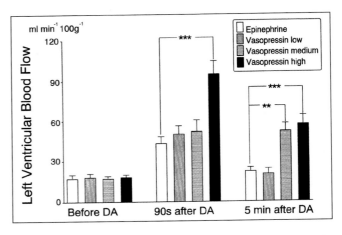

FIGURE 27-3 • Effects of different doses of arginine vasopressin versus high dose epinephrine on left ventricular blood flow. DA=drug administration (From Lindner KH, Prengel AW, Pfenninger EG, et al. Vasopressin improves vital organ blood flow during closed-chest cardiopulmonary resuscitation in pigs. *Circulation* 1995;91:215–221, with permission.)

Correspondingly, arginine vasopressin significantly improved cerebral oxygen delivery during CPR when compared with a maximum dose of epinephrine[41] (Fig. 27-4). Furthermore, the effects of arginine vasopressin on vital organ blood flow lasted longer after arginine vasopressin than after

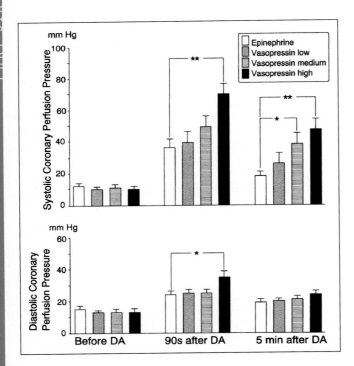

FIGURE 27-2 • Effects of different doses of arginine vasopressin versus high-dose epinephrine on systolic and diastolic blood pressure. DA=drug administration. (From Lindner KH, Prengel AW, Pfenninger EG, et al. Vasopressin improves vital organ blood flow during closed-chest cardiopulmonary resuscitation in pigs. *Circulation* 1995;91:215–221, with permission.)

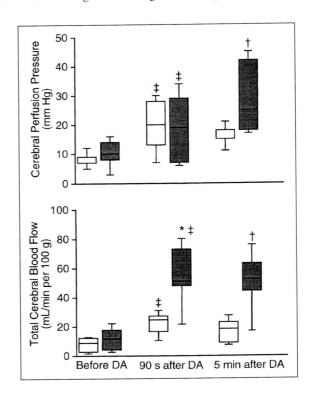

FIGURE 27-4 • Effects of different doses of arginine vasopressin versus high-dose epinephrine on total cerebral blood flow and cerebral perfusion pressure. DA=drug administration. (From Prengel AW, Lindner KH, Keller A. Cerebral oxygenation during cardiopulmonary resuscitation with epinephrine and vasopressin in pigs. *Stroke* 1996;27:1241–1248, with permission.)

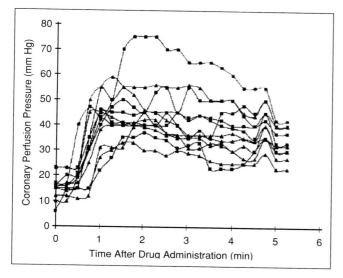

FIGURE 27-5 • Intravenous versus intraosseous arginine vasopressin during CPR. Individual coronary perfusion pressure tracings after intravenous arginine vasopressin (▲) and intraosseous arginine vasopressin (■) arginine vasopressin administration during CPR. No statistical analysis was performed for this figure. Some tracings may be superimposed on each other; defibrillation was performed approximately at 5 minutes and 15 seconds after drug administration. (From Wenzel V, Lindner KH, Augenstein S, et al. Intraosseous vasopressin improves coronary perfusion pressure rapidly during cardiopulmonary resuscitation in pigs. *Crit Care Med* 1999;27:1565–1569, with permission.)

epinephrine (~4 versus ~1.5 min); indeed, it was found that significantly more arginine vasopressin animals could be resuscitated.[42] The same dose of intravenous and endobronchial arginine vasopressin resulted in similar coronary perfusion pressures 4 minutes after drug administration.[43,44] Intraosseous versus intravenous arginine vasopressin administration led to comparable arginine vasopressin plasma levels, hemodynamic variables, coronary perfusion pressures, and rates of return of spontaneous circulation (ROSC)[45] (Fig. 27-5). Therefore, intraosseous arginine vasopressin might be a valuable alternative form of administration during CPR, when intravenous access is delayed or not available.

After repeated dosages of arginine vasopressin versus epinephrine were administered in a porcine model, coronary perfusion pressure increased only after the first of three epinephrine injections, but it increased after each of three arginine vasopressin injections.

After repeated dosages of arginine vasopressin versus epinephrine were administered in a porcine model, coronary perfusion pressure increased only after the first of three epinephrine injections, but it increased after each of three arginine vasopressin injections; accordingly, all arginine vasopressin animals survived, whereas all pigs resuscitated with epinephrine died[46] (Fig. 27-6). In the early postresuscitation phase of the same model, arginine vasopressin administra-

tion resulted in higher arterial blood pressure but a lower cardiac index; a reversible depressant but not critical effect on myocardial function by arginine vasopressin was observed when compared with epinephrine.[47] Renal and splanchnic perfusion may be impaired during[48] and after[49] successful resuscitation from cardiac arrest. Arginine vasopressin impaired mesenteric blood flow during CPR and in the early postresuscitation phase.[24] However, neither renal blood flow nor renal function was influenced by arginine vasopressin or epinephrine in this investigation.

In a model of prolonged advanced cardiac life support (22 minutes), all arginine vasopressin animals had ROSC, whereas all pigs in the epinephrine and saline placebo group died. Twenty-four hours after ROSC, the only neurologic deficit of pigs resuscitated with arginine vasopressin was an unsteady gait, which disappeared within 3 days. Subsequently performed magnetic resonance imaging revealed no cerebral cortical or subcortical edema, intraparenchymal hemorrhage, ischemic brain lesions, or cerebral infarction, indicating that pigs treated with arginine vasopressin but not those treated with epinephrine recovered fully from cardiac arrest, both anatomically and physiologically, even after prolonged CPR.[50]

In a model of advanced cardiac life support after 7 minutes of cardiac arrest, the administration of arginine vasopressin—compared with epinephrine or the combination of epinephrine and arginine vasopressin—did not improve the behavioral and cerebral histopathologic outcome.[51]

Clinical Trials of Vasopressin in Cardiac Arrest

In patients with refractory cardiac arrest, arginine vasopressin induced an increase in arterial blood pressure and, in some cases, ROSC, where standard therapy with chest compressions, ventilation, defibrillation, and epinephrine had failed.[52] In a small (n = 40) prospective randomized investigation of patients with shock-refractory out-of-hospital ventricular fibrillation, a significantly larger proportion of patients treated with arginine vasopressin were successfully resuscitated and survived 24 hours compared with patients treated with epinephrine.[53] In 1999, a Chinese study group reported a prospective randomized trial comparing two different dosages of arginine vasopressin and two different dosages of epinephrine in 83 patients with in-hospital cardiac arrest. Their findings indicated that high-dose arginine vasopressin (1 IU/kg) significantly increased the rate of ROSC and improved the survival rate compared with standard (1 mg) and high dosages (5 mg) of epinephrine.[54] In a large (n = 200) in-hospital CPR trial from Ottawa, Canada, comparable short-term survival was found in both groups treated with either arginine vasopressin or epinephrine, indicating that these drugs may be equipotent when response times of providers are short.[55] In another clinical evaluation in Detroit, Michigan, 4 of 10 patients responded to arginine vasopressin administration after ~45 minutes of unsuccessful advanced cardiac life support and had a mean increase in coronary perfusion pressure of 28 mm Hg.[56] This

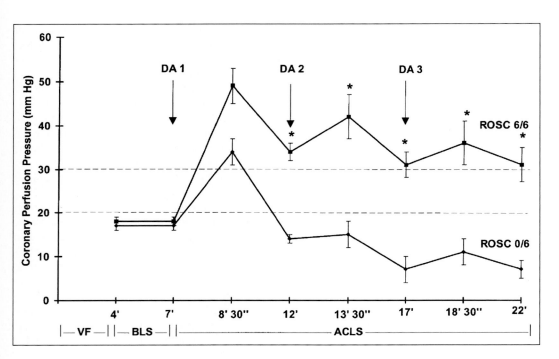

FIGURE 27-6 • Arginine vasopressin versus epinephrine during prolonged CPR. Administration of repeated doses of arginine vasopressin (■), but not epinephrine (♦) given early during basic life support CPR maintained mean ± SEM coronary perfusion pressure above the threshold of ~20 to 30 mm Hg (*dashed lines*), which is needed for successful defibrillation with ROSC. DA 1, drug administration of 0.4 U/kg arginine vasopressin versus 45 µg/kg epinephrine; DA 2, 0.4 U/kg arginine vasopressin versus 45 µg/kg epinephrine; DA 3, 0.8 U/kg arginine vasopressin versus 200 µg/kg epinephrine; *P <0.05 versus epinephrine; ROSC, return of spontaneous circulation; VF, ventricular fibrillation; ACLS, advanced cardiac life support. Time is given in minutes (') and seconds ("). (From Wenzel V, Lindner KH, Krismer AC, et al. Repeated administration of vasopressin but not epinephrine maintains coronary perfusion pressure after early and late administration during prolonged cardiopulmonary resuscitation in pigs. *Circulation* 1999;99:1379–1384, with permission.)

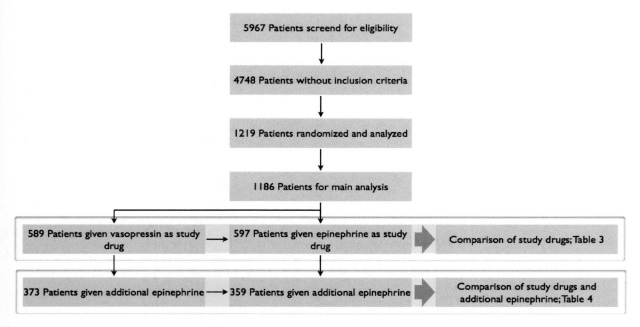

FIGURE 27-7 • Flowchart of the European multicenter study and analysis. (From Wenzel V, Krismer AC, Arntz HR, et al. A comparison of vasopressin and epinephrine for out-of-hospital cardiopulmonary resuscitation. *N Engl J Med* 2004;350:105–113, with permission.)

is surprising, since an arterial blood pressure increase with any drug after such a long period of ineffective CPR management is expected to be minimal.

From June 1999 to March 2002, we conducted a large multicenter trial in Austria, Germany, and Switzerland and randomized 1,219 out-of-hospital cardiac arrest patients to be treated with epinephrine or arginine vasopressin[57] (Fig. 27-7). Hospital admission and discharge rates were comparable between treatment arms for patients with ventricular fibrillation and for pulseless electrical activity, but patients with asystole were more likely to survive when primarily treated with arginine vasopressin (Table 27-1, Fig. 27-8). However, if patients could not be successfully resuscitated with two injections of arginine vasopressin, additional epinephrine significantly improved hospital admission ($P = 0.002$) and discharge rates ($P = 0.002$) when compared with patients who were treated with epinephrine alone (Table 27-2, Fig. 27-9). There was no difference in cerebral performance between groups for the entire trial.

These results could not confirm earlier data suggesting that arginine vasopressin was more effective than epinephrine as a first-line vasopressor drug in the treatment of ventricular fibrillation, pulseless electrical activity, or asystole.[40–42,46,50,53] Criticism has been raised that arginine vasopressin may improve coronary and cerebral perfusion pressures during CPR with refractory ventricular fibrillation

| TABLE 27-1 • European Multicenter Study: Data on Outcome in All Patients

	Vasopressin 589 of 1186	(49.7%)	Epinephrine 597 of 1186	(50.3%)	P	OR	CI
All Cardiac Rhythms							
ROSC after study drugs	145 of 589	(24.6%)	167 of 597	(28.0%)	19	12	0.9–1.5
Hospital admission	214 of 589	(36.3%)	186 of 597	(31.2%)	6	8	0.6–1.0
Hospital discharge	57 of 578	(9.9%)	58 of 588	(9.9%)	0.99	1	0.7–1.5
Ventricular Fibrillation							
ROSC after study drugs	82 of 223	(36.8%)	106 of 249	(42.6%)	0.2	1.3	0.9–1.8
Hospital admission	103 of 223	(46.2%)	107 of 249	(43.0%)	0.48	0.9	0.6–1.3
Hospital discharge	39 of 219	(17.8%)	47 of 245	(19.2%)	0.7	1.1	0.7–1.8
Pulseless Electrical Activity							
ROSC after study drugs	21 of 104	(20.2%)	17 of 82	(20.7%)	0.93	1	0.5–2.1
Hospital admission	35 of 104	(33.7%)	25 of 82	(30.5%)	0.65	0.8	0.5–1.6
Hospital discharge	6 of 102	(5.9%)	7 of 81	(8.6%)	0.47	1.4	0.5–4.7
Asystole							
ROSC after study drugs	42 of 262	(16.0%)	44 of 266	(16.5%)	0.87	1	0.7–1.6
Hospital admission	76 of 262	(29.0%)	54 of 266	(20.3%)	0.02	0.6	0.4–0.9
Hospital discharge	12 of 257	(4.7%)	4 of 262	(1.5%)	0.04	0.3	0.1–1.0
All Cardiac Rhythms-Cerebral Performance							
Good cerebral performance	15 of 46	(32.6%)	16 of 46	(34.8%)	0.99	...	...
Moderate cerebral disability	7 of 46	(15.2%)	12 of 46	(26.1%)	0.3	...	...
Severe cerebral disability	9 of 46	(19.6%)	7 of 46	(15.2%)	0.78	...	...
Coma	15 of 46	(32.6%)	11 of 46	(23.9%)	0.49	...	...

OR, odds ratio; 95% CI, 95% confidence interval; ROSC, return of spontaneous circulation.
P values are not adjusted for multiple comparisons.
Source: Wenzel V, Krismer AC, Arntz HR, et al. A comparison of vasopressin and epinephrine for out-of-hospital cardiopulmonary resuscitation. N Engl J Med 2004;350:105–113, with permission.

TABLE 27-2 • European Multicenter Study; Data On Outcome in Patients Who Initially Received Arginine Vasopressin or Epinephrine and Needed Additional Epinephrine

	Vasopressin 373 of 732	(51.0%)	Epinephrine 359 of 732	(49.0%)	P	OR	CI
All Cardiac Rhythms							
ROSC	137 of 373	(36.7%)	93 of 359	(25.9%)	0.002	0.6	0.4–0.8
Hospital admission	96 of 373	(25.7%)	59 of 359	(16.4%)	0.002	0.6	0.4–0.8
Hospital discharge	23 of 369	(6.2%)	6 of 355	(1.7%)	0.002	0.3	0.1–0.6
Ventricular Fibrillation							
ROSC	58 of 122	(47.5%)	40 of 122	(32.8%)	0.02	0.5	0.3–0.9
Hospital admission	37 of 122	(30.3%)	25 of 122	(20.5%)	0.08	0.6	0.3–1.1
Hospital discharge	13 of 121	(10.7%)	6 of 121	(5.0%)	0.09	0.4	0.2–1.2
Pulseless Electrical Activity							
ROSC	18 of 64	(28.1%)	14 of 56	(25.0%)	0.7	0.8	0.4–1.8
Hospital admission	17 of 64	(26.6%)	10 of 56	(17.9%)	0.25	0.6	0.2–1.4
Hospital discharge	3 of 64	(4.7%)	0 of 55	(0.0%)	0.1	...	...
Asystole							
ROSC	61 of 187	(32.6%)	39 of 181	(21.5%)	0.02	0.6	0.4–0.9
Hospital admission	42 of 187	(22.5%)	24 of 181	(13.3%)	0.02	0.5	0.3–0.9
Hospital discharge	7 of 184	(3.8%)	0 of 179	(0.0%)	0.008	...	...
All Cardiac Rhythms-Cerebral Performance							
Good cerebral performance	8 of 20	(40.0%)	2 of 5	(40.0%)	1	...	...
Moderate cerebral disability	2 of 20	(10%)	2 of 5	(40.0%)	0.17	...	...
Severe cerebral disability	2 of 20	(10%)	1 of 5	(20.0%)	0.5	...	...
Coma	8 of 20	(40%)	0 of 5	(0.0%)	0.14	...	...

OR, odds ratio; 95% CI, 95% confidence interval; ROSC, return of spontaneous circulation.
P values are not adjusted for multiple comparisons.
Source: Wenzel V, Krismer AC, Arntz HR, et al. A comparison of vasopressin and epinephrine for out-of-hospital cardiopulmonary resuscitation. N Engl J Med 2004;350:105–113, with permission.

and pulseless electrical activity, but that it will not improve outcome. Unfortunately we are unable to state whether this phenomenon may be similar to the observations described with high-dose epinephrine during CPR, when increasing epinephrine dosages were effective in the laboratory[58] but not in clinical practice.[59] It is clearly a principal problem to extrapolate laboratory CPR to the clinical setting, since species differences, comparing diseased patients with healthy laboratory animals, or differences in out-of-hospital CPR compared with laboratory conditions are hardly controllable factors of influence.

In the multicenter study, in contrast to its effects in individuals with ventricular fibrillation and pulseless electrical activity, arginine vasopressin improved the likelihood

that asystolic patients would reach the hospital alive by about 40% over epinephrine. A possible explanation may be profound ischemia, which is frequently present in asystolic patients. This is in accordance with an *in vitro* study where it was demonstrated that arginine vasopressin has vasoconstricting efficacy even in severe acidosis, when catecholamines are less potent.[21] Thus, arginine vasopressin seems to be more effective than epinephrine in asystolic patients, thereby resulting in better coronary perfusion pressure during cardiac resuscitation. Since improved coronary perfusion pressure during CPR improves survival,[60] arginine vasopressin may be a better option than epinephrine for asystolic patients, who normally have the worst chance of survival. Also, improvement in hospital discharge

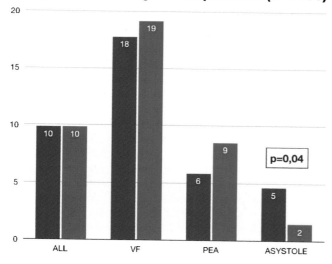

FIGURE 27-8 • Hospital discharge of all patients (n = 1,186) of the European multicenter study.

effects of epinephrine or vice versa, especially during prolonged ischemia.[61,62]

An observational prospective study of 598 patients with out-of hospital cardiac arrest found higher values of end-tidal carbon dioxide tension and mean arterial blood pressure in the combined arginine vasopressin/epinephrine group when compared to epinephrine therapy alone. Moreover, arginine vasopressin improved the restoration of spontaneous circulation, short-term survival, and neurologic outcome.[63]

In a recent in-hospital CPR study reporting comparable effects of arginine vasopressin and epinephrine, 87% of arginine vasopressin patients received additional epinephrine.[55] The concept of deliberate administration of arginine vasopressin combined with epinephrine during CPR is also supported by clinical observations that epinephrine followed by arginine vasopressin significantly improved coronary perfusion pressure,[56] ROSC,[52,62] and 24-hour survival rates.[64] It was also confirmed by a retrospective review that compared arginine vasopressin after epinephrine versus epinephrine

after treatment with epinephrine following arginine vasopressin may indicate that interactions among arginine vasopressin, epinephrine, and the underlying degree of ischemia during CPR may be more complex than previously thought. When prolonged asphyxia had depleted endogenous epinephrine levels and caused fundamental ischemia in pigs, arginine vasopressin combined with epinephrine tripled coronary perfusion pressure over either epinephrine or arginine vasopressin alone[61] (Fig. 27-10). This suggests that the presence of arginine vasopressin may enhance the

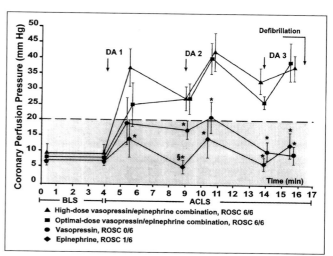

FIGURE 27-10 • Coronary perfusion pressure during CPR. Repeated doses of high-dose (▲) and optimal-dose (■) arginine vasopressin/epinephrine combinations, but not arginine vasopressin alone (●) or epinephrine alone (◆), maintained mean ± SEM coronary perfusion pressure at a level of 35 to 45 mm Hg, which makes successful defibrillation more likely. *$P < 0.05$ versus arginine vasopressin alone and epinephrine alone; §$P < 0.05$ versus epinephrine alone. BLS, basic life support; ACLS, advanced cardiac life support; DA 1, administration of 0.4 U/kg arginine vasopressin/45 µg/kg epinephrine combinations versus 0.4 U/kg arginine vasopressin alone versus 45 µg/kg epinephrine alone; DA 2, administration of 0.8 U/kg arginine vasopressin/200 µg/kg epinephrine combination versus 0.8 U/kg arginine vasopressin/45 µg/kg epinephrine combination versus 0.8 U/kg arginine vasopressin alone versus 200 µg/kg epinephrine alone; DA 3, administration of 0.8 U/kg arginine vasopressin/200 µg/kg epinephrine combination versus 0.8 U/kg arginine vasopressin/45 µg/kg epinephrine combination versus 0.8 U/kg arginine vasopressin alone versus 200 µg/kg epinephrine alone. Shaded area below 20 mm Hg indicates coronary perfusion pressure, which usually does not correlate with return of spontaneous circulation.

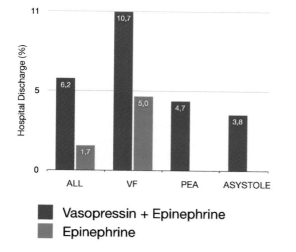

FIGURE 27-9 • In a subgroup analysis of the European multicenter study, patients treated with arginine–arginine vasopressin after epinephrine (n = 732) had a better long-term outcome than did patients treated with epinephrine only.

Vasopressors in Pittsburgh, Pennsylvania

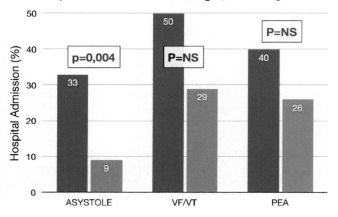

FIGURE 27-11 • Retrospective study comparing the effects of arginine vasopressin after epinephrine versus epinephrine only. Asystolic patients treated with arginine–arginine vasopressin after epinephrine had a better short-term survival than did patients treated with epinephrine only. (From Guyette FX, Guimond GE, Hostler D, et al. Vasopressin administered with epinephrine is associated with a return of a pulse in out-of-hospital cardiac arrest. *Resuscitation* 2004;63:277–282, with permission.)

only in a subset of patients with out-of-hospital cardiac arrest who did not respond to immediate therapy with epinephrine[62] (Fig. 27-11).

Although half of the survivors in the multicenter study with a good neurologic outcome received the combination of arginine vasopressin and epinephrine, this strategy also resulted in more, albeit not statistically significant, patients in coma than after epinephrine alone. This indicates that the combination of arginine vasopressin and epinephrine effectively resuscitated the heart but came too late to resuscitate the brain in some patients. When starting CPR, it is difficult to predict postresuscitation brain function.[65] Although our hospital discharge rate (9.7%) compares favorably with that in other reports, 2.2% of our patients had severe neurologic impairment. It must be stated that although the combination of arginine vasopressin and epinephrine improved survival rates, it resulted in an unfavorable neurologic outcome in some patients. In arginine vasopressin–treated patients, unfavorable neurologic outcomes were observed in 5 of 10 patients who were first found to be in asystole or pulseless electrical activity; in contrast, no patient with asystole or pulseless electrical activity receiving 3 mg epinephrine had an unfavorable neurologic outcome, since all died before discharge.

While an unfavorable ECG diagnosis upon starting CPR, such as asystole, may be one important surrogate for an unfavorable neurologic outcome, we ought not to forget that the duration of ischemia reflects injury to vital

organs and that the required vasopressor dosage reflects the organism's ability to respond to CPR. For example, both witnessed cardiac arrest and initiation of basic life support within 10 minutes was highly significant ($P < 0.001$) in predicting hospital admission in the European multicenter study. Patients who needed only one or two injections of the study drugs had a hospital discharge rate of 19.5%, while those requiring two injections of either of the study drugs and additional epinephrine had a hospital discharge rate of only 4%. In France, almost 3,000 patients have been randomized in a trial assessing effects of arginine vasopressin vs. arginine vasopressin combined with epinephrine. There were no differences between groups in survival, but about 85% of patients had in their initial ECG an asystole. (PY Gueugniaud, personal correspondence, 2008) Thus, it is possible that the underlying ischemia had a greater impact on survival than advanced cardiac life support drugs. Therefore, Arginine vasopressin is still a valuable drug if return of spontaneous circulation can not be restored with epinephrine alone. Future CPR trials need to determine when which vasopressor should be employed; due to lack of financial support, these trials are unlikely to be conducted. Therefore, a pragmatic extrapolation from the data available needs to be performed, again pointing at combining both Arginine vasopressin and epinephrine since none of these drugs has been proven to improve hospital discharge.

Clinical Uses for Arginine Vasopressin

Arginine Vasopressin during CPR—Limitations

The promising news about arginine vasopressin CPR studies cannot exclude the fact that many issues have not as yet been addressed. For example, there have still been no large clinical studies. This may be the reason why a recently conducted meta-analysis[66] could not show a statistically significant difference between arginine vasopressin and epinephrine in ROSC, hospital admission, and discharge rates (Tables 27-3 through 27-5). Another prospective randomized double-blind study of 325 patients with out-of hospital cardiac arrest found no change in short-term survival in the group receiving arginine vasopressin combined with epinephrine.[67] Further, extrapolating experience with arginine vasopressin from the adult to the pediatric setting is difficult and needs to be investigated.[68] Preliminary laboratory evidence suggests beneficial effects of a combination of arginine vasopressin with epinephrine in asphyctic cardiac arrest; however, this observation is inconsistent with reports in a postcountershock pulseless electrical activity preparation. Although preliminary experimental data suggest coronary vasodilatation after arginine vasopressin, this model may not reflect diffuse coronary artery disease of humans with possibly different physiology of the coronary

| TABLE 27-3 • Meta-analysis Comparing Arginine Vasopressin Against Epinephrine in Terms of Death Before Hospital Admission

Outcome: Study	Death before hospital admission Vasopressin n/N	Epinephrine n/N	RR (random) 95% CI	Weight %	RR (random) 95% CI
Lindner 1997	6/20	13/20		35.45	0.46 [0.22, 0.97]
Wenzel 2004	375/589	411/597		64.55	0.92 [0.85, 1.00]
Total (95% CI)	609	617		100.00	0.72 [0.38, 1.39]

Total events: 381 (vasopressin), 424 (epinephrine)
Test for heterogeneity: $Chi^2 = 3.36$, $df = 1$ ($P = 0.07$), $i^2 = 70.2\%$
Test for overall effect: $Z = 0.97$ ($P = 0.33$)

0.1 0.2 0.5 1 2 5 10
Favors vasopressin Favors epinephrine

Source: From Aung K, Htay T. Vasopressin for cardiac arrest: a systematic review and meta-analysis. *Arch Intern* Med 2005;165:17–24, with permission.

arteries.[69,70] Currently, we do not exactly know whether arginine vasopressin acts simply as a backup of the vasopressor epinephrine during life-threatening shock states, whether arginine vasopressin or epinephrine alone is better in certain situations, or whether these two hormones have unique adjunct features that we are only starting to understand. A better knowledge of these underlying mechanisms would likely save many patients—patients who at this point in time have relatively little chance of survival.[71]

Arginine Vasopressin during Hemorrhagic Shock

In 1990, about 5 million people died worldwide as a result of injury, and it seems likely that the global epidemic of deadly trauma is only beginning. By 2020, deaths from injury are expected to increase to 8 million worldwide,[72] and 30% of these fatalities will be attributable to uncontrolled hemorrhagic shock.[73] Resuscitation of patients in uncontrolled hemorrhagic shock remains one of the most challenging aspects of emergency care, and trauma patients with complete cardiovascular collapse have an extremely poor chance of survival. For example, in a 1993 study of 138

trauma patients requiring cardiopulmonary resuscitation at the accident scene or during transport, none of the initially successfully resuscitated patients survived to hospital discharge.[74] Accordingly, prevention of cardiac arrest has been considered to be the primary goal of trauma care.[75] Unfortunately, trauma-related cardiac arrest is only the tip of the iceberg. Because hemorrhage-induced hypotension in trauma patients is highly predictive of mortality and morbidity, managing prolonged hypotension aggressively may be equally important.

For hemodynamic stabilization of critically injured patients with uncontrolled hemorrhagic shock, current trauma guidelines recommend infusion of crystalloid or colloid solutions in addition to catecholamine vasopressors. In a large clinical study of penetrating torso trauma, patients receiving delayed fluid resuscitation had better survival rates than those receiving immediate fluid resuscitation.[76] Roberts et al.[77] further found no scientific evidence for the effectiveness of immediate fluid resuscitation in uncontrolled hemorrhagic shock. Also, a Cochrane review of randomized controlled trials found no evidence either for or against early or large-volume IV fluid administration in uncontrolled hemorrhage.[78] At present, therefore, we have no clearly proven fluid resuscitation strategy for uncontrolled hemorrhagic

| TABLE 27-4 • Meta-analysis Comparing Arginine Vasopressin Against Epinephrine in Terms of Death Within 24 hours

Outcome: Study	Death within 24 hours Vasopressin n/N	Epinephrine n/N	RR (random) 95% CI	Weight %	RR (random) 95% CI
Lindner 1997	8/20	16/20		41.40	0.50 [0.28, 0.89]
Stiell 2001	77/104	73/96		58.60	0.97 [0.83, 1.14]
Total (95% CI)	124	116		100.00	0.74 [0.38, 1.43]

Total events: 85 (vasopressin), 89 (epinephrine)
Test for heterogeneity: $Chi^2 = 4.99$, $df = 1$ ($P = 0.03$), $i^2 = 80.0\%$
Test for overall effect: $Z = 0.90$ ($P = 0.37$)

0.1 0.2 0.5 1 2 5 10
Favors vasopressin Favors epinephrine

Source: From Aung K, Htay T. Vasopressin for cardiac arrest: a systematic review and meta-analysis. *Arch Intern* Med 2005;165:17–24, with permission.

| TABLE 27-5 • Meta-analysis Comparing Arginine Vasoperssin Against Epinephrine in Terms of Death Before Hospital Discharge

Outcome: Study	Death before hospital discharge Vasopressin n/N	Epinephrine n/N	RR (random) 95% CI	Weight %	RR (random) 95% CI
Lindner 1997	12/20	17/20		5.25	0.71 [0.47, 1.06]
Li 1999	30/40	39/43		15.79	0.83 [0.68, 1.01]
Lee 2000	2/5	4/5		0.70	0.50 [0.16, 1.59]
Stiell 2001	92/104	83/96		31.64	1.02 [0.92, 1.14]
Wenzel 2004	521/578	530/588		46.62	1.00 [0.96, 1.04]
Total (95% CI)	747	752		100.00	0.96 [0.87, 1.05]

Total events: 657 (vasopressin), 673 (epinephrine)
Test for heterogeneity: $Chi^2 = 8.05$, df = 4 ($P = 0.09$), $i^2 = 50.3\%$
Test for overall effect: $Z = 0.92$ ($P = 0.36$)

0.1 0.2 0.5 1 2 5 10
Favors vasopressin   Favors epinephrine

Source: From Aung K, Htay T. Vasopressin for cardiac arrest: a systematic review and meta-analysis. *Arch Intern* Med 2005;165:17–24, with permission.

shock, and it seems expedient to consider alternative strategies to prevent immediate or delayed cardiac arrest in these patients. Moreover, during the late phase of hemorrhagic shock, when cardiac arrest may occur at any time, replacement of fluids and blood may become ineffective even when supported by conventional vasopressors such as norepinephrine.[79] In an experimental shock model in dogs, arginine vasopressin has been shown to effectively restore circulation in the late phase of hemorrhagic shock that was unresponsive to blood replacement and catecholamines.[79] Furthermore, arginine vasopressin enabled short- and long-term survival in a porcine model of uncontrolled hemorrhagic shock after penetrating liver trauma[80–84] (Fig. 27-12). Arginine vasopressin has also been used in a small number of nontrauma patients with upper gastrointestinal bleeding and subsequent shock that was unresponsive to volume replacement.[85] In the clinical setting, positive effects of arginine vasopressin were observed in some patients with life-threatening hemorrhagic shock with collapsing arterial blood pressure who were no longer responsive to adrenergic catecholamines and fluid resuscitation[86–89] (Fig. 27-13). Interestingly, all patients in these case reports received a combination of arginine vasopressin and catecholamines during the late phase of uncontrolled hemorrhagic shock, which may be more effective than either drug alone. This enhancing effect of a combination of arginine vasopressin and catecholamines is in agreement with our evidence in settings of severe shock, such as cardiac arrest and septic shock.[57,61,86,88,90] Furthermore, these case reports demonstrate that prolonged hemorrhagic shock with severe hypotension managed with arginine vasopressin can result in fully conscious patients with intact cardiocirculatory function and full neurologic recovery. This is in agreement with a case report[86] of a patient with multiple fractures of the pelvis, spine, and legs as well as a severe head trauma after a fall from a roof (fourth floor), resulting in uncontrolled hemorrhagic shock and severe hypotension that was refractory to massive infusion of fluids and norepinephrine. Subsequent infusion of arginine vasopressin prevented cardiocirculatory collapse, stabilized hemodynamic function, and enabled

emergency surgery. This patient made a full neurologic recovery.[86] (Fig. 27-13).

The case reports also provide valuable information, because the successful treatment of uncontrolled hemorrhagic shock with arginine vasopressin was reproducible and reported by different observers. We believe that in patients with uncontrolled hemorrhagic shock, infusing arginine vasopressin may be an option to stabilize cardiocirculatory function and prevent cardiac arrest. In the absence of randomized controlled trials investigating the role of arginine vasopressin in uncontrolled hemorrhagic shock today, even the currently limited clinical data available may support treatment decisions in selected patients who would otherwise quickly die. In the future, we need to assess whether the existing laboratory[80–84] and limited clinical data[86–89] on treating uncontrolled hemorrhagic shock successfully with arginine vasopressin can be confirmed in a randomized controlled clinical trial. In addition, the best timing of application and optimal dose of this form of therapy need to be addressed. Therefore, a multicenter trial to determine the role of arginine vasopressin in trauma patients who do not sufficiently respond to standard therapy with aggressive fluid resuscitation, intubation, mechanical ventilation, and catecholamine vasopressors will be conducted in Europe (www.vitris.at).[91]

Angiotensin II

Angiotensin II is a potent vasoconstricting octapeptide. As an intermediary in the renin-angiotensin-aldosterone system, angiotensin II has received much attention as a mediator of hypertension and congestive heart failure. Renin, on secretion by the renal juxtaglomerular cells, catalyzes the cleavage of angiotensinogen to angiotensin I, which is only a weak vasopressor.[92] Angiotensin II is formed by the cleavage of angiotensin I by angiotensin-converting enzyme. Angiotensin II is then converted to angiotensin III, which stimulates aldosterone release by the adrenal cortex. Angiotensin II has a very short serum half-life, as it is quickly

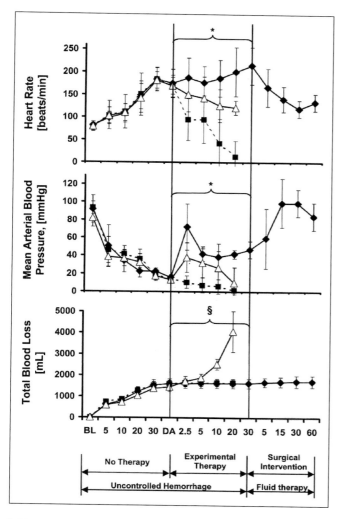

FIGURE 27-12 • Mean ± SD heart rate, mean arterial blood pressure, and total blood loss before, during, and after administration of a bolus dose of 0.4 U/kg followed by a continuous infusion of 0.08 U/kg/min of arginine vasopressin (*closed diamonds, continuous line*) versus fluid resuscitation (*closed triangles, continuous line*) with 25 mL/kg lactated Ringer's solution and 25 mL/kg of 3% gelatin solution versus saline placebo (*closed squares, dotted line*). BL = baseline; DA = drug administration; *$P < 0.05$ between groups for differences between all groups during the experimental protocol; §$P < 0.05$ for differences between the fluid resuscitation, and arginine vasopressin and saline placebo group during the experimental protocol. (From Stadlbauer KH, Wagner-Berger HG, Raedler C, et al. Vasopressin, but not fluid resuscitation, enhances survival in a liver trauma model with uncontrolled and otherwise lethal hemorrhagic shock in pigs. *Anesthesiology* 2003;98:699–704, with permission.)

converted to angiotensin III and broken down by serum and tissue peptidases.[92]

Angiotensin II has unique receptors, designated AT_1 and AT_2, of which AT_1 receptors mediate the vasopressor and chronotropic effects of angiotensin II.[93,94] The second-messenger system of the AT_1-receptor appears to involve activation of phospholipases C and D, leading to increased inositol phosphates.[92,94,95] This increase in inositol phosphates increases intracellular calcium and leads to smooth muscle contraction. The second-messenger system is distinct from that of the adrenergic system, which utilizes cyclic adenosine monophosphate (cAMP).

The vascular response to angiotensin II infusion is generalized vasoconstriction. On a molar basis, angiotensin II is approximately 30 times more potent than norepinephrine.[92] It produces a dose-dependent increase in blood pressure in humans and animals.[95–97] It acts in conjunction with the adrenergic system and arginine vasopressin to maintain mean arterial pressure during a variety of physiologic insults, including hemorrhage, sepsis, adrenal insufficiency, and other hypotensive states.[98–102]

Angiotensin II has been used experimentally as a vasopressor since the 1950s. The effect of pharmacologic doses of angiotensin II in the setting of hypotension and shock, however, has not been well studied. There are case reports of use of angiotensin II in individual patients but no comprehensive physiologic assessment. Much of the use of angiotensin II occurred before invasive hemodynamic monitoring became routine. The relative contribution of direct angiotensin II vasoconstriction compared to its effects on adrenal catecholamine release was not examined. The effects of angiotensin II on myocardial blood flow have been tested in a swine model of cardiac arrest with open-chest cardiac compressions. After administration of angiotensin II, myocardial blood flow was 118 mL/min per 100 g, which is near normal, compared with 56 mL/min per 100 g for the placebo group. Myocardial oxygen delivery and oxygen-extraction ratio were improved in the angiotensin II group.[48] Cerebral oxygen delivery and extraction ratios were also improved by angiotensin II in a porcine model of cardiac arrest.[103] A porcine study described the effects of angiotensin II (50 µg/kg) compared to epinephrine (20 µg/kg) and a group receiving the two agents in combination.[104] All groups had a significant increase in myocardial blood flow during CPR following drug administration. However, there was a trend toward higher flows in the epinephrine-treated animals. Furthermore, both groups that received epinephrine had significantly higher myocardial blood flow after ROSC when compared with angiotensin II.[104] Further studies will be needed to determine whether angiotensin II may have a role as a vasopressor in the therapy of cardiac arrest. At this point in time, there is not sufficient clinical evidence to support employment of angiotensin II during CPR.

Endothelin

Endothelin has been identified as a powerful vasoconstricting hormone secreted by endothelial cells.[105–107] DeBehnke et al.[108] reported that compared with endothelin or epinephrine, the combination of endothelin-1 plus epinephrine improved coronary perfusion pressure in a canine model of CPR. It was further shown that endothelin may significantly improve cerebral perfusion.[109,110] Another porcine model studied the effects of a combination of epinephrine and endothelin.[111] Although there was a greater ROSC in

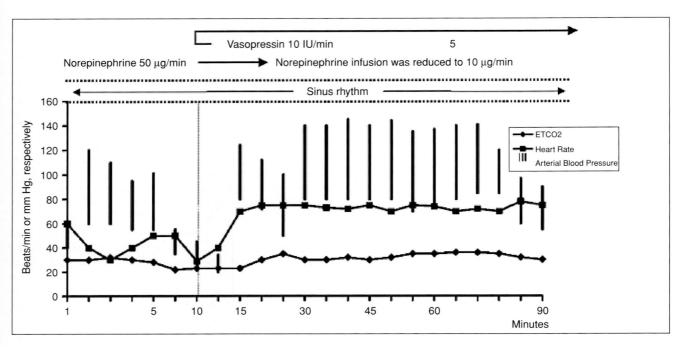

FIGURE 27-13 • A 41-year-old woman fell off a roof (height ~15 m) and was transported to the next county hospital. Because of an unstable pelvic fracture, the patient became hemodynamically unstable; therefore, an arterial cannula and a large-bore central venous catheter were placed and four units of packed red cells and coagulation factors were administered; the patient was then airlifted to a university hospital. After arrival in the emergency room of the level-one trauma center, hemodynamic stability could not be maintained despite massive infusion of fluids and norepinephrine (50 µg/min). The patient had a TRISS score predicted death rate of 84.9%. An infusion of arginine vasopressin was then started (10 IU/min), and blood pressure was stabilized, thus allowing emergent angiography and application of a pelvic clamp. Angiography revealed ruptured left internal iliac and left pudendal arteries; both blood vessels were successfully coiled and the patient was stabilized. Subsequent CT scanning revealed an injury pattern consisting of complex facial injuries, subdural hematomas, diffuse edema of the brain, spinal and rib fractures, hemothorax and hemomediastinum, rupture of the right bronchus, central hematoma of the liver, massive retroperitoneal hematoma, pelvic fractures, open fracture of the left femur, open fractures of both tibias, and fractures of both ankles and the right upper arm. The patient underwent several surgical procedures to repair the fractures, developed a systemic inflammatory response and a multiple organ dysfunction syndrome, but was discharged from the critical care unit to the ward without neurologic damage 39 days after the accident. (From Krismer AC, Wenzel V, Voelckel WG, et al. Employing vasopressin as an adjunct vasopressor in uncontrolled traumatic hemorrhagic shock. Three cases and a brief analysis of the literature. *Anaesthesist* 2005;54:220–224, with permission.)

the animals who received the combination of endothelin-1 plus epinephrine, the 1- and 24-hr survival rate were both less.[111] This was the result of a marked vasoconstricting effect of the combination of epinephrine and endothelin-1 in the doses used. There was a marked increase in coronary perfusion pressure but a dramatic narrowing of the pulse pressure and a marked drop in the end-tidal carbon dioxide level, indicating a marked decrease in forward blood flow. Results from a canine study suggested that endothelin-1 may contribute to the failure of cerebral circulation after cardiac arrest.[112]

In summary, it had been axiomatic that increased vasoconstriction during CPR improves coronary perfusion pressure and thereby immediate resuscitation success; however, data indicate that such vasoconstriction can be excessive. Postresuscitation left ventricular dysfunction is well documented and is a difficult-to-manage problem in the intensive care unit. Accordingly, the stunned left ventricle may be unable to tolerate the increased systemic vas-

cular resistance immediately after resuscitation. As a result, heart failure and malignant ventricular arrhythmias may occur. Accordingly, employing endothelin during CPR is not beneficial.

Practical Issues in Clinical Use:

Neither angiotensin II nor endothelin should be administered during CPR. According to new data from the European arginine vasopressin study,[57] we recommend first administering 1 mg of epinephrine followed alternately by 40 IU of arginine vasopressin and 1 mg of epinephrine every 3 minutes in adult victims of cardiac arrest regardless of the initial ECG rhythm (Fig. 27-14).

Hemorrhagic Shock Although observations made so far with arginine vasopressin in hemorrhagic shock and collapsing blood pressure both in the laboratory and in individual patients are promising, they need to be confirmed in future

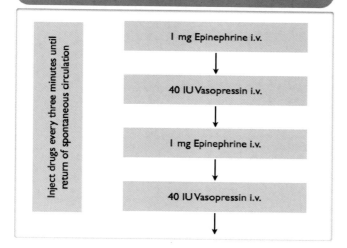

FIGURE 27-14 • Algorithm according to the new data from the European arginine vasopressin study.[57] In adult victims of cardiac arrest, we recommend administering first 1 mg of epinephrine followed alternately by 40 IU arginine vasopressin and 1 mg epinephrine every 3 minutes regardless of the initial ECG rhythm.

prospective randomized clinical trials. In selected patients with massive bleeding and intractable hemorrhagic shock resulting in collapsing blood pressure despite advanced trauma life support, 5 to 10 IU of arginine vasopressin may be injected; the cumulative dose should be titrated according to arterial blood pressure.

References

1. Ditchey RV, Lindenfeld J. Failure of epinephrine to improve the balance between myocardial oxygen supply and demand during closed-chest resuscitation in dogs. *Circulation* 1988;78:382–389.
2. Niemann JT, Haynes KS, Garner D, et al. Postcountershock pulseless rhythms: response to CPR, artificial cardiac pacing, and adrenergic agonists. *Ann Emerg Med* 1986;15:112–120.
3. Tang W, Weil MH, Gazmuri RJ, et al. Pulmonary ventilation/perfusion defects induced by epinephrine during cardiopulmonary resuscitation. *Circulation* 1991;84:2101–2107.
4. Tang WC, Weil MH, Sun SJ, et al. Epinephrine increases the severity of postresuscitation myocardial dysfunction. *Circulation* 1995;92:3089–3093.
5. Lindner KH, Strohmenger HU, Ensinger H, et al. Stress hormone response during and after cardiopulmonary resuscitation. *Anesthesiology* 1992;77:662–668.
6. Lindner KH, Haak T, Keller A, et al. Release of endogenous vasopressors during and after cardiopulmonary resuscitation. *Br Heart J* 1996;75:145–150.
7. Strohmenger HU, Lindner KH, Keller A, et al. Concentrations of prolactin and prostaglandins during and after cardiopulmonary resuscitation. *Crit Care Med* 1995;23:1347–1355.
8. Schultz CH, Rivers EP, Feldkamp CS, et al. A characterization of hypothalamic-pituitary-adrenal axis function during and after human cardiac arrest. *Crit Care Med* 1993;21:1339–1347.
9. Leng G, Brown CH, Russell JA. Physiological pathways regulating the activity of magnocellular neurosecretory cells. *Prog Neurobiol* 1999;57:625–655.
10. Sklar AH, Schrier RW. Central nervous system mediators of vasopressin release. *Physiol Rev* 1983;63:1243–1280.
11. Mutlu GM, Factor P. Role of vasopressin in the management of septic shock. *Intens Care Med* 2004;30:1276–1291.
12. Baumann G, Dingman JF. Distribution, blood transport, and degradation of antidiuretic hormone in man. *J Clin Invest* 1976;57:1109–1116.
13. Beardwell CG, Geelen G, Palmer HM, et al. Radioimmunoassay of plasma vasopressin in physiological and pathological states in man. *J Endocrinol* 1975;67:189–202.
14. Goldsmith SR. Baroreceptor-mediated suppression of osmotically stimulated vasopressin in normal humans. *J Appl Physiol* 1988;65:1226–1230.
15. Thrasher TN, Keil LC. Systolic pressure predicts plasma vasopressin responses to hemorrhage and vena caval constriction in dogs. *Am J Physiol Regul Integr Comp Physiol* 2000;279:R1035–R1042.
16. Berl T, Robertson GL. Pathophysiology of water metabolism. In Brenner BM, ed. *Brenner & Rector's The Kidney*. Philadelphia: Saunders, 2000:866–924.
17. Callahan MF, Ludwig M, Tsai KP, et al. Baroreceptor input regulates osmotic control of central vasopressin secretion. *Neuroendocrinology* 1997;65:238–245.
18. Kasting NW, Mazurek MF, Martin JB. Endotoxin increases vasopressin release independently of known physiological stimuli. *Am J Physiol* 1985;248:E420–E424.
19. Birnbaumer M. Vasopressin receptors. *Trends Endocrinol Metab* 2000;11:406–410.
20. Reid IA, Schwartz J. Role of vasopressin in the control of blood pressure. In Martini L, Ganong WF, eds. *Frontiers in Neuroendocrinology*. New York: Raven Press, 1976:177–197.
21. Fox AW, May RE, Mitch WE. Comparison of peptide and nonpeptide receptor-mediated responses in rat tail artery. *J Cardiovasc Pharmacol* 1992;20:282–289.
22. Garcia-Villalon AL, Garcia JL, Fernandez N, et al. Regional differences in the arterial response to vasopressin: role of endothelial nitric oxide. *Br J Pharmacol* 1996;118:1848–1854.
23. Moursi MM, van Wylen DG, D'Alecy LG. Regional blood flow changes in response to mildly pressor doses of triglycyl desamino lysine and arginine vasopressin in the conscious dog. *J Pharmacol Exp Ther* 1985;232:360–368.
24. Voelckel WG, Lindner KH, Wenzel V, et al. Effects of vasopressin and epinephrine on splanchnic blood flow and renal function during and after cardiopulmonary resuscitation in pigs. *Crit Care Med* 2000;28:1083–1088.
25. Martinez MC, Vila JM, Aldasoro M, et al. Relaxation of human isolated mesenteric arteries by vasopressin and desmopressin. *Br J Pharmacol* 1994;113:419–424.
26. Wallace AW, Tunin CM, Shoukas AA. Effects of vasopressin on pulmonary and systemic vascular mechanics. *Am J Physiol* 1989;257:H1228–H1234.
27. Okamura T, Ayajiki K, Fujioka H, et al. Mechanisms underlying arginine vasopressin-induced relaxation in monkey isolated coronary arteries. *J Hypertens* 1999;17:673–678.
28. Suzuki Y, Satoh S, Oyama H, et al. Vasopressin mediated vasodilation of cerebral arteries. *J Auton Nerv Syst* 1994;49 Suppl:S129–S132.
29. Russ RD, Walker BR. Role of nitric oxide in vasopressinergic pulmonary vasodilatation. *Am J Physiol* 1992;262:H743–H747.
30. Xu YJ, Gopalakrishnan V. Vasopressin increases cytosolic free [Ca2+] in the neonatal rat cardiomyocyte. Evidence for V1 subtype receptors. *Circ Res* 1991;69:239–245.
31. Fujisawa S, Iijima T. On the inotropic actions of arginine vasopressin in ventricular muscle of the guinea pig heart. *Jpn J Pharmacol* 1999;81:309–312.
32. Wuttke T. Endocrinology. In Schmidt RF, Thews G, eds. *Human Physiology*. Berlin, Heidelberg, New York: Springer, 1993:390–420.
33. Landry DW, Levin HR, Gallant EM, et al. Vasopressin pressor hypersensitivity in vasodilatory septic shock. *Crit Care Med* 1997;25:1279–1282.
34. Tsuneyoshi I, Yamada H, Kakihana Y, et al. Hemodynamic and metabolic effects of low-dose vasopressin infusions in vasodilatory septic shock. *Crit Care Med* 2001;29:487–493.

35. Holmes CL, Walley KR, Chittock DR, et al. The effects of vasopressin on hemodynamics and renal function in severe septic shock: a case series. *Intens Care Med* 2001;27:1416–1421.

36. Bilezikjian LM, Vale WW. Regulation of ACTH secretion from corticotrophs: the interaction of vasopressin and CRF. *Ann N Y Acad Sci* 1987;512:85–96.

37. Kornberger E, Prengel AW, Krismer A, et al. Vasopressin-mediated adrenocorticotropin release increases plasma cortisol concentrations during cardiopulmonary resuscitation. *Crit Care Med* 2000;28:3517–3521.

38. Dunser MW, Hasibeder WR, Wenzel V, et al. Endocrinologic response to vasopressin infusion in advanced vasodilatory shock. *Crit Care Med* 2004;32:1266–1271.

39. Lee B, Yang C, Chen TH, et al. Effect of AVP and oxytocin on insulin release: involvement of V1b receptors. *Am J Physiol* 1995;269:E1095–E1100.

40. Lindner KH, Prengel AW, Pfenninger EG, et al. Vasopressin improves vital organ blood flow during closed-chest cardiopulmonary resuscitation in pigs. *Circulation* 1995;91:215–221.

41. Prengel AW, Lindner KH, Keller A. Cerebral oxygenation during cardiopulmonary resuscitation with epinephrine and vasopressin in pigs. *Stroke* 1996;27:1241–1248.

42. Wenzel V, Lindner KH, Prengel AW, et al. Vasopressin improves vital organ blood flow after prolonged cardiac arrest with post-countershock pulseless electrical activity in pigs. *Crit Care Med* 1999;27:486–492.

43. Wenzel V, Lindner KH, Prengel AW, et al. Endobronchial vasopressin improves survival during cardiopulmonary resuscitation in pigs. *Anesthesiology* 1997;86:1375–1381.

44. Wenzel V, Prengel AW, Lindner KH. A strategy to improve endobronchial drug administration. *Anesth Analg* 2000;91:255–256.

45. Wenzel V, Lindner KH, Augenstein S, et al. Intraosseous vasopressin improves coronary perfusion pressure rapidly during cardiopulmonary resuscitation in pigs. *Crit Care Med* 1999;27: 1565–1569.

46. Wenzel V, Lindner KH, Krismer AC, et al. Repeated administration of vasopressin but not epinephrine maintains coronary perfusion pressure after early and late administration during prolonged cardiopulmonary resuscitation in pigs. *Circulation* 1999;99:1379–1384.

47. Prengel AW, Lindner KH, Keller A, et al. Cardiovascular function during the postresuscitation phase after cardiac arrest in pigs: a comparison of epinephrine versus vasopressin. *Crit Care Med* 1996;24:2014–2019.

48. Lindner KH, Brinkmann A, Pfenninger EG, et al. Effect of vasopressin on hemodynamic variables, organ blood flow, and acid-base status in a pig model of cardiopulmonary resuscitation. *Anesth Analg* 1993;77:427–435.

49. Prengel AW, Lindner KH, Wenzel V, et al. Splanchnic and renal blood flow after cardiopulmonary resuscitation with epinephrine and vasopressin in pigs. *Resuscitation* 1998;38:19–24.

50. Wenzel V, Lindner KH, Krismer AC, et al. Survival with full neurologic recovery and no cerebral pathology after prolonged cardiopulmonary resuscitation with vasopressin in pigs. *J Am Coll Cardiol* 2000;35:527–533.

51. Popp E, Vogel P, Teschendorf P, et al. Vasopressors are essential during cardiopulmonary resuscitation in rats: is vasopressin superior to adrenaline? *Resuscitation* 2007;72:137–144.

52. Lindner KH, Prengel AW, Brinkmann A, et al. Vasopressin administration in refractory cardiac arrest. *Ann Intern Med* 1996; 124:1061–1064.

53. Lindner KH, Dirks B, Strohmenger HU, et al. A Randomised comparison of epinephrine and vasopressin in patients with out-of-hospital ventricular fibrillation. *Lancet* 1997;349:535–537.

54. Li PF, Chen TT, Zhang JM. Clinical study on administration of vasopressin during closed-chest cardiopulmonary resuscitation. *Chin Crit Care Med* 1999;11:28–31.

55. Stiell IG, Hebert PC, Wells GA, et al. Vasopressin versus epinephrine for inhospital cardiac arrest: a randomised controlled trial. *Lancet* 2001;358:105–109.

56. Morris DC, Dereczyk BE, Grzybowski M, et al. Vasopressin can increase coronary perfusion pressure during human cardiopulmonary resuscitation. *Acad Emerg Med* 1997;4:878–883.

57. Wenzel V, Krismer AC, Arntz HR, et al. A comparison of vasopressin and epinephrine for out-of-hospital cardiopulmonary resuscitation. *N Engl J Med* 2004;350:105–113.

58. Babar SI, Berg RA, Hilwig RW, et al. Vasopressin versus epinephrine during cardiopulmonary resuscitation: a randomized swine outcome study. *Resuscitation* 1999;41:185–192.

59. Paradis NA, Wenzel V, Southall J. Pressor drugs in the treatment of cardiac arrest. *Cardiol Clin* 2002;20:61–78.

60. Paradis NA, Martin GB, Rivers EP, et al. Coronary perfusion pressure and the return of spontaneous circulation in human cardiopulmonary resuscitation. *JAMA* 1990;263:1106–1113.

61. Mayr VD, Wenzel V, Voelckel WG, et al. Developing a vasopressor combination in a pig model of adult asphyxial cardiac arrest. *Circulation* 2001;104:1651–1656.

62. Guyette FX, Guimond GE, Hostler D, et al. Vasopressin administered with epinephrine is associated with a return of a pulse in out-of-hospital cardiac arrest. *Resuscitation* 2004;63:277–282.

63. Mally S, Jelatancev A, Grmec S. Effects of epinephrine and vasopressin on end-tidal carbon dioxide tension and mean arterial blood pressure in out-of-hospital cardiopulmonary resuscitation: an observational study. *Crit Care* 2007;11:R39.

64. Grmec S, Mally S. Vasopressin improves outcome in out-of-hospital cardiopulmonary resuscitation of ventricular fibrillation and pulseless ventricular tachycardia: a observational cohort study. *Crit Care* 2006;10:R13.

65. Hypothermia After Cardiac Arrest Study Group. Mild therapeutic hypothermia to improve the neurologic outcome after cardiac arrest. *N Engl J Med* 2002;346:549–556.

66. Aung K, Htay T. Vasopressin for cardiac arrest: a systematic review and meta-analysis. *Arch Intern Med* 2005;165:17–24.

67. Callaway CW, Hostler D, Doshi AA, et al. Usefulness of vasopressin administered with epinephrine during out-of-hospital cardiac arrest. *Am J Cardiol* 2006;98:1316–1321.

68. Lienhart HG, John W, Wenzel V. Cardiopulmonary resuscitation of a near-drowned child with a combination of epinephrine and vasopressin. *Pediatr Crit Care Med* 2005;6:486–488.

69. Mayr VD, Wenzel V, Muller T, et al. Effects of vasopressin on left anterior descending coronary artery blood flow during extremely low cardiac output. *Resuscitation* 2004;62:229–235.

70. Wenzel V, Kern KB, Hilwig RW, et al. Effects of intravenous arginine vasopressin on epicardial coronary artery cross sectional area in a swine resuscitation model. *Resuscitation* 2005;64:219–226.

71. Wenzel V, Lindner KH. Employing vasopressin during cardiopulmonary resuscitation and vasodilatory shock as a lifesaving vasopressor. *Cardiovasc Res* 2001;51:529–541.

72. Murray CJ, Lopez AD. Alternative projections of mortality and disability by cause—1990–2020: Global Burden of Disease Study. *Lancet* 1997;349:1498–1504.

73. Deakin CD, Hicks IR. AB or ABC: pre-hospital fluid management in major trauma. *J Accid Emerg Med* 1994;11:154–157.

74. Rosemurgy AS, Norris PA, Olson SM, et al. Prehospital traumatic cardiac arrest: the cost of futility. *J Trauma* 1993;35:468–473; discussion 73–74.

75. Shoemaker WC, Peitzman AB, Bellamy R, et al. Resuscitation from severe hemorrhage. *Crit Care Med* 1996;24(Suppl):S12–S23.

76. Bickell WH, Wall MJ Jr, Pepe PE, et al. Immediate versus delayed fluid resuscitation for hypotensive patients with penetrating torso injuries. *N Engl J Med* 1994;331:1105–1109.

77. Roberts I, Evans P, Bunn F, et al. Is the normalisation of blood pressure in bleeding trauma patients harmful? *Lancet* 2001;357: 385–387.

78. Kwan I, Bunn F, Roberts I. Timing and volume of fluid administration for patients with bleeding. *Cochrane Database Syst Rev* 2003:CD002245.

79. Morales D, Madigan J, Cullinane S, et al. Reversal by vasopressin of intractable hypotension in the late phase of hemorrhagic shock. *Circulation* 1999;100:226–229.

80. Stadlbauer KH, Wagner-Berger HG, Raedler C, et al. Vasopressin, but not fluid resuscitation, enhances survival in a liver trauma model with uncontrolled and otherwise lethal hemorrhagic shock in pigs. *Anesthesiology* 2003;98:699–704.

81. Voelckel WG, Raedler C, Wenzel V, et al. Arginine vasopressin, but not epinephrine, improves survival in uncontrolled hemorrhagic shock after liver trauma in pigs. *Crit Care Med* 2003;31: 1160–1165.

82. Voelckel WG, von Goedecke A, Fries D, et al. Treatment of hemorrhagic shock. New therapy options. *Anaesthesist* 2004;53: 1151–1167.

83. Raedler C, Voelckel WG, Wenzel V, et al. Treatment of uncontrolled hemorrhagic shock after liver trauma: fatal effects of fluid resuscitation versus improved outcome after vasopressin. *Anesth Analg* 2004;98:1759–1766.
84. Feinstein AJ, Patel MB, Sanui M, et al. Resuscitation with pressors after traumatic brain injury. *J Am Coll Surg* 2005;201:536–545.
85. Shelly MP, Greatorex R, Calne RY, et al. The physiological effects of vasopressin when used to control intra-abdominal bleeding. *Intens Care Med* 1988;14:526–531.
86. Krismer AC, Wenzel V, Voelckel WG, et al. Employing vasopressin as an adjunct vasopressor in uncontrolled traumatic hemorrhagic shock. Three cases and a brief analysis of the literature. *Anaesthesist* 2005;54:220–224.
87. Sharma RM, Setlur R. Vasopressin in hemorrhagic shock. *Anesth Analg* 2005;101:833–834.
88. Haas T, Voelckel WG, Wiedermann F, et al. Successful resuscitation of a traumatic cardiac arrest victim in hemorrhagic shock with vasopressin: a case report and brief review of the literature. *J Trauma* 2004;57:177–179.
89. Yeh CC, Wu CT, Lu CH, et al. Early use of small-dose vasopressin for unstable hemodynamics in an acute brain injury patient refractory to catecholamine treatment: a case report. *Anesth Analg* 2003;97:577–579.
90. Dunser MW, Mayr AJ, Ulmer H, et al. The effects of vasopressin on systemic hemodynamics in catecholamine-resistant septic and postcardiotomy shock: a retrospective analysis. *Anesth Analg* 2001;93:7–13.
91. Lienhart HG, Wenzel V, Braun J, et al. [Vasopressin for therapy of persistent traumatic hemorrhagic shock: The VITRIS.at study]. *Anaesthesist* 2007;56:145–148, 150.
92. Garrison JC, Peach MJ. Renin and angiotensin. In Gilman AG, ed. *The Pharmacological Basis of Therapeutics*. Amsterdam: Pergamon Press, 1990:749–763.
93. Griendling KK, Murphy TJ, Alexander RW. Molecular biology of the renin-angiotensin system. *Circulation* 1993;87:1816–1828.
94. Vallotton MB, Capponi AM, Johnson EI, et al. Mode of action of angiotensin II and vasopressin on their target cells. *Horm Res* 1990;34:105–110.
95. Doursout MF, Chelly JE, Hartley CJ, et al. Regional blood flows and cardiac function changes induced by angiotensin II in conscious dogs. *J Pharmacol Exp Ther* 1988;246:591–596.
96. Scroop GC, Walsh JA, Whelan RF. A comparison of the effects of intra-arterial and intravenous infusions of angiotensin and noradrenaline on the circulation in man. *Clin Sci* 1965;29:315–326.
97. Heyndrickx GR, Boettcher DH, Vatner SF. Effects of angiotensin, vasopressin, and methoxamine on cardiac function and blood flow distribution in conscious dogs. *Am J Physiol* 1976;231:1579–1587.
98. Brooks VL. Vasopressin and ANG II in the control of ACTH secretion and arterial and atrial pressures. *Am J Physiol* 1989;256:R339–R347.
99. Downing SW, Edmunds LH Jr. Release of vasoactive substances during cardiopulmonary bypass. *Ann Thorac Surg* 1992;54:1236–1243.
100. Ishikawa S, Okada K, Saito T. Increases in cellular sodium concentration by arginine vasopressin and endothelin in cultured rat glomerular mesangial cells. *Endocrinology* 1992;131:1429–1435.
101. Paller MS, Linas SL. Role of angiotensin II, alpha-adrenergic system, and arginine vasopressin on arterial pressure in rat. *Am J Physiol* 1984;246:H25–H30.
102. Schaller MD, Waeber B, Nussberger J, et al. Angiotensin II, vasopressin, and sympathetic activity in conscious rats with endotoxemia. *Am J Physiol* 1985;249:H1086–H1092.
103. Little CM, Brown CG. Angiotensin II administration improves cerebral blood flow in cardiopulmonary arrest in swine. *Stroke* 1994;25:183–186.
104. Little CM, Angelos MG, Paradis NA. Compared to angiotensin II, epinephrine is associated with high myocardial blood flow following return of spontaneous circulation after cardiac arrest. *Resuscitation* 2003;59:353–359.
105. Luscher TF. Endothelin: systemic arterial and pulmonary effects of a new peptide with potent biologic properties. *Am Rev Respir Dis* 1992;146:S56–S60.
106. Luscher TF, Boulanger CM, Dohi Y, et al. Endothelium-derived contracting factors. *Hypertension* 1992;19:117–130.
107. Marsden PA, Brenner BM. Nitric oxide and endothelins: novel autocrine/paracrine regulators of the circulation. *Semin Nephrol* 1991;11:169–185.
108. DeBehnke DJ, Spreng D, Wickman LL, et al. The effects of endothelin-1 on coronary perfusion pressure during cardiopulmonary resuscitation in a canine model. *Acad Emerg Med* 1996;3:137–141.
109. DeBehnke D. The effects of graded doses of endothelin-1 on coronary perfusion pressure and vital organ blood flow during cardiac arrest. *Acad Emerg Med* 2000;7:211–221.
110. Holzer M, Sterz F, Behringer W, et al. Endothelin-1 elevates regional cerebral perfusion during prolonged ventricular fibrillation cardiac arrest in pigs. *Resuscitation* 2002;55:317–327.
111. Hilwig RW, Berg RA, Kern KB, et al. Endothelin-1 vasoconstriction during swine cardiopulmonary resuscitation improves coronary perfusion pressures but worsens postresuscitation outcome. *Circulation* 2000;101:2097–2102.
112. Takasu A, Yagi K, Okada Y. Role of endothelin-1 in the failure of cerebral circulation after complete global cerebral ischemia. *Resuscitation* 1995;30:69–73.
113. Schmittinger CA, Wenzel V, Herff H, et al. [Drug therapy during CPR]. *Anasthesiol Intensivmed Notfallmed Schmerzther* 2003;38:651–672; quiz 73–75.

Seven

Post–Cardiac Arrest Syndrome and Management

Chapter 28
Post–Cardiac Arrest Syndrome and Management

Robert W. Neumar and Jerry Nolan

Robert W. Neumar and Jerry P. Nolan for the ILCOR Post-Cardiac Arrest Syndrome Writing Group

Robert W. Neumar, Co-chair, Jerry P. Nolan, Co-chair, Christophe Adrie, Mayuki Aibiki, Bernd W. Bottiger, Robert A. Berg, Clifton W. Callaway, Robert S. B. Clark, Romergryko G. Geocadin, Edward C. Jauch, Karl B. Kern, Ivan Laurent, W. T. Longstreth, Jr, Laurie J. Morrison, Peter Morley, Raina M. Merchant, Vinay Nadkarni, Mary Ann Peberdy, Antonio Rodriguez-Nunez, Emanual P. Rivers, Christian Spaulding, Frank W. Sellke, Kjetil Sunde, and Terry Vanden Hoek.

- Mortality after ROSC is high. In published studies, average in-hospital mortality ranges from 50% to 90% after both out-of-hospital and in-hospital cardiac arrest.
- PCAS represents a unique combination of pathophysiolgic processes that are potentially reversible.
- Optimizing post–cardiac arrest care will improve survival with good neurologic outcome.
- Optimized post–cardiac arrest care is a complex, time-sensitive endeavor that is best performed by a well-coordinated multidisciplinary team.

See Web site for AHA Scientific Statement Post Circulatory Arrest Syndrome

Background

Originally the D in the ABCDs of cardiopulmonary resuscitation stood for "definitive therapy."[1] Definitive therapy includes management of the pathologies that result from cardiac arrest as well as those that cause it. PCAS is a unique and complex combination of pathophysiologic processes, including (1) post–cardiac arrest brain injury, (2) post–cardiac arrest myocardial dysfunction, and (3) a systemic ischemia–reperfusion response.[2] This state is often complicated by a fourth component: the unresolved pathology that caused the cardiac arrest. Extensive animal data have demonstrated that all components of PCAS are responsive to therapy. In humans, therapeutic hypothermia has provided the essential proof of concept that interventions initiated after ROSC can improve outcome.[3,4] It is clear that optimized post–cardiac arrest management requires a comprehensive multidisciplinary plan that can be executed reliably 24 hours a day, 7 days a week. This approach has already been shown to improve outcome at individual institutions when compared with historical controls.[5–7] In addition to an optimized therapeutic strategy, it is essential to develop a consistent, reliable, rational approach to limiting care in cases of futility and to consider the potential for organ donation.

Epidemiology of Post–Cardiac Arrest Syndrome

Early mortality of patients achieving ROSC after cardiac arrest varies dramatically between studies, countries, regions, and hospitals. The cause of these differences is multifactorial but includes variability in patient populations, reporting methods, and post–cardiac arrest care. In published studies, average in-hospital mortality ranges from 50% to 90% after both out-of-hospital and in-hospital cardiac arrest.[8–16] Of the patients who survive to hospital discharge, approximately 60% to 80% have a good neurologic outcome.[8,14,16] The reported incidence of clinical brain death in patients with sustained ROSC after cardiac arrest ranges from 8% to 16%.[17,18] A number of studies have reported that transplant outcomes using organs obtained from appropriately selected post–cardiac arrest patients do not differ from those using organs obtained from other brain-death donors.[18–20]

Pathophysiology of Post–Cardiac Arrest Syndrome

The high mortality of patients who initially achieve ROSC after cardiac arrest can be attributed to a unique pathophys-

The high mortality of patients who initially achieve ROSC after cardiac arrest can be attributed to a unique pathophysiologic process, involving multiple organs, which is often superimposed on the persistent, acute pathology that caused the cardiac arrest as well as underlying comorbidities.

iologic process, involving multiple organs, which is often superimposed on the persistent, acute pathology that caused the cardiac arrest as well as underlying comorbidities. The four key components of PCAS are (1) post–cardiac arrest brain injury, (2) post–cardiac arrest myocardial dysfunction, (3) a systemic ischemia–reperfusion response, and (4) persistent precipitating pathology (Table 28-1).[2] The severity of these disorders after ROSC will vary with the duration and cause of cardiac arrest, and they may be undetectable if cardiac arrest is brief.

Post–Cardiac Arrest Brain Injury

Post–cardiac arrest brain injury is a common cause of morbidity and mortality. In one study of patients surviving to ICU admission but subsequently dying in-hospital, brain damage was the cause of death in 68% after out-of-hospital cardiac arrest and in 23% after in-hospital cardiac arrest.[21] Clinical manifestations of post–cardiac arrest brain injury include coma, seizures, myoclonus, varying degrees of neurocognitive dysfunction (ranging from memory deficits to persistent vegetative state), and brain death (Table 28-1).[22–30] The unique vulnerability of the brain is attributed to its limited tolerance of ischemia as well as its unique response to reperfusion. The mechanisms of brain damage triggered by cardiac arrest and resuscitation are complex, and many pathways are executed over hours to days following ROSC.[31–33] The relatively protracted time course of injury cascades and histologic change suggests a broad therapeutic window for neuroprotective strategies following cardiac arrest.

Brain damage was the cause of death in 68% after out-of-hospital cardiac arrest and in 23% after in-hospital cardiac arrest.

Several postarrest factors can potentially exacerbate post–cardiac arrest brain injury. These include microcirculatory failure,[34–38] impaired autoregulation,[39–46] hyperoxia,[47–49] hypercarbia, pyrexia,[8,50,51] hyperglycemia,[8,52–57] and seizures.[30] Therapeutic strategies to limit these potential causes of secondary brain injury are discussed later in this chapter. There is limited evidence that brain edema or elevated intracranial pressure (ICP) directly exacerbates post–cardiac arrest brain injury. Although transient brain edema is observed early after ROSC, most commonly after asphyxial cardiac arrest, it is rarely associated with clinically relevant increases in ICP.[58–61] In contrast, delayed brain edema, occurring days to weeks after cardiac arrest has been attributed to delayed hyperemia; this is more likely the consequence rather than the cause of severe ischemic neurodegeneration.[59–61] There are no published prospective trials

| TABLE 28-1 • Post–Cardiac Arrest Syndrome: Pathophysiology, Clinical Manifestations, and Potential Treatments

	Pathophysiology	Clinical Manifestation	Potential Treatments
Post–cardiac arrest brain injury	Impaired cerebrovascular autoregulation Cerebral edema (limited) Postischemic neurodegeneration	Coma Seizures Myoclonus Cognitive dysfunction Persistent vegetative state Secondary parkinsonism Cortical stroke Spinal stroke Brain death	Therapeutic hypothermia[129] Early hemodynamic optimization Airway protection and mechanical ventilation Seizure control Controlled reoxygenation (SaO_2 94%–96%) Supportive care
Post–cardiac arrest myocardial dysfunction	Global hypokinesis (myocardial stunning) Acute coronary syndrome	Reduced cardiac output Hypotension Dysrhythmias Cardiovascular collapse	Early revascularization of AMI[90,92] Early hemodynamic optimization Intravenous fluid[63] Inotropes[63] Intra-aortic balloon pump[6,93] LVAD[223] ECMO[224]
Systemic ischemia/ reperfusion response	Systemic inflammatory response syndrome Impaired vasoregulation Increased coagulation Adrenal suppression Impaired tissue oxygen delivery and utilization Impaired resistance to infection	Ongoing tissue hypoxia/ ischemia Hypotension Cardiovascular collapse Pyrexia (fever) Hyperglycemia Multiorgan failure Infection	Early hemodynamic optimization Intravenous fluid Vasopressors High-volume hemofiltration[225] Temperature control Glucose control[166] Antibiotics
Persistent precipitating pathology	Cardiovascular disease (AMI/ACS, cardiomyopathy) Pulmonary disease (COPD, asthma) CNS disease (CVA) Thromboembolic disease (PE) Toxicologic (overdose, poisoning) Infection (sepsis, pneumonia) Hypovolemia (hemorrhage, dehydration)	Specific to etiology, but complicated by concomitant PCAS	Disease–specific interventions guided by patient condition concomitant PCAS

ACS, acute coronary syndrome; AMI, acute myocardial infarction; COPD, chronic obstructive disease; CVA, cerebrovascular accident; ECMO, extracorporeal membrane oxygenation; LVAD, left ventricular assist device; PCAS, post–cardiac arrest syndrome; PE, pulmonary embolism.

that examine the value of ICP monitoring and management in post–cardiac arrest patients.

Post–Cardiac Arrest Myocardial Dysfunction

Post–cardiac arrest myocardial dysfunction is a significant cause of morbidity and mortality after both in- and out-of-hospital cardiac arrest.[21,62,63] In swine studies, ejection fraction decreases from 55% to 20% and left ventricular end-diastolic pressure increases from 8 to 10 *to* 20 to 22 mm Hg as early as 30 minutes after ROSC.[64,65] In one series of 148 patients who underwent coronary angiography after cardiac arrest, 49% of subjects had myocardial dysfunction manifested by tachycardia and an elevated left ventricular end-diastolic pressure, followed approximately 6 hours later by

hypotension (mean arterial pressure <75 mm Hg) and a low cardiac output (cardiac index <2.2 L/min/m²).[63]

Existing preclinical and clinical evidence indicates that this phenomenon is both responsive to therapy and reversible.[63–68] In a swine model with no antecedent coronary or other features of left ventricular dysfunction, the time to recovery appeared to be somewhere between 24 and 48 hours.[65] Several case series have described transient myocardial dysfunction after human cardiac arrest. In one study, cardiac index values reached their nadir at 8 hours postresuscitation, improved substantially by 24 hours, and were almost uniformly back to normal by 72 hours in patients surviving out-of-hospital cardiac arrest.[63] More sustained depression of ejection fraction among in- and out-of-hospital post–cardiac arrest patients has been reported with continued recovery over weeks to months.[67] The responsiveness of post–cardiac arrest global myocardial dysfunction to inotropic drugs is well documented in animal studies.[64,66]

Systemic Ischemia–Reperfusion Response

Cardiac arrest represents the most severe shock state during which delivery of oxygen and metabolic substrates is halted abruptly and metabolites are no longer removed. Cardiopulmonary resuscitation (CPR) reverses this process only partially, achieving cardiac output and systemic oxygen delivery (DO_2) that is much less than normal. Inadequate tissue oxygen delivery can persist even following ROSC because of myocardial dysfunction, pressor-dependent hemodynamic instability, and microcirculatory failure. The whole-body ischemia–reperfusion of cardiac arrest with associated oxygen debt causes generalized activation of immunologic and coagulation pathways, thus increasing the risk of multiple organ failure and infection.[69–71] This condition has many features in common with sepsis.[72–76] In addition, activation of blood coagulation without adequate activation of endogenous fibrinolysis may also contribute to microcirculatory reperfusion disorders after cardiac arrest.[77,78] Finally, the stress of total-body ischemia–reperfusion appears to adversely affect adrenal function.[79,80] However, the relationship of adrenal dysfunction to outcome remains controversial.

Clinical manifestations of the systemic ischemia–reperfusion response include intravascular volume depletion, impaired vasoregulation, impaired oxygen delivery and utilization, and increased susceptibility to infection. In most cases these pathologies are both responsive to therapy and reversible. Data from clinical sepsis research suggest that outcomes are optimized when interventions are both goal-directed and initiated as early as possible.

Persistent Precipitating Pathology

PCAS is commonly associated with persisting acute pathology that caused or contributed to the cardiac arrest itself. The diagnosis and treatment of acute coronary syndrome, pulmonary diseases, hemorrhage, sepsis, and various toxidromes is often complicated in the setting of PCAS. However, early identification and effective therapeutic intervention is essential if optimal outcomes are to be achieved.

Therapeutic Strategies

Care of the post–cardiac arrest patient is time-sensitive, occurs in various locations both in and out of the hospital, and involves teams of health care providers from several disciplines. Ideally, a comprehensive clinical pathway tailored to available resources should be developed by relevant specialists.

Care of the post–cardiac arrest patient is time-sensitive, occurs in various locations both in and out of the hospital, and involves teams of health care providers from several disciplines. Ideally, a comprehensive clinical pathway tailored to available resources should be developed by relevant specialists. Treatment plans for post–cardiac arrest care must accommodate a spectrum of patients, ranging from the awake, hemodynamically stable survivor to the unstable comatose patient with persistent precipitating pathology. Such a plan enables physicians, nurses, and other health care professionals to optimize post–cardiac arrest care and prevent premature withdrawal of care before long-term prognosis can be established. This approach has been demonstrated to improve outcomes at individual institutions when compared with historical controls.[5,6,81]

Post–cardiac arrest patients generally require intensive care monitoring; this can be divided into three categories (Table 28-2): general intensive care monitoring, more advanced hemodynamic monitoring, and cerebral monitoring. General intensive care monitoring (Table 28-2) is the

| TABLE 28-2 • Post–Cardiac Arrest Syndrome: Monitoring Options

General intensive care monitoring
- Arterial catheter
- Oxygen saturation by pulse oximetry
- Continuous ECG
- Central venous pressure
- $ScvO_2$
- Temperature (bladder, esophagus)
- Urine output
- Arterial blood gases
- Serum lactate
- Blood glucose, electrolytes, CBC, and general blood sampling
- Chest radiograph

More advanced hemodynamic monitoring
- Echocardiography (daily for the first days)
- PA catheter or noninvasive cardiac output monitoring (several techniques are available)

Cerebral monitoring
- EEG (on indication/continuously): early seizure detection and treatment
- CT/MRI

CBC, complete blood count; CT, computed tomography; ECG, electrocardiography; EEG, electroencephalography; MRI, magnetic resonance imaging; PA, pulmonary artery; $ScvO_2$, central venous oxygen saturation.

minimal requirement; additional monitoring should be added depending on the status of the patient and local experience. The impact of specific monitoring techniques on outcome after cardiac arrest has not been studied prospectively.

Diagnosis and Treatment of Acute Coronary Syndromes

The majority of out-of-hospital cardiac arrest patients have coronary artery disease (CAD),[82-84] and an acute coronary syndrome (ACS) is the most common cause of sudden cardiac death in the adult.[84] Acute changes in coronary plaque morphology occur in 40% to 86% of cardiac arrest survivors and are found in 15% to 64% of autopsy studies.[85] Thus, early post–cardiac arrest coronary angiography with subsequent percutaneous coronary intervention (PCI) is appropriate not just for those patients with ST-segment elevation myocardial infarction (STEMI) but also for those who are suspected of having an ACS.[6,86-91] Several studies have evaluated the use of primary PCI for patients with ST elevation on their electrocardiograms (ECGs) following resuscitation from cardiac arrest, and the reported in-hospital mortality rates range from 20% to 45%.[89,90,92] These studies have included many patients who remain comatose after initial resuscitation and, when appropriate (see below), the combination of mild hypothermia and primary PCI resulted in better outcomes than PCI alone.[6,7,93] Chest pain and/or ST-segment elevation may be poor predictors of acute coronary occlusion in post–cardiac arrest patients;[86] prospective studies are needed to determine whether immediate coronary angiography should be performed on all patients who experience ROSC after out-of-hospital cardiac arrest.

If there are no facilities for immediate PCI, in-hospital thrombolysis is recommended for patients with ST-segment elevation who have not received prehospital thrombolysis.[94,95] Coronary artery bypass grafting is indicated in the postresuscitation phase for patients with left main stenosis or triple-vessel coronary artery disease if the cardiac arrest was thought to be caused by ischemic heart disease. In addition to acute reperfusion, management of ACS and CAD should follow standard guidelines (see Chapters 5 and 7).

Early Hemodynamic Optimization

Early hemodynamic optimization or early goal-directed therapy (EGDT) is an algorithmic approach to restoring and maintaining the balance between systemic oxygen delivery and demand. Monitoring and therapy are initiated as early as possible with the aim of achieving goals within hours of presentation. This involves optimizing preload, arterial oxygen content, afterload, contractility, and systemic oxygen utilization. EGDT has been studied in randomized prospective clinical trials of severe sepsis and in postoperative patients.[96–98] Goals in these studies have included a central venous pressure (CVP) of 8 to 12 mm Hg, mean arterial pressure (MAP) of 65 to 90 mm Hg, central venous oxygen saturation ($ScvO_2$) >70%, hematocrit >30% or Hb >8 g dL^{-1}, lactate $\leq$2 mmol/L, urine output $\geq$0.5 mL/kg/hr, and oxygen delivery index >600 mL/min/m^2. The goals are achieved with the use of intravenous fluids, inotropes, vasopressors, and blood transfusion as required. The benefits of EGDT include modulation of inflammation, reduction of organ dysfunction, and reduction of health care resource consumption.[96–98] In severe sepsis, EGDT has also been shown to reduce mortality.[96]

Early hemodynamic optimization or early goal-directed therapy (EGDT) is an algorithmic approach to restoring and maintaining the balance between systemic oxygen delivery and demand. Monitoring and therapy are initiated as early as possible with the aim of achieving goals within hours of presentation.

The systemic ischemia–reperfusion response and myocardial dysfunction of PCAS have many characteristics in common with sepsis.[72] Therefore, it has been hypothesized that early hemodynamic optimization might improve the outcome of post–cardiac arrest patients. However, the benefit of this approach has not been studied in randomized prospective clinical trials. Moreover, the optimal goals and strategies to achieve those goals could be different in PCAS, given the concomitant presence of post–cardiac arrest brain injury, myocardial dysfunction, and persistent precipitating pathologies.

Hemodynamic instability is common after cardiac arrest and manifests as dysrhythmias, hypotension, and a low cardiac index.[63] Underlying mechanisms include intravascular volume depletion, impaired vasoregulation, and myocardial dysfunction. Dysrhythmias are treated by maintaining normal electrolyte concentrations and using standard drug and electrical therapies. There is no evidence to support the prophylactic use of antiarrhythmic drugs after cardiac arrest. Dysrhythmias are commonly caused by focal cardiac ischemia, and early reperfusion treatment is probably the best antiarrhythmic therapy. Ultimately, survivors whose cardiac arrest is attributed to a primary dysrhythmia should be evaluated for pacemaker or an implantable or internal cardioverter defibrillator (ICD) placement.

The first-line intervention for hypotension is to optimize right heart filling pressures using intravenous fluid. In one study, 3.5 to 6.5 L intravenous crystalloid was required in the first 24 hours after out-of-hospital cardiac arrest to maintain right atrial pressures in the range of 8 to 13 mm Hg.[63] In one study, out-of-hospital post–cardiac arrest patients had a positive fluid balance of 3.5 ± 1.6 L in the first 24 hours, with a CVP goal of 8 to 12 mm Hg.[6] The appropriate CVP for individual patients is highly variable; for example, those with right heart dysfunction or pulmonary embolism will require a much higher CVP than a patient whose primary problem is severe left ventricular dysfunction.

The optimal MAP for post–cardiac arrest patients has not been defined by prospective clinical trials. These patients require an adequate MAP to perfuse the postischemic brain but without subjecting the postischemic heart to excessive afterload. The loss of cerebrovascular pressure autoregulation makes cerebral perfusion dependent on cerebral perfusion pressure (CPP = MAP − ICP). Since sustained elevation of the ICP during the early post–cardiac arrest phase is uncommon, cerebral perfusion is predominantly dependent on MAP. If fixed or dynamic cerebral microvascular dysfunction is present, an elevated MAP could theoretically increase cerebral oxygen delivery. In one human study, the MAP during the first 2 hours after ROSC correlated positively with neurologic outcome.[99] Good outcomes have been achieved in published studies where the MAP target was as low as 65 to 75 mm Hg[27] to as high as 90 to 100 mm Hg[4,5] for patients admitted after out-of-hospital cardiac arrest. The optimal MAP in the post–cardiac arrest period might be dependent on the duration of cardiac arrest, with higher pressures needed to overcome the potential noreflow phenomenon observed with >15 minutes of untreated cardiac arrest.[34,35,100] At the opposite end of the spectrum, a patient with an evolving acute myocardial infarction (AMI) or severe myocardial dysfunction might benefit from the lowest target MAP that will ensure adequate cerebral oxygen delivery.

Inotropes and vasopressors should be considered if hemodynamic goals are not achieved despite optimized preload. Post–cardiac arrest global myocardial dysfunction is common;[63,67,72] although it is generally reversible and responsive to inotropes, the severity and duration of the myocardial dysfunction will affect survival.[63] Early echocardiography will enable the extent of myocardial dysfunction to be quantified and may guide therapy. Impaired vasoregulation is also common in post–cardiac arrest patients; this may require treatment with vasopressors and is also reversible. Persistence of reversible vasopressor dependency has been reported for up to 72 hours after out-of-hospital cardiac arrest despite preload optimization and reversal of global myocardial dysfunction.[63] No individual drug or combination of drugs has been demonstrated to be superior in the treatment of post–cardiac cardiovascular dysfunction. The choice of inotrope and/or vasopressor can be guided by blood pressure, heart rate, echocardiographic estimates of myocardial dysfunction, and surrogate measures of tissue oxygen delivery such as $ScvO_2$, lactate clearance, and urine output. If a pulmonary artery catheter (PAC) or some form of noninvasive cardiac output monitor is being used, therapy can be further guided by cardiac index and systemic vascular resistance.

If volume expansion and treatment with vasoactive and inotropic drugs do not restore adequate organ perfusion, consider mechanical circulatory assistance.[101,102] This treatment can support the circulation for the period of transient severe myocardial dysfunction that often occurs after ROSC.[63] The intra-aortic balloon pump (IABP) is the most readily available device to augment myocardial perfusion; it is generally easy to insert with or without radiologic imaging, and its use after cardiac arrest is well documented.[6,93]

Monitoring of the balance between systemic oxygen delivery and consumption can be accomplished indirectly with SvO_2 (mixed venous oxygen saturation) or $ScvO_2$ (central venous oxygen saturation). However, use of PAC—required for the measurement of SvO_2—is diminishing, the optimal $ScvO_2$ goal for post–cardiac arrest patients has not been defined, and the value of continuous $ScvO_2$ monitoring is uncertain.

Urine output and lactate clearance are surrogates for oxygen delivery. Although two EGDT trials used a urine output target of ≥0.5 mL/kg/hr,[96,98] a higher urine output goal of >1 mL/kg/hr is reasonable in post–arrest patients treated with therapeutic hypothermia, because this intervention induces diuresis.[6] A limitation is that urine output can be misleading in the presence of acute or chronic renal insufficiency. Lactate concentrations are elevated early after ROSC because of the total-body ischemia caused by cardiac arrest. This limits the utility of a single measurement during early hemodynamic optimization. Lactate clearance is associated with outcome after out-of-hospital cardiac arrest;[103,104] however, lactate clearance can be impaired by hepatic insufficiency and hypothermia. The optimal goal for hemoglobin concentration in the post–cardiac arrest phase has not been defined.[6]

In summary, based on the limited available evidence, reasonable goals for post–cardiac arrest syndrome include a MAP of 65 to 100 mm Hg (taking into consideration the patient's normal blood pressure, the cause of the arrest, and the severity of any myocardial dysfunction), $ScvO_2$ >70%, urine output >1 mL/kg/hr, and a normal or decreasing serum lactate concentration. Goals for hemoglobin concentration during postresuscitation care remain to be defined.

Controlled Reoxygenation

Existing guidelines emphasize the use of an inspired oxygen concentration of 100% during CPR, and clinicians will frequently maintain ventilation with 100% oxygen for variable periods after ROSC. Although it is important to ensure that patients are not hypoxemic, a growing body of preclinical evidence suggests that hyperoxia during the early stages of reperfusion harms postischemic neurons by causing excessive oxidative stress.[47,48,105,106] Most relevant to post–cardiac arrest care, ventilation with 100% oxygen for the first hour after ROSC in dogs resulted in worse neurologic outcome compared with immediate adjustment of the fractional inspired oxygen concentration (FiO_2) to produce an arterial oxygen saturation of 94% to 96%.[49] Thus, based on preclinical evidence alone, it is advisable to avoid unnecessary arterial hyperoxia, especially during the initial post–cardiac arrest period. This can be achieved by adjusting the FiO_2 to produce an arterial oxygen saturation of 94% to 96%.

Ventilation

Although cerebral autoregulation is either absent or dysfunctional in most patients in the acute phase after cardiac arrest,[40] cerebrovascular reactivity to changes in arterial carbon dioxide tension seems to be preserved.[41,43,107,108] Cerebrovascular resistance may be elevated for at least 24 hours in comatose survivors of cardiac arrest.[43] There are no data to support the targeting of a specific $PaCO_2$ after resuscitation from cardiac arrest; however, extrapolation from studies of other cohorts suggest ventilation to normocarbia is appropriate. Studies in brain-injured patients have shown that the cerebral vasoconstriction caused by hyperventilation may produce potentially harmful cerebral ischemia.[109–111] Hyperventilation also increases intrathoracic pressure, which will decrease cardiac output during and after cardiopulmonary resuscitation.[112,113] Hypoventilation may also be harmful because hypoxemia and hypercarbia can increase intracranial pressure or compound metabolic acidosis, which is common shortly after ROSC.

High tidal volumes cause barotrauma, volutrauma,[114] and biotrauma[115] in patients with acute lung injury. Recent evidence indicates that normal lungs can also be injured by ventilation with high tidal volumes.[116] Although there are no data to support use of a specific tidal volume during postresuscitation care, it would seem reasonable, if patients are considered to be at risk of acute lung injury, to avoid tidal volumes >8 mL/kg. In inducing therapeutic hypothermia, additional blood gases may be helpful to guide adjustment of tidal volumes, because cooling will decrease metabolism and, therefore, the tidal volumes required.

Sedation and Neuromuscular Blockade

If patients do not show adequate signs of awakening within the first 5 to 10 minutes after ROSC, endotracheal intubation (if not already achieved), mechanical ventilation, and sedation will be required. Adequate sedation will reduce oxygen consumption, which is further reduced with therapeutic hypothermia. Use of published sedation scales for monitoring these patients (e.g., the Richmond or Ramsay scale) may be helpful.[117,118] Both opioids (analgesia) and hypnotics (e.g., propofol or benzodiazepines) should be used. In patients treated with therapeutic hypothermia, optimal sedation can prevent shivering, which is most prominent during the induction phase, and reduce the time taken to achieve target temperature. If shivering occurs despite deep sedation, neuromuscular blocking drugs (as an intravenous bolus or infusion) should be used with close monitoring of sedation and neurologic status (e.g., seizures). Because of the relatively high incidence of seizures after cardiac arrest, continuous electroencephalographic (EEG) monitoring should be considered for patients requiring sustained neuromuscular blockade.[119]

Therapeutic Hypothermia

A period of hyperthermia is common in the first 48 hours after cardiac arrest,[50,120,121] and the risk of a poor neurologic outcome increases for each degree of body temperature >37°C.[51] A retrospective study of patients admitted after out-of-hospital cardiac arrest reported that a maximal recorded temperature >37.8°C was associated with increased in-hospital mortality (OR 2.7; 95% CI 1.2–6.3).[8] If therapeutic hypothermia (see below) is not feasible or is contraindicated, then, at a minimum, pyrexia must be prevented.

A period of hyperthermia is common in the first 48 hours after cardiac arrest, and the risk of a poor neurologic outcome increases for each degree of body temperature >37°C. There is good animal and human evidence to indicate that mild hypothermia, even when induced after ROSC, is neuroprotective and improves outcome after a period of global cerebral hypoxia–ischemia.

There is good animal and human evidence to indicate that mild hypothermia, even when induced after ROSC, is neuroprotective and improves outcome after a period of global cerebral hypoxia–ischemia.[122,123] Cooling suppresses many of the pathways leading to delayed cell death. Hypothermia decreases the cerebral metabolic rate for oxygen ($CMRO_2$) by about 6% for each 1°C reduction in temperature,[124] and this may reduce the release of excitatory amino acids and free radicals.[122] Hypothermia blocks the intracellular consequences of excitotoxin exposure (high calcium and glutamate concentrations). Hypothermia may suppress apoptosis (programmed cell death) by blocking caspases, a family of cellular proteases that normally mediate this process.[123] Finally, hypothermia reduces the inflammatory response, which is a feature of the post–cardiac arrest period. Inflammatory mediators are thought to exacerbate delayed neurologic injury.

Two randomized clinical trials and a meta-analysis showed improved outcome in adults who remained comatose after initial resuscitation from out-of-hospital ventricular fibrillation (VF) cardiac arrest and were cooled within minutes to hours after ROSC.[3,4,125] Patients in these studies were cooled to 33°C or to the range of 32°C to 34°C for 12 to 24 hours. The Hypothermia After Cardiac Arrest (HACA) study included a small subset of patients with in-hospital cardiac arrest.[3] Four studies with historical control groups showed benefit after therapeutic hypothermia in comatose survivors of out-of-hospital cardiac arrest after non-VF arrest[126] and all rhythm arrests,[5,6,81] respectively. Other observational studies also indicate its possible benefit following cardiac arrest from other initial rhythms and in other settings.[127,128] Mild hypothermia is the only therapy given in the post–cardiac arrest setting that has been shown to increase survival, and it should be part of a standardized treatment strategy for comatose survivors of cardiac arrest.[6,129,130] The precise patients that may benefit from this treatment, the ideal induction technique (alone or in combination), target temperature, duration, and rewarming rate have yet to be established.

Animal studies demonstrate a benefit of very early cooling either during CPR or within 15 minutes of ROSC when cooling is maintained only for a short time (1–2 hours).[131,132] However, when prolonged cooling is used (>24 hours), less is known about the therapeutic window. The median time to achieve target temperature in the HACA trial was 8 hours (interquartile range [IQR] 6–26),[3] while in the Bernard study, average core temperature was reported to be 33.5°C within 2 hours of ROSC.[4] Clearly, additional clinical studies are needed to optimize this effective therapeutic strategy. At this time, each center should use a strategy that best suits its infrastructure, logistics, and treatment plan.

 See Web site for ILCOR Scientific Statement on Hypothermia

Practical Application of Therapeutic Hypothermia

The practical application of therapeutic hypothermia is divided into three phases: induction, maintenance, and rewarming. Induction can be achieved easily and inexpensively with intravenous ice-cold fluids (30 mL/kg of saline 0.9% or Ringer's lactate)[133–137] or traditional ice packs placed in the groins, armpits, and around the neck and head. Infusion of 30 mL/kg of 4°C crystalloid will reduce the core temperature by approximately 1.5°C. In most cases, it is easy to cool patients initially after ROSC because the temperature normally decreases within this first hour.[8,51] Initial cooling is facilitated by concomitant neuromuscular blockade and sedation, which will prevent shivering.[138] Magnesium sulphate, a naturally occurring NMDA receptor antagonist that reduces the shivering threshold slightly, can also be given.[139] Other potential benefits of magnesium are that it is a vasodilator, which will increase the cooling rate;[140] it is antiarrhythmic, and there are some animal data indicating that it offers additional neuroprotection in combination with hypothermia.[141] Magnesium sulphate 5 g can be infused over 5 hours, which will cover the period of induction of hypothermia. The shivering threshold can also be reduced by warming the skin; the shivering threshold is reduced by 1°C for every 4°C increase in skin temperature.[142] Application of a forced-air warming blanket will reduce shivering during intravascular cooling.[143]

If indicated, the patient can be transferred to the angiography laboratory with ongoing cooling using these methods.[6,7] Surface or internal cooling devices (described below) can also be used alone.[128,144]

In the maintenance phase, a cooling method with effective temperature monitoring that avoids temperature fluctuations is preferred. This is best achieved with external or internal cooling devices that include continuous temperature feedback to achieve a set target temperature. The temperature is typically monitored from a thermistor placed in the bladder and/or esophagus. Typical external devices are cooling blankets or pads with water-filled circulating systems or more advanced systems that include cooling tents (with cold air).[128,144–149] Typical internal cooling devices include intravascular cooling catheters, placed usually in the femoral or subclavian veins.[128] However, less sophisticated methods such as cold wet blankets on the torso and around the extremities or ice packs combined with ice cold fluids can also be effective; however, these methods may be more time-con-

suming for nursing staff, may result in greater temperature fluctuations, and do not enable controlled rewarming. Ice-cold fluids alone cannot be used to maintain hypothermia.[150] As yet, there are no data indicating that any specific cooling technique increases survival when compared with any other cooling technique; however, internal devices enable more precise temperature control compared with external techniques.[145] Overcooling and rebound hyperthermia are more likely to occur with external cooling techniques[152] because of the inevitable lag time between a change in the temperature setting of the external device and the core temperature.

The rewarming phase can be achieved with either external or internal cooling devices (if these are used) or with other heating systems. The optimal rate of rewarming is not known, but the consensus is currently about 0.25°C to 0.5°C of warming per hour.[127] Particular care should be taken during the cooling and rewarming phases because metabolic rate, plasma electrolyte concentrations, and hemodynamics may change rapidly.

Therapeutic hypothermia is associated with several complications in addition to the shivering, which has been discussed.[152] Mild hypothermia increases systemic vascular resistance, which reduces cardiac output. A variety of arrhythmias can be induced by hypothermia, but bradycardia is the most common to be documented in therapeutic hypothermia studies.[128] Hypothermia induces a diuresis, and any associated hypovolemia will compound hemodynamic instability. Hypothermia also causes electrolyte abnormalities such as hypophosphatemia, hypokalemia, hypomagnesemia, and hypocalcemia; these, in turn, can cause arrhythmias.[152,153] Hypothermia decreases insulin sensitivity and insulin secretion, which results in hyperglycemia.[4] This should be treated with insulin (see below). As a consequence of its effect on platelet and clotting function, mild hypothermia impairs coagulation and increases bleeding. Hypothermia can impair the immune system and increase infection rates.[154] In the HACA study, pneumonia was more common in the cooled group, but this did not reach statistical significance.[3] The serum amylase concentration is almost always increased during hypothermia, but the significance of this unclear. The clearance of sedative drugs and neuromuscular blockers is reduced by up to 30% at a temperature of 34°C.[155]

Relative contraindications to hypothermia include severe systemic infection, cardiogenic shock (systolic blood pressure <90 mm Hg despite inotropic drugs), established multiple organ failure, and preexisting medical coagulopathy. Although thrombolytic therapy is not considered a contraindication to therapeutic hypothermia, the interaction of these therapies when simultaneously administered has not been formally studied in post-cardiac arrest patients.

In summary, both preclinical and clinical evidence indicates that mild therapeutic hypothermia is an effective therapy for PCAS. Unconscious adult patients with spontaneous circulation after out-of-hospital VF cardiac arrest should be cooled to 32°C to 34°C for at least 12 to 24 hours.[129] Most experts recommend cooling for at least 24 hours. While data support cooling to 32°C to 34°C, the optimal temperature has not been determined. Induced hypothermia might also benefit unconscious adult patients with spontaneous circulation after out-of-hospital cardiac arrest from a nonshockable rhythm or cardiac arrest in hospital.[129] Although the optimal time to start cooling has not been defined clinically, it is reasonable to induce hypothermia as soon as possible. The therapeutic window, or time after ROSC at which therapeutic hypothermia is no longer beneficial, has also not been clinically defined. Rapid infusion of ice-cold fluid at 30 mL/kg is a very effective, simple method for initiating cooling. Shivering should be treated by ensuring adequate sedation and/or giving neuromuscular blocking drugs. Bolus doses of neuromuscular blockers are usually adequate, but infusions are occasionally necessary. Slow rewarming is recommended (0.25°C–0.5°C/hr), although the optimal rate for rewarming has not been clinically defined. If therapeutic hypothermia is not undertaken, any pyrexia occurring in the first 72 hours after cardiac arrest should be aggressively treated with antipyretics or active cooling.

Seizure Control and Prevention

Seizures and/or myoclonus occur in 5% to 15% of adult patients who achieve ROSC and in 10% to 40% of those who remain comatose.[22,30,156,157] Seizures increase cerebral metabolism by up to threefold.[158] There are no studies that directly address the use of prophylactic anticonvulsant drugs after cardiac arrest in adults. Anticonvulsants such as thiopental, and especially phenytoin, have been shown to be neuroprotective in experimental studies,[159–161] but a clinical trial of thiopental after cardiac arrest showed no benefit.[162] Myoclonus can be particularly difficult to treat; phenytoin is often ineffective. Clonazepam is the most effective antimyoclonic drug, but sodium valproate and levetiracetam may also be effective.[29] Effective treatment of myoclonus with propofol has been described.[163] With therapeutic hypothermia, survivors with good neurologic function have been reported, despite initially displaying severe postarrest status epilepticus.[164,165]

Glucose Control

Tight control of blood glucose (4.4–6.1 mmol/L or 80–110 mg/dL) using insulin reduced hospital mortality in critically ill adults in a surgical ICU[166] and appeared to protect the central and peripheral nervous system.[167] When the same group repeated this study in a medical ICU, the overall mortality was similar in the intensive insulin and control groups.[168] Among the patients with an ICU stay of 3 days or longer, intensive insulin therapy reduced the mortality from 52.5% (control group) to 43% (P = 0.009). Of the 1,200 patients in the medical ICU study, 61 had neurologic disease; the mortality among these patients was the same in the control and treatment groups (29% versus 30%).[168] In the United Kingdom, the median length of ICU stay for ICU survivors after admission following cardiac arrest is 3.4 days,[12] which is the same as that in Norway.[6]

In a study from Finland, 90 unconscious survivors of out-of-hospital VF cardiac arrest were cooled and randomized into two treatment groups: a strict glucose control group (SGC), with a blood glucose target of 4 to 6 mmol/L (27–108 mg/dL), and a moderate glucose control group (MGC), with a blood glucose target of 6 to 8 mmol/L (108–144 mg/dL).[169] Both groups were treated with an insulin infusion for 48 hours. Episodes of moderate hypoglycemia (<3.0 mmol/L or 54 mg/dL) occurred in 18% of the SGC group and 2% of the MGC group (P = 0.008); however, there were no episodes of severe hypoglycemia (<2.2 mmol/L or 40 mg/dL). There was no difference in mortality by day 30: 33% in the SGC group and 35% in the MGC group (P = 0.846). The upper glucose value of 8.0 mmol/L (144 mg/dL), which is significantly higher than the 6.1 mmol/L (110 mg/dL) recommended by van den Berghe,[166] has been suggested by others.[6,170,171] The lower glucose target range may not reduce mortality any further but instead may expose patients to the potentially harmful effects of hypoglycemia.[169] The incidence of severe hypoglycemia (glucose value <2.2 mmol/L or <40 mg/dL) in another recent study of intensive insulin therapy was 17%[172] and some authors have cautioned against its routine use in the critically ill.[173,174] Regardless of the chosen glucose target range, blood glucose must be measured frequently,[6,169] especially when insulin is started and during cooling and rewarming periods. The blood glucose concentration that triggers insulin therapy and the target range of blood glucose concentrations should be determined by local policy. Recent studies indicate that post–cardiac arrest patients may be treated optimally with a target range for blood glucose concentration of up to 8 mmol/L (144 mg/dL).[6,69,171]

Adrenal Dysfunction

The stress of total-body ischemia–reperfusion affects adrenal function. Although increased plasma cortisol levels occur in many patients after out-of-hospital cardiac arrest, relative adrenal insufficiency, defined as failure to respond to corticotrophin (i.e., <9 μg/dL increase in cortisol) is common.[79,80,175] Furthermore, basal cortisol levels measured within 6 to 36 hours after the onset of cardiac arrest were lower in patients who subsequently died from early refractory shock (median 27 μg/dL; IQR 15–47) than in those who died later from neurologic causes (median 52 μg/dL; IQR 28–72).[79] One small study has demonstrated increased ROSC when patients with out-of-hospital cardiac arrest were treated with hydrocortisone,[176] but the use of steroids has not been studied in the post–cardiac arrest phase. In a recent trial, hydrocortisone did not improve survival or reversal of shock in patients with septic shock.[177] Thus, the use of low-dose steroids, even in septic shock, where they are commonly given, remains controversial.[178,179] Although relative adrenal insufficiency may exist after ROSC, there is no evidence that treatment with steroids improves long-term outcomes, and their routine use after cardiac arrest is not recommended.

Post–Cardiac Arrest Prognostication

Appropriate prognostication of futility in an individual patient is an essential component of optimized post–cardiac arrest care. Recently several systematic reviews evaluated

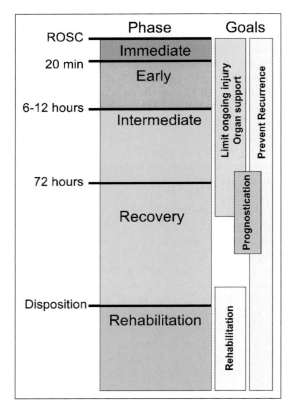

| FIGURE 28-1 • Phases of post-cardiac arrest syndrome.

predictors of poor outcome, including clinical circumstances of the cardiac arrest and resuscitation, patient characteristics, neurologic examination, electrophysiologic studies, biochemical markers, and neuroimaging.[180–182] Despite a large body of research in this area, the timing and optimal approach to prognostication of futility is controversial. However, it is clear that prearrest and intra-arrest factors cannot be used to accurately prognosticate futility in individual patients who achieve ROSC (Fig. 28-1). Furthermore, tests performed in the postarrest period have time-sensitive specificity that differs for each test. Finally, the impact of therapeutic hypothermia on the overall accuracy of clinical prognostication has undergone only limited prospective evaluation.

In patients not treated with therapeutic hypothermia, the bedside neurologic examination remains one of the most reliable and widely validated predictors of functional outcome after cardiac arrest.[22,180–182] The reliability and validity of neurologic examination as a predictor of poor outcome depends on the presence of neurologic deficits at specific time points after ROSC.[181,182] Absence of the pupillary light response, corneal reflex, or motor response to painful stimuli at day 3 provides the most reliable predictor of poor outcome (vegetative state or death).[157,180,182] Based on a systematic review of the literature, it was reported that absent brainstem reflexes or a Glasgow Coma Scale motor score ≤2 at 72 hours had a false-positive rate (FPR) of 0% (95% CI 0%–3%) for predicting poor outcome.[180] In a recent prospective trial, it was reported that absent pupillary or corneal reflexes at 72 hours had a 0% FPR (95% CI 0%–9%), while absent motor response at 72 hours had a 5% FPR (95% CI 2%–9%) for poor outcome.[157] In using

the neurologic examination as the basis for prognostication, it is important to consider that physiologic and pathologic factors (hypotension, shock, severe metabolic abnormalities) and interventions (paralytics, sedatives, and hypothermia) may influence the findings and lead to errors.[180] Use of the bedside neurologic examination can also be compromised by complications such as seizures and myoclonus which, if prolonged and repetitive, may carry their own grave prognosis.[180,183]

Of the electrophysiologic tools that have been studied, median nerve somatosensory evoked potentials (SSEP) appear to be the most reliable prognosticator of poor neurologic outcome.[157,182,184–186] SSEP tests the integrity of the neuronal pathways from a peripheral nerve, spinal cord, or brainstem to the cerebral cortex.[187,188] In unresponsive cardiac arrest survivors 24 hours to 1 week after ROSC, the bilateral absence of the N20 component of the median nerve SSEP reliably predicts poor outcome (FPR for poor outcome = 0.7%, 95% CI 0.1–3.7).[180–182] Other evoked potentials, such as brainstem auditory and visual and long-latency evoked potential tests, have not been thoroughly tested or widely replicated for their prognostic value after cardiac arrest.[189–192]

Electroencephalography (EEG) has been extensively studied as a prognostication tool after cardiac arrest. Malignant EEG patterns most reliably associated with poor functional outcome include generalized suppression to <20 μV, burst-suppression pattern with generalized epileptiform activity, and generalized periodic complexes on a flat background.[180] However, the predictive value of any one individual pattern is poorly understood, because most studies categorize a panel of patterns as malignant. A meta-analysis of studies reporting malignant EEG patterns within the first 3 days after ROSC calculated a FPR of 3% (95% CI 0.9%–11%).[180] Based on this result, the authors concluded that EEG alone was insufficient to prognosticate futility.

Biochemical markers derived initially from cerebrospinal fluid [creatine phosphokinase (CPK)-BB][193,194] or peripheral blood [neuron specific enolase (NSE) and S100β] have been used to prognosticate poor outcome after cardiac arrest. The clinical utility of these markers is limited by variability among studies in the cutoff value that achieves a 0% FPR for predicting poor neurologic outcome. For example, published cutoff values for the most reliable serum biomarker, neuron specific enolase (NSE), measured between 24 and 72 hours after ROSC range from >30 to >71 μg/L.[157,195–202]

Neuroimaging is performed to define structural brain injury related to cardiac arrest. The absence of a well-designed study has limited the use of neuroimaging in the prediction of outcome after cardiac arrest. At this time, the practical utility of neuroimaging, especially computed tomography scans, is limited to excluding intracranial pathologies such as hemorrhage or strokes.

Therapeutic hypothermia improves survival and functional outcome for 1 in every 6 comatose cardiac arrest survivors treated.[125] As a neuroprotective intervention, hypothermia alters the progression of neurologic injury and the evolution of recovery. Therefore, prognostication tools developed in patients not treated with hypothermia might not be accurate in those treated with hypothermia. There are no published studies examining the prognostic accuracy of bedside neurologic exam in post–cardiac arrest patients treated with hypothermia. Hypothermia may mask the neurologic examination or delay the clearance of exam-altering medications such as sedatives or neuromuscular blocking agents.[155,180,203] The prognostic accuracy of biochemical markers appears to be altered by therapeutic hypothermia.[197] In contrast, bilateral absence of cortical N20 responses predicted permanent coma with a FPR of 0% (95% CI, 0%–8%) in patients treated with hypothermia.[204] In summary, the concerns discussed above suggest that the approach to early prognostication might need to be modified when post–cardiac arrest patients are treated with therapeutic hypothermia. The recovery period after hypothermia therapy has not been defined clearly, and early withdrawal of life-sustaining therapies may not be in the best interest of patients and their families. Until more is known about the impact of therapeutic hypothermia, prognostication should probably be delayed, but the optimal time has yet to be determined.

Pediatrics: Special Considerations

Children who are successfully resuscitated from a cardiac arrest differ from adults because of anatomic, physiologic, and developmental differences and because the etiology and pathophysiology of their arrests are often different. In contrast to adults, children rarely develop sudden arrhythmogenic VF arrests from coronary artery disease. Pediatric cardiac arrests are caused typically by progressive respiratory failure and/or circulatory shock. Arrhythmogenic ventricular fibrillation/ventricular tachycardia (VF/VT) arrests occur in 5% to 20% of out-of-hospital pediatric cardiac arrests and ~10% of in-hospital pediatric arrests.[14,16,205–207] Outcomes are worse after asphyxial arrests than after VF/VT and much worse after ischemic arrests than asphyxial arrests, presumably because of the severity of the hypoxic–ischemic insult.[16] Although not well studied, it is likely that these factors affect the severity of the PCAS.

The decreased cardiovascular pulmonary reserve in infants and children compared with adults as well as transitional physiology for neonates certainly affect the pathophysiology and treatment of the PCAS in children. Many children who have an in-hospital cardiac arrest have preexisting underlying abnormalities, diseases, and other organ dysfunction; the effect of these on the PCAS are unknown. Finally, pediatrics is developmental medicine, and pediatric neurologic tools that are appropriate at one age may not be accurate or valid at another.

The impact of a child's death from a cardiac arrest is much greater than an adult's because of the potential years of life lost and the profound impact on the family. Coping with a sudden unexpected death is always difficult. When the victim is a child, the loss tends to be even more oppressive. These issues should have substantial effects on health care provision during the immediate postarrest phase.

As with adults, the post–cardiac arrest phase in children is a high-risk period for brain injury, ventricular arrhythmias, and other reperfusion injuries.[63,205,208–210] Therefore, interventions to restore organ function and limit cell damage are paramount and should be guided by the goals of preserving neurologic function and long-term quality of life.[211–215] Unfortunately there is a critical knowledge gap for postarrest interventions in children; therefore, recommendations are based on general principles of intensive care or extrapolation of evidence obtained from adults, newborns, and animal studies.[3–6,152,208,209,216–222]

Implementation Strategies

Implementation of optimized post–cardiac arrest care requires a multidisciplinary team with strong leadership. In the case of post–cardiac arrest care, this leadership is likely to be a senior critical care or emergency medicine physician.

Implementation of optimized post–cardiac arrest care requires a multidisciplinary team with strong leadership. In the case of post–cardiac arrest care, this leadership is likely to be a senior critical care or emergency medicine physician. Given the teamwork that is essential in the emergency department and critical care unit, a nurse–doctor partnership is ideal—each would carry the respect of colleagues. Implementation of post–cardiac arrest protocols in the prehospital environment will require a prehospital local champion; depending on the structure of the emergency medical services, this individual could be a paramedic or physician. Ideally, there should be a strong paramedic–doctor relationship that incorporates key in-hospital personnel.

A simple local treatment protocol should be developed with contributions from all the relevant disciplines;[2,6] this should then be disseminated to all relevant personnel, both out of hospital and in hospital. Everyone must understand that optimal post–cardiac arrest care requires good collaboration among doctors and nurses across several different specialities in multiple settings. Identification of weak links in the system may enable problems to be anticipated and resolved before there is any attempt to implement changes in practice. The importance and ease of interventions should be prioritized to enable, if necessary, phased implementation. Start with interventions that are both important and easy to implement.

Educational materials are a vital tool for implementing change; a formal education program should precede protocol implementation.[2] There should also be a formalized mechanisms for ongoing education. Any significant change in clinical practice is best initiated by undertaking a supportive pilot phase. At the end of the pilot phase, amendments can be made before further implementation.

All our clinical practice should be audited; this is particularly true when change is implemented. By measuring current performance against defined standards (e.g., time to achieve target temperature when using therapeutic hypothermia), it is possible to identify where local protocols and practice need to be modified. Process as well as clinical factors should be monitored as part of the quality program. The iterative process of reaudit and further change, as necessary, should enable optimal performance. Ideally, the standards against which local practice is audited are established at a national or international level. This type of benchmarking exercise is now common practice throughout many health care systems.

References

1. Cardiopulmonary resuscitation. *JAMA* 1966;198(4):372–379.
2. Neumar R, Nolan JP. AHA/ILCOR Post–Cardiac Arrest Statement of Science. *Circulation* 2008. In press.
3. Hypothermia After Cardiac Arrest Study Group. Mild therapeutic hypothermia to improve the neurologic outcome after cardiac arrest. *N Engl J Med* 2002;346(8):549–556.
4. Bernard SA, Gray TW, Buist MD, et al. Treatment of comatose survivors of out-of-hospital cardiac arrest with induced hypothermia. *N Engl J Med* 2002;346(8):557–563.
5. Oddo M, Schaller MD, Feihl F, et al. From evidence to clinical practice: effective implementation of therapeutic hypothermia to improve patient outcome after cardiac arrest. *Crit Care Med* 2006;34(7):1865–1873.
6. Sunde K, Pytte M, Jacobsen D, et al. Implementation of a standardised treatment protocol for post resuscitation care after out-of-hospital cardiac arrest. *Resuscitation* 2007;73(1):29–39.
7. Knafelj R, Radsel P, Ploj T, et al. Primary percutaneous coronary intervention and mild induced hypothermia in comatose survivors of ventricular fibrillation with ST-elevation acute myocardial infarction. *Resuscitation* 2007;74(2):227–234.
8. Langhelle A, Tyvold SS, Lexow K, et al. In-hospital factors associated with improved outcome after out-of-hospital cardiac arrest. A comparison between four regions in Norway. *Resuscitation* 2003;56(3):247–263.
9. Herlitz J, Engdahl J, Svensson L, et al. Major differences in 1-month survival between hospitals in Sweden among initial survivors of out-of-hospital cardiac arrest. *Resuscitation* 2006;70(3):404–409.
10. Stiell IG, Wells GA, Field B, et al. Advanced cardiac life support in out-of-hospital cardiac arrest. *N Engl J Med* 2004;351(7):647–656.
11. Keenan SP, Dodek P, Martin C, et al. Variation in length of intensive care unit stay after cardiac arrest: where you are is as important as who you are? *Crit Care Med* 2007;35(3):836–841.
12. Nolan JP, Laver SR, Welch CA, et al. Outcome following admission to UK intensive care units after cardiac arrest: a secondary analysis of the ICNARC Case Mix Programme Database. *Anaesthesia* 2007;62(12):1207–1216.
13. Mashiko K, Otsuka T, Shimazaki S, et al. An outcome study of out-of-hospital cardiac arrest using the Utstein template: a Japanese experience. *Resuscitation* 2002;55(3):241–246.
14. Young KD, Gausche-Hill M, McClung CD, et al. A prospective, population-based study of the epidemiology and outcome of out-of-hospital pediatric cardiopulmonary arrest. *Pediatrics* 2004;114(1):157–164.
15. Donoghue AJ, Nadkarni V, Berg RA, et al. Out-of-hospital pediatric cardiac arrest: an epidemiologic review and assessment of current knowledge. *Ann Emerg Med* 2005;46(6):512–522.
16. Nadkarni VM, Larkin GL, Peberdy MA, et al. First documented rhythm and clinical outcome from in-hospital cardiac arrest among children and adults. *JAMA* 2006;295(1):50–57.
17. Peberdy MA, Kaye W, Ornato JP, et al. Cardiopulmonary resuscitation of adults in the hospital: a report of 14720 cardiac arrests from the National Registry of Cardiopulmonary Resuscitation. *Resuscitation* 2003;58(3):297–308.
18. Adrie C, Haouache H, Saleh M, et al. An underrecognized source of organ donors: patients with brain death after successfully resuscitated cardiac arrest. *Intens Care Med* 2008;34(1):132–137.
19. Wilson DJ, Fisher A, Das K, et al. Donors with cardiac arrest: improved organ recovery but no preconditioning benefit in liver allografts. *Transplantation* 2003;75(10):1683–1687.
20. Ali AA, Lim E, Thanikachalam M, et al. Cardiac arrest in the organ donor does not negatively influence recipient survival after heart transplantation. *Eur J Cardiothorac Surg* 2007;31(5):929–933.
21. Laver S, Farrow C, Turner D, et al. Mode of death after admission to an intensive care unit following cardiac arrest. *Intensive Care Med* 2004;30(11):2126–2128.
22. Levy DE, Caronna JJ, Singer BH, et al. Predicting outcome from hypoxic-ischemic coma. *JAMA* 1985;253(10):1420–1426.
23. Pusswald G, Fertl E, Faltl M, et al. Neurological rehabilitation of severely disabled cardiac arrest survivors: Part II. Life situation of patients and families after treatment. *Resuscitation* 2000;47(3):241–248.
24. de Vos R, de Haes HC, Koster RW, et al. Quality of survival after cardiopulmonary resuscitation. *Arch Intern Med* 1999;159(3):249–254.
25. van Alem AP, de Vos R, Schmand B, et al. Cognitive impairment in survivors of out-of-hospital cardiac arrest. *Am Heart J* 2004;148(3):416–421.
26. Bass E. Cardiopulmonary arrest. Pathophysiology and neurologic complications. *Ann Intern Med* 1985;103(6, Pt 1):920–927.
27. Groswasser Z, Cohen M, Costeff H. Rehabilitation outcome after anoxic brain damage. *Arch Phys Med Rehabil* 1989;70(3):186–188.
28. Fertl E, Vass K, Sterz F, et al. Neurological rehabilitation of severely disabled cardiac arrest survivors. Part I. Course of post-acute inpatient treatment. *Resuscitation* 2000;47(3):231–239.
29. Caviness JN, Brown P. Myoclonus: current concepts and recent advances. *Lancet Neurol* 2004;3(10):598–607.
30. Krumholz A, Stern BJ, Weiss HD. Outcome from coma after cardiopulmonary resuscitation: relation to seizures and myoclonus. *Neurology* 1988;38(3):401–405.
31. Neumar RW. Molecular mechanisms of ischemic neuronal injury. *Ann Emerg Med* 2000;36(5):483–506.
32. Lipton P. Ischemic cell death in brain neurons. *Physiol Rev* 1999;79(4):1431–1568.
33. Bano D, Nicotera P. Ca^{2+} signals and neuronal death in brain ischemia. *Stroke* 2007;38(2 suppl):674–676.
34. Ames A III, Wright RL, Kowada M, et al. Cerebral ischemia: II. The no-reflow phenomenon. *Am J Pathol* 1968;52(2):437–453.
35. Wolfson SK Jr, Safar P, Reich H, et al. Dynamic heterogeneity of cerebral hypoperfusion after prolonged cardiac arrest in dogs measured by the stable xenon/CT technique: a preliminary study. *Resuscitation* 1992;23(1):1–20.
36. Fischer M, Bottiger BW, Popov-Cenic S, et al. Thrombolysis using plasminogen activator and heparin reduces cerebral no-reflow after resuscitation from cardiac arrest: an experimental study in the cat. *Intens Care Med* 1996;22(11):1214–1223.
37. Bottiger BW, Krumnikl JJ, Gass P, et al. The cerebral "no—reflow" phenomenon after cardiac arrest in rats-influence of low—flow reperfusion. *Resuscitation* 1997;34(1):79–87.
38. Sterz F, Leonov Y, Safar P, et al. Multifocal cerebral blood flow by Xe-CT and global cerebral metabolism after prolonged cardiac arrest in dogs. Reperfusion with open-chest CPR or cardiopulmonary bypass. *Resuscitation* 1992;24(1):27–47.
39. Nishizawa H, Kudoh I. Cerebral autoregulation is impaired in patients resuscitated after cardiac arrest. *Acta Anaesthesiol Scand* 1996;40(9):1149–1153.
40. Sundgreen C, Larsen FS, Herzog TM, et al. Autoregulation of cerebral blood flow in patients resuscitated from cardiac arrest. *Stroke* 2001;32(1):128–132.
41. Beckstead JE, Tweed WA, Lee J, MacKeen WL. Cerebral blood flow and metabolism in man following cardiac arrest. *Stroke* 1978;9(6):569–573.
42. Schaafsma A, de Jong BM, Bams JL, et al. Cerebral perfusion and metabolism in resuscitated patients with severe post-hypoxic encephalopathy. *J Neurol Sci* 2003;210(1–2):23–30.
43. Buunk G, van der Hoeven JG, Frolich M, et al. Cerebral vasoconstriction in comatose patients resuscitated from a cardiac arrest? *Intens Care Med* 1996;22(11):1191–1196.
44. Forsman M, Aarseth HP, Nordby HK, et al. Effects of nimodipine on cerebral blood flow and cerebrospinal fluid pressure after cardiac arrest: correlation with neurologic outcome. *Anesth Analg* 1989;68(4):436–443.
45. Michenfelder JD, Milde JH. Postischemic canine cerebral blood flow appears to be determined by cerebral metabolic needs. *J Cereb Blood Flow Metab* 1990;10(1):71–76.

46. Oku K, Kuboyama K, Safar P, et al. Cerebral and systemic arteriovenous oxygen monitoring after cardiac arrest. Inadequate cerebral oxygen delivery. *Resuscitation* 1994;27(2):141–152.

47. Vereczki V, Martin E, Rosenthal RE, et al. Normoxic resuscitation after cardiac arrest protects against hippocampal oxidative stress, metabolic dysfunction, and neuronal death. *J Cereb Blood Flow Metab* 2006;26(6):821–835.

48. Richards EM, Fiskum G, Rosenthal RE, et al. Hyperoxic reperfusion after global ischemia decreases hippocampal energy metabolism. *Stroke* 2007;38(5):1578–1584.

49. Balan IS, Fiskum G, Hazelton J, et al. Oximetry-guided reoxygenation improves neurological outcome after experimental cardiac arrest. *Stroke* 2006;37(12):3008–3013.

50. Takasu A, Saitoh D, Kaneko N, et al. Hyperthermia: is it an ominous sign after cardiac arrest? *Resuscitation* 2001;49(3):273–277.

51. Zeiner A, Holzer M, Sterz F, et al. Hyperthermia after cardiac arrest is associated with an unfavorable neurologic outcome. *Arch Intern Med* 2001;161(16):2007–2012.

52. Longstreth WT Jr, Inui TS. High blood glucose level on hospital admission and poor neurological recovery after cardiac arrest. *Ann Neurol* 1984;15(1):59–63.

53. Mullner M, Sterz F, Binder M, et al. Blood glucose concentration after cardiopulmonary resuscitation influences functional neurological recovery in human cardiac arrest survivors. *J Cereb Blood Flow Metab* 1997;17(4):430–436.

54. Skrifvars MB, Pettila V, Rosenberg PH, et al. A multiple logistic regression analysis of in-hospital factors related to survival at six months in patients resuscitated from out-of-hospital ventricular fibrillation. *Resuscitation* 2003;59(3):319–328.

55. Longstreth WT Jr, Diehr P, Inui TS. Prediction of awakening after out-of-hospital cardiac arrest. *N Engl J Med* 1983;308(23):1378–1382.

56. Longstreth WT Jr, Copass MK, Dennis LK, et al. Intravenous glucose after out-of-hospital cardiopulmonary arrest: a community-based randomized trial. *Neurology* 1993;43(12):2534–2541.

57. Calle PA, Buylaert WA, Vanhaute OA. Glycemia in the post-resuscitation period. The Cerebral Resuscitation Study Group. *Resuscitation* 1989;17(Suppl):S181–S188; discussion S199–S206.

58. Sakabe T, Tateishi A, Miyauchi Y, et al. Intracranial pressure following cardiopulmonary resuscitation. *Intens Care Med* 1987;13(4):256–259.

59. Morimoto Y, Kemmotsu O, Kitami K, et al. Acute brain swelling after out-of-hospital cardiac arrest: pathogenesis and outcome. *Crit Care Med* 1993;21(1):104–110.

60. Torbey MT, Selim M, Knorr J, et al. Quantitative analysis of the loss of distinction between gray and white matter in comatose patients after cardiac arrest. *Stroke* 2000;31(9):2163–2167.

61. Iida K, Satoh H, Arita K, et al. Delayed hyperemia causing intracranial hypertension after cardiopulmonary resuscitation. *Crit Care Med* 1997;25(6):971–976.

62. Herlitz J, Ekstrom L, Wennerblom B, et al. Hospital mortality after out-of-hospital cardiac arrest among patients found in ventricular fibrillation. *Resuscitation* 1995;29(1):11–21.

63. Laurent I, Monchi M, Chiche JD, et al. Reversible myocardial dysfunction in survivors of out-of-hospital cardiac arrest. *J Am Coll Cardiol* 2002;40(12):2110–2116.

64. Kern KB, Hilwig RW, Berg RA, et al. Postresuscitation left ventricular systolic and diastolic dysfunction. Treatment with dobutamine. *Circulation* 1997;95(12):2610–2613.

65. Kern KB, Hilwig RW, Rhee KH, et al. Myocardial dysfunction after resuscitation from cardiac arrest: an example of global myocardial stunning. *J Am Coll Cardiol* 1996;28(1):232–240.

66. Huang L, Weil MH, Tang W, et al. Comparison between dobutamine and levosimendan for management of postresuscitation myocardial dysfunction. *Crit Care Med* 2005;33(3):487–491.

67. Ruiz-Bailen M, Aguayo de Hoyos E, et al. Reversible myocardial dysfunction after cardiopulmonary resuscitation. *Resuscitation* 2005;66(2):175–181.

68. Cerchiari EL, Safar P, Klein E, et al. Cardiovascular function and neurologic outcome after cardiac arrest in dogs. The cardiovascular post-resuscitation syndrome. *Resuscitation* 1993;25(1):9–33.

69. Cerchiari EL, Safar P, Klein E, et al. Visceral, hematologic and bacteriologic changes and neurologic outcome after cardiac arrest in dogs. The visceral post-resuscitation syndrome. *Resuscitation* 1993;25(2):119–136.

70. Adams JA. Endothelium and cardiopulmonary resuscitation. *Crit Care Med* 2006;34(12 Suppl):S458–S465.

71. Esmon CT. Coagulation and inflammation. *J Endotoxin Res* 2003;9(3):192–198.

72. Adrie C, Adib-Conquy M, Laurent I, et al. Successful cardiopulmonary resuscitation after cardiac arrest as a "sepsis-like" syndrome. *Circulation* 2002;106(5):562–568.

73. Adrie C, Laurent I, Monchi M, et al. Postresuscitation disease after cardiac arrest: a sepsis-like syndrome? *Curr Opin Crit Care* 2004;10(3):208–212.

74. Gando S, Nanzaki S, Morimoto Y, et al. Out-of-hospital cardiac arrest increases soluble vascular endothelial adhesion molecules and neutrophil elastase associated with endothelial injury. *Intens Care Med* 2000;26(1):38–44.

75. Geppert A, Zorn G, Karth GD, et al. Soluble selectins and the systemic inflammatory response syndrome after successful cardiopulmonary resuscitation. *Crit Care Med* 2000;28(7):2360–2365.

76. Cavaillon JM, Adrie C, Fitting C, et al. Endotoxin tolerance: is there a clinical relevance? *J Endotoxin Res* 2003;9(2):101–107.

77. Bottiger BW, Motsch J, Bohrer H, et al. Activation of blood coagulation after cardiac arrest is not balanced adequately by activation of endogenous fibrinolysis. *Circulation* 1995;92(9):2572–2578.

78. Adrie C, Monchi M, Laurent I, et al. Coagulopathy after successful cardiopulmonary resuscitation following cardiac arrest: implication of the protein C anticoagulant pathway. *J Am Coll Cardiol* 2005;46(1):21–28.

79. Hekimian G, Baugnon T, Thuong M, et al. Cortisol levels and adrenal reserve after successful cardiac arrest resuscitation. *Shock* 2004;22(2):116–119.

80. Schultz CH, Rivers EP, Feldkamp CS, et al. A characterization of hypothalamic-pituitary-adrenal axis function during and after human cardiac arrest. *Crit Care Med* 1993;21(9):1339–1347.

81. Busch M, Soreide E, Lossius HM, et al. Rapid implementation of therapeutic hypothermia in comatose out-of-hospital cardiac arrest survivors. *Acta Anaesthesiol Scand* 2006;50(10):1277–1283.

82. Zheng ZJ, Croft JB, Giles WH, et al. Sudden cardiac death in the United States, 1989 to 1998. *Circulation* 2001;104(18):2158–2163.

83. Pell JP, Sirel JM, Marsden AK, et al. Presentation, management, and outcome of out of hospital cardiopulmonary arrest: comparison by underlying aetiology. *Heart* 2003;89(8):839–842.

84. Huikuri HV, Castellanos A, Myerburg RJ. Sudden death due to cardiac arrhythmias. *N Engl J Med* 2001;345(20):1473–1482.

85. Zipes DP, Wellens HJ. Sudden cardiac death. *Circulation* 1998;98(21):2334–2351.

86. Spaulding CM, Joly LM, Rosenberg A, et al. Immediate coronary angiography in survivors of out-of-hospital cardiac arrest. *N Engl J Med* 1997;336(23):1629–1633.

87. Bendz B, Eritsland J, Nakstad AR, et al. Long-term prognosis after out-of-hospital cardiac arrest and primary percutaneous coronary intervention. *Resuscitation* 2004;63(1):49–53.

88. Keelan PC, Bunch TJ, White RD, et al. Early direct coronary angioplasty in survivors of out-of-hospital cardiac arrest. *Am J Cardiol* 2003;91(12):1461–1463, A1466.

89. Quintero-Moran B, Moreno R, Villarreal S, et al. Percutaneous coronary intervention for cardiac arrest secondary to ST-elevation acute myocardial infarction. Influence of immediate paramedical/medical assistance on clinical outcome. *J Invas Cardiol* 2006;18(6):269–272.

90. Garot P, Lefevre T, Eltchaninoff H, et al. Six-month outcome of emergency percutaneous coronary intervention in resuscitated patients after cardiac arrest complicating ST-elevation myocardial infarction. *Circulation* 2007;115(11):1354–1362.

91. Nagao K, Hayashi N, Kanmatsuse K, et al. Cardiopulmonary cerebral resuscitation using emergency cardiopulmonary bypass, coronary reperfusion therapy and mild hypothermia in patients with cardiac arrest outside the hospital. *J Am Coll Cardiol* 2000;36(3):776–783.

92. Gorjup V, Radsel P, Kocjancic ST, et al. Acute ST-elevation myocardial infarction after successful cardiopulmonary resuscitation. *Resuscitation* 2007;72(3):379–385.

93. Hovdenes J, Laake JH, Aaberge L, et al. Therapeutic hypothermia after out-of-hospital cardiac arrest: experiences with patients treated with percutaneous coronary intervention and cardiogenic shock. *Acta Anaesthesiol Scand* 2007;51(2):137–142.

94. Antman EM, Anbe DT, Armstrong PW, et al. ACC/AHA guidelines for the management of patients with ST-elevation myocardial infarction-executive summary. A report of the American College of Cardiology/American Heart Association Task Force on Practice Guidelines (Writing Committee to revise the 1999 guidelines for the management of patients with acute myocardial infarction). *J Am Coll Cardiol* 2004;44(3):671–719.

95. Richling N, Herkner H, Holzer M, et al. Thrombolytic therapy vs primary percutaneous intervention after ventricular fibrillation cardiac arrest due to acute ST-segment elevation myocardial infarction and its effect on outcome. *Am J Emerg Med* 2007; 25(5): 545–550.

96. Rivers E, Nguyen B, Havstad S, et al. Early goal-directed therapy in the treatment of severe sepsis and septic shock. *N Engl J Med* 2001;345(19):1368–1377.

97. Polonen P, Ruokonen E, Hippelainen M, et al. A prospective, randomized study of goal-oriented hemodynamic therapy in cardiac surgical patients. *Anesth Analg* 2000;90(5):1052–1059.

98. Pearse R, Dawson D, Fawcett J, et al. Early goal-directed therapy after major surgery reduces complications and duration of hospital stay. A randomised, controlled trial [ISRCTN38797445]. *Crit Care* 2005;9(6):R687–693.

99. Mullner M, Sterz F, Binder M, et al. Arterial blood pressure after human cardiac arrest and neurological recovery. *Stroke* 1996; 27(1):59–62.

100. Shaffner DH, Eleff SM, Brambrink AM, et al. Effect of arrest time and cerebral perfusion pressure during cardiopulmonary resuscitation on cerebral blood flow, metabolism, adenosine triphosphate recovery, and pH in dogs. *Crit Care Med* 1999; 27(7):1335–1342.

101. Massetti M, Tasle M, Le Page O, et al. Back from irreversibility: extracorporeal life support for prolonged cardiac arrest. *Ann Thorac Surg* 2005;79(1):178–183; discussion 183–174.

102. Kurusz M, Zwischenberger JB. Percutaneous cardiopulmonary bypass for cardiac emergencies. *Perfusion* 2002;17(4):269–277.

103. Kliegel A, Losert H, Sterz F, et al. Serial lactate determinations for prediction of outcome after cardiac arrest. *Medicine (Baltimore)* 2004;83(5):274–279.

104. Donnino MW, Miller J, Goyal N, et al. Effective lactate clearance is associated with improved outcome in post–cardiac arrest patients. *Resuscitation* 2007;75(2):229–234.

105. Zwemer CF, Whitesall SE, D'Alecy LG. Cardiopulmonary–cerebral resuscitation with 100% oxygen exacerbates neurological dysfunction following nine minutes of normothermic cardiac arrest in dogs. *Resuscitation* 1994;27(2):159–170.

106. Liu Y, Rosenthal RE, Haywood Y, et al. Normoxic ventilation after cardiac arrest reduces oxidation of brain lipids and improves neurological outcome. *Stroke* 1998;29(8):1679–1686.

107. Roine RO, Launes J, Nikkinen P, et al. Regional cerebral blood flow after human cardiac arrest. A hexamethylpropyleneamine oxime single photon emission computed tomographic study. *Arch Neurol* 1991;48(6):625–629.

108. Buunk G, van der Hoeven JG, Meinders AE. Cerebrovascular reactivity in comatose patients resuscitated from a cardiac arrest. *Stroke* 1997;28(8):1569–1573.

109. Muizelaar JP, Marmarou A, Ward JD, et al. Adverse effects of prolonged hyperventilation in patients with severe head injury: a randomized clinical trial. *J Neurosurg* 1991;75(5):731–739.

110. Steiner LA, Balestreri M, Johnston AJ, et al. Sustained moderate reductions in arterial CO2 after brain trauma time-course of cerebral blood flow velocity and intracranial pressure. *Intens Care Med* 2004;30(12):2180–2187.

111. Coles JP, Fryer TD, Coleman MR, et al. Hyperventilation following head injury: effect on ischemic burden and cerebral oxidative metabolism. *Crit Care Med* 2007;35(2):568–578.

112. Aufderheide TP, Sigurdsson G, Pirrallo RG, et al. Hyperventilation-induced hypotension during cardiopulmonary resuscitation. *Circulation* 2004;109(16):1960–1965.

113. Aufderheide TP, Lurie KG. Death by hyperventilation: a common and life-threatening problem during cardiopulmonary resuscitation. *Crit Care Med* 2004;32(9 suppl):S345–S351.

114. The Acute Respiratory Distress Syndrome Network. Ventilation with lower tidal volumes as compared with traditional tidal volumes for acute lung injury and the acute respiratory distress syndrome. *N Engl J Med* 2000;342(18):1301–1308.

115. Plotz FB, Slutsky AS, van Vught AJ, et al. Ventilator-induced lung injury and multiple system organ failure: a critical review of facts and hypotheses. *Intens Care Med* 2004;30(10):1865–1872.

116. Wolthuis EK, Choi G, Dessing MC, et al. Mechanical ventilation with lower tidal volumes and positive end-expiratory pressure prevents pulmonary inflammation in patients without preexisting lung injury. *Anesthesiology* 2008;108(1):46–54.

117. Ely EW, Truman B, Shintani A, et al. Monitoring sedation status over time in ICU patients: reliability and validity of the Richmond Agitation-Sedation Scale (RASS). *JAMA* 2003; 289(22):2983–2991.

118. De Jonghe B, Cook D, Appere-De-Vecchi C, et al. Using and understanding sedation scoring systems: a systematic review. *Intens Care Med* 2000;26(3):275–285.

119. Rundgren M, Rosen I, Friberg H. Amplitude-integrated EEG (aEEG) predicts outcome after cardiac arrest and induced hypothermia. *Intens Care Med* 2006;32(6):836–842.

120. Takino M, Okada Y. Hyperthermia following cardiopulmonary resuscitation. *Intens Care Med* 1991;17(7):419–420.

121. Hickey RW, Kochanek PM, Ferimer H, et al. Induced hyperthermia exacerbates neurologic neuronal histologic damage after asphyxial cardiac arrest in rats. *Crit Care Med* 2003;31(2):531–535.

122. Gunn AJ, Thoresen M. Hypothermic neuroprotection. *NeuroRx* 2006;3(2):154–169.

123. Froehler MT, Geocadin RG. Hypothermia for neuroprotection after cardiac arrest: mechanisms, clinical trials and patient care. *J Neurol Sci* 2007;261(1–2):118–126.

124. McCullough JN, Zhang N, Reich DL, et al. Cerebral metabolic suppression during hypothermic circulatory arrest in humans. *Ann Thorac Surg* 1999;67(6):1895–1899; discussion 1919–1821.

125. Holzer M, Bernard SA, Hachimi-Idrissi S, et al. Hypothermia for neuroprotection after cardiac arrest: systematic review and individual patient data meta-analysis. *Crit Care Med* 2005;33(2):414–418.

126. Bernard SA, Jones BM, Horne MK. Clinical trial of induced hypothermia in comatose survivors of out-of-hospital cardiac arrest. *Ann Emerg Med* 1997;30(2):146–153.

127. Arrich J. Clinical application of mild therapeutic hypothermia after cardiac arrest. *Crit Care Med* 2007;35(4):1041–1047.

128. Holzer M, Mullner M, Sterz F, et al. Efficacy and safety of endovascular cooling after cardiac arrest: cohort study and Bayesian approach. *Stroke* 2006;37(7):1792–1797.

129. Nolan JP, Morley PT, Vanden Hoek TL, et al. Therapeutic hypothermia after cardiac arrest. An advisory statement by the Advancement Life support Task Force of the International Liaison committee on Resuscitation. *Resuscitation* 2003; 57(3): 231–235.

130. Soar J, Nolan JP. Mild hypothermia for post cardiac arrest syndrome. *BMJ* 2007;335(7618):459–460.

131. Kuboyama K, Safar P, Radovsky A, et al. Delay in cooling negates the beneficial effect of mild resuscitative cerebral hypothermia after cardiac arrest in dogs: a prospective, randomized study. *Crit Care Med* 1993;21(9):1348–1358.

132. Abella BS, Zhao D, Alvarado J, et al. Intra-arrest cooling improves outcomes in a murine cardiac arrest model. *Circulation* 2004;109(22):2786–2791.

133. Kliegel A, Losert H, Sterz F, et al. Cold simple intravenous infusions preceding special endovascular cooling for faster induction of mild hypothermia after cardiac arrest-a feasibility study. *Resuscitation* 2005;64(3):347–351.

134. Bernard S, Buist M, Monteiro O, et al. Induced hypothermia using large volume, ice-cold intravenous fluid in comatose survivors of out-of-hospital cardiac arrest: a preliminary report. *Resuscitation* 2003;56(1):9–13.

135. Virkkunen I, Yli-Hankala A, Silfvast T. Induction of therapeutic hypothermia after cardiac arrest in prehospital patients using ice-cold Ringer's solution: a pilot study. *Resuscitation* 2004;62(3):299–302.

136. Kim F, Olsufka M, Longstreth WT Jr, et al. Pilot randomized clinical trial of prehospital induction of mild hypothermia in out-of-hospital cardiac arrest patients with a rapid infusion of 4 degrees C normal saline. *Circulation* 2007;115(24):3064–3070.

137. Polderman KH, Rijnsburger ER, Peerdeman SM, et al. Induction of hypothermia in patients with various types of neurologic injury with use of large volumes of ice-cold intravenous fluid. *Crit Care Med* 2005;33(12):2744–2751.

138. Mahmood MA, Zweifler RM. Progress in shivering control. *J Neurol Sci* 2007;261(1–2):47–54.

139. Wadhwa A, Sengupta P, Durrani J, et al. Magnesium sulphate only slightly reduces the shivering threshold in humans. *Br J Anaesth* 2005;94(6):756–762.

140. Zweifler RM, Voorhees ME, Mahmood MA, et al. Magnesium sulfate increases the rate of hypothermia via surface cooling and improves comfort. *Stroke* 2004;35(10):2331–2334.

141. Zhu H, Meloni BP, Moore SR, et al. Intravenous administration of magnesium is only neuroprotective following transient global ischemia when present with post-ischemic mild hypothermia. *Brain Res* 2004;1014(1–2):53–60.

142. Cheng C, Matsukawa T, Sessler DI, et al. Increasing mean skin temperature linearly reduces the core-temperature thresholds for vasoconstriction and shivering in humans. *Anesthesiology* 1995; 82(5):1160–1168.

143. Guluma KZ, Hemmen TM, Olsen SE, et al. A trial of therapeutic hypothermia via endovascular approach in awake patients with acute ischemic stroke: methodology. *Acad Emerg Med* 2006; 13(8):820–827.

144. Haugk M, Sterz F, Grassberger M, et al. Feasibility and efficacy of a new non-invasive surface cooling device in post-resuscitation intensive care medicine. *Resuscitation* 2007;75(1):76–81.

145. Hoedemaekers CW, Ezzahti M, Gerritsen A, et al. Comparison of cooling methods to induce and maintain normo- and hypothermia in intensive care unit patients: a prospective intervention study. *Crit Care* 2007;11(4):R91.

146. Jordan JD, Carhuapoma JR. Hypothermia: comparing technology. *J Neurol Sci* 2007;261(1–2):35–38.

147. Mayer SA, Kowalski RG, Presciutti M, et al. Clinical trial of a novel surface cooling system for fever control in neurocritical care patients. *Crit Care Med* 2004;32(12):2508–2515.

148. Keller E, Imhof HG, Gasser S, et al. Endovascular cooling with heat exchange catheters: a new method to induce and maintain hypothermia. *Intens Care Med* 2003;29(6):939–943.

149. Al-Senani FM, Graffagnino C, Grotta JC, et al. A prospective, multicenter pilot study to evaluate the feasibility and safety of using the CoolGard System and Icy catheter following cardiac arrest. *Resuscitation* 2004;62(2):143–150.

150. Kliegel A, Janata A, Wandaller C, et al. Cold infusions alone are effective for induction of therapeutic hypothermia but do not keep patients cool after cardiac arrest. *Resuscitation* 2007;73(1):46–53.

151. Edelson DP, Abella BS, Kramer-Johansen J, et al. Effects of compression depth and pre-shock pauses predict defibrillation failure during cardiac arrest. *Resuscitation* 2006;71(2):137–145.

152. Polderman KH. Application of therapeutic hypothermia in the intensive care unit. Opportunities and pitfalls of a promising treatment modality: Part 2, practical aspects and side effects. *Intens Care Med* 2004;30(5):757–769.

153. Polderman KH, Peerdeman SM, Girbes AR. Hypophosphatemia and hypomagnesemia induced by cooling in patients with severe head injury. *J NeuroSurg* 2001;94(5):697–705.

154. Sessler DI. Complications and treatment of mild hypothermia. *Anesthesiology* 2001;95(2):531–543.

155. Tortorici MA, Kochanek PM, Poloyac SM. Effects of hypothermia on drug disposition, metabolism, and response: a focus of hypothermia-mediated alterations on the cytochrome P450 enzyme system. *Crit Care Med* 2007;35(9):2196–2204.

156. Snyder BD, Hauser WA, Loewenson RB, et al. Neurologic prognosis after cardiopulmonary arrest: III. Seizure activity. *Neurology* 1980;30(12):1292–1297.

157. Zandbergen EG, Hijdra A, Koelman JH, et al. Prediction of poor outcome within the first 3 days of postanoxic coma. *Neurology* 2006;66(1):62–68.

158. Ingvar M. Cerebral blood flow and metabolic rate during seizures. Relationship to epileptic brain damage. *Ann N Y Acad Sci* 1986;462:194–206.

159. Ebmeyer U, Safar P, Radovsky A, et al. Thiopental combination treatments for cerebral resuscitation after prolonged cardiac arrest in dogs. Exploratory outcome study. *Resuscitation* 2000; 45(2): 119–131.

160. Imaizumi S, Kurosawa K, Kinouchi H, et al. Effect of phenytoin on cortical Na(+)-K(+)-ATPase activity in global ischemic rat brain. *J Neurotrauma* 1995;12(2):231–234.

161. Taft WC, Clifton GL, Blair RE, et al. Phenytoin protects against ischemia-produced neuronal cell death. *Brain Res* 1989;483(1): 143–148.

162. Randomized clinical study of thiopental loading in comatose survivors of cardiac arrest. Brain Resuscitation Clinical Trial I Study Group. *N Engl J Med* 1986;314(7):397–403.

163. Wijdicks EF. Propofol in myoclonus status epilepticus in comatose patients following cardiac resuscitation. *J Neurol Neurosurg Psychiatry* 2002;73(1):94–95.

164. Sunde K, Dunlop O, Rostrup M, et al. Determination of prognosis after cardiac arrest may be more difficult after introduction of therapeutic hypothermia. *Resuscitation* 2006;69(1):29–32.

165. Hovland A, Nielsen EW, Kluver J, et al. EEG should be performed during induced hypothermia. *Resuscitation* 2006; 68(1):143–146.

166. van den Berghe G, Wouters P, Weekers F, et al. Intensive insulin therapy in the critically ill patients. *N Engl J Med* 2001;345(19): 1359–1367.

167. Van den Berghe G, Schoonheydt K, Becx P, et al. Insulin therapy protects the central and peripheral nervous system of intensive care patients. *Neurology* 2005;64(8):1348–1353.

168. Van den Berghe G, Wilmer A, Hermans G, et al. Intensive insulin therapy in the medical ICU. *N Engl J Med* 2006;354(5):449–461.

169. Oksanen T, Skrifvars MB, Varpula T, et al. Strict versus moderate glucose control after resuscitation from ventricular fibrillation. *Intens Care Med* 2007;33(12):2093–2100.

170. Finney SJ, Zekveld C, Elia A, et al. Glucose control and mortality in critically ill patients. *JAMA* 2003;290(15):2041–2047.

171. Losert H, Sterz F, Roine RO, et al. Strict normoglycaemic blood glucose levels in the therapeutic management of patients within 12h after cardiac arrest might not be necessary. *Resuscitation.* 2008; 76(2):214–220.

172. Brunkhorst FM, Engel C, Bloos F, et al. Intensive insulin therapy and pentastarch resuscitation in severe sepsis. *N Engl J Med* 2008;358(2):125–139.

173. Marik PE, Varon J. Intensive insulin therapy in the ICU: is it now time to jump off the bandwagon? *Resuscitation* 2007;74(1):191–193.

174. Watkinson P, Barber VS, Young JD. Strict glucose control in the critically ill. *BMJ* 2006;332(7546):865–866.

175. Pene F, Hyvernat H, Mallet V, et al. Prognostic value of relative adrenal insufficiency after out-of-hospital cardiac arrest. *Intensive Care Med* 2005;31(5):627–633.

176. Tsai MS, Huang CH, Chang WT, et al. The effect of hydrocortisone on the outcome of out-of-hospital cardiac arrest patients: a pilot study. *Am J Emerg Med* 2007;25(3):318–325.

177. Sprung CL, Annane D, Keh D, et al. Hydrocortisone therapy for patients with septic shock. *N Engl J Med* 2008;358(2):111–124.

178. Dellinger RP, Levy MM, Carlet JM, et al. Surviving Sepsis Campaign: International guidelines for management of severe sepsis and septic shock: 2008. *Crit Care Med* 2008;36(1):296–327.

179. Meyer NJ, Hall JB. Relative adrenal insufficiency in the ICU: can we at least make the diagnosis? *Am J Respir Crit Care Med* 2006;174(12):1282–1284.

180. Wijdicks EF, Hijdra A, Young GB, et al. Practice parameter: prediction of outcome in comatose survivors after cardiopulmonary resuscitation (an evidence-based review): report of the Quality Standards Subcommittee of the American Academy of Neurology. *Neurology* 2006;67(2):203–210.

181. Booth CM, Boone RH, Tomlinson G, et al. Is this patient dead, vegetative, or severely neurologically impaired? Assessing outcome for comatose survivors of cardiac arrest. *JAMA* 2004;291(7): 870–879.

182. Zandbergen EG, de Haan RJ, Stoutenbeek CP, et al. Systematic review of early prediction of poor outcome in anoxic-ischaemic coma. *Lancet* 1998;352(9143):1808–1812.

183. Wijdicks EF, Parisi JE, Sharbrough FW. Prognostic value of myoclonus status in comatose survivors of cardiac arrest. *Ann Neurol* 1994;35(2):239–243.

184. Bassetti C, Bomio F, Mathis J, et al. Early prognosis in coma after cardiac arrest: a prospective clinical, electrophysiological, and biochemical study of 60 patients. *J Neurol Neurosurg Psychiatry* 1996;61(6):610–615.

185. Rothstein TL, Thomas EM, Sumi SM. Predicting outcome in hypoxic-ischemic coma. A prospective clinical and electrophysiologic study. *Electroencephalogr Clin Neurophysiol* 1991;79(2): 101–107.

186. Zandbergen EG, de Haan RJ, Hijdra A. Systematic review of prediction of poor outcome in anoxic-ischaemic coma with biochemical markers of brain damage. *Intens Care Med* 2001;27(10):1661–1667.

187. Young GB. The EEG in coma. *J Clin Neurophysiol* 2000;17(5):473–485.

188. Rothstein TL. The role of evoked potentials in anoxic-ischemic coma and severe brain trauma. *J Clin Neurophysiol* 2000;17(5):486–497.

189. Sohmer H, Freeman S, Gafni M, et al. The depression of the auditory nerve-brain-stem evoked response in hypoxaemia—mechanism and site of effect. *Electroencephalogr Clin Neurophysiol* 1986;64(4):334–338.

190. Fischer C, Luaute J, Nemoz C, et al. Improved prediction of awakening or nonawakening from severe anoxic coma using tree-based classification analysis. *Crit Care Med* 2006;34(5):1520–1524.

191. Madl C, Kramer L, Domanovits H, et al. Improved outcome prediction in unconscious cardiac arrest survivors with sensory evoked potentials compared with clinical assessment. *Crit Care Med* 2000;28(3):721–726.

192. Zandbergen EG, Koelman JH, de Haan RJ, et al. SSEPs and prognosis in postanoxic coma: only short or also long latency responses? *Neurology* 2006;67(4):583–586.

193. Tirschwell DL, Longstreth WT Jr, Rauch-Matthews ME, et al. Cerebrospinal fluid creatine kinase BB isoenzyme activity and neurologic prognosis after cardiac arrest. *Neurology* 1997;48(2):352–357.

194. Longstreth WT, Jr., Clayson KJ, Sumi SM. Cerebrospinal fluid and serum creatine kinase BB activity after out-of-hospital cardiac arrest. *Neurology* 1981;31(4):455–458.

195. Grubb NR, Simpson C, Sherwood R, et al. Prediction of cognitive dysfunction after resuscitation from out-of-hospital cardiac arrest using serum neuron-specific enolase and protein S-100. *Heart* 2007;93(10):1268–1273.

196. Usui A, Kato K, Murase M, et al. Neural tissue-related proteins (NSE, G0 alpha, 28-kDa calbindin-D, S100b and CK-BB) in serum and cerebrospinal fluid after cardiac arrest. *J Neurol Sci* 1994;123(1–2):134–139.

197. Tiainen M, Roine RO, Pettila V, et al. Serum neuron-specific enolase and S-100B protein in cardiac arrest patients treated with hypothermia. *Stroke* 2003;34(12):2881–2886.

198. Roine RO, Somer H, Kaste M, et al. Neurological outcome after out-of-hospital cardiac arrest. Prediction by cerebrospinal fluid enzyme analysis. *Arch Neurol* 1989;46(7):753–756.

199. Prohl J, Rother J, Kluge S, et al. Prediction of short-term and long-term outcomes after cardiac arrest: a prospective multivariate approach combining biochemical, clinical, electrophysiological, and neuropsychological investigations. *Crit Care Med* 2007;35(5):1230–1237.

200. Martens P, Raabe A, Johnsson P. Serum S-100 and neuron-specific enolase for prediction of regaining consciousness after global cerebral ischemia. *Stroke* 1998;29(11):2363–2366.

201. Martens P. Serum neuron-specific enolase as a prognostic marker for irreversible brain damage in comatose cardiac arrest survivors. *Acad Emerg Med* 1996;3(2):126–131.

202. Karkela J, Bock E, Kaukinen S. CSF and serum brain-specific creatine kinase isoenzyme (CK-BB), neuron-specific enolase (NSE) and neural cell adhesion molecule (NCAM) as prognostic markers for hypoxic brain injury after cardiac arrest in man. *J Neurol Sci* 1993;116(1):100–109.

203. Fukuoka N, Aibiki M, Tsukamoto T, et al. Biphasic concentration change during continuous midazolam administration in brain-injured patients undergoing therapeutic moderate hypothermia. *Resuscitation* 2004;60(2):225–230.

204. Tiainen M, Kovala TT, Takkunen OS, et al. Somatosensory and brainstem auditory evoked potentials in cardiac arrest patients treated with hypothermia. *Crit Care Med* 2005;33(8):1736–1740.

205. Samson RA, Nadkarni VM, Meaney PA, et al. Outcomes of in-hospital ventricular fibrillation in children. *N Engl J Med* 2006;354(22):2328–2339.

206. Herlitz J, Engdahl J, Svensson L, et al. Characteristics and outcome among children suffering from out of hospital cardiac arrest in Sweden. *Resuscitation* 2005;64(1):37–40.

207. Tibballs J, Kinney S. A prospective study of outcome of in-patient paediatric cardiopulmonary arrest. *Resuscitation* 2006;71(3):310–318.

208. Morris MC, Nadkarni VM. Pediatric cardiopulmonary-cerebral resuscitation: an overview and future directions. *Crit Care Clin* 2003;19(3):337–364.

209. Hickey RW, Painter MJ. Brain injury from cardiac arrest in children. *Neurol Clin* 2006;24(1):147–158, viii.

210. Rodriguez-Nunez A, Lopez-Herce J, Garcia C, et al. Pediatric defibrillation after cardiac arrest: initial response and outcome. *Crit Care* 2006;10(4):R113.

211. Harrington DJ, Redman CW, Moulden M, et al. The long-term outcome in surviving infants with Apgar zero at 10 minutes: a systematic review of the literature and hospital-based cohort. *Am J Obstet Gynecol* 2007;196(5):463.

212. Jones S, Rantell K, Stevens K, et al. Outcome at 6 months after admission for pediatric intensive care: a report of a national study of pediatric intensive care units in the United Kingdom. *Pediatrics* 2006;118(5):2101–2108.

213. Lopez-Herce J, Garcia C, Rodriguez-Nunez A, et al. Long-term outcome of paediatric cardiorespiratory arrest in Spain. *Resuscitation* 2005;64(1):79–85.

214. Jayshree M, Singhi SC, Malhi P. Follow up of survival and quality of life in children after intensive care. *Indian Pediatr* 2003;40(4):303–309.

215. Taylor A, Butt W, Ciardulli M. The functional outcome and quality of life of children after admission to an intensive care unit. *Intens Care Med* 2003;29(5):795–800.

216. Azzopardi D, Robertson NJ, Cowan FM, et al. Pilot study of treatment with whole body hypothermia for neonatal encephalopathy. *Pediatrics* 2000;106(4):684–694.

217. Gluckman PD, Wyatt JS, Azzopardi D, et al. Selective head cooling with mild systemic hypothermia after neonatal encephalopathy: multicentre randomised trial. *Lancet* 2005;365(9460):663–670.

218. Wyatt JS, Gluckman PD, Liu PY, et al. Determinants of outcomes after head cooling for neonatal encephalopathy. *Pediatrics* 2007;119(5):912–921.

219. Wiklund L, Sharma HS, Basu S. Circulatory arrest as a model for studies of global ischemic injury and neuroprotection. *Ann N Y Acad Sci* 2005;1053:205–219.

220. Gunn AJ, Gluckman PD, Gunn TR. Selective head cooling in newborn infants after perinatal asphyxia: a safety study. *Pediatrics* 1998;102(4 Pt 1):885–892.

221. Fink EL, Marco CD, Donovan HA, et al. Brief induced hypothermia improves outcome after asphyxial cardiopulmonary arrest in juvenile rats. *Dev Neurosci* 2005;27(2–4):191–199.

222. Nozari A, Safar P, Stezoski SW, et al. Mild hypothermia during prolonged cardiopulmonary cerebral resuscitation increases conscious survival in dogs. *Crit Care Med* 2004;32(10):2110–2116.

223. Sung K, Lee YT, Park PW, et al. Improved survival after cardiac arrest using emergent autopriming percutaneous cardiopulmonary support. *Ann Thorac Surg* 2006;82(2):651–656.

224. Morris MC, Wernovsky G, Nadkarni VM. Survival outcomes after extracorporeal cardiopulmonary resuscitation instituted during active chest compressions following refractory in-hospital pediatric cardiac arrest. *Pediatr Crit Care Med* 2004;5(5):440–446.

225. Laurent I, Adrie C, Vinsonneau C, et al. High-volume hemofiltration after out-of-hospital cardiac arrest: a randomized study. *J Am Coll Cardiol* 2005;46(3):432–437.

Eight

Special Resuscitation Situations

Chapter 29
Toxicology in Emergency Cardiovascular Care

Allan R. Mottram and Timothy B. Erickson

When the responsible toxic agent is known, the clinical picture is often predictable and directed therapy can follow standard initial resuscitation. In patients who present with an unknown or multiple drug ingestion, the clinical picture can become clouded by inconsistent physical findings that do not fit a particular toxidrome. Regardless of etiology, the initial resuscitation is similar to that of other critically ill patients and is guided by clinical presentation. But, the critically ill poisoned patient with shock or cardiac arrest may not respond to usual therapies and often requires nonstandard approaches. For example, these patients may require prolonged durations of cardiopulmonary resuscitation, medications not commonly used in resuscitation, larger doses of commonly used drugs, and avoidance of certain drug therapies.

- ■ General approach to the poisoned patient
- ■ Specific considerations for emergency cardiovascular care (ECC) providers on cardiovascular toxicities of poisons
- ■ How to use a methodical approach focusing on aggressive supportive care to optimize care of the critically ill poisoned patient
- ■ Periarrest and arrest evidence-based alterations to the principles of advanced cardiac life support (ACLS) for patients with suspected poisoning

Introduction

Prescribed and illicit xenobiotics can cause direct and indirect cardiovascular and cardiopulmonary toxicity when taken in overdose. When the responsible agent is known, the clinical picture is often predictable, and directed therapy can follow standard initial resuscitation. In patients who present with an unknown or multiple drug ingestion, the clinical picture can become clouded by inconsistent physical findings that do not fit a particular toxidrome.

Regardless of etiology, the initial resuscitation is similar to that of other critically ill patients and is guided by clinical presentation. Following provision of this care, obtaining a detailed history, a thorough physical examination, and review of available laboratory and diagnostic information can narrow the differential diagnosis. Attention can then be directed toward minimizing bioavailability of unabsorbed toxin, enhancing elimination, use of antidotes, and obtaining toxicology consultation.

The approach to the critically ill poisoned patient is guided by available evidence in the literature. Considering this, it is important to understand the limitations of that evidence. The nature of poisoning and overdose does not lend itself to well constructed clinical trials. The heterogeneity and relative infrequency of life-threatening overdose limits the accumulation of useful data. As such, the majority of literature upon which guidelines are based include case reports, short case series, retrospective analyses, and animal studies. With an awareness of these limitations, this chapter discusses the differences in the approach to the acutely poisoned critically ill patient as compared with the nonpoisoned critically ill patient and reviews the most commonly encountered cardiotoxins, highlighting key diagnostic, pathophysiologic, and management issues.

Approach to the Poisoned Patient

Aggressive supportive care in an intensive care environment that adheres to the principles of ACLS is essential to the management of critically ill poisoned patients. However, drugs taken in overdose often do not follow standard pharmacologic parameters. Absorption, distribution, and elimination may be accelerated or delayed. Patients who appear critically ill may recover quickly with aggressive supportive care; conversely, patients who initially appear well may rapidly decompensate. A select group of patients may benefit from advanced decontamination and enhanced elimination procedures such as activated charcoal, whole-bowel irrigation, multiple-dose activated charcoal, urinary alkalinization, and hemodialysis. A few selected cardiotoxic agents have specific antidotes that may be indicated in critically ill patients, but this is the exception rather than the rule.

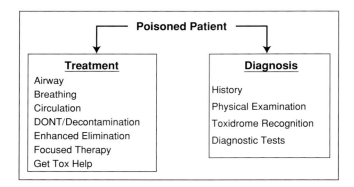

FIGURE 29-1 • Diagnosis and management of the poisoned patient. DONT stands for dextrose, oxygen, naloxone, and thiamine. (From Erickson TB, Thompson TM, Lu JJ. The approach to the patient with an unknown overdose. *Emerg Med Clin North Am* 2007;25[2]:249–281; abstract vii, with permission.)

The general approach to the diagnosis and management of the poisoned patient can be described using a two-pronged model as described in Figure 29-1.[1] In practice, the two prongs occur simultaneously. The left side of the diagram begins with basic emergency medical care directed at the ABCs (airway, breathing, circulation). The mnemonic DONT stands for dextrose, oxygen, naloxone, and thiamine. In most potentially poisoned patients, a rapid blood glucose measurement should be obtained and any derangements corrected. Supplemental oxygen, naloxone, and thiamine should be provided in appropriate cases. The various methods of decontamination should be considered in any poisoned patient. The exact method used should be based on each individual clinical situation. Once a poisoning has been identified, methods of enhanced elimination should be considered. Focused therapy involves antidote administration when appropriate, with aggressive supportive care tailored to the poison in question. Finally, in managing any poisoned patient, it is prudent to consider early consultation with a toxicology service or regional poison center for further guidance. The right side of the diagram focuses on obtaining the patient's history, performing a focused physical examination with attention to toxidrome recognition, and deciding on appropriate diagnostic testing. The two algorithms occur simultaneously and are integral to the diagnosis and management of the poisoned patient.[2,3]

In considering cardiotoxic xenobiotics, it is essential to obtain an electrocardiogram early following presentation. This step may uncover acute myocardial infarction related to cocaine, dysrhythmias related to cardioactive steroids, antihypertensives, or antidysrhythmic agents, and conduction abnormalities related to sodium, potassium, and calcium channel blockade. The remainder of this chapter reviews key presentations of poisoned patients, including the toxicologic differential diagnosis and appropriate interventions (see Sidebars 29-1 and 29-2). The chapter concludes with an in-depth review of specific commonly encountered drugs, poisons, and the appropriate treatments.

ACLS-ORIENTED DIFFERENTIAL DIAGNOSIS FOR THE POISONED PATIENT

Condition	Common Etiologies	
AMS ± respiratory compromise	Opioids Gammahydroxybutyrate Alcohols Benzodiazepines Barbiturates Hypoglycemics	Antidepressants Antipsychotics Cyanide Carbon monoxide Methemoglobinemia
Hypertension	Sympathomimetics Antihistamines Methylxanthines	Phencyclidine Withdrawal states
Tachycardia	Sympathomimetics Antihistamines Methylxanthines Phencyclidine Withdrawal states	Tricyclics Anticholinergics Carbon monoxide Cyanide Methemoglobinemia
ACS and chest pain	Cocaine	Methamphetamine
Ventricular dysrhythmias	Cocaine (QRS) Tricyclics (QRS) SSRI (QT)	Quinine (QRS) Cardiac glycosides
Bradycardia	Calcium channel antagonists Beta-blockers Alpha agonists Cardiac glycosides	Cholinergics Clonidine Nicotine
Shock	Calcium channel antagonists Beta-blockers Cardiac glucosides Cocaine Tricyclics	SSRI Nitrites Carbon monoxide Cyanide Methemoglobinemia
Seizure	INH Sympathomimetics Propoxyphene Hypoglycemics Tricyclics Methylxanthines	Propranolol Withdrawal states Lithium Lindane Local anesthetics Bupropion
Hyperthermia	Sympathomimetics NMS Serotonin syndrome	
Hypothermia	Sedatives Ethanol	
Cholinergic	Organophosphates Carbamates	
Anticholinergic	Atropine Antihistamines Tricyclics Antipsychotics	

ACS, acute coronary syndrome; AMS, altered mental status; INH, isoniazid; NMS, neuroleptic malignant syndrome; SSRI, selective serotonin reuptake inhibitor.

ACLS-ORIENTED INTERVENTIONS FOR THE POISONED PATIENT

Etiology	Potential Intervention	Avoid
Opioids	Naloxone	
Ethanol Benzodiazepines Barbiturates GHB	Supportive care Airway protection	Flumazenil
Toxic alcohols	Alcohol dehydrogenase antagonism Alcohol infusion Fomepizole	
Hypoglycemics	Dextrose Octreotide	
Sympathomimetics Methylxanthines Phencyclidine Withdrawal states	Benzodiazepines	Beta-blockers
Antihistamines Anticholinergics	Benzodiazepines Physostigmine	Antipsychotics Anticholinergics
Tricyclics	Sodium bicarbonate	Physostigmine
Cocaine	Benzodiazepines Aspirin Nitroglycerin Calcium channel antagonists Phentolamine Nitroprusside	Beta-blockers
Serotonin syndrome	Benzodiazepines Active cooling Cyproheptadine	
NMS	Benzodiazepines Active cooling Dantrolene	
Carbon monoxide	Oxygen Hyperbaric oxygen	
Methemoglobinemia	Methylene blue	Nitrites
Cyanide	Amyl nitrite Sodium nitrite Sodium thiosulfate Hydroxocobalamin	Methylene blue
Cardiac glycosides	Digoxin Immune FAB	Calcium
Calcium channel antagonists	Calcium Glucagon Vasopressors HIE	
Beta-blockers	Glucagon Vasopressors	
Cholinergic	Atropine Pralidoxime	
INH	Pyridoxine	Flumazenil

FAB, fragment, antigen binding; GHB, gammahydroxybutyrate; HIE, hyperinsulinemia-euglycemia; INH, isoniazid; NMS, neuroleptic malignant syndrome.

General Considerations for the Poisoned Patient

Approach to Advanced Cardiac Life Support

The general principles of ACLS apply to the poisoned patient; however, there are fundamental differences. The critically ill poisoned patient with shock or cardiac arrest may not respond to usual therapies and often requires nonstandard approaches. For example, these patients may require prolonged durations of cardiopulmonary resuscitation, medications not commonly used in resuscitation, larger doses of commonly used drugs, and avoidance of certain drug therapies. Early consideration of invasive therapies such as dialysis and circulatory assist devices may be warranted.[4]

See Web site for AHA ECC 2005 guidelines for CPR—toxicology.

Airway Control Airway control of the poisoned patient should be considered just as with nonpoisoned critically ill patients, with two caveats. In a patient with a clinically significant opioid overdose, the practice of routine endotracheal intubation before naloxone administration is not recommended.[4] When opioid overdose patients have respiratory insufficiency with a detectable pulse, an attempt at opioid reversal before tracheal intubation is warranted provided that adequate ventilatory support can be provided with bag-valve-mask. Patients with opioid-induced cardiac arrest or impending cardiac arrest should have aggressive airway management, including intubation prior to consideration of naloxone. Finally, patients in whom gastric lavage is being considered should not be intubated solely to facilitate this procedure.

Dextrose One of the most common causes of altered mental status is hypoglycemia. Prolonged hypoglycemia may result in significant morbidity, with permanent neurologic deficits. All patients with altered mental status require rapid bedside blood glucose determination and appropriate intervention. If rapid blood glucose testing is not available, it is acceptable to administer intravenous (IV) dextrose empirically. Following treatment of hypoglycemia, the blood glucose must be monitored for recurrence. This is a critical action in sedated or intubated patients, as they will not demonstrate the clinical clues that hypoglycemia has recurred.

Naloxone Naloxone is the preferred reversal agent for opioid toxicity even though it has a shorter duration of effect (45–60 minutes) than heroin (4–5 hours). There is debate over which route of administration is preferred; however, if IV access is possible, it should be utilized. The endpoint objectives for opioid reversal are adequate airway reflexes and ventilation, not complete arousal. Acute, abrupt opioid withdrawal may increase the likelihood of complications,

such as aspiration pneumonitis, pulmonary edema, ventricular arrhythmias, and severe agitation and hostility. Opioid-induced pulmonary edema occurs in 1% to 3% of patients with heroin overdose.[5–7] The etiology is unclear but may be attributable to opioid-induced capillary leak or a sympathetic surge in the setting of profound hypoxia. Sympathetic surge has been demonstrated in opioid-addicted patients following naloxone administration, and animal studies have demonstrated this surge from hypercapnia, which is exacerbated by naloxone.[5,6] This effect may be abated through ventilatory support prior to naloxone administration or by the use of graduated smaller doses of naloxone.[7]

When naloxone is given in incremental doses of 0.1 mg, the average naloxone reversal dose is 0.2 mg IV.[7] In emergencies, a slow, incremental rate of administration is less satisfactory. For these cases, the recommended initial dose of naloxone is 0.4 to 0.8 mg IV or 0.8 mg intramuscularly (IM) or subcutaneously (SQ). In communities where abuse of naloxone-resistant opioids is prevalent, larger initial doses of naloxone may be appropriate. When opioid overdose is strongly suspected or in locations where fentanyl or its derivatives are prevalent, titration to total naloxone doses of 6 to 10 mg may be necessary.[8] The majority of patients recover well following timely reversal of opioid intoxication with naloxone.[9–11] The duration of action of naloxone is shorter than that of most opioids, and a subset of patients may have recurrent symptoms.[12–14] Therefore, it is recommended that following arousal, all patients be observed beyond the duration of the naloxone effect to ensure their safety.

Flumazenil Flumazenil is a competitive benzodiazepine receptor antagonist of limited utility in the overdose setting. It is generally understood to have the potential to induce seizures in the unknown overdose, as these patients may be benzodiazepine-dependent, have coingested a proconvulsant drug, or have an underlying seizure disorder. Healthy volunteers have experienced mild withdrawal symptoms in an experimental setting after only 1 week of nightly doses of diazepam (15 mg/70 kg), as have chronic low-dose benzodiazepine users.[15,16] Animal studies have demonstrated withdrawal after 7 days, and seizure after 35 days, of daily benzodiazepine therapy followed by flumazenil.[17] The use of flumazenil is not effective from a cost or resource-utilization perspective.[18] In the undifferentiated comatose patient, flumazenil may resolve depressed mental status, but it carries a significant risk of seizure.[19–21] Pediatric ingestions have been considered appropriate situations in which to utilize flumazenil. However, the same caveats that apply to adults apply to children. The restricted indications for flumazenil include iatrogenic overdose (except when the benzodiazepine was given for seizure), pediatric accidental ingestion, and paradoxical reaction to benzodiazepines.

Activated Charcoal Activated charcoal is appropriate therapy within the first hour following ingestion for patients who have ingested a potentially toxic amount of drug and may be considered when such a patient presents beyond 1 hour postingestion, although efficacy decreases over time.[22]

It is generally considered safe and effective for gastrointestinal (GI) decontamination. However, routine administration in all ingestions is not indicated, as the administration of activated charcoal is not risk-free. Nausea, vomiting, aspiration, stercolith with intestinal perforation, and corneal abrasion have all been reported.[23,24] Aspiration is the most significant complication and is usually related to altered mental status or seizure. Activated charcoal should be avoided in patients with depressed mental status, unprotected airway, hydrocarbon exposure, or GI hemorrhage. Other contraindications to the use of charcoal include ingestions of pesticides, hydrocarbons, acids, alkalis, iron, lithium, and solvents, as these agents are not well adsorbed.[2]

There are multiple activated charcoal products on the market. These are available with and without a cathartic, and the concentration of cathartic varies. Multiple doses of activated charcoal containing sorbitol have resulted in severe hypernatremic dehydration in both adult and pediatric patients.[25-28] Therefore, in dosing activated charcoal in older children and adults, the first dose may contain sorbitol; subsequent doses should be sorbitol-free. Activated charcoal is commonly administered in a 50-g (or 1-g/kg) loading dose in adults. A more appropriate dose of charcoal is to provide at least a 10:1 ratio of activated charcoal to toxin.[29-31] If this ratio cannot be achieved in a single dose, serial dosing may be required. Note that serial doses of activated charcoal to achieve an adequate total dose differs from multiple-dose activated charcoal (MDAC), which is discussed below in the section on enhanced elimination.

Gastric Lavage Gastric lavage is an invasive procedure with significant inherent risk. There are appropriate indications for gastric lavage; however, one must weigh the risks and benefits carefully. Complications include aspiration, esophageal perforation, epistaxis, hypothermia, and death.[32] The amount of toxin removed is variable and less successful over time. Even when implemented within one hour, the clinical benefit is unclear.[33-37] Gastric lavage is contraindicated in patients with loss of airway protective reflexes, those with depressed mental status, following ingestion of corrosive agents or hydrocarbons, and those at risk for GI perforation or bleeding.[32] It should never be used as a punitive measure, for nontoxic overdoses, or forced on combative or uncooperative patients. Patients should not be intubated solely to facilitate gastric lavage.

Gastric lavage may be considered in patients with potentially life-threatening ingestions (digitalis, verapamil, amitriptyline) that can be lavaged within 60 minutes of ingestion. When utilized, the procedure requires use of a large-bore (36–40 Fr) orogastric tube. Because the lumen of a standard nasogastric tube is of insufficient diameter, such a tube should not be used. The patient should be placed in the left lateral head-down position and 250-mL aliquots of warm fluid, such as tap water or normal saline, used to irrigate.[2]

Whole-Bowel Irrigation Whole-bowel irrigation is based on the principle that large volumes of nonabsorbable polyethylene glycol traverse the length of the gut, decontaminating it by removing the gut contents via liquid stool.[38]

Volunteer studies show some evidence for decreased bioavailability and there are a number of case reports describing efficacy in the literature, although there are no well controlled clinical trials.[39-46] Whole-bowel irrigation may be effective for ingestions of iron, heavy metals, lithium, drugs poorly adsorbed by activated charcoal, sustained-release or enteric-coated products, and drug-filled packets or other potentially toxic foreign bodies. Contraindications to whole-bowel irrigation are hemodynamic instability, unprotected or compromised airway, intractable vomiting, ileus, GI hemorrhage, and bowel obstruction.[32] When whole-bowel irrigation is initiated, a polyethylene glycol solution is infused via nasogastric tube at a rate of 1 to 2 L/hr and continued until the rectal effluent is clear. In most cases, the gut should empty almost completely in 4 to 6 hours.[2]

Enhanced Elimination Enhanced elimination is the removal of a drug from the body after absorption has occurred. It includes multiple-dose activated charcoal, urinary alkalinization, and extracorporeal measures such as hemodialysis, hemofiltration, and hemoperfusion.

Multiple-dose activated charcoal has been shown in volunteer studies to reduce the elimination half-life of carbamazepine, dapsone, phenobarbital, quinine, and theophylline.[47] It has been evaluated for a number of other drugs and the data are either insufficient or indicate lack of efficacy. The mechanism is understood to be interruption of enteroenteral and enterohepatic circulation.[48] There are no controlled studies in poisoned patients to confirm efficacy in reducing morbidity and mortality. The initial dose should be 50 to 100 g followed by an average of 12.5 g/hr. This may be dosed as 12.5 g/hr, 25 g every 2 hours, or 50 g every 4 hours.[49] Sorbitol may be used in the first dose but not in subsequent doses due to the risk of severe electrolyte abnormality and dehydration.[25-28]

Alkalinization of urine promotes excretion of weakly acidic agents. It is the therapy of choice in salicylate toxicity for those who do not meet criteria for dialysis.[50] There is mixed evidence regarding the use of urinary alkalinization for phenobarbital. It does enhance elimination of phenobarbital, although it cannot be recommended as first-line therapy, as multiple-dose activated charcoal has been found to be superior.[50]

The traditionally proposed mechanism of alkalinization is ion trapping at the renal tubules; however, there are inconsistencies with this theory.[51,52] Regardless of mechanism, urinary alkalinization with sodium bicarbonate may be useful in salicylate overdoses. To alkalinize the urine, the nonalkalemic patient is bolused with 1 to 2 mEq/kg of sodium bicarbonate followed by a bicarbonate infusion. Alkalemic patients should not receive the bolus component. The infusion is prepared by adding 150 mEq sodium bicarbonate to 1 L D_5W with 20 to 40 mEq of potassium.[53] The infusion is started at 150 to 250 mL/hr and adjusted to reach a urinary pH of 7.5 to 8.0.[54] Serum potassium should be maintained in the high-normal range, as hypokalemia will prevent urinary alkalinization.[55] Patients should be monitored to avoid volume overload, especially the elderly and those with renal insufficiency or heart failure.

Extracorporeal measures for toxin removal include hemodialysis, hemofiltration, and hemoperfusion. Criteria that make a drug ideal for extracorporeal therapy include a small volume of distribution, low molecular weight, low protein binding, and water solubility. However, there is evidence that modern high-flux dialyzers are effective in removing larger molecules such as vancomycin as well as those which are significantly protein-bound, such as carbamazepine and valproic acid.[56–62] Charcoal hemoperfusion has traditionally been promoted for use in theophylline, barbiturate, and carbamazepine overdose. However, several factors have caused this modality to fall out of favor: the declining frequency of barbiturates and theophylline overdose; complications of hemoperfusion such as thrombocytopenia; and evidence that modern high-flux hemodialysis equipment is equally effective.[63] Hemofiltration following an initial hemodialysis session may be effective for drugs such as lithium and valproic acid to prevent a rebound effect.[64–66]

A common concern is that hemodynamically unstable patients are unsuitable for dialysis due to fluid shifts exacerbating hypotension. However, hypotension related to hemodialysis is caused by removal of volume and urea resulting in fluid shifts. Unlike the chronic dialysis patient, the toxic patient does not have a large urea burden and volume loss is minimal. The benefit of removing the toxin responsible for hypotension outweighs the concern of hypotension exacerbated by dialysis. Drugs or toxins with a large volume of distribution, such as lithium, can be difficult to dialyze.

Toxins that are commonly considered amenable to dialysis include salicylate, lithium, theophylline, methanol, and ethylene glycol. Prior to initiating dialysis, it should be clear that there are no effective alternative therapies and that the patient is unlikely to recover fully with supportive care alone.

Thermal Regulation Drug-induced hyperthermia may be secondary to sympathomimetic or anticholinergic syndrome, serotonin syndrome, or neuroleptic malignant syndrome. Drug intoxication alone can produce clinically significant hyperthermia.[67] When extremes of environmental temperatures are present, drug-related thermal dysregulation can exacerbate morbidity and mortality.[68] It is essential that patients with altered mental status have a core temperature recorded early and be cooled rapidly if they are hyperthermic. The preferred method of cooling is evaporative with water mist and high-power fans. In the absence of this modality, ice baths and ice packs should be utilized. Conversely, patients with alcohol- or sedative-related toxidromes may become hypothermic. Temperature measurement and appropriate warming methods are equally important in these settings.

Toxicology Consultation and Referral

Early consultation with a toxicologist or poison control center is strongly encouraged. In cases of known poisoning, such resources can assist in refining the treatment course. Patients with undifferentiated altered mental status or suspected poisoning can benefit from the expertise of these resources, especially for unusual or severe cases. Referral to regional centers with capability for specialized care should be pursued early in the course of critically ill patients, such as those who may require dialysis, specific antidote therapy, hyperbaric oxygen treatment, or consideration for organ transplantation.

Pharmaceuticals Causing Cardiovascular Toxicity

Beta-Adrenergic Blocking Agents

Toxicology

The case mortality rate following beta-blocker overdose is much lower than that for calcium channel antagonists or digoxin; but in terms of absolute numbers, they are the second leading cause of death from cardiovascular medications.[69] Beta$_1$- and beta$_2$-receptor antagonism, intrinsic sympathomimetic activity, and membrane-stabilizing activity are responsible for the clinical effects of these drugs. Alpha-antagonist activity is seen only with labetalol.[70]

The pharmacologic and toxicologic effects of beta-blocking drugs are mediated through indirect modulation of calcium secondary to inhibited adrenergic activation.[71] Beta$_1$ antagonism causes decreased cardiac contractility and conduction. Beta$_2$ antagonism causes increased smooth muscle tone, which manifests as bronchospasm, increased peripheral vascular tone, and increased gut motility. Although many beta-blockers are beta$_1$-selective at therapeutic doses, these drugs have both beta$_1$ and beta$_2$ effects in overdose.

Intrinsic sympathomimetic properties of some beta-blockers causes agonist–antagonist activity, which may blunt the bradycardic response in some patients.[70,72] Drugs with intrinsic sympathomimetic activity include acebutolol, carteolol, oxprenolol, penbutolol, and pindolol. The membrane-stabilizing activity characteristic of some beta-blockers is a quinidine-like effect, resulting in inhibition of fast sodium channels, decreased contractility, and ventricular arrhythmias.[73] This effect is additive to the beta$_1$ toxic effects.

Review of cases in the literature suggests that beta-blockers with increased intrinsic sympathomimetic activity and decreased membrane stabilizing properties demonstrate less toxicity. Conversely, those with increased membrane stabilizing properties show greater toxicity.[73–75] In fact, ingestion of a beta-blocker with membrane-stabilizing activity is second only to coingestion of a second cardioactive drug in predicting cardiovascular morbidity.[76] Propranolol, a drug with significant membrane-stabilizing properties, may induce seizures in overdose.[77] Additional drugs with membrane-stabilizing properties include acebutolol, betaxolol, and oxprenolol and to a lesser degree labetalol, metoprolol, and pindolol.[78]

Sotalol is a beta-blocker that has class III antiarrhythmic properties, and lacks intrinsic sympathomimetic or membrane stabilizing properties.[79] In overdose, it can prolong the QT interval via inhibition of the delayed rectifier potassium current. This may result in ventricular arrhythmias including torsades de pointes. Each different beta-blocker may have only some of the described activities, and the clinical manifestations may vary.

The absorption, distribution, and elimination of beta-blockers vary with the preparation. Beta-blockers are available in both immediate- and extended-release preparations. As with all extended-release preparations, the onset of toxic effects may be delayed. Beta-blockers are rapidly absorbed, with 30% to 90% bioavailability. The elimination half-life varies from 2 to 24 hours, depending on the drug. In many cases, the half-life is significantly increased in overdose. Due to the rapid absorption of many beta-blockers, the onset of symptoms may be as soon as 30 minutes after ingestion, but it most commonly occurs within 1 to 2 hours.

The clinical presentation of acute beta-blocker overdose is suppression of the cardiovascular system. Deaths from beta-blocker toxicity are associated with bradydysrhythmias and asystole; ventricular arrhythmias are less common. Respiratory compromise during beta-blocker overdose can result from cardiogenic shock, decreased respiratory drive, or beta$_2$-antagonist effects. Beta$_2$ blockade causes bronchospasm and usually affects patients with previously diagnosed bronchospastic disease. Patients may present with noncardiogenic pulmonary edema, cardiogenic pulmonary edema, or exacerbation of asthma. Hypoglycemia has been reported and may occur secondary to beta$_2$-mediated decrease in glycogenolysis and gluconeogenesis; however, it is not common unless the case is complicated by comorbidities or coingestants.[80] Central nervous system depression may be caused by direct toxicity, hypoxia, hypoglycemia, or shock and may result in seizure.

Electrocardiographic manifestations of toxicity include sinus bradycardia and prolongation of the PR interval, second and third-degree atrioventricular (AV) blockade, and junctional and interventricular conduction delays.[74,81] The QRS interval may be prolonged with ingestions of beta-blockers with membrane-stabilizing effects. Again, sotalol is unique among these agents in prolonging the QT interval via potassium channel effects. Propranolol and sotalol have been associated with ventricular arrhythmias.[81]

Management

Beta-blockers attenuate adrenergic tone and cAMP-dependent protein kinase pathways, resulting in disruption of cellular calcium flux. The consequences may range from negligible to life-threatening. Standard ACLS resuscitation followed by decontamination and enhanced elimination techniques apply, but attention must quickly turn to focused therapy.

Glucagon is the agent of choice for symptomatic beta-blocker ingestions resulting in hypotension or bradycardia.[82,83] Glucagon binds to its own receptor site, triggering cAMP signaling pathways, resulting in L-type calcium channel activation. Thus, glucagon bypasses the cellular problem at the beta receptor.[84] An initial bolus of glucagon is administered IV at a dose of 3 to 5 mg over 1 minute. If symptoms recur, a repeat bolus is given. An infusion may be started following the bolus dose, with the effective bolus dose being infused per hour. The initial effect is seen within several minutes, and should persist for 10 to 15 minutes. The pharmacodynamics of glucagon differ significantly from those of other commonly used adrenergic agents. This may be explained by compartmentalization of specific phosphodiesterases with different G-coupled receptors (i.e., glucagon receptor–coupled G proteins versus beta receptor–coupled G proteins), such that the cAMP generated by each receptor type is regulated in a unique way.[85] Note that nausea and vomiting are common side effects of glucagons, particularly if administered rapidly.

Sodium bicarbonate has narrow applicability in the setting of beta-blocker toxicity. With toxicity due to drugs with membrane-stabilizing properties, blockade of fast sodium channels may prolong the QRS duration. Although there is a paucity of case reports and a lack of prospective data to support its use, sodium bicarbonate may be effective in select cases.[86] It should be considered with QRS durations >120 ms and a suspected ingestion of a beta-blocking drug.[87]

Adrenergic agents are often effective in increasing heart rate, contractility, and peripheral vascular resistance. In cases of severe cardiovascular drug toxicity, large doses may be required.[87] If the response to glucagon is inadequate, epinephrine and dopamine may improve both heart rate and blood pressure.[77] Norepinephrine is effective in situations with low systemic vascular resistance; however, with the myocardial depression seen with severe beta blockade, alternative agents may be more efficacious.[87]

Hyperinsulinemia–euglycemia (HIE) therapy is an essential component of moderate to severe calcium channel blocker toxicity. Evidence supporting its use is derived from animal studies and a growing list of case reports and case series. Data supporting its use in beta-blocker toxicity is more limited. HIE has proven effective in both swine and dog models of propranolol toxicity.[88,89] However, there is a paucity of human case reports demonstrating efficacy.[90] Despite these limitations, HIE might be considered early in the course of resuscitation for patients with depressed myocardial function secondary to beta blockade who are refractory to other therapies.[78,87] Adverse reactions are predictable and treatable; they include hypoglycemia, hypokalemia, and hypophosphatemia.

Bradycardia and hypotension refractory to pharmacologic intervention may benefit from temporary pacing through improvement in heart rate, although this intervention will not reverse the cardiac depression of severe beta-blocker overdose.[91,92] Interventions such as intra-aortic balloon pump, extracorporeal membrane oxygenation (ECMO), or cardiac bypass are considerations for patients with toxicity refractory to all other therapy.[92,93] Hemodialysis, hemofiltration, and hemoperfusion are rarely useful in the setting of beta-blocker overdose. Most of the beta-blockers have a large volume of distribution and are highly protein-bound, making drug removal by hemodialysis impractical. A few drugs, such as nadolol, sotalol, atenolol, and acebutolol, can be dialyzed; but information is limited to case reports.[93–95] Hemodialysis can be considered in the setting of renal failure and hemodynamic instability due to a drug with low volume of distribution and low protein binding.

A patient with a history of immediate-release beta-blocker ingestion is observed on a cardiac monitor for 6 hours after ingestion.[76,96] Patients who have signs of cardiovascular, respiratory, or central nervous system (CNS) toxicity are admitted to an intensive care setting. Patients with a history of ingestion of extended-release preparations or sotalol are admitted and monitored for 24 hours. A patient who ingested an immediate-release beta-blocker can be medically cleared after the 6-hour observation period if there are no signs of toxicity found by clinical examination, electrocardiography (ECG), or cardiac monitoring.

Calcium Channel Antagonists

Toxicology

Calcium channel antagonists account for more poisoning deaths than any other cardiovascular medication.[69] This broad class of drugs is further classified as the dihydropyridines, phenylalkylamines, and benzothiazepines. Dihydropyridines include nifedipine, isradipine, amlodipine, felodipine, nimodipine, nisoldipine, and nicardipine. Verapamil is the sole phenylalkylamine, and diltiazem is the only benzothiazepine available.

The majority of available calcium channel antagonists work at the L-type calcium channel.[97] These channels affect automaticity at the sinoatrial node, conduction through the AV node, excitation–contraction coupling in cardiac and smooth muscle, as well as pancreatic insulin secretion.[71]

Their clinical effects differ due to variations in binding location on the alpha$_1$-receptor subunit, preferential binding at different resting cell membrane potentials, and as a function of channel state (activated, inactivated, resting).[98–100] This receptor selectivity has clinical implications in that the dihydropyridines primarily result in vasodilation, whereas the nondihydropyridines have a more pronounced effect on cardiac conduction. Specifically, verapamil affects both the myocardium and the peripheral arterioles, causing decreased contractility, AV-node conduction, and peripheral vascular resistance. Diltiazem has less effect on peripheral vasodilatation and myocardial contractility than verapamil. Diltiazem slows AV-node conduction and causes coronary artery dilatation. Nifedipine, representative of the dihydropyridine class, has the greatest effect on peripheral vascular resistance, and also decreases contractility, with minimal effect on AV-node conduction. The unique properties of each drug define their therapeutic and toxic effects. However, in overdose, any of these drugs can cause peripheral vasodilatation, decreased AV conduction, and decreased myocardial contractility.

The various calcium channel blockers have slightly different pharmacokinetic properties. In general, bioavailability ranges from 20% to 85%, they undergo hepatic metabolism with extensive first-pass effect, are extensively protein bound, and with the exception of nifedipine, nimodipine, and nicardipine, have a large volume of distribution.[97,101] The onset of action is 30 minutes and the half-life varies from 3 to 7 hours, but it can be greatly increased in the setting of overdose. It is important to be aware that sustained-release preparations can have a delayed onset of life-threatening effects due to their prolonged absorption time.

The clinical effects of calcium channel blocker overdose can be life-threatening. Slowing of the sinus node causes bradycardia. Slowing of conduction can cause heart blocks or asystole. Decreased contractility can cause heart failure and shock. Lowered peripheral vascular resistance leads to hypotension, which may exacerbate the hypotension associated with bradycardia, bradyarrhythmias, and heart failure. Hyperglycemia occurs frequently with significant overdoses and may correlate with the severity of poisoning.[102] Patients with cardiac disease and those on other medications that suppress heart rate and contractility may develop severe toxic effects after mild overdose, or even at therapeutic doses. Neurologic and respiratory findings are usually secondary to cardiovascular toxicity and shock. Respiratory effects include decreased respiratory drive, pulmonary edema, and acute respiratory distress syndrome. Neurologic sequelae include depressed sensorium, cerebral infarction, and seizures. Nausea, vomiting, and constipation can occur. The most important GI consequence to recognize is a concretion of sustained-release capsules. In addition to causing bowel obstruction, the concretion can be a source of continued toxicity. Evacuation of sustained-release capsules from the GI tract may decrease morbidity and mortality if performed early in the clinical course.

Management

To effectively manage calcium channel antagonist overdose, it is essential to understand the location of the cellular lesion. Calcium flux is the central component regulating cardiac conduction and excitation–contraction coupling. The majority of interventions used to combat calcium channel aberrancies focus on modulation of cellular processes proximal to the lesion at the calcium channel. These interventions may reduce vagal tone, increase calcium concentrations, augment alpha- and beta-adrenergic tone, or increase cAMP via phosphodiesterase inhibition, all in an effort to enhance calcium channel function.[90,103–105] However, when the calcium channel is severely poisoned, these upstream interventions will be minimally effective at best. Early consideration of HIE therapy in the nonresponding patient is essential.

Of the standard antidotes, IV calcium salts are readily available and easy to use. Increasing the extracellular calcium concentration may increase flux of calcium into the cell, thereby increasing cardiac conduction and contractility. Calcium is recommended as a first-line agent, although human data are mixed and the effect is inadequate in more severe poisonings.[90,105–111] Two calcium salts are available: calcium gluconate and calcium chloride. Both of these are supplied in 10% solutions, but each contains a different quantity of calcium. Calcium chloride contains 1.3 mEq/mL of calcium and calcium gluconate contains 0.45 mEq/mL of calcium. The dose is repeated in 10 to 15 minutes for patients with persistent hypotension or bradycardia.

Calcium salts primarily reverse hypotension due to vasodilation and may have little or no effect on heart rate or conduction.

For patients with symptomatic bradycardia or heart block, atropine may be helpful. However, accompanying hypotension is often related to peripheral vasodilation and will not respond to an increase in heart rate. Conversely, in a patient with stable blood pressure despite bradycardia, atropine will be of little benefit.

As with calcium salts and atropine, a trial of glucagon is indicated early in the course of resuscitation. However, in contrast to beta-blocker poisoning, glucagon does not bypass the cellular lesion but simply triggers cAMP signaling pathways in an attempt to overcome L-type calcium channel inactivation. The end result is that glucagon is not as effective in calcium channel antagonist poisoning as it is with beta-blocker poisoning. When used, the initial bolus is 3 to 5 mg IV over 1 minute. Clinical improvement will be seen in several minutes if it is going to be effective and will persist for 10 to 15 minutes. If symptoms recur, a repeat bolus and infusion may be used. Nausea and vomiting are frequent side effects of glucagons with rapid administration.

Vasopressors should be utilized early for patients who do not respond quickly to simple interventions such as IV fluid, calcium, atropine, and glucagon. Ideally, a vasopressor would be selected to counteract myocardial depression, vasodilation, or both, as determined by the patient's hemodynamics. In a resuscitation scenario, this is challenging to do; and an agent with combined alpha and beta effects, such as dopamine or norepinephrine, is a more logical approach. More than one agent may be required.

HIE therapy is a novel approach to treating calcium channel antagonist overdose. The efficacy of HIE therapy is likely attributable to the metabolic effects of insulin. Animal models of calcium channel antagonist toxicity have demonstrated hyperglycemia, insulin resistance, blunted insulin secretion, impaired fatty acid utilization, and lactic acidosis.[112–114] A shift in cardiovascular metabolism to favor glucose utilization seems to accompany marked improvements in hemodynamics, systolic and diastolic myocardial performance, and survival time.[115] In humans, the evidence in support of HIE therapy is limited to case reports and case series.[90,116–121] Despite this limitation, given the striking efficacy that has been observed with HIE, it should be utilized early in the course of resuscitation for severe calcium channel antagonist overdose.[87,117,122]

The therapy guideline for HIE is 1 U/kg of insulin as an IV bolus followed by 0.5 U/kg/hr as an IV infusion, with upward titration every 30 minutes as required.[87] An IV dextrose bolus of 25 g followed by an infusion of 0.5 g/kg/hr should accompany the insulin infusion. If the patient is markedly hyperglycemic, the bolus may be omitted. Serial blood sugar determinations should be followed and the dextrose infusion adjusted accordingly. Potassium should be monitored and replaced to maintain serum potassium levels at 2.8 to 3.2 mEq/L.

Interventions such as intra-aortic balloon pump, extracorporeal membrane oxygenation (ECMO), or cardiac bypass are considerations for patients with toxicity refractory to all other therapy.[123–125] However, it should be noted that the case reports in which these measures were used occurred prior to the advent of HIE therapy. Hemodialysis, hemofiltration, and hemoperfusion are not reported for calcium channel blocker overdose. Most calcium channel antagonists have a large volume of distribution, are highly protein-bound, and are subject to hepatic metabolism, making them poor candidates for extracorporeal removal.

Patients who have signs of cardiovascular, respiratory, or CNS compromise are admitted to an intensive care unit (ICU). Patients with a history of sustained-release ingestion are observed with cardiac monitoring for at least 24 hours. Those patients with no signs of toxicity, no history of sustained-release ingestion, and no ECG abnormalities can be observed for 6 to 8 hours after the time of ingestion. If they do not develop any signs of toxicity or ECG abnormalities during this period, they may be medically cleared.

Digoxin

Toxicology

Digoxin functions as a positive inotrope, increasing the force and velocity of myocardial contraction. In the failing heart, it can increase cardiac output, reduce pulmonary capillary wedge pressure, and decrease elevated ventricular end-diastolic pressures.[126] As with many cardiovascular medications, this effect is mediated through changes in intracellular calcium.[127]

Digoxin inhibits the Na/K/ATPase, resulting in increased intracellular sodium, which in turn inhibits calcium efflux through the Na/Ca exchanger.[128] Elevated intracellular calcium concentration resulting from supratherapeutic digoxin levels is likely responsible for the toxic effects.[129] This may lead to dysrhythmias and a decrease in conduction through the sinoatrial and AV nodes.[130] In addition, digoxin may augment parasympathetic stimulation, compounding the effect on sinoatrial and AV conduction.[131,132] There is evidence for a sympathoinhibitory effect in patients with heart failure, and a sympathoexcitatory effect in normal controls.[133]

Potassium balance is a critical component of digoxin toxicity. In chronic toxicity, hypokalemia increases the probability of digoxin binding to the Na/K/ATPase secondary to phosphorylation and resultant conformational changes, thus exacerbating toxic effects at a given digoxin level. Severe hypokalemia (2.5 mEq/L) compounds the effect by inhibiting ion flux.[128,134] In acute digoxin toxicity, the effects on the Na/K/ATPase predominate, with hyperkalemia resulting from inhibition of potassium influx.[135] Hypomagnesemia, hypercalcemia, and hypothyroidism may exacerbate these effects.[136]

The onset of action of digoxin is within 30 minutes for IV formulations, with the peak effect seen in 1.5 to 5 hours and a half-life of 36 to 48 hours.[137] It is primarily renally excreted, with limited gut metabolism. It is 23% protein-bound and has a large volume of distribution.[101]

Risk factors for digoxin toxicity vary based on age. Children are at risk from accidental ingestion, and dosing errors may occur when digoxin is taken therapeutically. The majority of adult patients will suffer toxicity related to an intentional ingestion.[138] The elderly are at risk for chronic toxicity due to age-related alterations in pharmacokinetics, drug interactions, and comorbidities. Specifically, age-related declines in volume of distribution, renal insufficiency, hypoalbuminemia, and diuretic-related hypokalemia may result in digoxin toxicity.[139]

The clinical signs and symptoms of chronic digoxin toxicity may be very subtle. Fatigue, anorexia, nausea, and vomiting are the most common presenting symptoms, followed by dizziness, visual disturbances, abdominal pain, and diarrhea.[140,141] Initial symptoms of an acute ingestion are typically nausea, vomiting, abdominal pain, weakness, confusion, and lethargy. Bradycardia, hyperkalemia, and vomiting are most predictive of significant ingestion in patients with acute digoxin intoxication.

It is important for the clinician to distinguish between the acute and chronic forms of toxicity. Acute toxicity generally responds well to therapy, while chronic toxicity is more refractory to treatment. The key is for the clinician to have a high index of suspicion. Chronic toxicity should be suspected in those patients presenting with vague, nonspecific symptoms who are taking or potentially taking digoxin. Malaise, headache, fatigue, and mild GI symptoms are subtle presenting symptoms commonly associated with digoxin toxicity.

Cardiovascular manifestations are the most important factor in determining morbidity and mortality. Symptoms include palpitations and dizziness, usually secondary to hypotension. A multitude of cardiac conduction aberrancies are commonly described. Ventricular ectopy and various AV blocks may be seen.[140–142] Although no rhythm is pathognomonic, additional rhythms that have been observed include junctional rhythms, sinus bradycardia, sinus pause, atrial fibrillation, paroxysmal atrial tachycardia, ventricular tachycardia, and ventricular fibrillation. The often cited pathognomonic bidirectional ventricular tachycardia has also been reported with aconite poisoning.[143]

Therapeutic digoxin levels are between 0.5 and 2 ng/mL. Levels are obtained upon admission and again at 6 hours after ingestion to account for full distribution of the drug. Serum digoxin concentrations obtained between 6 to 12 hours postingestion usually correlate with the clinical course of intoxication. However, even when distribution and acute versus chronic intoxication is accounted for, it is difficult to predict who will benefit from antidotal therapy solely based on a single serum digoxin level.[144] Given this difficulty, digoxin levels should be obtained for all patients who are or may be taking digoxin. The diagnosis of digoxin toxicity is considered if the serum level is >2 ng/mL in conjunction with clinical signs of toxicity. In the acute setting, the patient will have more dramatic clinical and laboratory findings than in the chronic setting. Patients with chronic toxicity will be more symptomatic, with lower corresponding digoxin serum levels. Key prognostic factors indicating increased risk for death are age >55, atrioventricular block, and potassium >4.5 mEq/L.[145]

Management

Patients with possible digoxin toxicity should be managed aggressively owing to the potential for morbidity and mortality.[144] All patients should have IV access, frequent assessment of vital signs, and continuous cardiac monitoring. If the patient's mental status is adequate, activated charcoal can be administered as a single dose. Multiple doses of charcoal have been reported to be of value for digitoxin or digoxin preparations and may be useful if antidotal therapy is not available.[146,147]

Digoxin immune Fab fragments are specific antidigoxin antibodies raised in sheep. Only the Fab fragment is used in order to decrease the risk of immunogenicity. This antidote has been used successfully in adults since the 1970s. Administration of the Fab fragments is indicated in cases of severe digitalis intoxication that is suspected by history, by a high level, or in those manifesting significant signs and symptoms of toxicity. Specific indications are based on absolute level, amount ingested, potassium level, and symptoms, as generated from case series and observational studies.[148–153] In general, those with potentially life-threatening dysrhythmias, significant GI symptoms, altered mental status, or a potassium >5 mEq/L in the setting of elevated digoxin levels are candidates for antidote administration. Markedly elevated 6-hour levels even in the absence of symptoms should also prompt consideration of antidotal therapy.

Most patients who respond to Fab fragment therapy do so within 1 hour and have a complete response by 4 hours.[149] Similarly, the effect on potassium concentration is delayed, which prompts the need for standard interventions for hyperkalemia in addition to Fab fragments. Glucose, insulin, and bicarbonate are appropriate. Calcium salts should be avoided because of the risk of exacerbating cardiotoxicity and precipitating cardiac arrest, although this risk has recently been disputed.[154,155]

Dosage of Fab fragments is based either on the acute ingestion of a known amount or on the steady-state serum concentration. Guidelines are available in the package insert or at http://us.gsk.com/products/assets/us_digibind.pdf. *It is important to note that following treatment with Fab total digoxin levels will be markedly elevated. Free digoxin levels may be obtained that will correlate with the amount of drug that is biologically active.*

Fab fragments are the cornerstone of therapy for the digoxin-toxic patient. However, the time to onset of Fab fragments mandates use of adjunctive therapies in the unstable patient. Atropine is appropriate for symptomatic bradycardia. The class Ib antiarrhythmics phenytoin and lidocaine may be effective. Phenytoin was first proposed as therapy for digoxin toxicity in the 1950s and was widely used until the advent of Fab fragments.[156,157] Both suppress ventricular automaticity without affecting conduction, and phenytoin improves AV conduction.[158]

Hypokalemia should be corrected with careful attention to avoiding overcorrection. Magnesium therapy has been reported as efficacious in refractory ventricular arrhythmias.[159,160] It should be repleted in deficient states, as hypomagnesemia may lead to refractory hypokalemia; but care should be taken in cases of renal insufficiency to avoid toxicity.

Cardiac pacing has not been shown to decrease mortality when compared with maximal medical therapy that includes Fab fragments, and it carries a high rate of complications.[152,161] Cardiac pacing should only be used as a therapy once other interventions have proven futile or are not available. Hemodialysis, hemofiltration, and hemoperfusion do not aid in the management of digoxin toxicity.

Patients who are asymptomatic, without dysrhythmias, or with minor ingestions or undetectable to therapeutic levels 6 hours after ingestion may be medically cleared. Any patient that has signs and symptoms of digoxin toxicity should be admitted to a monitored bed. All patients with significant signs and symptoms and in whom the use of Fab fragments is being considered should be admitted to an ICU. Consultation with the poison control center, toxicologist, or cardiologist familiar with the treatment of these cases is recommended.

Plants Containing Cardiac Glycosides

Foxglove (*Digitalis purpurea*), lily of the valley (*Convallaria majalis*), common oleander (*Nerium oleander*), and yellow oleander (*Thevetia peruviana*) all contain digitalis-like glycosides. Ingestion of yellow oleander results in the most significant degree of toxicity. Of all varieties of oleander, yellow oleander has been responsible for the greatest number of fatal poisonings worldwide. All parts of the plant contain several cardiac glycosides and can produce a syndrome similar to digoxin poisoning when ingested.

The patient may manifest abdominal pain, nausea, vomiting, and diarrhea as well as weakness, bradycardia, and AV block. Because some of the plant glycosides are structurally similar but not identical to digoxin, a serum digoxin level may not be accurate.

Treatment with digoxin immune Fab fragments is safe and effective for toxicity caused by yellow oleander.[162] The exact dose required is unknown, but a recent randomized controlled trial suggests that much higher doses may be needed than those used to treat digoxin overdose.[162] As with many modern therapeutic agents, a lack of availability in the developing world has resulted in increased morbidity from this treatable illness.[163] Fortunately, as an alternative, multiple-dose activated charcoal can be efficacious in this setting.[164]

Anticholinergic Agents

Toxicology

Acetylcholine is the neurotransmitter involved in the activation of both nicotinic and muscarinic cholinergic receptors. Nicotinic receptors are ligand-gated sodium and calcium channels. Muscarinic receptors are G protein–coupled.[165] Three of these muscarinic receptors are stimulatory, increasing cAMP and intracellular calcium; two are inhibitory, reducing cAMP and intracellular calcium.

The anticholinergic toxidrome results from competitive inhibition of acetylcholine at muscarinic receptors. Muscarinic receptors are found throughout the CNS and in sympathetic and parasympathetic ganglia. This toxidrome is quite common and may result from both pharmaceutical preparations and various plant species.

Anticholinergic or antimuscarinic toxicity may be divided into central and peripheral effects. Central effects include alteration in mental status including delirium, hallucinations, agitation, and seizures. Peripheral effects include mydriasis, tachycardia, flushing, dry skin and mucous membranes, urinary retention, and decreased GI motility.

The onset of anticholinergic toxicity varies depending on the particular toxin but usually occurs within several hours. Although central and peripheral anticholinergic effects are commonly seen simultaneously, the central effects may occasionally persist after the peripheral effects have resolved. An often-used mnemonic to remember the clinical manifestations of anticholinergic toxicity is "Hot as a hare, Blind as a bat, Dry as a bone, Red as a beet, Mad as a hatter."

The more significant components of anticholinergic toxicity is blockade of muscarinic receptors in the brain. The excessive CNS excitation that results clinically manifests as agitation, anxiety, delirium, lethargy, drowsiness, coma, and occasionally seizures. Peripheral blockade of muscarinic receptors also leads to cardiovascular effects such as tachycardia from antagonism of vagal tone, mydriasis with the inability to accommodate, decreased activity of sweat glands, hyperthermia, urinary retention, and reduced gut motility.

Drugs that may cause anticholinergic symptoms include antihistamines, antipsychotics, tricyclic antidepressants, and atropine. The antihistamine diphenhydramine is a common cause. In addition to its anticholinergic properties, it has type IA antidysrhythmic effects. A prolonged QRS interval with a subsequent prolonged QT may result, and severe cardiac dysrhythmias can occur.[166–168] Cases of torsades de pointes have also been reported.[169] Tricyclic antidepressants, which are discussed in a later section, behave similarly, although their cardiotoxic effects are more severe.

Serum drug concentrations are neither readily available nor helpful in the clinical setting. In overdoses, a screening acetaminophen level is indicated because products containing a combination of acetaminophen and antihistamine are common. Patients with severe psychomotor agitation and seizures should have a serum creatine kinase assessed because of the possibility of rhabdomyolysis. Patients who ingest the antihistamine doxylamine are particularly at risk for rhabdomyolysis.[170–172] Injury is likely due to direct drug injury to striated muscle.[173] Although most anticholinergic toxicity will result from ingestion, systemic anticholinergic toxicity has been reported from cutaneous absorption and from ocular exposure.[174,175]

Management

In most cases of anticholinergic toxicity, supportive care (i.e., benzodiazepines to treat agitation or seizures; cooling for hyperthermia) will be adequate therapy. Activated charcoal should be considered. Other associated complications, such as rhabdomyolysis from doxylamine, are also treated supportively with good outcome. However, cases of doxylamine-related renal failure requiring hemodialysis are reported.[173] Wide-complex cardiac dysrhythmias from severe diphenhydramine toxicity should be treated with boluses (1–2 mEq/kg) of IV sodium bicarbonate to reverse the sodium channel effects.[168,176,177]

For patients demonstrating profound central anticholinergic toxicity (delirium, hallucinations, tachydysrhythmias, or seizures) unresponsive to traditional doses of benzodiazepines, physostigmine may be used as antidotal therapy. Physostigmine is an anticholinesterase agent that antagonizes the effects of anticholinergic agents. It is sufficiently lipophilic to cross the blood–brain barrier and can counteract both peripheral and central effects. The onset of action is within several minutes, and the half-life of the drug is approximately 15 minutes. For agents that have a prolonged anticholinergic effect on the CNS, such as scopolamine, redosing may be necessary. Physostigmine has demonstrated efficacy for severe anticholinergic syndromes and has proven to be more effective than benzodiazepines.[178–181]

Physostigmine was a first-line agent for anticholinergic poisoning in the 1970s, even in cases of cyclic antidepressant ingestions.[182] In 1980, Pentel and Peterson published two cases of asystolic cardiac arrest following physostigmine use in the setting of tricyclic overdose; as a result, it became a rarely used drug.[183] Currently, physostigmine is considered appropriate therapy only in patients with anticholinergic syndromes who meet strict criteria: normal QRS and QTc intervals, clear historical evidence that tricyclic antidepressants have not been ingested, and absence of mechanical bowel and/or urogenital tract obstruction. Relative contraindications are reactive airways disease, seizure, cardiac conduction abnormalities, and peripheral vascular disease.[184]

Adverse effects of physostigmine include cholinergic crisis with increased bronchial secretions, bradycardia, and seizures. Although seizures have been reported with physostigmine, they are also a complication of severe anticholinergic syndrome. The association between physostigmine, tricyclic antidepressants, and seizures is well reported in the literature.[185–187] Controversy often results, as this is one of the CNS manifestations that physostigmine may resolve. Seizures occur more commonly in patients with QRS durations >100 ms, which may indicate more significant intoxication.[187] Rapid administration of physostigmine may induce seizure; therefore, it is imperative to use small doses, titrating upward to desired effect.[188] The patient should be closely monitored and the practitioner should be prepared for cholinergic toxicity with oral and laryngeal suction, endotracheal intubation, and atropine, as needed.

Patients who have significant anticholinergic toxicity and those treated with physostigmine should be admitted to an intensive care setting. Patients exposed to anticholinergic agents with additional toxicity (e.g., tricyclic antidepressants, phenothiazines) should also be closely observed for a minimum of 6 hours regardless of resolution of symptoms. Those with minimal anticholinergic toxicity from an ingestion without additional toxicity can be observed in the emergency department until symptoms resolve. Once symptoms resolve, they may be medically cleared.

Tricyclic Antidepressants

Toxicology

Antidepressants continue to represent a large portion of poison center referrals and poisoning fatalities in the United States. Historically, tricyclic antidepressants (TCAs) were the leading cause of poisoning fatalities. Owing to their superior efficacy, lower adverse-effects profile, and a reduced incidence of serious toxicity, selective serotonin reuptake inhibitors (SSRIs) and atypical antidepressants are currently prescribed more frequently than TCAs.

TCAs have a small therapeutic index, such that 10 to 20 mg/kg of most TCAs will cause significant toxicity. In infants or toddlers, this correlates to only one or two 100-mg tablets. Life-threatening exposures in adults are associated with ingestions >1,000 mg. TCAs are rapidly and easily absorbed in the intestine, although in overdose the anticholinergic effects may decrease gut motility, resulting in delayed absorption with prolonged or cyclic symptoms. TCAs and their metabolites are highly lipophilic and extensively protein-bound. Despite this, they have a large volume of distribution, resulting in a high tissue-to-plasma ratio.

In overdose, TCAs affect the cardiovascular system, the autonomic nervous system, and the CNS. This manifests as cardiac conduction delays, dysrhythmias, hypotension, altered mental status, and seizures. There are four main mechanisms by which TCAs manifest their toxic effects. Inhibition of norepinephrine and serotonin reuptake occurs at central presynaptic terminals and may result in early tachycardia and hypertension.[189] Peripheral and central antagonism of muscarinic acetylcholine receptors results in anticholinergic symptoms and tachycardia.[190] Sodium channel blockade causes a quinidine-like effect, prolonging the QRS interval, provoking atrial and ventricular arrhythmias, and perhaps ultimately resulting in bradycardia and hypotension.[191–193] Antagonism of peripheral alpha$_1$-adrenergic receptors may also cause hypotension.[189] TCAs can also prolong the QT interval due to potassium channel effects, and cases of torsades de pointes have been reported.[194–196] Altered mental status and CNS depression are due to central anticholinergic effects, but the pathophysiology of lowered seizure threshold is not fully understood. Possible explanations include an increased level of monoamines, antidopaminergic properties, inhibition of neuronal sodium channels, or interaction with CNS GABA receptors.

Clinical presentations consistent with TCA poisoning include lethargy, coma, seizures, cardiac dysrhythmias, and conduction delays. Clinical deterioration can be sudden and unpredictable, but patients with significant ingestions will typically demonstrate symptoms within 6 hours of presentation.[197,198]

Cardiovascular toxicity manifests as tachycardia, bradycardia, conduction delays, dysrhythmias, and hypotension. With the exception of sinus tachycardia and infrequent preventricular contractions (PVCs), ECG abnormalities are often associated with neurologic dysfunction.[199] QRS prolongation is a marker for serious toxicity, although absence of this finding does not rule it out.[200–202] In comparison to QRS prolongation, an R wave in AVR measuring >3 mm may be a more sensitive marker.[203–205] Physiologic consequences of tricyclic antidepressant overdose are dynamic, and the accompanying ECG changes may not manifest early in the clinical course. Therefore, serial ECGs and continuous cardiac monitoring are essential in the first 6 to 8 hours.[206]

CNS toxicity manifests as altered mental status, agitation, coma, and seizures. Seizures are more common in patients with ECG abnormalities.[187] They are usually generalized, brief, and tend to occur within the first few hours after presentation.[197,198] Other anticholinergic effects that are frequently seen are urinary retention, dry flushed skin, dry mouth, dilated pupils, and hyperthermia. Compared with the classic tricyclic antidepressants, the atypical agents amoxapine and maprotiline are associated with a higher incidence of seizures, but the argument that they have less cardiovascular toxicity is not supported in the literature.[187,196,207]

Management

Aggressive supportive care, GI decontamination when appropriate, and close observation are essential to the management of patients with TCA overdose. There is no role for enhanced elimination with hemodialysis, hemofiltration, or hemoperfusion because of the high volume of distribution and extensive protein binding of these agents.[101] Physostigmine should be avoided for reasons outlined in the prior section on anticholinergic toxicity.

Cardiovascular toxicity is treated with sodium bicarbonate, administered by IV bolus, as a first-line agent. The beneficial effects of sodium bicarbonate are clear, as indicated by numerous case reports and case series, although there are no randomized controlled trials.[208] Alkalinization has been shown to decrease heart rate, narrow QRS intervals, and increase blood pressure.[209,210] Sodium bicarbonate bolus has been demonstrated to reverse TCA-induced ventricular tachycardia despite preexisting alkalosis.[211] The exact mechanism is unclear, but is likely related to both sodium loading and reversal of acidosis. The exact QRS interval at which to initiate sodium bicarbonate therapy is debated, with both >100 ms being documented. Other indications for sodium bicarbonate include hypotension and compromising dysrhythmias. There is no evidence for prophylactic sodium bicarbonate use or with regard to utilizing a bicarbonate infusion following the bolus. However, acidosis should be avoided and the pH should be maintained below 7.55. Repeat boluses should be administered for recurrence of symptoms or ECG abnormalities. Hypotension is treated by volume expansion with isotonic saline. Vasopressors are utilized in cases refractory to volume expansion. Dopamine may be effective; however, owing to the depletion of endogenous norepinephrine seen in TCA overdose, norepinephrine infusion is preferred.[212] It offers the advantages of beta agonism for myocardial depression and alpha agonism for vasoconstriction.

Refractory dysrhythmias or hypotension despite alkalinization require additional therapy. Lidocaine, a class Ib antiarrhythmic, is considered second-line therapy for ventricular dysrhythmias in TCA poisoning; however, its use is poorly supported by the literature.[193] Lidocaine was found to be ineffective in a rat model of amitriptyline toxicity and transiently effective in a canine model; however, it also resulted in hypotension.[213,214]

Lidocaine has minimal effects on phase 0 of the action potential, which is likely the reason adverse effects have not been reported. Likewise, concerns that its sodium channel–blocking properties may be deleterious are not supported by the literature. Class Ia and Ic antiarrhythmics are contraindicated due to blockade of fast sodium channels. Class III antiarrhythmics have potassium channel–blocking effects and are, therefore, contraindicated owing to risk of prolonging the QT interval. Phenytoin, another class Ib antiarrhythmic and antiepileptic, has been considered as an agent to reverse TCA-induced dysrhythmias. It was generally ineffective in rabbits and found to be proarrhythmic in dogs.[215,216] Therefore, the use of phenytoin cannot be recommended.

There are conflicting animal data regarding the efficacy of magnesium sulfate for TCA toxicity.[213,217,218] Despite this, there are three case reports demonstrating efficacy in persistent ventricular dysrhythmias. Amitriptyline ingestions in two pediatric patients resulted in ventricular tachycardia that was refractory to standard measures. Following magnesium sulfate infusions, the patients converted to sinus rhythm.[219,220] Amitriptyline ingestion in an adult patient caused ventricular fibrillation refractory to standard measures. The patient converted to "stable regular heart rhythm" after magnesium sulfate infusion followed by "electroconversion" therapy.[221]

Seizures are usually brief and self-limited, but prolonged seizures can lead to acidosis, hyperthermia, rhabdomyolysis, and hypoxia, all of which can exacerbate cardiovascular toxicity. Benzodiazepines are first-line treatment, followed by barbiturates or propofol.[222] Phenytoin should be avoided out of concern for arrhythmogenicity and because it is generally ineffective for toxin-induced seizures.[216]

Patients who at presentation have signs of major toxicity, such as seizures, coma, dysrhythmia, hypotension, respiratory depression, or a QRS interval >100 ms, require admission to a monitored setting. Patients who have received appropriate GI decontamination, have no signs of major toxicity, have a QRS interval <100 ms, and are observed for 6 hours without change in clinical course or serial ECGs are unlikely to manifest symptoms.[197,198] These patients may be medically cleared.

Serotonin-Specific Reuptake Inhibitors and Atypical Antidepressants

Toxicology

The pharmacologic mechanism of SSRI medications, as the name suggests, is to inhibit serotonin reuptake. In overdose, the typical clinical manifestations are nausea, vomiting, sedation, and tachycardia; but QT prolongation and seizures also have been reported. SSRIs are better tolerated in overdose than tricyclic antidepressants and have far less cardiotoxicity.[223] In direct comparison to venlafaxine and tricyclic antidepressants, SSRIs were found to be less epileptogenic and cardiotoxic but to result in more serotonin toxicity.[224] This, however, did not translate into less ICU time or mortality. The more significant symptoms of QT prolongation and seizure are most often related to ingestions of citalopram and escitalopram.[225,226]

Citalopram is a racemic formulation of inactive R and active S enantiomers, whereas escitalopram contains solely the S enantiomer.[227] The R and S enantiomers undergo hepatic metabolism to their respective desmethylcitalopram products.[228] Desmethylcitalopram retains some of the pharmacologic activity of the parent compound. It also has affinity for alpha-adrenergic, dopamine, histamine, and muscarinic receptors.[229] This may explain the antimuscarinic effects that can be seen with citalopram in overdose. Desmethylcitalopram is further metabolized to didesmethylcitalopram, which may be responsible for the cardiotoxic effects of the drug.[230,231] However, this contention is based on limited animal work and remains controversial.[232]

Regardless of mechanism, QT prolongation related to citalopram overdose has been demonstrated in two case series.[225,233] These studies also showed an association with seizures in overdose. One case series documented an increased frequency of QRS prolongation and seizure with ingestions of >600 mg in comparison with smaller ingestions.[234] In this report, QT prolongation was not commented on. Additional publications of citalopram ingestions document delayed seizure, delayed QT prolongation, and torsades de pointes.[226,231,235–237]

Atypical antidepressants are neither tricyclics, MAOIs, or SSRIs; however, they tend to be derivatives of the SSRI class. They include mirtazapine, bupropion, venlafaxine, duloxetine, and trazodone. With the exception of mirtazapine, they have significantly more toxicity in overdose than the SSRIs, although they are less toxic than tricyclics.[238]

Bupropion is a unicyclic antidepressant that inhibits dopamine uptake, with a less significant effect on reuptake of serotonin and norepinephrine. Patients may exhibit tachycardia, hypertension, nausea, vomiting, drowsiness, and agitation. Seizure is common, occurring in over 10% of cases in one series.[239] Although rare, cardiotoxicity with prolonged QT, QRS, cardiogenic shock, and cardiac arrest has been reported with larger ingestions.[240–242]

Venlafaxine and duloxetine both block serotonin and norepinephrine reuptake and can be expected to have similar effects in overdose, although duloxetine is a more effective reuptake inhibitor.[243] An analysis of 235 consecutive venlafaxine overdoses demonstrated a significant occurrence of sympathomimetic syndrome, QTc prolongation, seizure, and rhabdomyolysis.[244,245] Venlafaxine has been shown to be more epileptogenic than tricyclics, to prolong the QRS in comparison to SSRIs, and to result in serotonin toxicity.[224]

Trazodone is an antidepressant with anxiolytic and hypnotic properties. It inhibits serotonin reuptake but differs from other atypical antidepressants by having antagonist activity at the 5-HT2A postsynaptic serotonin receptor. It has a high therapeutic index, being associated with few deaths as reported in the literature.[246] Sedation and ortho-static hypotension are the main findings in overdose.[247] Seizures are rare and where reported are related to marked hyponatremia.[248] There are several reports of QT prolongation; however, they are likely related to coingestants.[249–251]

Mirtazapine is a relatively new agent that increases neuronal serotonin and norepinephrine through inhibition of presynaptic alpha$_2$-adrenergic receptors and postsynaptic serotonin receptors. It appears to have less toxicity in overdose than other atypical antidepressants.[225] A retrospective review of 153 mirtazapine overdoses demonstrated mild clinical symptoms and no significant cardiotoxicity other than tachycardia.[252] Altered mental status and CNS depression may be effects of mirtazapine overdose; however, it is difficult to distinguish a true effect from that of coingestant based on the available literature. There are no documented cases of significant cardiotoxicity.

Management

The clinical presentation of an acute SSRI overdose with the most commonly used agents is that of nausea, vomiting, dizziness, blurred vision, CNS depression, tremor, sinus tachycardia, and mydriasis. Serotonin syndrome only rarely follows isolated SSRI overdose but should be monitored for closely in the symptomatic patient. SSRI poisoning should be suspected in any patient with lethargy, coma or seizures, and no significant cardiotoxicity.

No readily available laboratory tests or clinical parameters identify and predict the course of SSRI and atypical antidepressant exposures. A decision tool has been developed to assist in management of citalopram-related QT prolongation, but it has not been adequately validated and its clinical utility is undetermined.[233] Qualitative and quantitative testing will not help in the acute setting. An early ECG is essential owing to the risk of coingested medicines and to evaluate for QT prolongation, but sinus tachycardia is often the only ECG finding. SSRIs and atypical antidepressants rarely manifest the severe toxicity common with tricyclics.

Treatment includes appropriate use of activated charcoal, supportive care, and close observation. Charcoal may be effective in reducing citalopram-related QT prolongation.[253] In cases of serotonin syndrome, aggressive cooling and benzodiazepines are essential, and cyproheptadine may be effective. There is no role for extracorporeal therapies. Seizures, hypotension, and conduction disturbances can be managed as for TCA overdose and are guided by ECG findings. Cases with prolonged QT intervals should prompt optimization of potassium, magnesium, and calcium levels. In the case of torsades de pointes, a 2- to 5-g IV magnesium bolus is indicated. Intralipid infusion has been utilized in a case of severe bupropion and lamotrigine overdose refractory to standard measures.[254] Serotonin syndrome should be treated with cessation of the offending agent, supportive care, and measures to decrease muscle rigidity and control hyperthermia.

No disposition algorithm for SSRI and atypical antidepressant exposure has been studied or established. In general, admission is not required in the absence of symptoms or an abnormal ECG after an adequate observation period extending through the peak absorption and distribution period. Exceptions to this rule are in the case of citalopram, escitalopram, bupropion, venlafaxine, duloxetine, or extended-release preparations, where admission is warranted because of the potential for delayed onset of QT prolongation or seizure.

Antipsychotics

Toxicology

Antipsychotic drugs are effective and widely utilized. It is convenient to classify them as either typical or atypical agents. Typical agents are useful in ameliorating positive symptoms such as aggression, hallucinations, delusions, and paranoia. Atypical agents have the additional benefit of combating such negative symptoms as social withdrawal and flat affect.

In overdose, antipsychotics may cause CNS depression, antimuscarinic symptoms, acute dystonia, akathisia, and hypotension mediated through alpha$_1$-adrenergic blockade. Lower-potency drugs such as thioridazine and chlorpromazine result in more sedation and cardiotoxic effects.[255,256] Seizures may occur, are dose-dependent, and occur more commonly with clozapine and chlorpromazine.[257] Cardiotoxicity with QRS prolongation is discussed for typical agents, although there is limited support for this effect. QT prolongation is more common with typical antipsychotics; however, a significant effect is also seen with ziprasidone. Neuroleptic malignant syndrome, while rare, is life-threatening. Symptoms consistent with this syndrome are altered mental status, hyperthermia, autonomic instability, and "lead pipe" rigidity.[258]

The cardiotoxicity of antipsychotics is related to their effect on fast sodium channels and delayed rectifier potassium channels. In psychiatric patients on therapeutic doses of antipsychotics, thioridazine—followed by ziprasidone, haloperidol, quetiapine, and risperidone—was found to have the greatest effect on QT prolongation.[259] The effect on QT prolongation may be exacerbated by concurrent therapy with antidepressants, other drugs known to prolong the QT interval, inhibitors of select p450 enzymes, hypokalemia, hypomagnesemia, hypocalcemia, female gender, and comorbid disease.[260–262]

Prolonged QT intervals may trigger torsades de pointes. Blockade of the delayed rectifier potassium channel shifts phase 3 of the cardiac action potential, delaying recovery of phase 4, and creating a circumstance where a premature action potential could result in this dysrhythmia.[263] There are numerous case reports of torsades de points related to the use of antipsychotic medications.[264–268] Many are complicated by coingestants or comorbidities, making a clear causal relationship difficult to establish. However, this fact reinforces the importance of concurrent risk factors as a cause of this malignant rhythm.

Typical antipsychotics have effects on fast sodium channels, which manifest as prolongation of the QRS interval. *In vitro* work has shown the ability of haloperidol to block sodium channels in guinea pig myocytes.[269] A retrospective study demonstrated increased risk of prolonged QT duration, QRS duration, and ventricular arrhythmias with thioridazine overdose.[255] Case reports identify instances of wide-complex arrhythmias related to mesoridazine and risperidone; however, there are also cases related to ziprasidone/bupropion and meperidine/promethazine/chlorpromazine combinations in overdose.[270–274] Asystolic cardiac arrest has been reported with haloperidol.[275,276]

Management

Aggressive supportive care, GI decontamination where appropriate, and close observation are indicated. Patients with underlying depression, bipolar disease, or schizophrenia are often on multiple psychotropic medications, so attention to possible coingestants is essential. There is no role for enhanced elimination with hemodialysis, hemofiltration, or hemoperfusion.

Antipsychotic cardiovascular toxicity is treated as it is for SSRIs and TCAs. Following initial resuscitation, an ECG should be obtained early in the clinical course to guide therapy. IV magnesium, sodium bicarbonate, or both may be indicated in addition to standard ACLS interventions. Hypotension is managed with crystalloid infusion, and vasopressors are utilized if the hypotension is refractory. Agents with direct alpha effects, such as norepinephrine, are preferred over dopamine. As with SSRIs and tricyclics, seizures are usually brief and self-limited but may require intervention to avoid exacerbating cardiovascular toxicity. Benzodiazepines constitute the first-line treatment, followed by barbiturates or diprivan.[222] Phenytoin should be avoided out of concern for arrhythmogenicity and because it is generally ineffective for toxin-induced seizures.[216]

Patients with signs of major toxicity, such as seizures, coma, dysrhythmia, hypotension, respiratory depression, or ECG abnormalities, require admission to a monitored setting. Patients who have received appropriate GI decontamination, have no signs of major toxicity, have a normal ECG, and are observed beyond the peak absorption and distribution times of the ingested drug are unlikely to develop symptoms. These patients may be medically cleared.

Drugs of Abuse Commonly Causing Toxicity in Overdose

Amphetamines and Amphetamine Derivatives

Toxicology

In 2005, there were 10,921 exposures to amphetamine and 3,456 exposures to methamphetamine reported to poison conrol centers nationwide.[69] These resulted in 16 and 37 deaths, respectively. In 2004, some 1.4 million people reported methamphetamine use in the preceding year, and 583,000 reported use within the prior month. These statistics make methamphetamine the most abused amphetamine in the United States.[277]

Methamphetamine is also known as "speed," "meth," "chalk," "crystal," "crank," and "ice." The ice preparation is precipitated in a purified crystalline form that is less likely to be adulterated. It can be smoked, injected, or nasally insufflated. Effects persist up to 24 hours. Auditory hallucinations, paranoid reactions, delirium, and violent behavior are reported to be more frequent with ice than with other forms of amphetamine.

The pharmacologic properties of amphetamines parallel those of endogenous catecholamines. However, depending on substitution, amphetamines may be sympathomimetic, anorectic, or hallucinogenic. Pharmacologic activity is classically described as being indirect and occurring by three distinct mechanisms: triggering neurotransmitter release at the cell membrane by exchange diffusion, diffusing across the cell membrane and interacting with the neurotransmitter storage vesicle membrane, and diffusing through the cell and vesicle membrane and inducing neurotransmitter release via alkalinization.[278] Abuse of the substituted varieties of amphetamine is a significant problem, as these drugs can cause both neurotoxicity and cardiotoxicity that may not be reversible.[279–281]

Methamphetamine is a substituted amphetamine that has numerous central and peripheral effects resulting in mood elevation, psychomotor activation, and with chronic use or overdose, psychotic and violent behavior. The cardiovascular effects result from alpha-adrenergic agonist properties resulting in stimulation of vascular smooth muscle and vasoconstriction. Methamphetamine stimulates both cortical and medullary centers in the CNS to increase sympathomimetic outflow. Peripherally, methamphetamine causes release of norepinephrine, stimulating both alpha- and beta-adrenergic receptors. Beta-adrenergic activity increases cardiac contractility and heart rate. Methamphetamines may also inhibit endogenous catecholamine breakdown via inhibition of monoamine oxidase. With intoxicated patients, these sympathomimetic effects are exaggerated. It is common for abusers to use the drug several times within a short period, which may exacerbate the cardiotoxic effects.[279]

The substituted amphetamine 3,3-methylene dioxymethamphetamine (MDMA, or "ecstasy") has similar characteristics; however, it also has affinity for serotonergic neurons. This may explain the hallucinations seen in both recreational use and in toxicity. Ecstasy intoxication will, therefore, result in both sympathomimetic and serotonergic syndromes. The clinical syndrome associated with amphetamine toxicity consists of vasoconstriction, tachycardia, and hypertension, which are associated with agitation and CNS excitation. In acute toxicity, cardiovascular and CNS complications require immediate intervention.

Cardiovascular complications of amphetamine use include chest pain and acute coronary syndrome (ACS), aortic dissection, and sudden death.[282,283] Ischemic and hemorrhagic stroke are both reported and often occur in association with marked hypertension.[284] Carotid artery dissection may present with neurologic deficits with or without neck pain.[285]

The respiratory tract is vulnerable following either nasal insufflation or smoking of amphetamines. Complications include nasal septal perforation, barotrauma, pulmonary edema, pneumothorax, pneumomediastinum, and pneumonia.[286,287] Long-term use may result in pulmonary hypertension.[288]

Mild amphetamine-induced hyperthermia is common in overdose and likely relates to agitation. Hypertonicity due to dehydration may be present. However, acute nontraumatic cerebral edema associated with hyponatremia is reported as a complication of the use of MDMA.[289,290] Severe hyperthermia (40°C) is of multifactorial origin, with dopamine and serotonin dysregulation, increased metabolic demands, and psychomotor agitation all being involved.[291–293] It is associated with hepatic necrosis, rhabdomyolysis, and shock.

Amphetamine toxicity should be suspected in any patients who exhibit signs and symptoms consistent with sympathomimetic toxidrome. They will present with CNS excitation, mydriasis, tachycardia, hypertension, and hyperthermia. This must be distinguished from anticholinergic toxidrome, which will have the characteristic features of dry skin and mucous membranes, hypoactive bowel sounds, and urinary retention.

Management

Less severe cases of intoxication with amphetamines or amphetamine derivatives will present with agitation, mild tachycardia, and hypertension. Benzodiazepine sedation, often with large doses, may be all that is required to resolve these clinical manifestations.

In patients with marked hypertension that requires intervention, vasodilators such as nitroprusside or nitroglycerin are appropriate. Phentolamine, an alpha-adrenergic antagonist, may also be utilized. If rate control is required, diltiazem is preferred. Beta-blockers, including labetalol, should be avoided while the patient is in the hyperadrenergic state, as unopposed alpha stimulation may cause or exacerbate a hypertensive crisis. There is little information guiding therapy for amphetamine-related chest pain and ACS. Given the similarities between cocaine and methamphetamine toxicity, these complications should be treated similarly.[294]

Seizures should be controlled with benzodiazepines; second-line agents are propofol and phenobarbital. Phenytoin is not useful for drug-induced seizures. Severely intoxicated patients with hyperthermia or seizures should have hepatic enzymes, bilirubin, coagulation parameters, creatinine kinase, and urine myoglobin assayed. Marked hyperpyrexia may lead to acute hepatic failure, disseminated intravascular coagulopathy, and rhabdomyolysis, similar to that seen in environmental heat stroke. Rhabdomyolysis is treated with volume diuresis. Alkalinization of the urine may also be required.

Variable protein binding and large volumes of distribution hinder hemodialysis or other means of extracorporeal elimination. Asymptomatic or mild cases of amphetamine toxicity can adequately be observed for 4 to 6 hours in the emergency department until sympathomimetic signs and symptoms normalize. Patients with moderate to severe symptoms are admitted to a monitored setting.

Cocaine

Toxicology

Cocaine, also known as benzoylmethylecgonine, is a naturally occurring anesthetic and sympathomimetic. The drug can be purified into crystalline cocaine hydrochloride, producing a concentrated formulation that is rapidly absorbed from mucous membranes, lung tissue, and, somewhat less rapidly, the GI tract. Cocaine hydrochloride is heat-labile and undergoes pyrolytic degradation. Conversely, cocaine that has been precipitated from an alkaline medium crystallizes as the alkaloid "free base," which is heat-stable when smoked.

The physiologic effects of cocaine are both sympathomimetic and membrane-stabilizing.[295] Presynaptic reuptake of biogenic amines such as norepinephrine, serotonin, and dopamine is inhibited, resulting in CNS stimulation and heightened adrenergic tone.[281,296,297] The membrane-stabilizing effects exacerbate cardiotoxicity and may result in QRS prolongation; QT prolongation is seen and may be related to potassium channel blockade.[298]

Cocaine-induced myocardial infarction is well documented.[299] Cocaine causes coronary vasoconstriction, is thrombogenic, and increases myocardial work.[300-304] It occurs in young patients, in those without preexisting coronary artery disease, and with an incidence as high as 6% in those presenting with cocaine-related chest pain.[305-308]

The epileptogenic property of cocaine is multifactorial; it is related to the sympathomimetic toxidrome, increases in neuroexcitatory chemicals, and reduction in GABAergic tone.[309-311] Cocaine's membrane-stabilizing effects may compound the probability of seizures. Coadministration of cocaine with lidocaine, another membrane-stabilizing drug, has been shown to lower the seizure threshold in animals.[312,313] The primary target organs are the CNS, cardiovascular system, lungs, GI tract, skin, and thermoregulatory center, although all physiologic systems are at risk.

The clinical manifestations of acute cocaine toxicity may be mild, with transient anxiety, tachycardia, and hypertension. With more significant ingestions, marked cardiovascular and neurologic abnormalities will be observed.

Chest pain is common, and select cases may be related to an acute coronary event, aortic dissection, or pulmonary complication. Pulmonary complications include cardiogenic and noncardiogenic pulmonary edema, pulmonary hemorrhage, pneumothorax, pneumomediastinum, and pneumopericardium.[286,287]

Vascular complications in the GI and genitourinary tracts are less common but include mesenteric ischemia and renal infarction.[314,315] Orally ingested cocaine can cause ischemic complications in the GI tract, including acute abdominal pain, hemorrhagic diarrhea, and shock from mesenteric ischemia. However, ingestions of large amounts of cocaine, as in the case of "body stuffers" or "body packers," is more likely to result in marked systemic cocaine toxicity than focal abdominal complaints.

Hyperthermia related to cocaine intoxication may be severe. Peripheral vasoconstriction and lack of heat perception limit heat loss, while psychomotor agitation increases heat production.[316] Increased ambient temperatures exacerbate these phenomena and increase mortality from cocaine overdose.[317] Complications include disseminated intravascular coagulation and fulminant hepatic necrosis. Severe hyperthermia (40°C) correlates with mortality and should be treated aggressively.[318,319] Rhabdomyolysis occurs both in the presence and absence of hyperthermia.

Cocaine toxicity is likely in patients who exhibit signs and symptoms consistent with sympathomimetic stimulation. They often present with CNS excitation, mydriasis, tachycardia, hypertension, and hyperthermia. As with amphetamines, this must be distinguished from an anticholinergic toxidrome, which will have the characteristic features of dry skin and mucous membranes, hypoactive bowel sounds, and urinary retention.

Management

Less severe cases of cocaine intoxication will present with agitation, mild tachycardia, and hypertension. Benzodiazepine sedation, often with large doses, may be all that is required to resolve these clinical findings. In patients with marked hypertension requiring intervention, vasodilators such as nitroprusside or nitroglycerin are appropriate. Phentolamine, an alpha-adrenergic antagonist, may also be utilized. If rate control is required, diltiazem is preferred. Beta-blockers, including labetalol, should be avoided while the patient is in the hyperadrenergic state. They have been found to be detrimental in an animal model and may induce unopposed alpha stimulation, causing or exacerbating a hypertensive crisis.[320] All patients with significant toxicity should have an ECG early in the evaluation.

Activated charcoal adsorbs unpackaged or poorly packaged orally ingested cocaine and is useful for gastric decontamination. The majority of cocaine intoxications involve IV injection, insufflations, or inhalation, limiting the utility of activated charcoal. Variable protein binding and large volumes of distribution hinder hemodialysis or other means of extracorporeal elimination.

Cocaine-associated ACS in the hyperadrenergic patient should be managed as with noncocaine-associated ACS, with several caveats. Benzodiazepines should be utilized as first-line sympatholytic agents. Nitroglycerin is indicated for hypertension and coronary vasodilation in the setting of chest pain and may be more effective when used in combination with benzodiazepines.[321,322] Calcium channel blockers may be useful for alleviating coronary vasospasm, hypertension, and tachycardia.[294] Beta-blockers, including labetalol, do not reduce coronary vasospasm and may actually exacerbate it.[304,323,324] For this reason in conjunction with the reasons outlined above, this class of medications should be avoided.

The cardiovascular toxicity of cocaine is not limited to ACS. Severe intoxications may result in QT prolongation, QRS prolongation, or more malignant rhythms. These aberrancies are in part rate- and pH-dependent. They are exacerbated by seizures and the resultant acidosis, tachycardia, and hypoxia. Prolonged QRS duration related to fast sodium channel blockade is ominous. It should be aggressively treated with sodium bicarbonate, administered by IV bolus. Animal studies have demonstrated a clear beneficial effect by reversing QRS prolongation in acute cocaine-induced dysrhythmias.[325–327] Case reports confirm the salutary effect in human cases.[328,329] The benefit of a sodium bicarbonate infusion following bolus therapy is not clear; however, it may be useful to avoid recurrent acidosis. Marked alkalosis should be avoided, with a pH goal below 7.55. Repeat boluses should be administered for recurrence of symptoms or ECG abnormalities.

In the setting of refractory ventricular arrhythmias poorly responsive to sodium bicarbonate, lidocaine is considered the second-line antiarrhythmic. However, its utility is not clear. *In vitro* work indicates that it may be effective in treating wide-complex dysrhythmias, although it may also prolong QT intervals.[330–332] Animal work demonstrates a clear increased rate of seizures and a mixed effect on mortality.[312,313,333]

Prolonged QT intervals leading to torsades de pointes are related to potassium channel blockade. Prolonged QT intervals should prompt optimization of potassium, magnesium, and calcium levels. In the case of torsades de pointes, a 2- to 5-g IV magnesium bolus is indicated.

Refractory cocaine toxicity that results in hypotension should be treated with volume expansion using isotonic saline. Vasopressors are utilized as second-line agents.

Seizures should be controlled with benzodiazepines; second-line agents are propofol or phenobarbital. Phenytoin is not useful for toxin-induced seizures. Severely intoxicated patients with hyperthermia or seizures should have hepatic enzymes, bilirubin, coagulation parameters, creatinine kinase, and urinary myoglobin assayed. Marked hyperpyrexia may lead to acute hepatic failure, and disseminated intravascular coagulopathy, and rhabdomyolysis, similar to that seen in environmental heat stroke. Rhabdomyolysis is treated with volume diuresis and urinary alkalinization as indicated.

Body stuffers may swallow cocaine in an attempt to avoid prosecution when confronted by the police. Body packers intentionally swallow or pack body orifices with drug in an attempt to conceal and illegally transport the product. Body packing often entails very elaborate methods of packaging so as to make rupture less likely.[334] Conversely, body stuffing implies poorly wrapped cocaine, which is likely to become bioavailable.[335] Even carefully packaged packets can rupture, and this setting typically involves potentially lethal doses of cocaine. Types of packages most likely to rupture are paper, aluminum foil, or poorly secured plastic bags.

The physician may be able to gather enough information regarding the amount of cocaine ingested and the type of packaging to assess the potential for toxicity. Abdominal radiographs are generally not useful for body stuffers but may be more helpful with body packers. A Gastrografin swallow or CT scan of the abdomen with contrast may reveal ingested packets in cases where plain radiographs are negative but suspicion of ingestion is high.

In body stuffers and packers, gastric lavage is contraindicated, as it may cause rupture of the packets. Conservative therapy utilizing polyethylene glycol whole-bowel irrigation is recommended in asymptomatic patients.[45,336] It is important to ensure that all ingested packets pass before the patient is discharged, which may require repeat imaging. Body packers who are symptomatic or have a bowel obstruction should have a surgical consultation. Laparotomy may be a necessary lifesaving intervention to remove leaking packets.[337]

Asymptomatic or mild cases of cocaine toxicity should be observed for 4 to 6 hours in the emergency department until sympathomimetic signs and symptoms normalize. Patients with moderate to severe symptoms are admitted to a monitored setting.

Inhalants

Toxicology

Inhalant abuse includes the practices of sniffing, huffing, and bagging. Sniffing entails the inhalation of a volatile substance directly from a container, as occurs with airplane glue or rubber cement. Huffing involves pouring a volatile liquid onto fabric (e.g., a rag or sock) and placing it over the mouth and nose while inhaling. Huffing is the method used by over half of those who abuse volatile substances. "Bagging" refers to spraying a solvent into a plastic or paper bag and rebreathing from the bag several times; spray paint is among the agents commonly used.

A multitude of inhalational substances are abused, most being volatile hydrocarbons. Commonly inhaled hydrocarbons include gasoline, spray paints, lighter fluid, and glue. In many cases, the class of the substance is identified rather than the specific chemical. Since exact components may vary between products, this method is often inaccurate and imprecise.

The volatile hydrocarbons can be further divided into aliphatic hydrocarbons, aromatic hydrocarbons, halogenated hydrocarbons, and alkyl nitrites. The alkyl nitrites include amyl, butyl, and isobutyl nitrite and are sold in shops dealing in sex and drug paraphernalia. Amyl nitrite is contained in small glass capsules known as "poppers." When covered in gauze and crushed, the capsules release the nitrite and make a characteristic sound. Amyl, butyl, and isobutyl nitrites are sold as room deodorizers or liquid incense in small vials typically containing 10 to 30 mL.

The most commonly used nonhydrocarbon inhalant is nitrous oxide. Nitrous oxide, or "laughing gas," is used therapeutically as an inhalational anesthetic. Cartridges of the compressed gas, known as "whippets," are sold for commercial use in whipped cream dispensers. These battery-sized metal containers of compressed gas are punctured using a "cracker" and the escaping gas is either inhaled directly or collected in a balloon and then inhaled.

Inhalants are highly lipophilic agents that readily gain entrance into the CNS. Early CNS effects include euphoria, visual and auditory hallucinations, as well as headache and dizziness. As intoxication progresses, CNS depression worsens and patients may develop slurred speech, confusion, tremor, and weakness. Further CNS depression is marked by ataxia, lethargy, seizures, coma, respiratory depression, and death. The mechanism of inhalant effects on the CNS is poorly studied, although some generalizations can be made.

Volatile alkyl nitrites likely mediate their effects through cGMP-mediated vasodilation, although it is unclear if they have direct CNS effects.[338,339] Nitrous oxide may inhibit excitatory NMDA receptors and affect dopaminergic activity.[340,341] Volatile solvents and fuels such as toluene and trichloroethane produce effects similar to those of CNS depressants such as ethanol and barbiturates, likely mediated through GABA receptors.[339] Toluene is also thought to have NMDA antagonist activity.[342,343]

Cardiotoxicity, in its most abrupt form, results in the "sudden sniffing death." History surrounding these events indicates that the user, while intoxicated, was startled immediately prior to death. Although mechanism is not clear, these findings implicate catecholamine surge in the setting of inhalant-induced cardiac channelopathy as a mechanism.

This effect has been studied in children undergoing halothane (a halogenated hydrocarbon) anesthesia for dental procedures.[344] During dental extraction or emergence, the children were noted to have an increased rate of ventricular arrhythmias in comparison to those on sevoflurane anesthesia. The effective use of halothane–epinephrine for generating animal models of ventricular arrhythmias supports this concept.[345] Potassium channel blockade is suspected, as this correlates with the QT prolongation that has been documented following volatile anesthetic administration.[346] The rapid delayed rectifier potassium channel is often implicated in drug-induced myocardial sensitization; it is particularly sensitive to the effects of hydrophobic (aromatic or halogenated) hydrocarbons.[347] An animal model of toluene toxicity demonstrated loss of R-wave height, broadening of the R wave, inverted T waves, and ST-segment depression, an effect that may have been related to hypoxia, or toluene intoxication.[348] Sodium channel blockade by toluene has been demonstrated *in vitro*, although this mechanism is less substantiated.[349]

Pulmonary toxicity associated with volatile hydrocarbons is often due to aspiration following attempted ingestion of a liquid hydrocarbon. Asphyxiation may be ascribed to the inhalant or to suffocation from a plastic bag utilized for inhalant delivery.[350] Volatile hydrocarbons are pulmonary irritants that may induce coughing, dyspnea, bronchospasm, and pneumonitis. Hydrocarbon pneumonitis is characterized by rales or rhonchi on lung auscultation, tachypnea, fever, leukocytosis, and radiographic abnormalities.[351]

Cardiac and pulmonary toxicities are effects of volatile hydrocarbons, and toxicity to other organ systems is unique to the specific chemical. Hepatoxicity has been associated with carbon tetrachloride and other halogenated hydrocarbons, including chloroform, trichloroethane, trichloroethylene, and toluene.

Inhalation of toluene, which is often found in spray paints and glues, may cause a distal renal tubule acidosis (RTA) and hypokalemia. Although distal RTAs are associated with a hyperchloremic metabolic acidosis and a normal anion gap, some patients have been found to have an increased anion gap following toluene inhalation.

Methylene chloride, most commonly found in paint removers and degreasers, differs from other halogenated hydrocarbons in that it is metabolized by cytochrome P450 to carbon monoxide. Carboxyhemoglobin levels may be significantly elevated and may not rise for several hours after exposure because of the time required for metabolism. Inhalation of amyl, butyl, and isobutyl nitrites may induce methemoglobinemia. These agents also cause peripheral vasodilatation and can result in orthostatic hypotension and syncope.

The clinical presentation of inhalant use varies widely among individuals. In general, symptoms will resolve within 2 hours of exposure. Following acute exposure, there may be a distinct odor of the abused substance on the patient's breath or clothing. Depending on the agent used and the method, there may be discoloration of the skin around the nose and mouth. Mucous membrane irritation may cause sneezing, coughing, and tearing. Patients may complain of dyspnea and palpitations. GI complaints include nausea, vomiting, and abdominal pain. After an initial period of euphoria, patients may have headache and dizziness.

Syncope is one of the more serious clinical events that may occur with inhalant abuse. Patients may present with a persistent altered level of consciousness or in cardiac arrest. The most common causes of such events are hypoxia from simple asphyxiation, profound respiratory depression, and malignant dysrhythmia. Determining the exact cause of syncope or death is difficult, as most events are unwitnessed. Clinical testing and autopsy generally reveal little confirmatory information.

Management

In the vast majority of patients, symptoms will resolve quickly and hospitalization will not be required. Agitation, either from acute effects of the inhalant or from withdrawal, is safely managed with benzodiazepines. Regardless of severity, consultation with a regional poison control center is appropriate to assist with identification of the toxin and specific management issues.

Mild pulmonary symptoms such as wheezing are adequately treated with oxygen and nebulized albuterol. Respiratory distress prompts consideration of chemical pneumonitis and the addition of continuous cardiorespiratory monitoring, ECG, chest radiography, screening for electrolyte abnormalities, and, in severe cases, intubation and mechanical ventilation. Neither prophylactic antibiotics nor steroids have proven beneficial.

Symptomatic patients with a history of alkyl nitrite use should be screened for methemoglobinemia. Methylene chloride induces carboxyhemoglobinemia, which may be delayed. Initial screening for this complication is warranted, and should be repeated in several hours if the patient remains symptomatic or worsens. Treatment with high-flow oxygen is generally sufficient.

Cardiac dysrhythmias associated with inhalant abuse carry a poor prognosis. There appears to be no premonitory signal to the user, and the effect of the inhalant on the myocardium lingers after inhalation has stopped. There are no evidence-based treatment guidelines for the management of inhalant-induced cardiac dysrhythmias; standard ACLS protocols should be followed.

Animal work and studies of dysrhythmias under halogenated hydrocarbon anesthesia indicate increased morbidity with elevated sympathomimetic tone.[344,345] It is recommended that use of sympathomimetic agents be minimized, although it is understood that this may not be possible in cases of respiratory distress, shock, or cardiac arrest. Agents with beta-blocking activity may be cardioprotective in the hydrocarbon-sensitized myocardium. Esmolol has been shown to both prevent and suppress halothane–epinephrine induced ventricular arrhythmias in an animal model.[352] In a similar model, propranolol was shown to abolish ventricular arrhythmias.[353] There are case reports of both esmolol and propranolol resolving trichloroethylene-induced ventricular arrhythmias.[354,355] Considering this evidence, beta-blockers should be considered in the setting of hydrocarbon-induced ventricular arrhythmias.

Opioids

Toxicology

Opioid agonists bind to a family of inhibitory G protein–coupled receptors, namely the mu, kappa, and delta receptors. They inhibit adenylate cyclase, which reduces the formation of cAMP, close calcium channels decreasing neurotransmitter release, and open potassium channels inducing cell hyperpolarization. The physiologic effects depend on which receptor subtype is involved and the location of the receptor.

The important clinical effects from a toxicological perspective are a result of activity at the μ receptor. μ1 Receptors mediate sedation, analgesia, and euphoria. μ2 Receptors mediate respiratory depression and bradycardia, among other effects. The etiology of miosis is unclear.

The clinical presentation of opioid intoxication is primarily that of depressed mental status and respiratory insufficiency. Miosis will likely be present, but may be absent in patients ingesting meperidine, pentazocine, propoxyphene, tramadol, heroin mixed with adulterants or cocaine, or diphenoxylate/atropine. CNS depression ranges from mild sedation to stupor and coma. Patients may be hypotensive, hypothermic, bradycardic, and hyporeflexic. Vomiting may occur, and when coupled with respiratory depression and a diminished gag reflex, places the patient at risk for aspiration.

Additional pulmonary effects may include bronchospasm due to histamine release or pulmonary irritation induced by insufflating or inhaling opioids cut with impurities or adulterants. In massive overdoses, the pulmonary toxicity can also cause severe hypoxia, hypercarbia, and acute lung injury.

Opioid-induced pulmonary edema occurs in 1% to 3% of patients with heroin overdose.[14,356,357] The etiology is unclear but may involve opioid-induced capillary leak and sympathetic surge in the setting of profound hypoxia.

Seizure in the setting of opioid overdose is often related to hypoxia. However, some opioids are proconvulsant. The meperidine metabolite normeperidine has a longer half-life than its parent compound. In patients receiving large doses or in those with renal insufficiency, it may accumulate and result in seizure activity.[358] Tramadol is a weak agonist at the mu opioid receptor and an inhibitor of monoamine uptake. Supratherapeutic doses have been shown to induce seizures in animal models, an effect that is well described in humans.[359,360] Seizures have been reported with pentazocine (Talwin)/tripelennamine, although this seems to be less commonly abused than in past years.[69,361]

Propoxyphene is a weak opioid agonist that is metabolized to nordextropropoxyphene. It may cause CNS depression, seizures, and cardiotoxicity among other adverse effects, even at therapeutic doses.[362] In a case series of 222 patients, 10% had seizures, 45% had respiratory failure, and 48% had cardiotoxicity.[363] Overall mortality was 8%. Cardiotoxicity resulting from propoxyphene is complex and may be mediated through both sodium and potassium channels.[364,365] Significant toxicity is associated with prolonged QRS complexes.[364,366,367]

Management

In a patient with a clinically significant opioid overdose, the practice of routine intubation before naloxone administration is not recommended.[4] When opioid overdose patients have respiratory insufficiency with a detectable pulse, an attempt at opioid reversal before tracheal intubation is warranted provided that adequate ventilatory support can be given with bag-valve-mask.

Patients with opioid-induced cardiac arrest or impending cardiac arrest should have aggressive airway management, including intubation, prior to consideration of naloxone. The endpoint objectives for opioid reversal are adequate airway reflexes and ventilation, not complete arousal. Acute, abrupt opioid withdrawal may increase the likelihood of severe complications, such as aspiration pneumonitis, pulmonary edema, ventricular arrhythmias, and severe agitation and hostility.[8]

Compared with longer-acting opioid antagonists, naloxone is preferred, despite having a shorter duration of effect (45–60 minutes) than most opioids. Repeat doses may be required, particularly in dealing with opioids with longer durations of action, such as oxycodone, methadone, and diphenoxylate–atropine (Lomotil). A continuous IV infusion of naloxone can be instituted. The drip rate can be calculated by using two-thirds of the initial dose required to reverse the patient's respiratory depression and administering this amount hourly. There is debate over which route of administration is preferred; however, if IV access is possible, it should be established and utilized. Alternate routes include endotracheal, SQ, or IM administration and administration by nebulizer with a comparably rapid onset of action.

Seizures resulting from meperidine, tramadol, pentazocine, or propoxyphene should be managed as are other toxin-induced seizures. Benzodiazepines are the drug of choice, with second-line agents being propofol and phenobarbital. Phenytoin is not useful for drug-induced seizures.

Similarities between the cardiotoxicity of propoxyphene and TCAs indicate that propoxyphene dysrhythmias should respond to the same therapy. Case reports have demonstrated efficacy of both IV sodium bicarbonate and lidocaine for QRS prolongation in this setting.[366,367]

Patients who present as body packers or stuffers of heroin or opioid-containing drugs may require GI decontamination with whole-bowel irrigation using polyethylene glycol solution to enhance the elimination of drug packets. Contraindications to whole-bowel irrigation include unstable vital signs, respiratory compromise, and lack of bowel sounds or gut motility. Activated charcoal should be given prior to whole-bowel irrigation to adsorb any leaking drug from the packets. Charcoal noted in the rectal effluent indicates successful whole-bowel irrigation. In contrast to cases involving cocaine, a less aggressive approach to surgical intervention is warranted with heroin. Supportive care and antidotal therapy with naloxone should be effective in the case of leaking packets. In the case of bowel obstruction, surgical consultation is indicated.

Patients presenting with CNS depression from opioid overdose who respond to naloxone administration can be medically cleared after 4 to 6 hours of observation. Patients who continue to demonstrate respiratory compromise or require repeated doses of naloxone should be observed for a longer period of time.

Agents with a prolonged half-life, such as methadone, are much more likely to cause recurrence of CNS and respiratory depression. The toxicity of diphenoxylate–atropine (Lomotil) may be delayed or prolonged due to anticholinergic effects.[368] Therefore, these patients should be observed in a monitored setting for at least 24 hours.

Environmental, Occupational, and Iatrogenic Toxins

Carbon Monoxide and Carboxyhemoglobin

Toxicology

Carbon monoxide is among the most common environmental toxins and a leading cause of death by poisoning. It is colorless, tasteless, odorless, and nonirritating yet highly toxic. The diagnosis may be obvious when there is a history of fire, combustion appliances, or automobiles utilized in an enclosed space; however, the diagnosis may be unrecognized. Symptoms are typically vague or present like other common disorders. A high index of suspicion and careful attention to historical clues, such as multiple symptomatic patients or animals from the same dwelling, is essential.

Readily absorbed upon inhalation, carbon monoxide binds avidly to hemoglobin with an affinity >200 times greater than that of oxygen.[369] Carbon monoxide binding to hemoglobin has the effect of increasing the affinity of the remaining binding sites for oxygen, thus shifting the oxyhemoglobin dissociation curve to the left.[370,371] Carbon monoxide also binds to myoglobin and cytochrome oxidase, resulting in cytotoxicity and cardiotoxicity.[372,373]

In a series of 230 patients with moderate to severe carbon monoxide poisoning, ischemic ECG changes were found in 30%, and 35% had elevated cardiac biomarkers.[374] Echocardiographic evidence of myocardial dysfunction has been documented.[375]

CNS dysfunction is multifactorial, with hypotension, hypoxia, cytotoxicity, and lipid peroxidation all likely involved. Certain brain regions are more sensitive to carbon monoxide toxicity, such as the cortical rather than subcortical areas, basal ganglia, and Purkinje cells in the cerebellum.[373] Carbon monoxide poisoning may be associated with delayed neurologic sequelae, which is the basis of the argument for hyperbaric oxygen therapy.

The clinical presentation of carbon monoxide toxicity is widely varied. Signs and symptoms range from headache, nausea, vomiting, weakness, and decreased mental status to syncope, seizures, coma, myocardial dysfunction, and arrhythmias. Severe cases can present in shock and cardiac arrest.

Elevated carboxyhemoglobin levels document exposure, although a normal level does not exclude the possibility that exposure has occurred. Carbon monoxide levels are usually measured using arterial blood, although venous blood levels are comparable. Standard oximeters cannot quantify carboxyhemoglobin percentage and typically give normal readings in carbon monoxide poisoning. Cooximeters are able to make the distinction between these species and quantify the percentage of carboxyhemoglobin. In mild to moderate toxicity, laboratory testing other than a carboxyhemoglobin level is rarely helpful. A mild metabolic (lactic) acidosis may be present; however, this is very nonspecific and does not guide therapy. A markedly elevated lactate and significant symptoms in house fire victims is suggestive of concomitant cyanide poisoning.

Management

The initial resuscitation of patients with carbon monoxide toxicity is similar to that for other critically ill patients. Careful assessment of the airway for burns should occur in the patient presenting from a fire. First, 100% oxygen by face mask or endotracheal intubation if required is essential. Carboxyhemoglobin half-life, as measured in volunteers, averages 5 hours.[376,377] This drops to approximately 90 minutes in those receiving 100% oxygen therapy.[378,379] Oxygen therapy should be continued for 4 to 6 hours to ensure the elimination of carbon monoxide. In the pregnant patient, oxygen therapy should be administered approximately five times longer once the mother has normalized so as to ensure adequate carbon monoxide clearance from the fetus.

Considerable controversy exists regarding the utility of hyperbaric oxygen in carbon monoxide toxicity. A number of large trials have attempted to evaluate the efficacy of this therapy; however, the results are conflicting and not without criticism.[380–383] Despite a lack of clear, evidence-based guidelines, hyperbaric therapy is generally felt to be indicated for patients with altered mental status, syncope, coma, seizure, focal neurologic deficit, or an absolute carboxyhemoglobin level >25% (15% in pregnancy, or with signs of fetal distress). More recent work has identified patients >36 years of age and those with exposure intervals ≥24 hours as being at risk of delayed neurologic sequelae and likely to benefit from hyperbaric oxygen therapy.[384] Critically ill patients present an additional complication in that they must be stable enough to withstand the duration of therapy in an isolating hyperbaric chamber. If a local chamber is not available, patients should be stabilized prior to transfer.

Patients exposed to carbon monoxide who have low documented levels, are asymptomatic, and are without evidence of subtle neuropsychiatric dysfunction may be medically cleared. Carbon monoxide–poisoned patients whose symptoms resolve with normobaric oxygen may be medically cleared but should be seen in follow-up as outpatients to assess for delayed neuropsychiatric sequelae. Any patient requiring hyperbaric therapy, with coma, altered mental status, or other evidence of end-organ involvement should be admitted to the ICU. When the fetus is viable following treatment with hyperbaric oxygen, obstetric consultation with fetal monitoring is warranted for carbon monoxide poisoning in pregnancy.

Methemoglobinemia The oxidation of reduced hemoglobin (Fe^{2+}) transforms the iron moiety from a ferrous to a ferric state. Methemoglobin (Fe^{3+}) results, and this oxidized molecule is unable to bind and transport oxygen. Typically, methemoglobinemia is induced by oxidizing medications or toxins. The list of inducers is extensive as indicated in Table 29-1. The more commonly reported methemoglobin inducers include nitrates and nitrites. The source may be food, well water contaminated with nitrogenous waste, or medications, which have a more pronounced effect. Topical anesthetics are often implicated, as are dapsone and phenazopyridine. Of 198 benzocaine-related adverse events reported to the U.S. Food and Drug Administration between 1997 and 2002, a total of 132 were attributed to methemoglobinemia.[386] Of these, 107 were considered serious and there were two deaths. In a retrospective review of 138 cases at two teaching hospitals, dapsone was the most common offending agent.[385]

Under normal physiologic conditions, NADH derived from the glycolytic pathway relieves this oxidant stress. The reaction is catalyzed by NADH methemoglobin reductase, which converts methemoglobin (Fe^{3+}) to hemoglobin (Fe^{2+}). Patients with hereditary methemoglobinemia are at risk for additional toxicity due to a preexisting deficiency of this enzyme.[387] Alternatively, methemoglobin is reduced via NADPH generated by the hexose monophosphate shunt. This reaction predominantly occurs in the presence of methylene blue and is catalyzed by NADPH methemoglobin reductase. Patients with G6PD deficiency are at risk for hemolysis when treated with methylene blue as it competes

TABLE 29-1 • Methemoglobin Inducers
Amyl nitrite
Aniline dyes
Butyl nitrite
Benzocaine
Cetacaine
Chloroquine
Dapsone
EMLA
Flutamide
Herbicides
Isobutyl nitrite
Isosorbide dinitrate
Lidocaine
Metoclopramide
Naphthalene
Nitrates
Nitric oxide
Nitrous oxide
Nitrobenzene
Nitroethane
Pesticides
Petrol octane booster
Phenazopyridine
Prilocaine
Primiquine
Pyridium
Riluzole
Sulfonamides
Silver nitrate
Sodium nitate
Trinitrotoluene

Source: Ash-Bernal R, Wise R, Wright SM. Acquired methemoglobinemia: a retrospective series of 138 cases at 2 teaching hospitals. *Medicine (Baltimore)* 2004;83(5):265–273.

for an already limited supply of NADPH. These risks aside, methylene blue is the first-line therapy for methemoglobinemia and has proven efficacy.

The clinical presentation of methemoglobinemia varies. With levels of up to 15%, patients may be asymptomatic, although mild cyanosis and abnormal pulse oximetry are likely. Above 15%, cyanosis will be readily apparent and the blood may appear chocolate-brown. At levels of 20%, patients will develop symptoms such as headache, dyspnea, fatigue, and light-headedness. As the methemoglobin level approaches 50%, patients will appear critically ill, with tachypnea, CNS depression, seizures, metabolic acidosis, and dysrhythmias.[388] Those with underlying comorbidities such as coronary and pulmonary disease will be symptomatic at lower levels and are more likely to become critically ill.

Pulse oximetry decreases with rising methemoglobin levels. In dogs, oxygen saturation measured by pulse oximeter was found to drop steadily with rising methemoglobin levels until it reached a plateau of 85%, corresponding to a methemoglobin level of 30% to 35%.[389] Prior to reaching this plateau, the pulse oximeter overestimated oxygen saturation; at higher methemoglobin levels, the relationship was nonlinear. The recent development of cooximeters that have the ability to measure both methemoglobin and carboxyhemoglobin will likely aid in diagnosis, although experience is limited at this time.[390]

Management

The initial resuscitation of patients with methemoglobinemia should proceed as with other critically ill patients. Careful attention to airway management is essential. Supplemental oxygen by face mask or endotracheal intubation if required should be provided. Physical exam findings and pulse oximetry findings may clarify the diagnosis, as will a history of methemoglobin-inducing drug ingestion. An arterial or venous blood gas level should be ordered early to assess for methemoglobin and carboxyhemoglobin levels. Mild symptoms with levels <25% may be treated with supplemental oxygen.[385] Those with moderate to severe symptoms, or levels >25% (regardless of symptoms) should receive IV methylene blue 1 mg/kg.[385] The dose should be repeated for recurrence of symptoms.

Dapsone-induced methemoglobinemia is unique in that this agent has a half-life of approximately 30 hours and is more likely to cause recurrence.[101] Refractory patients who are markedly symptomatic may respond to exchange transfusion or hyperbaric therapy. Asymptomatic patients and those with levels that drop to <15% without therapy may be medically cleared. Persistently symptomatic patients and those who require methylene blue should be admitted to an intensive care setting.

Cyanide

Toxicology

Cyanide poisoning is unusual in the United States, although its contribution to toxicity and death may be underestimated in victims of smoke inhalation. Cyanide exposure by this route is known to be a major cause of toxicity among fire victims; however, it is often not considered in the critically ill fire victim.[391] Combustion of wool, silk, synthetic fabrics, and building materials may form hydrogen cyanide. The increasing use of synthetic building materials compounds the risk of cyanide toxicity resulting from building fires. Underscoring this risk is work by Baud et al.[392] Of 109 residential fire victims, the 43 who died had a mean cyanide concentration of 3.14 mg/L.[392] This was sixfold higher than cyanide levels in the 66 survivors, although there was considerable variability within both groups.

Workplace exposures to hydrogen cyanide gas are rare but do occur.[393] Risk factors are industrial settings where chemicals are stored or used, as in electroplating or precious metal extraction.[394,395] Hydrogen cyanide gas is rapidly absorbed in the lungs and may cause profound toxicity within seconds. Intentional ingestions of cyanide salts, such as sodium cyanide and potassium cyanide, are more likely in knowledgeable health care or laboratory workers who have access to such chemicals.[396] They are rapidly absorbed across the gastric mucosa and may result in toxicity within minutes.

There are a number of other sources of cyanide toxicity. Acetonitrile is a component of nail glue remover. It is used to remove artificial nails and should not be confused with nail polish remover, which typically contains acetone. Acetonitrile undergoes microsomal oxidation to liberate cyanide; the rate and severity of toxicity are dependent on this conversion.[397] The clinical implication of this *in vivo* liberation of cyanide is that toxicity may be delayed for several hours. Clinically significant cyanide levels have been documented as far out as 12 to 72 hours postingestion and may recur following treatment due to the prolonged half-life of acetonitrile.[398]

Laetrile, or vitamin B_{17}, was developed in the 1950s and promoted as an antineoplastic agent, although it has no efficacy against malignancies.[399] It is similar to the naturally occurring cyanogenic molecule amygdalin with the exception of one less sugar moiety. When ingested, intestinal beta glucosidase converts it to glucose, aldehyde, and cyanide. It is available on the Internet, making it readily available to the public.[400–402]

Cyanogenic plants include cassava, and those of the *Prunus* species among others. Linamarin is the predominant naturally occurring cyanogen found in cassava. It is commonly ingested in the tropics and is safe if prepared properly. Prunus species include choke cherries, black cherries, plums, bitter almonds, peaches, and apricots. Exposures to cyanogenic plants are fairly common and outcomes are less severe, although significant toxicity is reported.[403,404] Finally, the antihypertensive agent sodium nitroprusside may result in cyanide toxicity. In general, it occurs in patients on prolonged infusions and those with renal failure.[405]

The mechanism of cyanide toxicity is disruption of the cytochrome oxidase system, resulting in cellular hypoxia. Cyanide has a high affinity for the ferric iron (Fe^{3+}) moiety of cytochrome a3. When it binds, it disrupts the mitochondrial respiration, reduces ATP production, and results in lactic acidosis. The critical targets of cyanide are those organs most dependent on oxidative phosphorylation, namely the brain and heart.

The body has endogenous detoxification mechanisms for cyanide. Approximately 80% is detoxified by sulfurtransferase which, in the presence of thiosulfate, converts cyanide to nontoxic thiocyanate. Thiocyanate is renally excreted. Thiosulfate is rapidly depleted in cyanide poisoning, thus limiting this endogenous mechanism. Alternatively, a limited amount of cyanide is converted to nontoxic cyanocobalamin in the presence of hydroxocobalamin. The reported elimination half-life in humans is highly variable, and treatment should be guided by clinical condition rather than predicted toxicokinetics.

The clinical presentation depends on the route and dose of exposure. Inhalation of cyanide gas causes loss of consciousness within seconds, whereas symptoms from an oral exposure develop anywhere from 30 minutes to several hours from the time of ingestion. Toxicity will initially manifest in the central nervous and the cardiovascular systems. Initial symptoms in victims not experiencing rapid loss of consciousness include headache, anxiety, confusion, blurred vision, palpitations, nausea, and vomiting. With progression of toxicity, patients may experience a feeling of neck constriction, suffocation, and unsteadiness.

Early clinical signs of cyanide poisoning are CNS stimulation or depression, tachycardia or bradycardia, hypertension, and dilated pupils. Funduscopy may reveal bright red retinal veins. Late signs of poisoning are seizures, coma, apnea, cardiac arrhythmias, and cardiovascular collapse. The characteristic musty smell of "bitter almonds" may be detected in some cases. Although cyanide poisoning causes cellular hypoxia, the presence of cyanosis is a relatively late finding. The absence of cyanosis in the presence of clinical evidence of severe hypoxia should prompt the examiner to consider the diagnosis of cyanide poisoning.

Whole blood cyanide levels <0.5 μg/mL are considered nontoxic; those >3 μg/mL are lethal without treatment. Arterial blood gas measurements indicate metabolic acidosis with chemistry results reflecting an anion-gap metabolic acidosis, both secondary to lactate accumulation. When venous blood gas results are available, comparison with the arterial specimen may reveal a reduced arterial–venous oxygen difference due to reduced oxygen extraction. The ECG may demonstrate tachycardia, bradycardia, conduction defects, or ischemic changes, all dependent on the degree of cellular hypoxia and underlying comorbidities.

Management

The management of cyanide poisoning requires immediate supportive care as well as specific antidotal therapy. Oxygen is immediately administered and rapid sequence intubation may be necessary. Fluid resuscitation is initiated in patients with hypotension. Sodium bicarbonate should be considered in profound acidosis. Standard decontamination procedures should be followed in order to limit any further absorption by the patient and any absorption by health care personnel, although contamination of health care providers away from the scene is unlikely. Gastric decontamination with activated charcoal may be considered only in a patient who arrives with minimal symptoms soon after an oral exposure.

The traditional antidote available in the United States for cyanide poisoning is a kit containing amyl nitrite, sodium nitrite, and sodium thiosulfate. The nitrite components are oxidizing agents, converting hemoglobin to methemoglobin (Fe^{3+}). Cyanide has a higher affinity for methemoglobin than cytochrome a3, such that they bind and form the relatively nontoxic cyanomethemoglobin. Cyanomethemoglobin production displaces cyanide from cytochrome a3 and allows resumption of oxidative phosphorylation and aerobic metabolism.

Clinical improvement following nitrite administration occurs within minutes, yet nitrite-induced methemoglobinemia is known to be a relatively slow process. This has prompted alternative theories regarding nitrite reversal of cyanide toxicity, with the focus on the effects of nitrite-induced nitric oxide.

Nitrite is a potent vasodilator, which is likely related to its reduction to nitric oxide by deoxyhemoglobin.[406] This may partially ameliorate cyanide-induced circulatory dysfunction and contribute to the rapid antidotal efficacy of sodium nitrite. More likely, the effect is at the mitochondrial level.

Endogenous nitric oxide has been found to augment cyanide binding to cytochrome a3, whereas high exogenous levels, such as that induced by IV sodium nitrite, paradoxically inhibit cyanide binding.[407] This would explain the rapid effect of sodium nitrite in the absence of significant methemoglobinemia.

Hydroxocobalamin is an effective cyanide antidote, infusions of which are associated with transient but clinically significant hypertension. The proposed mechanism underlying this hypertension is nitric oxide scavenging.[408] This complicates the previously mentioned theories regarding early efficacy of nitrites being mediated through nitric oxide. Nevertheless, cyanide binding to methemoglobin or hydroxocobalamin is the key mechanism, with the effects of nitric oxide being variable and likely less significant.

When the traditional cyanide antidote kit is used, amyl nitrite is administered first. The ampules are crushed in gauze and held near the nose and mouth for 30 seconds, which should produce a methemoglobin level of 3% to 7%. Once an IV line is established and sodium nitrite administered, amyl nitrite may be discontinued. In critically ill or comatose patients, amyl nitrite will have little utility. Sodium nitrite is administered as 300 mg (10 mL of a 3% solution) at a rate of 2.5 to 5 mL/min. In an unstable hypotensive patient, the dose may be given over 30 minutes. With the slower rate of infusion, the methemoglobin level peaks in 35 to 70 minutes and rises to roughly 10% to 15%. Side effects of nitrite administration include headache, blurred vision, nausea, vomiting, and hypotension. High methemoglobin levels result in similar symptoms and impair oxygen delivery. Therefore, methemoglobin levels should be monitored closely.

Following sodium nitrite, 12.5 g of sodium thiosulfate should always be administered. It provides a sulfur donor for the sulfurtransferase-mediated conversion of cyanide to thiocyanate, augmenting the nitrate-induced effect. Thiosulfate has minimal side effects; however, thiocyanate levels >10 mg/dL may be associated with nausea, vomiting, arthralgias, and confusion. Thiocyanate is renally excreted, so these symptoms may be exacerbated in the setting of renal failure.

Typically, symptoms and signs of cyanide poisoning begin to respond within minutes of the administration of nitrites. When symptoms recur following antidote administration, both the sodium nitrite and sodium thiosulfate may be given again at half the original doses. In a situation in which cyanide poisoning is being considered but the diagnosis is uncertain, the use of sodium thiosulfate alone may be considered. This has particular utility in fire victims. These patients may have cyanide toxicity; however, inducing methemoglobinemia in a critically ill, hypoxic, potentially carbon monoxide–poisoned patient prior to documenting a clear need is controversial.

Hydroxocobalamin was recently approved by the U.S. Food and Drug Administration for treatment of known or suspected cyanide poisoning. Hydroxocobalamin complexes with cyanide to form nontoxic cyanocobalamin, which is excreted in the urine. It is an attractive alternative to the traditional cyanide antidote kit, as it is not associated with hypotension or methemoglobinemia. It has a mild side-effect profile, although chromaturia and skin redness are common.[409] Clinically significant increases in systolic and diastolic blood pressure are seen, as well as mild decreases in heart rate correlating with the hypertension.[409]

Hydroxocobalamin has been used in France for over 30 years in both the hospital and prehospital settings and has been evaluated as an antidote for cyanide poisoning related to smoke inhalation in two observational studies.[410,411] Case series and retrospective chart reviews document efficacy in cyanide poisoning unrelated to smoke inhalation.[402,412–414] A lack of controlled trials establishing clear superiority of hydroxocobalamin is the remaining criticism. Despite this, there is strong evidence in support of its use. Hydroxocobalamin is a safe and effective first-line therapy for cyanide toxicity and should be carefully considered as empiric therapy for victims of smoke inhalation when cyanide toxicity is likely.

Patients who are asymptomatic and whose exposure has apparently been minimal are observed for several hours. Those who have ingested cyanogenic glycosides are observed for at least 6 hours for evidence of toxicity. Those ingesting acetonitrile-containing compounds are observed for 12 to 24 hours. Patients requiring antidotal treatment are admitted to an ICU, where vital signs, mental status, arterial blood gases, methemoglobin, and carboxyhemoglobin levels can be checked frequently. Following recovery, patients are observed for 24 to 48 hours.

Organophosphates and Carbamates

Toxicology

Unintentional pesticide poisonings, including those attributed to organophosphates and carbamates, have declined significantly over the past decade.[415] Despite this fact, these agents remain a significant source of toxicity, with almost 10,000 combined cases reported to U.S. poison centers in 2005.[69] The cholinergic toxidrome is identical to that of the chemical weapons sarin, soman, tabun, and VX, although these agents are markedly more potent in comparison.

Organophosphates are well absorbed in the lungs and GI system as well as through mucous membranes and skin. They inhibit acetylcholinesterase, resulting in accumulation of acetylcholine in nicotinic and cholinergic nerve terminals. The central and autonomic nervous system as well as neuromuscular junctions in skeletal muscle are affected.

Under normal conditions, acetylcholinesterase cleaves acetylcholine into acetic acid and choline, with choline undergoing reuptake into the presynaptic nerve terminal. Organophosphates phosphorylate the active hydroxyl group of acetylcholinesterase, rendering it inactive. During this period the inactivated enzyme undergoes slow hydrolysis. The addition of pralidoxime enhances this reaction. "Aging" occurs after a delay of 24 to 72 hours; one of the aromatic or aliphatic groups bound to the central phosphorus leaves and the enzyme is permanently inactivated. The initial process is similar for carbamates; however, aging does not occur. Enzymes that have undergone carbamylation slowly hydrolyze and the enzyme is reactivated.

The clinical presentation of the cholinergic toxidrome is classically described as defecation, urination, miosis, bronchospasm, bronchorrhea, emesis, lacrimation, and salivation (DUMBBELS). This acronym reflects the muscarinic component of toxicity, which may not be uniformly present. Nicotinic stimulation results in muscle fasciculations, twitching, and weakness.

Significant CNS and cardiac complications are common with severe poisonings. CNS manifestations include anxiety, confusion, seizure, and coma.[416] Cardiac manifestations are less prominent than with other direct cardiotoxins; however, hypertension, hypotension, PR and QT prolongation, ST-segment and T-wave abnormalities, atrial fibrillation, ventricular tachycardia, and ventricular fibrillation have been observed.[417] Onset of symptoms may be acute and usually occurs within <12 hours.[416] Longer delays are seen with compounds that require *in vivo* activation and those that are very lipid-soluble.

Management

Aggressive supportive care and thorough decontamination with appropriate protection for health-care workers is essential to the management of cholinergic toxins. Attention to life-threatening manifestations takes precedence. Respiratory failure from bronchorrhea and respiratory muscle weakness should be managed with early endotracheal intubation.

Seizures are treated with benzodiazepines and phenobarbital unless they are brief and self-limited. Vasopressors are indicated for hypotension that does not respond to atropine. Following the initial resuscitation, attention is turned to managing muscarinic symptoms. Atropine competitively antagonizes acetylcholine at muscarinic receptors and is the treatment of choice. Unlike standard ACLS-recommended doses of atropine, the initial dose is 1 to 5 mg, with subsequent doses doubled and administered every 2 to 3 minutes as needed.[418] The endpoint of treatment is improvement of pulmonary symptoms, which may require large doses.

Pralidoxime is effective in regenerating acetylcholinesterase that has been inactivated by an organophosphate. It should be considered even in late presentations. Bound enzyme that has not undergone the aging process is liberated when the nucleophilic oxime attacks the phosphorus atom of the bound organophosphate. The increase in acetylcholinesterase should ameliorate both muscarinic and nicotinic symptoms, whereas atropine is effective only for muscarinic symptoms. It is not considered useful for carbamates; however, it is generally not contraindicated and should be utilized when it is unclear whether an organophosphate or carbamate is involved.

Patients who are asymptomatic or who have mild symptoms that resolve without treatment may be discharged home. Patients with persistent symptoms should be admitted. Those requiring treatment should be closely observed for recurrence and have red blood cell cholinesterase levels assayed. They may be medically cleared once they have been asymptomatic for 24 to 48 hours and their red blood cell cholinesterase levels are stable.

Conclusion

Utilizing a methodical approach that focuses on aggressive supportive care and the principles of ACLS optimizes care of the critically ill poisoned patient. Consideration must be given to nonstandard absorption, distribution, and elimination when drugs are taken in overdose. Attention to clinical clues and laboratory findings can narrow the differential diagnosis. The focus can then turn to advanced decontamination, enhanced elimination, and antidotal therapy.

Synthesis of basic science and clinical research is essential for continued optimal advanced care of the poisoned patient. Examples of such advances are hydroxocobalamin for cyanide toxicity, HIE therapy for poisoning with a calcium channel antagonist, and the emerging utility of intralipid. This work has expanded therapeutic options and is important for the management of these common yet potentially complicated cardiotoxic patients.

References

1. Erickson TB, Thompson TM, Lu JJ. The approach to the patient with an unknown overdose. *Emerg Med Clin North Am* 2007;25(2):249–281; abstract vii.
2. Aks SE, et al. Toxicology update: A rational approach to managing the poisoned patient. *Emerg Med Pract* 2001;3(8).
3. Erickson TB, Aks S, Gussow L. Diagnosis and management of the overdosed patient: a rational approach to the toxic patient. *EM Practice* 2001;1–25.
4. Part 102: Toxicology in ECC. *Circulation* 2005;112(24 Suppl):IV-126–IV-132.
5. Kienbaum P, et al. Profound increase in epinephrine concentration in plasma and cardiovascular stimulation after mu-opioid receptor blockade in opioid-addicted patients during barbiturate-induced anesthesia for acute detoxification. *Anesthesiology* 1998;88(5):1154–1161.
6. Mills CA, et al. Narcotic reversal in hypercapnic dogs: comparison of naloxone and nalbuphine. *Can J Anaesth* 1990;37(2):238–244.
7. Osterwalder JJ. Naloxone—for intoxications with intravenous heroin and heroin mixtures—harmless or hazardous? A prospective clinical study. *J Toxicol Clin Toxicol* 1996;34(4):409–416.
8. Toxicology in Emergency Cardiovascular Care 2005
9. Moss ST, et al. Outcome study of prehospital patients signed out against medical advice by field paramedics. *Ann Emerg Med* 1998;31(2):247–250.
10. Vilke GM, et al. Are heroin overdose deaths related to patient release after prehospital treatment with naloxone? *Prehosp Emerg Care* 1999;3(3):183–186.
11. Vilke GM, et al. Assessment for deaths in out-of-hospital heroin overdose patients treated with naloxone who refuse transport. *Acad Emerg Med* 2003;10(8):893–896.
12. Sporer KA, Dorn E. Heroin-related noncardiogenic pulmonary edema: a case series. *Chest* 2001;120(5):1628–1632.
13. Sporer KA, Firestone J, Isaacs SM. Out-of-hospital treatment of opioid overdoses in an urban setting *Acad Emerg Med* 1996;3(7):660–667.
14. Sporer KA. Acute heroin overdose. *Ann Intern Med* 1999; 130(7):584–590.
15. Mintzer MZ, Griffiths RR. Flumazenil-precipitated withdrawal in healthy volunteers following repeated diazepam exposure. *Psychopharmacology (Berl)* 2005;178(2–3):259–267.
16. Mintzer MZ, Stoller KB, Griffiths RR. A controlled study of flumazenil-precipitated withdrawal in chronic low-dose benzodiazepine users. *Psychopharmacology (Berl)* 1999;147(2):200–209.
17. Lukas SE, Griffiths RR. Precipitated withdrawal by a benzodiazepine receptor antagonist (Ro 15-1788) after 7 days of diazepam. *Science* 1982;217(4565):1161–1163.
18. Barnett R, et al. Flumazenil in drug overdose: randomized placebo-controlled study to assess cost effectiveness. *Crit Care Med* 1999;27(1):78–81.
19. Gueye PN, et al. Empiric use of flumazenil in comatose patients: limited applicability of criteria to define low risk. *Ann Emerg Med* 1996;27(6):730–735.
20. Haverkos GP, DiSalvo RP, Imhoff TE. Fatal seizures after flumazenil administration in a patient with mixed overdose. *Ann Pharmacother* 1994;28(12):1347–1349.
21. Spivey WH. Flumazenil and seizures: analysis of 43 cases. *Clin Ther* 1992;14(2):292–305.
22. Chyka PA, et al. Position paper: single-dose activated charcoal. *Clin Toxicol (Phila)* 2005;43(2):61–87.
23. Gomez HF, et al. Charcoal stercolith with intestinal perforation in a patient treated for amitriptyline ingestion. *J Emerg Med* 1994;12(1):57–60.
24. Seger D. Single-dose activated charcoal-backup and reassess. *J Toxicol Clin Toxicol* 2004;42(1):101–110.
25. Allerton JP, Strom JA. Hypernatremia due to repeated doses of charcoal-sorbitol. *Am J Kidney Dis* 1991;17(5):581–584.
26. Farley TA. Severe hypernatremic dehydration after use of an activated charcoal-sorbitol suspension. *J Pediatr* 1986;109(4):719–722.
27. Gazda-Smith E, Synhavsky A. Hypernatremia following treatment of theophylline toxicity with activated charcoal and sorbitol. *Arch Intern Med* 1990;150(3):689–692.
28. Moore CM. Hypernatremia after the use of an activated charcoal-sorbitol suspension. *J Pediatr* 1988;112(2):333.
29. Chin L, et al. Optimal antidotal dose of activated charcoal. *Toxicol Appl Pharmacol* 1973;26(1):103–108.
30. Levy G, Tsuchiya T. Effect of activated charcoal on aspirin absorption in man: Part I. *Clin Pharmacol Ther* 1972;13(3):317–322.
31. Levy G, Houston JB. Effect of activated charcoal on acetaminophen absorption. *Pediatrics* 1976;58(3):432–435.
32. Gastric lavage (The AACT/EAPCCT position statements on gastrointestinal decontamination). *J Toxicol Clin Toxicol* 1997;(9):711.
33. Merigian KS, et al. Prospective evaluation of gastric emptying in the self-poisoned patient. *Am J Emerg Med* 1990;8(6):479–483.
34. Kulig K, et al. Management of acutely poisoned patients without gastric emptying. *Ann Emerg Med* 1985;14(6):562–567.
35. Tenenbein M. Inefficacy of gastric emptying procedures. *J Emerg Med* 1985;3(2):133–136.
36. Tenenbein M, Cohen S, Sitar DS. Efficacy of ipecac-induced emesis orogastric lavage and activated charcoal for acute drug overdose. *Ann Emerg Med* 1987;16(8):838–841.
37. Grierson R, et al. Gastric lavage for liquid poisons. *Ann Emerg Med* 2000;35(5):435–439.
38. Tenenbein M. Whole bowel irrigation as a gastrointestinal decontamination procedure after acute poisoning. *Med Toxicol Adverse Drug Exp* 1988;3(2):77–84.
39. Position paper: whole bowel irrigation. *J Toxicol Clin Toxicol* 2004;42(6):843–854.
40. Palatnick W, Tenenbein M. Safety of treating poisoning patients with whole bowel irrigation. *Am J Emerg Med* 1988 6(2):200–201.
41. Traub SJ, et al. Pediatric "body packing." *Arch Pediatr Adolesc Med* 2003;157(2):174–177.

42. Clifton JC II, et al. Acute pediatric lead poisoning: combined whole bowel irrigation succimer therapy and endoscopic removal of ingested lead pellets. *Pediatr Emerg Care* 2002;18(3):200–202.

43. Kaczorowski JM, Wax PM. Five days of whole-bowel irrigation in a case of pediatric iron ingestion. *Ann Emerg Med* 1996;27(2):258–263.

44. Roberge RJ, Martin TG. Whole bowel irrigation in an acute oral lead intoxication. *Am J Emerg Med* 1992;10(6):577–583.

45. Hoffman RS, Smilkstein MJ, Goldfrank LR. Whole bowel irrigation and the cocaine body-packer: a new approach to a common problem. *Am J Emerg Med* 1990;8(6):523–527.

46. Burkhart KK, Kulig KW, Rumack B. Whole-bowel irrigation as treatment for zinc sulfate overdose. *Ann Emerg Med* 1990;19(10):1167–1170.

47. Vale JA. Position statement and practice guidelines on the use of multi-dose activated charcoal in the treatment of acute poisoning. American Academy of Clinical Toxicology; European Association of Poisons Centres and Clinical Toxicologists. *J Toxicol Clin Toxicol* 1999;37(6):731–751.

48. Bradberry SM, Vale JA. Multiple-dose activated charcoal: a review of relevant clinical studies. *J Toxicol Clin Toxicol* 1995;33(5):407–416.

49. Ilkhanipour K, Yealy DM, Krenzelok EP. The comparative efficacy of various multiple-dose activated charcoal regimens. *Am J Emerg Med* 1992;10(4):298–300.

50. Proudfoot AT, Krenzelok EP, Vale JA. Position paper on urine alkalinization. *J Toxicol Clin Toxicol* 2004;42(1):1–26.

51. Proudfoot AT, et al. Does urine alkalinization increase salicylate elimination? If so why? *Toxicol Rev* 2003;22(3):129–136.

52. Macpherson CR, Milne MD, Evans BM. The excretion of salicylate. *Br J Pharmacol Chemother* 1955;10(4):484–489.

53. Flomenbaum NE. Salicylates. In Flomenbaum NE, Goldfrank LR, Hoffman RS, et al, eds. *Goldfrank's Toxicologic Emergencies*, 8th ed. New York: McGraw–Hill, 2007.

54. Temple AR. Acute and chronic effects of aspirin toxicity and their treatment. *Arch Intern Med* 1981;141(3 Spec No):364–369.

55. Yip L, Dart RC, Gabow PA. Concepts and controversies in salicylate toxicity. *Emerg Med Clin North Am* 1994;12(2):351–364.

56. Tapolyai M, et al. Hemodialysis is as effective as hemoperfusion for drug removal in carbamazepine poisoning. *Nephron* 2002;90(2):213–215.

57. Schuerer DJ, et al. High–efficiency dialysis for carbamazepine overdose. *J Toxicol Clin Toxicol* 2000;38(3):321–323.

58. Kielstein JT, et al. High–flux hemodialysis—an effective alternative to hemoperfusion in the treatment of carbamazepine intoxication. *Clin Nephrol* 2002;57(6):484–486.

59. Kielstein JT, et al. Efficiency of high–flux hemodialysis in the treatment of valproic acid intoxication. *J Toxicol Clin Toxicol* 2003;41(6):873–876.

60. Kay TD Playford HR, Johnson DW. Hemodialysis versus continuous veno-venous hemodiafiltration in the management of severe valproate overdose. *Clin Nephrol* 2003;59(1):56–58.

61. Hicks LK, McFarlane PA. Valproic acid overdose and haemodialysis. *Nephrol Dial Transplant* 2001;16(7):1483–1486.

62. Kane SL, et al. High-flux hemodialysis without hemoperfusion is effective in acute valproic acid overdose. *Ann Pharmacother* 2000;34(10):1146–1151.

63. Shalkham AS, et al. The availability and use of charcoal hemoperfusion in the treatment of poisoned patients. *Am J Kidney Dis* 2006;48(2):239–241.

64. Al Aly Z, Yalamanchili P, Gonzalez E. Extracorporeal management of valproic acid toxicity: a case report and review of the literature. *Semin Dial* 2005;18(1):62–66.

65. Meyer RJ, et al. Hemodialysis followed by continuous hemofiltration for treatment of lithium intoxication in children. *Am J Kidney Dis* 2001;37(5):1044–1047.

66. van Bommel EF, Kalmeijer MD, Ponssen HH. Treatment of life-threatening lithium toxicity with high-volume continuous venovenous hemofiltration. *Am J Nephrol* 2000;20(5):408–411.

67. Rosenberg J, et al. Hyperthermia associated with drug intoxication. *Crit Care Med* 1986;14(11):964–969.

68. Martinez M, et al. Drug-associated heat stroke. *South Med J* 2002;95(8):799–802.

69. Lai MW, et al. 2005 Annual Report of the American Association of Poison Control Centers' national poisoning and exposure database. *Clin Toxicol (Phila)* 2006;44(6–7):803–932.

70. Frishman WH. Clinical differences between beta-adrenergic blocking agents: implications for therapeutic substitution. *Am Heart J* 1987;113(5):1190–1198.

71. Katz AM. Selectivity and toxicity of antiarrhythmic drugs: molecular interactions with ion channels. *Am J Med* 1998;104(2):179–195.

72. Frishman WH. Clinical significance of beta 1–selectivity and intrinsic sympathomimetic activity in a beta-adrenergic blocking drug. *Am J Cardiol* 1987;59(13):33F–37F.

73. Henry JA, Cassidy SL. Membrane stabilising activity: a major cause of fatal poisoning. *Lancet* 1986;1(8495):1414–1417.

74. Love JN, et al. Electrocardiographic changes associated with beta-blocker toxicity. *Ann Emerg Med* 2002:40(6):603–610.

75. Frishman W, et al. Clinical pharmacology of the new beta-adrenergic blocking drugs: Part 8. Self-poisoning with beta-adrenoceptor blocking agents: recognition and management. *Am Heart J* 1979;98(6):798–811.

76. Love JN, et al. Acute beta blocker overdose: factors associated with the development of cardiovascular morbidity. *J Toxicol Clin Toxicol* 2000;38(3):275–281.

77. Weinstein RS. Recognition and management of poisoning with beta–adrenergic blocking agents *Ann Emerg Med* 1984;13(12):1123–1131.

78. Brubacher J. Beta-adrenergic agonists. In Flomenbaum NE, Howland M, Goldfrank LR, et al, eds. *Goldfrank's Toxicologic Emergencies*, 8th ed. New York: McGraw–Hill, 2007.

79. Hohnloser SH, Woosley RL. Sotalol. *N Engl J Med* 1994;331(1):31–38.

80. Reith DM, et al. Relative toxicity of beta blockers in overdose. *J Toxicol Clin Toxicol* 1996;34(3):273–278.

81. Delk C, Holstege CP, Brady WJ. Electrocardiographic abnormalities associated with poisoning. *Am J Emerg Med* 2007;25(6):672–687.

82. Pollack CV Jr. Utility of glucagon in the emergency department. *J Emerg Med* 1993;11(2):195–205.

83. Taboulet P, et al. Pathophysiology and management of self–poisoning with beta blockers. *J Toxicol Clin Toxicol* 1993;31(4):531–551.

84. Yagami T. Differential coupling of glucagon and beta-adrenergic receptors with the small and large forms of the stimulatory G protein. *Mol Pharmacol* 1995;48(5):849–854.

85. Rochais F, et al. A specific pattern of phosphodiesterases controls the cAMP signals generated by different Gs-coupled receptors in adult rat ventricular myocytes. *Circ Res* 2006;98(8):1081–1088.

86. Donovan KD, Gerace RV, Dreyer JF. Acebutolol-induced ventricular tachycardia reversed with sodium bicarbonate. *J Toxicol Clin Toxicol* 1999;37(4):481–484.

87. Kerns W II. Management of beta-adrenergic blocker and calcium channel antagonist toxicity. *Emerg Med Clin North Am* 2007;25(2):309–331; abstract viii.

88. Kerns W, et al. Insulin improves survival in a canine model of acute beta-blocker toxicity. *Ann Emerg Med* 1997;29(6):748–757.

89. Holger JS, et al. Insulin versus vasopressin and epinephrine to treat beta-blocker toxicity. *Clin Toxicol (Phila)* 2007;45(4):396–401.

90. Yuan TH, et al. Insulin–glucose as adjunctive therapy for severe calcium channel antagonist poisoning. *J Toxicol Clin Toxicol* 1999;37(4):463–474.

91. Kenyon CJ, et al. Successful resuscitation using external cardiac pacing in beta adrenergic antagonist–induced bradyasystolic arrest. *Ann Emerg Med* 1988;17(7):711–713.

92. Lane AS, Woodward AC, Goldman MR. Massive propranolol overdose poorly responsive to pharmacologic therapy: use of the intra-aortic balloon pump. *Ann Emerg Med* 1987;16(12):1381–1383.

93. Rooney M, et al. Acebutolol overdose treated with hemodialysis and extracorporeal membrane oxygenation. *J Clin Pharmacol* 1996;36(8):760–763.

94. Saitz R, Williams BW, Farber HW. Atenolol-induced cardiovascular collapse treated with hemodialysis. *Crit Care Med* 1991;19(1):116–118.

95. Salhanick SD, Wax PM. Treatment of atenolol overdose in a patient with renal failure using serial hemodialysis and hemoperfusion and associated echocardiographic findings. *Vet Hum Toxicol* 2000;42(4):224–225.

96. Love JN. Beta blocker toxicity after overdose: when do symptoms develop in adults? *J Emerg Med* 1994;12(6):799–802.

97. Pitt B. Diversity of calcium antagonists. *Clin Ther* 1997;19(Suppl A):3–17.

98. Taira N. Differences in cardiovascular profile among calcium antagonists. *Am J Cardiol* 1987;59(3):24B–29B.

99. Barrett TD, et al. Mechanism of tissue-selective drug action in the cardiovascular system. *Mol Intervent* 2005;5(2):84–93.

100. Hondeghem LM, Katzung BG.Antiarrhythmic agents: the modulated receptor mechanism of action of sodium and calcium channel–blocking drugs. *Annu Rev Pharmacol Toxicol* 1984;24:387–423.

101. Leikin JB, Palouchek FP, eds. *Poisoning and Toxicology Handbook*, 3rd ed. Hudson, OH: Lexi-Comp, 2002.

102. Levine M, et al. Assessment of hyperglycemia after calcium channel blocker overdoses involving diltiazem or verapamil. *Crit Care Med* 2007;35(9):2071–2075.

103. Caulfield MP, Birdsall NJ. International Union of Pharmacology XVII Classification of muscarinic acetylcholine receptors. *Pharmacol Rev* 1998;50(2):279–290.

104. Wolf LR, Spadafora MP, Otten EJ. Use of amrinone and glucagon in a case of calcium channel blocker overdose. *Ann Emerg Med* 1993;22(7):1225–1228.

105. Haddad LM. Resuscitation after nifedipine overdose exclusively with intravenous calcium chloride. *Am J Emerg Med* 1996;14(6): 602–603.

106. Lam YM, Tse HF, Lau CP. Continuous calcium chloride infusion for massive nifedipine overdose. *Chest* 2001;119(4):1280–1282.

107. Luscher TF, et al. Calcium gluconate in severe verapamil intoxication. *N Engl J Med* 1994;330(10):718–720.

108. Spiller HA, et al. Delayed onset of cardiac arrhythmias from sustained-release verapamil. *Ann Emerg Med* 1991;20(2):201–203.

109. Perkins CM. Serious verapamil poisoning: treatment with intravenous calcium gluconate. *Br Med J* 1978;2(6145):1127.

110. Crump BJ, Holt DW, Vale JA. Lack of response to intravenous calcium in severe verapamil poisoning. *Lancet* 1982;2(8304): 939–940.

111. Horowitz BZ, Rhee KJ. Massive verapamil ingestion: a report of two cases and a review of the literature. *Am J Emerg Med* 1989; 7(6):624–631.

112. Kline JA, Leonova E, Raymond RM. Beneficial myocardial metabolic effects of insulin during verapamil toxicity in the anesthetized canine. *Crit Care Med* 1995;23(7):1251–1263.

113. Kline JA, et al. Myocardial metabolism during graded intraportal verapamil infusion in awake dogs. *J Cardiovasc Pharmacol* 1996; 27(5):719–726.

114. Kline JA, et al. The diabetogenic effects of acute verapamil poisoning. *Toxicol Appl Pharmacol* 1997;145(2):357–362.

115. Kline JA, et al. Insulin improves heart function and metabolism during non-ischemic cardiogenic shock in awake canines. *Cardiovasc Res* 1997;34(2):289–298.

116. Boyer EW, Shannon M. Treatment of calcium-channel-blocker intoxication with insulin infusion. *N Engl J Med* 2001;344(22): 1721–1722.

117. Boyer EW, Duic PA, Evans A. Hyperinsulinemia/euglycemia therapy for calcium channel blocker poisoning. *Pediatr Emerg Care* 2002;18(1):36–37.

118. Rasmussen L, Husted SE, Johnsen SP. Severe intoxication after an intentional overdose of amlodipine. *Acta Anaesthesiol Scand* 2003;47(8):1038–1040.

119. Marques ME, et al. Treatment of calcium channel blocker intoxication with insulin infusion: case report and literature review. *Resuscitation* 2003;57(2):211–213.

120. Harris NS. Case records of the Massachusetts General Hospital Case 24–2006. A 40-year-old woman with hypotension after an overdose of amlodipine. *N Engl J Med* 2006;355(6):602–611.

121. Ortiz-Munoz L, Rodriguez-Ospina LF, Figueroa-Gonzalez M. Hyperinsulinemic–euglycemic therapy for intoxication with calcium channel blockers. *Bol Asoc Med P R* 2005;97(3 Pt 2):182–189.

122. Lheureux PE, et al. Bench-to-bedside review: hyperinsulinaemia/euglycaemia therapy in the management of overdose of calcium-channel blockers. *Crit Care* 2006; 10(3):212.

123. Holzer M, et al. Successful resuscitation of a verapamil-intoxicated patient with percutaneous cardiopulmonary bypass. *Crit Care Med* 1999;27(12):2818–2823.

124. Frierson J, et al. Refractory cardiogenic shock and complete heart block after unsuspected verapamil-SR and atenolol overdose. *Clin Cardiol* 1991;14(11):933–935.

125. Hendren WG, Schieber RS, Garrettson LK. Extracorporeal bypass for the treatment of verapamil poisoning. *Ann Emerg Med* 1989;18(9):984–987.

126. Gheorghiade M, Adams KF Jr, Colucci WS.Digoxin in the management of cardiovascular disorders. *Circulation* 2004;109(24): 2959–2964.

127. Hauptman PJ, Garg R, Kelly RA. Cardiac glycosides in the next millennium. *Prog Cardiovasc Dis* 1999;41(4):247–254.

128. Levi AJ, Boyett MR, Lee CO. The cellular actions of digitalis glycosides on the heart. *Prog Biophys Mol Biol* 1994;62(1):1–54.

129. Dvela M, et al. Diverse biological responses to different cardiotonic steroids. *Pathophysiology* 2007;14(3–4):159–166.

130. Antman EM, Smith TW. Digitalis toxicity. *Annu Rev Med* 1985; 36:357–367.

131. Quan KJ, et al. Endocardial stimulation of efferent parasympathetic nerves to the atrioventricular node in humans: optimal stimulation sites and the effects of digoxin. *J Intervent Cardiol Electrophysiol* 2001;5(2):145–152.

132. Krum H, et al. Effect of long–term digoxin therapy on autonomic function in patients with chronic heart failure. *J Am Coll Cardiol* 1995;25(2):289–294.

133. Ferguson DW, et al. Sympathoinhibitory responses to digitalis glycosides in heart failure patients. Direct evidence from sympathetic neural recordings. *Circulation* 1989;80(1):65–77.

134. Kelly RA, Smith TW. Recognition and management of digitalis toxicity. *Am J Cardiol* 1992;69(18):108G–118G; discussion 118G–119G.

135. Clausen T. Clinical and therapeutic significance of the Na+K+ pump. *Clin Sci (Lond)* 1998;95(1):3–17.

136. Bigger JT Jr, Sahar DI. Clinical types of proarrhythmic response to antiarrhythmic drugs. *Am J Cardiol* 1987;59(11):2E–9E.

137. Smith TW, et al. Digitalis glycosides: mechanisms and manifestations of toxicity: Part I. *Prog Cardiovasc Dis* 1984;26(5):413–458.

138. Hack JB, Lewin NA. Cardioactive steroids. In Flomenbaum NE, Goldfrank LR, Hoffman RS, et al, eds. *Goldfrank's Toxicologic Emergencies*, 8th ed. New York: McGraw–Hill, 2006.

139. Wofford JL, Ettinger WH. Risk factors and manifestations of digoxin toxicity in the elderly. *Am J Emerg Med* 1991;9(2 Suppl 1): 11–15.

140. Mahdyoon H, et al. The evolving pattern of digoxin intoxication: observations at a large urban hospital from 1980 to 1988. *Am Heart J* 1990;120(5):1189–1194.

141. Lely AH, van Enter CH. Large–scale digitoxin intoxication. *Br Med J* 1970;3(5725):737–740.

142. Irons GV Jr, Orgain ES. Digitalis-induced arrhythmias and their management. *Prog Cardiovasc Dis* 1966;8(6):539–569.

143. Smith SW, et al. Bidirectional ventricular tachycardia resulting from herbal aconite poisoning. *Ann Emerg Med* 2005;45(1):100–101.

144. Ordog GJ, et al. Serum digoxin levels and mortality in 5100 patients. *Ann Emerg Med* 1987;16(1):32–9.

145. Dally S, et al. [Prognostic factors in acute digitalis poisoning (author's transl)]. *Nouv Presse Med* 1981;10(27):2257–2260.

146. Critchley JA, Critchley LA. Digoxin toxicity in chronic renal failure: treatment by multiple dose activated charcoal intestinal dialysis. *Hum Exp Toxicol* 1997;16(12):733–735.

147. Lalonde RL, et al. Acceleration of digoxin clearance by activated charcoal. *Clin Pharmacol Ther* 1985;37(4):367–371.

148. Hickey AR, et al. Digoxin Immune Fab therapy in the management of digitalis intoxication: safety and efficacy results of an observational surveillance study. *J Am Coll Cardiol* 1991;17(3): 590–598.

149. Antman EM, et al. Treatment of 150 cases of life-threatening digitalis intoxication with digoxin-specific Fab antibody fragments. Final report of a multicenter study. *Circulation* 1990;81(6): 1744–1752.

150. Smith TW, et al. Treatment of life–threatening digitalis intoxication with digoxin-specific Fab antibody fragments: experience in 26 cases. *N Engl J Med* 1982;307(22):1357–1362.

151. Smolarz A, et al. Digoxin specific antibody (Fab) fragments in 34 cases of severe digitalis intoxication. *J Toxicol Clin Toxicol* 1985; 23(4–6):327–340.

152. Taboulet P, et al. Acute digitalis intoxication—is pacing still appropriate? *J Toxicol Clin Toxicol* 1993;31(2):261–273.

153. Smith TW, et al. Reversal of advanced digoxin intoxication with Fab fragments of digoxin-specific antibodies. *N Engl J Med* 1976;294(15):797–800.

154. Van Deusen SK, Birkhahn RH, Gaeta TJ. Treatment of hyper-kalemia in a patient with unrecognized digitalis toxicity. *J Toxicol Clin Toxicol* 2003;41(4):373–376.

155. Hack JB, et al. The effect of calcium chloride in treating hyper-kalemia due to acute digoxin toxicity in a porcine model. *J Toxicol Clin Toxicol* 2004;42(4):337–342.

156. Rumack BH, Wolfe RR, Gilfrich H. Phenytoin (diphenylhydan-toin) treatment of massive digoxin overdose. *Br Heart J* 1974;36(4):405–408.

157. Harris AS, Kokernot RH. Effects of diphenylhydantoin sodium (dilantin sodium) and phenobarbital sodium upon ectopic ventricular tachycardia in acute myocardial infarction. *Am J Physiol* 1950;163(3):505–516.

158. Mason DT, et al. Current concepts and treatment of digitalis toxicity. *Am J Cardiol* 1971;27(5):546–559.

159. Reisdorff EJ, Clark MR, Walters BL. Acute digitalis poisoning: the role of intravenous magnesium sulfate. *J Emerg Med* 1986;4(6):463–469.

160. French JH, et al. Magnesium therapy in massive digoxin intoxication. *Ann Emerg Med* 1984;13(7):562–566.

161. Bismuth C, et al. Acute digitoxin intoxication treated by intracardiac pacemaker: experience in sixty-eight patients. *Clin Toxicol* 1977;10(4):443–456.

162. Eddleston M, et al. Anti-digoxin Fab fragments in cardiotoxicity induced by ingestion of yellow oleander: a randomised controlled trial. *Lancet* 2000;355(9208):967–972.

163. Eddleston M, et al. Deaths due to absence of an affordable anti-toxin for plant poisoning. *Lancet* 2003;362(9389):1041–1044.

164. de Silva HA, et al. Multiple-dose activated charcoal for treatment of yellow oleander poisoning: a single-blind randomised placebo-controlled trial. *Lancet* 2003;361(9373):1935–1938.

165. Durieux ME. Muscarinic signaling in the central nervous system. Recent developments and anesthetic implications. *Anesthesiology* 1996;84(1):173–189.

166. Thakur AC, et al. QT interval prolongation in diphenhydramine toxicity. *Int J Cardiol* 2005;98(2):341–343.

167. Krenzelok EP, Anderson GM, Mirick M. Massive diphenhydramine overdose resulting in death. *Ann Emerg Med* 1982;11(4):212–213.

168. Clark RF Vance MV. Massive diphenhydramine poisoning resulting in a wide–complex tachycardia: successful treatment with sodium bicarbonate. *Ann Emerg Med* 1992;21(3):318–321.

169. Pratt CM, et al. Risk of developing life-threatening ventricular arrhythmia associated with tefenadine in comparison with over-the-counter antihistamines ibuprofen and clemastine. *Am J Cardiol* 1994;73(5):346–352.

170. Soto LF, Miller CH, Ognibere AJ. Severe rhabdomyolysis after doxylamine overdose. *Postgrad Med* 1993;93(8):227–232.

171. Frankel D, Dolgin J, Murray BM. Non-traumatic rhabdomyolysis complicating antihistamine overdose. *J Toxicol Clin Toxicol* 1993;31(3):493–496.

172. Leybishkis B, Fasseas P, Ryan KF. Doxylamine overdose as a potential cause of rhabdomyolysis. *Am J Med Sci* 2001;322(1): 48–49.

173. Koppel C, Ibe K, Oberdisse U. Rhabdomyolysis in doxylamine overdose. *Lancet* 1987;1(8530):442–443.

174. Reilly JF Jr, Weisse ME. Topically induced diphenhydramine toxicity. *J Emerg Med* 1990;8(1):59–61.

175. Reilly KM, et al. Systemic toxicity from ocular homatropine. *Acad Emerg Med* 1996;3(9):868–871.

176. Sharma AN, et al. Diphenhydramine-induced wide complex dys-rhythmia responds to treatment with sodium bicarbonate. *Am J Emerg Med* 2003;21(3):212–215.

177. Farrell M, Heinrichs M, Tilelli JA. Response of life threatening dimenhydrinate intoxication to sodium bicarbonate administration. *J Toxicol Clin Toxicol* 1991;29(4):527–535.

178. Burns MJ, et al. A comparison of physostigmine and benzodiazepines for the treatment of anticholinergic poisoning. *Ann Emerg Med* 2000;35(4):374–381.

179. Ceha LJ, et al. Anticholinergic toxicity from nightshade berry poisoning responsive to physostigmine. *J Emerg Med* 1997;15(1): 65–69.

180. Teoh R, Page AV, Hardern R. Physostigmine as treatment for severe CNS anticholinergic toxicity. *Emerg Med J* 2001;18(5):412.

181. Richmond M, Seger D. Central anticholinergic syndrome in a child: a case report. *J Emerg Med* 1985;3(6):453–456.

182. Suchard JR. Assessing physostigmine's contraindication in cyclic antidepressant ingestions. *J Emerg Med* 2003;25(2):185–191.

183. Pentel P, Peterson CD. Asystole complicating physostigmine treatment of tricyclic antidepressant overdose. *Ann Emerg Med* 1980;9(11):588–590.

184. Frascogna N. Physostigmine: is there a role for this antidote in pediatric poisonings? *Curr Opin Pediatr* 2007;19(2):201–205.

185. Newton CR, Delgado JH, Gomez HF. Calcium and beta receptor antagonist overdose: a review and update of pharmacological principles and management. *Semin Respir Crit Care Med* 2002;23(1):19–25.

186. Walker WE, Levy RC, Hanenson IB. Physostigmine—its use and abuse. *JACEP* 1976;5(6):436–439.

187. Knudsen K, Heath A. Effects of self poisoning with maprotiline. *Br Med J (Clin Res Ed)* 1984;288(6417):601–603.

188. Shannon M. Toxicology reviews: physostigmine. *Pediatr Emerg Care* 1998;14(3):224–226.

189. Benowitz NL, Rosenberg J, Becker CE. Cardiopulmonary catastrophes in drug-overdosed patients. *Med Clin North Am* 1979;63(1):267–296.

190. Thorstrand C. Cardiovascular effects of poisoning by hypnotic and tricyclic antidepressant drugs. *Acta Med Scand Suppl* 1975; 583:1–34.

191. Kantor SJ, et al. The cardiac effects of therapeutic plasma concentrations of imipramine *Am J Psychiatry* 1978;135(5):534–538.

192. Bigger JT, et al. Cardiac antiarrhythmic effect of imipramine hydrochloride. *N Engl J Med* 1977;296(4):206–208.

193. Kolecki PF, Curry SC. Poisoning by sodium channel blocking agents. *Crit Care Clin* 1997;13(4):829–848.

194. Vieweg WV, Wood MA. Tricyclic antidepressants. QT interval prolongation and torsades de pointes. *Psychosomatics* 2004;45(5): 371–377.

195. Yap YG, Camm AJ. Drug induced QT prolongation and torsades de pointes. *Heart* 2003;89(11):1363–1372.

196. Darpo B. Spectrum of drugs prologing QT interval and the incidence of torsades de pointes. *Eur Heart J* 2001; (Suppl 3): K70–K80.

197. Callaham M, Kassel D. Epidemiology of fatal tricyclic antidepressant ingestion: implications for management. *Ann Emerg Med* 1985;14(1):1–9.

198. Ellison DW, Pentel PR. Clinical features and consequences of seizures due to cyclic antidepressant overdose, *Am J Emerg Med* 1989;7(1):5–10.

199. Fasoli RA Glauser FL. Cardiac arrhythmias and ECG abnormalities in tricyclic antidepressant overdose. *Clin Toxicol* 1981;18(2): 155–163.

200. Foulke GE, Albertson TE. QRS interval in tricyclic antidepressant overdosage: inaccuracy as a toxicity indicator in emergency settings. *Ann Emerg Med* 1987;16(2):160–163.

201. Foulke GE. Identifying toxicity risk early after antidepressant overdose. *Am J Emerg Med* 1995;13(2):123–126.

202. Boehnert MT, Lovejoy FH Jr. Value of the QRS duration versus the serum drug level in predicting seizures and ventricular arrhythmias after an acute overdose of tricyclic antidepressants. *N Engl J Med* 1985;313(8):474–479.

203. Niemann JT, et al. Electrocardiographic criteria for tricyclic antidepressant cardiotoxicity. *Am J Cardiol* 1986;57(13):1154–1159.

204. Wolfe TR, Caravati EM, Rollins DE. Terminal 40-ms frontal plane QRS axis as a marker for tricyclic antidepressant overdose. *Ann Emerg Med* 1989;18(4):348–351.

205. Liebelt EL, Francis PD, Woolf AD. ECG lead aVR versus QRS interval in predicting seizures and arrhythmias in acute tricyclic antidepressant toxicity. *Ann Emerg Med* 1995;26(2):195–201.

206. Liebelt EL, et al. Serial electrocardiogram changes in acute tricyclic antidepressant overdoses. *Crit Care Med* 1997;25(10):1721–1726.

207. Wedin GP, et al. Relative toxicity of cyclic antidepressants. *Ann Emerg Med* 1986;15(7):797–804.

208. Blackman K, Brown SG, Wilkes GJ. Plasma alkalinization for tricyclic antidepressant toxicity: a systematic review. *Emerg Med (Fremantle)* 2001;13(2):204–210.

209. Hoffman JR, McElroy CR. Bicarbonate therapy for dysrhythmia and hypotension in tricyclic antidepressant overdose. *West J Med* 1981;134(1):60–64.

210. Hoffman JR, et al. Effect of hypertonic sodium bicarbonate in the treatment of moderate-to-severe cyclic antidepressant overdose. *Am J Emerg Med* 1993;11(4):336–341.

211. Molloy DW, et al. Use of sodium bicarbonate to treat tricyclic antidepressant-induced arrhythmias in a patient with alkalosis. *Can Med Assoc J* 1984;130(11):1457–1459.

212. Teba L, et al. Beneficial effect of norepinephrine in the treatment of circulatory shock caused by tricyclic antidepressant overdose. *Am J Emerg Med* 1988;6(6):566–568.

213. Knudsen K, Abrahamsson J. Effects of magnesium sulfate and lidocaine in the treatment of ventricular arrhythmias in experimental amitriptyline poisoning in the rat. *Crit Care Med* 1994;22(3):494–498.

214. Nattel S, Mittleman M. Treatment of ventricular tachyarrhythmias resulting from amitriptyline toxicity in dogs. *J Pharmacol Exp Ther* 1984;231(2):430–435.

215. Mayron R, Ruiz E. Phenytoin: does it reverse tricyclic-antidepressant-induced cardiac conduction abnormalities? *Ann Emerg Med* 1986;15(8):876–880.

216. Callaham M, Schumaker H, Pentel P. Phenytoin prophylaxis of cardiotoxicity in experimental amitriptyline poisoning. *J Pharmacol Exp Ther* 1988;245(1):216–220.

217. Knudsen K, Abrahamsson J. Effects of epinephrine norepinephrine magnesium sulfate and milrinone on survival and the occurrence of arrhythmias in amitriptyline poisoning in the rat. *Crit Care Med* 1994;22(11):1851–1855.

218. Kline JA, et al. Magnesium potentiates imipramine toxicity in the isolated rat heart. *Ann Emerg Med* 1994;24(2):224–232.

219. Sarisoy O, et al. Efficacy of magnesium sulfate for treatment of ventricular tachycardia in amitriptyline intoxication. *Pediatr Emerg Care* 2007;23(9):646–648.

220. Citak A, et al. Efficacy of long duration resuscitation and magnesium sulphate treatment in amitriptyline poisoning. *Eur J Emerg Med* 2002;9(1):63–66.

221. Knudsen K, Abrahamsson J. Magnesium sulphate in the treatment of ventricular fibrillation in amitriptyline poisoning. *Eur Heart J* 1997;18(5):881–882.

222. Merigian KS, Browning RG, Leeper KV. Successful treatment of amoxapine–induced refractory status epilepticus with propofol (diprivan). *Acad Emerg Med* 1995;2(2):128–133.

223. Isbister GK, et al. Relative toxicity of selective serotonin reuptake inhibitors (SSRIs) in overdose. *J Toxicol Clin Toxicol* 2004;42(3):277–285.

224. Whyte IM, Dawson AH, Buckley NA. Relative toxicity of venlafaxine and selective serotonin reuptake inhibitors in overdose compared to tricyclic antidepressants. *Q J Med* 2003;96(5):369–374.

225. Kelly CA, et al. Comparative toxicity of citalopram and the newer antidepressants after overdose. *J Toxicol Clin Toxicol* 2004;42(1):67–71.

226. Engebretsen KM, Harris CR, Wood JE. Cardiotoxicity and late onset seizures with citalopram overdose. *J Emerg Med* 2003;25(2):163–166.

227. Holmgren P, et al. Enantioselective analysis of citalopram and its metabolites in postmortem blood and genotyping for CYD2D6 and CYP2C19. *J Anal Toxicol* 2004;28(2):94–104.

228. Greiner C, et al. Determination of citalopram and escitalopram together with their active main metabolites desmethyl(es-)citalopram in human serum by column-switching high performance liquid chromatography (HPLC) and spectrophotometric detection. *J Chromatogr B Analyt Technol Biomed Life Sci* 2007;848(2):391–394.

229. Deupree JD, Montgomery MD, Bylund DB. Pharmacological properties of the active metabolites of the antidepressants desipramine and citalopram. *Eur J Pharmacol* 2007;576(1–3):55–60.

230. von Moltke LL, et al. Escitalopram (S-citalopram) and its metabolites in vitro: cytochromes mediating biotransformation inhibitory effects and comparison to R-citalopram. *Drug Metab Dispos* 2001;29(8):1102–1109.

231. Catalano G, et al. QTc interval prolongation associated with citalopram overdose: a case report and literature review. *Clin Neuropharmacol* 2001;24(3):158–162.

232. Rasmussen SL, Overo KF, Tanghoj P. Cardiac safety of citalopram: prospective trials and retrospective analyses. *J Clin Psychopharmacol* 1999;19(5):407–415.

233. Isbister GK, Friberg LE, Duffull SB. Application of pharmacokinetic-pharmacodynamic modelling in management of QT abnormalities after citalopram overdose. *Intens Care Med* 2006;32(7):1060–1065.

234. Personne M, Sjoberg G, Persson H. Citalopram overdose—review of cases treated in Swedish hospitals. *J Toxicol Clin Toxicol* 1997;35(3):237–240.

235. Meuleman C, et al. [Citalopram and torsades de pointes. A case report]. *Arch Mal Coeur Vaiss* 2001;94(9):1021–1024.

236. Tarabar AF, Hoffman RS, Nelson LS. Citalopram overdose: late presentation of torsades de pointes (TdP) with cardiac arrest [abstract]. *J Toxicol Clin Toxicol* 2003;41(5):676.

237. Wilting I, et al. QTc prolongation and torsades de pointes in an elderly woman taking fluoxetine. *Am J Psychiatry* 2006;163(2):325.

238. Deshauer D. Venlafaxine (Effexor): concerns about increased risk of fatal outcomes in overdose. *CMAJ* 2007;176(1):39–40.

239. Shepherd G, Velez LI, Keyes DC. Intentional bupropion overdoses. *J Emerg Med* 2004;27(2):147–151.

240. Shrier M, Diaz JE, Tsarouhas N. Cardiotoxicity associated with bupropion overdose. *Ann Emerg Med* 2000;35(1):100.

241. Tracey JA, et al. Bupropion (Zyban) toxicity. *Ir Med J* 2002;95(1):23–24.

242. Givens ML, Gabrysch J. Cardiotoxicity associated with accidental bupropion ingestion in a child. *Pediatr Emerg Care* 2007;23(4):234–237.

243. Bymaster FP, et al. Comparative affinity of duloxetine and venlafaxine for serotonin and norepinephrine transporters in vitro and in vivo human serotonin receptor subtypes and other neuronal receptors. *Neuropsychopharmacology* 2001;25(6):871–880.

244. Howell C, Wilson AD, Waring WS. Cardiovascular toxicity due to venlafaxine poisoning in adults: a review of 235 consecutive cases. *Br J Clin Pharmacol* 2007;64(2):192–197.

245. Wilson AD, Howell C, Waring WS. Venlafaxine ingestion is associated with rhabdomyolysis in adults: a case series. *J Toxicol Sci* 2007;32(1):97–101.

246. Martinez MA, et al. Investigation of a fatality due to trazodone poisoning: case report and literature review. *J Anal Toxicol* 2005;29(4):262–268.

247. Cohn KE, Agmon J, Gamble OW. The effect of glucagon on arrhythmias due to digitalis toxicity. *Am J Cardiol* 1970;25(6):683–689.

248. Vanpee D, Laloyaux P, Gillet JB. Seizure and hyponatraemia after overdose of trazodone. *Am J Emerg Med* 1999;17(4):430–431.

249. Mazur A, et al. QT prolongation and polymorphous ventricular tachycardia associated with trasodone–amiodarone combination. *Int J Cardiol* 1995;52(1):27–29.

250. Levenson JL. Prolonged QT interval after trazodone overdose. *Am J Psychiatry* 1999;156(6):969–970.

251. Dattilo PB, Nordin C/ Prolonged QT associated with an overdose of trazodone. *J Clin Psychiatry* 2007;68(8):1309–1310.

252. Waring WS, Good AM, Bateman DN. Lack of significant toxicity after mirtazapine overdose: a five–year review of cases admitted to a regional toxicology unit. *Clin Toxicol (Phila)* 2007;45(1):45–50.

253. Isbister GK, et al. Activated charcoal decreases the risk of QT prolongation after citalopram overdose. *Ann Emerg Med* 2007;50(5):593–600.

254. Sirianni AJ, et al. Use of lipid emulsion in the resuscitation of a patient with prolonged cardiovascular collapse after overdose of bupropion and lamotrigine. *Ann Emerg Med* 2008;51(4):412–415.

255. Buckley NA, Whyte IM, Dawson AH. Cardiotoxicity more common in thioridazine overdose than with other neuroleptics. *J Toxicol Clin Toxicol* 1995;33(3):199–204.

256. Buckley N, McManus P. Fatal toxicity of drugs used in the treatment of psychotic illnesses. *Br J Psychiatry* 1998;172:461–464.

257. Pisani F, et al. Effects of psychotropic drugs on seizure threshold. *Drug Saf* 2002;25(2):91–110.

258. Reilly TH, Kirk MA. Atypical antipsychotics and newer antidepressants. *Emerg Med Clin North Am* 2007;25(2):477–497; abstract x.

259. Harrigan EP, et al. A randomized evaluation of the effects of six antipsychotic agents on QTc in the absence and presence of metabolic inhibition. *J Clin Psychopharmacol* 2004;24(1):62–69.

260. Sala M, et al. QT interval prolongation related to psychoactive drug treatment: a comparison of monotherapy versus polytherapy. *Ann Gen Psychiatry* 2005;4(1):1.

261. Stollberger C, Huber JO, Finsterer J. Antipsychotic drugs and QT prolongation. *Int Clin Psychopharmacol* 2005;20(5):243–251.

262. Liu BA, Juurlink DN. Drugs and the QT interval—caveat doctor. *N Engl J Med* 2004;351(11):1053–1056.

263. Testai L, et al. Torsadogenic cardiotoxicity of antipsychotic drugs: a structural feature potentially involved in the interaction with cardiac HERG potassium channels. *Curr Med Chem* 2004;11(20):2691–706.

264. Vieweg WV, Schneider RK, Wood MA. Torsade de pointes in a patient with complex medical and psychiatric conditions receiving low-dose quetiapine. *Acta Psychiatr Scand* 2005;112(4):318–322; author reply 322.

265. Tei Y, et al. Torsades de pointes caused by a small dose of risperidone in a terminally ill cancer patient. *Psychosomatics* 2004;45(5):450–451.

266. O'Brien JM, Rockwood RP, Suh KI. Haloperidol-induced torsade de pointes. *Ann Pharmacother* 1999;33(10):1046–1050.

267. Denvir MA, et al. Thioridazine diarrhoea and torsades de pointe. *J R Soc Med* 1998;91(3):145–147.

268. Heinrich TW, Biblo LA, Schneider J. Torsades de pointes associated with ziprasidone. *Psychosomatics* 2006;47(3):264–268.

269. Ogata N, Narahashi T. Block of sodium channels by psychotropic drugs in single guinea-pig cardiac myocytes. *Br J Pharmacol* 1989;97(3):905–913.

270. Ravin DS, Levenson JW. Fatal cardiac event following initiation of risperidone therapy. *Ann Pharmacother* 1997;31(7–8):867–870.

271. Vertrees JE, Siebel G. Rapid death resulting from mesoridazine overdose. *Vet Hum Toxicol* 1987;29(1):65–67.

272. Biswas AK, et al. Cardiotoxicity associated with intentional ziprasidone and bupropion overdose. *J Toxicol Clin Toxicol* 2003; 41(2):101–104.

273. Niemann JT, et al. Cardiac conduction and rhythm disturbances following suicidal ingestion of mesoridazine. *Ann Emerg Med* 1981;10(11):585–8

274. Brown ET, Corbett SW, Green SM. Iatrogenic cardiopulmonary arrest during pediatric sedation with meperidine promethazine and chlorpromazine. *Pediatr Emerg Care* 2001;17(5):351–353.

275. Johri S, et al. Cardiopulmonary arrest secondary to haloperidol. *Am J Emerg Med* 2000;18(7):839.

276. Huyse F, van Schijndel RS. Haloperidol and cardiac arrest. *Lancet* 1988;2(8610):568–569.

277. Substance Abuse and Mental Health Services Administration. Results from the 2004 National Survey on Drug Use and Health: National Findings. NSDUH Series H–28. DDHS Publication No SMA 05-4062. Rockville, MD: Office of Applied Studies, 2005.

278. Seiden LS, Sabol KE, Ricaurte GA. Amphetamine: effects on catecholamine systems and behavior. *Annu Rev Pharmacol Toxicol* 1993:33:639–677.

279. Varner KJ, et al. Cardiovascular responses elicited by the "binge" administration of methamphetamine. *J Pharmacol Exp Ther* 2002; 301(1):152–159.

280. Quinton MS, Yamamoto BK. Causes and consequences of methamphetamine and MDMA toxicity. *AAPS J* 2006;8(2): E337–E347.

281. Fleckenstein AE, Gibb JW, Hanson GR. Differential effects of stimulants on monoaminergic transporters: pharmacological consequences and implications for neurotoxicity. *Eur J Pharmacol* 2000;406(1):1–13.

282. Turnipseed SD, et al. Frequency of acute coronary syndrome in patients presenting to the emergency department with chest pain after methamphetamine use. *J Emerg Med* 2003;24(4):369–373.

283. Kaye S, et al. Methamphetamine and cardiovascular pathology: a review of the evidence. *Addiction* 2007;102(8):1204–11

284. Perez JA Jr, Arsura EL, Strategos S. Methamphetamine-related stroke: four cases. *J Emerg Med* 1999;17(3):469–471.

285. McIntosh A, et al. Carotid artery dissection and middle cerebral artery stroke following methamphetamine use. *Neurology* 2006;67(12):2259–2260.

286. Cruz R, et al. Pulmonary manifestations of inhaled street drugs. *Heart Lung* 1998;27(5):297–305; quiz 306–307.

287. Gotway MB, et al. Thoracic complications of illicit drug use: an organ system approach. *Radiographics* 2002;22(Spec No):S119–S135.

288. Chin KM, Channick RN, Rubin LJ. Is methamphetamine use associated with idiopathic pulmonary arterial hypertension? *Chest* 2006;130(6):1657–1663.

289. Kalantar-Zadeh K, et al. Fatal hyponatremia in a young woman after ecstasy ingestion. *Nat Clin Pract Nephrol* 2006;2(5):283–288; quiz 289.

290. Cherney DZ, Davids MR, Halperin ML. Acute hyponatraemia and "ecstasy": insights from a quantitative and integrative analysis. *QJM* 2002;95(7):475–483.

291. Wallace ME, Squires R. Fatal massive amphetamine ingestion associated with hyperpyrexia. *J Am Board Fam Pract* 2000;13(4): 302–304.

292. Prosser JM, Naim M, Helfaer MA. A 14-year-old girl with agitation and hyperthermia. *Pediatr Emerg Care* 2006;22(9):676–679.

293. Numachi Y, et al. Methamphetamine-induced hyperthermia and lethal toxicity: role of the dopamine and serotonin transporters. *Eur J Pharmacol* 2007;572(2–3):120–128.

294. Anderson JL, et al. ACC/AHA 2007 guidelines for the management of patients with unstable angina/non ST-elevation myocardial infarction: a report of the American College of Cardiology/American Heart Association Task Force on Practice Guidelines (Writing Committee to Revise the 2002 Guidelines for the Management of Patients With Unstable Angina/Non ST-Elevation Myocardial Infarction): developed in collaboration with the American College of Emergency Physicians the Society for Cardiovascular Angiography and Interventions and the Society of Thoracic Surgeons: endorsed by the American Association of Cardiovascular and Pulmonary Rehabilitation and the Society for Academic Emergency Medicine. *Circulation* 2007;116(7): e148–e304.

295. Kloner RA, et al. The effects of acute and chronic cocaine use on the heart. *Circulation* 1992;85(2):407–19.

296. Billman GE. Cocaine: a review of its toxic actions on cardiac function. *Crit Rev Toxicol* 1995;25(2):113–32.

297. Muller CP, et al. Serotonin and psychostimulant addiction: focus on 5–HT1A–receptors. *Prog Neurobiol* 2007;81(3):133–178.

298. Kobayashi T, et al. Inhibition by cocaine of G protein–activated inwardly rectifying K+ channels expressed in Xenopus oocytes. *Toxicol In Vitro* 2007;21(4):656–664.

299. Mittleman MA, et al. Triggering of myocardial infarction by cocaine. *Circulation* 1999;99(21):2737–2741.

300. Vongpatanasin W, Lange RA, Hillis LD. Comparison of cocaine-induced vasoconstriction of left and right coronary arterial systems. *Am J Cardiol* 1997;79(4):492–493.

301. Lange RA, et al. Cocaine-induced coronary–artery vasoconstriction. *N Engl J Med* 1989;321(23):1557–1562.

302. Brogan WC III, et al. Recurrent coronary vasoconstriction caused by intranasal cocaine: possible role for metabolites. *Ann Intern Med* 1992;116(7):556–561.

303. Heesch CM, et al. Cocaine activates platelets and increases the formation of circulating platelet containing microaggregates in humans. *Heart* 2000;83(6):688–695.

304. Shannon RP, et al. Cholinergic modulation of the coronary vasoconstriction induced by cocaine in conscious dogs. *Circulation* 1993;87(3):939–949.

305. Amin M, Gabelman G, Buttrick P. Cocaine-induced myocardial infarction. A growing threat to men in their 30s. *Postgrad Med* 1991;90(4):50–55.

306. Hollander JE, et al. Prospective multicenter evaluation of cocaine-associated chest pain. Cocaine Associated Chest Pain (COCHPA) Study Group. *Acad Emerg Med* 1994;1(4):330–339.

307. Weber JE, et al. Cocaine-associated chest pain: how common is myocardial infarction? *Acad Emerg Med* 2000;7(8):873–877.

308. Feldman JA, et al. Acute cardiac ischemia in patients with cocaine–associated complaints: Results of a multicenter trial. *Ann Emerg Med* 2000;36(5):469–476.

309. Smith JA, et al. Cocaine increases extraneuronal levels of aspartate and glutamate in the nucleus accumbens. *Brain Res* 1995;683(2): 264–269.

310. Sizemore GM, Co C, Smith JE. Ventral pallidal extracellular fluid levels of dopamine serotonin gamma amino butyric acid and glutamate during cocaine self-administration in rats. *Psychopharmacology (Berl)* 2000;150(4):391–398.

311. Ikeda M, Dohi T, Tsujimoto A. Inhibition of gamma-aminobutyric acid release from synaptosomes by local anesthetics. *Anesthesiology* 1983;58(6):495–499.

312. Derlet RW, Albertson TE, Tharratt RS. Lidocaine potentiation of cocaine toxicity. *Ann Emerg Med* 1991;20(2):135–138.

313. Barat SA, Abdel-Rahman MS. Cocaine and lidocaine in combination are synergistic convulsants. *Brain Res* 1996;742(1–2): 157–162.

314. Myers SI, et al. Chronic intestinal ischemia caused by intravenous cocaine use: report of two cases and review of the literature. *J Vasc Surg* 1996;23(4):724–729.

315. Bemanian S, Motallebi M, Nosrati SM. Cocaine-induced renal infarction: report of a case and review of the literature. *BMC Nephrol* 2005;6:10.

316. Crandall CG, Vongpatanasin W, Victor RG. Mechanism of cocaine-induced hyperthermia in humans. *Ann Intern Med* 2002; 136(11):785–791.

317. Marzuk PM, et al. Ambient temperature and mortality from unintentional cocaine overdose. *JAMA* 1998;279(22):1795–800.

318. Guinn MM, Bedford JA, Wilson MC. Antagonism of intravenous cocaine lethality in nonhuman primates. *Clin Toxicol* 1980; 16(4): 499–508.

319. Catravas JD, Waters IW. Acute cocaine intoxication in the conscious dog: studies on the mechanism of lethality. *J Pharmacol Exp Ther* 1981;217(2):350–356.

320. Smith M, Garner D, Niemann JT. Pharmacologic interventions after an LD50 cocaine insult in a chronically instrumented rat model: are beta-blockers contraindicated? *Ann Emerg Med* 1991;20(7):768–771.

321. Brogan WC III, et al. Alleviation of cocaine-induced coronary vasoconstriction by nitroglycerin. *J Am Coll Cardiol* 1991;18(2): 581–586.

322. Honderick T, et al. A prospective randomized controlled trial of benzodiazepines and nitroglycerine or nitroglycerine alone in the treatment of cocaine-associated acute coronary syndromes. *Am J Emerg Med* 2003;21(1):39–42.

323. Boehrer JD, et al. Influence of labetalol on cocaine-induced coronary vasoconstriction in humans. *Am J Med* 1993;94(6):608–610.

324. Lange RA, et al. Potentiation of cocaine-induced coronary vasoconstriction by beta-adrenergic blockade. *Ann Intern Med* 1990;112(12):897–903.

325. Beckman KJ, et al. Hemodynamic and electrophysiological actions of cocaine. Effects of sodium bicarbonate as an antidote in dogs. *Circulation* 1991;83(5):1799–1807.

326. Parker RB, et al. Comparative effects of sodium bicarbonate and sodium chloride on reversing cocaine-induced changes in the electrocardiogram. *J Cardiovasc Pharmacol* 1999;34(6):864–869.

327. Wilson LD, Shelat C. Electrophysiologic and hemodynamic effects of sodium bicarbonate in a canine model of severe cocaine intoxication. *J Toxicol Clin Toxicol* 2003;41(6):777–788.

328. Kerns W II, Garvey L , Owens J. Cocaine-induced wide complex dysrhythmia. *J Emerg Med* 1997;15(3):321–329.

329. Wang RY. pH-dependent cocaine-induced cardiotoxicity. *Am J Emerg Med* 1999;17(4):364–369.

330. Winecoff AP, et al. Reversal of the electrocardiographic effects of cocaine by lidocaine: Part 1. Comparison with sodium bicarbonate and quinidine. *Pharmacotherapy* 1994;14(6):698–703.

331. Grawe JJ, et al. Reversal of the electrocardiographic effects of cocaine by lidocaine: Part 2. Concentration–effect relationships. *Pharmacotherapy* 1994;14(6):704–711.

332. Liu D, Hariman RJ, Bauman JL. Cocaine concentration–effect relationship in the presence and absence of lidocaine: evidence of a competitive binding between cocaine and lidocaine. *J Pharmacol Exp Ther* 1996;276(2):568–577.

333. Heit J, Hoffman RS, Goldfrank LR. The effects of lidocaine pretreatment on cocaine neurotoxicity and lethality in mice. *Acad Emerg Med* 1994;1(5):438–442.

334. June R, et al. Medical outcome of cocaine bodystuffers. *J Emerg Med* 2000;18(2):221–224.

335. Roberts JR, et al. The bodystuffer syndrome: a clandestine form of drug overdose. *Am J Emerg Med* 1986;4(1):24–27.

336. Olmedo R, et al. Is surgical decontamination definitive treatment of "body-packers"? *Am J Emerg Med* 2001;19(7):593–596.

337. Schaper A, et al. Surgical treatment in cocaine body packers and body pushers. *Int J Colorectal Dis* 2007;22(12):1531–1535.

338. Murad F. Cyclic guanosine monophosphate as a mediator of vasodilation. *J Clin Invest* 1986;78(1):1–5.

339. Balster RL. Neural basis of inhalant abuse. *Drug Alcohol Depend* 1998;51(1–2):207–214.

340. Jevtovic–Todorovic V, et al. Nitrous oxide (laughing gas) is an NMDA antagonist, neuroprotectant, and neurotoxin. *Nat Med* 1998;4(4):460–463.

341. Murakawa M, et al. Activation of the cortical and medullary dopaminergic systems by nitrous oxide in rats: a possible neuro-chemical basis for psychotropic effects and postanesthetic nausea and vomiting. *Anesth Analg* 1994;78(2):376–381.

342. Cruz SL, et al. Effects of the abused solvent toluene on recombinant N-methyl-D-aspartate and non-N-methyl-D-aspartate receptors expressed in Xenopus oocytes. *J Pharmacol Exp Ther* 1998;286(1):334–340.

343. Cruz SL, et al. Effects of inhaled toluene and 111-trichloroethane on seizures and death produced by N-methyl-D-aspartic acid in mice. *Behav Brain Res* 2003;140(1–2):195–202.

344. Blayney MR, Malins AF, Cooper GM. Cardiac arrhythmias in children during outpatient general anaesthesia for dentistry: a prospective randomised trial. *Lancet* 1999;354(9193):1864–1866.

345. Noda Y, Hashimoto K. Development of a halothane–adrenaline arrhythmia model using in vivo guinea pigs. *J Pharmacol Sci* 2004;95(2):234–239.

346. Guler N, et al. The effects of volatile anesthetics on the Q-Tc interval. *J Cardiothorac Vasc Anesth* 2001;15(2):188–191.

347. Nelson LS. Toxicologic myocardial sensitization. *J Toxicol Clin Toxicol* 2002;40(7):867–879.

348. Ikeda N, et al. The course of respiration and circulation in "toluene–sniffing." *Forens Sci Int* 1990;44(2–3):151–158.

349. Cruz SL, et al. Inhibition of cardiac sodium currents by toluene exposure. *Br J Pharmacol* 2003;140(4):653–660.

350. Kringsholm B. Sniffing-associated deaths in Denmark. *Forens Sci Int* 1980;15(3):215–225.

351. Eade NR, Taussig LM, Marks MI. Hydrocarbon pneumonitis. *Pediatrics* 1974;54(3):351–357.

352. Dimich I, et al. Esmolol prevents and suppresses arrhythmias during halothane anaesthesia in dogs. *Can J Anaesth* 1992;39(1): 83–86.

353. Sharma PL. Effect of propranolol on catecholamine-induced arrhythmias during nitrous oxide–halothane anaesthesia in the dog. *Br J Anaesth* 1966;38(11):871–877.

354. Gindre G, et al. [Late ventricular fibrillation after trichloroethylene poisoning.] *Ann Fr Anesth Reanim* 1997;16(2):202–203.

355. Mortiz F, et al. Esmolol in the treatment of severe arrhythmia after acute trichloroethylene poisoning. *Intens Care Med* 2000; 26(2):256.

356. Flacke JW, Flacke WE, Williams GD. Acute pulmonary edema following naloxone reversal of high-dose morphine anesthesia. *Anesthesiology* 1977;47(4):376–378.

357. Schwartz J, Koenigsberg M. Naloxone-induced pulmonary edema. *Ann Emerg Med* 1987;16(11):1294–1296.

358. Armstrong PJ, Bersten A. *Normeperidine toxicity. Anesth Analg* 1986;65(5):536–538.

359. Potschka H, Friderichs E, Loscher W. Anticonvulsant and proconvulsant effects of tramadol its enantiomers and its M1 metabolite in the rat kindling model of epilepsy. *Br J Pharmacol* 2000;131(2):203–212.

360. Jovanovic–Cupic V, Martinovic Z, Nesic N. Seizures associated with intoxication and abuse of tramadol. *Clin Toxicol (Phila)* 2006; 44(2):143–146.

361. Poklis A. Pentazocine/tripelennamine (T's and blues) abuse: a five-year survey of St Louis, Missouri. *Drug Alcohol Depend* 1982; 10(2–3):257–267.

362. Barkin RL, Barkin SJ, Barkin DS. Propoxyphene (dextro-propoxyphene): a critical review of a weak opioid analgesic that should remain in antiquity. *Am J Ther* 2006;13(6):534–542.

363. Sloth Madsen P, et al. Acute propoxyphene self-poisoning in 222 consecutive patients. *Acta Anaesthesiol Scand* 1984;28(6):661–665.

364. Lund-Jacobsen H. Cardio-respiratory toxicity of propoxyphene and norpropoxyphene in conscious rabbits. *Acta Pharmacol Toxicol (Copenh)* 1978;42(3):171–178.

365. Ulens C, Daenens P, Tytgat J.Norpropoxyphene-induced cardiotoxicity is associated with changes in ion-selectivity and gating of HERG currents. *Cardiovasc Res* 1999;44(3):568–578.

366. Stork CM, et al. Propoxyphene-induced wide QRS complex dysrhythmia responsive to sodium bicarbonate—a case report. *J Toxicol Clin Toxicol* 1995;33(2):179–183.

367. Whitcomb DC, et al. Marked QRS complex abnormalities and sodium channel blockade by propoxyphene reversed with lidocaine. *J Clin Invest* 1989;84(5):1629–1636.

368. Thomas TJ, Pauze D, Love JN. Are one or two dangerous? Diphenoxylate–atropine exposure in toddlers. *J Emerg Med* 2008;34(1):71–75.

369. Douglas CG, Haldane JS, Haldane JB. The laws of combination of haemoglobin with carbon monoxide and oxygen. *J Physiol* 1912;44(4):275–304.

370. Roughton FJW, Darling RC. The effect of carbon monoxide on the oxyhemoglobin dissociation curve. *Am J Physiol* 1944;141(1): 17–31.

371. Okada Y, et al. Effect of carbon monoxide on equilibrium between oxygen and hemoglobin. *Am J Physiol* 1976;230(2):471–475.

372. Ball EG, Strittmatter CF, Cooper O. The reaction of cytochrome oxidase with carbon monoxide. *J Biol Chem* 1951;193(2):635–647.

373. Prockop LD, Chichkova RI. Carbon monoxide intoxication: an updated review. *J Neurol Sci* 2007;262(1–2):122–130.

374. Satran D, et al. Cardiovascular manifestations of moderate to severe carbon monoxide poisoning. *J Am Coll Cardiol* 2005;45(9): 1513–1516.

375. Kalay N, et al. Cardiovascular effects of carbon monoxide poisoning. *Am J Cardiol* 2007;99(3):322–324.

376. Pace N, Strajman E, Walker EL. Acceleration of carbon monoxide elimination in man by high pressure oxygen. *Science* 1950; 111(2894):652–654.

377. Peterson JE, Stewart RD. Absorption and elimination of carbon monoxide by inactive young men. *Arch Environ Health* 1970;21(2): 165–171.

378. Jay GD, et al. Portable hyperbaric oxygen therapy in the emergency department with the modified Gamow bag. *Ann Emerg Med* 1995;26(6):707–711.

379. Weaver LK, et al. Carboxyhemoglobin half–life in carbon monoxide–poisoned patients treated with 100% oxygen at atmospheric pressure. *Chest* 2000;117(3):801–808.

380. Raphael JC, et al. Trial of normobaric and hyperbaric oxygen for acute carbon monoxide intoxication. *Lancet* 1989;2(8660): 414–419.

381. Thom SR, et al. Delayed neuropsychologic sequelae after carbon monoxide poisoning: prevention by treatment with hyperbaric oxygen. *Ann Emerg Med* 1995;25(4):474–480.

382. Scheinkestel CD, et al. Hyperbaric or normobaric oxygen for acute carbon monoxide poisoning: a randomized controlled clinical trial. *Undersea Hyperb Med* 2000;27(3):163–164.

383. Weaver LK, et al. Hyperbaric oxygen for acute carbon monoxide poisoning. *N Engl J Med* 2002;347(14):1057–1067.

384. Weaver LK, Valentine KJ, Hopkins RO. Carbon monoxide poisoning: risk factors for cognitive sequelae and the role of hyperbaric oxygen. *Am J Respir Crit Care Med* 2007;176(5):491–497.

385. Ash-Bernal R, Wise R, Wright SM. Acquired methemoglobinemia: a retrospective series of 138 cases at 2 teaching hospitals. *Medicine (Baltimore)* 2004;83(5):265–273.

386. Moore TJ, Walsh CS, Cohen MR. Reported adverse event cases of methemoglobinemia associated with benzocaine products. *Arch Intern Med* 2004;164(11):1192–1196.

387. Borgese N, Pietrini G, Gaetani S. Concentration of NADH–cytochrome b5 reductase in erythrocytes of normal and methemoglobinemic individuals measured with a quantitative radioimmunoblotting assay. *J Clin Invest* 1987;80(5):1296–1302.

388. Price D. Methemoglobin inducers. In Flomenbaum NE, Goldfrank LR, Hoffman RS, et al, eds. *Goldfrank's Toxicologic Emergencies*, 8th ed. New York: McGraw–Hill, 2006.

389. Barker SJ, Tremper KK, Hyatt J. Effects of methemoglobinemia on pulse oximetry and mixed venous oximetry. *Anesthesiology* 1989;70(1):112–117.

390. Barker SJ, et al. Measurement of carboxyhemoglobin and methemoglobin by pulse oximetry: a human volunteer study. *Anesthesiology* 2006;105(5):892–897.

391. Eckstein M, Maniscalco PM. Focus on smoke inhalation—the most common cause of acute cyanide poisoning. *Prehosp Disaster Med* 2006;21(2 Suppl 2):s49–s55.

392. Baud FJ, et al. Elevated blood cyanide concentrations in victims of smoke inhalation. *N Engl J Med* 1991;325(25):1761–1766.

393. Lam KK, Lau FL. An incident of hydrogen cyanide poisoning. *Am J Emerg Med* 2000;18(2):172–175.

394. Piccinini N, et al. Risk of hydrocyanic acid release in the electroplating industry. *J Hazard Mater* 2000;71(1–3):395–407.

395. Blanc P, et al. Cyanide intoxication among silver–reclaiming workers. *JAMA* 1985;253(3):367–371.

396. Binder L, Fredrickson L. Poisonings in laboratory personnel and health care professionals. *Am J Emerg Med* 1991;9(1):11–15.

397. Tanii H, Hashimoto K. Studies on the mechanism of acute toxicity of nitriles in mice. *Arch Toxicol* 1984;55(1):47–54.

398. Michaelis HC, et al. Acetonitrile serum concentrations and cyanide blood levels in a case of suicidal oral acetonitrile ingestion. *J Toxicol Clin Toxicol* 1991;29(4):447–358.

399. Unproven methods of cancer management. Laetrile. *CA Cancer J Clin* 1991;41(3):187–192.

400. Beamer WC, Shealy RM, Prough DS. Acute cyanide poisoning from laetrile ingestion. *Ann Emerg Med* 1983;12(7):449–451.

401. O'Brien B, Quigg C, Leong T. Severe cyanide toxicity from "vitamin supplements." *Eur J Emerg Med* 2005;12(5):257–258.

402. Bromley J, et al. Life-threatening interaction between complementary medicines: cyanide toxicity following ingestion of amygdalin and vitamin C. *Ann Pharmacother* 2005;39(9):1566–1569.

403. Hall AH, Rumack BH. Clinical toxicology of cyanide. *Ann Emerg Med* 1986;15(9):1067–1074.

404. Suchard JR, Wallace KL, Gerkin RD. Acute cyanide toxicity caused by apricot kernel ingestion. *Ann Emerg Med* 1998;32(6):742–744.

405. Hollenberg SM. Vasodilators in acute heart failure. *Heart Fail Rev* 2007;12(2):143–147.

406. Cosby K, et al. Nitrite reduction to nitric oxide by deoxyhemoglobin vasodilates the human circulation. *Nat Med* 2003;9(12): 1498–1505.

407. Leavesley HB, et al. Interaction of cyanide and nitric oxide with cytochrome c oxidase: implications for acute cyanide toxicity. *Toxicol Sci* 2008;101(1):101–111.

408. Gerth K, et al. Nitric oxide scavenging by hydroxocobalamin may account for its hemodynamic profile. *Clin Toxicol (Phila)* 2006;44(Suppl 1):29–36.

409. Uhl W, et al. Safety of hydroxocobalamin in healthy volunteers in a randomized placebo-controlled study. *Clin Toxicol (Phila)* 2006;44(Suppl 1):17–28.

410. Fortin JL, et al. Prehospital administration of hydroxocobalamin for smoke inhalation–associated cyanide poisoning: 8 years of experience in the Paris Fire Brigade. *Clin Toxicol (Phila)* 2006;44(Suppl 1):37–44.

411. Borron SW, et al. Prospective study of hydroxocobalamin for acute cyanide poisoning in smoke inhalation. *Ann Emerg Med* 2007;49(6):794–801.

412. Weng TI, et al. Elevated plasma cyanide level after hydroxocobalamin infusion for cyanide poisoning. *Am J Emerg Med* 2004;22(6):492–493.

413. Fortin JL, et al. Hydroxocobalamin for poisoning by ingestion of potassium cyanide: A case study. *Clin Toxicol* 2005;43(6):731.

414. Borron SW, et al. Hydroxocobalamin for severe acute cyanide poisoning by ingestion or inhalation. *Am J Emerg Med* 2007;25(5):551–558.

415. Blondell JM. Decline in pesticide poisonings in the United States from 1995 to 2004. *Clin Toxicol (Phila)* 2007;45(5):589–592.

416. Namba T, et al. Poisoning due to organophosphate insecticides. Acute and chronic manifestations. *Am J Med* 1971;50(4):475–492.

417. Saadeh AM, Farsakh NA, al-Ali MK. Cardiac manifestations of acute carbamate and organophosphate poisoning. *Heart* 1997;77(5):461–464.

418. Clark RF. Insecticides: organic phosphorus compounds and carbamates. In Flomenbaum NE, Goldfrank LR, Hoffman RS, et al, eds. *Goldfrank's Toxicologic Emergencies*, 8th ed. New York: McGraw–Hill, 2006.

Chapter 30
Drowning

David Szpilman, Anthony J. Handley, Joost Bierens, Linda Quan, and Rafael Vasconcellos

Drowning is an injury whose treatment may involve many layers of personnel from laypersons, lifeguards, and prehospital care providers to highly specialized hospital staff. Care of the drowning victim is unique in that bystanders or rescuers need specific skills that allow them to help the victim without becoming victims themselves. However, prevention, not resuscitation, is the primary objective with regard to drowning and adequate supervision of children is the most important preventative goal.

- Updated definition- Drowning is progressive respiratory impairment from submersion in a liquid
- The majority of drownings while accidental are due to negligence and failure of supervision
- The most effective intervention for drowning is prevention
- Additional medications may include antihistamines, corticosteroids, and glucagon.
- Use a drowning algorithm for triage, treatment and prognosis

Introduction

On a sunny weekend day, a family was invited to a barbecue at a friend's swimming pool. Suddenly, the mother noticed that her 4-year-old boy was missing. After about 7 minutes, he was found at the bottom of the pool and brought up to the pool's edge. He appeared dead and no one knew what to do.

This scenario is usual in many countries and transforms a happy time into a very dramatic moment and a future for everyone involved not only of profound loss and grief but also guilt for failure to protect the victim or even intense anger at those who did not provide adequate supervision or medical care.

Drowning is an injury whose treatment may involve many layers of personnel, from laypersons, lifeguards, and prehospital care providers to highly specialized hospital staff. Care of the drowning victim is unique in that bystanders or rescuers need specific skills that allow them to help the victim without becoming victims themselves. Furthermore, the rescuers' role is critical, since the chance for a good outcome rests almost entirely with care provided at the scene. If rescue and first aid from bystanders fail, delayed medical treatment cannot compensate for hypoxic injuries, even when more advanced therapies are initiated.

Interest in drowning rescue and resuscitation has existed for hundreds of years and drove the development of the first resuscitation instruments, research, protocols, education, and systems. In the past as well as today, drowning is among the most frequent causes of traumatic death. While the main focus of the current resuscitation community is on those with cardiac disease, this chapter advocates that the resuscitation of drowning victims should also be of importance to the resuscitation community, at least for those who are concerned with aquatic environments, which constitute 80% of the earth's surface. Although drowning has often been a neglected public health problem,[1] it has recently begun to receive the attention it deserves.

At both the medical and societal levels, it must be recognized that every drowning-related death or hospitalization signals the failure of prevention.

Epidemiology

Each year, drowning is responsible for more than 500,000 deaths worldwide.[2] This number is an underestimate of the real figure. Especially in developing countries, many drowning deaths are unreported (Table 30-1).[3] Statistics on drowning vary widely depending on different geographic, cultural, and economic resources. In some European countries, many drowning deaths are intentional injuries due to suicide, while in Australia, the United States, and Brazil, the majority of drowning deaths are unintentional. In the United States, an estimated 40% to 45% of drowning deaths occur during swimming.[4] Mortality and, less frequently, hospitalization following drowning

| TABLE 30-1 • Global Coverage of Death Registration Data: WHO Presentation: "Mortality and Causes of Death"

	Developed Countries	Sub-Saharan Africa	Latin America	Middle East	Asia and Pacific	Total
Data available	55	4	29	9	18	115
Data not available	2	42	4	12	17	77
Total	57	46	33	21	35	192

Source: From International Life Saving Federation. World drowning report. *Int J Aquatic Res Educ* 2007;1:381–401, with permission.

are the most commonly reported indicators of drowning injury.

Age, gender, alcohol use, socioeconomic status (income, education, and ethnicity), exposure, risk behavior, and lack of supervision are key risk factors in drowning. Considering all ages, males die five times more often from drowning than females. Young children, teenagers, and older adults are at highest risk of drowning. Worldwide, drowning is the leading cause of death in males between 5 and 14 years of age and the fifth leading cause among females.[5] It is the leading killer of children 1 to 17 years of age in Asia.[6]

In the United States, drowning is the seventh leading cause of unintentional traumatic death for all ages and the second leading cause of all traumatic deaths among children 1 to 14 years of age.

Many of these injuries occur in recreational settings, including pools, spas/hot tubs, and natural outdoor settings (e.g., lakes, rivers, and oceans). During 2001 to 2002, an estimated 4,174 persons, on average, were treated in the United States emergency departments (EDs) for nonfatal, unintentional drowning injuries in recreational settings and 3,372 persons died of drowning in 2001. Children below the age of 4 years of age accounted for nearly 50% of such ED visits, and children aged 5 to 14 years accounted for an additional 25%. An estimated 75% of nonfatal injuries occurred in pools, whereas 70% of the fatalities occurred in natural outdoor settings. Approximately 53% of ED-treated patients required hospitalization or transfer to a hospital offering specialized care.[8]

In Brazil, with a population of 176 million inhabitants in 2003, a total of 6,688 died (3.8 per 100,000 inhabitants) by drowning, the second leading cause of death among those aged 1 to 14 years. Most of these drowning deaths, or 88%, were unintentional. Fatal drowning involved mostly 20- to 29-year-old individuals (22%), followed by those aged 15 to 19 (16%), 30 to 39 (15%), 10 to 14 (11%), 40 to 49 (9%), 1 to 4 (8%), and 5 to 9 (7%). There was no sex distinction in death rates under 1 year of age, but among those between the ages of 20 and 29, males drowned 8.7 times more often.[9]

As one of the largest year-round aquatic recreational areas in the world, Brazil provides a model for the development of a first-responder system for drowning, to be compared with emergency medical services (EMS) systems in other countries. In 1984, the emphasis on lifesaving increased significantly when firefighters assumed the role of lifeguarding the beaches and inland water spots, with many more professionals also on duty. The development of a large cadre of these professionals guarding the beaches led to the creation, in 1995, of the Brazilian Lifesaving Society, supported by the International Lifesaving Federation (ILS)—the largest world water safety organization. A recent study analyzed the drowning trends from 1979 to 2003 in Brazil.[10] The effect of this initiative was a 30% reduction in rates of drowning death from 1979 (5.42 per 100,000) to 2003 (3.78 per 100,000). Most of this occurred from 1995 (4.91 per 100,000) to 2003 (3.78 per 100,000), suggesting that two interventions associated with maturation of the system—more lifeguards on duty and prevention campaigns—led to the dramatic decrease in drowning deaths (Fig. 30-1).

On Rio de Janeiro's beaches, predisposing conditions are discernible in 13% of all drowning cases; the most common is use of alcohol (37%); followed by convulsions (18%); trauma, including boating accidents (16.3%); cardiopulmonary diseases (14.1%); skin and SCUBA diving (3.7%); diving resulting in head or spinal cord injuries; and others (e.g., homicide, suicide, syncope, cramps, or immersion syndrome: 11.6%).[11]

These statistics highlight the fact that 87% of drownings occur with no reasons other than negligence by adults, regarding either themselves or their children.

Drowning: Definition and Terminology

The definition of drowning has been a significant problem for a long time. Until recently there has been no consensus either in the literature, among the various water safety and health organizations, among experts in the field, or among laypersons.[12] Terms and definitions were awkward and confusing, including sudden death, hypothermia, and diseases occurring in water. At the same time, some definitions excluded true cases of drowning due to complications of drowning, such as pneumonia, acute respiratory distress syndrome (ARDS), or ischemic encephalopathy. Therefore, the global scope of drowning has been wrongly measured not only through imprecise national statistics, but also through inadequate terms and definitions.

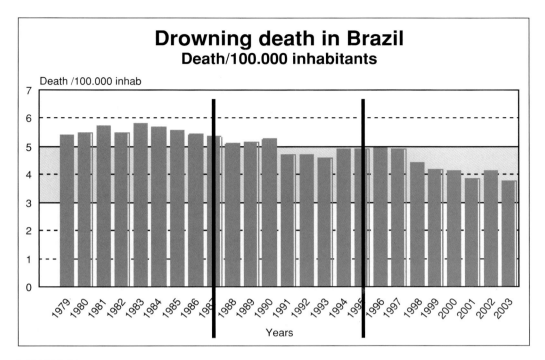

Drowning death in Brazil
Death/100.000 inhabitants

FIGURE 30-1 • Drowning death trends in Brazil from 1979 to 2003, selecting three different periods. (From Szpilman D, Goulart PM, Mocellin O, et al. 12 years of Brazilian Lifesaving Society (Sobrasa) - Did we make any difference? World Water Safety, Matosinhos- Portugal 2007.

Based on this problem, a Task Force on Epidemiology of Drowning (TFED) was established in 1998 within the framework of the World Congress on Drowning (WCOD). Following a discussion over several years, with contributions from many experts around the world, the TFED in 2002 adopted the following definition:

Drowning is the process of experiencing respiratory impairment from submersion or immersion in liquid.

According to this new definition, the drowning process is a continuum beginning with respiratory impairment—for example, when the patient's airway is below the surface of the liquid or when there is a splashing of waves in the face. A patient can be rescued at any time during the process and given appropriate resuscitative measures, in which case the process of drowning is interrupted. Any submersion or immersion incident without evidence of liquid aspiration or respiratory impairment should be considered a water rescue and not a drowning. The terms "near-drowning," "dry drowning," "secondary drowning," and "delayed onset of respiratory distress" are eliminated. Immersion or submersion is a way of drowning and not the name of a disease. [13]

Pathophysiology of Drowning

Drowning may occur in fresh or salt water. A 2-year-old toddler may fall into a swimming pool, where he will disappear without any sign of distress, or a young, athletic swimmer may be caught by a rip current and, after an exhausting struggle, finally succumb. Despite some differences between drowning in fresh versus salt water, from a clinical and therapeutic perspective, there are no important differences in humans. The common significant pathophysiologic mechanism in any case of drowning is hypoxia.[14]

Despite some differences between drowning in fresh water versus salt water, from a clinical and therapeutic perspective, there are no important differences in humans.

Process of Drowning

Initially the victim is typically in an upright posture, with eyes just above the water surface, arms extended laterally, and thrashing and slapping on the water surface in an effort to get her airway above the water. Exhaustion will render the victim unable to scream for help. Children who cannot swim struggle for only 10 to 20 seconds before final submersion, while adults may be able to struggle for up to 60 seconds. When there is no way of keeping the airway out of the water, intentional breath-holding is the first automatic response. Water in the mouth is spit out or swallowed. When, after some time, a breath is taken, the result may be a first involuntary aspiration of water and consequent coughing or rarely laryngospasm, leading to hypoxia. If laryngospasm occurs, the onset of hypoxia will terminate it rapidly. If not, water is gradually but quickly aspirated into the lungs, rendering them unable to absorb oxygen. Consciousness deteriorates and is eventually lost.

Progressive hypoxia leads to apnea, followed by cardiac arrest. In the early stages of drowning, while the victim is still able to inhale some air, hyperventilation may lead to apnea and loss of consciousness as a result of a very low carbon dioxide level. The more intense the hyperventilation, the longer the apnea will persist. The victim may then stop struggling and slip below the water. This entire course of events may last from 1 minute to as long as hours.

Since the term "drowning" refers to a continuum that may or may not be fatal, a victim can be rescued at any time during the drowning process. The victim may not require any intervention at all or may receive appropriate resuscitative measures, in which case the drowning process is interrupted. Permanent brain damage generally occurs only in cases of cardiac arrest. The development of posthypoxic encephalopathy with or without cerebral edema is the most common sequela of cardiac arrest in resuscitated drowning victims. However, all organ systems can be involved in the postdrowning period, with complications including disseminated intravascular coagulation (DIC), acute tubular necrosis (ATN), and ARDS.

Physiologic Consequences of Drowning

The pulmonary damage of drowning is a function not of the water composition but of the pulmonary response to the water aspirated.

The aspiration of either fresh or salt water can produce, depending on the amount, surfactant destruction, alveolitis, and noncardiogenic pulmonary edema, resulting in an increased intrapulmonary shunting and hypoxia.[15] In animal research, the aspiration of 2.2 mL/kg of water decreases the arterial oxygen pressure (PaO_2) to approximately 60 mm Hg within 3 minutes.[16] In humans, aspiration of as little as 1 to 3 mL/kg of water produces profound alterations in pulmonary gas exchange and decreases pulmonary compliance by 10% to 40%.[15] Humans rarely aspirate sufficient water to provoke significant electrolyte disturbances and victims usually do not require initial correction of electrolytes.[17]

Decreased cardiac output, arterial hypotension, increased pulmonary arterial pressure, and pulmonary vascular resistance are the results of hypoxia. Ventricular fibrillation (VF) in drowning is not common. When it occurs, the victim is usually older, with a history of coronary artery disease. VF is due to hypoxia and acidosis and not to hemolysis and hyperkalemia. VF may also occur during resuscitation, mainly owing to the use of epinephrine.

The more common scenario is hypoxia producing a well-established sequence of cardiac deterioration, with tachycardia followed by bradycardia, pulseless electrical activity (PEA), and finally asystole.[15]

Drowning Chain of Survival (Fig. 30-2)

Prevention

Despite the emphasis on immediate treatment, the most effective intervention for drowning is prevention.

Prevention programs are estimated to be potentially effective in preventing >85% of current annual drownings.[20,21] Drowning prevention is multifaceted and involves education, technology, and legislation. In high-income countries, children below the age of 5 years have the highest drowning rates; they drown in swimming pools into which they fall while being unsupervised. The most effective intervention to prevent drowning in this age group is to fence in all swimming pools with four-sided, inclimbable fences with self-closing, self-latching gates. Legislation requiring installation of such barriers has been adopted in several countries.

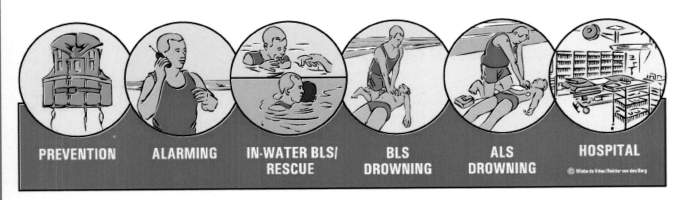

FIGURE 30-2 • Drowning chain of survival. (From Szpilman D, Morizot-Leite L, Vries W, et al. First aid courses for the aquatic environment. In Bierens J, ed. *Handbook on Drowning: Prevention, Rescue, and Treatment.* Berlin: Springer-Verlag, 2005, with permission.)

However, enforcement of these laws is key to maximizing their effectiveness. Adequate supervision of children is the most important preventative goal. Supervision must be defined as the complete attention of an adult who is unimpaired by alcohol, drugs, or distraction and is capable of rescue.

Prevention of drowning in open water is more problematic, as it involves older children and adults engaged in a wide variety of activities. The prevention of such drowning has received less attention, since its victims usually die without medical interface. In the United States and Canada, >85% to 90% of boat-related drowning deaths involve people without life jackets. Some countries have legislation requiring children to wear life jackets while on small boats. However, adult males in small boats are the most common victims, and they are generally not required to wear life jackets.

Swimming or water survival skills may also enable potential victims to avoid drowning. Recent efforts in low-income countries to teach school-age children to dog paddle for a few yards has been helpful. Another subpopulation at risk of drowning comprises those who are subject to seizures. Most such drownings occur in the bathtub or during recreational swimming. Prevention for this group would be to shower instead of using the tub and to swim where there is a lifeguard. (See preventive measures in Table 30-2.)[22]

Alarming (Recognition and Activation of Emergency Medical Services)

Contrary to popular opinion, the victim generally does not wave or call for help and usually drowns unnoticed. Bystanders may not recognize that the victim is struggling and may assume that the victim is playing and splashing in the water.

The key initial step in the treatment of drowning is to recognize that someone is drowning. Contrary to popular opinion, the victim generally does not wave or call for help and usually

| TABLE 30-2 • Drowning Preventive Measures

Watch children carefully; 84% of child drownings occur because of poor adult supervision.

Begin swimming lessons from 2 years old but be very careful at this age.

Avoid inflatable swimming aids such as "floaties." They can give a false sense of security. Use a lifejacket!

Never try to help rescue someone without knowing how to do it. Many people have died trying to do so.

Avoid drinking alcohol and eating before swimming.

Do not dive into shallow water; this can lead to spinal injury.

Beaches	Pools, Spas, and Hot Tubs
• Always swim in a lifeguard-supervised area.	• Over 65% of deaths occur in fresh water, even on the coast.
• Ask the lifeguard for safe places to swim or play.	
• Read and follow warning signs posted on the beach.	• Fence off your pool and include a gate. Recommended approved fencing can decrease drowning by 50% to 70%.
• Do not overestimate your swimming ability; 45% of drowning victims thought they knew how to swim.	• Avoid toys around the pool; they are very attractive to children.
• Swim away from piers, rocks, and stakes.	• Whenever infants or toddlers are in or around water, be within arm's length, providing "touch supervision."
• Take lost children to the nearest lifeguard tower.	
• Over 80% of drownings occur in rip currents (the rip is usually the most falsely calm deep place between two sandbars). If caught in a rip, swim transversally to the sand bar or let it take you away without fighting and wave for help.	• Turn off motor filters when using the pool.
	• Always use portable phones in pool areas, so that you are not called away to answer.
• If you are fishing on rocks, be cautious about waves that may sweep you into the ocean.	• Do not try to increase your submersion time by hyperventilating.
• Keep away from marine animals.	• Use warning signs of deep water in the pool.
	• Learn CPR. Over 42% of pools owners are not knowledgeable about first aid techniques. Be careful!

Source: From Szpilman D, Orlowski JP, Bierens J. Drowning. In Fink M, Abraham E, Vincent JL, Kochanek P, eds. *Textbook of Critical Care*, 5th ed.Philadelphia: Elsevier Science, 2004:699–706, with permission.

drowns unnoticed.[23] A typical victim who drowns while swimming is a male young adult who may initially be embarrassed to cry for help and whose decision to ask for help is made too late, when his arms and legs are exhausted. While drowning, the victim is typically in an upright posture, with eyes just above the water surface, arms extended laterally, and thrashing and slapping on the water surface in an effort to get his airway above the water. Exhaustion will lead to the inability to scream for help. Bystanders may not recognize that the victim is struggling and may assume that he is playing and splashing in the water. The victim may submerge and surface several times during this struggle. Children who cannot swim struggle for only 10 to 20 seconds before final submersion, while adults may be able to struggle for up to 60 seconds.[23]

In swimming pools, the victim usually goes unnoticed until he or she is observed to be under the water. This can happen in spite of good surveillance by pool lifeguards. The most effective method of pool surveillance still remains unclear and is currently under scientific investigation. Legally compulsory fencing and drowning detection systems can help to reduce the number of pool drownings.

The moment a drowning is recognized, it is essential to activate the emergency system to dispatch lifeguards and prehospital medical personnel to the scene and to take immediate action.

Rescue and Basic Water Life Support (BWLS)

Rescuers should be careful to not become additional victims.

Rescuers should be careful to not become additional victims. If possible, potential rescuers should stay out of the water and use techniques like "throw before you go" and "reach with a long object before you assist." The rescuer can advise the victim on how to get out of the situation (i.e., choosing a better path of escape or reassuring the victim that assistance is coming).

The decision of how to provide BWLS[18] is based on the victim's level of consciousness. The victim who is panicking and struggling to breathe can drown the would-be rescuer. It is always best to approach a struggling victim with an intermediary object or from the back. Lifeguards use rescue or torpedo buoys, which can also be used as flotation devices to keep the victim's head and airway out of the water.[23] Other objects, such as a plastic food cooler, a foam car seat, or any other object that floats, can be used in those situations. For the conscious victim, rescue involves bringing the victim to land without further medical care.[24]

The most important step in BWLS is the immediate institution of ventilation, which has usually ceased by the time the victim becomes unconscious.

Cardiac arrest ensues within minutes if apnea is not corrected. In-water resuscitation, providing ventilation only, can increase a victim's chance of survival without sequelae by

more than threefold—assuming adequate support once out of the water. Rescuers should check the airway and ventilation and, if necessary, attempt to provide mouth-to-mouth ventilation for 1 minute. Victims with only respiratory arrest usually respond after a few artificial breaths. If there is no response, the victim should be assumed to be in cardiac arrest and the rescuer should immediately take the victim out of the water. Assessment for pulse in the water does not serve a purpose. External cardiac compression cannot be performed effectively in the water and must be delayed until the victim is out of the water.[24]

A few studies have described the frequency of in-water cervical spine injury (CSI). A retrospective evaluation of over 46,000 water rescues on sand beaches demonstrated an incidence of CSI of 0.009%.[25] In another retrospective survey of more than 2,400 drownings, <0.5% had a CSI. All who were injured had a history of obvious trauma from diving, falling from a height, or a motor vehicle accident.[26] Valuable time spent immobilizing the cervical spine of an unconscious victim with no signs of trauma could lead to a hypoxia and cardiopulmonary deterioration and ultimately death.

Considering the reported low incidence of cervical spine injury and the risk of wasting precious time, routine cervical spine immobilization during water rescue without strong evidence of a traumatic injury is not recommended.

Rescuers who do suspect a spinal cord injury should float the supine victim in a horizontal position, allowing the airway to be out of the water, and check for spontaneous breathing. If there is no spontaneous breathing, the airway is opened and mouth-to-mouth ventilation is started while maintaining the head in a neutral position as much as possible. It should be remembered that the jaw thrust has been shown to allow some movement of the cervical spine. If there is spontaneous breathing, the hands of the rescuer can be used to stabilize the victim's neck in a neutral position. If possible, the victim is kept floating with the help of a back support before being moved to a dry place. Alignment and support of the head, neck, chest, and body should be maintained if the victim must be moved or turned.[14]

On-Land Basic Drowning Life Support (BDLS)

The technique of removing a victim from the water depends on the circumstances where the drowning has occurred and the victim's level of consciousness. Preferably a vertical position should be adopted to prevent vomiting and further airway complications. If the victim is exhausted, confused, or unconscious, transport should be in as near a horizontal position as possible but with the head still maintained above body level to minimize the risk of aspiration. An exception is cold-water immersion, when the victim should be kept as horizontal as possible to avoid hypotension due to vasodilation during rewarming. The airway must be kept open.[27]

When on the land, the first procedure is to place the victim in a position parallel to the water line or with the head higher than the feet so as to avoid regurgitation from the stomach and consequently further aspiration. The victim should be supine and far enough away from the water to avoid incoming waves but not so far as to waste time on transportation. If conscious, the victim should be repositioned supine with the head up. If breathing and unconscious, the victim should be placed in the lateral decubitus position to avoid aspiration.[27] In a 10-year Australian study, vomiting occurred in more than 65% of victims who needed rescue breathing and in 86% of those who required both rescue breathing and chest compressions.[28] Even in victims who required no interventions after water rescue, vomiting occurred in 50% once the victims had reached shore. The presence of vomit in the airway can result in further aspiration and impairment of oxygenation by obstruction of the airways; it can also discourage rescuers from attempting mouth-to-mouth resuscitation.[28] Positive-pressure ventilation will force water from the airways into the pulmonary circulation, where it is absorbed; this appropriate intervention will simultaneously provide what the victim needs: ventilation and oxygenation.

Specific efforts to expel water from the airway and lungs are hazardous.

The abdominal thrust Heimlich maneuver should never be used as a means of expelling water from the lungs; it is ineffective and carries significant risks of vomiting and other injuries. Attempts at active drainage by placing the victim head down increases the risk of vomiting more than fivefold and leads to a significant increase in mortality (19%) when compared with keeping the victim in a horizontal position.[27] If vomiting occurs, the victim's mouth should be turned to the side and the vomitus removed with a finger sweep, cloth, or suction.

A lifeguard or emergency health professional must make a number of difficult decisions in order to treat a drowning victim appropriately. The most life-threatening situations, cardiopulmonary or isolated respiratory arrest, comprise only 0.5% of all rescues.[11] Most cases are less dramatic and many potential interventions can be considered. The questions to be addressed include: Should rescuers administer oxygen? Should an ambulance be called? Should the drowned person be transported to a hospital or observed for a time at the site?

To address these questions, a classification system was developed in Rio de Janeiro in 1972 to assist lifeguards, ambulance personnel, and physicians at the scene (see below). The update of the classification system in 1997[11] was based on an analysis of 41,279 rescues between 1972 and 1991, of which 2,304 (5.5%) were drownings that needed medical attention. The classification system was revalidated in 2001 by a 10-year study of 46,080 rescues.[29] This classification allows determination of needed levels of support and treatment from the scene to the hospital and shows the likelihood of death based on the severity of injury (Fig. 30-3).[11]

The severity of the drowning injury is assessed by the on-scene rescuer, emergency medical technician (EMT) or physician using clinical variables and by the emergency physician once the victim has arrived at the hospital.

Advanced Drowning Life Support (ADLS)

Depending on the distance involved, the best recommendation for drowning may be to bring the medical equipment to the victim instead of the victim to the ambulance in order to decrease time to intervention. Advanced medical treatment is given according to the drowning classification (Fig. 30-3).[11]

Dead Body

Such a victim has had a submersion time of more than an hour in non-icy waters or has obvious physical evidence of death (rigor mortis, putrefaction, or dependent lividity). The recommendation here is not to start resuscitation.

Grade 6: Cardiopulmonary Arrest

Resuscitation started by a layperson or lifeguard should be continued on scene by advanced life support (ALS) personnel. An exception to prolonged resuscitation at the scene is the moderately or severely hypothermic victim, who should rapidly be transported (while receiving resuscitation) to a hospital, where advanced warming measures can be implemented.

Cardiopulmonary resuscitation (CPR) with high-flow oxygen should be continued until a cuffed orotracheal tube can be inserted. Suctioning is usually necessary to visualize the glottis for intubation, and a cricoid pressure Sellick maneuver may help prevent aspiration. Once intubated, victims can be oxygenated and ventilated effectively despite copious pulmonary edema fluid. In spite of massive foam production after intubation, additional suctioning is not needed because foam usually does not disturb oxygenation, as does aspiration after intubation. If possible, positive end-expiratory pressure (PEEP) should be used at the beginning for better oxygenation.

Hypothermia Complicating Drowning If the victim is hypothermic ($<34°C$), CPR should continue even if in asystole (see also Chapter 31). The axiom "not dead until warm and dead" has validity in this clinical situation. Tympanic temperature measurement may be helpful if available. Although VF is uncommon in drowning, adults may develop VF as a consequence of coronary artery disease or ALS therapies, such as epinephrine.

Peripheral venous access is the preferred route for drugs. If a peripheral line cannot be established, intraosseous (IO) is preferred over endotracheal administration if equipment is available. Although some drugs can be administered endotracheally, drug doses and absorption in the setting of copious pulmonary edema fluid may be highly variable.[23] The epinephrine dose for endotracheal

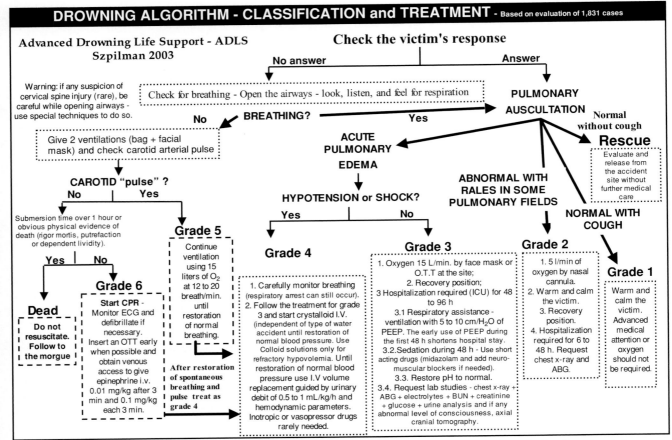

DROWNING ALGORITHM - CLASSIFICATION and TREATMENT - Based on evaluation of 1,831 cases

Advanced Drowning Life Support - ADLS
Szpilman 2003

Check the victim's response

Algorithm: Do not spend time trying to drain water from the lungs; this will only increase the risk of vomiting and complication. Do not aspirate foam while ventilating. Do not use diuretics or water restriction to treat pulmonary edema. Do not use antibiotics before 48 h except if thea accident occurred in an area of high water bacterial colonization (CFU > 10^{20}). Do not use steroids except in case of refractory bronchospasm; Always treat hypothermia. Do not stop CPR until body temperature rises to 34°C. There is no difference in ALS support between different kinds of water. Abbreviations: CPR (Cardio-pulmonary resuscitation); CPA(Cardiopulmonary Arrest); OTT(Oro-tracheal Tube); PEEP(Positive End Expiratory pressure); Recovery position (lateral decubitus position).

| FIGURE 30-3 • Drowning algorithm—classification and treatment. Based on the evaluation of 1,831 cases.

administration remains controversial, perhaps even more so in drowning.

Grade 5: Respiratory Arrest

Respiratory arrest is usually reversed with a few mouth-to-mouth ventilations. The protocol for grade 4 is then appropriate. If the victim remains apneic, mechanical ventilatory support is required.

Grade 4: Acute Pulmonary Edema With Hypotension

Oxygen with positive-pressure ventilation is the first-line therapy. Initially some of these victims will be able to maintain adequate oxygenation through an abnormally high respiratory rate or effort. But early intubation and mechanical ventilation are indicated, as the patient is consuming large amounts of energy and is likely to tire.[23] Oxygen should be administered by face mask with 15 L/min until a cuffed orotracheal tube can be inserted by rapid sequence induction.

Following intubation, patients should be kept sedated with drugs (sedative, analgesic, and muscular blockers as needed) in order to tolerate intubation and artificial mechanical ventilation. A tidal volume of at least 5 mL/kg of body weight should be used. Inspired oxygen (FiO_2) can start at 100% but as soon as possible should be reduced to 45% or less. Positive end-expiratory pressure (PEEP) should be added initially at a level of 5 cm H_2O and increased in increments of 2 to 3 cm H_2O until the desired intrapulmonary shunt (QS:QT) of ≤20% or PaO_2:FiO_2 of ≥250 is achieved.

If low blood pressure is not corrected after the administration of oxygen and mechanical ventilation, a rapid crystalloid infusion (regardless of type of drowning) should be administered.[15,23]

Grade 3: Acute Pulmonary Edema Without Hypotension

Some victims (28%) can maintain their arterial oxygen saturation above 90% with high-flow oxygen and noninvasive ventilatory support. Most, however (72%), need intubation and mechanical ventilation, in which case the protocols for grade 4[11] should be followed.

Grade 2: Abnormal Auscultation With Rales in Some Pulmonary Fields

Most victims (93%) need only 5 L of oxygen by nasal cannula.

Grade 1: Coughing With Normal Lung Auscultation

Victims do not require any oxygen or respiratory assistance.

Rescue: No Coughing, Foam, or Difficulty Breathing

These people can be evaluated and released from the accident site without further medical care if there is no associated disease or condition.

Hospital

Immediate Treatment

In severe cases (grades 5 and 6) survival to hospital is possible only if adequate and prompt basic life support (BLS) and ALS were available at the scene. Inpatient hospitalization is recommended for grades 2 to 6. Decision making in the ED about admission to an intensive care unit (ICU) or hospital bed versus observation in an ED or discharge home should include a thorough history of the drowning incident and previous illness, a physical examination, and a few diagnostic studies, including chest radiography and measurement of

arterial blood gases. Electrolytes, blood urea nitrogen, creatinine, and hemoglobin should also be assessed serially, although perturbations in these laboratory tests are unusual. For adolescents and adults, a toxicologic screen for suspected alcohol or drug ingestion may also be warranted. Grade 3 to 6 victims should be admitted to an ICU for close observation and therapy. Grade 2 patients can be observed in the ED for 6 to 24 hours, but grade 1 and rescue cases with no complaints or associated illness should be released home. Table 30-3 shows rates of hospitalization, overall mortality, and in-hospital mortality for each grade of severity.[11]

Central Nervous System Assessment and Interventions

The most important long-term complication of drowning injury is the anoxic–ischemic cerebral insult that occurs in survivors of cardiac arrest. Most late deaths and long-term sequelae of drowning are neurologic in origin.[32] Although the highest priority is restoration of spontaneous circulation, every effort in the early stages after rescue should be directed at resuscitating the brain and preventing further neurologic damage. These steps include all measures to provide adequate oxygenation ($StO_2 > 92\%$) and cerebral perfusion (mean arterial pressure around 100 mm Hg).

Any victim who remains comatose and unresponsive after successful CPR or deteriorates neurologically should undergo careful and frequent assessment of neurologic function for the development of cerebral edema. Helpful measures include elevating the head of the bed to 30 degrees (if there is no hypotension); avoiding jugular vein compression and situations that could provoke the Valsalva maneuver; securing good mechanical ventilation without the patient fighting the respirator; performing appropriate respiratory toilet without provoking hypoxia; treating convulsions;

| TABLE 30-3 • Rates of Mortality and Hospitalization (n = 1,831[a])

Grade	No.	Overall Mortality (%)	Admission to Hospital (%)	Hospital Mortality (%)
Rescue	38.976	0 (0.0%)	0 (0.0%)	0 (0.0%)
1	1,189	0 (0.0%)	35 (2.9%)	0 (0.0%)
2	338	2 (0.6%)	50 (14.8%)	2 (4.0%)
3	58	3 (5.2%)	26 (44.8%)	3 (11.5%)
4	36	7 (19.4%)	32 (88.9%)	7 (19.4%)
5	25	11 (44%)	21 (84%)[c]	7 (33.3%)
6	185	172 (93%)	23 (12.4%)[c]	10 (43.5%)
Total	1,831[b]	195 (10.6%)	187 (10.2%)[d]	29 (15.5%)
		$P < 0.0001$		

[a]Overall mortality was 10.6%.
[b]The rescue cases were excluded.
[c]A total of 4 patients of grade 5 and 162 of grade 6 were pronounced dead and thus taken directly to the morgue.
[d]Need of overall hospitalization (10.2%) in ND/D cases in association with grade and mortality. Mortality in the hospital was 15.5%.

avoiding sudden metabolic corrections; preventing anything that would increase intracranial pressure (ICP) such as urinary retention, pain, or hypotension; and maintaining normal serum glucose levels.[8]

Continuous monitoring of core temperature is important in the ED and ICU. Drowning victims with restoration of adequate spontaneous circulation who remain comatose should not be actively rewarmed to temperature values >32°C to 34°C. If core temperature exceeds 34°C, hypothermia (32°C–34°C) should be achieved as soon as possible and sustained for 12 to 24 hours. Hyperthermia should be prevented at all times in the acute recovery period. Unfortunately, studies that have evaluated the results of cerebral resuscitation measures in drowning victims have failed to demonstrate that therapies directed at controlling intracranial hypertension and maintaining cerebral perfusion pressure (CPP) improve outcome. These studies have shown poor outcomes (i.e., death or moderate to profound neurologic sequelae) when the intracranial pressure was ≥20 mm Hg and the CPP was ≤60 mm Hg despite therapies directed at controlling and improving these pressures. More research is needed to evaluate the specific efficacy of neuroresuscitative therapies in drowning victims.[31]

New therapeutic interventions for drowning victims, such as extracorporeal membrane oxygenation, artificial surfactant, nitric oxide, liquid lung ventilation, and early initiation of mild hypothermia, are still at the investigational stage.

Pulmonary Assessment and Interventions

Grade 4 to 6 patients who have received prehospital ALS care usually arrive in the ED with mechanical ventilation and acceptable oxygenation. If not, PEEP should be instituted. Once the desired oxygenation is achieved at a given level of positive airway pressure, that level of PEEP should be maintained unchanged for 48 hours before attempting to decrease it, in order to allow adequate surfactant regeneration. During that time, if the patient begins to breathe adequately on his or her own, extubation may proceed, but with continuous positive airway pressure (CPAP) plus ventilatory pressure support mode (PSV). In selected cases, CPAP may be provided initially by mask or nasal cannula (in infants who are obligate nasal breathers), but usually this is not tolerated by older patients, and pulmonary edema generally necessitates intubation.

After the airway is secured, nasogastric tube placement reduces gastric distention and prevents further aspiration.

A clinical picture very similar to ARDS is common after significant drowning (grades 3–6). The difference is that the acute respiratory distress seen with drowning has a much faster time to recovery and usually no pulmonary sequelae. Management is similar to that of other patients with ARDS, including efforts to minimize volutrauma and barotrauma. However, lung salvage involving permissive hypercapnia probably is not suitable for grade 6 drowning victims with significant hypoxic–ischemic brain injury. Instead, mild to moderate hyperventilation, aiming for a $PaCO_2$ in the range of 30 to 35 mm Hg, is probably indicated, together with other therapeutic measures to control cerebral edema.

Barotrauma The clinician must be aware of and constantly vigilant for potential complications of therapy and underlying pulmonary injury, namely, volutrauma and barotrauma.[32] Spontaneous pneumothoraces are common (10%) secondary to positive-pressure ventilation and local areas of hyperinflation. Any sudden change in hemodynamic stability during mechanical ventilation should be considered a pneumothorax or other barotrauma until proven otherwise.

Cardiovascular Assessment and Interventions

In patients who are hemodynamically unstable or have severe pulmonary dysfunction (grades 4–6), pulmonary artery catheterization or noninvasive techniques may improve the ability to assess and treat the victim. Colloid solutions are controversial and should be used only for refractory hypovolemia when replacement with crystalloid was not enough to restore blood pressure promptly. No evidence exists to support the routine administration of hypertonic solutions and blood transfusions for freshwater drowning or the use of hypotonic solutions in saltwater drowning.[15,23] Pulmonary artery catheterization or other less invasive techniques also enable the clinician to monitor cardiac function, pulmonary function, and adequacy of tissue oxygenation and perfusion as well as to assess the response of these parameters to various therapies. Echocardiography to assess cardiac function and ejection fraction can help guide the clinician in deciding on inotropic agents, vasopressors, or both if crystalloid volume replacement has failed. Some studies have shown that early cardiac dysfunction with low cardiac output is common following severe drowning (grades 4–6).[15] Important supportive measures include Foley catheter placement to monitor urine output. Low cardiac output is associated with high pulmonary capillary occlusion pressure, high central venous pressure, and high pulmonary vascular resistance; it can persist for days after reoxygenation and reperfusion. The result is the addition of cardiogenic pulmonary edema to the noncardiogenic pulmonary edema. Despite a depressed cardiac output, furosemide therapy is not a good idea. One study has even suggested that volume infusion benefits drowning victims. Other studies suggest that dobutamine infusion to improve cardiac output is the most logical and potentially beneficial therapy.[19]

Metabolic acidosis occurs in 70% of patients arriving at the hospital.[17] Correction should be considered only when pH is <7.2 or the bicarbonate <12 mEq/L if the victim has adequate ventilatory support.[10] Significant depletion of bicarbonate is rarely present in the first 10 to 15 minutes of CPR, contraindicating its use initially.[30]

Infection

Pools and beaches usually do not have sufficiently high bacterial counts to cause pneumonia soon after the incident.[32] However, if the victim has needed mechanical respiratory assistance, the incidence of secondary pneumonia increases from 34% to 52% by the third or fourth day of hospitalization, when pulmonary edema usually is nearly resolved.[33] Vigilance not only for pulmonary infection but also for other septic complications is important. Prophylactic antibiotics are of doubtful value and tend only to select out more resistant and aggressive organisms. An abnormal chest x-ray should not automatically be interpreted as pneumonia, because it is usually the result of pulmonary edema and aspirated water in the alveoli and bronchi. A preferable approach is daily monitoring of tracheal aspirates with Gram's stain, culture, and sensitivity. Prolonged fever, sustained leukocytosis, persistent or new pulmonary infiltrates, and leukocyte response in the tracheal aspirate all suggest pneumonia, which usually occurs after the first 48 to 72 hours. Empiric antibiotic therapy is then initiated, with definitive therapy based on culture and sensitivity results. Fiberoptic bronchoscopy may be useful for obtaining sputum for culture, for determining the extent and severity of airway injury in cases of solid aspiration, and, on rare occasions, for therapeutic clearing of sand, gravel, and others solids. Corticosteroids for pulmonary injury are at best of doubtful value and probably should not be used except for bronchospasm. A persistent systemic inflammatory response has been reported in the first 24 hours after successful resuscitation and explains the very common refractory low-grade fever often seen during this period.

Renal System Assessment and Interventions

Renal insufficiency or failure is rare in drowning victims but can occur secondary to anoxia, shock, or hemoglobinuria. Serial electrolytes and renal function studies are monitored in indicated patients.

Outcome and Scoring Systems

Almost all (95%) grade 1 to 5 drowning victims return home safely without sequelae,[11] although grade 3 to 6 drownings have the potential to provoke multisystem organ failure.[17] Grade 6 victims are, of course, at major risk. Difficult questions arise, such as: Which victims should be resuscitated? How long should CPR be continued? What treatment should be performed postresuscitation? And what quality of life can be expected after successful resuscitation? Unfortunately, no single indicator for grade 6 drowning can reliably predict outcome, either at the rescue site or in the hospital.[34]

Indications for starting and prolonging resuscitation vary. Multiple studies have suggested that outcome is almost solely determined by a single factor: duration of submersion (Table 30-4).[11,24,28,32,35–39] However, the effect of rapidly induced hypothermia may alter the value of submersion time as an outcome predictor. Body-heat exchange occurs very quickly in the water environment, when a large body surface area comes in contact with water whose temperature is usually lower than that of the victim Moreover, the water is often flowing, so that conductive cooling is enhanced.

TABLE 30-4 • Probability of Neurologically Intact Survival to Hospital Discharge Based on Duration of Submersion

Duration of Submersion (minutes)	Death or Severe Neurologic Impairment
0–5 minutes	10%
5–10 minutes	56%
10–25 minutes	88%
>25 minutes	100%

Note in these data how 5 more minutes of submersion in the 5- to 10-minute group increases mortality almost six times compared with the group submerged for <5 minutes.

Based on one reported case of a victim who had the longest submersion time (66 minutes) with recovery,[23] the recommendation is to initiate resuscitation without delay for every victim without a carotid palpable pulse who has been submerged for <1 hour in very cold or icy water and who does not present obvious physical evidence of death (rigor mortis, putrefaction, or dependent lividity). However, the concept that successful resuscitation after a lengthy submersion is possible only in cold or icy water has been challenged by several anecdotal reports of drownings in warm water followed by survival without sequelae.[11,35,36]

BLS and ALS enable victims to achieve the best outcome possible given the duration of cardiopulmonary arrest submersion time. Based on a report of a drowning victim successfully resuscitated after 2 hours of CPR,[32] effort should stop only if asystole persists after the victim has been rewarmed above 34°C. "No one is dead until warm and dead."[43] However, in the northern United States, where drowning most often occurs in cold but not icy waters, one large study of 194 hospitalized children and adolescents (an age group most easily cooled during a submersion) reported no survivors who required >25 minutes of CPR by EMS.[40]

Regardless of core temperature, however, a serum potassium level of 10 mEq/L in nonhemolyzed blood is generally accepted as an indication of irreversible death.

After successful CPR, it is crucial to stratify the severity of neurologic injury, which will allow comparison of different therapeutic approaches. Various prognostic scoring systems have been developed to predict which patients will do well with standard therapy and which are likely to have a significant anoxic encephalopathy requiring aggressive measures to protect the brain. The most powerful predictor of outcome is the consciousness level as measured by the Glasgow Coma Scale in the period immediately after the first hour of resuscitation. Alert patients should survive; most comatose patients will die (Table 30-5).

Because of 2- to 6-hour delays between rescue and transfer from the scene to an outlying emergency facility or an ICU, many patients with severe anoxic–ischemic cerebral insults and coma have had multiple determinations of neurologic status and level of consciousness before definitive therapy is begun. In the comatose patient, clinical and laboratory indicators of

TABLE 30-5 • Conn & Modell Neurologic Classification and Clinical Prognostic Score for the Immediate Period Following Successful CPR, Based on Glasgow Coma Scale Score

A: First hour	B: After 5 to 8 hours
Alert, 10	Alert, 9.5
Confused, 9	Confused, 8
Stupor, 7	Torpor, 6
Coma with normal brainstem, 5	Coma with normal brainstem, 3
Coma with abnormal brainstem, 2	Coma with abnormal brainstem, 1

A + B: Recovery Without Sequelae	
Excellent, 0 (≥13)	≥95%
Very good, 10–12	75%–85%
Good, 8	40%–60%
Fair, 5	10%–30%
Poor, 3	≥5%

brainstem death, such as absent papillary reflex and lack of spontaneous breathing or severe acidosis and severe hyperglycemia, predict death or severe neurologic sequelae, including persistent vegetative state.[40] Prognostic variables are important in counseling family members of drowning victims soon after the incident, and they are particularly crucial in deciding which patients are likely to have a good outcome with standard supportive therapy and which should be candidates for more aggressive cerebral resuscitation therapies.[37]

Uniform Clinical Reporting of Drowning

Standardization of definition, terminology, nomenclature, and classification of drowning is extremely important in distinguishing different pathologies resulting from drowning, including the severity and grading of drowning (Fig. 30-4). Standardization allows comparisons of statistics from different parts of the world by any lifeguard service, prehospital system, or hospital facility.

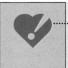 See Web site for ILCOR advisory statement on uniform reporting of drowning, Utstein style.

A Final Comment

Drowning represents, a tragedy that all too often is preventable. Perhaps the majority of such deaths are the end result of commonsense violations, alcohol consumption, and neglect of responsible child care. This picture needs a radical preventive intervention.

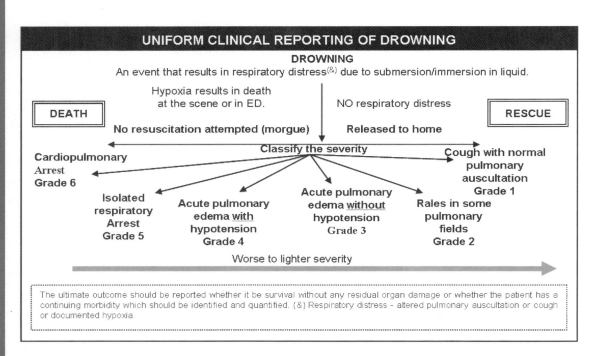

FIGURE 30-4 • Guidelines for uniform clinical reporting of drowning. (Unpublished data, Szpilman, 2002.)

References

1. Murray CJL. Quantifying the burden of disease: the technical basis for disability-adjusted life years. *Bull WHO* 1994;72:429–445.
2. Peden M, McGee K, Sharma K. *The Injury Chart Book: A Graphical Overview of the Global Burden of Injuries.* Geneva: World Health Organization, 2002.
3. International Life Saving Federation. World drowning report. *Int J Aquatic Res Educ* 2007;1:381–401.
4. Branche CM. What is really happening with drowning rates in the United States? In Fletemeyer JR, Freas SJ, eds. *Drowning: New Perspectives on Intervention and Prevention.* Boca Raton, FL: CRC Press, 1998:31–42.
5. World Health Organization. Bulletin report on A Injury-a leading cause of the global burden of disease @.Geneva: WHO, 1998.
6. Peden MM, McGee K. The epidemiology of drowning worldwide. *Injury Control Safety Promotion* 2003;10(4):195–199.
7. CDC. Web-based Injury Statistics Query and Reporting System (WISQARS). Available at http://www.cdc.gov/ncipc/wisqars.
8. Gilchrist J, Gotsch K, Ryan G. Nonfatal and fatal drownings in recreational water settings: United States, 2001–2002. National Center for Injury Prevention and Control. *MMWR* 2004;53(21):447–452.
9. Szpilman D. Drowning in Brazil—179,000 deaths in 25 years—are we stepping down? World Water Safety Congress, Porto, Portugal, September 2007.
10. Szpilman D, Goulart PM, Mocellin O, et al. 12 years of Brazilian Lifesaving Society (Sobrasa) – Did we make any difference? World Water Safety, Matosinhos – Portugal 2007, Book of Abstracts, ISBN: 978-989-95519-0-9, :207–208.
11. Szpilman D. Near-drowning and drowning classification: a proposal to stratify mortality based on the analysis of 1831 cases. *Chest* 1997; 112(3):660–665.
12. Szpilman D, Orlowski, JP, Cruz-Filho FES, et al. Near-drowning: you've been messing up our minds! In Amsterdam: Book of Abstract of World Congress on Drowning, 2002:114.
13. Szpilman D. Definition of drowning and other water-related injuries. June 2002. Available at "http://www.drowning.nl" www.drowning.nl
14. The International Liaison Committee on Resuscitation in collaboration with the American Heart Association. Guidelines 2000 for Cardiopulmonary Resuscitation and Emergency Cardiovascular Care. Part 8: Advanced Challenges in Resuscitation: Section 3: Special Challenges in ECC 3B: Submersion or Near-Drowning. Resuscitation 2000;46:273–277.
15. Orlowski JP, Abulleil MM, Phillips JM. The hemodynamic and cardiovascular effects of near-drowning in hypotonic, isotonic, or hypertonic solutions. *Ann Emerg Med* 1989;18:1044–1049.
16. Modell JH, Moya F, Newby EJ, et al. The effects of fluid volume in seawater drowning. *Ann Intern Med* 1967;67:68–80.
17. Szpilman D. Afogamento. *Revista Bras Med Esporte* 2000;6(4):131–144.
18. Szpilman D, Morizot-Leite L, Vries W, et al. First aid courses for the aquatic environment. In Bierens J, ed. *Handbook on Drowning: Prevention, Rescue, and Treatment.* Berlin: Springer-Verlag, 2005:342–347.
19. Donoghue AJ, Nadkarni V, Berg RA, et al. Out-of-hospital pediatric cardiac arrest: an epidemiologic review and assessment of current knowledge. *Ann Emerg Med* 2005;46(6):512–522.
20. Quan L, Liller K, Bennett E. Water related injuries of children and adolescents. In Liller K, ed. *Injury Prevention for Children and Adolescents: Research, Practice, and Advocacy.* Washington DC: American Public Health Association, 2006.
21. Quan L, Bennett E, Branche CM. Interventions to prevent drowning. In Doll LS, Bonzo SE, Sleet DA et al, eds. *Handbook of Injury and Violence Prevention.* New York: Springer, 2007:81–96.
22. Szpilman D, Orlowski JP, Bierens J. Drowning. In Fink M, Abraham E, Vincent JL, Kochanek P, eds. *Textbook of Critical Care,* 5th ed. Philadelphia: Elsevier Science, 2004:699–706.
23. Orlowski JP, Szpilman D. Drowning: rescue, resuscitation, and reanimation. Pediatric critical care: a new millennium. *Pediatr Clin North Am* 2001;48(3):627–646.
24. Szpilman D, Soares M. In-water resuscitation—is it worthwhile? *Resuscitation* 2004;63:25–31.
25. Wernick P, Fenner P, Szpilman D. Immobilization and extraction of spinal injuries. In Bierens J, ed. *Handbook on Drowning: Prevention, Rescue, and Treatment.* Berlin: Springer-Verlag, 2005:291–295.
26. Watson RS, Cummings P, Quan L, et al. Cervical spine injuries among submersion victims. *J Trauma* 2001;51:658–662.
27. Szpilman D, Handley A. Positioning the drowning victim. In Bierens J, ed. *Handbook on Drowning: Prevention, Rescue, and Treatment.* Berlin: Springer-Verlag, 2005:336–341.
28. Manolios N, Mackie I. Drowning and near-drowning on Australian beaches patrolled by life-savers: a 10-year study, 1973–1983. *Med J Aust* 1988;148:165–167, 170–171.
29. Szpilman D, Elmann J, Cruz-Filho RES. Drowning classification: a revalidation study based on the analysis of 930 cases over 10 years. In Bierens J, ed. *Handbook on Drowning: Prevention, Rescue, and Treatment.* Berlin: Springer-Verlag, 2005:66.
30. Guidelines for cardiopulmonary resuscitation and emergency cardiac care (ECC). *Circulation* 2000;102(8):129.
31. Nichter MA, Everett PB. Childhood near-drowning: is cardiopulmanry resuscitation always indicated? *Crit Care Med* 1989;17:993–995.
32. Orlowski JP. Drowning, near-drowning, and ice water submersion. *Pediatr Clin North Am* 1987;34:92.
33. Berkel M, Bierens J, Lerlk C, et al. Pulmonary oedema, pneumonia and mortality in submersions victims: a retrospective study in 125 patients. *Int C Md* 1996;22:101–107.
34. Bierens J, Velde EA, Berkel M, et al. Submersion in the Netherlands: prognostic indicators and results of resuscitation. *Ann Emerg Med* 1990;19:1390–1395.
35. Szpilman D. A case report of 22 minutes submersion in warm water without sequelae. In Bierens J, ed. *Handbook on Drowning: Prevention, Rescue, and Treatment.* Berlin: Springer-Verlag, 2005:375–376.
36. Allman FD, Nelson WB, Gregory AP, et al. Outcome following cardiopulmonary resuscitation in severe near-drowning. *Am J Dis Child* 1986;140:571–575.
37. Orlowski JP. Prognostic factors in pediatric cases of drowning and near-drowning. *J Coll Emerg Physicians* 1979;8:176–179.
38. Cummings P, Quan L. Trends in unintentional drowning: the role of alcohol and medical care. *JAMA* 1999;281:2198–2202.
39. Cummins RO, Szpilman D. Submersion. In Cummins RO, Field JM, Hazinski MF, eds. *ACLS: The Reference Textbook:* vol II. *ACLS for Experienced Providers.* Dallas: American Heart Association, 2003:97–107.
40. Graf WD, Cummings P, Quan L, et al. Predicting outcome in pediatric submersion victims. *Ann Emerg Med* 1995;26:312–319.
41. Modell JH. Drowning: current concepts. *N Engl J Med* 1993;328(4):253–256.
42. Conn AW, Modell JH. Current neurological considerations in near-drowning (editorial). *Can Anaesth Soc J* 1980;27:197.
43. Southwick FS, Dalglish PH. Recovery after prolonged asystolic cardiac arrest in profound hypothermia. *JAMA* 1980;243:1250–1253.

Chapter 31
Hypothermia

Eric A. Weiss

Severe hypothermia (body temperature <30°C [86°F]) is associated with marked depression of critical body functions, which may make the victim appear clinically dead during the initial assessment. In some cases hypothermia may exert a protective effect on the brain and organs in cardiac arrest, and intact neurologic recovery may be possible after prolonged periods of cardiac arrest in the hypothermic victim. Therefore, lifesaving procedures should not be withheld on the basis of clinical presentation.

- Severely hypothermic victims require careful handling because they are prone to develop ventricular fibrillation (VF) or asystole with handling.
- Meaningful rewarming of a severely hypothermic patient in the field is difficult; a pre–hospital care goal involves the use of rewarming modalities to stabilize the victim's body temperature, prevent further cooling, and facilitate immediate transport to an appropriate facility.
- If a severely hypothermic victim has any signs of life, chest compressions should not be initiated as they may precipitate VF.
- If VF or pulseless ventricular tachycardia (VT) is detected, it should be treated with one shock until core temperature rises to between 30°C and 32°C.

Introduction

Unintentional hypothermia is classically defined as a decrease in core body temperature to below 35°C (95°F).[1] Victims of accidental hypothermia present year-round and in all climates. The progressive lowering of core body temperature produces a predictable pattern of organ dysfunction and associated clinical manifestations (Table 31-1). Recognition of the relationship between core temperature and physiologic manifestations is important, as it provides a blueprint and foundation for management decisions that are often unique to hypothermic victims. Cardiopulmonary resuscitation (CPR) and emergency care of hypothermic patients differ in several important respects from that of normothermic patients.

Severe hypothermia (body temperature <30°C [86°F)]) is associated with marked depression of critical body functions, which may make the victim appear clinically dead during the initial assessment.[2,3] In some cases, hypothermia may exert a protective effect on the brain and organs in cardiac arrest.[4,5] Intact neurologic recovery may be possible after prolonged periods of cardiac arrest in the hypothermic victim, although those with nonasphyxial arrest have a better prognosis than those with asphyxia-associated hypothermic arrest.[6–8] Therefore, lifesaving procedures should not be withheld on the basis of clinical presentation.[2,7] Victims should be transported as soon as possible to a center where monitored rewarming is possible.

Classification of Hypothermia

Several different classification systems for hypothermia have been proposed based on core temperature.[7,9,10] For purposes of emergency management and resuscitation, hypothermia can best be characterized as either mild or severe. In mild hypothermia (core temperature 35°C–31°C [95°F–87.8°F]), the victim is conscious, still shivering, and generally not prone to developing cardiac dysrhythmias. In severe hypothermia (core temperature below 31°C [87.8°F]), the victim has an altered level of consciousness, diminished or absent shivering, and is prone to develop cardiac dysrhythmias.[9]

Since mildly hypothermic victims are still able to generate heat through shivering, they do well without invasive rewarming. Severely hypothermic victims have markedly diminished or absent thermogenesis owing to the cessation of shivering and require active internal (invasive) rewarming during resuscitation. Active internal rewarming methods include extracorporeal blood rewarming, inhalation therapy, peritoneal lavage, thoracic cavity lavage, and thoracotomy with mediastinal irrigation.

| TABLE 31-1 • Classification of Hypothermia: Signs, Physical Findings and Cardiac Characteristics

Stage	°C	°F	Characteristics
Mild hypothermia			
	37.6	99.6 ± 1	Normal rectal temperature
	37.0	98.6 ± 1	Normal oral temperature
	36.0	96.8	Increase in metabolic rate and blood pressure
	35.0	95.0	Maximum shivering thermogenesis
	34.0	93.2	Dysarthria and poor judgment develop, maladaptive behavior; normal blood pressure, maximum respiratory stimulation, tachycardia and then progressive bradycardia
Severe hypothermia			
	30.0	86.0	Extinguished shivering thermogenesis, atrial fibrillation and other arrhythmias develop, cardiac output two thirds of normal
	29.0	85.2	Progressive decrease in level of consciousness, pulse, and respiration; pupils dilated; paradoxical undressing occurs
	28.0	82.4	Decreased ventricular fibrillation threshold, 50% decrease in oxygen consumption and pulse
	26.0	78.8	Major acid-base disturbances, no reflexes or response to pain
	25.0	77.0	Cerebral blood flow one third of normal, loss of cerebrovascular autoregulation, cardiac output 45% of normal, pulmonary edema may develop
	23.0	73.4	No corneal or oculocephalic reflexes, areflexia
	22.0	71.6	Maximum risk of ventricular fibrillation, 75% decrease in oxygen consumption
	20.0	68.0	Lowest resumption of cardiac electromechanical activity, pulse 20% of normal
	19.0	66.2	Electroencephalographic silencing
	18.0	64.4	Asystole
	13.7	56.8	Lowest adult accidental hypothermia survival
	15.0	59.2	Lowest infant accidental hypothermia survival
	10.0	50.0	92% decrease in oxygen consumption
	9.0	48.2	Lowest therapeutic hypothermia survival

Source: Adapted from Auerbach PS, Weiss EA, Donner H. *Field Guide to Wilderness Medicine.* Philadelphia: Mosby, 2003, with permission.

Cardiovascular Manifestations

Cold stress initially stimulates tachycardia and peripheral vasoconstriction, both of which increase systemic blood pressure and cardiac afterload.[11,12] There is a resultant increase in myocardial oxygen demand. As the core temperature drops, there is a linear decrease in pulse rate. At 28°C (82.4°F) there is a 50% decrease in heart rate.[11–13] This bradycardia is caused by decreased spontaneous depolarization of the pacemaker cells and is, therefore, refractory to atropine administration.[10]

During hypothermic bradycardia, unlike normothermia, systole is prolonged longer than diastole. In addition, the conduction system is much more sensitive to cold than is the myocardium, so the cardiac cycle is lengthened.[13]

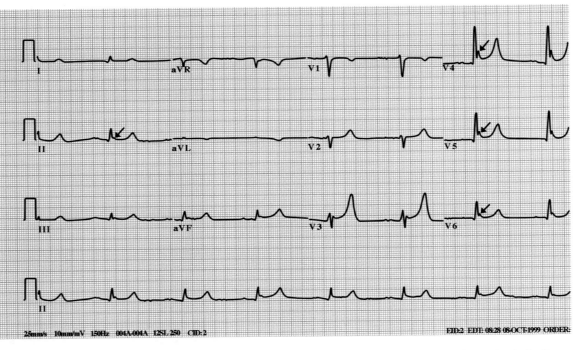

FIGURE 31-1 • A 12-lead ECG obtained at core body temperature of 85°F. Note Osborn waves and an extra deflection at the end of the QRS complex (*arrows*). (From Alhaddad IA, Khalil M, Brown EJ Jr. Osborn waves of hypothermia. *Circulation* 2000;101[25]27:e233–e234, with permission.)

Hypothermia progressively decreases mean arterial pressure and cardiac index. Cardiac output drops to about 45% of normal at 25°C. Even after rewarming, cardiovascular function may remain temporarily depressed, with impaired myocardial contractility and peripheral vascular function.[14]

Characteristic electrocardiographic alterations and conduction abnormalities occur as hypothermia progresses. First the PR, then the QRS, and finally the QT intervals become prolonged.[10] The J wave (Osborn wave or hypothermic hump) occurs at the junction of the QRS complex and the ST segment at temperatures below 32°C[15,16] (Fig. 31-1). Osborn waves are typically seen in leads II and V3 to V6. They are neither prognostic nor specific to hypothermia.

Below 30°C, atrial and ventricular arrhythmias are common. Hypothermia-induced VF and asystole often occur spontaneously below 25°C.[17] The VF threshold and the transmembrane resting potential are decreased. VF and asystole may both result from rough handling or jostling of the victim or from sudden vertical positioning.[10]

Prehospital Treatment of Mild Hypothermia

The priority in the prehospital setting is to prevent further heat loss and facilitate rewarming. The rescuer should remove all wet clothing, replace it with dry clothing, and insulate the victim with sleeping bags, blankets, extra clothing, or other suitable material. Use adequate insulation underneath the victim as well as on top. If the victim is capable of purposeful swallowing (will not aspirate), encourage drinking of warm and sugary drinks.

Prehospital Treatment of Severe Hypothermia

Severely hypothermic victims require careful handling because they are prone to develop VF or asystole with handling. If in the back country, consider helicopter transport to prevent the jostling that would occur with an overland evacuation. Because of autonomic dysfunction, victims should be kept in a horizontal position whenever possible to minimize orthostatic hypotension (see also hypothermia associated with drowning in Chapter 30).[9]

Oxygen should be provided by nasal cannula or face mask or, if necessary, bag-valve-mask ventilation or endotracheal intubation. The indications for endotracheal intubation in hypothermia are identical to those in normothermia.[18] Endotracheal intubation should be performed without concern for inducing VF. In a multicenter survey, endotracheal intubation was performed on 117 patients by multiple clinicians in various settings. No induced arrhythmias occurred in any of the patients.[19] Fiberoptic intubation or cricothyroidotomy may be required to secure the airway when cold-induced trismus prevents direct laryngoscopy. Rapid sequence intubation with paralytic agents may not be productive, as paralytic agents will not be able to overcome the trismus produced by profound hypothermia.

Overinflation of the endotracheal tube cuff with cold air should be avoided, as the air inside the cuff will expand as the victim rewarms and potentially kink the tube or rupture the cuff.[18]

Administration of at least 500 mL of heated (37°C–41°C [98.6°F–105.8°F]) intravenous (IV) normal saline or 5% dextrose in normal saline may help to stabilize the conduction system of the heart and begin to reverse dehydration. Lactated Ringer's solution should be avoided because a cold liver metabolizes lactate poorly. Intraosseous infusion provides an excellent alternative pathway for fluid replacement in a severely hypothermic patient when peripheral vessels have collapsed and are unable to be cannulated.

Meaningful rewarming of a severely hypothermic patient in the field is difficult; the goal in prehospital care should thus be to use rewarming modalities to stabilize the victim's body temperature and prevent further cooling. Warmed IV solutions, heated humidified oxygen, and externally applied heat provide only a small amount of heat input. Hot water bottles or heat packs can be placed in the axillae and groin area and alongside the neck, where large blood vessels course near the surface. Hot water bottles should be wrapped with insulation to prevent thermal burns.

Ventricular Arrhythmias

Transient ventricular arrhythmias are common in severe hypothermia and should generally be left untreated.[20] Class IA (i.e., procainamide) and class IB (i.e., lidocaine) ventricular antiarrhythmics have not been shown to be effective in reversing or preventing VF in hypothermic victims.[21,22] The class III agent bretylium tosylate was effective in preventing VF when administered to dogs prior to induction of hypothermia, but it was not therapeutic in reversing VF after it occurred.[23,24] There are no human studies to validate its use in hypothermic patients and it is not commercially available at present. In a canine model of severe hypothermic VF, amiodarone did not improve conversion to sinus rhythm or survival.[24] In summary, there are no commercially available ventricular antiarrhythmics proven safe and effective for use in hypothermic victims.

Atrial Arrhythmias

Atrial arrhythmias, including atrial fibrillation, are common in victims with temperature below 32°C. They usually convert spontaneously during rewarming and should be considered innocent. Treatment is directed toward rewarming and correcting fluid needs and electrolyte abnormalities rather than administering atrial antiarrhythmics.

Cardiopulmonary Resuscitation

Severe hypothermia is associated with marked depression of critical body functions, which may make a "live" victim appear clinically dead during the initial assessment. Breathing may be difficult to detect if tidal volume and ventilatory rate are significantly depressed. The rescuer should listen and feel carefully around the nose and mouth and use a glass object or mirror to detect a "vapor trail." Palpation of peripheral pulses is often difficult in vasoconstricted and bradycardic patients. The rescuer should auscultate and palpate for at least 1 minute to detect a pulse. This is best done at the carotid or femoral arteries.[10] Rapid cardiac ultrasound of patients with pulseless electrical activity (PEA) can be successfully integrated into the ACLS response to assist in confirming the presence of cardiac asystole (see Chapter 8).[25]

If a hypothermic victim has any sign of life, chest compressions should not be initiated, as they may precipitate VF.[19] If the victim is without any sign of life, begin standard CPR. A single rescuer who is fatigued may continue at slower rates of compression and rescue breathing, as these may be adequate because of the protective effects of hypothermia.[26]

If a cardiac monitor is available, use maximal amplification to search for QRS complexes. If VT or VF is present, defibrillation should be attempted. The energy requirement for defibrillation does not increase in hypothermia. Automated external defibrillators (AEDs) may be used for these patients. If VF or pulseless VT is detected, it should be treated with one shock, as outlined in the AHA ECC "Guidelines for Management of Cardiac Arrest" in patients with hypothermia (Fig. 31-2). If the victim does not respond to one shock, further defibrillation attempts should be deferred until the victim has been rewarmed to at least 30°C (86°F). Defibrillation rarely succeeds below a core temperature of 30°C (86°F).[3,27] In the prehospital setting, warming and CPR should be continued until the victim either responds with a return of pulse or arrives at a hospital or the rescuer cannot continue because of fatigue or danger to the rescuer.

See Web site for AHA ECC 2005 guidelines for CPR: hypothermia.

More force is often needed to depress the chest wall during CPR in a severely hypothermic victim due to decreased chest wall elasticity. Myocardial and pulmonary compliance are also markedly reduced in hypothermia. During hypothermic cardiac arrest in swine, the cardiac output, cerebral blood flow, and myocardial blood flow averaged 50%, 55%, and 31%, respectively, of those achieved during normothermic closed-chest compressions.[27]

In a multicenter survey of 428 cases, 9 of the 27 patients receiving CPR initiated in the field survived, as did 6 of 14 patients with ED-initiated CPR.[19] Based on these cases and other reports in the literature, CPR is recommended in the prehospital setting unless any of the following exist: do-not-resuscitate status, obviously lethal injuries, impossibility of chest wall depression, any sign of life, or danger to the rescuers.[10,19] Apparent rigor mortis, dependent lividity, and fixed, dilated pupils are not reliable criteria for withholding CPR.[10] Intermittent CPR is preferable to no CPR. One patient recovered after 6½ hours of intermittent closed-chest compressions.[28]

Initial therapy for all patients
- Remove wet garments
- Protect against heat loss and wind chill
  (use blankets and insulating equipment)
- Maintain horizontal position
- Avoid rough movement and excess activity
- Monitor core temperature
- Monitor cardiac rhythm[1]

Assess responsiveness, breathing, and pulse

Pulse and breathing present

What is core temperature?

>34°C (>93.2°F)
Mild hypothermia
- Passive rewarming
- Active external rewarming

30°C to 34°C (86°F to 93.2°F)
Moderate hypothermia
- Passive rewarming
- Active external rewarming of truncal
  areas only[2,3]

<30°C (86°F)
Severe hypothermia
- Active internal rewarming sequence (see
  below)

Pulse or breathing absent

- Start CPR
- Give 1 Shock
  — Manual biphasic: device specific (typically 120 to 200 J)
    If unknown, use 200 J
  — AED, device specific
  — Monophasic: 360 J
- Resume CPR immediately
- Attempt, confirm, secure airway
- Ventilate with warm, humid *oxygen* (42°C to 46°C [108°F to 115°F])[2]
- Establish IV access
- Infuse warm NS (42°C to 44°C [108°F to 111.2°F])[2]

What is core temperature?

<30°C (86°F)   **>30°C (86°F)**

- Continue CPR
- Withhold IV medications
- Limit to one shock for
  VF/VT
- Transport to hospital

- Continue CPR
- Give IV medications as
  indicated (but space at
  longer than standard
  intervals)
- Repeat defibrillation
  for VF/VT as core
  temperature rises

Active internal rewarming[2]
- Warm IV fluids (43°C [109°F])
- Warm, humid *oxygen* (42°C to 46°C [108°F to 115°F])
- Peritoneal lavage (KCI-free fluid)
- Extracorporeal rewarming
- Esophageal rewarming tubes[4]

Continue internal rewarming until
- Core temperature >35°C (95°F) or
- Return of spontaneous circulation or
- Resuscitative efforts cease

© 2008 American Heart Association

| FIGURE 31-2 • AHA Hypothermia algorithm, revised 2008.

Epinephrine or vasopressin is not recommended for hypothermic cardiac arrest below 30°C. There is no evidence that repeated or high-dose epinephrine during hypothermic cardiac arrest improves outcome.[29,30] Low-dose dopamine (1–5 μg/kg/min) should be reserved for severe hypotension that does not respond to administration of IV fluids and rewarming.[31]

Rewarming Modalities

Mild hypothermia is best treated with noninvasive external rewarming. If vigorous shivering is present, drying the patient and providing insulation is sufficient. The use of a forced-air surface warming system such as the Bair Hugger is ideal and generally available at most primary care centers. Rewarming rates with this modality average 1°C to 2°C/hr.[32,33]

It is not uncommon to observe a continued decline in core temperature after a hypothermic patient is removed from the cold environment and external rewarming is initiated. This phenomenon, referred to as "core temperature afterdrop," can be attributed to two main factors. The primary factor is the temperature gradient that exists between the cooler periphery and the warmer core. When the surface is rewarmed, the gradient starts to reverse, but there is continued equilibration between the warmer core and the cooler periphery, resulting in continued lowering of the core temperature.[9] The other contributing factor is peripheral vasodilatation secondary to external rewarming, with increased flow of blood to the previously hypoperfused and colder extremities resulting in further cooling of the core.[9,34]

Afterdrop may be clinically important in patients who are bordering on severe hypothermia and likely to develop cardiovascular deterioration with a small further drop in core temperature. In such patients, it may be preferable to utilize active internal core rewarming methods.

Active internal core rewarming modalities should also be considered for patients with severe hypothermia, cardiovascular instability, or cardiac arrest. The most effective internal core rewarming modalities are peritoneal lavage with warmed fluids; pleural lavage with warm saline through chest tubes; and extracorporeal blood warming with hemodialysis, venovenous rewarming, continuous arteriovenous rewarming, or cardiopulmonary bypass (Table 31-2).[35-56]

Heated intravenous fluids and inspired air help to prevent further heat loss, but provide only a very limited amount of heat toward rewarming. For example, if 1 L of 42°C saline is infused into a 70-kg patient with a core temperature of 25°C, the heat transfer would be 17 kcal, which would raise the core temperature only 0.29°C.[57] The rewarming rate of heated inspired air is approximately 0.5°C to 1°C/hr.[38,57-60]

Gastrointestinal irrigation (stomach, colon) and bladder irrigation with warm fluid provides negligible heat transfer, as these cavities have a small mucosal surface area and there is splanchnic vasoconstriction in patients with severe hypothermia.

Cessation of Resuscitative Efforts

Hypothermia victims have survived prolonged periods of cardiopulmonary resuscitation, and recovered after more than an hour of submersion in cold water.[61-63] Dramatic recoveries after prolonged submersion in cold water are due largely to the protective effects of hypothermia. Hypothermia increases the tolerance of the brain to ischemia; it slows metabolic processes and reduces oxygen consumption.[64] At a core temperature of 20°C, cardiac arrest is tolerated for up to 30 minutes without clinically significant neurologic or neuropsychological deficits.[65,66] This knowledge, combined with the observation that a dead victim may be clinically indistinguishable from one who is profoundly hypothermic and alive, has led to the adage that "no one should be pronounced dead until they are warm and dead." Attempting to rewarm someone who is cold and dead can be difficult without extracorporeal blood warming and requires a tremendous amount of time and resources.

A clinical marker for irreversible injury and death that would preclude the need to rewarm a victim of severe hypothermia prior to declaring death is desirable. A serum potassium level >10 mmol/L in a nonhemolyzed specimen

| TABLE 31-2 • Active Internal Rewarming Modalities and Rewarming Rates

Rewarming Method	Rewarming Rate	Comments
Peritoneal lavage	1°C–3°C/hr	Widely available and not technically difficult
Thoracic lavage	3°C–5°C/hr	Direct warming of the myocardium may allow for more rapid cardioversion.
Continuous arteriovenous rewarming	3°C–4°C/hr	Rapid initiation Anticoagulation not required Requires blood pressure of >60
Venovenous	2°C–3°C/hr	Limited by profound hypotension
Hemodialysis	2°C–3°C/hr	Widely available Anticoagulation not required Requires adequate blood pressure
Cardiopulmonary bypass	7°C–9.5°C/hr	Full circulatory support

has been proposed as a reasonable ceiling for viability. In two series involving victims of avalanche and climbing accidents, the nonsurvivors all had serum potassium levels >10 mmol/L.[67,68] In situations where the serum potassium is <10 mmol/L, it is prudent to rewarm a hypothermic victim who is in cardiac arrest to at least 32°C before declaring death and withdrawing life support.

References

1. Kempainen R, Brunette D. The evaluation and management of accidental hypothermia. *Respir Care* 2004;49(2):192–205.
2. Steinman AM. Cardiopulmonary resuscitation and hypothermia. *Circulation* 1986;74(Pt 2):IV29–IV32.
3. Southwick FS, Dalglish PH Jr. Recovery after prolonged asystolic cardiac arrest in profound hypothermia: a case report and literature review. *JAMA* 1980;243:1250–1253.
4. Holzer M, Behringer W, Schorkhuber W, et al. Mild hypothermia and outcome after CPR. Hypothermia for Cardiac Arrest (HACA) study group. *Acta Anaesthesiol Scand Suppl* 1997;111:55–58.
5. Sterz F, Safar P, Tisherman S, et al. Mild hypothermic cardiopulmonary resuscitation improves outcome after prolonged cardiac arrest in dogs. *Crit Care Med* 1991;19:379–389.
6. Farstad M, Andersen KS, Koller ME, et al. Rewarming from accidental hypothermia by extracorporeal circulation: a retrospective study. *Eur J Cardiothorac Surg* 2001;20:58–64.
7. Schneider SM. Hypothermia: from recognition to rewarming. *Emerg Med Rep* 1992;13:1–20.
8. Gilbert M, Busund R, Skagseth A, et al. Resuscitation from accidental hypothermia of 13.7°C with circulatory arrest. *Lancet* 2000;355:375–376.
9. Giesbrecht GG, Bristow GK. Recent advances in hypothermia research. *Ann N Y Acad Sci* 1997;813:676.
10. Danzl DF. Accidental hypothermia. In Auerbach PS, ed. *Wilderness Medicine*. St. Louis: Mosby, 2007:125–160.
11. Lauri T. Cardiovascular responses to an acute volume load in deep hypothermia. *Eur Heart J* 1996;17:606.
12. Lauri T, Leskinen M, Timisjarvi J, et al. Cardiac function in hypothermia. *Arctic Med Res* 1991;50:63.
13. Maaravi AY, Weiss AT. The effect of prolonged hypothermia on cardiac function in a young patient with accidental hypothermia. *Chest* 1990;98:1019.
14. Tveita T, Mortensen E, Hevroy O, et al. Hemodynamic and metabolic effects of hypothermia and rewarming. *Arctic Med Res* 1991;50:48.
15. Graham CA, McNaughton GW, Wyatt JP. The electrocardiogram in hypothermia. *Wilderness Environ Med* 2001;12:232.
16. Osborn JJ. Experimental hypothermia respiratory and blood pH changes in relation to cardiac function. *Am J Physiol* 1953;175:389.
17. Duguid H, Simpson RG, Stowers JM. Accidental hypothermia. *Lancet* 1961;2:1213.
18. Danzl DF. Hypothermia. *Semin Resp Crit Care Med* 2002;23:57.
19. Danzl DF, Pozos RS, Auerbach PS, et al. Multicenter hypothermia survey. *Ann Emerg Med* 1987;16:1042–1055.
20. Rankin AC, Rae AP. Cardiac arrhythmias during rewarming of patients with accidental hypothermia. *Br Med J (Clin Res Ed)* 1984;289:874–877.
21. Wong KC. Physiology and pharmacology of hypothermia. *West J Med* 1983;138:227.
22. Reuler JB. Hypothermia: pathophysiology, clinical settings, and management. *Ann Intern Med* 1978;89:519–527.
23. Elenbaas RM, Mattson K, Cole H, et al. Bretylium in hypothermia-induced ventricular fibrillation in dogs. *Ann Emerg Med* 1984;13:994.
24. Stoner J, Martin G, O'Mara K, et al. Amiodarone and bretylium in the treatment of hypothermic ventricular fibrillation in a canine model. *Acad Emerg Med* 2003;10:187–191.
25. Durrer B, Brugger H, Syme D. International Commission for Mountain Emergency Medicine: The medical on-site treatment of hypothermia: ICAR-MEDCOM recommendation. *High Alt Med Biol* 2003;4:99–103.
26. Niendorff DF, Rassias AJ, Palac R, et al. Rapid cardiac ultrasound of inpatients suffering PEA arrest performed by nonexpert sonographers. *Resuscitation* 2005;67(1):81–87.
27. DaVee TS, Reineberg EJ. Extreme hypothermia and ventricular fibrillation. *Ann Emerg Med* 1980;9:100.
28. Maningas PA, DeGuzman LR, Hollenbach SJ. Regional blood flow during hypothermic arrest. *Ann Emerg Med* 1986;15:390.
28a. Lexow K. Severe accidental hypothermia: Survival after 6 hours 30 minutes of cardiopulmonary resuscitation. *Arctic Med Res* 1991;50:112.
29. Kornberger E, Lindner KH, Mayr VD, et al. Effects of epinephrine in a pig model of hypothermic cardiac arrest and closed-chest cardiopulmonary resuscitation combined with active rewarming. *Resuscitation* 2001;50:301.
30. Krismer AC, Lindner KH, Kornberger R, et al. Cardiopulmonary resuscitation during severe hypothermia in pigs: does epinephrine or vasopressin increase coronary perfusion pressure? *Anesth Analg* 2000;90:69.
31. Oung CM, English M, Chiu RC, et al. Effects of hypothermia on hemodynamic responses to dopamine and dobutamine. *J Trauma* 1992;33:671.
32. Steele MT, Nelson MJ, Sessler DI, et al. Forced air speeds rewarming in accidental hypothermia. *Ann Emerg Med* 1996;27:479.
33. Goheen MS, Ducharme MB, Kenny GP, et al. Efficacy of force-air and inhalation rewarming by using a human model for severe hypothermia. *J Appl Physiol* 1997;83(5):1635–1640.
34. Giesbrecht GG, Johnston CE, Bristow GK. The convective afterdrop component during hypothermic exercise decreased with delayed exercise onset. *Aviat Space Environ Med* 1998;69:17.
35. Aslam AF, et al. Hypothermia: evaluation, electrocardiographic manifestations, and management. *Am J Med* 2006;119(4):297–301.
36. Iversen RJ, Atkin SH, Jaker MA, et al. Successful CPR in a severely hypothermic patient using continuous thoracostomy lavage. *Ann Emerg Med* 1990;19(11):1335–1337.
37. Hall KN, Syverud SA. Closed thoracic cavity lavage in the treatment of severe hypothermia in human beings. *Ann Emerg Med* 1990;19(2):204–206.
38. Otto RJ, Metzler MH. Rewarming from experimental hypothermia: comparison of heated aerosol inhalation, peritoneal lavage, and pleural lavage. *Crit Care Med* 1988;16(9):869–875.
39. Terba JA. Efficacy and safety of prehospital rewarming techniques to treat accidental hypothermia. *Ann Emerg Med* 1991;20(8):896–901.
40. Brunette DD, Sterner S, Robinson EP, et al. Comparison of gastric lavage and thoracic cavity lavage in the treatment of severe hypothermia in dogs. *Ann Emerg Med* 1987;16(11):1222–1227.
41. Brunette DD, Biros M, Mlinek EJ, et al. Internal cardiac massage and mediastinal irrigation in hypothermic cardiac arrest. *Am J Emerg Med* 1992;10(1):32–34.
42. Brunette DD, McVaney K. Hypothermic cardiac arrest: an 11 year review of ED management and outcome. *Am J Emerg Med* 2000;18(4):418–422.
43. Davis FM, Judson JA. Warm peritoneal dialysis in the management of accidental hypothermia: report of five cases. *N Z Med J* 1981;94(692):207–209.
44. Jessen K, Hagelsten JO. Peritoneal dialysis in the treatment of profound accidental hypothermia. *Aviat Space Environ Med* 1978;49(2):426–429.
45. Reuler JB, Parker RA. Peritoneal dialysis in the management of hypothermia. *JAMA* 1978;240(21):2289–2290.
46. Davies DM, Millar EJ, Miller IA. Accidental hypothermia treated by extracorporeal blood warming. *Lancet* 1967;1(7498):1036–1037.
47. Vretenar DF, Urschel JD, Parrott JC, et al. Cardiopulmonary bypass resuscitation for accidental hypothermia. *Ann Thorac Surg* 1994;58(3):895–898.
48. Splittgerber FH, Talbert JG, Sweezer WP, et al. Partial cardiopulmonary bypass for core rewarming in profound accidental hypothermia. *Am Surg* 1986;52(8):407–412.
49. Letsou GV, Kopf GS, Elefteriades JA, et al. Is cardiopulmonary bypass effective for treatment of hypothermic arrest due to drowning or exposure? *Arch Surg* 1992;127(5):525–528.
50. Gentilello LM, Cobean RA, Offner PJ, et al. Continuous arteriovenous rewarming: rapid reversal of hypothermia in critically ill patients. *J Trauma* 1992;32(3):316–325.
51. Gregory JS, Bergstein JM, Aprahamian C, et al. Comparison of three methods of rewarming from hypothermia: advantages of

extracorporeal blood warming. *J Trauma* 1991;31(9):1247–1251; discussion 1251–1252.

52. Van der Maten J, Schrijver G. Severe accidental hypothermia: rewarming with CVVHD. *Neth J Med* 1996;49(4):160–163.

53. Brauer A, Wrigge H, Kersten J, et al. Severe accidental hypothermia: rewarming strategy using a veno-venous bypass system and a convective air warmer. *Intens Care Med* 1999;25(5):520–523.

54. Brodersen HP, Meurer T, Bolzenius K, et al. Hemofiltration in very severe hypothermia with favorable outcome. *Clin Nephrol* 1996;45(6):413–415.

55. Higley RR. Continuous arteriovenous hemofiltration: a case study. *Crit Care Nurse* 1996;16(5):37–40, 43.

56. Spooner K, Hassani A. Extracorporeal rewarming in a severely hypothermic patient using venovenous haemofiltration in the accident and emergency department. *J Accid Emerg Med* 2000;17(6):422–424.

57. Fildes J, Sheaff C, Barrett J. Very hot intravenous fluid in the treatment of hypothermia. *J Trauma* 1993;35(5):683–686; discussion 686–687.

58. Goheen MS, Ducharme MB, Kenny GP, et al. Efficacy of forced-air and inhalation rewarming by using a human model for severe hypothermia. *J Appl Physiol* 1997;83(5):1635–1640.

59. Steele MT, Nelson MJ, Sessler DI, et al. Forced air speeds rewarming in accidental hypothermia. *Ann Emerg Med* 1996;27(4):479–484.

60. Frank SM, Hesel TW, El-Rahmany HK, et al. Warmed humidified inspired oxygen accelerates postoperative rewarming. *J Clin Anesth* 2000;12(4):283–287.

61. Perk L, Borger Van de BF, Berendsen HH, et al. Full recovery after 45 min accidental submersion. *Intens Care Med* 2002;28(4):524.

62. Siebke H, Rod T, Breivik H, et al. Survival after 40 minutes submersion without cerebral sequelae. *Lancet* 1975;(7919):1275–1277.

63. Young RSK, Zalneraitis EL, Dooling EC. Neurological outcome in cold water drowning. *JAMA* 1980;244:1233–1235.

64. Rosomoff HL. Pathophysiology of the central nervous system during hypothermia. *Acta Neurochir Suppl (Wien)* 1964;131:11–22.

65. Griepp EB, Griepp RB. Cerebral consequences of hypothermic circulatory arrest in adults. *J Card Surg* 1992;7:134–155.

66. Beat H, Beyhan N, et al. Outcome of survivors of accidental deep hypothermia and circulatory arrest treated with extracorporeal blood warming. *N Engl J Med* 1997;337;1500–1505.

67. Schaller MD, Fischer AP, Perret CH. Hyperkalemia: a prognostic factor during acute severe hypothermia. *JAMA* 1990;264:1842.

68. Hauty MG, Esrig BC, Hill JG, et al. Prognostic factors in severe accidental hypothermia: experience from the Mt. Hood tragedy. *J Trauma* 1987;27:1107.

Chapter 32
Electrical Current and Lightning Injury

Mary Ann Cooper, Christopher J. Andrews, and Ronald L. Holle

Electrical current can be a great force for good in the community. Our society has become dependent on electric power for heating and cooling, cooking and food preservation, motive force, and the multitude of electronic gadgets that make our lives easier, more enjoyable, and more productive. Nonetheless, uncontrolled electrical current causes severe injuries when it enters the body accidentally. There are two major ways by which this occurs: technical electrical current and lightning current.

- Prevention of electrical and lightning injuries, like that of drowning, is the most cost-effective approach to these devastating injuries.
- Aggressive resuscitation is indicated after first attention to rescuer safety.
- Injuries can be profound, but some cardiac functional recovery may occur. With rare exceptions, hypoxic brain injury seldom recovers to any great extent.
- Emergency department (ED) assessment and attention to noncardiac electrical trauma is important for patient survival and long-term functional recovery.

Introduction

Electrical current can be a great force for good in the community. Our society has become dependent on electric power for heating and cooling, cooking and food preservation, motive force, and the multitude of electronic gadgets that make our lives easier, more enjoyable, and more productive.

Electrical current offers many therapeutic opportunities in modern medicine. With defibrillation, cardiac arrhythmias can be treated and life-threatening rhythms terminated. With stimulation, bone growth can be facilitated. Physical therapies rely on many means of electrical stimulation. Even in psychiatry, electroconvulsive therapy has a body of support.

Nonetheless, uncontrolled electrical current causes severe injuries when it enters the body accidentally. There are two major types of electricity that may do this: technical electrical current and lightning current.

Technical Electrical Current

Technical electrical current can cause massive, deep injury and not infrequently death. Devastating internal burning may be seen, and some victims experience tetanic skeletal muscle contractions and "lock" to the source of current, prolonging exposure and multiplying the injury (Fig. 32-1). This "no let go" phenomenon has also been linked to symptoms of posttraumatic stress disorder.[1] Current passing through on the heart can induce physical injury (burning, bruising, and physical disruption, for example) and arrhythmias, of which asystole and ventricular fibrillation (VF) cause cardiac arrest and death unless immediate resuscitation is initiated. A period of pulseless electrical activity can lead to hemodynamic impairment and cardiopulmonary arrest. Even low-voltage sources can cause cardiac arrest, often with little external evidence, as in a bathtub incident. In these cases skin resistance is lowered to such an extent that no skin burns occur but the current affects the heart maximally.

Lightning Current

Lightning current presents a unique injury constellation of its own quite different from that seen in technical electrical injury. Burns are of minimal concern; and although cardiac injury is significant, central; nervous system and autonomic nervous system injury can be marked. Both types of injury carry a similar, severe long-term psychiatric legacy.[2]

Blunt trauma and blunt head injury may be caused by both types of current because of muscle contraction or falls, a blast effect from arcing and explosions, or the concussive effects of being close to the point of a lightning strike. Long-term neurocognitive damage with chronic pain, sometimes termed

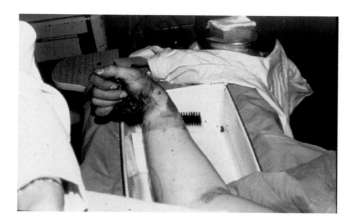

FIGURE 32-1 • High-voltage burn with arcing to median nerve/wrist area. Note the dusky fingers, which will need amputation. Also note the "kissing" burns in the antecubital fossa area. (Courtesy of Mary Ann Cooper, MD.)

"post–electric shock syndrome," has been consistently identified. This syndrome contributes to marked long-term disability and dysfunction.

INJURIES FROM TECHNICAL ELECTRICAL CURRENT AND LIGHTNING CURRENT

Technical electrical current:
- Physical injuries such as burns, fractures, and contusions
- Arrhythmias, including VF and asystole
- Fatal cardiac contractile impairment
- Pulseless electrical activity

Lightning current:
- Most lightning-strike patients have minimal cardiac injury; but when more injury is present, it may involve significant sequelae.
- Marked central nervous system and autonomic nervous system injury.
- Burns are of minimal concern.

Both types of current:
- Blunt trauma
- Blunt head injury
- Long-term neurocognitive damage with chronic pain (*post–electric shock syndrome*)

Epidemiology

Electrical Injury

Various groups are at particular risk for electrical injury. The purpose of identifying them is to identify circumstances where protective strategies and procedures may be concentrated.

A recent study from Sweden identified patterns of injury in a wide population of 285 cases.[3] Results are pre-

sented in Table 32-1, along with the results of two U.S. studies.[4,5] It is surprisingly difficult to obtain comprehensive epidemiologic analyses of electric shocks for a particular country. Furthermore, it is difficult to obtain exactly corresponding data from different reports to compare studies.

The Swedish study[3] is perhaps the most comprehensive to date and is, therefore, important. In this study the investigators defined electrocution as a *cause of death*[*][1] that included death from electric shock, from burns caused by arcs, and from falls from a height due to electric shock. It must be remembered that falls should prompt a search for injury beyond those due to electrical current.

The vast majority of the injured were male (94%); 132 incidents (46%) occurred in an industrial situation and 151 (53%) during recreation (two cases unknown). Over the total period, industrial and recreational deaths tended to parallel each other in a decreasing trend. Similarly, deaths due to high-voltage current (>1,000 V), as compared with deaths due to low-voltage current (≥1,000 V) decreased, the former by a larger percentage. There were 36 adolescent deaths (13%). Approximately 20% of cases involved alcohol.

RISK GROUPS FOR ELECTROCUTION

Various groups are at particular risk for electrocution:[3]
- Males
- Adolescents
- Utility, agricultural, and construction workers

The following activities are significantly dangerous:
- Performing unauthorized repairs
- Using alcohol while working with electricity
- Overlooking overhead power lines
- Employing poor judgment

Neglect of proper use of protective devices and procedures is a significant contributor to electrocution in work-related cases.

The most dangerous situation remains accidental contact with aerial power lines, and these deaths were roughly equally distributed between recreational and industrial deaths. Such incidents accounted for 40% of the total. Of these, the most dangerous location was railway lines (61 of 113, or 54%), followed by forest and field lines (23 of 113, or 20%) and public roads (7 of 113, or 6%). The remaining 22 deaths due to contact with a power line occurred in substations, farms, over watercourses, and in other minor locations.[3]

Carelessness, including the lifting of ladders, media truck satellite probes, metal poles, and other long metal apparatus into overhead lines, is commonly involved in such

*Loose terminology might refer to any electric shock as an "electrocution." But "electrocution" refers specifically to a *death* from electrical current. Otherwise the victim suffers an "electrical current injury" or an "electric shock injury."

TABLE 32-1 • Epidemiology of Electrical Injury

	Sweden[3]		United States[4]	United States[5]
Years of study	1975–2000		1977–1985	1960–1980
Accidental deaths per year, n	2,422–3,929			
Electrical deaths	0.15%–0.52%			0.78/100,000
Cases	285		277 (196 occupational)	220
Male:female, n	269:16			
Deaths	285		0.9–1.15/100,000 Seasonal (May–September) Biased to Monday and Thursday	Most occurred June–October
Inpatient cases	9			
Inpatient days	277			
Age, years, mean (median)	38 (35)		31 (29)	
Trends				
Deaths per year in 5-year blocks	Decrease from 17.4 to 5.8		Slight decrease	
All accidental deaths	Decrease from 3,823 to 2,510			
Occupational vs. recreational deaths	8:9.5 vs 1.3:4			
HV deaths (end study)	Decreased by 73% (to 46%)			
LV deaths (end study)	Decreased by 55% (to 54%)			
Illicit drugs	2/135			
Alcohol	47/231			
Mechanism of death				
Arrhythmia	79%		85%	
Burns	9% (usually caused by HV shock)		5%	
Location of incident	Occupational	Leisure		
Railway site	23/64	41/64		
Residential	6/53	49/53		
Substation	25/30	5/30		
Farmhouse	19/25	6/25		
Garden	0/21	21/21		
Workshop	15/18	3/18		
Construction site	15/16	1/16		
Power pole	12/15	3/15		
Water area	1/11	10/11		
Other	16/32	12/32		
	132/285ª	**151/285ª**		
Nature of incident				
Alcohol-positive (224 tested; with blood or urine tests, some both)	5/104	42/120	Rare (industrial)	
Climbing on railway carriage		20/47		
Alcohol level >1.5 g/L		19/47		
HV:LV	71:61	59:92	130:44	93:108
Personal contribution to injury	80/123	99/144		
Electricians	47/56			
Occupations				
Electric linesman	31/132			
Electrical fitters	19/132		22/95	
Professional (electrical)	6/132			
Equipment operators	5/132			
Construction, general laborer			24/95	
Construction, special trades			34/95	
Nonelectrical	71/132			
Industry[b]				
Utilities			10	
Mining			5.9	
Construction			3.9	
Agriculture			2.9	
Transportation			1.3	
Mechanism of injury				
HV				
Touched intact conductor				25/29
Conductor fouled on overhead line	113/285			38/52
Touched fallen line				0/8
LV				
Tools and appliances at work				29/36
Wiring at work				16/29
Faulty energized item				4/14

HV, high voltage; LV, low voltage.
ªIn two cases the classification of death (occupational versus leisure) was unknown.
bNumbers are per 100,000 employees per year.
cFigures given are industrial; the remainder are domestic

injuries. Nor can one ignore the role of illegal activities in these incidents, such as unauthorized entry into railway property. The findings of the Swedish study emphasize the importance of staying clear of fallen lines as well as the necessity of keeping domestic electrical apparatus in good repair.

Locations for shock give little cause for complacency; railway locations (22%), the interiors of residential properties (19%), substations (11%), farms (9%), and gardens (7%) are common sites for these incidents and represent areas in which we all move.

Childhood and adolescent electrocutions illustrate a foolhardiness that we should all attempt to counter. For example, 20 of the 36 adolescents who died (56%) were electrocuted while climbing on railway carriages, mostly by touching overhead lines.

Occupational deaths (132) were not restricted to electrical workers (only 46%). Agricultural workers were next (14%) with construction workers (11%) following. Neglect of proper use of protective devices and procedures was considered to be a significant contributor to 65% of these deaths.

Alcohol was a significant factor in more than one third of deaths that occurred during leisure pursuits (35%); almost half of these cases involved illegal activities like climbing on railway carriages or entering power substations, often, in developing countries, for theft of copper.[6] Performing unauthorized repairs, using alcohol, overlooking overhead power lines, or simply employing poor judgment, were found to be significantly dangerous factors for electrocution.

Identification of the risk factors described above allows the rational introduction of protective measures (e.g., circuit breaker closure and reclosure apparatus, earthing/grounding, residual current devices, and insulation strategies), procedures for behavior to avoid shocks (e.g., workplace protection, access protocols, and equipment construction standards), and legal measures to prevent risky behavior.

By far the most common mechanism of fatal injury was fatal cardiac arrhythmia (79%). Although accidental death is an undoubted tragedy, it must be remembered that survivors of electrical injury demonstrate tremendous ongoing disability,[7] which is important for both the victim and society.

Lightning Injury

Cloud-to-ground lightning strikes the surface of the United States about 25 million times each year. Figure 32-2, from the National Lightning Detection Network, which has operated continuously over the continental United States since 1989, shows the locations of these flashes.[8] The largest number of cloud-to-ground flashes per area occur in central Florida between Tampa and Orlando.[9,10] Other regions of Florida and across the Gulf Coast also have high flash densities. This high frequency is due to the warm, humid air at the surface and coastal sea breezes, which fuel thunderstorm growth during most afternoons of the 6-month thunderstorm season. Some flash densities in equatorial Africa,

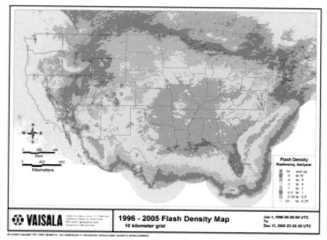

FIGURE 32-2 • Cloud-to-ground flashes per square kilometer per year in the United States, 1996–2005. (Courtesy of Vaisala Inc., Tucson, AZ.)

South America, and Asia are much greater than those in the United States.

Cloud-to-ground flash densities decrease to the north and west away from the Gulf and Atlantic regions. Additional important maxima and minima are found in and around the regions in the western United States, where there are mountains and large slopes in terrain.[11] The West Coast has minimal lightning because the ocean offshore is so cold that updrafts are not strong enough to reach altitudes where lightning forms, as it does at temperatures colder than freezing in the presence of water mixed with ice particles.

Two thirds of cloud-to-ground lightning occurs during June, July, and August in most parts of the United States. Nearly half of all lightning in the United States occurs between 3 P.M. and 6 P.M., although some Plains states have later maxima. Lightning is at a maximum in the afternoon, because the updrafts necessary for thunderstorm formation are strongest when surface temperatures are highest, resulting in the greatest vertical instability. In addition, for every cloud-to-ground flash, another three to five flashes remain in the clouds.

Lightning Casualties

During many recent years, lightning has been second to only floods and flash floods as a cause of storm-related deaths in the United States. In some years, deaths due to tornadoes or hurricanes exceed lightning deaths. Florida leads the nation in the number of lightning deaths (Fig. 32-3A, top); Colorado is second. When population is taken into account (Fig. 32-3B, bottom), the highest death rates are clustered in the Southeast and Rocky Mountain states. The western mountain maximum is attributed to more people being out of doors at the time of year when thunderstorms occur as well as to the less intense rain associated with lightning, which provides an impression of a less dangerous situation than is the case.

Two thirds of lightning casualties occur between noon and 6 P.M. in the summer months. Males are much more

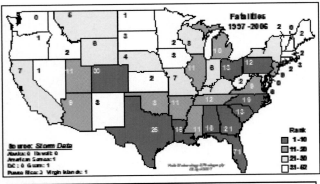

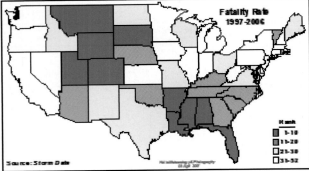

FIGURE 32-3 • Lightning deaths in the continental United States, 1997–2006. **Top**. Deaths per state. **Bottom**. Deaths weighted by state population. (Updated from Curran EB, Holle RL, López RE. *Lightning Fatalities, Injuries, and Damage Reports in the United States from 1959–1994.* Silver Spring, MD: National Oceanic and Atmospheric Administration, 1997.)

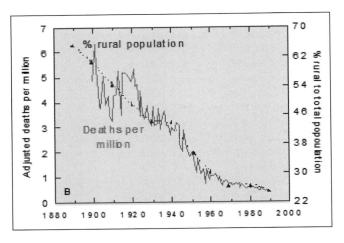

FIGURE 32-4 • Adjusted yearly lightning deaths normalized by population (*red*) and percentage of population in rural areas (*blue*). (From López RE, Holle RL. Changes in the number of lightning deaths in the United States during the twentieth century. *J Climate* 1998;11:2070, with permission.)

often victims of lightning strikes than females.[12] This is because males spend more time outdoors in work and recreational activities and tend to underestimate the dangers of lightning. Other possible contributors to the higher risk for males are more risk-taking behaviors as well as aversion to changing activities already started.

Lightning deaths are tracked more carefully than injuries because deaths are reported more completely.[13] A ratio of 10 injuries per death is considered to be the most reasonable estimate over the long term.[14] One reason for the difficulty in reporting lightning casualties is that about 90% of all deaths and injuries occur to one person at a time. For many reasons these events may never be recorded in hospital admission data or coroner or newspaper accounts, all sources of data in assessing the impact. Nonfatal injuries are notoriously underreported because a significant number of victims do not seek immediate medical care or do not need to be admitted for care.

The number of lightning deaths is determined from the monthly publication *Storm Data*, which is prepared by National Weather Service. The current fatality total is between 40 and 60 per year. (In the early 20th century, the death total often exceeded 400 per year.) The currently recorded injuries amount to 400 to 600 per year. The fatality rate has dropped by more than an order of magnitude in recent decades in the United States, from 6 per 1 million during some years in the early 20th century to <0.5 per 1 million in recent years. A similar drop has been documented in other developed countries, but the decrease is much less apparent in developing regions of the world.

The reduced lightning fatality rate has been attributed to the large decrease in the percentage of the population working and living in rural areas. A concomitant factor is the very large increase during the 20th century in the quality of construction, making it safe from lightning. Most people in developed regions live and work in large enclosed buildings that are safe from lightning because of the "Faraday cage effect" of wiring and plumbing. Other factors include better awareness of weather, better medical care and communications, and the availability of metal-topped, fully enclosed vehicles for safety. In parts of the world where people work in labor-intensive agriculture and live in unsafe structures, an estimated 24,000 deaths and 240,000 injuries occur annually.[15]

An analysis of entries in *Storm Data* 100 years ago and in recent years showed a number of changes in the circumstances surrounding lightning deaths (Fig. 32-4).[16,17] In the 1890s, rural deaths were much more frequent than urban deaths. Indoor fatalities were the most frequent, accounting for 23% of all deaths due to lightning. Outdoor and agricultural incidents were the next most frequent types of lightning incidents. But in the 1990s, rural settings and agricultural incidents were much less frequent, and only 2% of current-day lightning deaths occur indoors. Outdoor incidents have become the most frequent type, with victims often standing under trees. A high percentage also occur during recreation, especially during beach, water, and camping activities. Incidents during sports such as soccer, baseball and softball, golf, camping, and hiking are more common today than they were a century ago.[18,19] Rural casualties are now half as frequent as urban ones.

Literature Review: Cardiac Effects of Electrical Current and Lightning Shock

Arrhythmias

The greatest danger for death from electrical or lightning shock is the induction of arrhythmias. The arrhythmias of most importance are those capable of causing cardiac arrest. These range from asystole, which is thought to occur more commonly in lightning strike as a presenting arrhythmia, to VF, thought to occur in "lesser" shocks such as technical electrical shock. Because VF deteriorates to asystole, these observations may be related more to the timing of discovery or rescue of the victim than real. The consequences of asystole and VF are cardiac arrest and peripheral ischemia.

Electrical shock can also induce atrial tachycardia and fibrillation, ventricular tachycardia, and atrial and ventricular ectopy. These arrhythmias do not necessarily lead to immediate death, so the literature concentrates largely on induction of VF.

A current of around 20 µA applied directly to the heart is sufficient to induce an asystolic state or VF. Conversely, this level of current can act as a defibrillating current when applied directly.

Most standards for electrical technologies such as power generation, transmission to home appliances, and so on are written in terms of the current required via external application pathways to induce VF. These are empirically determined and are statistically distributed in a given population. Presumably they represent currents externally applied via a given pathway that, when all the internal tissues are navigated, result in approximately 20 µA of current at the heart. The statistical variation takes into account different tissue constitutions for individual people and the variability in the threshold of a fibrillating heart.

Although arrhythmia induction is the most serious consequence of electrical shock for cardiac function, other abnormalities have been reported in the myocardium. Neural dysfunction and burns are other major overall injuries.

Direct Damage to Myocardial Tissue

Commonsense reasoning assumes that because nervous tissue is by nature electrical in function, it must be particularly susceptible to electrical stimulation and injury. This view assumes that neural membranes are immediately available to the passage of current. But nerve trunks are enclosed in a protective sheath of highly fatty and relatively resistant tissue, so electrical current may not have immediately deleterious effects on nerve function. The commonsense view also ignores electrical field, electroporation, and thermal effects, although these topics are beyond the scope of this chapter.

Tissue—and myocardial tissue is no exception—may be damaged by burns. Burn damage produces a stunned area of myocardium not unlike that seen in ischemia and infarction, and this area becomes a potential site of myocardial rupture. The analogy to a stunned area of myocardium after prolonged ischemia is not unreasonable considering the consequences of an electrical burn: electrical current most often travels from hand to foot, so burn damage is usually seen inferiorly. This damage may be reflected in the electrocardiogram (ECG).

Electrocardiogram

This type of damage and an ECG pattern typical of infarction have been reported by several authors. Romero et al.,[20] for example, reported severe anteroapical myocardial necrosis in a healthy 22-year-old man who sustained an electrical current injury. The findings on the ECG, enzyme studies, scintigraphy, and a scan by single photon emission computed tomography (SPECT), suggest necrosis; but the echocardiogram indicated only minor anteroapical dysfunction. In such cases one must also consider the effects of catecholamine excess and hypertension—which can develop from inotropic and vascular changes—on the damaged heart.

Cardiac monitoring and a 12-lead ECG is mandatory for the detection and diagnosis of arrhythmias. In lightning injury, the QTc interval is particularly important.[21]

Echocardiogram

Homma et al.[22] have described echocardiographic findings in two patients with acute electrical injury. Although for some years it was thought that survival with almost complete restoration of myocardial function was the norm, these authors observed, in their patients, persistent ventricular dysfunction that did not resolve. They proposed that the two mechanisms of damage seen in electrical injury are heat-induced myocardial tissue burn and hypotension induced by arrhythmia, with the latter being most important in their patients. In contrast, Rivera et al.[23] reported severe congestive heart failure and myocardial stunning in a 42-year-old woman struck by lightning. Their novel treatment included administration of levosimendan, which increases intracellular sensitivity to calcium, a mechanism that is impaired in stunned myocardium. The authors postulated that in the absence of direct electrofulguration, cytosolic overload of calcium, release of free radicals, and proteolysis of contractile elements, may contribute to myocardial stunning.

It may well be that the degree of electrical insult (i.e., the current–time profile, or the amount and duration of exposure) is an operative parameter in myocardial tissue damage. For example, Chandra et al.[23] found that the best clinical predictors of myocardial damage were the extent of surface burns and a pathway of current involving the heart, which they define as one where the entry and exit points are, respectively, superior and inferior to the heart. It is known that skin burns are very dependent on the current–time profile.[24]

Prognosis

The common belief is that once a patient survives the acute event, the ECG changes and myocardial damage caused by electrical injury resolve. But the studies described above cast doubt on this. Furthermore, Xenopoulos et al.[25] described the case of a patient with rapid resolution of ECG changes but profound and ongoing echocardiographic dysfunction that continued until cardiac arrest occurred and the patient died. The myocardium at autopsy showed dramatic hemorrhage but normal patent coronary circulation. Many histologic signs of failure and inotropic therapy, such as contraction bands, were evident on microscopic examination. These changes led to a marked heterogeneity of viable and nonviable muscle. This and the above-described studies indicate that resolution of ECG changes and enzyme levels alone are insufficient to assure recovery of the myocardium. Consequent pulmonary edema secondary to failing myocardium is well known and not especially an electrical phenomenon.

A valuable overview of these issues is given by Fish,[26] although it is cautioned that the comments regarding the preferential susceptibility of nervous tissue may not reflect the true pathophysiology. Fish goes on to give a very useful resume of cardiac pathology. The mechanisms of arrhythmia induction have also been well outlined by Bridges et al.[24] and Geddes et al.[27]

Lightning injury seems to be more straightforward. It is commonly agreed and seems supported that although many different ECG patterns can be seen acutely, full recovery of function with resolution of signs is the norm.

Monitoring and Discharge

A clinical phenomenon that remains controversial is the delayed induction of arrhythmias within the first few days to 1 to 2 weeks after recovery from electric shock. There is little discussion of this observation in the literature. Bailey et al. are among the few to address the problem.[28] In a paper with wider conclusions, they suggest that no patient considered to be at risk of "late" arrhythmias actually developed them up to 24 hours (their cutoff for "late"). Even so, enigmatically, they suggest that arrhythmias can occur after this period, and that if they do, medical advice should be sought. This may not be a helpful comment for any lethal late arrhythmia. Fatovich[29] joins the discussion, suggesting that even in those who were said to have later arrhythmias after discharge, the arrhythmias in fact were not unequivocally connected to the shock. He suggests that later arrhythmias are "exceptionally rare." One difficulty, for example, raised by the present authors is that no shock can be said to have no transthoracic component.

In light of these findings the further question of how long a person should be monitored after an electric shock is raised. Fatovich and Bailey et al. are proponents of an aggressive view. Bailey et al. suggest that where there is no perceived cardiac risk to the electric shock (no transthoracic current path, no tetany, no loss of consciousness, and an applied voltage $\leq 1,000$ V), monitoring is unnecessary. Fatovich holds that if a patient is asymptomatic and has a normal ECG, cardiac monitoring is not necessary. A conservative course seems to be to monitor such a person for 24 hours and, in the absence of complications, to discharge thereafter. Any complication that develops should be treated appropriately before discharge. While there is little repeated evidence yet to support either view, Bailey's study is a worthy one and bears repeating. Until evidence is reproduced, a prudent course may be to monitor for 6–24 hours based on clinical judgement, and if there is no rhythm abnormality or other complication discharge to appropriate follow-up.

Pathophysiology

Pathophysiology involves us in the description of the way in which current affects the body, which requires prediction of the amount of current flowing at a particular moment and some attempt to describe its consequences. It is readily admitted that our knowledge of what occurs at the cellular and tissue levels is limited.

Electrical Injury

The main endeavor of electrical current research is to attempt to predict the current flowing in a particular pathway. The use of a standard such as those developed by the International Electrotechnical Commission (IEC)[30] in Geneva is essential. Use of a standard allows prediction of the total amount of current entering the body and subsequently prediction of the amount that traverses the heart. From these predictions, the probability of induction of VF, and hence the danger of the current, can be estimated.

Basic Physics

In determining the amount of current traversing a conductor, the physical principle used is Ohm's law. Electrons are "pushed" down a conductor from a source of electrons by a force known as electromotive force, which is measured in volts (this is sometimes loosely called the "voltage" of the source). The number of electrons per second traversing the conductor (i.e., the current) can be increased by increasing the forcing pressure, or voltage, of the source. Within reason, this voltage can be varied under external control. However, the degree to which the conductor resists this flow is a physical property of the conductor: it is a "given" of the system. The resulting current is directly proportional to the voltage and inversely proportional to the resistance.

Little is known about how this current affects individual cells. Most of our understanding comes from examining the phenomenon of electroporation,[31] a technique used in molecular biology in which electrical current is

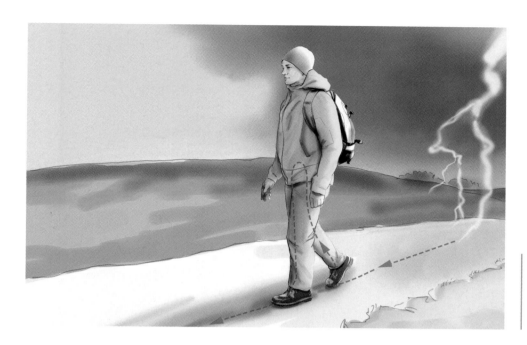

FIGURE 32-5 • Ground potential. Lightning hits the ground at a distance from the person; the current is then injected into the ground and flows radially from the struck point.

applied to a cell plasma membrane (or other living surface, such as skin) to increase its electrical conductivity and permeability. With exposure to current, pores will form in the membrane, allowing the introduction of a substance such as a drug or coding DNA. If the voltage and duration of exposure are appropriate, these pores will reseal in a short time with no long-term damage to the cell. But if the voltage is too high or exposure too long, the cell will become unstable and progress to lysis. It is thought that this same process occurs in victims of electric shock.

Lightning Injury

There are five mechanisms by which electrical current in a lightning strike may affect a person:[32,33]

1. Direct strike—self-explanatory and not nearly as common as it appears in the press: <10% of such injuries are thought highly dangerous, possibly accounting for the largest number of deaths.
2. Side flash or splash ("flashover")—when a person is standing next to a struck object and a portion of current jumps to the individual: 25% to 40% of injuries.
3. Contact potential—when a person is touching a struck object and a portion of the current is diverted through the individual: 3% to 10% of injuries.
4. Ground potential (step voltage, stride potential)—when lightning hits the ground at a distance from the person, current is injected into the ground and flows radially from the struck point (Fig. 32-5). Injury to a person in contact with the ground at two separate points follows as the current is diverted through the person or as it arcs radially across an irregular surface: 30% to 60% of injuries.

5. Upward streamer (Fig. 32-6)—the electrical field in a thundercloud induces opposite charges and "upward streamers" that may pass through anything in the field, including people. Even when the streamer fails to contact the lightning channel to complete the stroke, the current

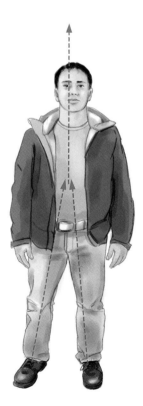

FIGURE 32-6 • Upward streamer. The electrical field in a thundercloud induces opposite charges and "upward streamers" that may pass through anything in the field, including people.

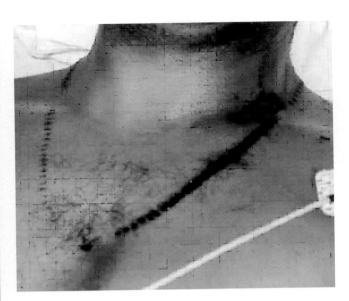

FIGURE 32-7 • Necklace burned into skin. (Courtesy of Mary Ann Cooper, MD.)

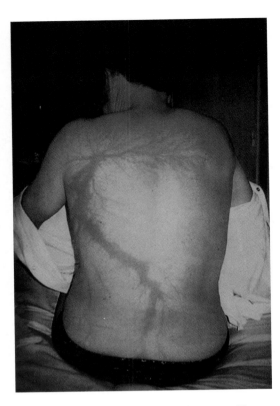

FIGURE 32-8 • Lichtenberg figures or "ferning." This aftereffect of lightning injury is thought to be caused by the rupture of small capillaries under the skin and is not a true burn. (From the *New England Journal of Medicine,* with permission.)

can be significant enough to cause serious injury or death: 10% to 25% of injuries.

Each mechanism has a range of severity of injury and likelihood of cardiac arrest. Although common sense suggests that a direct strike is more likely to cause fatalities, this belief has never been substantiated by clinical or laboratory studies. The physics of lightning is incredibly complex; lightning is a current phenomenon, not the voltage phenomenon of generated electricity with which we are more familiar. This difference accounts for a further difference between lightning injury and electrical injury.

Lightning injury is not scalable; one cannot use experience with generated electricity to predict findings or outcomes in a lightning-injured victim. For instance, lightning injury, despite the tremendous energy involved, rarely includes deep burns (Figs. 32-7 and 32-8). Part of the reason for this is that lightning is so short-lived that it may not transmit sufficient energy during a short exposure to heat the skin enough to cause a burn.[24,34] In addition, although a small portion of lightning energy may go "through" a victim, the vast majority of energy from a direct strike (and perhaps other mechanisms) flashes around the person, a phenomenon called "flashover" (Figs. 32-9 and 32-10). It is not known how much current goes through or around a person in any of these mechanisms, although numbers can be modeled.[35–39] Postulated magnetic field effects are probably negligible.[40,41]

An animal study has shown that a portion of the current may enter the body at various cranial ports of entry (eye, mouth, nose, ears).[42] Once diverted internally, the pathway to deep structures, including the brainstem and hypothalamus, is short. The same study showed preferential damage to the brainstem's respiratory centers.

Acutely, both respiratory and cardiac arrest may follow a lightning injury. The etiology of cardiac arrest from lightning injury has not been well studied; but arrest may arise from central nervous system injury, autonomic injury, injury to the sinoatrial node, atrioventricular node, or other conducting pathways as current traverses them; or other hypothetical causes. Certainly autonomic injury has been reported both clinically and in laboratory studies.[43–46]

Although inherent automaticity may restart the myocardium, ventilation does not always recommence, and a secondary hypoxic cardiac arrest may follow. Whether ventilation and oxygenation at this point may be restorative or whether the respiratory arrest signifies a more severe and perhaps irrecoverable injury has not been studied. But this sequence of events highlights the importance of cardiopulmonary resuscitation (CPR) and airway management as interventions.

Out-of-Hospital Management

Electrical Injury

Out-of-hospital management initially is first aid on site at the point of shock. The most important consideration is not to convert a situation with one victim into a situation with multiple victims. Safety is the top priority.

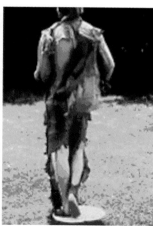

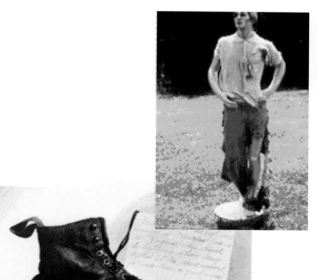

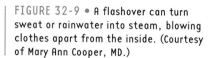

FIGURE 32-9 • A flashover can turn sweat or rainwater into steam, blowing clothes apart from the inside. (Courtesy of Mary Ann Cooper, MD.)

The first task is extrication of the victim. It is most important to know—and this is entirely different from lightning-injured persons—that *a victim remaining in contact with electrical current is dangerous to touch*. A rescuer who touches a victim before the source of current is turned off may well be shocked.

The first step is to break the connection between the person and the current source. For incidents involving a utility worker atop a pole, the specific protocols for pole-top rescue must be followed, and all workers should be well trained in these procedures. *Only rescuers specifically trained to execute such tasks should attempt them.*

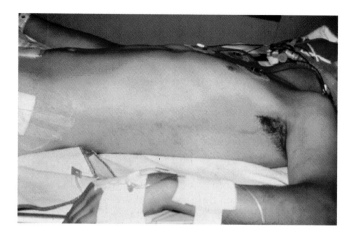

FIGURE 32-10 • Steam burns along sweat lines. This pattern of burn injury occurs when a flashover turns sweat into steam. (Courtesy of Mary Ann Cooper, MD.)

For incidents occurring during recreational activities, the following procedure can be used:

1. Safely switch off the power to the apparatus or line that is thought to be the source of the shock, either at a switch or by pulling the plug. This must be done safely—with *no contact with any conductor*. A wise policy is to do this with one hand only and with no other environmental body contact.
2. If an immediate disconnection is not possible, switch off a circuit breaker or pull the appropriate fuse at the switchboard.
3. Alternatively, turn off the whole installation at the main switch.

Alternative methods of removing a victim from the source of current have been proposed. These methods include dragging the victim away with insulated hands or a belt and using a dry pole as a lever to move the victim. These methods should be used with extreme caution.

Once removed from the source of current, the victim is safe to touch. Waiting until the power supply is turned off may mean that the victim has prolonged contact with current and dies. Although this scenario is highly distressing for rescuers, the loss of two lives is a worse consequence. Once the victim is separated from the source of current, assessment follows the standard principles of CPR.

Lightning Injury

Victims of lightning strike will not be connected to the source of electricity when rescuers arrive, but if weather conditions are still inclement, the scene remains dangerous.

Rescuers should remove the victim from the lightning-prone area to a safer shelter or emergency medical services (EMS) vehicle as soon as possible and provide basic life support (BLS) and advanced cardiac life support (ACLS) as described below. Spinal precautions should be used when moving the victim.

Basic Life Support for Electrical Current and Lightning Injury

If immediate resuscitation is provided, survival from cardiac arrest caused by lightning strike is higher than that reported following cardiac arrest from other non-VF causes. The goal is to oxygenate the heart and brain adequately until cardiac activity resumes. Victims in respiratory arrest may require only ventilation and oxygenation to avoid secondary hypoxic cardiac arrest.

Once the victim is separated from the source of current and the scene is safe, determine cardiorespiratory status. Immediately after electrocution, respiration, circulation, or both may fail. If spontaneous respiration or circulation is absent, immediately initiate BLS, including activation of the EMS system, prompt provision of CPR, and use of an automated external defibrillator (AED) when available. Immediate provision of ventilations and compressions (if needed) is essential. Use the AED to identify and treat ventricular tachycardia or VF.

Maintain spinal stabilization throughout extrication and treatment if there is a likelihood of head or neck trauma. Both lightning and electrical trauma often cause multiple trauma, including injury to the spine and musculature, internal injuries from being thrown, and fractures caused by the tetanic response of skeletal muscles. Do not remove smoldering clothing, shoes, and belts as this may cause further damage.

Vigorous resuscitative measures are indicated even for those who appear dead on initial evaluation. Because many victims are young and without preexisting cardiopulmonary disease, they have a good chance of survival if immediate support of cardiopulmonary function is provided.

The Concept of Reverse Triage for Lightning Injury

In multiple-casualty emergencies, especially from traumatic events, victims in cardiac arrest are given the lowest priority. The harsh but evidence-based principle is that these victims have a very low probability of survival even with aggressive resuscitative efforts. Emergency personnel, especially if they are limited in number, will save more lives if they support victims who are not in cardiac arrest.

But in a multicasualty lightning strike event, the victim who develops immediate cardiac arrest has a high probability of survival and recovery if BLS is provided without delay. When multiple victims suffer simultaneous lightning strike, rescuers should give highest priority to victims who are in respiratory or cardiac arrest. Survival is high when victims with cardiac or respiratory arrest receive immediate resusci-

tation. This is true even when the presenting rhythm is asystole or prolonged efforts are required. Victims of lightning strike who do not suffer immediate cardiopulmonary arrest are unlikely to do so. They have an excellent chance of acute recovery with little additional treatment, although they may have permanent disabling sequelae.

"REVERSE TRIAGE" FOR MULTIPLE VICTIMS OF LIGHTNING STRIKE

In a multicasualty lightning-strike event, the victim who develops immediate cardiac arrest has a high probability of survival and recovery if BLS is provided without delay. When multiple victims suffer simultaneous lightning strike, highest priority should be given to victims who are in respiratory or cardiac arrest. Victims of lightning strike who do not suffer immediate cardiopulmonary arrest are unlikely to do so. They have an excellent chance of recovery with little additional treatment.

Advanced Cardiovascular Life Support for Electrical Current and Lightning Injury

In treating electrical current and lightning injuries, rescuers must first be sure that the scene is safe. Patients who are unresponsive after an electrical injury may be in either respiratory or cardiac arrest. Airway control, prompt CPR, and attempts at defibrillation (if indicated) are critically important. Treat VF, asystole, and other serious arrhythmias with the ACLS techniques outlined in this text. Quickly start CPR and attempt defibrillation at the scene if needed. Then take steps to manage the airway, including early placement of an advanced airway (e.g., endotracheal intubation). It may be difficult to establish an airway in patients with electrical burns of the face, mouth, or anterior neck. Because extensive soft tissue swelling may develop rapidly, complicating airway control measures, early intubation should be performed for patients with evidence of extensive burns even if he or she has begun to breathe spontaneously. ACLS providers should be prepared to provide respiratory support in case respiratory arrest persists even after the return of spontaneous circulation.

Initial support of cardiovascular function requires treatment of arrest rhythms and then treatment of any life-threatening arrhythmias. Once spontaneous perfusion is restored, the victim may require fluid therapy and inotropic or vasopressor support. Victims with technical electric injuries have greater fluid requirements than those with thermal burns and will need rapid intravascular fluid administration to replace ongoing fluid losses and prevent hemodynamic compromise. For victims with hypovolemic shock or significant tissue destruction, rapid intravenous fluid administration is indicated to counteract shock and correct ongoing fluid losses due to third spacing. Fluid administration should be adequate to maintain a brisk diuresis. Fluid replacement will facilitate renal excretion of myoglobin, potassium, and other by-products of tissue destruction (this is particularly true for patients with electrical injury). Since the majority of lightning victims do not have substantial burns, fluid replacement should usually be limited to avoid increasing brain edema.

Emergency Department Management

Electrical Injury

The general ED evaluation and management of patients with electrical injury is initially similar to that of other patients with possible multisystem trauma. There is no evidence that cardiopulmonary arrest from electrical trauma requires management different from that for cardiac arrest due to other traumatic mechanisms. Most victims are young, with little cardiac risk. But if the patient is in cardiac arrest, the reestablishment of perfusion, with continued high-quality BLS and ACLS including inotropic agents and antiarrhythmics, is paramount. This care is continued into the intensive care unit. The arrested myocardium takes first priority; but if the myocardium is functioning adequately, other injuries may take priority.

If severe deep burns are present, major fluid shifts resulting in hypotension and electrolyte disturbances, myoglobinuric renal toxicity, and release of potential intracellular toxins from massive muscle and tissue injuries, are considerations. Volume and fluid resuscitation is preferentially initiated out of hospital to treat hypotension and provide prophylaxis for renal damage due to myoglobinuria. Later, alkaline diuresis for myoglobinuria is a consideration to prevent or attenuate acute renal failure. If anesthesia is anticipated or required in patients who have sustained significant muscle injury, serum potassium and creatinine should be monitored closely. A systemic inflammatory state can also occur and complicate hypotension due to the release of cytokines and other factors (loosely identified as intracellular toxins) released, such as tumor necrosis factor.

For less severe injuries, tissue injury may be less of a concern and cardiac issues are more of a priority. Many arrhythmias have been reported, but in reality few are unstable or life-threatening. The major question most clinicians will have is how long an otherwise "normal" person with an unremarkable ECG should be monitored. Provided that there has been no loss of consciousness, confusion, dyspnea, chest pain, dizziness, arrhythmia on the ECG, or other red flags, the vast majority of patients can be sent home after their other injuries (e.g., burns, fractures, or pain) have been treated.

Lightning-Strike Injury

ED management of victims of lightning strikes varies tremendously but is supportive and guided by the patient's injuries.

The *only* cause of death in the lightning-strike victim is cardiac arrest at the immediate time of injury. AEDs have been useful in several cases. But other than providing standard resuscitation, there is nothing that the rescuer or emergency physician can do to *prevent* a cardiac arrest because the die has been cast by the time rescue arrives at the scene. Management of the cardiac arrest is standard, involving ventilatory support, monitoring, cardiac compression, and standard drugs. There is no research to suggest that some drugs are more effective than others for victims of lightning strike.

Cardiac arrest or death does not occur minutes to days after the injury unless other injuries, such as trauma from a fall or exposure, are present.

Early Subspecialty Involvement and Transfer

As significant as the external injuries may appear after electrothermal shock, the underlying tissue damage may be far more extensive, and survivors may have permanent neurologic and cardiac sequelae. Early consultation with or transfer to a physician and a facility (e.g., burn center) familiar with treatment of these injuries is critical. For lightning injuries involving few substantial burns, this is much less likely to apply.

EARLY CONSULTATION AND TRANSFER

As significant as the external injuries may appear after electrothermal shock, the underlying tissue damage may be far more extensive, and survivors may have permanent neurologic and cardiac sequelae. Early consultation with or transfer to a physician and a facility (e.g., burn center) familiar with the treatment of these injuries is critical. For lightning injuries involving few substantial burns, this is much less likely to apply.

Prevention

Electrical Current Protection

Several useful strategies have been developed to help prevent purely electrical injuries. These include building construction techniques and codes to require insulation of conductors in overhead cable swings so that they are insulated where contact might be likely to occur.

The adoption of standards for safe equipment manufacture has led to the development of closure and reclosure apparatus for circuit breakers, semi-insulated cable plugs, and molded integrated plugs and sockets to prevent tampering and unauthorized repair. A significant advance is the development of residual current devices. These devices compare the current flowing to and from a device, which should be equal. If the device detects an imbalance, it is assumed that the imbalance is caused by diversion of current through a person and the power is disconnected.

Many companies have adopted workplace codes, safe procedures, and specific protocols for responding to accidents. Because adoption of such codes and procedures necessitates a significant amount of employee training, it provides a pool of skilled workers more attuned to safety.

Prevention of Lightning Injury

Lightning safety is not convenient, but then neither are other forms of safety. The prevention of lightning injury is by and large an individual responsibility unless large venues such as summer camps or sports stadiums are involved.

Prevention requires familiarity with the following safety guidelines:

1. Know the weather forecast before starting an activity.
2. If bad weather is predicted, make alternate plans.
3. Know the weather patterns in the area where you plan to be. Be off of mountains, golf courses, and other lightning-prone areas before the time of maximum lightning exposure, generally the afternoon hours.
4. Have a "weather eye"—watch the sky for signs of unexpected storms.
5. At the first sound of thunder, which can rarely be heard more than 10 miles away (and often a lot less), danger already exists and evacuation to a safer shelter, such as a substantial (habitable) building with plumbing and wiring or a fully enclosed metal vehicle with the windows closed, is required.
6. Outdoor activities should not be resumed until at least 30 minutes after the last thunder is heard or the last lightning is seen.

Information about lightning protection for larger venues is available from the National Weather Service (www.lightningsafety.noaa.gov) and other sources.[47-49]

References

1. Kelley KM, Tkachenko TA, Pliskin NH, et al. Life after electrical injury. Risk factors for psychiatric sequelae. *Ann N Y Acad Sci* 1999;888:356–363.
2. Pliskin NH, Ammar AN, Fink JW, et al. Neuropsychological changes following electrical injury. *J Int Neuropsychol Soc* 2006;12:17–23.
3. Lindstrom R, Bylund PO, Eriksson A. Accidental deaths caused by electricity in Sweden, 1975–2000. *J Forens Sci* 2006;51:1383–1388.
4. Jones JE, Armstrong CW, Woolard CD, Miller GB Jr. Fatal occupational electrical injuries in Virginia. *J Occup Med* 1991;33:57–63.
5. Wright RK, Davis JH. The investigation of electrical deaths: a report of 220 fatalities. *J Forens Sci* 1980;25:514–521.
6. Blumenthal R. A retrospective descriptive study on the pathology of trauma of high-voltage electrocution fatality cases in Gauteng, 2001–2004. In *International Conference on Lightning and Static Electricity*. Paris, 2007.
7. Cooper MA, Andrews CJ. Disability, not death, is the issue in lightning injury. In *International Conference on Lightning and Static Electricity*. Seattle, 2005.
8. Cummins KL, et al. A combined TOA/MDF technology upgrade of the U.S. National Lightning Detection Network. *J Geophys Res* 1998;103:9035.
9. Huffines GR, Orville RE. Lightning ground flash density and thunderstorm duration in the contiguous United States: 1989–1996. *J Appl Meteorol* 1999;38:1013.
10. Orville RE, Huffines GR, Burrows WR, et al. The North American Lightning Detection Network (NALDN)—first results: 1998–2000. *Mon Wea Rev* 2002;130:2098.
11. López RE, et al. Spatial and temporal distributions of lightning over Arizona from a power utility perspective. *J Appl Meteorol* 1997;36:825.
12. Curran EB, Holle RL, López RE. *Lightning Fatalities, Injuries, and Damage Reports in the United States from 1959–1994*. Silver Spring, MD: National Oceanic and Atmospheric Administration, 1997.
13. López RE. The underreporting of lightning injuries and deaths in Colorado. *Bull Am Meteorol Soc* 1993;74:2171.
14. Cherington M, et al. Closing the gap on the actual numbers of lightning casualties and deaths. In *11th Conference on Applied Climatology*. Dallas, 1999.
15. Holle RL, López RE. A comparison of current lightning death rates in the U.S. with other locations and times. In *International Conference on Lightning and Static Electricity*. Blackpool, UK, 2003.
16. Holle RL, López RE, Navarro BC. Deaths, injuries, and damages from lightning in the United States in the 1890s in comparison with the 1990s. *J Appl Meteorol* 2005;44:1563–1573.
17. López RE, Holle RL. Changes in the number of lightning deaths in the United States during the twentieth century. *J Climate* 1998;11:2070.
18. Holle RL. Activities and locations of recreation deaths and injuries from lightning. In *International Conference on Lightning and Static Electricity*. Blackpool, UK, 2003.
19. Holle RL. Lightning-caused deaths and injuries during hiking and mountain climbing. In *International Conference on Lightning and Static Electricity*. Seattle, 2005.
20. Romero B, Candell-Riera J, Gracia RM, et al. Myocardial necrosis by electrocution: evaluation of noninvasive methods. *J Nucl Med* 1997;38:250–251.
21. Andrews CJ, Colquhoun D. The QT interval in lightning injury with implications for the 'cessation of metabolism' hypothesis. *J Wilderness Med* 1993;4:155–166.
22. Homma S, Gillam LD, Weyman AE. Echocardiographic observations in survivors of acute electrical injury. *Chest*. 1990;97:103–105.
23. Rivera J, Romero KA, Gonzalez-Chon O, et al. Severe stunned myocardium after lightning strike. *Crit Care Med* 2007;35: 280–285.
24. Bridges JE et al, eds. *Electrical Shock Safety Criteria: Proceedings of the First International Symposium on Electrical Shock Safety Criteria*. New York: Pergamon Press, 1985.
25. Xenopoulos N, Movahed A, Hudson P, et al. Myocardial injury in electrocution. *Am Heart J* 1991;122:1481–1484.
26. Fish R. Electric shock: Part II. nature and mechanisms of injury. *J Emerg Med* 1993;11:457–462.
27. Geddes LA, Bourland JD, Ford G. The mechanism underlying sudden death from electric shock. *Med Instrum* 1986;20:303–315.
28. Bailey B, Gaudreault P, Thivierge RL. Cardiac monitoring of high-risk patients after an electrical injury: a prospective multicentre study. *Emerg Med J* 2007;24:348–352.
29. Fatovich DM. Delayed lethal arrhythmia after an electrical injury. *Emerg Med J* 2007;24:743.
30. *Effects of Current on Human Beings and Livestock*. Technical specification 60479. Geneva: International Electrotechnical Commission, 2005.
31. Lee RC. Cell injury by electric forces. *Ann N Y Acad Sci* 2005; 1066:85–91.
32. Cooper MA. A fifth mechanism of lightning injury. *Acad Emerg Med* 2002;9:172–174.
33. Cooper MA, Andrews CJ, Holle RL. Distribution of lightning injury mechanisms. In *International Lightning Detection Conference*. Tucson, AZ, 2006.
34. Cooper MA. Lightning burns are usually minor, superficial, and less common than expected. In *International Lightning Detection Conference*. Tucson, AZ, 2006.
35. Andrews CJ, Darveniza M. New models of the electrical insult in lightning strike. In *Proceedings of the 9th International Conference on Atmospheric Physics*. St Petersburg, 1992.

36. Cooper MA, Andrews CJ, Holle RL. Lightning injuries. In Auerbach PS, ed. *Wilderness Medicine: Management of Wilderness and Environmental Emergencies*. 5th ed. Philadelphia: Mosby-Elsevier, 2007.
37. Kitigawa N, Turumi S, Ishikawa T, et al. The nature of lightning discharges on human bodies and the basis for safety and protection. In *18th International Conference on Lightning Protection*. Berlin: VDE-Verlag, 1985:435–438.
38. Ohashi M, Kitagawa N, Ishikawa T. Lightning injury caused by discharges accompanying flashovers: a clinical and experimental study of death and survival. *Burns Incl Therm Inj* 1986;12:496–501.
39. Kitigawa N. Response address for the Kitigawa Medal in Keraunomedicine. In *Royal Aeronautical Society International Conference on Lightning and Static Electricity*. Blackpool, UK, 2003.
40. Cherington M, Wachtel H, Yarnell PR. Could lightning injury be magnetically induced? *Lancet* 1998; 351:1788.
41. Andrews CJ, Cooper MA, Kotsos T, et al. Magnetic effects of lightning strikes. *Electr J Lightning Res* 2007.
42. Andrews C. Structural changes after lightning strike, with special emphasis on special sense orifices as portals of entry. *Semin Neurol* 1995;15:296–303.
43. Grubb BP, Karabin B. New onset postural tachycardia syndrome following lightning injury. *Pacing Clin Electrophysiol* 2007;30:1036–1038.
44. Weeramanthri TS, Puddey IB, Beilin LJ. Lightning strike and autonomic failure: coincidence or causally related? *J R Soc Med* 1991;84:687–688.
45. Cooper MA, Kotsos T, Gandhi MV, et al. Acute autonomic and cardiac effects of simulated lightning strike in rodents. In *International Bioengineering Symposium*. Chicago, 2000.
46. Cooper MA. The acute effects of simulated lightning strike on the cardiac and autonomic nervous system in an animal model. In *International Conference on Lightning and Static Electricity*. Blackpool, UK, 2003.
47. Andrews CJ. Crowd protection strategies: experience from Sydney Olympic Games, 2000. In *Royal Aeronautical Society International Conference on Lightning and Static Electricity*. Blackpool, UK, 2003.
48. Gratz J. Lightning safety and outdoor stadiums. In *American Meteorol Society Conference on Meteorological Applications of Lightning Data*. San Diego, CA, 2005.
49. Makdissi M, Brukner P. Recommendations for lightning protection in sport. *Med J Aust* 2002;177:35–37.

Chapter 33
Severe, Life–Threatening Asthma

Jill M. Baren

Asthma is responsible for >2 million emergency department (ED) visits in the U.S. each year, and approximately 1 in 4 (~500,000) of these visits resulted in an admission in recent years. Patients with severe, life-threatening asthma are challenging for emergency providers. The immediate goal is to prevent deterioration to respiratory or cardiopulmonary arrest. The provider must make difficult decisions about noninvasive ventilation, endotracheal intubation, and mechanical ventilation. Severe asthma exacerbations are prone to be fatal when combined with one or more asthma-related complications. These complications include tension pneumothorax (often bilateral), pneumomediastinum, pneumonia, lobar atelectasis (from mucous plugging, often of larger airways), cardiac dysfunction, and pulmonary edema.

- Pathophysiology of severe, life-threatening asthma
- Early management and assessment prior to intubation and respiratory arrest
- Key concepts and pitfalls in management
- Update on the 2007 recommendations from the National Heart, Lung and Blood Institute (NHLBI) for the management of severe asthma

Overview and Epidemiology

Asthma is a common, worldwide disease affecting 300 million people, with its highest prevalence in industrialized countries.[1] An estimated 30 million Americans (approximately 7% of adults) have been diagnosed with asthma within their lifetimes according to a 2004 National Health Interview Survey.[2,3] Asthma is responsible for >2 million ED visits in the U.S. each year, and approximately 1 in 4 (~500,000) of these visits resulted in an admission.[4] The economic burden of asthma is excessive at over $12 billion annually, with over $7 billion in direct medical costs.[5]

Most patients with asthma have mild to moderate disease that can be well controlled with a combination of anti-inflammatory drugs, although they may experience intermittent exacerbation of symptoms.[6] Exacerbations are acute worsening of disease of approximately 3 or more days' duration, need for unscheduled health care, reduction or cessation of normal activities, and increase in treatment.[6] The majority of these exacerbations, fortunately, are mild or moderate; however, all asthma patients are at risk for developing a severe exacerbation.[4]

A subgroup of patients with acute, severe asthma do not respond to conventional therapy and often progress rapidly to respiratory failure. Acute, severe asthma is considered to be a distinct entity or subtype of asthma that is sometimes referred to as "near-fatal asthma" or "life-threatening asthma."[2,4] These terms are used interchangeably throughout this chapter. Near-fatal and fatal asthma represent the most severe clinical presentations of asthma. There are no universally agreed upon definitions, but near fatal asthma is almost always associated with the presence of hypercapnia, acidemia, altered mental status, the need for endotracheal intubation and mechanical ventilation, and a high incidence for cardiopulmonary arrest.[7] Patients with near-fatal asthma, despite optimal treatment, typically have at least one asthma exacerbation in the year prior to the severe episode.[7]

Acute, severe asthma accounts for approximately 2% to 20% of admissions to intensive care units, with up to one third of these patients requiring intubation and mechanical ventilation.[8] Of every 100 admissions, approximately 1 will die (5,000 deaths).[9] Death from asthma is, therefore, not common, but there are approximately 5,000 to 6,000 deaths annually; many occur in the prehospital setting. About 1% to 7% of all patients with severe asthma will die each year; of those who survive an episode of near-fatal asthma, 17% will subsequently die from another acute severe episode.[4]

Over the last few decades guidelines developed by the National Asthma Education and Prevention Program of the NHLBI and the Global Initiative for Asthma have focused on the recognition and management of acute asthma and may have contributed to a rise in outpatient visits, a concomitant fall in hospitalizations, and improved outcomes.[1,10,11] The latest asthma mortality data indicate that in 2003 there were just over 4,000 deaths, a 12% reduction from 1999. Gender-specific death rates still show a female preponderance (1.8:1), and asthma death rates for blacks are approximately 2.7 per 100,000 compared with 1.2 for whites.[2]

Experts believe that >50% of fatal asthma may not be recognized as such because the deaths occur at home or during transport to the hospital. Most acute episodes resulting in death are related to severe underlying disease, inadequate baseline management, and acute exacerbations of inflammation.

LATEST GUIDELINES

Several consensus groups have developed excellent practice guidelines for the diagnosis and treatment of asthma. These groups include the National Asthma Education and Prevention Program of the National Institutes of Health,[10,12] the Global Initiative for Asthma,[11] and the Canadian Association of Emergency Physicians and the Canadian Thoracic Society.[13,14]

- National Asthma Education and Prevention Program: http://www.nhlbi.nih.gov/about/naepp/
- Global Initiative for Asthma: http://www.ginasthma.com/
- CAEP: http://www.caep.ca/

Life-Threatening and Fatal Asthma

Pathophysiology

Asthma represents a spectrum of disease characterized by a cascade of inflammatory mediators. The pathophysiology of asthma consists of three key abnormalities:

- Bronchoconstriction
- Airway inflammation
- Mucous impaction

Severe exacerbations of asthma can rapidly lead to death. Cardiac arrest in patients with asthma has been linked to a variety of pathophysiologic mechanisms that complicate exacerbations of asthma, but the most likely cause is thought to be bronchospasm with subsequent plugging of the narrowed airways by mucus.[9] Marked airway thickening and rapid infiltration of neutrophils into the airways are consistent findings in acute, severe asthma and may differentiate these patients from those with milder disease. In fatal cases, a 25- to 30-fold greater degree of thickening of the airways has been noted.[4] At autopsy, these patients display marked mucous plugging, airway edema, exudation of plasma proteins, hypertrophy of airway smooth muscle, and cellular activation, with increased production and activation of inflammatory mediators.[15–17] Some patients experience a sudden, severe onset of bronchospasm that responds rapidly to inhaled beta$_2$ agonists.[18] This observation suggests that marked bronchiolar smooth muscle spasm is the major component in at least some cases of fatal asthma.

Acute, severe asthma results in hypoxemia secondary to the processes of hyperinflation and regional ventilation/perfusion mismatch. Carbon dioxide retention does not typically occur until FEV$_1$ falls below 25% of predicted.[4] Airway occlusion due to smooth muscle bronchoconstriction, airway edema, inflammation, and formation of mucous plugs forms the pathologic basis of the gas-exchange abnormalities observed in acute, severe asthma, and leads to the development of extensive intrapulmonary shunting. Metabolic lactic acidosis may also coexist at later stages of the disease.[7]

Bronchoconstriction and airway obstruction from mucous plugging cause hyperinflation and increased airway resistance (Fig. 33-1). As a consequence, the work of breath-

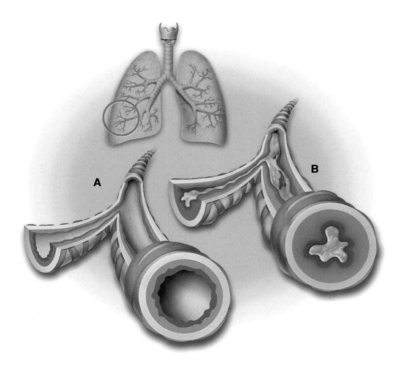

FIGURE 33-1 • Asthma occurs in the setting of underlying inflammation. Diffuse bronchospasm occurs, causing air passages to constrict. Hypersecretion of mucous leads to plugs, which block oxygenation and ventilation. **A.** Normal healthy bronchus **B.** Bronchiole during asthma attack.

ing increases dramatically. For example, at an FEV_1 of 50% of predicted, the work of breathing increases to 10 times normal. At an FEV_1 of <25% of predicted, severe respiratory muscle fatigue can contribute to the development of respiratory arrest and death unless urgent treatment is provided.

Severe asthma exacerbations are prone to be fatal when combined with other asthma-related complications. These complications include tension pneumothorax (often bilateral), pneumomediastinum, pneumonia, lobar atelectasis (from mucous plugging, often of larger airways), cardiac dysfunction, and pulmonary edema. Previous suspicion that fatal cardiac arrhythmias occur from the use (or misuse) of beta-adrenergic agonists is unfounded.[16,17] In reviews of asthma-related deaths, several authors were unable to document an association between these drugs and fatal arrhythmias.[18–20]

Signs and Symptoms

Significant risk factors affecting the severity of asthma include environmental exposures, genetic polymorphisms, and especially prior asthma-related events (Table 33-1).[2] A history of prior hospitalization, especially if mechanical ventilation was required, is considered the greatest predictor of an episode of near-fatal asthma.[7]

Asthma Triggers

Just as patient profiles and risk factors for asthma can be identified, so too can triggers for exacerbations in many individuals. Some of these are unavoidable, but they should still be identified if possible. Some can be avoided in the future if patients and their families are aware. In other instances, they must be treated concomitantly with the asthma exacerbation (Table 33-2).

Viruses are responsible for triggering the vast majority of asthma exacerbations. They are accompanied by lower airway neutrophilia and have been linked to asthma mortality. Although patients with severe asthma do not seem to have more viral infections than patients without asthma or those with mild asthma, the effect of viruses on their lower airways seems to be more substantial.[6] Certain bacteria (e.g., *Chlamydia pneumoniae* and *Mycoplasma pneumoniae*) are also associated with asthma exacerbations and, in the case of patients with severe asthma, also lead to a more intense inflammatory response than is seen in asthma patients without such infections.[6]

Aeroallergens and pollutants are other triggers for asthma exacerbation and are all associated with increased rates of hospitalization and health care expenditures.[6]

Allergen exposure is also an important environmental factor in triggering asthma exacerbations: dust mites, cockroaches, and fungi such as *Alternaria* have all been strongly implicated.[21] Cigarette smoke is another widely cited trigger

TABLE 33-1 • Risk Factors for Fatal, Near-Fatal, or Life-Threatening Asthma[2]

- History of sudden severe exacerbation
- Prior asthma exacerbation requiring intubation and mechanical ventilation
- Prior admission to intensive care unit
- Two or more hospitalizations for asthma exacerbation in the past year
- Three or more emergency care visits for asthma exacerbation in the past year
- Hospitalization or emergency care visit for asthma within the past month
- Use of more than two canisters per month of inhaled short acting β_2- agonist
- Current use or recent withdrawal from systemic corticosteroids
- Lack of a written asthma action plan
- Lack of adherence to or compliance with therapy such as inhaled corticosteroids within the past 2 weeks
- Lack of regular assessment using objective measurements of airflow obstruction
- Difficulty perceiving airflow obstruction or its severity
- Other comorbidity: cardiovascular, chronic obstructive pulmonary disease
- Psychological problems or psychiatric disease
- Low socioeconomic status
- Urban/inner-city residence
- Illicit drug use
- Sensitivity to fungi such as *Alternaria*

TABLE 33-2 • Triggers of Fatal and Near Fatal Asthma Exacerbations

1. Environment:
   - extremes of temperature
   - high humidity and dew points
   - episodic contaminants (smoke, cigarette smoke)
2. Upper respiratory infections (viruses and bacteria)
3. Allergens (pollens and molds)
4. Exercise (cold-induced)
5. Other medical conditions (COPD, GE reflux)
6. Drugs (aspirin, beta-blockers, nonsteroidal anti-inflammatory medications)

COPD, chronic obstructive pulmonary disease; GE, gastroesophageal.

for an asthma exacerbation. Sinusitis episodes are common triggering events as well.[21] Drugs such as aspirin, beta-blockers, and nonsteroidal anti-inflammatory agents may predispose to asthma exacerbations. In the subset of asthma patients who require mechanical ventilation, almost 10% have aspirin use as a precipitating factor. Heroin, cocaine, and alcohol intoxication are also frequently reported in association with asthma death.[7]

ASTHMA FACTS

The number of patients with severe asthma exacerbations who present to the ED at night is ten times greater than the number who present during the day; 2% of patients with acute asthma who present at night require intubation. Most deaths from asthma occur at home or during transport to an ED.

Those groups at increased risk for near-fatal and fatal asthma include:

- Patients who fail to recognize the severity of their exacerbation
- Patients who attempt to treat themselves during an exacerbation without notifying their primary provider
- Patients with a high level of denial about their disease on psychological evaluation
- Patients who receive suboptimal treatment from their primary care provider
- Patients who are depressed or anxious
- Patients whose asthma was diagnosed when they were <5 years of age

Based on studies of risk factors, the patient with near-fatal asthma has a somewhat stereotypical picture of non-compliance, inadequate medication regimen, and denial. But that stereotype is inaccurate for about half of life-threatening asthma events.[22] Nearly half of near-fatal and fatal asthma episodes occur suddenly and unexpectedly, outside the hospital, in stable, younger, atopic patients who are reportedly compliant with their medical plan of care, using inhaled corticosteroids on a daily basis.[22]

Based on clinical presentation, there seem to be two distinct phenotypes of acute, severe asthma. Type 1, or slowly progressive asthma, is characterized by a prolonged, slow onset of symptoms with late arrival for medical care. This type is more common and represents about 80% to 85% of acute, severe asthma patients; it is generally considered to be preventable. These patients have excess mucous plugging and tend to perceive symptoms early despite delay in seeking treatment, and they also tend to have a slow response to treatment. Type 2, or sudden asphyxic asthma, is characterized by the rapid onset of symptoms with sudden, severe deterioration; it is seen in the remaining 15% to 20%. Such patients are characterized by a history of unstable disease that is partially responsive to treatment. They have hyperacute or acute asphyxic symptoms leading to the development of respiratory failure within 2 hours of symptom onset. These patients also tend to have massive allergen exposure as well as emotional distress. The airways tend to be empty of secretions and there is a late perception of symptoms but an often rapid response to treatment if the patient is able to get to emergency medical care.[2,7]

Signs and Symptoms: Assessing Severity

Asthma exacerbations are acute or subacute episodes of progressively worsening shortness of breath, cough, wheezing, or chest tightness or a combination of several of these symptoms. The hallmark finding that characterizes an asthma exacerbation is a decrease in expiratory airflow that can be documented by spirometry or peak expiratory flow measurement. It is important to use these objective measures to more reliably gauge the severity of an exacerbation (Table 33-3).

 See Web site for NHLBI National Asthma Education and Prevention Program guidelines for the diagnosis and management of asthma.

Clinical evaluation of severe asthma must occur immediately, and the medical history should not differ substantially from that of patients with a less severe presentation other than the fact that those who are severely ill may be too dyspneic to provide much information prior to initial therapy. Common symptoms reported are dyspnea, cough, and wheezing, but presentations are variable and dyspnea can be absent in up to 18% of cases.[2] Wheezing can be a poor indicator of functional impairment.

The patient's report of subjective symptoms is often an inaccurate gauge of asthma severity. Reported severity correlates poorly with objective severity scoring systems. Some patients with severe, life-threatening asthma have an impaired response to hypercapnia and hypoxia. Their perception of dyspnea appears to be blunted. These patients may present with severe abnormalities of oxygenation as well as with respiratory acidosis.[23]

WHEEZING AND ASTHMA SEVERITY

In severe asthma, the severity of wheezing provides a poor indicator of airflow or adequacy of gas exchange.

- A patient with severe bronchospasm and obstruction may not move air and may not wheeze at all.[24,25]
- The "silent" chest in an asthma patient is an ominous sign.

Treatment that results in the return of wheezes on auscultation in this situation can be considered effective.

The priority of the clinical examination is to confirm the diagnosis of asthma and to assess its severity. Most of the relevant physical examination can be determined from the vital signs and by direct observation of the patient. Physical signs and symptoms include tachypnea, tachycardia, wheezing, accessory muscle use, diaphoresis, cyanosis, and altered mental status. Auditory wheezing or wheezing heard through auscultation is present in almost all cases with the exception of those patients who have severely diminished air movement; in such cases, the chest is "quiet" and may represent severe obstruction. Although physical examination findings do not always correlate well with severity, they

	Mild	Moderate	Severe	Subset: Respiratory Arrest Imminent
Symptoms				
Breathlessness	While walking	While at rest (infant—softer, shorter cry, difficulty feeding)	While at rest (infant—stops feeding)	
	Can lie down	Prefers sitting	Sits upright	
Talks in	Sentences	Phrases	Words	
Alertness	May be agitated	Usually agitated	Usually agitated	Drowsy or confused
Signs				
Respiratory rate	Increased	Increased	Often >30/minute	
		Guide to rates of breathing in awake children: *Age* — *Normal rate* <2 months — <60/minute 2–12 months — <50/minute 1–5 years — <40/minute 6–8 years — <30/minute		
Use of accessory muscles; suprasternal retractions	Usually not	Commonly	Usually	Paradoxical thoracoabdominal movement
Wheeze	Moderate, often only end expiratory	Loud; throughout exhalation	Usually loud; throughout inhalation and exhalation	Absence of wheeze
Pulse/minute	<100	100–120	>120	Bradycardia
		Guide to normal pulse rates in children: *Age* — *Normal rate* 2–12 months — <160/minute 1–2 years — <120/minute 2–8 years — <110/minute		
Pulsus paradoxus	Absent <10 mm Hg	May be present 10–25 mm Hg	Often present >25 mm Hg (adult) 20–40 mm Hg (child)	Absence suggests respiratory muscle fatigue
Functional Assessment				
PEF percent predicted or percent personal best	≥70 percent	Approx. 40–69 percent or response lasts <2 hours	<40 percent	<25 percent Note: PEF testing may not be needed in very severe attacks
PaO$_2$ (on air)	Normal (test not usually necessary)	≥60 mm Hg (test not usually necessary)	<60 mm Hg: possible cyanosis	
and/or PcO$_2$	<42 mm Hg (test not usually necessary)	<42 mm Hg (test not usually necessary)	≥42 mm Hg possible respiratory failure (See pages 393–394, 399)	
SaO$_2$ percent (on air) at sea level	>95 percent (test not usually necessary)	90–95 percent (test not usually necessary)	<90 percent	

Hypercapnia (hypoventilation) develops more readily in young children than in adults and adolescents.

Key Pao$_2$, arterial oxygen pressure; Pco$_2$, partial pressure of carbon dioxide; PEF, peak expiratory flow; SaO$_2$, oxygen saturation.

Notes:
• The presence of several parameters, but not necessarily all, indicates the general classification of the exacerbation.
• Many of these parameters have not been systematically studied, especially as they correlate with each other. Thus, they serve only as general guides.
From the National Heart, Lung, and Blood Institute National Asthma Education and Prevention Program Expert Panel Report 3: Guidelines for the Diagnosis and Management of Asthma, 2007.

should be used as a guide to determining severity. For example, an asthmatic patient who is sitting upright to breathe and using accessory inspiratory muscles in the neck and chest, is at risk for sudden respiratory failure. Somnolence, mental confusion, and a moribund or exhausted appearance are ominous signs that respiratory arrest is imminent.

Vital signs during an acute, severe asthma exacerbation typically show tachypnea >30 breaths per minute and tachycardia. Blood pressure can fluctuate depending on the degree of hemodynamic compromise secondary to lung hyperinflation and on the degree of dehydration.[4] Increasing heart rate has close correlation with worsening asthma severity; do not assume that tachycardia is only due to beta-agonist treatment, because studies have shown that adequate bronchodilator response has been associated with a decrease in heart rate.[26]

The assessment of severity and prediction of treatment requirements, including the need for hospitalization, depends on repeated clinical assessments. In adults, repeated objective measures of lung function are helpful; but in children, this type of monitoring will depend on age. Many clinical scoring systems to gauge the severity of asthma have been developed, but none are 100% predictive for hospitalization. The benefit of using clinical asthma severity scores is primarily to highlight the importance of regular comprehensive assessments.

Close monitoring includes serial measurement of lung function. Every effort should be made to obtain objective measures of lung function. These include forced expiratory volume in 1 second (FEV_1) and peak expiratory flow rate (PEFR), which are useful for predicting the need for hospitalization in adults. FEV_1 is preferred but usually less available in EDs than PEFR. The PEFR and FEV_1 are not equivalent in terms of the percentage of predicted values; FEV_1 is on average about 5 to 10 points lower than the PEFR (FEV_1 of 30% is equivalent to a PEFR of 35%–40%).[26] The only patients who do not warrant a peak flow or FEV_1 measurement are those with life-threatening exacerbations, during which the clinical assessment should suffice. Otherwise the FEV_1 or PEFR should be obtained initially and then 30 to 60 minutes after initial treatment (NHLBI). An FEV_1 or PEFR that is <25% of predicted, that improves only <10% after treatment, or that shows very wide fluctuation, is a potential indication for admission to an intensive care unit (ICU); such patients should be very carefully observed.[10] Some patients can appear deceptively well despite the presence of severe airflow obstruction; this underscores the importance of objective lung function measurements.[26]

For children >5 years of age, either FEV_1 or PEFR may be useful; but neither may be feasible during an exacerbation.[10] Only 65% of children 5 to 18 years of age and virtually no children <5 years can perform these tests.[27]

A peak flow meter provides a quick, accurate, and reproducible measure of PEFR in cooperative adults and children; it is also not influenced by the person supervising the test.[28] EDs should consider PEFR as a vital sign for an asthma patient. Store the PEFR device with a small box of disposable mouthpieces and a copy of the expected normal flow rate values for men, women, and children.

Pulse oximetry has been shown to be useful in infants and children in determining the severity of an exacerbation but not for predicting hospitalization unless repeated.[10] Measurement of pulse oximetry should be made in all patients with severe asthma. Arterial oxygen desaturation and hypercarbia occurring concurrently may indicate the need for endotracheal intubation and may portend a life-threatening situation.[26]

OXYGEN SATURATION CAN BE MISLEADING

Oxygen saturation (SaO_2) levels may not reflect progressive alveolar hypoventilation, particularly if O_2 is being administered. Note that the SaO_2 may initially fall during therapy because beta agonists produce both bronchodilation and vasodilation and may initially increase intrapulmonary shunting.

Most often, other diagnostic tests will not be necessary. Even if specific laboratory tests are deemed necessary, they should not delay treatment. The primary purpose of diagnostic testing in the setting of asthma is to hasten the detection of respiratory failure or confirm suspected complications of asthma exacerbations, such as pneumonia. The following laboratory tests can be considered.

Arterial blood gases are not necessary for most patients but can provide information about respiratory reserve, metabolic disturbances, and degree of hypoxemia. The most common abnormality is respiratory alkalosis, but as lung function drops, hypercarbia and respiratory acidosis develop, with a subset of patients also having metabolic acidosis; the latter is thought to be due to accumulating lactate from respiratory muscle fatigue and tissue hypoxia.[4]

Chest radiography is also not routinely needed for the assessment and management of all asthma patients. Abnormalities other than hyperinflation and atelectasis are rarely found (<5%).[4] In acute, severe asthma, where barotrauma is a significant consideration, more frequent use of chest radiography is justified.[4] About one third of chest radiographs in one series of admitted asthma patients were found to indicate major abnormalities that needed intervention.[4] Most of these were cases of pneumonia treated with antibiotics. The same principle applies to children, where the clinical significance of a chest radiograph during the first presenting episode of asthma was very limited.[29]

Complete blood count may be useful in patients with fever and/or the presence of purulent sputum to support the diagnosis of infection as a trigger of asthma.[7] Some of the electrocardiographic (ECG) changes noted in acute, severe asthma are right axis deviation and evidence of right ventricular hypertrophy, which usually resolves with effective therapy.

Differential Diagnosis

When a patient presents with wheezing, it must be determined if the patient has acute asthma. When a patient presents with extreme dyspnea, it may not be possible to obtain a confirmatory history of asthma. It will be possible to identify most patients with acute, severe asthma; but in adults with no prior history of asthma, a number of mimicking conditions must be immediately considered (Table 33-4).

TABLE 33-4 • Asthma: Differential Diagnosis—Other Primary Pulmonary and Systemic Conditions

- Obliterative bronchiolitis
- Vocal cord dysfunction
- Cystic fibrosis
- Bronchiectasis
- Endobronchial lesion
- Inhaled foreign body
- Recurrent aspiration
- Congestive heart failure episode
- Tracheobronchomalacia
- Upper airway obstruction
- Allergic bronchopulmonary aspergillosis
- Pulmonary eosinophilic syndromes
- Pneumonia
- Acute allergic bronchospasm or anaphylaxis (aspirin, foods, or idiopathic)
- Pulmonary embolism

Prehospital Clinical Deterioration, Imminent Respiratory Arrest, and Cardiopulmonary Arrest

Patients with severe, life-threatening asthma pose a challenge to emergency providers. The immediate goal is to prevent deterioration to respiratory or cardiopulmonary arrest. The provider must make difficult decisions about noninvasive ventilation, endotracheal intubation, and mechanical ventilation.

Immediate Actions

Start supplementary oxygen at once; use a nonrebreathing mask with high-flow oxygen or a bag and mask. Administer epinephrine 0.3 mg subcutaneously (SQ) as quickly as possible. A total dose of 0.01 mg/kg can be given in divided doses approximately 20 minutes apart, based on patient response. Potential side effects of epinephrine are small relative to the risk of cardiopulmonary arrest. Immediately administer an inhaled beta$_2$ agonist if respiratory effort is adequate or if SQ epinephrine has improved airflow. Administer the first dose with a metered-dose inhaler (MDI) with spacer or nebulizer, whichever can be assembled more quickly. The NHLBI guidelines strongly advocate for all emergency medical services (EMS) providers to have a standing order allowing them to provide albuterol to patients with asthma exacerbations. Both nebulizers and MDI with spacer/holding chamber are acceptable prehospital methods of drug delivery. Transport should not be delayed in any circumstances but treatment can be repeated en route as necessary.[10] In systems with a long transport time, ambulance services should consider the development of prehospital protocols that allow for the addition of ipratropium bromide and oral corticosteroids.

Evaluate Immediate Response

Evaluate how well the patient responds in the first 10 to 20 minutes to oxygen, epinephrine, and inhaled beta$_2$ agonists. There should be unequivocal and significant objective improvement (e.g., improvement in oxygenation and clinical appearance, a change in PEFR from a severe degree of obstruction of <100 L/min to 150–200 L/min).

If the patient deteriorates, proceed to rapid sequence intubation (RSI) if resources and skilled EMS personnel are available and support ventilations with bag-mask while preparations are immediately initiated.

DO NOT HYPERVENTILATE

Do not hyperventilate the patient during bag-mask ventilation. Hyperventilation may compromise cardiac output (see below). Overly rapid breaths cause increased intrathoracic pressure and inadequate exhalation in some patients.

Primary Therapy and Reassessment in the Emergency Department

Clinicians should pay special attention to patients who are at high risk of asthma-related death and institute early therapy. Severe exacerbations are potentially life-threatening; therefore, care must be prompt. Approximately 10% to 25% of ED patients will require hospitalization. Initial assessment is composed of a brief history and physical examination and objective measures of lung function. Asthma patients should be immediately triaged and placed in a clinical care area so that treatment can begin instantly, particularly when the exacerbation is moderate to severe. The length of ED treatment before a disposition decision can be made is usually about 4 to 6 hours. About 75% of patients will resolve their bronchospasm within 2 hours, and the remaining patients will likely need at least 24 hours of observation or admission.

Patients who have a partial response where the FEV_1 is still <60% predicted after 2 hours of therapy should be admitted to a general medical ward; those who fail to respond to therapy (PEFR improved by <10%–20%) or with persistent hypercapnia, tachypnea, or altered mental status should be admitted to the ICU.[7]

Primary Therapy

Management of a primary exacerbation includes the following therapies: oxygen, short-acting selective beta$_2$ agonists and ipratropium bromide, systemic corticosteroids, and consideration of adjunctive treatments, such as IV magnesium or heliox, and continuous monitoring.[10] These therapeutic agents are discussed individually below. The Expert Panel Report 3 from the National Asthma Education and Prevention Program is the first comprehensive update on asthma management in 10 years from the NHLBI. It represents consensus expert opinion on the best available evidence for the treatment of acute asthma.[10]

Oxygen

A major treatment goal is correction of significant hypoxemia by administering supplemental oxygen. Oxygen should be started for all patients with acute, severe asthma either by mask or nasal cannula, whichever is tolerated best. The immediate endpoint is to maintain SaO_2 above 90% (95% in pregnant women and patients with heart disease).[10] Start supplementary oxygen before or simultaneously with initial inhaled beta$_2$ agonists. Oxygen saturation should be monitored until there is a clearly established response to bronchodilator therapy.

Inhaled Beta$_2$ Agonists

Another goal of treatment is rapid reversal of airflow obstruction using repetitive or continuous administration of a short-acting beta$_2$ agonist. This is the most effective way to reverse airflow obstruction.[10]

Albuterol and salbutamol are equivalent beta$_2$-selective beta agonists that act by relaxing bronchial smooth muscles. These drugs provide rapid, dose-dependent, short-acting reduction in bronchospasm with minimal adverse effects. Albuterol has gained almost universal acceptance as the therapeutic bronchodilator for acute asthma. Inhaled albuterol (0.5 mL diluted in 2–2.5 mL normal saline) is delivered through a nebulizer or MDI. Because the administered dose depends on the patient's lung volume and inspiratory flow rates, the same dose can be used in most patients regardless of age or size.

Metered-Dose Inhalers Versus Nebulizers Studies have shown no difference in the effects of continuous versus intermittent administration of nebulized albuterol; continuous administration was more effective in a subset of patients with severe exacerbations of asthma, and it was more cost-effective in a pediatric trial.[30–32] A Cochrane meta-analysis showed no overall difference between the effects of albuterol delivered by MDI-spacer or nebulizer, but MDI-spacer administration can be difficult in patients in severe distress; therefore, nebulizers are often preferred for patients who are unable to cooperate with the use of an MDI because of age, agitation, or the severity of the exacerbation.[33] Delivery by nebulizer has become the most common ED treatment for acute asthma, but a number of studies suggest that MDIs with spacers have several advantages over nebulizers, although the technique of administration must be precise. MDI-spacer administration is less expensive, starting treatment is faster and easier, and there is more efficient use of staff time.[34–37]

ADMINISTRATION OF BETA$_2$-SELECTIVE BETA AGONISTS

There is no overall difference whether albuterol is administered by continuous or intermittent dosing or by MDI-spacer or nebulizer, but:

- Continuous administration was more effective in the subset of patients with severe exacerbations of asthma and severe airflow limitation.
- MDI-spacer administration can be difficult in patients in severe distress.

Initial therapy with albuterol by nebulizer is between 2.5 and 7.5 mg every 15 to 20 minutes intermittently or by continuous nebulization (adults) in a dose of 10 to 15 mg/hr. Continuous therapy may be more effective for patients with severe airflow obstruction. "Aggressive dosing" for more severe cases calls for higher amounts of agents at shorter intervals. The typical initial therapy with albuterol by MDI-spacer is 4 to 8 puffs every 20 minutes for three doses up to 4 hours in adults. Continue dosing every 1 to 4 hours as needed. The MDI should be used in conjunction with a volume holding chamber for all patients and with the addition of a mask for children <4 to 5 years of age.

There are no data describing the toxicity of continuous bronchodilator therapy, but it is reasonable to consider additional monitoring with ECG and oximetry or alternative therapy for patients at higher risk of cardiovascular complications, such as those with known ischemic heart disease.[3]

Levalbuterol is the R isomer of albuterol. It has recently become available in the United States for the treatment of acute asthma. Conventional albuterol is an equal mixture of the R and S isomers and may exaggerate airway hyperresponsiveness through the effects of the S isomer, previously thought to be an inert compound. However, most studies have shown equivalent safety and efficacy between levalbuterol and racemic albuterol, with possible slight improvement in bronchodilation when compared with albuterol in the ED.[29,38–40] However, the relative benefits of levalbuterol—which is more expensive than albuterol—have not been determined.[41] If levalbuterol is used, the MDI dose is 0.075 mg/kg (minimum 1.25 mg/dose, range 1.25–2.5 mg) every 20 minutes for three doses, then 5 mg every 1 to

4 hours as needed. The dose by nebulization has not been evaluated.

Corticosteroids

In conjunction with short-acting selective beta$_2$ agonists, administer systemic corticosteroids early to patients with moderate to severe exacerbations or those who fail to respond promptly and completely to bronchodilator therapy.[10] Systemic corticosteroids are the only proven treatment for the inflammatory component of asthma and help speed the resolution of airflow obstruction. However, the onset of their anti-inflammatory effects can be as long as 6 to 12 hours after administration, although it is more likely to be between 2 and 6 hours.[10] The early use of systemic steroids reduces hospitalization.[42] In addition, reduction of inflammation and bronchial edema decreases length of hospital stay, in-hospital complications, readmissions, and return visits to the ED.[43,44]

Health care providers should administer steroids as early as possible to all asthma patients but should not expect effects for several hours. Although there is no difference in clinical effects between oral and IV formulations of corticosteroids, the oral route is usually preferred for most patients.[45] The IV route is preferable in patients with severe, acute asthma since they may vomit or be unable to swallow.[46] A typical initial dose of IV methylprednisolone is 125 mg (dose range: 40–250 mg).

The weight-based dose is 2 mg/kg IV, which can be repeated every 6 hours. The question of dose provokes debate, and optimal dosing has not been well established in the literature. Some clinicians prescribe as little as 40 mg of IV methylprednisolone in the ED. Others use doses as high as 250 mg IV or the equivalent.

Inhaled Steroids Use of inhaled steroids in lieu of systemic steroids is not recommended at this time. However, a Cochrane meta-analysis of seven randomized trials (four adult and three pediatric) of inhaled corticosteroids concluded that they significantly reduced the likelihood of admission to the hospital, particularly in patients who were not receiving concomitant systemic steroids. There is mounting evidence that multiple high doses of inhaled steroids in the ED in adults are beneficial, but there is insufficient evidence that inhaled corticosteroids alone are as effective as systemic steroids.[43]

Anticholinergics

Ipratropium bromide is an anticholinergic bronchodilator that is pharmacologically related to atropine. It can produce a clinically modest improvement in lung function compared with albuterol alone.[47,48] The nebulizer dose is 0.025 to 0.5 mg every 20 minutes for three doses then as needed or four to eight puffs by MDI every 20 minutes as needed up to 3 hours. It has a slow onset of action (approximately 20 minutes), with peak effectiveness at 60 to 90 minutes and few systemic side effects. It is typically given only once because

of its prolonged onset of action, but some studies have shown clinical improvement with repeated doses.[49] Given the few side effects, ipratropium should be considered an important first-line therapy that is synergistic with albuterol in certain patients. Tiotropium is a new, longer-acting anticholinergic that is currently undergoing clinical testing for use in acute asthma.[50]

Pharmacology Ipratropium inhibits vagally mediated constriction of bronchial smooth muscles. The result is local, site-specific bronchodilation. Ipratropium bromide produces less bronchodilation than inhaled beta$_2$ agonists, and it has a slower onset of action (about 20 minutes longer).[48,51]

Use for Severe, Life-Threatening Asthma There is a role for ipratropium bromide *in combination* with inhaled beta agonists for acute events. This beneficial effect appears to occur specifically in cases of severe, life-threatening asthma. The only age groups with relevant studies are children and adolescents, but the results are frequently applied to adults.[52] When added to albuterol in children and adolescents with moderately severe asthma (FEV$_1$ <55% of predicted), multiple doses of ipratropium improved pulmonary function and reduced the rate of hospitalization by 30%.[52,53] This benefit was not observed when the asthma exacerbation was mild. In trials limited to adults, there was an observed modest benefit from ipratropium combined with beta$_2$ agonists (7% improvement in FEV$_1$, 22% improvement in PEFR).[54] Adding multiple doses of ipratropium bromide to short-acting beta agonists produces additional bronchodilation, especially among those with severe airflow obstruction.

Magnesium Sulfate

IV magnesium sulfate can modestly improve pulmonary function in patients with asthma when combined with nebulized beta-adrenergic agents and corticosteroids.[55] Magnesium causes bronchial smooth muscle relaxation independent of the serum magnesium level, with only minor side effects (flushing, light-headedness). A Cochrane meta-analysis of seven studies concluded that IV magnesium sulfate improves pulmonary function and reduces hospital admissions, particularly for patients with the most severe exacerbations of asthma.[56]

Pharmacology The exact mechanism of action is unknown but may be similar to the tocolytic effects on smooth muscle. A number of clinical trials have reported that magnesium sulfate improves bronchodilation in patients who are persistently symptomatic after inhaled adrenergic agents and corticosteroids.[55–59]

Dose Magnesium sulfate should be considered for use in all patients who have a severe or life-threatening asthma exacerbation. Consideration of use typically occurs after the first hour of conventional therapy when there is a suboptimal response, but it can be considered for earlier administration as well. The typical dose is 25 to 75 mg/kg (about 1–2 g in adults) IV given over 20 minutes. When given with a beta$_2$ agonist, nebulized magnesium sulfate also improved pulmonary function during an acute asthma attack but does not reduce rate of hospitalization.[60]

Parenteral Epinephrine or Terbutaline

IV beta-agonist administration is still considered to be an unproven treatment with no obvious benefits demonstrated compared with aerosolized beta$_2$ agonist; however, decreased tidal volume and airway obstruction may preclude the use of aerosolized therapy.[29]

Epinephrine and terbutaline are adrenergic agents that can be given SQ to patients with acute, severe asthma. Epinephrine is an effective bronchial smooth muscle dilator with a rapid onset of action. The dose of SQ epinephrine (concentration of 1:1,000) is 0.01 mg/kg divided into three doses of approximately 0.3 mg given at 20-minute intervals. The nonselective adrenergic properties of epinephrine may cause an increase in heart rate, myocardial irritability, and oxygen demand. But its use (even in patients >35 years of age) is well tolerated.[61] Terbutaline is given in a dose of 0.25 mg SQ and can be repeated in 30 to 60 minutes. These drugs are more commonly administered to children with acute asthma. Terbutaline is the current IV beta agonist agent of choice in the United States. Although most studies have shown these drugs to be equally efficacious, one study concluded that terbutaline was superior.[62]

Pharmacology   Epinephrine is a nonselective beta agonist that requires parenteral (SQ or intravenous [IV]) administration. The nonselective properties of epinephrine also produce tachycardia, acute blood pressure elevation, and myocardial irritability. Epinephrine will increase myocardial oxygen demand.

Use in Severe, Life-Threatening Asthma   SQ epinephrine is often omitted in patients with severe asthma, but some experts suggest that the subcutaneous administration of epinephrine or terbutaline should be used in patients unresponsive to continuous nebulized beta agonists and in those unable to cooperate owing to alteration in mental status or an inability to tolerate oral therapy. SQ epinephrine may also be delivered to intubated patients not responding to inhaled therapy during mechanical ventilation.[7] Patients with severe airflow obstruction, where wheezing cannot be heard on auscultation, are those most likely to benefit from epinephrine, and they cannot effectively inhale beta$_2$ agonists through an MDI or nebulizer. As the patient deteriorates, the inspiratory flow rate decreases and compromises delivery of inhaled medications. There is little evidence for withholding epinephrine (even if it must be given IV) from patients with severe, life-threatening asthma solely because of age.

Parenteral Terbutaline

Terbutaline is a selective beta$_2$ agonist with pharmacologic and adverse effects similar to those of albuterol. In the ED,

terbutaline is given by SQ injection or IV infusion. Compared with epinephrine, terbutaline has a slower onset of action (5–30 minutes), a longer time to peak effect (1–2 hours), and a much longer duration of action (3–6 hours). As an alternative to epinephrine, terbutaline has little role to play in adults with severe, life-threatening asthma because of its slow onset of action and longer time to peak effects. But in children, at least one ED study has found terbutaline to be more efficacious than epinephrine for reversal of wheezing.[63] The dose of terbutaline is 0.25 mg SQ, which can be repeated once in 30 to 60 minutes. The total dose should not exceed 0.5 mg every 4 hours. Dosing for IV infusion starts at 0.05 to 0.1 μg/kg/min and has been used predominantly in pediatric patients.

The adverse effects of IV beta agonists are mainly cardiovascular in nature: tachycardia, increased QT interval, dysrhythmias, hyper- and hypotension. Dysrhythmias may result from induced hypokalemia. A single study demonstrated that there was no clinically significant cardiac toxicity in pediatric patients receiving IV terbutaline, and it remains the IV agent of choice in this population.[29]

Ketamine

Ketamine is a parenteral dissociative anesthetic that has both sedative and bronchodilatory properties. A single randomized trial published to date showed no benefit of the routine administration of ketamine to standard care.[64] Ketamine stimulates copious bronchial secretions, which may further complicate asthma. Ketamine is also recommended as a preferred sedative during RSI of the asthma patient owing to the properties discussed above.[46]

Other Agents

Heliox   Heliox is a mixture of helium and oxygen (usually a 60:40 or 70:30 helium-to-oxygen ratio mix) that is less dense than ambient air and has been hypothesized to improve gas exchange in patients with airway obstruction. Heliox has been shown to improve the delivery and deposition of nebulized albuterol.[65] Although multiple small studies have been conducted with conflicting results, a meta-analysis of six clinical trials did not support the use of heliox in the initial treatment of patients with acute asthma.[66] There may be some benefit for patients who are refractory to conventional therapy.[67] The heliox mixture requires at least 70% helium for effect, so if the patient requires >30% oxygen, the heliox mixture cannot be used.

Antileukotrienes   Leukotriene antagonists improve lung function and decrease the need for short-acting beta agonists during long-term asthma therapy, but their effectiveness during acute exacerbations of asthma is unproven. One study in patients with moderate to severe asthma demonstrated improvement in lung function with the addition of IV montelukast to standard therapy, but further research is needed before widespread use can be recommended.[68]

Inhaled Anesthetics Case reports in adults and children suggest a benefit of inhalation anesthetics for patients with status asthmaticus unresponsive to maximal conventional therapy.[69,70] These anesthetic agents may work directly as bronchodilators and may have indirect effects by enhancing patient–ventilator synchrony and reducing oxygen demand and carbon dioxide production. This therapy, however, requires an ICU setting, and there have been no randomized studies to evaluate its effectiveness.

Additional Therapies Neither antibiotics, aggressive hydration, chest physical therapy, mucolytics, nor sedation is recommended in the setting of acute asthma. None of these have demonstrated benefit and some may be potentially harmful.[10]

Posttreatment/ Resuscitation Care

Response to Initial Treatment

Clinical decision making for severe, life-threatening asthma is determined by the patient's response to initial treatment. Patients should be assessed after the initial dose of a short-acting bronchodilator and again after three doses. Response to treatment, as opposed to the initial level of exacerbation severity, is superior in predicting the need for hospitalization.[10] A patient's own assessment of symptoms and a physician's assessment of the physical examination, objective measures of lung function, pulse oximetry, and occasionally arterial blood gas results are important components of reassessment. The decision to hospitalize a patient should be based on the following factors: duration and severity of symptoms, severity of airflow obstruction, response to ED treatment, severity of prior exacerbations, medication use at the time of the exacerbation, access to medical care, support, home environment, and presence of psychiatric illness.

Clinical Improvement

FEV$_1$ or PEFR >70% of Predicted After 1 to 3 Hours of Treatment: Consider Discharge Home Most patients who improve clinically and are breathing room air with adequate oxygenation (oxyhemoglobin saturation of ≥95%) and FEV$_1$ or PEFR >70% of predicted after 1 to 3 hours of inhaled beta$_2$ agonists, anticholinergics, and corticosteroids can be discharged home.[8,9] This disposition may need to be modified on the basis of the identified risk factors discussed in this chapter. Observe patients for at least 1 hour after they reach >70% of predicted FEV$_1$ or PEFR to ensure their stability. Review the discharge medications closely. Studies confirm the value of continued inhaled or oral steroids and of inhaled beta$_2$ agonists after an ED visit for acute asthma. These medications significantly reduce the need for return ED visits and subsequent hospitalizations.

Some Clinical Improvement
FEV$_1$ or PEFR 50% to 70% of Predicted After 4 Hours of Intensive Treatment: Incomplete Responders

Risk Stratification for Incomplete Responders Patients who achieve some clinical improvement but have persistent signs of moderate to severe asthma with improved oxygenation (oxyhemoglobin saturation of 90%–95%) and FEV$_1$ or PEFR 50% to 70% of predicted after 4 hours of intensive treatment are classified as *incomplete responders*. They require careful triage. Concurrent comorbidity—such as insulin-dependent diabetes, coronary artery disease, cerebrovascular disease, chronic obstructive pulmonary disease, or acute pneumonia—should almost always prompt further inpatient monitoring and therapy.

Low-Risk Incomplete Responders Some incomplete responders are at low risk for continued deterioration and may be discharged conditionally. Appropriate discharge requires that patients have adequate discharge medications, home resources, access to follow-up care, and a detailed discharge care plan.

High-Risk Incomplete Responders Incomplete responders with one or more of the following risk factors should be hospitalized (with occasional individual exceptions):

- History of intubation and mechanical ventilation for acute, life-threatening asthma.
- Recent (within 2–4 weeks) hospitalization for asthma.
- Recurrent ED visits (i.e., patient was evaluated and treated in an ED in the previous 24–48 hours), also known as relapse patients.
- Duration of exacerbation symptoms is 1 week or longer.
- Current use of oral steroids (steroid-dependent); studies have not yet established whether patients currently using inhaled steroids should be stratified as being at high risk.
- Inadequate home care resources.
- Known or suspected poor compliance.

Inadequate Clinical Improvement
FEV$_1$ or PEFR 25% to 50% of Predicted After 4 Hours of Intensive Treatment: Hospital Admission and Noninvasive Assisted Ventilation Admit these patients to the hospital and consider the use of noninvasive positive-pressure ventilation (NPPV). NPPV is rapidly emerging as an effective ED technique and is discussed in more detail below. The initiation of NPPV is not to prevent hospital admission. The major clinical purpose is to prevent endotracheal intubation. These techniques are judged "effective" only if the patient avoids endotracheal intubation.

No Clinical Improvement
FEV$_1$ or PEFR <25% of Predicted After 4 Hours of Intensive Treatment: ICU Admission and Assisted Ventilation These patients need intensive monitoring and care. Endotracheal intubation and mechanical ventilation

may be necessary if a patient continues to be unresponsive to therapy.

Indications for ICU Admission In addition to an FEV_1 or PEFR $<25\%$ of predicted, other objective signs and clinical symptoms indicate the need for ICU admission and probable intubation:

- PaO_2 <65 mm Hg with 40% inspired oxygen (oxyhemoglobin saturation $<90\%$)
- $PaCO_2$ >40 mm Hg (especially if rising during treatment in the ED)
- Altered level of consciousness
- Extreme dyspnea (patient can speak only one or two words at a time)
- Inability to lie in the supine position
- Increasing fatigue

Noninvasive Assisted Ventilation

NPPV may offer short-term support to patients with acute respiratory failure and may delay or eliminate the need for endotracheal intubation.[71] This therapy requires an alert patient with adequate spontaneous respiratory effort. Bilevel positive airway pressure (BiPAP), the most common way of delivering NPPV, allows for separate control of inspiratory and expiratory pressures.

Description

The decision to intubate a patient with asthma is difficult. Noninvasive assisted ventilation techniques are emerging as an effective way for patients with severe, life-threatening asthma to avoid the need for intubation and mechanical ventilation.[72] Noninvasive positive-pressure ventilation uses a mechanical ventilation device to deliver positive-pressure ventilation through a mask to assist the patient's spontaneous respiratory efforts. The mask may cover a patient's mouth, nose, or both. It must fit with a relatively tight seal.

Benefits

These devices are intended for patients who are refractory to bronchodilators and steroids. In the past, such patients almost always required endotracheal intubation and mechanical ventilation. If it can prevent intubation, this technique conveys numerous benefits. NPPV can enable support of ventilation without the need for and hazards of endotracheal tube placement. The patient, however, must have effective spontaneous respiratory effort and adequate airway protective mechanisms (Table 33-5).

Evidence for the use of NPPV in the setting of asthma is weaker than for other conditions leading to respiratory failure. Large, randomized controlled trials are needed before

TABLE 33-5 • Criteria and Contraindications for the Use of Noninvasive Positive-Pressure Ventilation

Critical Requirements:

- Alert and able to protect airway
- Cooperative
- Demonstrating effective spontaneous respirations

Contraindications: Noninvasive assisted ventilation techniques are contraindicated for patients who are

- Severely hypoxemic: PaO_2 <60 mm Hg or O_2 saturation $<90\%$ on rebreathing mask
- Deteriorating steadily or rapidly
- Confused, somnolent, moribund, or uncooperative
- Unable to protect the airway
- Hypotensive (BP <90 mm Hg)
- Known to have ischemic heart disease
- Having ventricular arrhythmias
- In cardiopulmonary/respiratory arrest
- Severe encephalopathy
- Hemodynamic instability
- Facial deformity/surgery
- High risk for aspiration
- Nonrespiratory organ failure
- Severe upper gastrointestinal bleeding
- Upper airway obstruction

NPPV can be recommended for widespread use in status asthmaticus.[73] Only a few small, prospective randomized trials, one in children, have been completed using NPPV in patients with severe asthma. Both suggested that in selected patients with severe asthma, NPPV can improve lung function and possibly reduce the need for hospitalization.[74] One must be particularly cautious in using NPPV in pediatric patients, where the margin of safety is narrow.[74] Nevertheless, experienced clinicians often recommend NPPV for patients who do not respond satisfactorily to aggressive first-line therapy.[75,76] Initial steps and sample setting are as follows:

- Secure a face mask with head straps over the nose and mouth, ensuring a tight seal.
- Connect the ventilator to the face mask by using either a conventional mechanical ventilator or one made specifically for NPPV.
- Start with continuous positive airway pressure (CPAP) set to 0 cm H_2O; then slowly increase to maintain positive end-expiratory pressure even during spontaneous inspiration.

- Set positive-pressure support (inspiratory pressure) of ventilation at 10 cm H_2O and adjust on the basis of arterial blood gases; do not exceed 25 cm H_2O.
- Set tidal volume at 500 mL or 7 mL/kg.
- Set ventilation rate at <25 breaths per minute.
- Continue to administer nebulized medications through the system.

Bilevel Positive Airway Pressure

Bilevel positive airway pressure (BiPAP) has proven to be the most effective type of NPPV for life-threatening asthma. The BiPAP ventilator is a variable-flow device that offers separate control of the inspiratory positive airway pressure and expiratory positive airway pressure. BiPAP devices reduce the work of breathing more than any other noninvasive respiratory support technique by reducing the force required for exhalation and increasing the work of inspiration. Most experts begin with an inspiratory positive airway pressure of 8 to 10 cm H_2O and an expiratory airway pressure of 3 to 5 cm H_2O.[77]

Endotracheal Intubation for Life-Threatening Asthma

Ventilation is frequently lifesaving, and about 11% of patients admitted with acute asthma are admitted to an ICU, intubated, or both. Compared to standard admissions, patients who are intubated are more likely to die, with about a 60- to 90-fold higher in-hospital mortality rate compared to patients with a standard asthma hospitalization.[5] Once it is considered necessary, there should be no delay in intubation. Respiratory failure is characterized by an inability to speak, altered mental status, severe accessory muscle use, fatigue, and elevated or rising Pco_2. Early recognition and treatment are paramount to reversing the process. Waiting to reassess such a patient after adjunctive medications should never occur. Patients who are comatose or apneic should be intubated immediately. Progressive exhaustion despite maximal therapy together with altered level of consciousness are indications for intubation.[78]

Endotracheal intubation does not solve the problem of bronchoconstriction in patients with severe asthma. In addition, intubation and positive-pressure ventilation can trigger further bronchoconstriction and complications such as breath stacking (auto-PEEP positive end-expiratory pressure) and barotrauma. Although endotracheal intubation introduces risks, it should be performed if the patient deteriorates despite aggressive management.

Intubation in the setting of severe asthma has the potential to be very complicated; all patients should be intubated by a physician with extensive experience in airway management and all should be managed in an ICU setting or transferred to a facility that has this capability. RSI is the technique of choice. The provider should use the largest endotracheal tube available (usually 8 or 9 mm) so as to decrease airway resistance. Immediately after intubation, confirm endotracheal tube placement by clinical examination and a CO_2 detection device and obtain a chest radiograph.

Indications

The major indications for rapid endotracheal intubation in life-threatening asthma are:

- Failure to improve after 4 hours of NPPV.
- Continued deterioration despite aggressive first-line therapy.
- Association with anaphylaxis.
- Deterioration with exhaustion.
- Altered level of consciousness, confusion, or somnolence.
- A rising $Paco_2$ (>40 mm Hg) with a falling pH. These values are particularly worrisome in association with clinical signs of altered mental status, somnolence, and poor muscle tone. They suggest the presence of exhaustion and respiratory failure. Isolated hypercarbia does not always require immediate endotracheal intubation and should be interpreted within the clinical context of the patient.
- Pao_2 <50 mm Hg on a nonrebreathing mask, especially when associated with clinical signs of hypoxemia. These signs include severe agitation, confusion, and fighting against the oxygen mask.[79]

Rapid Sequence Intubation (See also Chapter 18)

Precautions

Rapid sequence intubation (RSI) is the technique of choice for endotracheal intubation in patients with severe, life-threatening asthma.[41] Other techniques, especially nasotracheal intubation, have high failure rates.

- The most experienced laryngoscopist should perform the procedure, since excess airway stimulation with a laryngoscope blade can provoke severe laryngospasm and reflex bronchoconstriction.
- It may be impossible to provide effective bag-mask ventilation when acute severe asthma is present. In patients with severe, life-threatening asthma, most of the air delivered with a bag and mask will divert away from the high-resistance airways and into the stomach. This can produce gastric distention, a further decrease in effective ventilation, regurgitation, and aspiration.
- Use the largest endotracheal tube possible. The larger the tube diameter, the less the airway resistance. Suctioning of the airway secretions can be handled better with large-diameter tubes.

Sedation and Anesthesia

Ketamine is an effective sedative, analgesic, and dissociative anesthetic. Many experts recommend ketamine as the IV anesthetic of choice for patients with severe asthma.

Ketamine possesses strong bronchodilator properties.[64] It potentiates catecholamines and relaxes bronchiolar smooth muscle. Ketamine does not cause vasodilatation, circulatory collapse, or myocardial depression. A dose of 2 mg/kg IV (1–4 mg/kg pediatrics) induces anesthesia in 30 seconds and lasts 10 to 15 minutes. Because ketamine increases bronchial secretions, many experts also premedicate with atropine (0.01 mg/kg; minimum dose of 0.1 mg) when using ketamine.

Propofol is another sedative with bronchodilator properties.[75] It is effective for both intubation and maintenance of sedation during mechanical ventilation. A dose of 2 to 2.5 mg/kg induces anesthesia in approximately 40 seconds and lasts 3 to 5 minutes. This drug may cause hypotension and lactic acidosis.

Etomidate is an acceptable induction agent, although it lacks bronchodilator properties.[80] Etomidate is ultra–short-acting and has a safer hemodynamic profile than either ketamine or propofol. A dose of 0.2 to 0.4 mg/kg induces anesthesia in 60 seconds and lasts 3 to 5 minutes. This drug has no analgesic properties.

Inhaled Volatile Anesthetics Volatile anesthetics are powerful bronchial smooth muscle relaxants. Enflurane and ether have been used successfully in the treatment of acute, severe asthma refractory to other treatments.[81] Use these agents with extreme caution because they are also vasodilators and myocardial depressants. Some of these anesthetics sensitize the myocardium to catecholamines, leading to life-threatening arrhythmias. They are rarely available in the ED and hence rarely used there.

Paralysis

Two agents are commonly used for paralysis. Succinylcholine, at a dose of 1 to 2 mg/kg, is the paralytic agent of choice for RSI in patients with severe asthma and no contraindications to the drug. Rocuronium, at a dose of 0.6 to 1.2 mg/kg, is a good alternative. Its rapid onset of action is similar to that of succinylcholine, but it has a longer duration of action. There is a higher incidence of complications induced by neuromuscular blocking agents in mechanically ventilated asthma patients.[78] Diffuse paresis can last from a few hours to months after cessation of these drugs, which can delay ventilator weaning. Many of these cases follow combined treatment with corticosteroids. It is recommended that neuromuscular blocking agents be given as intermittent boluses rather than as a continuous infusion to help avoid this complication.[78]

Immediately After Intubation

Endotracheal intubation does not solve the problem of airway obstruction. Patients with severe, life-threatening asthma may be extremely difficult to oxygenate prior to intubation, even with bag-mask ventilation. In addition, hypercarbia may cause respiratory acidosis. Problems with oxygenation and ventilation may persist even after intubation.

• **Continue inhaled beta₂ agonists after intubation.** Since breathing efforts may not have been adequate, the patient may not have had adequate distribution of beta₂ agonists prior to intubation. Immediately after intubation administer 2.5 to 5 mg of albuterol directly into the endotracheal tube.

• **Ventilate the patient slowly with 100% oxygen:** When severe asthma is present, significant obstruction to airflow persists even after intubation. In fact, if there is no significant obstruction to airflow immediately after intubation, reevaluate the diagnosis of acute asthma and consider the possibility that the resistance to airflow was present in the upper airway (e.g., vocal cord dysfunction, tumor, or a foreign body).

Slowly ventilate at a rate of only 8 to 10 breaths per minute, allowing adequate time for exhalation between delivered breaths. This slow respiratory rate and adequate exhalation time can minimize the development of auto-PEEP and its serious consequences of hypotension and pneumothorax.

Mechanical Ventilation in Patients with Severe Asthma

The main goal of mechanical ventilation is to support gas exchange until bronchodilators and steroids improve airflow.

Difficulties and Complications

Mechanical ventilation in patients with severe, life-threatening asthma is challenging and may produce several significant complications.

SUDDEN DETERIORATION IN A VENTILATED PATIENT

If the patient with asthma deteriorates or is difficult to ventilate, verify endotracheal tube position, eliminate tube obstruction (eliminate any mucous plugs and kinks), and rule out (or decompress) a pneumothorax. Only experienced providers should perform needle decompression or insertion of a chest tube for pneumothorax.

Check the ventilator circuit for leaks or malfunction. High end-expiratory pressure can be quickly reduced by separating the patient from the ventilator circuit; this will allow PEEP to dissipate during passive exhalation.

• To minimize auto-PEEP, if present, decrease inhalation time (this increases exhalation time), decrease the respiratory rate by two breaths per minute, and reduce the tidal volume to 3 to 5 mL/kg.
• Continue treatment with inhaled albuterol.

Volume-controlled mode is the preferred mode of ventilation. Pressure-controlled mode is not ideal because of fluctuation in airflow resistance and auto-PEEP levels, leading to variable tidal volume and hypo- and hyperventilation.

Critical Concepts: Troubleshooting Problems in the Intubated, Ventilator-Dependent Asthmatic Patient

Auto-PEEP

Clinicians who provide mechanical ventilatory support for patients with severe asthma must understand the concept of auto-PEEP. Although asthma patients experience some obstruction of inspiration, they experience *marked* obstruction of expiration. As resistance to exhalation increases, the inevitable result will be air trapping and "breath stacking" (inspired air enters and then cannot exit). Gas trapping occurs because the low expiratory flow rates mandate long expiratory times if the entire inspired volume is to be exhaled. If the next breath interrupts exhalation, gas trapping results[74] (Fig. 33-2). Because gas is trapped in the lungs, there is additional pressure at the end of expiration (auto- or intrinsic PEEP), which leads to dynamic hyperinflation. These terms are frequently used interchangeably.[74] Dynamic hyperinflation is defined as the failure of the lung to return to its relaxed volume or functional residual capacity at end-exhalation.[74] Excessive dynamic hyperinflation has been shown to predict the development of hypotension and barotrauma during mechanical ventilation of severe asthma.[74]

With severe airway obstruction, the duration of spontaneous expiration increases. But during mechanical ventilation, expiratory time is set. If expiratory time is inadequate, this can lead to "self-produced" or "autoproduced" PEEP. In this case, end-expiratory pressure increases without addition of PEEP to the mechanical ventilatory circuit. Increased intrathoracic pressure from auto-PEEP can reduce venous return to the heart. Reduced venous return can lead to reduced cardiac output, hemodynamic compromise, and hypotension. Note that hyperinflation and increased intrathoracic pressure can also produce barotrauma, such as a tension pneumothorax.

Use a slower respiratory rate (6–10 breaths per minute) with smaller tidal volumes (6–8 mL/kg), shorter inspiratory time (adult inspiratory flow rate 80–100 mL/min), and longer expiratory time (inspiratory to expiratory ratio 1:4 or 1:5) than would typically be provided to ventilated patients who do not have asthma.[41]

Ventilation with "Permissive Hypercapnia"

Strategies to limit the potential for ventilator-associated adverse events in severe asthma include permissive hypercapnia, also called controlled hypoventilation. This technique can provide adequate oxygenation and ventilation while reducing the risk of barotrauma.[76] Ventilatory support is controlled, so that there is gradual development (over 3–4 hours) of hypercarbia (PaCO$_2$ levels may rise to 70–90 mm Hg). Acidemia also develops, with pH values in the range of 7.2 to 7.3, but the level is controlled by controlling the rise in PaCO$_2$. Within 24 to 48 hours, the patient's serum pH will be restored to near-normal levels because the kidneys will reabsorb bicarbonate to compensate for the respiratory acidosis.

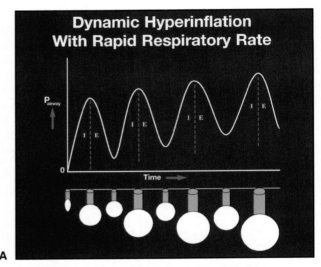

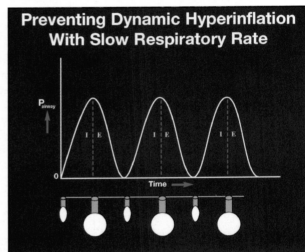

FIGURE 33-2 • Dynamic hyperinflation. Bronchospasm and endobronchiole secretions delay alveolar emptying. Increased ventilatory rates cause air trapping and increased alveolar volume, leading to decreased compliance or lung stiffness. Figure 33-2A depicts air trapping at high ventilatory rates. Figure 33-2B depicts decreased rate of ventilation, allowing the alveolus more time to empty.

Permissive hypercapnia is typically well tolerated except in the patient with increased intracranial pressure or severe myocardial depression who otherwise does not need to be treated. One can maximally reduce CO$_2$ production by the use of sedation, analgesia, and antipyretics.[78] If these methods do not work, muscle relaxants can be considered. One very significant clinical challenge arises in the setting of cardiopulmonary arrest secondary to severe asthma with postanoxic brain injury. Here the clinician faces the therapeutic dilemma of brain protection versus ventilator-induced lung injury. Blood alkalinization could be considered in this context, using a slow infusion of sodium bicarbonate and recognizing that this may transiently raise the arterial P_{CO_2} and worsen intracellular and cerebrospinal acidosis.[78]

Adequate oxygenation is relatively easy to achieve with mechanical ventilation in patients with severe asthma. It includes reducing respiratory rates, relieving expiratory flow resistance with frequent suctioning, administration of bronchodilators and steroids, the use of large-bore endotracheal tubes, and reducing the inspiratory time by increasing the inspiratory flow rate and reducing the need for high minute ventilation by decreasing carbon dioxide production with sedation, paralysis, and control of fever and pain.[74] Sedation and analgesia also allow the clinician to avoid patient–ventilator asynchrony.

Deep sedation is best accomplished through the use of benzodiazepines, which are safe and well tolerated. Propofol, a bronchodilator, is an alternative but carries the risk of hypotension, especially in hypovolemic patients.

Patient Is Difficult to Ventilate

When ventilation is difficult or inadequate, clinical assessment and evaluation may be difficult and elusive in patients with severe refractory asthma. The lack of audible breath sounds comes from poor airflow and hyperinflation of the chest wall.

If the patient is extremely "tight" (with limited airflow) and difficult to ventilate, perform the following procedures *in order* until ventilation is adequate:

1. Ensure that the patient is adequately sedated and paralyzed so that there is patient–ventilator synchrony.
2. Check the endotracheal tube for patency. Look for obstruction from kinking, mucous plugging, or biting. Suction the tube.
3. You may need to increase the time for exhalation, shorten the time for inhalation, and markedly increase the limit of peak inspiratory pressure to ensure that the patient is receiving the set tidal volume.
4. Reduce the respiratory rate to 6 to 8 breaths per minute to reduce auto-PEEP to 15 mm Hg.
5. Reduce the tidal volume to 3 to 5 mL/kg to reduce auto-PEEP to 15 mm Hg.
6. Increase peak flow to >60 L/min (90–120 L/min is commonly used) to further shorten inspiratory time and increase exhalation time.

Hypoxia or Hypotension After Intubation

The most frequently reported complication of mechanical ventilation is hemodynamic instability manifesting as hypotension. This usually occurs at the initiation of ventilation and is related to decreased venous return caused by worsening of hyperinflation. This can be verified by temporarily disconnecting the ventilator and documenting an increase in blood pressure. Ventilation can be resumed at a lower tidal volume and respiratory rate accompanied by volume expansion. If the decrease in blood pressure does not respond to ventilator disconnection, tension pneumothorax should be suspected.[78]

There are four common causes of significant hypoxia or hypotension immediately after intubation: incorrect placement of the endotracheal tube, obstruction of the endotracheal tube, significant auto-PEEP buildup, and tension pneumothorax.

Incorrect Placement of the Endotracheal Tube With any drop in oxygen saturation or exhaled CO_2, reconfirm tube position immediately. Do this even if correct tube position was initially verified. Check that the endotracheal tube has not been inserted too far. It may be located in either the right (most likely) or left main bronchus. If you suspect incorrect placement of the endotracheal tube, evaluate the tube placement *immediately*. Do not take time to obtain a chest radiograph.

Note that patients with acute severe asthma can demonstrate false-negative results with the esophageal detector device. When the endotracheal tube is in the esophagus of the patient with severe asthma, the detector bulb may reexpand immediately, suggesting endotracheal tube placement. Providers must be aware that severe asthma may cause erroneous results with the esophageal detector device; they should use exhaled CO_2 detectors as an alternate confirmation device.

Obstruction of the Endotracheal Tube If the patient is difficult to ventilate manually, check for patency of the tube. If the tube is patent, attempt to suction the tube and check for tube obstructions from kinking, mucous plugging, or biting.

Critical Auto-PEEP Buildup The most common cause of profound hypotension after intubation is a significant buildup of auto-PEEP. If auto-PEEP is suspected, stop ventilating the patient for a brief time (20–40 seconds). This pause allows the auto-PEEP to dissipate. Monitor the patient's oxygenation and resume ventilation after auto-PEEP dissipates or if the patient develops significant hypoxemia or clinical signs of further deterioration.

Tension Pneumothorax Evidence of a tension pneumothorax includes decreased chest expansion and decreased breath sounds on the side of the pneumothorax, shifting of the trachea away from the side of the pneumothorax, or the development of SQ emphysema. The immediate lifesaving treatment is needle decompression to release air from the pleural space. This procedure is followed by placement of a chest tube.

Final Interventions to Consider

Consultation with a pulmonologist or critical care specialist is always appropriate for patients with refractory, severe asthma. Evidence from anecdotal case reports and surveys of chest radiographs suggest that unrecognized bilateral tension pneumothoraces may underlie some cases of fatal asthma. There are insufficient published data to support a recommendation for empiric attempts at bilateral needle decompression in such instances. The critical point is to consider whether unrecognized pneumothoraces may have precipitated an asthma-related cardiac arrest. There are increasing reports of success with extracorporeal membrane oxygenation (ECMO) in mechanically ventilated patients who could not be adequately oxygenated.[82] Additional therapies such as "lung massage" have been reported to benefit some patients.[79,82] These complex therapies should be considered only on a case-by-case basis.

Prognosis

The mortality rate of patients with near-fatal asthma has declined in the last several years but can still be as high as 20%. About 10% to 30% of patients with life-threatening asthma need mechanical ventilation; therefore, early recognition and extremely close observation of high-risk patients is paramount and may avert fatalities. Severe asthma remains a significant health problem that is often underdiagnosed and treated.[7] Hypervigilance and rapid action on the part of health care providers in response to a near-fatal episode will provide the best chance of improved outcome.

References

1. Moore WC, Peters SP. Severe asthma: an overview. *J Allergy Clin Immunol* 2006;117:487–494.
2. Kaza V, Bandi V, Guntupalli KK. Acute severe asthma: recent advances. *Curr Opin Pulm Med* 2007;13:1–7.
3. Peters SG. Continuous bronchodilator therapy. *Chest* 2007;131:286–289.
4. Kenyon N, Albertson TE. Status asthmaticus. *Clin Rev Allergy Immunol* 2001;20:271–292.
5. Pendergraft TB, Stabford RH, BEasley R, et al. Rates and characteristics of intensive care unit admissions and intubations among asthma-related hospitalizations. *Ann Allergy Asthma Immunol* 2004;93:29–35.
6. Holgate ST, Polosa R. The mechanisms, diagnosis, and management of severe asthma in adults. *Lancet* 2006; 368:780–793.
7. Restrepo RD, Peters J. Near-fatal asthma: recognition and management. *Curr Opin Pulm Med* 2008;14:13–23.
8. Division of Data Services. New asthma estimates: tracking prevalence, health care, and mortality. In. Hyattsville, MD: National Center for Health Statistics; 2001.
9. Molfino NA, Nannini LJ, Martelli AN, et al. Respiratory arrest in near-fatal asthma. *N Engl J Med* 1991;324:285–288.
10. National Asthma Education and Prevention Program. Expert panel report-3: Guidelines for the diagnosis and management of asthma. US Department of Health and Human Services, August 2007.
11. GINA. *Global Strategy for Asthma Management and Prevention*, Global Initiative for Asthma (GINA) 2007. Available from: http://www.ginasthma.org.
12. Emond SD, Camargo CA Jr, Nowak RM. 1997 National Asthma Education and Prevention Program guidelines: a practical summary for emergency physicians. *Ann Emerg Med* 1998;31:579–589.
13. Alvey Smaha D. Asthma emergency care: national guidelines summary. *Heart Lung* 2001;30:472–474.
14. Beveridge RC, Grunfeld AF, Hodder RV, et al. Guidelines for the emergency management of asthma in adults. CAEP/CTS Asthma Advisory Committee. Canadian Association of Emergency Physicians and the Canadian Thoracic Society. *CMAJ* 1996;155:25–37.
15. Reid LM. The presence or absence of bronchial mucus in fatal asthma. *J Allergy Clin Immunol*. 1987;80:415–416.
16. Robin ED, McCauley R. Sudden cardiac death in bronchial asthma, and inhaled b-adrenergic agonists. *Chest* 1992;101:1699–702.
17. Robin ED, Lewiston N. Unexpected, unexplained sudden death in young asthmatic subjects. *Chest* 1989;96:790–793.
18. Kallenbach JM, Frankel AH, Lapinsky SE, et al. Determinants of near fatality in acute severe asthma. *Am J Med* 1993;95:265–272.
19. Abramson MJ, Bailey MJ, Couper FJ, et al. Are asthma medications and management related to deaths from asthma? *Am J Respir Crit Care Med* 2001;163:12–18.
20. McFadden ER Jr, Warren EL. Observations on asthma mortality. *Ann Intern Med* 1997;127:142–147.
21. Wenzel S. Severe asthma in adults. *Am J Respir Crit Care Med* 2005;172:149–160.
22. Hannaway PJ. Demographic characteristics of patients experiencing near-fatal and fatal asthma: results of a regional survey of 400 asthma specialists. *Ann Allergy Asthma Immunol* 2000;84:587–593.
23. Kikuchi Y, Okabe S, Tamura G, et al. Chemosensitivity and perception of dyspnea in patients with a history of near-fatal asthma. *N Engl J Med* 1994;330:1329–1334.
24. Nowak RM, Pensler MI, Sarkar DD, et al. Comparison of peak expiratory flow and FEV$_1$ admission criteria for acute bronchial asthma. *Ann Emerg Med* 1982;11:64–69.
25. Shim CS, Williams MH Jr. Evaluation of the severity of asthma: patients versus physicians. *Am J Med* 1980;68:11–13.
26. Aldington S, Beasley R. Asthma exacerbations: assessment and management of severe asthma in adults in hospital. *Thorax* 2007;62:447–458.
27. Gorelick MH, Stevens MW, Schultz T, et al. Difficulty in obtaining peak expiratory flow measurements in children with acute asthma. *Pediatr Emerg Care* 2004;20(1):22–26.
28. Mannix R, Bachur R. Status asthmaticus in children. *Curr Opin Pediatr* 2007;19:281–287.
29. Levin E, Gold MI. The mini-Wright expiratory peak flow meter. *Can Anaesth Soc J* 1981;28:285–287.
30. Lin RY, Sauter D, Newman T, et al. Continuous versus intermittent albuterol nebulization in the treatment of acute asthma. *Ann Emerg Med* 1993;22:1847–1853.
31. Rudnitsky GS, Eberlein RS, Schoffstall JM, et al. Comparison of intermittent and continuously nebulized albuterol for treatment of asthma in an urban emergency department. *Ann Emerg Med* 1993;22:1842–1846.
32. Khine H, Fuchs SM, Saville AL. Continuous vs intermittent nebulized albuterol for emergency management of asthma. *Acad Emerg Med* 1996;3:1019–1024.
33. Newman KB, Milne S, Hamilton C, et al. A comparison of albuterol administered by metered-dose inhaler and spacer with albuterol by nebulizer in adults presenting to an urban emergency department with acute asthma. *Chest* 2002;121:1036–1041.
34. Bowton DL. Metered-dose inhalers versus hand-held nebulizers: some answers and new questions. *Chest* 1992;101:298–299.
35. Bowton DL, Goldsmith WM, Haponik EF. Substitution of metered-dose inhalers for hand-held nebulizers: success and cost savings in a large, acute-care hospital. *Chest* 1992;101:305–308.
36. Colacone A, Afilalo M, Wolkove N, et al. A comparison of albuterol administered by metered dose inhaler (and holding chamber) or wet nebulizer in acute asthma. *Chest* 1993;104:835–841.
37. Idris AH, McDermott MF, Raucci JC, et al. Emergency department treatment of severe asthma: metered-dose inhaler plus holding chamber is equivalent in effectiveness to nebulizer. *Chest* 1993;103:665–672.
38. Gawchik SM, Saccar CL, Noonan M, et al. The safety and efficacy of nebulized levalbuterol compared with racemic albuterol and placebo in the treatment of asthma in pediatric patients. *J Allergy Clin Immunol* 1999;103:615–621.
39. Nelson HS, Bensch G, Pleskow WW, et al. Improved bronchodilation with levalbuterol compared with racemic albuterol in patients with asthma. *J Allergy Clin Immunol* 1998;102:943–952.
40. Nelson HS. Clinical experience with levalbuterol. *J Allergy Clin Immunol* 1999;104(2 Pt 2):S77–S84.
41. Marik PE, Varon J, Fromm R Jr. The management of acute severe asthma. *J Emerg Med* 2002;23:257–268.

42. Gibbs MA, Camargo CA Jr, Rowe BH, et al. State of the art: therapeutic controversies in severe acute asthma. *Acad Emerg Med* 2000;7:800–815.

43. Rowe BH, Spooner CH, Ducharme FM, et al. Early emergency department treatment of acute asthma with systemic corticosteroids. *Cochrane Database Syst Rev* 2000:CD002178.

44. Rowe BH, Keller JL, Oxman AD. Effectiveness of steroid therapy in acute exacerbations of asthma: a meta-analysis. *Am J Emerg Med* 1992;10:301–310.

45. Ratto D, Alfaro C, Sipsey J, et al. Are intravenous corticosteroids required in status asthmaticus? *JAMA* 1988;260:527–529.

46. Biarant D. Therapeutic strategies in near fatal asthma in children. *Pediatr Pulm* 2001;23S:90–93.

47. Aaron SD. The use of ipratropium bromide for the management of acute asthma exacerbation in adults and children: a systematic review. *J Asthma* 2001;38:521–530.

48. Rodrigo G, Rodrigo C. Ipratropium bromide in acute asthma: small beneficial effects? *Chest* 1999;115:1482.

49. Plotnick LH, Ducharme FM. Acute asthma in children and adolescents: should inhaled anticholinergics be added to beta(2)-agonists? *Am J Respir Med* 2003;2:109–115.

50. Keam SJ, Keating GM. Tiotropium bromide. A review of its use as maintenance therapy in patients with COPD. *Treat Respir Med* 2004;3:247–268.

51. Rodrigo G, Rodrigo C, Burschtin O. A meta-analysis of the effects of ipratropium bromide in adults with acute asthma. *Am J Med* 1999;107:363–370.

52. Qureshi F, Zaritsky A, Lakkis H. Efficacy of nebulized ipratropium in severely asthmatic children. *Ann Emerg Med* 1997;29:205–211.

53. Plotnick LH, Ducharme FM. Combined inhaled anticholinergic agents and b_2-agonists for initial treatment of acute asthma in children. *Cochrane Database Syst Rev* 2000:CD000060.

54. Stoodley RG, Aaron SD, Dales RE. The role of ipratropium bromide in the emergency management of acute asthma exacerbation: a meta-analysis of randomized clinical trials. *Ann Emerg Med* 1999;34:8–18.

55. Silverman RA, Osborn H, Runge J, et al. IV magnesium sulfate in the treatment of acute severe asthma: a multicenter randomized controlled trial. *Chest* 2002;122:489–497.

56. Rowe BH, Bretzlaff JA, Bourdon C, et al. Intravenous magnesium sulfate treatment for acute asthma in the emergency department: a systematic review of the literature. *Ann Emerg Med* 2000;36:181–190.

57. Schiermeyer RP, Finkelstein JA. Rapid infusion of magnesium sulfate obviates need for intubation in status asthmaticus. *Am J Emerg Med* 1994;12:164–166.

58. Rowe BH, Bretzlaff JA, Bourdon C, et al. Systematic review of magnesium sulfate in the treatment of acute asthma. *Cochrane Database Syst Rev* 1998;4.

59. Rowe BH, Edmonds ML, Spooner CH, et al. Evidence-based treatments for acute asthma. *Respir Care* 2001;46:1380–1390; discussion 1390–1391.

60. Blitz M, Blitz S, Beasely R, et al. Inhaled magnesium sulfate in the treatment of acute asthma. *Cochrane Database Syst Rev* 2005: CD003898.

61. Cydulka R, Davison R, Grammer L, et al. The use of epinephrine in the treatment of older adult asthmatics. *Ann Emerg Med* 1988; 17:322–326.

62. Victoria MS, Battista CJ, Nangia BS. Comparison between epinephrine and terbutaline injections in the acute management of asthma. *J Asthma* 1989;26:287–290.

63. Safdar B, Cone DC, Pham KT. Subcutaneous epinephrine in the prehospital setting. *Prehosp Emerg Care* 2001;5:200–207.

64. Howton JC, Rose J, Duffy S, et al. Randomized, double-blind, placebo-controlled trial of intravenous ketamine in acute asthma. *Ann Emerg Med* 1996;27:170–175.

65. Hess DR, Acosta FL, Ritz RH, et al. The effect of heliox on nebulizer function using a beta-agonist bronchodilator. *Chest* 1999;115:184–189.

66. Rodrigo GJ, Rodrigo C, Pollack CV, et al. Use of helium–oxygen mixtures in the treatment of acute asthma: a systematic review. *Chest* 2003;123:891–896.

67. Reuben AD, Harris AR. Heliox for asthma in the emergency department: a review of the literature. *Emerg Med J* 2004;21:131–135.

68. Camargo CA Jr, Smithline HA, Malice MP, et al. A randomized controlled trial of intravenous montelukast in acute asthma. *Am J Respir Crit Care Med* 2003;167:528–533.

69. Schultz TE. Sevoflurane administration in status asthmaticus: a case report. *AANA J* 2005;73:35–36.

70. Wheeler DS, Clapp CR, Ponaman ML, et al. Isoflurane therapy for status asthmaticus in children: a case series and protocol. *Pediatr Crit Care Med* 2000;1:55–59.

71. Soroksky A, Stav D, Shpirer I. A pilot prospective, randomized, placebo-controlled trial of bilevel positive airway pressure in acute asthmatic attack. *Chest* 2003;123:1018–1025.

72. Meduri GU, Cook TR, Turner RE, et al. Noninvasive positive pressure ventilation in status asthmaticus. *Chest* 1996;110:767–774.

73. Hill NS, Brennan J, Garpestad E, et al. Noninvasive ventilation in acute respiratory failure. *Crit Care Med* 2007;35:2402–2407.

74. Stather DR, Stewart TE. Clinical review: mechanical ventilation in severe asthma. *Crit Care* 2005;9:581–558.

75. Eames WO, Rooke GA, Wu RS, et al. Comparison of the effects of etomidate, propofol, and thiopental on respiratory resistance after tracheal intubation. *Anesthesiology* 1996;84:1307–1311.

76. Mazzeo AT, Spada A, Pratico C, et al. Hypercapnia: what is the limit in paediatric patients? A case of near-fatal asthma successfully treated by multipharmacological approach. *Paediatr Anaesth* 2004;14:596–603.

77. Shapiro MB, Kleaveland AC, Bartlett RH. Extracorporeal life support for status asthmaticus. *Chest* 1993;103:1651–1654.

78. Oddo M, Feihl F, Schaller M, et al. Management of mechanical ventilation in acute severe asthma: practical aspects. *Intens Care Med* 2006;32:501–510.

79. Van der Touw T, Tully A, Amis TC, et al. Cardiorespiratory consequences of expiratory chest wall compression during mechanical ventilation and severe hyperinflation. *Crit Care Med* 1993;21:1908–1914.

80. Bergen JM, Smith DC. A review of etomidate for rapid sequence intubation in the emergency department. *J Emerg Med* 1997;15:221–230.

81. Saulnier FF, Durocher AV, Deturck RA, et al. Respiratory and hemodynamic effects of halothane in status asthmaticus. *Intens Care Med* 1990;16:104–107.

82. Van der Touw T, Mudaliar Y, Nayyar V. Cardiorespiratory effects of manually compressing the rib cage during tidal expiration in mechanically ventilated patients recovering from acute severe asthma. *Crit Care Med* 1998;26:1361–1367.

Chapter 34
Anaphylaxis

Michael E. Winters

Anaphylaxis is widely recognized by emergency care providers as an acute, severe, potentially life-threatening allergic reaction.

- Anaphylaxis is a potentially life-threatening allergic reaction.
- Circulatory collapse and/or respiratory failure are the major concerns.
- Treatment involves securing an adequate airway, ventilation and oxygenation, aggressive fluid resuscitation, and judicious use of epinephrine.
- Additional medications may include antihistamines, corticosteroids, and glucagon.
- Other modalities may involve intravenous epinephrine, mechanical ventilation, vasopressor medications, inotropic support, transcutaneous pacing, or intra-aortic balloon pump counterpulsation.

Introduction

Since its original description in 1902 by Richet and Portier,[1] much has been published regarding the epidemiology, pathophysiology, clinical presentation, diagnosis, and treatment of anaphylaxis. Although significant questions remain, it is imperative that emergency care providers be able to promptly recognize and appropriately treat patients with anaphylaxis. Any delay in recognition or initiation of therapy may contribute to unnecessary increases in patient morbidity and mortality. This chapter serves to educate and update the emergency care provider about the assessment and management of patients with anaphylaxis.

While upper airway obstruction and/or bronchospasm may be prominent features of anaphylaxis in many patients, emphasis here is placed on the management of patients with impending cardiovascular collapse and circulatory arrest due to anaphylaxis.

Overview

Definition and Diagnostic Criteria

Anaphylaxis may be defined as "a serious allergic reaction that is rapid in onset and may cause death.

Currently, there is no universally accepted definition of anaphylaxis.[2–6] As a result, the literature is replete with varying opinions and interpretations regarding many aspects of the assessment and management of patients with anaphylaxis. In an effort to develop a universal definition, the National Institute of Allergy and Infectious Disease along with the Food Allergy and Anaphylaxis Network gathered experts and representatives from numerous professional, governmental, and lay organizations. In 2006, recommendations from the Second Symposium on the Definition and Management of Anaphylaxis were published. As a part of their recommendations, the consensus panel proposed that anaphylaxis be defined as "a serious allergic reaction that is rapid in onset and may cause death."[3]

In addition to the lack of a universal definition, there is also a lack of formal diagnostic criteria that reliably and accurately identify patients with anaphylaxis. To this end, participants at the Second Symposium on the Definition and Management of Anaphylaxis also put forth a set of diagnostic criteria designed to provide an easy and rapid means of identifying patients with anaphylaxis. Participants at this symposium felt that these criteria are "likely to capture 95% of cases."[3]

The proposed diagnostic criteria for anaphylaxis are listed in Table 34-1. Although these diagnostic criteria require prospective validation, they provide an important framework for the emergency care provider to successfully identify patients with this potentially deadly disorder.

Epidemiology

Each year, anaphylaxis accounts for nearly 1% of all U.S. emergency department (ED) visits and is estimated to cause approximately 1,500 fatal reactions.

A recent review of studies from North America, Europe, and Australia reported the lifetime prevalence of anaphylaxis to be approximately 0.05% to

| TABLE 34-1 • Diagnostic Criteria for Anaphylaxis

Anaphylaxis is highly likely when any ONE of the following three criteria are fulfilled:

1. Acute onset of an illness (minutes to hours) with involvement of the skin, mucosal tissue, or both AND AT LEAST ONE OF THE FOLLOWING:
   a. Respiratory compromise
   b. Reduced blood pressure or associated symptoms of end-organ dysfunction

2. TWO or more of the following that occur rapidly after exposure to a _likely allergen for that patient_ (minutes to hours)
   a. Skin and/or mucosal tissue involvement
   b. Respiratory compromise
   c. Reduced blood pressure or associated symptoms of end-organ dysfunction
   d. Persistent gastrointestinal symptoms

3. Reduced blood pressure after exposure to a _known allergen for that patient_ (minutes to hours)
   a. Adults: systolic blood pressure <90 mm Hg or a decrease of >30% from the baseline blood pressure
   b. Infants and children: age-specific low systolic blood pressure or >30% decrease from the baseline blood pressure

Source: Adapted from Sampson HA et al. Second symposium on the definition and management of anaphylaxis: summary report. Second National Institute of Allergy and Infectious Disease/Food Allergy and Anaphylaxis Network symposium. _J Allergy Clin Immunol_ 2006;117(2):391–397, with permission.

2.0%.[7] Despite an often frightening clinical presentation, death from anaphylaxis is uncommon. The mortality rate reported by most studies on anaphylaxis is approximately 1%.[8–12] In the United States, it is estimated that 1.2% to 15% of the population is at risk for anaphylaxis.[10] Each year, anaphylaxis accounts for nearly 1% of all U.S. ED visits[13] and is estimated to cause approximately 1,500 fatal reactions.[10]

Unfortunately, anaphylaxis is not a reportable disease. As a result, current morbidity and mortality statistics are likely an underestimate of the true impact of the disease. In addition, incidence and prevalence rates from current studies are hampered by varying patient populations, varying methods of patient identification and classification, and small sample sizes.[14] Although current studies provide important epidemiologic information, it should be noted that the exact incidence of anaphylaxis remains unknown.[15,16]

Etiologies

Any agent or condition that results in the release of mediators from mast cells and/or basophils can cause anaphylaxis.

Foods, medications, insect stings, and immunotherapy injections account for the majority of identifiable causes.[9,17–20] In the United States, food is the leading identifiable cause of anaphylaxis.[21] In fact, as many as 2% of the U.S. population are reported to have a food allergy.[7,22] In children, peanuts and tree nuts are the most common foods implicated in cases of anaphylaxis.[7,23] For adults, shellfish, peanuts, and tree nuts account for the most severe reactions.[7,21] Additional foods commonly implicated in cases of food anaphylaxis include fish, eggs, milk, soy, and wheat.[7,21] Antibiotics (especially penicillin) and nonsteroidal anti-inflammatory drugs account for the majority of cases of medication-induced anaphylaxis.[5] Anaphylaxis caused by insects is due to stings from members of the order Hymenoptera. Insects in this order include wasps, yellow jackets, hornets, honeybees, and fire ants. In the United States, yellow jackets account for the majority of cases of anaphylaxis due to insects.[20] Additional identifiable etiologies of anaphylaxis are listed in Table 34-2. In as many as one-third of cases, the etiology is undetermined.[17] Patients with an undetermined etiology are diagnosed as having idiopathic anaphylaxis.

Clinical Manifestations

Anaphylaxis is a multisystem disorder that can have a myriad of clinical manifestations. Importantly, the symptoms of anaphylaxis occur along a continuum and are dependent upon the type, route, and quantity of antigen exposure. Symptom onset can range anywhere from several minutes to hours after exposure to an antigen.[24] In general, the more rapid the onset of symptoms, the more likely the reaction is to be life-threatening.[25,26] Cutaneous symptoms such as urticaria and angioedema are the most common manifestation of anaphylaxis, occurring in over 90% of patients.[5,16–18,27]

Respiratory symptoms occur in 40% to 70%,[5,27] whereas cardiovascular manifestations are seen in 30% to 35%[5] of patients.

Up to 40% of patients present with gastrointestinal signs and symptoms.[5,27] Neurologic manifestations, such as headache and seizures, occur in <10% of patients with anaphylaxis.[5]

| TABLE 34-2 • Identifiable Etiologies of Anaphylaxis

- Foods
  - Peanuts
  - Tree nuts
  - Shellfish
  - Fish
  - Milk
  - Eggs
  - Wheat
  - Soy
- Medications
  - Antibiotics
  - Nonsteroidal anti-inflammatory drugs
  - Opioids
  - Muscle relaxants
  - Protamine
  - Insulin
  - Hormones
- Insect venom
- Immunotherapy injections
- Latex
- Physical factors
  - Exercise
  - Temperature
- Radiocontrast media
- Transfusion of blood products
- Intravenous immunoglobulin
- Animal or human proteins
- Colorants
- Enzymes
- Polysaccharides
- Psychogenic (factitious)

Sources: Adapted from Stevenson DD. Anaphylactic and anaphylactoid reactions to aspirin and other nonsteroidal antiiflammatory drugs. *Immunol Allergy Clin North Am* 2001;21:745–768. and Kemp SF, Lockey RF. Anaphylaxis: a review of causes and mechanisms. *J Allergy Clin Immunol* 2002;110(3):341–348, with permission.

| TABLE 34-3 • Clinical Manifestations of Anaphylaxis

General
- Impending sense of doom
- Generalized weakness
- Diaphoresis

Cutaneous
- Urticaria
- Angioedema
- Flushing
- Pruritus
- Periorbital edema

Respiratory
- Upper airway
  - Rhinitis
  - Oropharyngeal edema
  - Laryngeal edema
  - Dysphonia
  - Stridor
- Lower airway
  - Tachypnea
  - Dyspnea
  - Bronchospasm
  - Cough

Cardiovascular
- Tachy- or bradyarrhythmias
- Hypotension
- Palpitations
- Syncope or near-syncope
- Myocardial ischemia

Gastrointestinal
- Nausea
- Vomiting
- Abdominal pain
- Diarrhea

Neurologic
- Headache
- Seizure

Ocular
- Conjunctivitis
- Lacrimation

Genitourinary
- Pelvic pain in women secondary to uterine contractions

Table 34-3 lists the clinical manifestations of anaphylaxis according to organ system. As a rule of thumb, children more often have respiratory involvement, whereas adults more commonly have cardiovascular and cutaneous manifestations.[28,29]

Differential Diagnosis

Given the variety of clinical presentations, it is not surprising that the differential diagnosis of anaphylaxis is extensive. Vasovagal reaction is reported to be the most common condition confused with anaphylaxis.[16] Importantly, vasovagal reactions lack the cutaneous findings usually seen in patients with anaphylaxis. Table 34-4 provides a representative list of the differential diagnosis according to the predominant organ system involved. Potentially life-threatening conditions to consider early in the assessment of patients with suspected anaphylaxis include hypoglycemia, asthma exacerbation, pulmonary embolism, and other forms of shock (septic, cardiogenic, hypovolemic).

Current and Evolving Pathophysiologic Concepts

Anaphylaxis begins with antigen exposure and the activation of mast cells and basophils. Regardless of the mechanism, once activated, these cells generate and release numerous chemical mediators. Preformed mediators released within seconds of activation include histamine,

| TABLE 34-4 • Differential Diagnosis of Anaphylaxis

Cutaneous symptoms (flushing, urticaria)
- Carcinoid syndrome
- Systemic mastocytosis
- Postprandial syndromes
  - Monosodium glutamate ingestion
  - Sulfite ingestion
  - Scombroidosis
  - Alcohol ingestion
- Pheochromocytoma
- Gastrointestinal tumors (vasoactive polypeptide-secreting tumors)
- Niacin
- "Red-man syndrome" (vancomycin)
- Hematologic malignancies (leukemia)

Cardiovascular collapse
- Cardiogenic shock
- Septic shock
- Pulmonary embolism
- Hypovolemic shock
- Acute coronary syndrome
- Arrhythmias

Respiratory compromise
- Asthma exacerbation
- Pulmonary embolism
- Foreign body aspiration
- Vocal cord dysfunction

Neurologic involvement (loss of consciousness)
- Seizure
- Hypoglycemia
- Vasovagal reaction
- Arrhythmias

Source: Modified from Ellis AK, Day JH. Diagnosis and management of anaphylaxis. *CMAJ* 2003;169(4):307–311 and Lieberman P, et al. The diagnosis and management of anaphylaxis: an updated practice parameter. *J. Allergy Clin Immunol* 2005;115(3 Suppl 2);S483–S523, with permission.

heparin, tryptase, chymase, and tumor necrosis factor-alpha (TNF-α).[30]

Within several minutes, mast cells and basophils generate and release additional mediators, namely platelet-activating factor, TNF-α, prostaglandin D2, leukotriene B4, and the cysteinyl leukotrienes C4, D4, and E4.[30] Over the course of several hours, cells release granulocyte-macrophage colony stimulating factor and a number of interleukins.[30] Termed the "mast cell–leukocyte–cytokine cascade," these mediators provide for significant positive feedback pathways, thereby propagating and potentially augmenting the clinical symptoms.[30] In cases of severe anaphylaxis, these mediators may also activate components of the complement system, coagulation cascade, and the contact (kallikrein–kinin) system.

Distributive and Hypovolemic Shock

While both the arterial and venous circulations are affected in anaphylaxis, the key vascular pathophysiologic features appear to be a profound reduction in both venous tone and vascular permeability.[30] It is believed that these effects are primarily mediated by histamine, the most well studied of the preformed mediators.[16] In fact, plasma histamine levels have been shown to correlate with the duration and severity of cardiovascular symptoms in patients with anaphylaxis.[31] Histamine, through stimulation of endothelial cells and the production of nitric oxide, results in vasodilation (primarily reduced venous tone) and increased vascular permeability, both of which reduce venous return to the heart. Surprisingly, according to one study, up to 35% of the effective circulating volume can be extravasated into the peripheral tissues within 10 minutes of the onset of anaphylaxis.[32] The reductions in venous tone and venous return result in shock that is both distributive and hypovolemic.

Is the Heart a Target Organ in Anaphylaxis?

Recent literature has focused on the heart as a possible target organ in anaphylaxis. It is known that cardiac mast cells are concentrated around coronary vessels and in the right atrium, near the sinoatrial node.[33] Histamine can not only induce coronary artery vasospasm but also increase myocardial oxygen demand through increases in both heart rate and contractility. A number of recent case reports have detailed the presence of severe myocardial depression along with nonspecific electrocardiographic (ECG) changes in patients with severe anaphylaxis.[29,33,34] In some cases, patients have had ECG and laboratory evidence of an acute myocardial infarction.[35] In many patients with evidence of severe myocardial depression, cardiac catheterization has revealed normal coronary arteries.[34] Furthermore, those with severe myocardial depression and no preexisting cardiac disease often have a gradual return to their baseline cardiac function following resolution of anaphylaxis. At present, it is unclear whether the severe myocardial depression observed in some cases is due to either a direct mediator effect, a profound decrease in venous return, existing myocardial dysfunction, or the high level of circulating catecholamines commonly encountered during anaphylaxis.

General Care for All Victims of Anaphylaxis

Regardless of whether the patient is first encountered in the prehospital setting or the ED, the general care of all victims of anaphylaxis should focus on maintaining adequate oxygenation, restoring effective circulatory volume, and administering epinephrine.

A rapid assessment of the airway and breathing should be immediately performed. A low threshold for emergent intubation should be maintained for any patient with respiratory distress, stridor, significant oropharyngeal and/or laryngeal edema, hypoxemia, or altered mentation. If intubation is required, a large-bore endotracheal tube is preferred. This will lessen airway resistance when instituting mechanical ventilation. Any patient who requires intubation but who cannot be successfully intubated should undergo emergent cricothyroidotomy. Patients who do not need immediate intubation or cricothyroidotomy should receive supplemental oxygen, initially via a nonrebreather mask. Continuous pulse oximetry should be used to monitor oxygenation.

Circulatory evaluation begins with an assessment of blood pressure, pulse, peripheral perfusion, and mentation. Patients with anaphylaxis should be placed in the supine position. This recommendation stems from the observation that cardiac arrest has been reported in some patients within seconds of being moved to an upright posture.[36] Recall that as much as 35% of the effective circulating volume may be extravasated into the interstitial tissues within the first several minutes of anaphylaxis.[32] As such, peripheral intravenous access with a large-bore catheter should be obtained as soon as possible. Fluid resuscitation should begin as soon as intravenous access is obtained. For adults, 5 to 10 mL/kg should be administered within the first several minutes.[3,5,37] For children, 30 mL/kg should be given in the first hour of treatment.[3,5] In general, isotonic crystalloids are recommended. All patients should be placed on continuous cardiac monitor with frequent blood pressure recordings.

Epinephrine remains the drug of choice for anaphylaxis.

Although based primarily on clinical observation and animal data, epinephrine remains the drug of choice for anaphylaxis.[3,5,38] Epinephrine stimulates alpha, beta$_1$, and beta$_2$ adrenergic receptors. Alpha-adrenergic stimulation causes peripheral vasoconstriction, resulting in improved blood pressure, improved coronary artery perfusion, and a reduction in angioedema.[37–39] Stimulation of beta$_1$ receptors results in increased inotropy and chronotropy, while stimulation of beta$_2$ receptors reverses bronchospasm and suppresses further mediator release from mast cells and basophils.[37–39] Although epinephrine is listed in every guideline on anaphylaxis, it is well reported that its use is underutilized.[4,38,40] In fact, underutilization, delayed dosing, inappropriate dosing, and inappropriate route of epinephrine administration have contributed to deaths from anaphylaxis.[16] Importantly, there are no absolute contraindications to epinephrine use in anaphylaxis.

It appears that reversal of symptoms, and possibly survival, are dependent upon rapidly achieving high plasma and tissue levels of epinephrine.[40]

The initial recommended dose for adults is 0.3 mg to 0.5 mg of aqueous epinephrine (1:1,000) injected intramuscularly into the lateral thigh.

For children, the dose of aqueous epinephrine is 0.01 mg/kg, with a maximum dose of 0.3 mg. Intramuscular injection

into the lateral thigh is recommended based upon studies that demonstrate more rapid peak plasma epinephrine concentrations when compared with intramuscular and subcutaneous injections into the deltoid.[41,42] It is important to note, however, that these studies were conducted on healthy volunteers. To date, no study has examined the optimal intramuscular route, dose, or outcome in patients with anaphylaxis. Intramuscular epinephrine injections may be repeated every 5 to 15 minutes based upon clinical response.

Additional therapy (discussed below) is based upon the response to intravenous fluids and epinephrine.

Important ACLS Considerations and Prehospital Care

The majority of deaths in anaphylaxis are due to circulatory and/or respiratory failure.

As such, advanced cardiac life support (ACLS) providers should pay particular attention to these two organ systems. Given the potential for the rapid development of oropharyngeal or laryngeal edema, the need for endotracheal intubation or cricothyroidotomy must always be anticipated. Airway equipment, sedative and paralytic medications, and surgical airway equipment should be readily available. All patients should be placed on cardiac monitoring and continuous pulse oximetry, and provided with supplemental oxygen. Intravenous access should be attempted and, if successful, isotonic crystalloid fluids should be administered. Importantly, intramuscular injection of epinephrine, as described above, should not be delayed. Depending on transport time, a second injection may be required for patients with an incomplete response to the initial dose. Patients should be placed in the recumbent position during transfer to the ED.

 See Web site for AHA/ECC guidelines for CPR—cardiac arrest associated with anaphylaxis.

Initial ED Management

ED management of the patient with anaphylaxis begins with an assessment of the airway, breathing, circulation, and mentation. Intramuscular epinephrine should be given as soon as possible. All patients should be placed on a cardiac monitor with continuous pulse oximetry. Initially, high-flow supplemental oxygen should be given through a nonrebreather mask. Once intravenous access is obtained, aggressive fluid resuscitation with isotonic crystalloids should begin.

Additional medications are given based upon the initial response to intravenous fluids and epinephrine.

Antihistamines

Antihistamines are typically administered in the ED treatment of anaphylaxis. Importantly, antihistamines should be considered "second-line" medications and never used as monotherapy to treat patients with anaphylaxis.[5] In fact, a recent review found no good evidence to recommend either for or against the routine use of H_1 antihistamines in anaphylaxis.[27] Antihistamines are useful for relieving the cutaneous symptoms of anaphylaxis. Unfortunately they have little to no effect on reversing cardiovascular, pulmonary, or gastrointestinal manifestations.[3,37] If given to alleviate cutaneous symptoms, the combination of an H_1 and H_2 blocker has been shown to be superior to therapy with an H_1 blocker alone.[3,43,44] Most guidelines recommend the use of diphenhydramine (25–50 mg for adults) along with ranitidine. There are no studies, however, that demonstrate the superiority of any one H_2 blocker over another.[5]

Corticosteroids

Corticosteroids are frequently administered along with antihistamines in patients with anaphylaxis. Recall that corticosteroids have a relatively slow onset of action. As such, they are not useful in the acute management of anaphylaxis. It is believed by many that corticosteroids prevent recurrent reactions and attenuate protracted episodes. This belief, however, is based on an extrapolation of data on their effectiveness in other acute illnesses, such as asthma. To date, the effectiveness of corticosteroids in the management of anaphylaxis has not been proven.[3,5] Nevertheless, corticosteroids do appear in many current guidelines pertaining to the acute management of anaphylaxis. If given, 1 to 2 mg/kg of methylprednisolone every 6 hours is recommended.[3]

Glucagon

Glucagon is recommended in the treatment of patients with anaphylaxis who are taking beta-blocker medications. Although anaphylaxis has not been shown to occur more frequently in these patients,[2,5] it may occur with greater severity.[45] Increased severity of anaphylaxis is possibly secondary to a blunted response to epinephrine, although this has not been proven.[5] Glucagon has positive inotropic, chronotropic, and vasoactive effects that are independent of the beta receptor.[24] It is believed that glucagon reverses hypotension and bronchospasm by bypassing the beta receptor and directly activating intracellular adenylate cyclase.[2,5] The dose of glucagon for adults with anaphylaxis is 1 to 5 mg intravenously over 5 minutes, followed by an infusion of 5 to 15 µg/min. For children, the recommended dose is 20 to 30 µg/kg to a maximum dose of 1 mg. It is important to note that the predominant side effect of glucagon is emesis.

In patients with upper airway involvement who require glucagon, emesis may further compromise the airway.

Albuterol

Patients with anaphylaxis who exhibit bronchospasm should be given a nebulized solution of albuterol. This can be achieved by adding 2.5 or 5 mg of albuterol to 3 mL of normal saline. Albuterol treatments can be given as frequently as needed.

The Unstable Patient

Patients who remain hemodynamically unstable despite aggressive fluid resuscitation and intramuscular epinephrine injections should receive intravenous epinephrine.

To date, there is no established dose or regimen for giving intravenous epinephrine.[5] Depending upon the publication, recommendations vary between intermittent bolus dosing and titration of a continuous infusion. Intermittent dosing can be achieved by adding 0.1 mL of 1:1,000 to 10 mL of normal saline.[5] This provides a solution of 1:10,000, which can be given slowly over several minutes and repeated every 5 to 15 minutes as necessary.[5] Great caution should be used with intermittent bolus dosing of intravenous epinephrine. The majority of adverse events, such as myocardial infarction, reported with intravenous epinephrine tend to be associated with intermittent dosing. These adverse events are most often due to rapid administration, inadequate dilution, or excessive dosing.[39]

Perhaps the safest way to administer epinephrine intravenously is by a low-dose continuous infusion.[3] As an example, 1.0 mg of 1:1,000 epinephrine can be added to 500 mL of D_5W, creating a concentration of 2 mg/mL. This can then be infused at a rate of 1 µg/min and titrated to 10 µg/min based upon the clinical response.[5] Alternative routes of epinephrine administration—such as inhalational, sublingual, and conjunctival—have been investigated. To date, there are not enough data to support the administration of epinephrine via these routes,[5] although epinephrine can be administered through an endotracheal tube if intravenous access is delayed or not achievable.

Vasopressor medications can be used in the hemodynamically unstable patient who is unresponsive to intravenous fluids and epinephrine.

Dopamine (in the alpha-adrenergic range beginning at 10 µg/min) has been advocated by some as the vasopressor of choice; however, there are no randomized, controlled studies that demonstrate the superiority of any vasopressor in the setting of anaphylaxis. Additional vasopressor medications that have been used in anaphylaxis include norepinephrine, metaraminol, vasopressin, glucagon, amrinone, and milrinone. The choice of any particular vasopressor medication should be based upon the individual patient and clinical scenario. Importantly, aggressive fluid resuscitation should continue while administering vasopressor medications.

Atropine (0.02 mg/kg) and/or transcutaneous pacing are recommended for the unstable patient with hypotension and severe bradycardia.[5,29,30,37]

Post–Circulatory Arrest Management

Management of anaphylactic patients who are resuscitated from circulatory arrest is challenging. Similar to the initial care of anaphylaxis, postarrest management should focus on optimizing oxygenation and perfusion pressure. In nearly every patient who has sustained a circulatory arrest, the airway is secured either with cricothyroidotomy or endotracheal intubation. Therefore oxygenation is optimized through the use of mechanical ventilation. Mechanically ventilating the patient with anaphylaxis, however, can be fraught with peril. Barotrauma and worsening hemodynamic compromise are recognized complications of mechanical ventilation in anaphylaxis. Essentially, increased intrathoracic pressure from overinflation decreases venous return and further impairs cardiac output. To limit these complications, tidal volumes of 6 to 7 mL/kg delivered over 1.5 to 2 seconds are recommended.[37] Plateau pressures should be followed and ideally kept below 30 to 35 cm H_2O.

To restore adequate perfusion after circulatory arrest, intravenous fluids should be continued. In some patients, up to 7 L of crystalloid fluid may be needed.[37] In addition to continued intravenous fluids, an emergent bedside echocardiogram should be considered.[29] Those with severely depressed myocardial function require additional hemodynamic support. To date, case reports have detailed the successful use of glucagon, amrinone, and intra-aortic balloon counterpulsation in patients with depressed cardiac function.[30,34,45,46] If continued fluid resuscitation, epinephrine, and inotropic support fail to improve perfusion pressure, patients should be started on vasopressor medication. As discussed, there are currently no good data to routinely recommend any one vasopressor medication over the others in the setting of anaphylaxis.

Termination of Resuscitative Efforts

Prolonged resuscitative efforts are recommended for the patient with circulatory arrest secondary to anaphylaxis.[5] More often, these patients are younger and lack significant preexisting cardiac disease as compared with the typical victims of cardiac arrest. Therefore survival with a reasonable chance of neurologic recovery is more likely.

Summary

Anaphylaxis is a potentially life-threatening allergic reaction that requires prompt recognition and treatment by the emergency care provider. The tenets of treatment, regardless of the setting, include ensuring adequate oxygenation, aggressive fluid resuscitation, and judicious use of epinephrine. It is recommended that the initial dose of epinephrine be given intramuscularly into the lateral thigh. Additional medical therapies are then administered based upon the response to intravenous fluids and epinephrine. Patients who remain unstable despite intravenous fluids and epinephrine require intensive treatment that may include intravenous epinephrine, mechanical ventilation, vasopressor medications, inotropic support, transcutaneous pacing, or intra-aortic balloon pump counterpulsation.

References

1. Portier P. De l'action anaphylactique de certains venins. *Soc Biol (Paris)* 1902;54: 170–172.
2. Sampson HA, et al. Symposium on the definition and management of anaphylaxis: summary report. *J Allergy Clin Immunol* 2005;115(3): 584–591.
3. Sampson HA, et al. Second symposium on the definition and management of anaphylaxis: summary report. Second National Institute of Allergy and Infectious Disease/Food Allergy and Anaphylaxis Network symposium. *J Allergy Clin Immunol* 2006;117(2):391–397.
4. Lieberman P, et al. SAFE: a multidisciplinary approach to anaphylaxis education in the emergency department. *Ann Allergy Asthma Immunol* 2007;98(6):519–523.
5. The diagnosis and management of anaphylaxis: an updated practice parameter. *J Allergy Clin Immunol* 2005;115(3 Suppl 2):S483–S523.
6. Lane RD, Bolte RG. Pediatric anaphylaxis. *Pediatr Emerg Care* 2007;23(1):49–56; quiz 57–60.
7. Lieberman P, et al. Epidemiology of anaphylaxis: findings of the American College of Allergy Asthma, and Immunology. Epidemiology of Anaphylaxis Working Group. *Ann Allergy Asthma Immunol* 2006;97(5):596–602.
8. Valentine M, Friedland L, et al. Allergic emergencies. In *Asthma and Other Allergic Diseases*. Bethesda, MD: National Institutes of Health, 1979:467–507.
9. Yocum MW, et al. Epidemiology of anaphylaxis in Olmsted County: A population-based study. *J Allergy Clin Immunol* 1999;104(2 Pt 1):452–456.
10. Neugut AI, Ghatak AT, Miller RL. Anaphylaxis in the United States: an investigation into its epidemiology. *Arch Intern Med* 2001;161(1):15–21.
11. Simons FE, Peterson S, Black CD. Epinephrine dispensing for the out-of-hospital treatment of anaphylaxis in infants and children: a population-based study. *Ann Allergy Asthma Immunol* 2001;86(6): 622–626.
12. Simons FE, Peterson S, Black CD. Epinephrine dispensing patterns for an out-of-hospital population: a novel approach to studying the epidemiology of anaphylaxis. *J Allergy Clin Immunol* 2002;110(4):647–651.
13. Gaeta TJ, et al. National study of US emergency department visits for acute allergic reactions, 1993 to 2004. *Ann Allergy Asthma Immunol* 2007;98(4):360–365.
14. Clark S, Camargo CA Jr. Epidemiology of anaphylaxis. *Immunol Allergy Clin North Am* 2007;27(2):145–163, v.
15. Lieberman P. Anaphylaxis and anaphylactoid reactions. In Adkinson NF (ed) *Allergy: Principles and Practice*. Philadelphia: Mosby, 2003:1497–1522.
16. Lieberman P. Anaphylaxis. *Med Clin North Am* 2006; 90(1):77–95, viii.

17. Kemp SF, Lockey RF. Anaphylaxis: a review of causes and mechanisms. *J Allergy Clin Immunol* 2002;110(3):341–348.

18. Brown AF, McKinnon D, Chu K. Emergency department anaphylaxis: a review of 142 patients in a single year. *J Allergy Clin Immunol* 2001;108(5):861–866.

19. Stewart GE II, Lockey RF. Systemic reactions from allergen immunotherapy. *J Allergy Clin Immunol* 1992;90(4 Pt 1):567–578.

20. Chiu AM Kelly KJ. Anaphylaxis: drug allergy, insect stings, and latex. *Immunol Allergy Clin North Am* 2005;25(2):389–405, viii.

21. Sampson HA. Anaphylaxis and emergency treatment. *Pediatrics* 2003;111(6 Pt 3):1601–1608.

22. Sicherer SH, et al. Prevalence of peanut and tree nut allergy in the US determined by a random digit dial telephone survey. *J Allergy Clin Immunol* 1999;103(4):559–562.

23. Yocum MW, Khan DA. Assessment of patients who have experienced anaphylaxis: a 3-year survey. *Mayo Clin Proc* 1994;69(1):16–23.

24. Ellis AK, Day JH. Diagnosis and management of anaphylaxis. *CMAJ* 2003;169(4):307–311.

25. James LP Jr, Austen KF. Fatal systemic anaphylaxis in man. *N Engl J Med* 1964;270:597–603.

26. Lockey RF, et al. Fatalities from immunotherapy (IT) and skin testing (ST). *J Allergy Clin Immunol* 1987;79(4):660–677.

27. Sheikh A, et al. H_1-antihistamines for the treatment of anaphylaxis. *Cochrane Syst Rev Allergy* 2007;62(8): 830–837.

28. Brown SG, Mullins RJ, Gold MS. Anaphylaxis: diagnosis and management. *Med J Aust* 2006;185(5):283–289.

29. Brown SG. Anaphylaxis: clinical concepts and research priorities. *Emerg Med Australas* 2006;18(2):155–169.

30. Brown SG. The pathophysiology of shock in anaphylaxis. *Immunol Allergy Clin North Am* 2007;27(2):165–175, v.

31. Simons FE, et al. Risk assessment in anaphylaxis: current and future approaches. *J Allergy Clin Immunol* 2007;120(1 Suppl):S2–S24.

32. Fisher MM. Clinical observations on the pathophysiology and treatment of anaphylactic cardiovascular collapse. *Anaesth Intens Care* 1986;14(1):17–21.

33. Bani D, et al. Cardiac anaphylaxis: pathophysiology and therapeutic perspectives. *Curr Allergy Asthma Rep* 2006;6(1):14–19.

34. Raper RF, Fisher MM. Profound reversible myocardial depression after anaphylaxis. *Lancet* 1988;1(8582):386–388.

35. Kounis NG. Kounis syndrome (allergic angina and allergic myocardial infarction): a natural paradigm? *Int J Cardiol* 2006;110(1):7–14.

36. Pumphrey RS. Fatal posture in anaphylactic shock. *J Allergy Clin Immunol* 2003;112(2):451–552.

37. Oswalt ML Kemp SF. Anaphylaxis: office management and prevention. *Immunol Allergy Clin North Am* 2007;27(2):177–191, vi.

38. Lieberman P. Use of epinephrine in the treatment of anaphylaxis. *Curr Opin Allergy Clin Immunol* 2003; 3(4):313–318.

39. McLean-Tooke AP, et al. Adrenaline in the treatment of anaphylaxis: what is the evidence? *BMJ* 2003;327(7427): 1332–1335.

40. Simons FE. First-aid treatment of anaphylaxis to food: focus on epinephrine. *J Allergy Clin Immunol* 2004;113(5):837–844.

41. Simons FE, et al. Epinephrine absorption in children with a history of anaphylaxis. *J Allergy Clin Immunol* 1998;101(1 Pt 1): 33–37.

42. Simons FE, Gu X, Simons KJ. Epinephrine absorption in adults: intramuscular versus subcutaneous injection. *J Allergy Clin Immunol* 2001;108(5):871–873.

43. Simons FE. Advances in H_1-antihistamines. *N Engl J Med* 2004;351(21):2203–2217.

44. Lin RY, et al. Histamine and tryptase levels in patients with acute allergic reactions: an emergency department–based study. *J Allergy Clin Immunol* 2000;106(1 Pt 1):65–71.

45. Thomas M, Crawford I. Best evidence topic report. Glucagon infusion in refractory anaphylactic shock in patients on beta-blockers. *Emerg Med J* 2005;22(4):272–273.

46. Zaloga GP, et al. Glucagon reversal of hypotension in a case of anaphylactoid shock. *Ann Intern Med* 1986;105(1):65–66.

Chapter 35
Cardiopulmonary Resuscitation in Pregnancy

Carolyn M. Zelop and Edward P. Grimes

Cardiopulmonary resuscitation of the pregnant victim is surprisingly similar in many respects to advanced cardiac life support (ACLS) protocols for nonpregnant patients. However, the unique physiologic changes of pregnancy require special consideration and necessitate some modification of standard algorithms. There are two patients, and pregnancy also requires a multidisciplinary approach and coordination of specialties: emergency medicine, obstetrics including perinatology, neonatology, and possibly cardiothoracic surgery.

- Causes of cardiac arrest include those found in nonpregnant patients as well as those unique to pregnancy.
- Pregnancy results in a myriad of physiologic, anatomic, and metabolic changes.
- Cardiopulmonary resuscitation (CPR) involves a number of modifications, including the left lateral uterine displacement position and removal of all fetal monitoring leads prior to defibrillation.
- Any medication that would be utilized in the nonpregnant patient should be utilized in the pregnant cardiopulmonary arrest patient.
- Emergent delivery of the fetus, open-chest cardiac massage, and cardiopulmonary bypass.

The Setting

You are a physician called to the emergency department to help evaluate a pregnant patient involved in a motor vehicle accident.

Paramedics at the scene noticed blood on her clothing, apparently from her groin, as they secured her neck in a cervical spine collar. They reported the following: HR, 140; BP, 80/palp; RR, 24; SaO$_2$, 96%. Abdominal exam revealed marked diffuse tenderness. Several dark clots are passed per vagina. For volume replacement, a second large-bore IV is placed, infusing lactated Ringers (LR) as the patient is transported. Upon arrival at the hospital, assessment continues. In the emergency department (ED), fetal monitoring is initiated, revealing a fetal heart rate in the 130s with no decelerations. Fundal height is consistent with 32 weeks' gestation. The obstetric and neonatology services are called STAT. BP now falls to 60/palp and the patient becomes unresponsive. Shallow respirations are noted after 100% O$_2$ is administered by face mask. Rapid sequence intubation is performed using succinylcholine and cricoid pressure. A cardiac monitor attached to this patient reveals sinus tachycardia. BP can no longer be measured, pulses are found to be absent. Cardiopulmonary resuscitation (CPR) is initiated after moving the patient into left lateral uterine displacement. Cardiac monitors reveal deterioration into a wide-complex rhythm consistent with ventricular tachycardia, which progresses quickly to ventricular fibrillation. After fetal monitors are removed, defibrillation sequence is attempted at 200, 300, and 360 J. Cardiac rhythm returns to sinus tachycardia after the third attempt at defibrillation, but pulses are still not palpable. CPR continues. Epinephrine 1 mg is given using IV above the groin. Vital signs do not improve. With no response to resuscitation, an emergency cesarean section is performed by the obstetric team at the bedside. With continued volume replacement and incremental doses of epinephrine, peripheral pulses become palpable. The mother improves hemodynamically and is transferred to the intensive care unit. Although the fetus requires intubation, the neonatology staff report improving hemodynamic and metabolic parameters.

This clinical vignette describes the rare but catastrophic occurrence of cardiopulmonary arrest during pregnancy. The complexity of dealing with altered physiology and the unique clinical scenario of treating two patients simultaneously often paralyzes the clinician when time is of the essence. This chapter should enable the clinician to generate a differential diagnosis and to modify ACLS protocols to respond appropriately to this specialized rescue situation.

Epidemiology and Clinical Spectrum

The differential diagnosis of cardiopulmonary arrest is expansive. The etiologies are related to causes found in the nonpregnant population as well as conditions unique to the pregnant state.

Maternal mortality has been increasing during the new millennium. In 2004, maternal deaths in the United States reached a new high with 13.1 deaths per 100,000 live births.[1-4] Reportedly, the prevalence of maternal cardiac arrest is estimated to be 1 per 30,000; however, this figure may be rising.[5,6] Advances in medical technology open the door to reproductive options for women with chronic illness who previously could not consider pregnancy. The escalating cesarean birth rate will give rise to increased rates of accreta and other obstetric conditions, which elevate the risk of maternal hemorrhage.[7] The obesity epidemic is rampant, especially during pregnancy, leading to medical and surgical complications in the mother and fetus which can become life-threatening.[8]

The differential diagnosis of cardiopulmonary arrest is expansive. The etiologies are related to causes found in the nonpregnant population as well as conditions unique to the pregnant state. The clinician assessing the pregnant patient with sudden cardiopulmonary collapse must consider hemorrhage, embolism, and other unique etiologies (Table 35-1).[9-12]

Physiologic Changes of Pregnancy and Their Impact on Cardiovascular Collapse

Pregnancy results in a myriad of physiologic, anatomic, and metabolic changes that allow successful maternal adaptation to the fetal–placental unit.

Pulmonary and Airway Changes

Estrogen induced hyperemia and edema of the upper airway may alter the usual anatomic landmarks of the pharynx and larynx. The level of the diaphragm rises 4 cm, but the excursion remains normal. Thoracic compliance, however, decreases, especially in the third trimester, although respiratory muscle function remains unchanged. The rise in the diaphragm leads to a 20% decrease in functional residual capacity, mainly due to a decrease in residual volume. Lung volume changes result in a more rapid oxygen desaturation in the setting of oxygen deprivation. Progesterone-induced

| TABLE 35-1 • Causes of Cardiopulmonary Arrest in Pregnancy

Pulmonary
  Embolism
    Thrombotic
    Amniotic
  Asthma

Trauma
  Domestic violence
  Motor vehicle accident

Hemorrhagic complications
  Abruption
  Atony
  Abnormally adherent placentation

Preeclampsia/eclampsia
  Stroke
  Hypertensive crisis

Medication-related
  Tocolytic complications
  Illicit drug use
  Hypermagnesemia
  Anaphylaxis

Anesthetic-related
  Failed intubation
  Intravascular injections of local anesthetics
  Aspiration

Infection/sepsis

Cardiac
  Arrhythmias
  Cardiomyopathy of pregnancy
  Congenital cardiac disease
  Myocardial infarction

increase in minute ventilation, mainly due to increased tidal volume, produces a respiratory alkalosis accompanied by a compensatory renally induced metabolic acidosis. While this facilitates excretion of fetal CO_2, decreased serum bicarbonate renders the pregnant woman less capable of neutralizing the acid load that may arise during anaerobic respiration. The increased metabolic rate requires that oxygen consumption increase by 20% to 40%. The parameters are different for interpreting a normal arterial blood gas in pregnancy: PH, 7.40 to 7.45; Pco_2, 28 to 32; Po_2, 101 to 106; and HCO_3^-, 18 to 21.

Gastrointestinal Changes

Progesterone decreases the motility of the gastrointestinal tract and weakens the competency of the lower esophageal sphincter. Therefore, upon loss of consciousness, the pregnant patient has a higher risk of aspiration.

Hematologic Changes

There is a 40% increase in blood volume beginning at 6 weeks and plateauing at 30 weeks of gestation. Erythropoietin and reticulocyte count increase at a slower rate but contribute to the overall expansion of the red cell mass. The increased circulatory volume protects the mother against hypotension and hemorrhage. It perfuses the expanded vascular system created by the vasodilation and low resistance of the uteroplacental unit. The disproportionate increase in volume over red cell mass creates the physiologic anemia of pregnancy.

Cardiovascular Changes

Cardiac output increases 40% starting as early as the first trimester. This increase in cardiac output is primarily due to an increase in stroke volume. However, increased heart rate does contribute secondarily. One of the primary functions of the increase in the cardiac output is to perfuse the uteroplacental unit, which requires 20% of the overall cardiac output, and to sustain the increased metabolic requirements of tissue throughout the body during pregnancy.

Paradoxically, the enlarging uteroplacental unit mechanically compresses the great vessels, thereby decreasing venous return from the inferior vena cava and increasing afterload through compression of the aorta. This physiologic aberration, due to the enlarging uterus, begins at about 20 weeks and is exacerbated with increasing uterine distention, which would be magnified in certain clinical settings such as multiple gestations. These cardiopulmonary changes render the pregnant patient more vulnerable to any cardiopulmonary insult and require special consideration during any resuscitation sequence.[15,16]

The ABCs of Resuscitation become ABCDs ("D" for Delivery)

Cardiopulmonary resuscitation of the pregnant victim is surprisingly similar in many respects to ACLS protocols for nonpregnant patients (Table 35-2).[17–21] However, the unique physiologic changes outlined above require special consideration and necessitate some modification of standard algorithms, as detailed below.

 See Web site for AHA ECC guidelines for CPR—cardiac arrest associated with pregnancy.

| TABLE 35-2 • Modifications to CPR in Pregnancy

Unmodified by Pregnancy	Modifications in Pregnancy
Support of ventilation	Aggressive airway management
Closed chest compressions (somewhat more cephalad than usual)	Left lateral uterine displacement
Defibrillation (remove internal and external fetal monitors)	Consideration of delivery
Pharmacologic therapy Pressors Antiarrhythmics	Intravenous access above the groin

Source: Adapted from Dildy GA, Clark SL. Cardiac arrest during pregnancy. *Obstet Gynecol Clin North Am* 1995;22(2):303–314.

Pregnancy also requires a multidisciplinary approach and coordination of specialties: emergency medicine, obstetrics (including perinatology), neonatology, and possibly cardiothoracic surgery.

Assessment of the pregnant unconscious victim begins with acquiring vital signs and securing the airway if necessary with rapid sequence intubation using succinylcholine (1.5 mg/kg) accompanied by cricoid pressure and use of 100% oxygen. The size of the endotracheal tube required in pregnancy is often smaller than in the nonpregnant adult female. While considering the differential diagnosis outlined above, the gestational age must also be ascertained. Prenatal care history may not be available. Real-time transabdominal ultrasound may confirm fetal well-being by demonstrating fetal cardiac activity and could be used to estimate gestational age. However, in the interest of time, physical exam can be used to obtain an estimate of fetal gestational age. The fetus is at 20 weeks of gestation when the uterus is at the umbilicus. Every centimeter above the umbilicus roughly corresponds to another week of gestation, such that the total distance from the pubic symphysis to the top of the fundus in centimeters corresponds to the gestational age in weeks.. Special situations such uterine fibroids or multiple gestations might overestimate the fetal gestational age; however, the size of the uterus will correspond to the degree of aortocaval compression, which will affect the success of early interventions.

SUMMARY OF RESCUE SEQUENCE FOR CARDIAC ARREST

- Call maternal CODE BLUE
- Manual uterine displacement
- ABCs
- At 4 minutes, begin to perform perimortem cesarean section.
- At 15 minutes, consider open cardiac massage.
- At 20 minutes, consider cardiopulmonary bypass.

Later in the algorithm, the gestational age of the fetus will play a pivotal role in the resuscitation schema.[11]

In addition to assessment of gestational age, the question arises as to whether to perform continuous fetal monitoring to assess fetal well-being. In general, if the status of the mother is not reassuring, the status of the fetus will be further compromised. Thus, while fetal monitoring may be instituted to gain information regarding fetal well-being, in general the status of mother will direct further resuscitation during cardiopulmonary arrest.

Fetal monitors should be removed to avoid electrocution injury if defibrillation is required.

Intravenous access should be placed above the groin in pregnancy. Lines placed below the groin will be much less effective because aortocaval compression will prevent medications from reaching the central circulation.

Prior to the initiation of CPR, it is necessary to place the unconscious pregnant patient in left lateral uterine displacement because of the aortocaval compression described previously.

Prior to the initiation of CPR, it is necessary to place the unconscious pregnant patient in left lateral uterine displacement due to the aortocaval compression described previously (Fig. 35-1).

This can be accomplished in several ways, including manual displacement supported by the lap of a rescuer, lateral tilting of the operating room table, or placement of a wedge such as the Cardiff [22,23] resuscitation wedge, which maintains the patient at a 30-degree angle. Rees et al.[22] analyzed the maximum chest compression force generated as a function of the angle of inclination. At an angle of 27 degrees, 80% of the compression force achieved in the supine position can be generated. Although higher angles would better

relieve aortocaval compression, the effectiveness of CPR would be dramatically diminished. Closed-chest CPR generally produces about the equivalent of 30% of cardiac output. Therefore, at best during pregnancy, 24% can be produced through CPR, while 20% is required by the uteroplacental unit, which further complicates the resuscitative efforts.

During pregnancy, closed-chest compressions should be performed slightly higher than in the nonpregnant patient owing to upward displacement of the diaphragm by the gravid uterus.

Laceration of the liver and spleen, hemoperitoneum, and hemopericardium may occur at higher frequency when CPR is performed during pregnancy.[17]

The 5-Minute Rule and Consideration of Delivery

If initial resuscitation efforts prove unsuccessful, cesarean delivery becomes the next strategy to rescue both mother and fetus. When normal cardiac and respiratory function cease, there is only a short time before anoxic damage ensues. If emergency care is instituted within 4 minutes of cardiac arrest, recovery may be good. If emergency care is instituted within 4 to 6 minutes, survival is possible, but with deficits. After 6 minutes, irreversible anoxic brain trauma occurs. In their landmark publication in 1986, Katz et al.[24] reviewed the history of perimortem cesarean birth and concluded that delivery by 5 minutes after maternal cardiac arrest optimized the outcome for both mother and fetus. These investigators reported a 70% infant survival rate when delivery was accomplished by 5 minutes, which decreased to 3.3% after 21 minutes. They also cited several case reports published in the anesthesia literature in the 1980s, clearly demonstrating that cesarean delivery

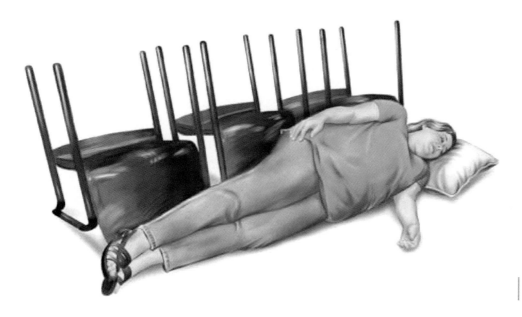

FIGURE 35-1 • Left lateral uterine displacement position.

dramatically improved the mother's condition, restoring hemodynamic stability following cardiac arrest.[25,26] A more recent review published by Katz et al. in 2005 substantiated these initial recommendations.[27]

At what gestational age is delivery a reasonable consideration? The gestational age for viability is currently 24 weeks. However, some neonatal units report survivability at 22 to 23 weeks. The literature seems to suggest that aortocaval compression affecting maternal hemodynamics begins as early as 20 weeks of gestation. Johnson et al.,[11] therefore, suggest hysterotomy to decompress the uterus during cardiopulmonary resuscitation, using the 20-week rule if maternal resuscitation was not successful by 4 minutes.

Delivery Logistics

The cesarean delivery can be performed anywhere, and time should not necessarily be spent moving the patient to an operating room. A vertical skin incision should be used to provide the most exposure and the fastest access and to allow for other options that may be necessary in the resuscitation sequence (e.g., direct cardiac massage; see below). Broadspectrum antibiotics should be administered. Following delivery of the fetus, the placenta should be extracted and the hysterotomy be closed. Relative hypoperfusion may conceal bleeders, so technique is important. Uterotonics may be necessary later to facilitate uterine hemostasis.

Defibrillation in Pregnancy

For cardiac rhythms that require defibrillation or cardioversion, care should be taken to remove internal and external fetal monitors so as to avoid electrocution injury to mother, fetus, and staff.

Do the physiologic changes in pregnancy affect defibrillation energy requirements? The increased blood volume and alterations in lung volumes may theoretically alter transthoracic impedance. Nanson et al.[28] compared transthoracic impedance measured in 45 patients at term compared to 42 patients who were 6 to 8 weeks postpartum. These researchers reported no statistical differences. Therefore, they recommended no change in the energy levels utilized for defibrillation in pregnancy.

Use of Drugs in Cardiopulmonary Arrest during Pregnancy

Although there is a reluctance to use pharmacologic therapy in pregnancy, the severity of cardiopulmonary arrest transcends this dictum; therefore, any medication that would be utilized in the nonpregnant patient should be utilized in the pregnant patient with cardiopulmonary arrest.

There are two medications that deserve a more detailed commentary. First, sodium bicarbonate has been deemphasized in recent ACLS protocols. In pregnancy, sodium bicarbonate should be considered only for documented severe acidosis during resuscitation. Use of bicarbonate may actually worsen fetal acidosis, since rapid overcorrection of maternal acidosis may cause pooling of CO_2 in the fetus.[17] Second, calcium gluconate (10 mL of 10% solution) should be used early in the resuscitation of suspected magnesium toxicity. This may occur following magnesium sulfate administration for tocolysis or seizure prophylaxis in preeclampsia. Magnesium toxicity can lead to cardiopulmonary arrest when the maternal serum concentration exceeds 12 mEq/L.[29]

Consideration of Open-Chest Massage

Troiano et al.[30] question the continued efficacy of closed-chest cardiac massage during resuscitation of the pregnant patient. They emphasize that decreased intrathoracic compliance interferes with the phasic fluctuations in intrathoracic pressure that are required for the forward movement of blood to vital organs. Lee et al.[31] suggest, therefore, that open-chest massage through a thoracotomy be considered after 15 minutes of unsuccessful closed-chest CPR. Alternatively, direct cardiac massage may be performed by accessing the heart through the abdominal incision used for cesarean delivery. Using an electrical simulation model, Babbs et al.[32] demonstrated the superiority of open-chest CPR in which near-normal systemic perfusion could be generated throughout the entire compression cycle. In contrast, in this same model, closed-chest CPR generated lower perfusion pressures that were confined mostly to the diastolic phase of the compression cycle, thus lessening the overall effectiveness of cranial blood flow.

Consideration of Cardiopulmonary Bypass for Resuscitation of the Pregnant Patient

The widespread availability of cardiothoracic surgery and perfusionist teams perhaps offers alternative strategies to continued resuscitation during cardiopulmonary arrest in pregnancy. Based upon several case reports,[33,34] cardiopulmonary bypass (CPB) may be particularly successful in the setting of pulmonary embolism, local anesthetic toxicity, illicit drug overdose, amniotic fluid embolism, and pulseless electrical activity. Johnson et al.[11] suggested that CPB be considered after 20 minutes of unsuccessful resuscitation of the pregnant patient with cardiac arrest.

Acknowledgment

Special thanks to Elizabeth Legassie for manuscript preparation.

References

1. Save the Children. State of the World's Mothers 2000. Available at: http://www.savethechildren.org/jump.jsp?path=/publications/mothers/2000/sowm2000.pdf. Accessed May 16, 2008.
2. Hoyert DL. Maternal mortality and related concepts. National Center for Health Statistics. *Vital Health Stat* 2007;33:1–13.
3. Poole JH, Long J. Maternal mortality—a review of current trends. *Crit Care Nurs Clin North Am* 2004;16:227–231.
4. Lewis G, ed. *Why Mothers Die, 2000–2002*. London: RCOG Press, 2004.
5. Doan-Wiggins L. Resuscitation of the pregnant patient suffering sudden death. In Braems G, Ramirez MM, eds. *Cardiac Arrest: The Science & Practice of Resuscitation Medicine*. Turrentine, MA: Wilkins & Wilkins, 1997:812–819.
6. Fillion DN. Being prepared for a pregnant code blue. *MCN Am J Matern Child Nurs* 1998;23(5):240–245.
7. Herbert W, Zelop CM. Postpartum hemorrhage. ACOG Practice Bulletin. *Obstet Gynecol* 2006;108:1039–1047.
8. Catalano PM. Management of obesity in pregnancy. *Obstet Gynecol* 2007;109(2):419–433.
9. Whitty JE. Maternal cardiac arrest in pregnancy. *Clin Obstet Gynecol* 2002;45(2):377–392.
10. Luppi CJ. Cardiopulmonary resuscitation in pregnancy. *ACCN Clinical Issues* 1997;8(4):574–585.
11. Johnson MD, Luppi CJ, Over DC. Cardiopulmonary resuscitation. In Gambling DR, Douglas MJ, eds. *Obstetric Anesthesia and Uncommon Disorders*. Philadelphia: Saunders, 1998:50–73.
12. Lapinsky SE. Cardiopulmonary complications of pregnancy. *Crit Care Med* 2005;33(7):1616–1622.
13. Conklin KA, Backus AM. Physiologic changes of pregnancy. In Chestnut DH, ed. *Obstetric Anesthesia*, 2nd ed. St. Louis: Mosby, 1999:17–32.
14. Shapiro JM. Critical care of the obstetric patient. *J Intens Care Med* 2006;21:278–286.
15. Ueland K, Novy MJ, et al. Maternal cardiovascular dynamics. *Am J Obstet Gynecol* 1969;104(6):856–864.
16. Kerr MG. The mechanical effects of the gravid uterus in late pregnancy. *J Obstet Gynaecol Br Commonw* 1965;(72):513–529.
17. Cummins RO, Hazinski MF, Zelop CM. Cardiac arrest associated with pregnancy. In Cummins R, Hazinski M, Field J, eds. *ACLS: The Reference Textbook*. Dallas: American Heart Association, 2005:143–151.
18. Dildy GA, Clark SL. Cardiac arrest during pregnancy. *Obstet Gynecol Clin North Am* 1995;22(2):303–314.
19. Schimmelpfennig K, Stanfill T. Preparing for maternal cardiac arrest. *AWHONN Lifelines* 2006;10(4):307–311.
20. American Heart Association. Advanced challenges in resuscitation. *Resuscitation* 2000;46:293–295.
21. Morris S, Stacey M. Resuscitation in pregnancy. *BMJ* 2003;327:1277–1279.
22. Rees GAD, Willis BA. Resuscitation in late pregnancy. *Anesthesia* 1988;43:347–349.
23. Campbell LA, Klocke RA. Update in nonpulmonary critical care: implications for the pregnant patient. *Am J Respir Crit Care Med* 2001;163:1051–1054.
24. Katz VL, Dotters DJ, Droegemueller W. Perimortem cesarean delivery. *Obstet Gynecol* 1986;68 (4):571–576.
25. Marx GF. Cardiopulmonary resuscitation of late-pregnant women (letter). *Anesthesiology* 1982;56:156.
26. Lindsay SL, Hanson GC. Cardiac arrest in near-term pregnancy. *Anesthesia* 1987;42:1074–1077.
27. Katz V, Balderston K, DeFreest M. Perimortem cesarean delivery: were our assumptions correct? *Am J Obstet Gynecol* 2005;192:1916–1921.
28. Nanson J, Elcock D, Williams M, et al. Do physiological changes in pregnancy change defibrillation energy requirements? *Br J Anaesth* 2001;87(2):237–239.
29. Repke JT. Pre-eclampsia and hypertension. In Repke JT, ed. *Intrapartum Obstetrics*. New York: Churchill Livingstone, 1996:153–273.
30. Troiano NH. Cardiopulmonary resuscitation of the pregnant woman. *J Perinat Neonat Nurs* 1989;3(2):1–13.
31. Lee RV, Rodgers BD, et al. Cardiopulmonary resuscitation of pregnant women. *Am J Med* 1986; 81:311–318.
32. Babbs CF. Hemodynamic mechanisms in CPR: a theoretical rationale for resuscitative thoracotomy in non-traumatic cardiac arrest. *Resuscitation* 1987;15(1):37–50.
33. Marty AT, Hilton FL, et al. Postcesarean Pulmonary Embolism, Sustained Cardiopulmonary Resuscitation, Embolectomy, and near-death experience. *Obstet Gynecol* 2005;106(5):1153–1155.
34. Stanten RD, Iverson LI, et al. Amniotic fluid embolism causing catastrophic pulmonary vasoconstriction: diagnosis by transesophageal echocardiogram and treatment by cardiopulmonary bypass. *Obstet Gynecol* 2003;102(3):496–498.

Nine

Stroke

Chapter 36
Stroke

Edward C. Jauch and Todd J. Crocco

Health care providers, hospitals, and communities must develop stroke systems to increase the efficiency and effectiveness of stroke care. Emergency medical services (EMS) use is strongly associated with decreased time to initial physician assessment, computed tomography (CT) imaging for stroke, and neurologic evaluation. Once a patient with probable stroke is identified, EMS personnel should transport the patient to the nearest, most appropriate facility. Prearrival notification of the facility is key, decreasing time to examination by a physician, CT imaging, and reperfusion therapy. An ambulance may bypass a hospital that does not have the resources or the institutional commitment to treat patients with a stroke if a more appropriate hospital, preferably a stroke center, is available within a reasonable transport interval.

■ Minimizing disability from stroke starting with dispatch
■ Priority transport to an appropriate facility for stroke care
■ Identification of patients with ischemic stroke for reperfusion therapy
■ Update of 2007 AHA/ASA ischemic stroke guidelines

Key Points from AHA ASA 2007 Ischemic Stroke Update

- EMS activation and transport result in faster hospital arrival and decreased emergency department (ED) evaluation time.
- EMS dispatchers can identify 50% of patients with stroke.
- Public education programs result in sustained identification and treatment of stroke patients.
- Designation of *primary stroke centers* for emergency stroke care is strongly recommended.
- Patients should be transported to the nearest stroke center for evaluation and care if a stroke center is located within a reasonable transport distance and transport time.

See Web site for AHA/ASA guidelines update for management of patients with ischemic stroke.

Introduction

Each year in the United States over 780,000 people suffer a new or repeat stroke. On average a new stroke occurs every 40 seconds. More than 180,000 of these people will die, making stroke the third leading cause of death in the United States.[1] Many advances have been made in stroke prevention, treatment, and rehabilitation.[2,3] For example, fibrinolytic therapy can limit the extent of neurologic damage from stroke and improve outcome, but the time available for treatment is limited.[3,4]

STROKE FACTS[1]

On average, someone in the United States has a stroke every 40 seconds.

- On average, someone dies of a stroke every 3 to 4 minutes.
- Each year over 780,000 people experience a new or recurrent stroke. About 600,000 of these are first strokes and 180,000 are recurrent strokes.
- Men's stroke incidence rates are greater than women's at younger ages but not at older ages. Each year approximately 60,000 more women than men have a stroke.
- Blacks have almost twice the risk of first-ever stroke compared with whites.
- Silent strokes are a common occurrence, increasing in prevalence from 11% for ages 55 to 64 and 43% over age 85.

Approximately 15% of strokes are heralded by transient ischemic attacks (TIAs).

Health care providers, hospitals, and communities must develop systems to increase the efficiency and effectiveness of stroke care. The seven "Ds" of stroke care—detection, dispatch, delivery, door (arrival and urgent triage in the ED), data, decision, and drug administration—highlight the major steps in diagnosis and treatment and the key points at which delays can occur.[5,6]

This chapter summarizes the management of acute stroke in the adult patient, including out-of-hospital care through the first hours of treatment; this early management focuses on the rapid identification of acute ischemic stroke while allowing evaluation for reperfusion therapy. Highlights from and updates of the 2007 ischemic stroke guidelines are included. For additional information about the management of acute ischemic stroke and these guidelines, see the American Heart Association (AHA)/American Stroke Association (ASA) guidelines for the early management of adults with ischemic stroke.[7,8]

AHA/ASA GUIDELINES UPDATE

- Activation of the 911 system is strongly supported because it speeds treatment of stroke.
- Educational programs to increase public awareness are encouraged because they increase the number of patients evaluated and treated for stroke.
- Brief EMS assessment and transport of potential stroke patients to the closest facility providing emergency stroke care are recommended (class I).

Although reperfusion therapy in patients using tissue plasminogen activator (tPA) is presented in the context of early identification and management, other reperfusion methods may be available for selected patients in specialized stroke centers. These include intra-arterial administration of a fibrinolytic agent in carefully selected patients,[9–13] angioplasty and stenting,[14] mechanical clot distruption,[15] and clot extraction.[16]

The Stroke Chain of Survival

The AHA and ASA have developed a community-oriented "stroke chain of survival" that links specific actions to be taken by patients and family members with recommended actions by out-of-hospital health care responders, ED personnel, and in-hospital specialty services (Fig. 36-1):

- Rapid recognition and reaction to stroke warning signs
- Rapid start of prehospital care
- Rapid EMS transport and hospital prenotification
- Rapid diagnosis and treatment in hospital

The 7 D's of Stroke Survival

In ST-segment elevation myocardial infarction (STEMI), time is muscle. When acute ischemic stroke occurs, time is brain, so the reperfusion concept was expanded to include not only patients with acute coronary syndromes (STEMI) but also highly selected stroke patients.[5] Hazinski was the first to describe an analogous series of linked actions to guide advanced cardiac life support (ACLS) stroke care.[17] Borrowing from the "door-to-drug" theme of the National Heart Attack Alert Program for fibrinolytic treatment of STEMI,[18] the seven "Ds" of ACLS stroke care begin each step with the letter D: detection, dispatch, delivery, door, data, decision, and drug. Table 36-1 lists the seven steps of stroke care plus the major actions in each step. At each step, care must be organized and efficient in order to avoid needless delays.

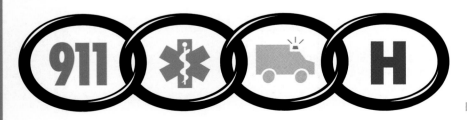

| FIGURE 36-1 • The stroke chain of survival.

TABLE 36-1 • The 7 "D's" of Stroke Care in the Reperfusion Era

7 "D's"	Major Actions
✔ Detection	• Early recognition—onset of stroke signs and symptoms
✔ Dispatch	• Activation of the EMS system and prompt EMS response
✔ Delivery	• Transportation, with prearrival notification, to receiving hospital • Provision of appropriate prehospital assessment and care
✔ Door	• Immediate general and neurologic assessment in the ED • Aim for predefined evaluation targets
✔ Data	• CT scan • Serial neurologic exams • Review for tPA exclusions • Review patient data
✔ Decision	• Patient remains candidate for tPA therapy? If "yes," then: — Review risks and benefits with patient and family — Obtain informed consent for tPA therapy
✔ Drug	• Begin tPA treatment within 3-hour time limit

Definitions

Acute ischemic stroke (AIS), refers to an abrupt or rapidly developing neurologic impairment lasting >24 hours that is attributable to a focal vascular cause and results in an interruption of the blood supply to a region of the brain. The *sudden onset of focal brain dysfunction* is the hallmark of stroke.[19] Experts and clinicians most often classify strokes as either *hemorrhagic* or *ischemic*. Hemorrhagic stroke occurs when a blood vessel within the brain ruptures. Ischemic stroke occurs when a blood vessel becomes blocked, typically by plaque and/or clot, interrupting flow to a region of the brain. If blood flow is interrupted long enough, irreversible infarction of brain tissue often ensues. Although the causes of stroke are numerous, the distinction between ischemic and hemorrhagic types is important, since therapy differs significantly based on stroke type (Fig. 36-2).

Ischemic Stroke

Definition and Categories of Ischemic Stroke

In an ischemic stroke (87% of all strokes[1]), interruption in the blood supply is caused by occlusion of an artery to a region of the brain. Ischemic strokes can be defined on the basis of etiology and duration of symptoms. With the more widespread use of modern brain imaging, many patients with symptoms lasting ≤24 hours are found to have an infarction. The most recent definition of stroke for clinical trials has required either symptoms lasting >24 hours or imaging of an acute, clinically relevant brain lesion in patients with rapidly vanishing symptoms.

Ischemic stroke is classified into categories based upon the presumed mechanism of stroke and the type and local-

ization of the vascular lesion.[20] Strokes are generally subdivided into the following categories:[20]

- **Thrombotic stroke (large artery atherosclerotic stroke):** An acute thrombus that occludes an artery is superimposed on chronic arterial narrowing, acutely altered endothelial lining, or both. This pathophysiology parallels that for acute coronary syndromes (ACS), where a ruptured or eroded plaque is the proximate cause of most episodes of ACS. The artery may be extracranial or intracranial.
- **Embolic stroke:** Intravascular material, most often a blood clot, separates from a proximal source and flows through an artery until it occludes a distal site. Many of these events are cardioembolic—originating from the heart—in patients with atrial fibrillation, valvular heart disease, acute MI, or rarely endocarditis. Cardiogenic

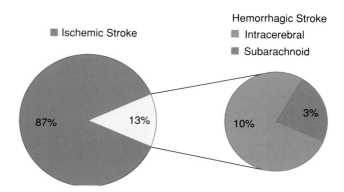

FIGURE 36-2 • Type of stroke. Some 87% of strokes are ischemic and potentially eligible for fibrinolytic therapy if patients otherwise qualify; 13% of strokes are hemorrhagic, and the majority of these are intracerebral. Men have 1.25 times the number of strokes as women, and blacks have almost twice the risk of first-ever stroke compared with whites.[11]

cerebral embolism is responsible for about 20% of ischemic strokes. There is a history of nonvalvular atrial fibrillation (AF) in about half of these patients, valvular heart disease in one fourth, and left ventricular (LV) thrombus in almost one third.[21]

- **Other causes:** These include small-vessel disease and other causes such as sickle cell disease, hypercoagulable states, and arterial dissection, resulting in a more global pattern of brain infarction. This is typically due to periods of significant systemic hypotension and inadequate cerebral perfusion that cannot support the metabolic demands of the brain tissue. Hypoperfusion stroke often occurs in patients who recover cardiac function after sudden cardiac arrest.
- **Undetermined**

Transient Ischemic Attack

By conventional clinical definitions, if the neurologic symptoms continue for 24 hours, a person is diagnosed with stroke; otherwise a focal neurologic deficit lasting ≤24 hours is defined as a TIA. However, approximately one third of all TIAs would be classified as stroke based on diffusion-weighted magnetic resonance imaging,[22] and new diagnostic techniques have shown that up to 60% of patients with a TIA have definite radiographic evidence of brain infarction.[23] A proposed new definition of TIA is a "brief episode of neurologic dysfunction caused by a focal disturbance of brain or retinal ischemia, with clinical symptoms typically lasting <1 hour, and without evidence of infarction."[24]

The distinction between TIA and ischemic stroke has become less important in recent years because many of the preventive approaches are applicable to both groups. TIA and stroke share pathogenetic mechanisms; prognosis may vary, depending on their severity and cause; and definitions are dependent on the timing and degree of the diagnostic evaluation.

TIAs, however, are an important determinant of stroke, with 90-day risks of stroke reported as high as 10.5% and the greatest stroke risk apparent in the first week.[25,26] Risk scores have been developed and validated to allow risk stratification of patients with TIA, including duration of symptoms.[25,27–29]

Classification by Vascular Supply

Strokes are also classified by vascular supply and anatomic location:

- **Anterior circulation (carotid artery territory) stroke:** Stroke that results from occlusion of branches of the *carotid artery*. Such strokes usually involve the cerebral hemispheres.
- **Posterior circulation (vertebrobasilar artery territory) stroke:** Stroke that follows occlusion of branches of the *vertebral or basilar arteries*. These strokes usually involve the brainstem or cerebellum.

Hemorrhagic Stroke

Hemorrhagic strokes (13% of all strokes) occur when a blood vessel in the brain suddenly ruptures, with hemor-

rhage into the surrounding tissue. Damage typically results from direct trauma to brain cells; expanding hematoma effects leading to elevated intracranial pressure; release of damaging neurotoxic mediators; local vascular spasm; and loss of blood supply to brain tissue downstream from the ruptured vessel.

There are two types of hemorrhagic stroke, based on the location of the arterial rupture:[30]

- **Intracerebral hemorrhagic stroke (10%):** Occurs when blood ruptures directly into the brain parenchyma, usually from small intracerebral arterioles pathologically altered by chronic hypertension.
  - Hypertension is the most common cause of intracerebral hemorrhage.[31]
  - Among the elderly, amyloid angiopathy appears to play a major role in intracerebral hemorrhage.
- **Subarachnoid hemorrhagic stroke (3%):** Occurs when blood leaks from a cerebral vessel into the subarachnoid space. If the rupture occurs in a cerebral artery, the blood is released at systemic arterial pressure, causing sudden, painful, and dramatic neurologic symptoms.
  - Aneurysms cause most subarachnoid hemorrhages.
  - Arteriovenous malformations cause approximately 5% of subarachnoid hemorrhages.

Pathophysiology

Concept of the Evolving "Ruptured Plaque"

The "ruptured plaque" pathophysiologic concept of ACS is also applicable to many ischemic strokes (see Chapter 1, Figures 1-1 and 1-5).[32–34] An ulcerated ruptured plaque is the key mechanism of most thrombotic and embolic strokes in patients without valvular heart disease or atrial fibrillation. In thrombotic stroke, complete occlusion typically develops at an atherosclerotic plaque.[35,36] In embolic stroke, the developing thrombus breaks off and floats downstream, ultimately lodging in and obstructing a smaller arterial vessel. A thrombotically active carotid plaque associated with high inflammatory infiltrate was observed in about 75% of patients with ipsilateral major stroke. In addition, ruptured plaques of these patients affected by stroke were characterized by the presence of a more severe inflammatory infiltrate—comprising monocytes, macrophages, and T lymphocytes—compared with those observed in the TIA and asymptomatic groups.[37] Ruptured plaques may occur not only in the intracranial branches of the carotid and vertebrobasilar arteries but also in the extracranial portions of the carotid arteries and in the aorta.

Vessel occlusion results from the interaction between blood vessels, activated coagulation components of blood, inflammatory cells, and chemical mediators of inflammation. The pathology of recently symptomatic carotid plaques is similar to that of culprit coronary plaques, with strong correlations between macrophage infiltration and plaque instability.[34]

- The most common cause of acute ischemic stroke is atherosclerosis of the carotid or vertebrobasilar artery.

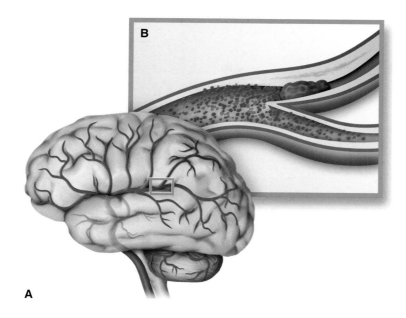

FIGURE 36-3 • Occlusion in a artery due to cerebral embolism at the arterial bifurcation. **A.** Area of infarction surrounding immediate site and distal portion of brain tissue after occlusion. **B.** Area of ischemic penumbra [ischemic but not yet infarcted (dead) brain tissue] surrounding areas of infarction. This ischemic penumbra tissue is alive but dysfunctional because of altered membrane potentials. The dysfunction is potentially reversible. Current stroke treatment attempts to keep the area of permanent brain infarction as small as possible by preventing the areas of reversible brain ischemia in the penumbra from transforming into larger areas of irreversible brain infarction. [Reprinted with permission of Genentech, Inc, from the Internet Stroke Center (www.strokecenter.org). Copyright Genentech, Inc.]

Varying degrees of inflammation in vulnerable atherosclerotic plaques predispose these arteries to endothelial erosion, plaque rupture, and platelet activation as well as aggregation.

- The ensuing development of a thrombus—composed of platelets, fibrin, and other elements of coagulation—can completely occlude an artery already narrowed by atherosclerosis. This occlusion of blood flow first leads to ischemia and ultimately to infarction of downstream brain tissue, producing a thrombotic stroke.
- The thrombus, either before or immediately after it becomes completely occlusive, may dislodge and travel to more distal cerebral arteries, producing an embolic stroke (Fig. 36-3).

Postocclusion Dynamics

Downstream from the thrombotic or embolic obstruction, brain cells begin to die and necrosis occurs. With persistent occlusion, an area of irreversible brain damage (infarction or necrosis) develops.

- Surrounding the central area of necrosis or infarction is an area of ischemia called the *ischemic penumbra*.
- This area of "threatened" but still viable brain tissue is an area of *potentially reversible* brain injury.[38–40]

"TIME IS BRAIN"

The recently coined term "brain attack" and the phrase "time is brain" convey the sense of urgency in stroke care. Once restriction of blood flow occurs as a result of occlusion, an ever-increasing amount of brain tissue becomes irreversibly injured over time. There is only a limited amount of time available to recognize and treat reversible brain ischemia.[41–43]

Other Pathophysiologic Processes

Atrial Fibrillation

Atrial fibrillation remains the most frequent cause of cardioembolic stroke.[44]

- The noncontracting walls of the fibrillating left atrium and left atrial appendage serve as both a stimulus and a reservoir for small emboli.
- The risk of stroke in patients with nonvalvular atrial fibrillation averages 5% per year, two to seven times that of people without atrial fibrillation.[45–47]

Hypertension

Hypertension causes a thickening of the walls of small cerebral arteries, leading to reduced flow and a predisposition to thrombosis.

- Lacunar infarcts exemplify the type of thrombotic stroke caused by chronic hypertension. They are thought to result from occlusion of a small perforating artery to the subcortical areas of the brain.
- The major cerebrovascular burden imposed by chronic hypertension is hemorrhagic stroke.

Stroke Risk Factors

Risk factors can be identified in most stroke patients.[48] Primary and secondary stroke prevention requires identification of a patient's risk factors, followed by elimination, control, or treatment of as many factors as possible:

- Elimination (e.g., smoking)
- Control (e.g., hypertension, diabetes mellitus)
- Treatment (e.g., antiplatelet therapy, carotid endarterectomy when indicated)

Table 36-2 lists the major modifiable stroke risk factors.

| TABLE 36-2 • Stroke Risk: Factors That Can Be Modified

Risk Factor	Comments
Hypertension	• One of the most important modifiable risk factors for ischemic and spontaneous hemorrhagic stroke[26,27] • Risk of hemorrhagic stroke increases markedly with elevations in systolic pressure • Control of hypertension significantly decreases the risk of stroke[26,28,29]
Cigarette Smoking	• All of the following smoking effects have been linked to stroke: — Accelerated atherosclerosis — Transient elevations in blood pressure — Release of toxic enzymes (linked to formation of aneurysms) — Altered platelet function and reduced platelet survival[30,31] • Cessation of cigarette smoking reduces the risk of stroke[32,33]
Transient Ischemic Attack	• Highly significant indicator of a person at increased risk for stroke[5,34] • 25% of stroke patients have had a previous TIA[35] • 10% of patients presenting to an ED with TIA will have a completed stroke within 90 days; half of these within the first 2 days[36] • Antiplatelet agents (e.g., aspirin, ticlopidine) can reduce the risk of stroke in patients with TIA
Heart Disease	• Coronry artery disease and heart failure double the risk of stroke[37] • Atrial fibrillation increases the risk of embolic stroke • Prophylactic warfarin, given to patients with atrial fibrillation, reduces the risk of embolic stroke[38-40]
Diabetes Mellitus	• Highly associated with accelerated atherosclerosis • Careful monitoring and control of hyperglycemia reduce the risk of microvascular complications due to diabetes, and reduction of microvascular complications reduces stroke risk
Hypercoagulopathy	• Any hypercoagulative state (e.g., protein S or C deficiency, cancer, pregnancy) increases the risk of stroke
High RBC Count and Sickle Cell Anemia	• A moderate increase in RBC count increases the risk of stroke • Increases in RBC count can be treated by removing blood and replacing it with IV fluid or by administering an anticoagulant • Sickle cell anemia increases the risk of stroke because "sickled" red blood cells can clump, causing arterial occlusion. Stroke risk from sickle cell anemia may be reduced by maintaining adequate oxygenation and hydration and by providing exchange transfusions
Carotid Bruit*	• Carotid bruits often indicate partial obstruction (atherosclerosis) of an artery indicating vascular disease and associated stroke risk • This risk is reduced by surgical endarterectomy but only in symptomatic patients with >70% stenosis[41] • Some evidence suggests that carotid endarterectomy is beneficial in selected asymptomatic patients with high-grade stenosis[42]

*Absence of a bruit does not preclude vascular disease.
RBC, red blood cell; TIA, transient ischemic attack.

PHYSICAL ACTIVITY REDUCES THE RISK OF STROKE

• A meta-analysis of reports of 31 observational studies conducted mainly in the United States and Europe found that moderate and high levels of leisure-time and occupational physical activity protected against total stroke, hemorrhagic stroke, and ischemic stroke.[23]

• Physical activity reduces stroke risk. Results from the Physicians' Health Study showed a lower stroke risk associated with vigorous exercise among men.[24,25] The Harvard Alumni Study also showed a decrease in total stroke risk in men who were highly physically active.

Stroke Management

Stroke treatment begins with the recognition of the symptoms of stroke. An important component in this initial step is education—of the patient, family, community, 911 dispatcher, prehospital care provider, and health care provider. Once recognition of potential stroke symptoms occurs, management involves expeditious transfer of the patient to an appropriate facility for further assessment and care. Stroke centers are important because they focus on the integration of multidisciplinary care helping ensure appropriate hemodynamic management, optimal glucose control, prevention of aspiration, and rehabilitation. Figure 36-4 is the suspected stroke algorithm, which identifies treatment goals for these patients.

Signs and Symptoms of Ischemic Stroke

The warning signs of an ischemic stroke or TIA may be varied, subtle, and transient, but they represent a potentially life-threatening neurologic illness (Fig. 36-4, Box 1). Like the symptoms of an ACS, symptoms of ischemic stroke can be misinterpreted and denied by patients. Emergency health care providers should recognize the importance of these symptoms and respond quickly with effective interventions in stroke management. The signs and symptoms of a stroke may be subtle and include:

- Sudden numbness or weakness of the face, arm, or leg, especially on one side of the body
- Sudden confusion, trouble speaking or understanding speech
- Sudden trouble seeing in one or both eyes
- Sudden trouble walking, dizziness, loss of balance or coordination
- Sudden severe headache with no known cause

Out-of-Hospital Management: The Important Role of the Community EMS System in Stroke Care (Fig. 36-4, Box 2)

See Web site for AHA/ASA guidelines for implementation strategies, EMS services, and stroke systems of care.

Three of the four links in the stroke chain of survival and the first three of the seven Ds of stroke care (detection, dispatch, and delivery) require effective operation of the EMS system. For this reason the *2005 AHA Guidelines for Cardiopulmonary Resuscitation and Emergency Cardiovascular Care* and the 2007 AHA/ASA guidelines for the early management of adults with ischemic stroke strongly emphasize the important role of these personnel and services.[8] Recent data show that 29% to 65% of patients with signs and symptoms of stroke contact local EMS, but only

14% to 32% of them arrive within 2 hours of symptom onset.[52,53] EMS use is strongly associated with decreased time to initial physician assessment, computed tomography (CT) imaging for stroke, and neurologic evaluation.[54,55]

TIME TO STROKE TREATMENT

EMS use is strongly associated with *decreased* time to

- Initial physician assessment
- CT imaging for stroke
- Neurologic evaluation

✔ *Detection: Early Recognition of Stroke Signs and Symptoms*

Early treatment of stroke depends on the patient, family members, or other bystanders recognizing the event. Patients often ignore the initial signs and symptoms of a stroke and delay access to care for several hours after the onset of symptoms. Because of these time delays, many patients with ischemic stroke may not benefit from time-dependent therapies such as intravenous fibrinolytic treatment, which must be started within 3 hours of symptom onset.

In one study of 100 stroke patients, only 8% had received information about the signs of stroke, yet nearly half had previously had a prior TIA or stroke.[48] Unlike many acute myocardial infarctions in which chest pain can be a dramatic and unrelenting symptom, a stroke may have a subtle presentation with only mild facial paralysis or speech difficulty. Mild signs or symptoms may go unnoticed or be denied by the patient or bystander. Strokes that occur while the patient is asleep or when he or she is alone further hamper prompt recognition and action.

✔ *Dispatch: Call 911 and Priority EMS Dispatch*

Stroke patients and their families must understand the need to call 911 and activate the EMS system as soon as they suspect stroke signs or symptoms. The EMS system provides the safest and most efficient method for transporting the patient to the hospital.[56]

EMS Assessments and Actions

EMS assessments and actions for patients with suspected stroke include the following steps:

- Rapid identification of patients with signs and symptoms of acute stroke (through the performance of a prehospital stroke assessment tool)
- Support of vital functions
- Prearrival notification of the receiving facility
- Rapid transport of the patient to the most appropriate receiving facility (often a primary stroke center)
- Whenever possible, EMS should bring a witness with the patient to the receiving facility.

Emergency medical dispatchers play a critical role in the timely treatment of potential stroke patients. Data show that dispatchers correctly identify stroke symptoms on the basis

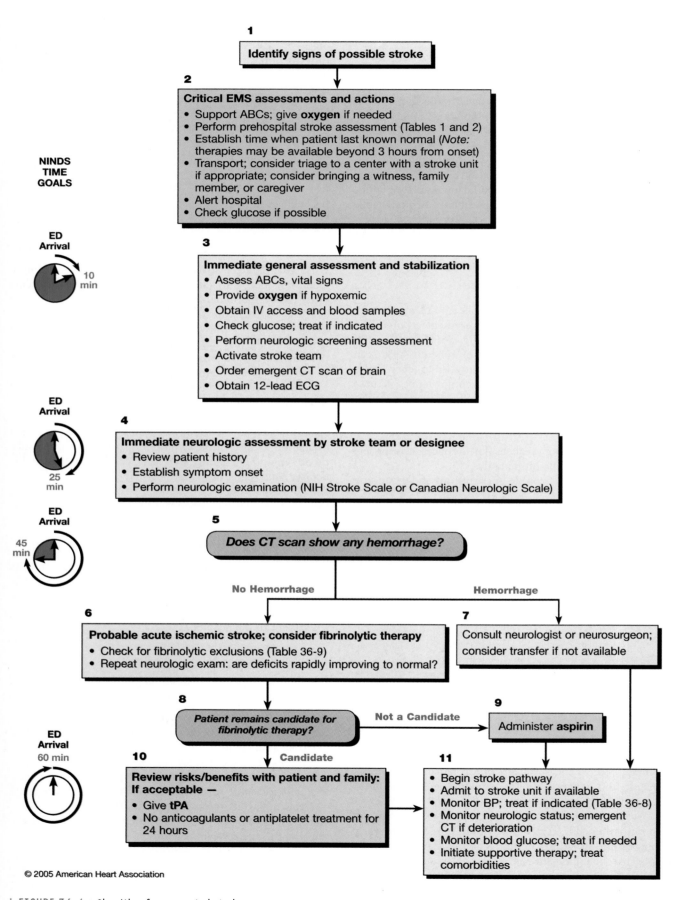

NINDS TIME GOALS

ED Arrival 10 min

ED Arrival 25 min

ED Arrival 45 min

ED Arrival 60 min

1 Identify signs of possible stroke

2 Critical EMS assessments and actions
- Support ABCs; give **oxygen** if needed
- Perform prehospital stroke assessment (Tables 1 and 2)
- Establish time when patient last known normal (*Note:* therapies may be available beyond 3 hours from onset)
- Transport; consider triage to a center with a stroke unit if appropriate; consider bringing a witness, family member, or caregiver
- Alert hospital
- Check glucose if possible

3 Immediate general assessment and stabilization
- Assess ABCs, vital signs
- Provide **oxygen** if hypoxemic
- Obtain IV access and blood samples
- Check glucose; treat if indicated
- Perform neurologic screening assessment
- Activate stroke team
- Order emergent CT scan of brain
- Obtain 12-lead ECG

4 Immediate neurologic assessment by stroke team or designee
- Review patient history
- Establish symptom onset
- Perform neurologic examination (NIH Stroke Scale or Canadian Neurologic Scale)

5 *Does CT scan show any hemorrhage?*

No Hemorrhage   Hemorrhage

6 Probable acute ischemic stroke; consider fibrinolytic therapy
- Check for fibrinolytic exclusions (Table 36-9)
- Repeat neurologic exam: are deficits rapidly improving to normal?

7 Consult neurologist or neurosurgeon; consider transfer if not available

8 *Patient remains candidate for fibrinolytic therapy?*   Not a Candidate

9 Administer **aspirin**

10 Review risks/benefits with patient and family: If acceptable —
- Give **tPA**
- No anticoagulants or antiplatelet treatment for 24 hours

Candidate

11
- Begin stroke pathway
- Admit to stroke unit if available
- Monitor BP; treat if indicated (Table 36-8)
- Monitor neurologic status; emergent CT if deterioration
- Monitor blood glucose; treat if needed
- Initiate supportive therapy; treat comorbidities

| FIGURE 36-4 • Algorithm for suspected stroke.

| TABLE 36-3 • Key Components of a Focused Stroke Patient History

Onset of symptoms
Recent events
　Stroke
　Myocardial infarction
　Trauma
　Surgery
　Bleeding
Comorbid diseases
　Hypertension
　Diabetes mellitus
Use of medications
　Anticoagulants
　Insulin
　Antihypertensives

Source: AHA/ASA Ischemic Stroke Guidelines.

of just the initial phone description in more than half of all stroke cases.[52,57] Dispatchers can triage emergencies over the telephone and prioritize calls to ensure a rapid response by the EMS system. Specific dispatch educational efforts about stroke are encouraged, and stroke dispatch should be given a priority, like that for acute myocardial infarction and trauma.

✔ *Delivery: Prompt Transport and Prearrival Notification to Hospital*

Leaders in EMS and emergency medicine must develop training programs and patient care protocols to guide the actions of prehospital care providers. After the basic life support (BLS) primary and ACLS secondary surveys and appropriate actions have been performed for airway, breathing, and circulation, EMS providers should immediately obtain a focused history and patient assessment (Table 36-3).

A key component of the patient's history is the *time of symptom onset or when the patient was last known to be normal.*

The history *must* include this information. The provider may need to obtain this and other details of the patient's history from family or the appropriate bystander. Preferably this person should be transported with the patient. Prehospital providers can help establish the precise time of stroke onset or the last time the patient was noted to be neurologically normal. This time point is viewed as "time zero," a starting point that is critical for time-dependent treatments.

Out-of-Hospital Stroke Scales for Early Detection and Delivery

The assessment includes a brief and focused examination for stroke. Providers can conduct a rapid neurologic assessment using validated prehospital stroke assessment tools such as the Cincinnati Prehospital Stroke Scale[58,59] or the Los Angeles Prehospital Stroke Screen.[60,61] Studies have confirmed the sensitivity and specificity of these two scales for prehospital identification of patients with ischemic stroke.

Cincinnati Prehospital Stroke Scale (CPSS)　The CPSS (Table 36-4) is based on physical examination only, and it can be completed in 30 to 60 seconds.[58] The EMS responder checks for three physical findings:

- Facial droop (Fig. 36-5)
- Arm weakness
- Speech abnormalities

Los Angeles Prehospital Stroke Screen (LAPSS)　The LAPSS (Table 36-5) requires the examiner to rule out other causes of altered level of consciousness (e.g., history of seizures, severe hyperglycemia or hypoglycemia) and then identify asymmetry (right versus left) in any of three exam categories:

- Facial smile or grimace
- Grip
- Arm strength (Fig. 36-6)

The LAPSS builds on the physical findings of the CPSS, adding criteria for age, history of seizures, symptom duration, blood glucose level, and ambulation. A person with positive findings for all six criteria has a 97% probability of stroke.

| TABLE 36-4 • The Cincinnati Prehospital Stroke Scale

Test	Findings
Facial Droop: Have the patient show teeth or smile (Figure 36-5)	• **Normal**—both sides of face move equally • **Abnormal**—one side of face does not move as well as the other side
Arm Drift: Patient closes eyes and extends both arms straight out. with palms up, for 10 seconds (Figure 36-6)	• **Normal**—both arms move the same or both arms do not move at all (other findings, such as pronator drift, may be helpful) • **Abnormal**—one arm does not move or one arm drifts down compared with the other
Abnormal Speech: Have the patient say "you can't teach an old dog new tricks"	• **Normal**—patient uses correct words with no slurring • **Abnormal**—patient slurs words, uses the wrong words, or is unable to speak

Source: Kothari R, Hall K, Brott T, et al. Early stroke recognition: developing an out-of-hospital NIH stroke scale. *Acad Emerg Med* 1997;4:986–990.

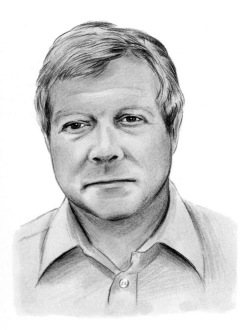 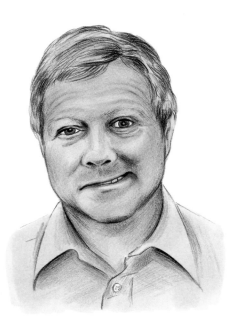

| FIGURE 36-5 • Facial droop.

Out-of-hospital stroke scales provide objective, validated methods for early detection of stroke and enable appropriate triage and prearrival notification to the receiving hospital. When EMS personnel discover findings consistent with stroke on either the CPSS or the LAPSS, they should notify the receiving hospital that they have a patient with possible acute stroke. This information allows the hospital to activate stroke protocols before the patient arrives to ensure rapid patient evaluation and therapy. Advanced planning and collaboration allow medical control physicians to direct EMS providers to transport the patient to a hospital designated and organized to provide the full range of acute stroke care.

| TABLE 36-5 • Los Angeles Prehospital Stroke Screen

For *evaluation of acute, noncomatose, nontraumatic neurlogic complaint.* If items 1 through 6 are *all **checked "Yes"*** (or "Unknown"), provide prearrival notification to hospital of potential stroke patient. If any item is checked "No," return to appropriate treatment protocol. *Interpretation:* 93% of patients with stroke will have a positive LAPSS score (sensitivity = 93%), and 97% of those with a positive LAPSS score will have a stroke (specificity = 97%). Note that the patient may still be experiencing a stroke if LAPSS criteria are not met.

Criteria	Yes	Unknown	No
1. Age >45 years	☐	☐	☐
2. History of seizures of epilepsy absent	☐	☐	☐
3. Symptom duration <24 hours	☐	☐	☐
4. At baseline, patient is not wheelchair bound or bedridden	☐	☐	☐
5. Blood glucose between 60 and 400	☐	☐	☐
6. Obvious asymmetry (right vs left) in *any* of the following 3 exam categories **(must be unilateral):**	☐	☐	☐

	Equal	R Weak	L Weak
Facial smile/grimace	☐	☐ Droop	☐ Droop
Grip	☐	☐ Weak grip ☐ No grip	☐ Weak grip ☐ No grip
Arm strength	☐	☐ Drifts down ☐ Falls rapidly	☐ Drifts down ☐ Falls rapidly

Sources: Kidwell CS, Saver JL, Schubert GB, et al. Design and retrospective analysis of the Los Angeles prehospital stroke screen (LAPSS). *Prehosp Emerg Care* 1998;2:267–273. Kidwell CS, Starkman S, Eckstein M, et al. Identifying stroke in the field: prospective validation of the Los Angeles Prehospital Stroke Screen (LAPSS). *Stroke.* 2000;31:71–76.

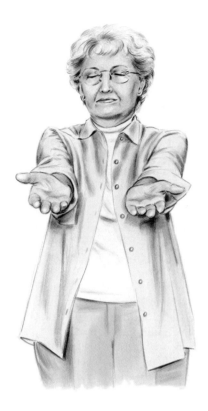
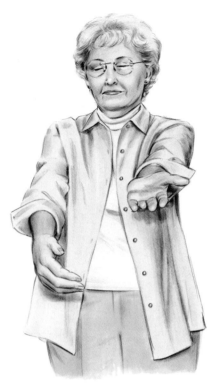

FIGURE 36-6 • One-sided motor weakness (right arm).

Destination Hospital Protocols

Once a patient with probable stroke is identified, EMS personnel should transport him or her to the nearest *most appropriate* facility. Prearrival notification of the facility is key and allows for decreasing time to examination by a physician, CT imaging, and reperfusion therapy. An ambulance may bypass a hospital that does not have the resources or the institutional commitment to treat patients with stroke if a more appropriate hospital is available within a reasonable transport interval.

Air medical transport appears to be beneficial, but studies are limited. Helicopters' ability to rapidly transport patients to appropriate facilities may improve the opportunity for reperfusion therapy in more rural areas.[62–66] Helicopter transfer of patients has been shown to be cost-effective.[65]

HOSPITAL BYPASS

An ambulance may bypass a hospital if
- The facility does not have the resources for acute stroke care.
- The facility lacks an institutional commitment to treat patients with stroke.
- A more appropriate hospital is available within a reasonable transport interval.

 See Web site for AHA/ASA recommendations for comprehensive stroke centers.

Prehospital Initial Studies

Prehospital care and assessment beyond initial management should be completed during patient transport and should not delay transport to the hospital. Prehospital intervention in potential stroke patients includes establishing intravenous (IV) access with normal saline, ensuring adequate oxygenation and ventilation, hemodynamic support if necessary, avoiding glucose-containing fluids unless hypoglycemia is strongly suspected or present (hyperglycemia [blood glucose >200] is associated with worse outcomes in stroke patients[67–71]), checking and treating abnormal blood glucose levels, and initiating cardiac monitoring. Obtain a 12-lead electrocardiogram (ECG) if the patient has symptoms concerning for ACS.

In-Hospital Management

Collaborative stroke protocols should be employed in the ED to minimize delay to definitive diagnosis and therapy.[72] Diagnostic studies ordered in the ED are aimed at:

- Excluding other nonstroke causes of the patient's symptoms (hypoglycemia, etc.)
- Establishing stroke as the cause of the patient's symptoms
- Differentiating ischemic from hemorrhagic stroke
- Rapidly providing stroke therapy to appropriate patients with ischemic stroke, which may include intravenous tPA if no contraindications are present

✔ *Door: Immediate ED Triage*

Immediate General Assessment and Stabilization (Fig. 36-4, Box 3)

ED Arrival

10 min

As a goal, ED personnel should assess the patient with suspected stroke within 10 minutes of arrival in the ED. The ED physician, typically the first member of the stroke team to evaluate the patient, should ensure respiratory and hemodynamic stability, perform a neurologic screening assessment, order an emergent CT scan of the brain if stroke is believed possible, coordinate with the other members of the stroke team, or arrange consultation with a stroke expert if available. General care includes assessment and support of airway, breathing, and circulation and evaluation of baseline vital signs. Oxygen should be administered to hypoxemic patients or those with unknown oxygen saturation. Clinicians may consider giving oxygen to patients who are not hypoxemic. High-flow oxygen therapy in a small clinical trial of patients without hypoxia was associated with transient improvement in clinical deficits and abnormalities on magnetic resonance imaging (MRI), but large scale clinical trials are not available.[73,74] Oxygen saturation should be monitored and maintained at ≥92%. Establish (or confirm) IV access and obtain blood samples for baseline studies (blood count, coagulation studies, blood glucose, electrolytes, etc.). Hypoglycemia should be treated immediately if present.

A 12-lead ECG and other ancillary studies do not routinely take priority over the CT scan of the brain. However, the ECG may ultimately identify a recent acute myocardial infarction or arrhythmia (e.g., atrial fibrillation) as the cause of a cardioembolic stroke and is recommended early in the evaluation of patients with stroke.[75] If the patient is hemodynamically stable, immediate treatment of arrhythmias prior to CT scan—including bradycardia, premature atrial or ventricular contractions, or abnormal atrioventricular conduction—may be unnecessary.[76]

✔ *Data: ED Evaluation, Prompt Laboratory Studies, CT Imaging*

Immediately initiate diagnostic studies in all patients to assess for conditions that may mimic stroke and comorbid problems that can complicate management. Consider the need for additional studies and perform them in selected patients. See Table 36-6.

Establish Time of Onset (<3 Hours Required for Intravenous tPA) Protocols for EMS personnel should direct them to ask the patient and family about when they

---

DO NOT DELAY CT IMAGING OR FIBRINOLYTIC THERAPY

Ancillary diagnostic studies should not delay CT imaging or time-dependent stroke therapies such as fibrinolysis when indicated unless contraindications to such therapies exist:

1. There is clinical suspicion of a bleeding disorder.
2. The patient has recently received heparin or warfarin.
3. Hypertension requires control.

| TABLE 36-6 • ED Evaluation and Diagnostic Studies

All Patients	Selected Patients
• Noncontrast brain CT or MRI	• Chest x-ray
• Blood glucose	• Hepatic function
• Serum electrolytes	• Blood alcohol and
• Renal function	toxicology screen
• CBC and platelet count	• Arterial blood gas
• Coagulation studies	• Lumbar puncture
(PTT, PT, INR)	• EEG
• Oxygen saturation	• Pregnancy test
• ECG	

CBC, complete blood count; CT, computed tomography; ECG, electrocardiogram; EEG, electroencephalogram; INR, international normalized ratio; MRI, magnetic resonance imaging; PT, prothrombin time; PTT, partial thromboplastin time.

---

first noted any stroke symptoms. Neither the patient nor family members may recall the exact hour and minute, but they may be able to relate the onset of symptoms to other events, such as a television or radio program that was playing, a telephone call, or someone's arrival or departure. Be aware that time of onset is difficult to establish for patients who are discovered unconscious, are unable to communicate, or awaken from sleep with neurologic abnormalities. In these cases the time of onset is considered the last time the patient was seen normal.

Inability to establish the time of symptom onset with accuracy is a contraindication to tPA therapy! If prehospital care personnel cannot reliably determine a specific time, ED personnel should continue the inquiries. Call or speak directly to a family member, coworker, or bystander.

Immediate Neurologic Screening Assessment The clinical status of stroke patients often fluctuates. Health care providers should perform serial focused neurologic examinations to detect any deterioration or improvement.

Immediate Neurologic Assessment by Stroke Team or Designee

ED Arrival

25 min

The patient's history and physical examination findings should be reviewed by a physician who is part of the stroke team, or, in the absence of a formal stroke team, a physician with expertise in the evaluation and management of acute stroke patients. Remote stroke expertise may also be helpful to the evaluation and care of such patients. (Fig. 36-4, Box 4). This may require interviewing out-of-hospital providers, witnesses, and family members to establish the time that the patient was last known to be normal. Neurologic assessment is performed incorporating either the National Institutes of Health (NIH) Stroke Scale or Canadian Neurologic Scale (see the ASA Web site: www.strokeassociation.org).

Determine Severity of Stroke (NIH Stroke Scale) The NIH Stroke Scale (NIHSS) is a validated measure of stroke severity based on a detailed neurologic physical examination.[41] The NIH Stroke Scale allows nurses, midlevel providers, nursing staff, and physicians to perform standardized neurologic evaluations of a patient.[41,77] The score correlates with long-term outcome in patients with ischemic stroke[77–79] and is designed to provide a reliable,[80] valid, and easy-to-perform alternative to the standard neurologic examination. The NIH Stroke Scale can be performed in <7 minutes. This instrument received further validation during the National Institute of Neurological Disorders and Stroke (NINDS) trial of tPA for acute ischemic stroke.[4] The NIHSS is associated with final size of infarct volume, prognosis, and hemorrhagic risk and potential response to fibrinolytic therapy.[81]

The total score ranges from 0 (normal) to 42 points. The scale covers the following major areas:[82]

- Level of consciousness: alert, drowsy; knows month, age; performs tasks correctly
- Visual assessment: follows finger with or without gaze palsy, forced deviation; hemianopsia (none, partial, complete, bilateral)
- Motor function: face, arm, leg strength
- Sensation: pinprick to face, arm, trunk, leg; compare side after side; neglect (extinction and inattention).
- Cerebellar function: finger to nose, heel to shin
- Language: aphasia (name items, describe a picture, read sentences); dysarthria (evaluate speech clarity by having patient repeat listed words)

An NIH Stroke Scale score of <4 usually indicates more limited neurologic deficits, such as sensory losses, dysarthria, or some manual clumsiness. Fibrinolytic agents are generally not recommended for these patients because treatment offers minimal benefits relative to the risks. Some disabling neurologic deficits, such as isolated severe aphasia (score of 3) or the visual field losses of hemianopsia (score of 2 or 3), can be associated with a low score on the NIH Stroke Scale. Patients with these more significant deficits may be exceptions to the recommendation against fibrinolytic agents for patients with an NIH Stroke Scale score of <4 (Table 36-7).

Severe deficits (score >22) indicate large areas of ischemic damage. Patients with such deficits face an increased risk of brain hemorrhage.[83] In general the use of fibrinolytic treatment in these patients should follow careful discussion with the patient, the patient's spouse and family, and the admitting physicians to ensure that everyone understands the risk and benefits. A favorable risk–benefit ratio varies from patient to patient. The responsible clinician should always evaluate therapeutic decisions on an individual basis in close collaboration with the patient and family.

Management of Hypertension Management of hypertension in the stroke patient is controversial. For patients eligible for fibrinolytic therapy, however, control of blood pressure is required to reduce the risk of bleeding. If a patient who is otherwise eligible for treatment with tPA has elevated blood pressure, providers can try to lower it to a systolic pressure of <185 mm Hg and a diastolic blood pressure of <110 mm Hg. Since the maximum interval from onset of stroke until effective treatment of stroke with tPA is limited, many patients with sustained hypertension above these levels (i.e., systolic blood pressure >185 mm Hg or diastolic blood pressure >110 mm Hg) may not be eligible for treatment with IV tPA (Table 36-8).[84,85]

*Fibrinolytic-**Ineligible** Patients* In patients who are not candidates for fibrinolytic therapy, more permissive hypertension is recommended. Pending more data, the consensus of the AHA ASA stroke panel is that emergency administration of antihypertensive agents should be withheld unless the diastolic blood pressure is >120 mm Hg or the systolic blood pressure is >220 mm Hg. The panel recognizes that no data show that these values are especially dangerous and emergency treatment is needed. However, the panel remains concerned by the evidence that aggressive lowering of blood pressure among patients may cause neurologic worsening, and the goal is to avoid overtreating blood pressure in patients with stroke until definitive data are available.

FIBRINOLYTIC-ELIGIBLE PATIENTS

Treatment of hypertension in acute ischemic stroke remains controversial. Administration of tPA with hypertension is associated with excess intracerebral hemorrhage.

- Data suggest that prompt treatment should be initiated when systolic blood pressure exceeds 180 mm Hg or diastolic blood pressure exceeds 105 mm Hg in patients who are otherwise eligible for tPA.
- A sustained blood pressure >185 mm Hg systolic or >110 mm Hg diastolic is a contraindication for administration of tPA.
- If blood pressure >185 mm Hg systolic or >105 mm Hg diastolic develops during or after tPA administration, begin immediate treatment.

Brain and Vascular Imaging

ED Arrival

45 min

The most commonly obtained brain imaging test is a noncontrast-enhanced CT scan, but some centers can now obtain an MRI scan as quickly and efficiently as a CT. The noncontrast CT scan accurately identifies most cases of acute intracranial hemorrhage and helps identify nonvascular causes of neurologic symptoms mimicking stroke (e.g., brain tumor). Ongoing research is evaluating advanced MRI, magnetic resonance angiography, and multimodal CT, which includes noncontrast CT, perfusion CT, and CT angiographic studies.

Ideally the CT scan should be completed within 25 minutes of the patient's arrival in the ED and should be read within 45 minutes of ED arrival (Fig 36-4, Box 5). Emergent CT or MRI scans of patients with suspected stroke should be promptly evaluated by a physician with expertise in the interpretation of these studies.[86,87] During the first few hours of an ischemic stroke, the noncontrast CT scan may not show signs of brain ischemia.

Category	Description	Score	Baseline Date/Time	Date/Time
1a. Level of consciousness (LOC) *(Alert, drowsy, etc)*	Alert	0		
	Drowsy	1		
	Stuporous	2		
	Coma	3		
1b. LOC questions *(Month, age)*	Answers both correctly	0		
	Answers 1 correctly	1		
	Incorrect	2		
1c. LOC commands *(Open, close eyes; make fist, let go)*	Obeys both correctly	0		
	Obeys 1 correctly	1		
	Incorrect	2		
2. Best gaze *(Eyes open—patient follows examiners's finger or face)*	Normal	0		
	Partial gaze palsy	1		
	Forced deviation	2		
3. Visual *(Introduce visual stimulus/threat to patient's visual field quadrants)*	No visual loss	0		
	Partial hemianopia	1		
	Complete hemianopia	2		
	Bilateral hemianopia	3		
4. Facial palsy *(Show teeth, raise eyebrows, and squeeze eyes shut)*	Normal	0		
	Minor	1		
	Partial	2		
	Complete	3		
5a. Motor arm—left *(Elevate extremity to 90° and score drift/movement)*	No drift	0		
	Drift	1		
	Can't resist gravity	2		
	No effort against gravity	3		
	No movement	4		
	Amputation, joint fusion (explain)	9		
5b. Motor arm—right *(Elevate extremity to 90° and score drift/movement)*	No drift	0		
	Drift	1		
	Can't resist gravity	2		
	No effort against gravity	3		
	No movement	4		
	Amputation, joint fusion (explain)	9		
6a. Motor leg—left *(Elevate extremity to 30° and score drift/movement)*	No drift	0		
	Drift	1		
	Can't resist gravity	2		
	No effort agaisnt gravity	3		
	No movement	4		
	Amputation, joint fusion (explain)	9		
6b. Motor leg—right *(Elevate extremity to 30° and score drift/movement)*	No drift	0		
	Drift	1		
	Can't resist gravity	2		
	No effort against gravity	3		
	No movement	4		
	Amputation, joint fusion (explain)	9		
7. Limb ataxia *(Finger-nose, heel down shin)*	Absent	0		
	Present in 1 limb	1		
	Present in 2 limbs	2		
8. Sensory *(Pinprick to face, arm, trunk, and leg—compare side to side)*	Normal	0		
	Partial loss	1		
	Severe loss	2		
9. Best language *(Name items, describe a picture, and read sentences)*	No aphasia	0		
	Mild to moderate aphasia	1		
	Severe aphasia	2		
	Mute	3		
10. Dysarthria *(Evaluate speech clarity by patient repeating listed words)*	Normal articulation	0		
	Mild to moderate dysarthria	1		
	Near to unintelligible or worse	2		
	intubated or other physical barrier	9		
11. Extinction and inattention *(Use information from prior testing to identify neglect or double simultaneous stimuli testing)*	No neglect	0		
	Partial neglect	1		
	Complete neglect	2		

Individual administering scale:

Source: Adapted from Spilker J, Kongable G. The NIH Stroke Scale: its importance and practical application in the clinical setting. *Stroke Intervent* 2000;2:7–13. For further information, please refer to the Web site *www.stroke-site.org.*

| TABLE 36-8 • Approach to Arterial Hypertension in Acute Ischemic Stroke in Fibrinolytic Eligible Patients

Eligible for Treatment with Intravenous rtPA or Other Acute Reperfusion Intervention

- Blood pressure level:
  Systolic >185 mm Hg or diastolic >110 mm Hg
    Labetalol 10 to 20 mg IV over 1 to 2 minutes, may repeat x1;
      or
    Nitropaste 1 to 2 inches;
      or
    Nicardipine infusion, 5 mg/hr, titrate up by 2.5 mg/hr at 5- to 15-minute intervals, maximum dose 15 mg/hr; when desired blood pressure attained, reduce to 3 mg/hr
- If blood pressure does not decline and remains >185/110 mm Hg, do not administer rtPA

During or After Treatment

- Monitor blood pressure every 15 minutes during treatment and then for another 2 hours, then every 30 minutes for 6 hours, and then every hour for 16 hours
- Blood pressure level:
  Systolic 180 to 230 mm Hg or diastolic 105 to 120 mm Hg
    Labetalol 10 mg IV over 1 to 2 minutes, may repeat every 10 to 20 minutes, maximum dose of 300 mg;
      or
    Labetalol 10 mg IV followed by an infusion at 2 to 8 mg/min
  Systolic >230 mm Hg or diastolic 121 to 140 mm Hg
    Labetalol 10 mg IV over 1 to 2 minutes, may repeat every 10 to 20 minutes, maximum dose of 300 mg;
      or
    Labetalol 10 mg IV followed by an infusion at 2 to 8 mg/min;
      or
    Nicardipine infusion, 5 mg/hr, titrate up to desired effect by increasing 2.5 mg/hr every 5 minutes to maximum of 15 mg/hr
- If blood pressure not controlled, consider sodium nitroprusside

Source: AHA/ASA guidelines for early management of adults with ischemic stroke. *Stroke* 2007;38:1671.

The CT scan is central to the triage and treatment of the stroke patient. If the CT scan shows no evidence of hemorrhage, the patient may be a candidate for fibrinolytic therapy (Fig. 36-4, Boxes 6 and 8).

A NORMAL CT = CANDIDATE FOR FIBRINOLYTIC THERAPY

An important point to remember is that a completely normal CT scan—no sign of hemorrhage, and no hypodense areas—is supportive of tPA administration in a stroke patient who otherwise meets the criteria for fibrinolytic therapy.

Ischemic Stroke   During the first few hours of a thrombotic or embolic stroke, the noncontrast CT scan will generally appear *normal*. Brain structures without normal blood flow appear initially the same as structures with good blood flow on the CT scan. For this reason the CT scan will continue to appear "normal" for a few hours after blood flow is obstructed or reduced to an area of the brain. A well-defined area of hypodensity, purported to be caused by lack of blood flow past an occlusion, will rarely develop within the first

3 hours of a stroke. If the brain tissue downstream of an occlusion is indeed ischemic, it soon begins to swell with edema and inflammation.

After 6 to 12 hours, the edema and swelling are sufficient to produce a hypodense area that is usually visible on a CT scan. This well-defined hypodensity rarely develops within the 3-hour limit required for administration of tPA. In fact, the time since stroke onset is likely to be >3 hours if a well-defined hypodensity is present on the CT scan. For this reason a large hypodense area on the CT scan generally excludes a patient from fibrinolytic therapy. Changes of early ischemia and infarction from ischemic stroke may cause CT changes, but these changes are often subtle, such as obscuring of the gray–white matter junction, loss of the insular ribbon, sulcal effacement, or early hypodensity.

Hemorrhagic Stroke   If the initial noncontrast CT scan shows intracerebral or subarachnoid hemorrhage, the treating physician should immediately consult a neurosurgeon or neurointerventionalist to initiate appropriate actions for acute hemorrhage (see below and Fig. 36-4, Boxes 7 and 11).

✔*Decision: Diagnosis and Decision: Appropriate Therapy*

TABLE 36-9 • Fibrinolytic Checklist

Use of tPA in Patients With Acute Ischernic Stroke

All boxes must be checked before tPA can be given.
Note: The following checklist includes FDA-approved indications and contraindictions for tPA administration for acute ischemic stroke. A physician with expertise in acute stroke care may modify this list.

Inclusion Criteria (all YES boxes in this section must be checked):

Yes
☐ Age 18 years or older?
☐ Clinical diagnosis of ischemic stroke with a measurable neurologic deficit?
☐ Time of symptom onset (when patient was last seen normal) well established as <180 minutes (3 hours) before treatment would begin?

Exclusion Criteria (all No boxes in "Contraindications" section must be checked):
Contraindications:

No
☐ Evidence of intracranial hemorrhage on pretreatment noncontrast head CT?
☐ Clinical presentation suggestive of subarachnoid hemorrhage even with normal CT?
☐ CT shows multilobar infarction (hypodensity greater than one third cerebral hemisphere)?
☐ History of intracranial hemorrhage?
☐ Uncontrolled hypertension: At the time treatment should begin. systolic pressure remains >185 mm Hg or diastolic pressure remains >110 mm Hg despite repeated measurements?
☐ Known arteriovenous malformation, neoplasm, or aneurysm?
☐ Active internal bleeding or acute trauma (fracture)?[b]
☐ Acute bleeding diathesis, including but not limited to
  • Plalet count <100 000/mm^3?
  • Heparin received within 48 hours, resulting in an activated partial thromboplastin time (aPTT) that is greater than upper limit of normal for laboratory?
  • Current use of anticoagulant (e.g., warfarin sodium) that has produced an elevated international normalized ratio (INR) >1.7 or prothombin time (PT) >15 seconds?[a]
☐ Within 3 months of intracranial or intraspinal surgery, serious head trauma, or previous stroke?
☐ Arterial puncture at a noncompressible site within past 7 days?

Relative Contraindications/Precautions:
Recent experience suggests that under some circumstances—with careful consideration and weighing of risk-to-benefit ratio—patients may receive fibrinolytic therapy despite one or more relative contraindications. Consider the pros and cons of tPA administration carefully if any of these relative contraindications is present:
• Only minor or rapidly improving stroke symptoms (clearing spontaneously)
• Within 14 days of major surgery or serious trauma
• Recent gastrointestinal or urinary tract hemorrhage (within previous 21 days)
• Recent acute myocardial infarction (within previous 3 months)
• Postmyocardial infarction pericarditis
• Abnormal blood glucose level (<50 or >400 mg/dl [<2.8 or >22.2 mmol/L])

[a]In patients without recent use of oral anticoagulants or heparin, treatment with tPA can be initiated before availability of coagulation study results but should be discontinued if the international normalized ratio (INR) is >1.7 or the partial thromboplastin time is elevated by local laboratory standards.
[b]Note: AHA/ASA 2007 Ischemic Stroke Update: Seizures at onset is now a **relative contraindication.**

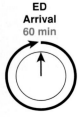

ED Arrival 60 min

Risk Assessment and Administration of IV tPA (Fig. 36-4, Boxes 6, 8, and 10)

When the CT scan shows no hemorrhage, the stroke team or physician expert should review the inclusion and exclusion criteria for IV fibrinolytic therapy (Table 36-9) and perform a repeat the neurologic examination (incorporating the NIH Stroke Scale or Canadian Neurological Scale). If the patient's neurologic signs are spontaneously improving (i.e., function is rapidly improving toward normal) and are near baseline, fibrinolytic administration is not recommended (Fig. 36-4, Box 6).

Risk–Benefit of tPA Therapy The administration of IV tPA has been controversial since its initial approval by the FDA in 1996 but is now generally accepted in carefully selected patients with ischemic stroke.[88] In the Canadian Stroke Registry, only 8.9% of patients received tPA.[89] This treatment rate is due to several factors, most importantly treatment time from symptom onset. Of all stroke patients, only 10% to 20% are eligible within the 3-hour time window and half of these are not treated for other reasons.[89,90] New imaging techniques such as MRI may identify a subgroup of patients eligible beyond the 3-hour window.[91] Triage to a stroke center may also allow additional patients to be treated up to 6 hours with intra-arterial fibrinolysis, although this is not yet approved by the FDA, or mechanical reperfusion modalities.

Benefit—Improved Neurologic Outcome Without Increased Mortality Several studies have documented a higher likelihood of good to excellent functional outcome when intravenous tPA is administered to adults with acute ischemic stroke within 3 hours of symptom onset.[4,92,93] Such results are obtained when intravenous tPA is administered by physicians in hospitals with a stroke protocol that rigorously adheres to the eligibility criteria and therapeutic regimen of the NINDS study protocol. These results have been supported by a subsequent 1-year follow-up study,[94] reanalysis of the NINDS data,[95] and a meta-analysis.[96] Evidence from prospective, randomized studies in adults also documents a greater likelihood of benefit the earlier treatment is begun. Many physicians have emphasized imbalances in the NINDS trials.[97,98] However additional analyses of the original NINDS data by an independent group of investigators[95] confirmed the validity of the results, verifying that improved outcomes in the IV tPA treatment arm persist even after imbalances in baseline stroke severity among treatment groups were corrected.[99]

Major Risk—Intracranial Hemorrhage and Death Like all medications, fibrinolytics have potential adverse effects. The physician must verify that there are no exclusion criteria, consider the risks and benefits to the patient, and be prepared to monitor and treat any potential complications. The major complication of IV tPA for stroke is symptomatic intracranial hemorrhage. This complication occurred in 6.4% of the 312 patients treated in the NINDS trial[4] and 4.6% of the 1,135 patients treated in 60 Canadian centers.[100] A meta-analysis of 15 published case series on the open-label use of tPA for acute ischemic stroke in general clinical practice shows a symptomatic hemorrhage rate of 5.2% among 2,639 patients treated.[101] Other complications include orolingual angioedema (occurs in about 1.5% of patients), acute hypotension, and systemic bleeding. In one large prospective registry, major systemic bleeding was uncommon (0.4%) and usually occurred at the site of femoral groin puncture for acute angiography.[100,102] Despite these risks, when administered in accordance with the NINDS study protocol, tPA is both safe and effective.

The American College of Emergency Physicians (ACEP) has a developed policy statement on use of tPA in ischemic stroke. This document provides additional insight and guidance on risk stratification and selection of patients for tPA administration.

See Web site for ACEP policy statement and policy resource and education paper on intravenous tPA for the management of acute stroke in the emergency department.

How to Minimize Risks and Maximize Benefits of Intravenous tPA for Acute Stroke In the NINDS trial, fatal intracranial hemorrhage occurred in approximately 3 of every 100 patients treated with intravenous tPA (3%) but only 3 of every 1,000 (0.3%) receiving placebo. This means that the risk of fatal bleeding into the brain was 10 times greater in the tPA-treated patients. But it is important to note that overall mortality was not increased in the tPA-treated group (17% versus 21% for the placebo group). For a perspective on this risk, consider that the rate of fatal hemorrhagic stroke in patients given tPA within 12 hours of acute coronary artery occlusion averages <1%. To minimize the risks and maximize the benefits, responsible clinicians must adhere strictly to the inclusion and exclusion criteria (Table 36-9). Intravenous tPA therapy is acceptable only with strict adherence to these criteria.

Strategies for Success

Administration of IV tPA to patients with acute ischemic stroke who meet the NINDS eligibility criteria is recommended if tPA is administered by physicians in the setting of a clearly defined protocol, a knowledgeable team, institutional commitment, and the patient's informed consent. It is important to note that the superior outcomes reported in both community and tertiary care hospitals in the NINDS trials have been difficult to replicate in hospitals with less experience in and institutional commitment to acute stroke care.[103,104] Failure to adhere to protocol is associated with an increased rate of complications, particularly the risk of symptomatic intracranial hemorrhage.[105,106] There is also strong evidence to avoid all delays and treat patients as soon as possible.

Community hospitals have reported outcomes comparable to the results of the NINDS trials after implementing a stroke program with a focus on quality improvement.[100,107,108] The experience of the Cleveland Clinic system is instructive.[104,108] A quality improvement program increased compliance with the tPA treatment protocol in nine community hospitals, and the rate of symptomatic intracerebral hemorrhage fell from 13.4% to 6.4%.[108]

There is a relationship between violations of the NINDS treatment protocol and increased risk of symptomatic intracerebral hemorrhage and death.[101] In Germany there was an increased risk of death after administration of tPA for acute ischemic stroke in hospitals that treated five or fewer patients per year, which suggests that clinical experience is an important factor in ensuring adherence to protocol.[102] The addition of a dedicated stroke team to a community hospital can increase the number of patients with acute stroke treated with fibrinolytic therapy and produce excellent clinical outcomes.[109] These findings show that it is important to have an institutional commitment to ensure optimal patient outcomes.

To provide standardized and comprehensive stroke care, the Brain Attack Coalition published criteria for primary stroke centers (PSC) and comprehensive stroke centers (CSC). A PSC has resources to care for many of the patients with uncomplicated stroke. A CSC provides comprehensive and specialized care for patients with a complicated stroke and those requiring specialized care, such as surgery or stroke intensive care.[110]

STROKE GUIDELINES UPDATE

New recommendations for stroke care include:

- Transport to closest facility with resources to care for stroke patients (i.e., hospital bypass)
- Development of primary stroke centers—strongly recommended
- Certification of stroke centers by external agency—strongly encouraged

✔ *Drug: Administration of tPA When Indicated and Other Therapies*

Additional Actions Before Fibrinolytic Therapy

Review for CT Exclusions: Are Any Observed?

- Hemorrhage, either intracerebral or subarachnoid, must be excluded. Failure to identify a small area of hemorrhage could be a **fatal error.**
- Large areas of well-defined hypodensity are generally CT exclusions because they indicate either that >3 hours have passed since the infarction or that a large area of the brain is threatened. Larger brain infarctions are prone to undergo hemorrhagic transformation, exposing a patient receiving a fibrinolytic agent to the risk of fatal intracerebral hemorrhage. A knowledgeable stroke expert must carefully weigh risk–benefit ratios in consultation with the patient.

Review Fibrinolytic Exclusions: Are Any Observed?

- Table 36-9 lists the major exclusions for the use of fibrinolytics. Such a checklist, in a form suitable for inclusion in a patient's medical record, should be available wherever stroke patients might be treated with fibrinolytics.

Review Patient Data: Is Time Since Symptom Onset Now ≥3 Hours?

- This step reminds the clinician to make one last review of all the information gathered during the patient assessments. In particular, the estimated length of time that

has passed since the onset of the stroke must be documented.

- IV infusion of the fibrinolytic agent must begin within 180 minutes of the beginning of stroke symptoms.

ANTICOAGULANTS AND ANTIPLATELET THERAPY

Neither anticoagulants nor antiplatelet treatment should be administered for 24 hours after administration of tPA, typically until a follow-up CT scan at 24 hours shows no hemorrhage (Fig. 36-4, Box 10).

- If the patient has brain hemorrhage, DO NOT GIVE ASPIRIN (Fig. 36-4, Box 7).
- If the patient has ischemic stroke but is not a candidate for tPA, consider aspirin.
- DO NOT administer heparin (unfractionated or low molecular weight). Heparin is associated with an increased risk of bleeding within the first 24 hours.

✔ *Drug: Administration and Monitoring of tPA Infusion*

IV fibrinolytic therapy is a class I recommendation for a highly selected, well-defined subset of ischemic stroke patients. Treatment with IV tPA within 3 hours of the onset of ischemic stroke improved clinical outcome at 3 months. ED- or hospital-based stroke specialists should aim to start the initial bolus within 60 minutes of arrival in the ED. Ten percent of a total dose of 0.9 mg/kg (maximum 90 mg) is given by bolus administration and the remainder infused over 60 minutes.

During tPA infusion:

- Monitor neurologic status; if any signs of deterioration develop, stop the IV tPA and obtain an emergent CT scan.
- Monitor blood pressure, which may increase during fibrinolytic treatment. Initiate antihypertensive treatment with any increase over 180 mm Hg systolic or over 105 mm Hg diastolic (see above and Table 36-8).
- Admit patient to the critical care unit, stroke unit, or other skilled facility capable of careful observation, frequent neurologic assessments, and cardiovascular monitoring.
- Avoid anticoagulant or antiplatelet treatment for the next 24 hours.

Intra-arterial tPA

For patients with acute ischemic stroke who are not candidates for standard IV fibrinolysis, administration of intra-arterial fibrinolysis within 6 hours from symptom onset (class I, level of evidence B) or mechanical embolectomy (class IIb, level of evidence B) in centers that have the resources and expertise available may be considered within the first few hours after the onset of symptoms.[7] Intra-arterial administration of tPA has not yet been approved by the FDA.

Transition to Critical Care

General Stroke Care

Additional stroke care includes support of the airway, oxygenation and ventilation, and nutritional support. Normal saline is administered at approximately 75 to 100 mL/hr to maintain euvolemia if needed. The reported frequency of seizures during the first days of stroke ranges from 2% to 23%.[111–114] Most seizures occur during the first day and can recur. Seizure prophylaxis is not recommended. Treatment of acute seizures followed by administration of anticonvulsants to prevent further seizures is recommended, consistent with the established management of seizures.[7] Monitor the patient for signs of increased intracranial pressure. Continued control of blood pressure is required to reduce the risk of bleeding in patients who have received tPA.

Hyperglycemia

Hyperglycemia is present in about one third of patients admitted with stroke. Hyperglycemia is associated with worse clinical outcome in patients with acute ischemic stroke than is normoglycemia, but there is no direct evidence that active glucose control improves clinical outcome.[115,116] There is evidence that insulin treatment of hyperglycemia in other critically ill patients improves survival rates. For this reason administration of IV or subcutaneous insulin may be considered to lower blood glucose in patients with acute ischemic stroke when the serum glucose level is >10 mmol/L (>~200 mg/dL).[117,118]

Temperature Control

Increased temperature in stroke is associated with poor neurologic outcome. No data have demonstrated that lowering temperature improves outcome, but fever >37.5°C (99.5°F) should be treated and the source of fever identified and treated if possible.

Induced hypothermia may exert neuroprotective effects after a stroke.[119–123] Hypothermia has been shown to improve survival and functional outcome in patients following resuscitation from ventricular fibrillation sudden cardiac arrest, but it has not been shown in controlled human trials to be effective for acute ischemic stroke. In some small human pilot studies and in animal models, hypothermia (33°C to 36°C [91.4°F to 96.8°F]) for acute ischemic stroke has been shown to be relatively safe and feasible.[122,124,125] Although effects of hypothermia on both global and focal cerebral ischemia in animals have been promising, cooling to ≤33°C (91.4°F) appears to be associated with increased complications, including hypotension, cardiac arrhythmias, cardiac failure, pneumonia, thrombocytopenia, and a rebound increase in intracranial pressure during rewarming.[120,121,123,126,127] At present there is insufficient scientific evidence to recommend for or against the use of hypothermia in the treatment of acute ischemic stroke.[7]

Stroke Units

Patients should be admitted to a stroke unit (if available) for careful observation, including monitoring of blood pressure and neurologic status and treatment of hypertension if indicated. If the patient's neurologic status deteriorates, order an emergent CT scan to determine if cerebral edema or hemorrhage is responsible for the deterioration and treat if possible.

All patients with stroke should be screened for dysphagia before anything is given by mouth. A simple bedside screening evaluation involves asking the patient to sip water from a cup. If the patient can sip and swallow without difficulty, he or she is asked to take a large gulp of water and swallow. If there are no signs of coughing or aspiration after 30 seconds, it is safe for the patient to have a thickened diet until he or she is formally assessed by a speech pathologist.[7] Medications may be given in applesauce or jam. Any patient who fails a swallow test may be given medications such as aspirin rectally or, if appropriate, via the IV, intramuscular, or subcutaneous route.

Summary

As in the management of the patient with an ACS, the patient with ischemic stroke requires a time-dependent therapy and a coordinated interdisciplinary system of care. Rapid recognition of stroke symptoms and activation of EMS speeds patient assessment and management and may result in earlier reperfusion, stroke volume reduction, and improved short- and long-term prognosis.

Stroke centers provide many of the hospital-based elements of this system of care, including stroke units, written care protocols for stroke health care professional interdisciplinary teams, neurologic expertise, and coordinated comprehensive consultation and support. When properly integrated, these centers and systems are associated with improved outcomes for stroke patients.[110,128] Stroke center certification is progressing, and the Joint Commission on Accreditation of Healthcare Organizations (JCAHO) began a formal process for certification of Primary Stroke Centers (PSC) in 2004. At present, >200 hospitals have been certified as stroke centers. Use of destination hospital protocols routing acute stroke patients to a PSC has increased the number of patients receiving tPA.[129] Although initial reperfusion of ischemic stroke patients has focused on the use of IV fibrinolytic therapy (tPA), stroke centers are now evaluating the use of other reperfusion methods including intra-arterial tPA and mechanical reperfusion methods for patients ineligible for pharmacologic agents. It is possible that these evolving methods combined with neuroprotection will, in the future, extend the time window for salvage of ischemic brain in stroke patients.

References

1. Rosamond W, Flegal K, Furie K, et al. Heart disease and stroke statistics—2008 update: a report from the American Heart Association

Statistics Committee and Stroke Statistics Subcommittee. *Circulation* 2008;117(4):e25–e146.

2. Schwamm LH, Pancioli A, Acker JE III, et al. Recommendations for the establishment of stroke systems of care: recommendations from the American Stroke Association's Task Force on the Development of Stroke Systems. *Circulation* 2005;111(8):1078–1091.

3. Dobkin BH. Clinical practice. Rehabilitation after stroke. *N Engl J Med* 2005;352(16):1677–1684.

4. Tissue plasminogen activator for acute ischemic stroke. The National Institute of Neurological Disorders and Stroke rt-PA Stroke Study Group. *N Engl J Med* 1995;333(24):1581–1587.

5. Hazinski M. D-mystifying recognition and management of stroke. *Curr Emerg Cardiac Care* 1996;7:8.

6. Acute stroke: current treatment and paradigms. In: Cummins R, Field J, Hazinski M, eds. *ACLS: Principles and Practice.* Dallas: American Heart Association, 2003:437–482.

7. Adams HP Jr, del Zoppo G, Alberts MJ, et al. Guidelines for the early management of adults with ischemic stroke: a guideline from the American Heart Association/American Stroke Association Stroke Council, Clinical Cardiology Council, Cardiovascular Radiology and Intervention Council, and the Atherosclerotic Peripheral Vascular Disease and Quality of Care Outcomes in Research Interdisciplinary Working Groups: The American Academy of Neurology affirms the value of this guideline as an educational tool for neurologists. *Circulation* 2007;115(20):e478–e534.

8. Acker JE III, Pancioli AM, Crocco TJ, et al. Implementation strategies for emergency medical services within stroke systems of care: a policy statement from the American Heart Association/American Stroke Association Expert Panel on Emergency Medical Services Systems and the Stroke Council. *Stroke* 2007;38(11):3097–3115.

9. Furlan A, Higashida R, Wechsler L, et al. Intra-arterial prourokinase for acute ischemic stroke. The PROACT II study: a randomized controlled trial. Prolyse in Acute Cerebral Thromboembolism. *JAMA* 1999;282(21):2003–2011.

10. Furlan AJ. Acute ischemic stroke: new strategies for management and prevention. Interview by Wayne Kuznar. *Geriatrics* 1999;54(8):47–52; quiz 54.

11. Katzan IL, Masaryk TJ, Furlan AJ, et al. Intra-arterial thrombolysis for perioperative stroke after open heart surgery. *Neurology* 1999;52(5):1081–1084.

12. Ducrocq X, Bracard S, Taillandier L, et al. Comparison of intravenous and intra-arterial urokinase thrombolysis for acute ischaemic stroke. *J Neuroradiol* 2005;32(1):26–32.

13. Macleod MR, O'Collins T, Horky LL, et al. Systematic review and meta-analysis of the efficacy of melatonin in experimental stroke. *J Pineal Res* 2005;38(1):35–41.

14. Brekenfeld C, Remonda L, Nedeltchev K, et al. Endovascular neuroradiological treatment of acute ischemic stroke: techniques and results in 350 patients. *Neurol Res* 2005;27(Suppl 1):S29–S35.

15. Noser EA, Shaltoni HM, Hall CE, et al. Aggressive mechanical clot disruption: a safe adjunct to thrombolytic therapy in acute stroke? *Stroke* 2005;36(2):292–296.

16. Schumacher HC, Meyers PM, Yavagal DR, et al. Endovascular mechanical thrombectomy of an occluded superior division branch of the left MCA for acute cardioembolic stroke. *Cardiovasc Intervent Radiol* 2003;26(3):305–308.

17. Hazinski M. Demystifying the recognition and management of stroke. *Curr Emerg Card Care* 1996;7:8–9.

18. Emergency department: rapid identification and treatment of patients with acute myocardial infarction. National Heart Attack Alert Program Coordinating Committee, 60 Minutes to Treatment Working Group. *Ann Emerg Med* 1994;23(2):311–329.

19. Kothari RU, Brott T, Broderick JP, et al. Emergency physicians. Accuracy in the diagnosis of stroke. *Stroke* 1995;26(12):2238–2241.

20. Sacco RL, Adams R, Albers G, et al. Guidelines for prevention of stroke in patients with ischemic stroke or transient ischemic attack: a statement for healthcare professionals from the American Heart Association/American Stroke Association Council on Stroke: co-sponsored by the Council on Cardiovascular Radiology and Intervention: the American Academy of Neurology affirms the value of this guideline. *Stroke* 2006;37(2):577–617.

21. Cardiogenic brain embolism. The second report of the Cerebral Embolism Task Force. *Arch Neurol* 1989;46(7):727–743.

22. Ovbiagele B, Kidwell CS, Saver JL. Epidemiological impact in the United States of a tissue-based definition of transient ischemic attack. *Stroke* 2003;34(4):919–924.

23. Rovira A, Rovira-Gols A, Pedraza S, et al. Diffusion-weighted MR imaging in the acute phase of transient ischemic attacks. *AJNR Am J Neuroradiol* 2002;23(1):77–83.

24. Albers GW, Caplan LR, Easton JD, et al. Transient ischemic attack—proposal for a new definition. *N Engl J Med* 2002;347(21):1713–1716.

25. Johnston SC, Gress DR, Browner WS, et al. Short-term prognosis after emergency department diagnosis of TIA. *JAMA* 2000;284(22):2901–2906.

26. Rothwell PM, Warlow CP. Timing of TIAs preceding stroke: time window for prevention is very short. *Neurology* 2005;64(5):817–820.

27. Lovett JK, Dennis MS, Sandercock PA, et al. Very early risk of stroke after a first transient ischemic attack. *Stroke* 2003;34(8):e138–e140.

28. Rothwell PM, Giles MF, Flossmann E, et al. A simple score (ABCD) to identify individuals at high early risk of stroke after transient ischaemic attack. *Lancet* 2005;366(9479):29–36.

29. Johnston KC, Wagner DP, Wang XQ, et al. Validation of an acute ischemic stroke model: does diffusion-weighted imaging lesion volume offer a clinically significant improvement in prediction of outcome? *Stroke* 2007;38(6):1820–1825.

30. National Heart, Lung and Blood Institute. *Incidence and Prevalence: 2006 Chart Book on Cardiovascular and Lung Disease.* Bethesda, MD: NHLBI, 2006.

31. Ferro JM. Update on intracerebral haemorrhage. *J Neurol* 2006;253(8):985–999.

32. Carr S, Farb A, Pearce WH, et al. Atherosclerotic plaque rupture in symptomatic carotid artery stenosis. *J Vasc Surg* 1996;23(5):755–765; discussion 765–766.

33. Spagnoli LG, Mauriello A, Sangiorgi G, et al. Extracranial thrombotically active carotid plaque as a risk factor for ischemic stroke. *JAMA* 2004;292(15):1845–1852.

34. Redgrave JN, Lovett JK, Gallagher PJ, et al. Histological assessment of 526 symptomatic carotid plaques in relation to the nature and timing of ischemic symptoms: the Oxford plaque study. *Circulation* 2006;113(19):2320–2328.

35. Carr SC, Cheanvechai V, Virmani R, et al. Histology and clinical significance of the carotid atherosclerotic plaque: implications for endovascular treatment. *J Endovasc Surg* 1997;4(4):321–325.

36. Carr S, Farb A, Pearce WH, et al. Atherosclerotic plaque rupture in symptomatic carotid artery stenosis. *J Vasc Surg* 1996;23(5):755–765; discussion 765–756.

37. Spagnoli LG, Mauriello A, Sangiorgi G, et al. Extracranial thrombotically active carotid plaque as a risk factor for ischemic stroke. *JAMA* 2004;292(15):1845–1852.

38. Prabhakaran S, Zarahn E, Riley C, et al. Inter-individual variability in the capacity for motor recovery after ischemic stroke. *Neurorehabil Neural Repair* 2008;22(1):64–71.

39. Redgrave JN, Schulz UG, Briley D, et al. Presence of acute ischaemic lesions on diffusion-weighted imaging is associated with clinical predictors of early risk of stroke after transient ischaemic attack. *Cerebrovasc Dis* 2007;24(1):86–90.

40. Redgrave JN, Coutts SB, Schulz UG, et al. Systematic review of associations between the presence of acute ischemic lesions on diffusion-weighted imaging and clinical predictors of early stroke risk after transient ischemic attack. *Stroke* 2007;38(5):1482–1488.

41. Brott T, Adams HP Jr, Olinger CP, et al. Measurements of acute cerebral infarction: a clinical examination scale. *Stroke* 1989;20(7):864–870.

42. Brott T, Haley EC Jr, Levy DE, et al. Urgent therapy for stroke: Part I. Pilot study of tissue plasminogen activator administered within 90 minutes. *Stroke* 1992;23:632–640.

43. Zachariah BS, Pepe PE. The development of emergency medical dispatch in the USA: a historical perspective. *Eur J Emerg Med* 1995;2(3):109–112.

44. Wolf PA, Abbott RD, Kannel WB. Atrial fibrillation as an independent risk factor for stroke: the Framingham Study. *Stroke* 1991;22(8):983–988.

45. Risk factors for stroke and efficacy of antithrombotic therapy in atrial fibrillation. Analysis of pooled data from five randomized controlled trials. *Arch Intern Med* 1994;154(13):1449–1457.

46. Flegel KM, Hutchinson TA, Groome PA, et al. Factors relevant to preventing embolic stroke in patients with non-rheumatic atrial fibrillation. *J Clin Epidemiol* 1991;44(6):551–560.

47. Flegel KM, Shipley MJ, Rose G. Risk of stroke in non-rheumatic atrial fibrillation. *Lancet* 1987;1(8532):526–529.

48. Feldmann E, Gordon N, Brooks JM, et al. Factors associated with early presentation of acute stroke. *Stroke* 1993;24(12):1805–1810.

49. Wendel-Vos GC, Schuit AJ, Feskens EJ, et al. Physical activity and stroke. A meta-analysis of observational data. *Int J Epidemiol* 2004;33(4):787–798.

50. Lee IM, Hennekens CH, Berger K, et al. Exercise and risk of stroke in male physicians. *Stroke* 1999;30(1):1–6.

51. Lee IM, Paffenbarger RS Jr. Physical activity and stroke incidence: the Harvard Alumni Health Study. *Stroke* 1998;29(10):2049–2054.

52. Handschu R, Poppe R, Rauss J, et al. Emergency calls in acute stroke. *Stroke* 2003;34(4):1005–1009.

53. Williams JE, Rosamond WD, Morris DL. Stroke symptom attribution and time to emergency department arrival: the Delay in Accessing Stroke Healthcare Study. *Acad Emerg Med* 2000;7(1):93–96.

54. Morris DL, Rosamond W, Madden K, et al. Prehospital and emergency department delays after acute stroke: the Genentech Stroke Presentation Survey. *Stroke* 2000;31(11):2585–2590.

55. Schroeder EB, Rosamond WD, Morris DL, et al. Determinants of use of emergency medical services in a population with stroke symptoms: the Second Delay in Accessing Stroke Healthcare (DASH II) Study. *Stroke* 2000;31(11):2591–2596.

56. Barsan WG, Brott TG, Broderick JP, et al. Time of hospital presentation in patients with acute stroke. *Arch Intern Med* 1993;153(22):2558–2561.

57. Kothari R, Barsan W, Brott T, et al. Frequency and accuracy of prehospital diagnosis of acute stroke. *Stroke* 1995;26(6):937–941.

58. Kothari RU, Pancioli A, Liu T, et al. Cincinnati Prehospital Stroke Scale: reproducibility and validity. *Ann Emerg Med* 1999;33(4):373–378.

59. Kothari R, Hall K, Brott T, et al. Early stroke recognition: developing an out-of-hospital NIH stroke scale. *Acad Emerg Med* 1997;4(10):986–990.

60. Kidwell CS, Saver JL, Schubert GB, et al. Design and retrospective analysis of the Los Angeles Prehospital Stroke Screen (LAPSS). *Prehosp Emerg Care* 1998;2(4):267–273.

61. Kidwell CS, Starkman S, Eckstein M, et al. Identifying stroke in the field. Prospective validation of the Los Angeles prehospital stroke screen (LAPSS). *Stroke* 2000;31(1):71–76.

62. Chalela JA, Kasner SE, Jauch EC, et al. Safety of air medical transportation after tissue plasminogen activator administration in acute ischemic stroke. *Stroke* 1999;30(11):2366–2368.

63. Conroy MB, Rodriguez SU, Kimmel SE, et al. Helicopter transfer offers a potential benefit to patients with acute stroke. *Stroke* 1999;30(12):2580–2584.

64. Silbergleit R, Scott PA. Thrombolysis for acute stroke: the incontrovertible, the controvertible, and the uncertain. *Acad Emerg Med* 2005;12(4):348–351.

65. Silbergleit R, Scott PA, Lowell MJ, et al. Cost-effectiveness of helicopter transport of stroke patients for thrombolysis. *Acad Emerg Med* 2003;10(9):966–972.

66. Crocco TJ, Grotta JC, Jauch EC, et al. EMS management of acute stroke—prehospital triage (resource document to NAEMSP position statement). *Prehosp Emerg Care* 2007;11(3):313–317.

67. Alvarez-Sabin J, Molina CA, Montaner J, et al. Effects of admission hyperglycemia on stroke outcome in reperfused tissue plasminogen activator–treated patients. *Stroke* 2003;34(5):1235–1241.

68. Auer RN. Insulin, blood glucose levels, and ischemic brain damage. *Neurology* 1998;51(3 Suppl 3):S39–S43.

69. Baird TA, Parsons MW, Phanh T, et al. Persistent poststroke hyperglycemia is independently associated with infarct expansion and worse clinical outcome. *Stroke* 2003;34(9):2208–2214.

70. Bruno A, Biller J, Adams HP Jr, et al. Acute blood glucose level and outcome from ischemic stroke. Trial of ORG 10172 in Acute Stroke Treatment (TOAST) Investigators. *Neurology* 1999;52(2):280–284.

71. Bruno A, Levine SR, Frankel MR, et al. Admission glucose level and clinical outcomes in the NINDS rt-PA Stroke Trial. *Neurology* 2002;59(5):669–674.

72. A systems approach to immediate evaluation and management of hyperacute stroke. Experience at eight centers and implications for community practice and patient care. The National Institute of Neurological Disorders and Stroke (NINDS) rt-PA Stroke Study Group. *Stroke* 1997;28(8):1530–1540.

73. Singhal AB, Benner T, Roccatagliata L, et al. A pilot study of normobaric oxygen therapy in acute ischemic stroke. *Stroke* 2005;36(4):797–802.

74. Singhal AB, Ratai E, Benner T, et al. Magnetic resonance spectroscopy study of oxygen therapy in ischemic stroke. *Stroke* 2007;38(10):2851–2854.

75. Adams HJ, Brott T, Crowell R, et al. Guidelines for the management of patients with acute ischemic stroke: a statement for healthcare professionals from a special writing group of the Stroke Council, American Heart Association. *Stroke* 1994;25:1901–1914.

76. Oppenheimer SM, Cechetto DF, Hachinski VC. Cerebrogenic cardiac arrhythmias: cerebral electrocardiographic influences and their role in sudden death. *Arch Neurol* 1990;47(5):513–519.

77. Lyden P, Rapp K, Babcock T, et al. Ultra-rapid identification, triage, and enrollment of stroke patients into clinical trials. *J StrokeCerebrovasc Dis* 1994;2:106–113.

78. Brott T. Utility of the NIH stroke scale. *Cerebrovasc Dis* 1992;2:241–242.

79. Lyden P, Lu M, Jackson C, et al. Underlying structure of the National Institutes of Health Stroke Scale: results of a factor analysis. NINDS tPA Stroke Trial Investigators. *Stroke* 1999;30(11):2347–2354.

80. Goldstein LB, Bertels C, Davis JN. Interrater reliability of the NIH stroke scale. *Arch Neurol* 1989;46(6):660–662.

81. Spilker J, Kongable GL. The NIH Stroke Scale: its importance and practical application in the clinical setting. *Stroke Intervent* 2000;2:7–14 (for further information refer to Web site *http://www.stroke-site.org*).

82. Spilker J, Kongable GL. The NIH Stroke Scale: its importance and practical application in the clinical setting. *Stroke Intervent* 2000;2:7–14. (For further information refer to *http://www.stroke-site.org*).

83. Intracerebral hemorrhage after intravenous t-PA therapy for ischemic stroke. The NINDS t-PA Stroke Study Group. *Stroke* 1997;28(11):2109–2118.

84. Adams H, Adams R, Del Zoppo G, et al. Guidelines for the early management of patients with ischemic stroke: 2005 guidelines update a scientific statement from the Stroke Council of the American Heart Association/American Stroke Association. *Stroke* 2005;36(4):916–923.

85. Adams HP Jr, Adams RJ, Brott T, et al. Guidelines for the early management of patients with ischemic stroke: A scientific statement from the Stroke Council of the American Stroke Association. *Stroke* 2003;34(4):1056–1083.

86. Connors JJ III, Sacks D, Furlan AJ, et al. Training, competency, and credentialing standards for diagnostic cervicocerebral angiography, carotid stenting, and cerebrovascular intervention: a joint statement from the American Academy of Neurology, American Association of Neurological Surgeons, American Society of Interventional and Therapeutic Radiology, American Society of Neuroradiology, Congress of Neurological Surgeons, AANS/CNS Cerebrovascular Section, and Society of Interventional Radiology. *Radiology* 2005;234(1):26–34.

87. Schriger DL, Kalafut M, Starkman S, et al. Cranial computed tomography interpretation in acute stroke: physician accuracy in determining eligibility for thrombolytic therapy. *JAMA* 1998;279(16):1293–1297.

88. Lyden P. *Thrombolytic Therapy for Acute Stroke*, 2nd ed. Totowa NJ: Humana Press, 2005.

89. Nadeau JO, Shi S, Fang J, et al. TPA use for stroke in the Registry of the Canadian Stroke Network. *Can J Neurol Sci* 2005;32(4):433–439.

90. Hills NK, Johnston SC. Why are eligible thrombolysis candidates left untreated? *Am J Prev Med* 2006;31(6 Suppl 2):S210–S216.

91. Albers GW. Expanding the window for thrombolytic therapy in acute stroke. The potential role of acute MRI for patient selection. *Stroke* 1999;30(10):2230–2237.

92. Hacke W, Donnan G, Fieschi C, et al. Association of outcome with early stroke treatment: pooled analysis of ATLANTIS, ECASS, and NINDS rt-PA stroke trials. *Lancet* 2004;363(9411):768–774.

93. Hill MD, Buchan AM. Thrombolysis for acute ischemic stroke: results of the Canadian Alteplase for Stroke Effectiveness Study. Canadian Alteplase for Stroke Effectiveness Study (CASES) Investigators. *CMAJ* 2005;172(10)(10):1307.

94. Kwiatkowski TG, Libman RB, Frankel M, et al. Effects of tissue plasminogen activator for acute ischemic stroke at one year. National Institute of Neurological Disorders and Stroke Recombinant Tissue Plasminogen Activator Stroke Study Group. *N Engl J Med* 1999;340(23):1781–1787.

95. Ingall TJ, O'Fallon WM, Asplund K, et al. Findings from the reanalysis of the NINDS tissue plasminogen activator for acute ischemic stroke treatment trial. *Stroke* 2004;35(10):2418–2424.

96. Wardlaw JM, Zoppo G, Yamaguchi T, et al. Thrombolysis for acute ischaemic stroke. *Cochrane Database Syst Rev* 2003(3): CD000213.

97. Mann J. Truths about the NINDS study: setting the record straight. *West J Med* 2002;176(3):192–194.

98. Lindley RI. Further randomized controlled trials of tissue plasminogen activator within 3 hours are required. *Stroke* 2001; 32(11):2708–2709.

99. Kwiatkowski T, Libman R, Tilley BC, et al. The impact of imbalances in baseline stroke severity on outcome in the National Institute of Neurological Disorders and Stroke Recombinant Tissue Plasminogen Activator Stroke Study. *Ann Emerg Med* 2005;45(4):377–384.

100. Hill MD, Buchan AM. Thrombolysis for acute ischemic stroke: results of the Canadian Alteplase for Stroke Effectiveness Study. Canadian Alteplase for Stroke Effectiveness Study (CASES) Investigators. *CMAJ* 2005;172(10):1307–1312.

101. Graham GD. Tissue plasminogen activator for acute ischemic stroke in clinical practice: a meta-analysis of safety data. *Stroke* 2003;34(12):2847–2850.

102. Heuschmann PU, Berger K, Misselwitz B, et al. Frequency of thrombolytic therapy in patients with acute ischemic stroke and the risk of in-hospital mortality: the German Stroke Registers Study Group. *Stroke* 2003;34(5):1106–1113.

103. Bravata DM, Kim N, Concato J, et al. Thrombolysis for acute stroke in routine clinical practice. *Arch Intern Med* 2002;162(17): 1994–2001.

104. Katzan IL, Furlan AJ, Lloyd LE, et al. Use of tissue-type plasminogen activator for acute ischemic stroke: the Cleveland area experience. *JAMA* 2000;283(9):1151–1158.

105. Katzan IL, Hammer MD, Hixson ED, et al. Utilization of intravenous tissue plasminogen activator for acute ischemic stroke. *Arch Neurol* 2004;61(3):346–350.

106. Lopez-Yunez AM, Bruno A, Williams LS, et al. Protocol violations in community-based rTPA stroke treatment are associated with symptomatic intracerebral hemorrhage. *Stroke* 2001;32(1): 12–16.

107. Asimos AW, Norton HJ, Price MF, et al. Therapeutic yield and outcomes of a community teaching hospital code stroke protocol. *Acad Emerg Med* 2004;11(4):361–370.

108. Katzan IL, Hammer MD, Furlan AJ, et al. Quality improvement and tissue-type plasminogen activator for acute ischemic stroke: a Cleveland update. *Stroke* 2003;34(3):799–800.

109. Lattimore SU, Chalela J, Davis L, et al. Impact of establishing a primary stroke center at a community hospital on the use of thrombolytic therapy: the NINDS Suburban Hospital Stroke Center experience. *Stroke* 2003;34(6):e55–e57.

110. Alberts MJ, Hademenos G, Latchaw RE, et al. Recommendations for the establishment of primary stroke centers. Brain Attack Coalition. *JAMA* 2000;283(23):3102–3109.

111. Kilincer C, Asil T, Utku U, et al. Factors affecting the outcome of decompressive craniectomy for large hemispheric infarctions: a prospective cohort study. *Acta Neurochir (Wien)* 2005; 147(6): 587–594; discussion 594.

112. Burn J, Dennis M, Bamford J, et al. Epileptic seizures after a first stroke: the Oxfordshire Community Stroke Project. *BMJ* 1997;315(7122):1582–1587.

113. Davalos A, Cendra E, Genis D, et al. The frequency, characteristics and prognosis of epileptic seizures at the onset of stroke. *J Neurol Neurosurg Psychiatry* 1988;51(11):1464.

114. Kilpatrick CJ, Davis SM, Hopper JL, et al. Early seizures after acute stroke. Risk of late seizures. *Arch Neurol* 1992;49(5): 509–511.

115. Scott JF, Robinson GM, French JM, et al. Glucose potassium insulin infusions in the treatment of acute stroke patients with mild to moderate hyperglycemia: the Glucose Insulin in Stroke Trial (GIST). *Stroke* 1999;30(4):793–799.

116. Gray CS, Hildreth AJ, Alberti GK, et al. Poststroke hyperglycemia: natural history and immediate management. *Stroke* 2004;35(1):122–126.

117. Van den Berghe G, Wouters PJ, Bouillon R, et al. Outcome benefit of intensive insulin therapy in the critically ill: insulin dose versus glycemic control. *Crit Care Med* 2003;31(2):359–366.

118. Van den Berghe G, Wouters P, Weekers F, et al. Intensive insulin therapy in the critically ill patients. *N Engl J Med* 2001;345(19): 1359–1367.

119. De Georgia MA, Krieger DW, Abou-Chebl A, et al. Cooling for Acute Ischemic Brain Damage (COOL AID): a feasibility trial of endovascular cooling. *Neurology* 2004;63(2):312–317.

120. Georgiadis D, Schwarz S, Aschoff A, et al. Hemicraniectomy and moderate hypothermia in patients with severe ischemic stroke. *Stroke* 2002;33(6):1584–1588.

121. Georgiadis D, Schwarz S, Kollmar R, et al. Endovascular cooling for moderate hypothermia in patients with acute stroke: first results of a novel approach. *Stroke* 2001;32(11):2550–2553.

122. Wang H, Olivero W, Lanzino G, et al. Rapid and selective cerebral hypothermia achieved using a cooling helmet. *J Neurosurg* 2004;100(2):272–277.

123. Schwab S, Schwarz S, Spranger M, et al. Moderate hypothermia in the treatment of patients with severe middle cerebral artery infarction. *Stroke* 1998;29(12):2461–2466.

124. Kammersgaard LP, Rasmussen BH, Jorgensen HS, et al. Feasibility and safety of inducing modest hypothermia in awake patients with acute stroke through surface cooling: A case-control study: the Copenhagen Stroke Study. *Stroke* 2000;31(9):2251–2256.

125. Knoll T, Wimmer ML, Gumpinger F, et al. The low normothermia concept—maintaining a core body temperature between 36 and 37 degrees C in acute stroke unit patients. *J Neurosurg Anesthesiol* 2002;14(4):304–308.

126. Schwab S, Georgiadis D, Berrouschot J, et al. Feasibility and safety of moderate hypothermia after massive hemispheric infarction. *Stroke* 2001;32(9):2033–2035.

127. Krieger DW, De Georgia MA, Abou-Chebl A, et al. Cooling for acute ischemic brain damage (cool aid): an open pilot study of induced hypothermia in acute ischemic stroke. *Stroke* 2001;32(8): 1847–1854.

128. Alberts MJ, Latchaw RE, Selman WR, et al. Recommendations for comprehensive stroke centers: a consensus statement from the Brain Attack Coalition. *Stroke* 2005;36(7):1597–1616.

129. Wojner-Alexandrov AW, Alexandrov AV, Rodriguez D, et al. Houston paramedic and emergency stroke treatment and outcomes study (HoPSTO). *Stroke* 2005;36(7):1512–1518.

Ten

Ethics

**Chapter 37
Ethics in Emergency
Cardiovascular Care**

Kenneth V. Iserson

*While the idea of applying ethics to and during cardiopulmonary resuscitation (CPR) may seem
daunting, the basic principle is quite easy to understand: the patient's value system is paramount.*

- Patient values should guide resuscitation decisions.
- In emergency care, adequate information about the patient and the prognosis is required
  if treatment is to be withheld.
- Advance directives and surrogate decision makers are used if the patient lacks decision-
  making capacity.
- A patient's decision-making capacity is a clinical determination made at the bedside.
- Family members may be allowed to observe resuscitation attempts.
- Trained personnel must be provided to notify and care for survivors.

Basic Principles

Three ethical issues surround emergency cardiovascular care:

- Who makes treatment decisions?
- On what basis are these decisions made?
- How should clinicians interact with families during and after cardiac resuscitations?

While the idea of applying ethics to cardiopulmonary resuscitation issues may seem
daunting, the basic principle is quite easy to understand: the patient's value system is paramount. It determines his or her goals of therapy and willingness to assume treatment burdens to achieve a certain outcome. The only exceptions are when the patient lacks the
capacity to make a decision or when it is not possible to honor his or her treatment
requests or when they are not consistent with the possible goals of medicine.

Patient and Societal Values

The patient's values, which are sometimes expressed through surrogate decision makers
or advance directives, incorporate many personal factors, such as religious and cultural
beliefs, social relationships, learned behaviors, and self-image. Even though patients may
not be able to verbalize the factors they consider in making their health care decisions,

PART TEN • ETHICS

the decisions themselves express their values. In pluralistic societies, clinicians treat multiple individuals with many different value systems, so they must be sensitive to others' beliefs and traditions.

People learn their values from the culture in which they live, through observation, and through secular (including professional) and religious education. One common source of personal values is organized religion, which helps to mold and maintain societal values. Although various religions may appear dissimilar, most teach the Golden Rule: "Do unto others as you would have them do unto you." This meshes with, and was probably the source of, commonly accepted secular principles, such as beneficence and nonmaleficence. Problems surface in trying to apply religion-based rules to specific bioethical situations. For example, although the ethical proscription "Do not kill" is generally accepted, interpretations vary on which activities constitute "killing:" active or passive euthanasia, terminal sedation, or other end-of-life palliative medical care.[1]

Although each individual is entitled to have a personal system of values, certain values have become generally accepted by the medical community, courts, legislatures, and society at large (Table 37-1). Although some groups disagree about each of the generally accepted values, this dissension has not affected their application to medical care in many western countries.[2]

Principle of Autonomy (Self-Determination)

Patient *autonomy*, or self-determination, has long been the overarching professional and societal bioethical value (as well as the key value in health care law). Autonomy recognizes an adult individual's right to accept or reject recommendations for medical care, even to the extent of refusing all care, if that individual has appropriate decision-making capacity.[3] This is the counterweight to the medical profession's long-practiced *paternalism* (or parentalism), wherein

medical care was based on whatever the practitioner determined was "good" for the patient regardless of whether the patient agreed. Coercion to influence behavior or choice through the force of authority is often coupled with paternalism. The joining of the august figure in white with implied or explicit threats has been and still is a potent force for counteracting any potential patient autonomy. However, the thrust of modern bioethics is to respect patients by honoring their autonomy.[2]

Health Care Professionals' Values

CPR and other resuscitation measures should be used only when they may benefit the patient. They should never be used when they merely prolong the dying process. In emergency situations, when information about patients, their wishes, and their medical conditions are unknown, clinicians must assume that resuscitation is warranted until clinical signs demonstrate that further intervention will not be effective.

Health care workers, both in the prehospital arena and in health care facilities, have specific goals for their interventions. Most entered the healing professions to help others, a principle termed *beneficence*; they dislike intervening when it will not benefit the patient.

Some practitioners have a conflict with specific professional or societal values on a religious, philosophic, or practical basis.[4] When such a conflict exists in a practitioner's mind, it is deemed morally and legally acceptable, within certain constraints, for the individual to follow a course of action based on a personal value system. When conflicts between the practitioner's and the patient's values exist, however, it is essential for the practitioner to recognize the patient's identity, dignity, and autonomy and to avoid the

| TABLE 37-1 • Commonly Accepted Societal and Bioethical Values

Autonomy	Self-determination. A person's ability to make personal decisions, including those affecting personal medical care. Autonomy is the opposite of paternalism.
Beneficence	Doing good. A duty to confer benefits. Production of benefit.
Confidentiality	The presumption that what the patient tells the physician will not be revealed to any other person or institution without the patient's permission.
Distributive justice	Fairness in the allocation of resources and obligations. This value is the basis of and is incorporated into societywide health care policies.
Nonmaleficence	Not doing harm, prevention of harm, and removal of harmful conditions.
Personal integrity	Adhering to one's own reasoned and defensible set of values and moral standards.
Privacy	Controlling the extent, timing, and circumstances of sharing oneself (physically, behaviorally, or intellectually) with others.

Source: Adapted from: Iserson KV. Bioethics. In Marx JA, Hockberger RS, Walls RM, et al, eds. *Rosen's Emergency Medicine: Concepts and Clinical Practice*, 6th ed. Philadelphia: Mosby, 2006:3127–3139, with permission.

error of blindly imposing one's own values on another. Even when the physician plans to follow a treatment course consistent with accepted societal values, it is desirable to review the case's specific circumstances and the hierarchical importance of the values involved. In each case, the ethical analysis must recognize all practicable courses of action and the benefits and detriments of each, while at the same time respecting the patient's values.[5]

For emergency cardiovascular care, the key to this analysis is to recognize that the goals are to preserve life, restore health, relieve suffering, limit disability, and reverse clinical death.[6] CPR and other resuscitation measures should be used only when they may benefit the patient. They should never be used when they merely prolong the dying process. "Benefit" means attempting to meet the patient's goals of therapy. In emergency situations, when information about patients, their wishes, and their medical conditions are unknown, clinicians must assume that resuscitation is warranted until clinical signs demonstrate that further intervention will not be effective.

Patient self-determination may not apply when insufficient resources exist to provide the desired intervention. This often occurs in disasters and in less developed nations. In these situations, the ethical principle of comparative, or distributive, justice comes into play. Health care policy based on this principle requires that individuals and groups with similar problems should receive similar (generally an equitable, not necessarily an equal) distribution of available resources. Such a public health policy should be triggered by specific events; it should not be applied ad hoc by individual clinicians at the bedside.[2,7]

Clinicians often attempt to use legal justifications for their actions or inactions in end-of-life care, including cardiac resuscitation. In general, physicians' legal knowledge is often incorrect, only partially true, or applied incorrectly.[8] Patients and health care providers are best served if the patient's values and goals of therapy guide the physician's course of action.

 See Web site for ACEP policy statement on ethical issues for resuscitation.

Withholding and Withdrawing CPR

Differing levels of knowledge about patients, their medical conditions, and their desire for resuscitation require the use of separate approaches to withholding and withdrawing CPR in the prehospital, emergency department, and inpatient settings. Inpatients may also have ongoing treatments withdrawn.

Prehospital Considerations

Resuscitative efforts should not be withheld or withdrawn on the basis of DNAR (do not attempt resuscitation) tattoos or other nonstandard requests that do not involve discussions with patients or their legal surrogate decision makers.

Bystander CPR

In the prehospital setting, what is known about patients in cardiopulmonary arrest can vary greatly depending upon the setting and the nature of bystanders' knowledge. Given the general paucity of facts and the wide range of skill levels among those who may be in a position to initiate CPR, the standard for withholding life-sustaining treatments in the prehospital setting is much higher and more specific than that for other settings. Based on the assumption that most people in cardiopulmonary arrest would want resuscitation, lay-rescuers and bystanders normally *should* initiate CPR. There are only three exceptions to this rule: (1) when a person has obvious clinical signs of irreversible death (e.g., rigor mortis, dependent lividity, injuries incompatible with life, decomposition, or burned beyond recognition), (2) when performing CPR would place the rescuer at risk, and (3) when an available and interpretable advance directive specifies that the individual does not desire resuscitation.[6] Advance directives may not apply in cases of a failed suicide attempt.[9–11]

INDICATIONS FOR WITHHOLDING PREHOSPITAL BASIC LIFE SUPPORT

1. Clinical signs of irreversible death
2. Risk of injury or death to rescuer
3. Available and interpretable advance directive

Resuscitative efforts should not be withheld or withdrawn on the basis of DNAR (do not attempt resuscitation) tattoos or other nonstandard requests that do not involve discussions with patients or their legal surrogate decision makers.[12,13] They should also not be withheld or withdrawn based on the patient's age, socioeconomic status, insurance coverage, cultural background, or relationship to the criminal justice system.

Having begun, those performing CPR should continue until one of the following occurs:

- Effective, spontaneous circulation and ventilation are restored.
- Care is transferred to a more senior-level emergency medical professional.
- Reliable criteria indicating irreversible death are present.
- The rescuer is unable to continue due to exhaustion or the presence of dangerous environmental hazards or because

continuation of resuscitative efforts places other lives in jeopardy.
- A valid and interpretable DNAR order is presented to rescuers. [6,14]

 See Web site for ACEP policy statement on DNAR in the out-of-hospital setting.

Emergency Medical Services

Emergency medical services (EMS) providers have a higher level of training and more experience than lay-people, resulting in a greater awareness of when to refrain from resuscitative efforts. EMS providers may also have the emotional distance and clinical expertise to know when to stop CPR. The ability to provide advanced cardiac life support (ACLS) interventions, do electrocardiograms, and contact a base station for medical direction helps them make these decisions. However, neither lay-rescuers nor EMS personnel should make judgments about the present or future quality of life of a cardiac arrest victim on the basis of current or anticipated neurologic status. Such snap judgments are often inaccurate. Quality of life should never be used by EMS personnel as a criterion to withhold CPR, because conditions such as irreversible brain damage or brain death cannot reliably be assessed or predicted. [15–20]

EMS Termination of Resuscitation Efforts

The most powerful discriminatory criterion on the appropriateness of CPR is knowledge of the time of onset of CPR (i.e., witnessed cardiac arrest).

When, then, should EMS personnel cease resuscitative efforts? Although there are no scientifically valid clinical criteria that accurately predict the futility of CPR, the most powerful discriminatory criterion on whether CPR is appropriate are whether the cardiac arrest was witnessed and whether the rescuer knows the time of onset of the arrest. [21–25] Most commonly, patients with an unwitnessed cardiac arrest are persons who died and were later discovered. [26] Another useful criterion to cease CPR is the absence of a "shockable" rhythm on the defibrillator after an adequate trial of CPR, even if ACLS providers are not available. [6]

The American Heart Association (AHA) has affirmed that "emergency transportation of patients requiring continuing CPR after ACLS-level care in the field is rarely indicated or successful. Any such transportation for reasons other than to benefit the patient is unethical." [26] Unless patients are suffering from rare, specific pathologic conditions (e.g., hypothermia or drug overdose), there are no in-hospital interventions that will successfully resuscitate those who fail out-of-hospital efforts. [27] Studies have consistently shown that <1% of patients who continue to receive CPR while being transported to the hospital will survive to hospital discharge, but EMS personnel in the United States continue to transport them, usually "Code 3," posing an unnecessary risk to themselves and others. [6,22,24,28–30] This may be due to rules within the EMS system or to their discomfort with having to stop efforts in a victim's home, which they may see as publicly acknowledging "failure." [31] In addition, both family and EMS personnel are often uncomfortable in leaving a body at the scene.

 See Web site for AHA ECC 2005 guidelines for cardiopulmonary resuscitation—ethical issues.

To end these unnecessary, wasteful, and potentially dangerous transports, it is vital that EMS systems establish protocols for death pronouncement in out-of-hospital settings in a manner consistent with state and national regulations. The AHA, American College of Emergency Physicians (ACEP), and National Association of EMS Physicians support this. [31] Even where a death pronouncement protocol exists, there may be significant variability among base hospitals in the rate with which they pronounce deaths using online medical control. [30] Additionally, even with protocols in place, paramedics may be reluctant to terminate resuscitation efforts in children in the prehospital setting. [32]

 See Web site for ACEP policy statement on discontinuation of resuscitation orders in the out-of-hospital setting.

Emergency Department

In emergency medicine, a significant difference *rightfully* persists between the withholding and the withdrawal of life-sustaining medical treatment. The justification for this stems in part from the nature of emergency medical practice and the unique manner in which clinicians apply many ethical principles. Because emergency physicians often lack vital information about their patients' identities, medical conditions, and goals for medical treatment, withholding emergency medical treatment is more problematic than is later withdrawing unwanted or useless interventions. Owing to the nature of emergency medicine, both in the prehospital and the emergency department settings, higher standards are required to withhold than to withdraw medical treatment. [33]

Physicians should begin or continue resuscitation of those patients who arrive at the emergency department without sufficient evidence to determine that the resuscitation effort will be unsuccessful. The only reason to *withhold* CPR is when the physician has clear evidence (e.g., a standard advance directive) indicating that the patient did not wish this done. Without this information, the presumption must be to intervene.

The only reason to withhold CPR is clear evidence (e.g., a standard advance directive) indicating that the patient did not wish resuscitation to be initiated.

Once the emergency physician obtains information confirming a patient's wish not to be resuscitated or about a medical condition not amenable to resuscitation, resuscitative efforts and other medical treatment may appropriately be withdrawn. This information may be obtained from an advance directive, patient surrogate, recent documentation in the medical chart, or medics detailing the failed results of the ongoing resuscitative effort. With rare exceptions, such as after failed suicide attempts, resuscitative efforts should be withdrawn when information is provided either that the patients did not want such efforts or that their medical condition precludes success.[11,14]

Many factors influence the potential success of resuscitative efforts, including time to CPR; time to defibrillation, IV line, and first epinephrine dose; time to insertion of first advanced airway device; comorbid disease; prearrest state; and initial arrest rhythm. No combination of these factors, though, clearly predicts the outcome.[26,34] The most important factor associated with poor outcome is the *duration* of unsuccessful resuscitative efforts.

The possibility of a successful resuscitation becomes clearer as time progresses: a patient's chance of being discharged from the hospital alive and neurologically intact diminishes if spontaneous circulation does not return after 10 minutes of intensive resuscitative efforts.[20,35–37] Malpractice concerns have led some physicians to prolong all resuscitation attempts until they reach the point at which there have been no survivors.[26] In reality, cardiac resuscitation with properly executed ACLS interventions and documented asystole should not last >30 minutes and should usually end much sooner except in unusual circumstances, as with prearrest hypothermia, after some drug-induced events, following lightning or electrical shocks, or in infants or children with refractory ventricular fibrillation (VF) or ventricular tachycardia (VT).[26,37–40] Indeed, without these mitigating factors, prolonged resuscitative efforts are unlikely to be successful.[41]

Cardiac resuscitation with properly executed ACLS interventions and documented asystole should not last >30 minutes and should usually end much sooner except in unusual circumstances, as with prearrest hypothermia, after some drug-induced events, following lightning or electrical shocks, or in infants or children with refractory VF or VT.

Three special situations should be noted. (1) Cardiac arrest from blunt trauma is nearly uniformly fatal, so there is little benefit from doing chest compressions for any extended length of time after the airway is secured.[42] (2) When health care resources are limited, as during disasters, available resources (i.e., time, personnel, and equipment) should be devoted to those patients with the greatest chance of benefiting. This may lead to withholding or more rapid discontinuation of resuscitative efforts than is standard in normal practice. (3) It is unethical to prolong resuscitative efforts to practice or teach procedures or to complete research protocols.[14]

In the Hospital

In health care institutions, staff generally know or have medical records showing their patients' medical condition, prognosis, wishes regarding resuscitation, and goals for medical treatment. Resuscitation attempts should be consistent with these goals and medical conditions. As the AHA notes, "It is inappropriate to start CPR when survival is not expected or the patient is expected to survive without the capacity for meaningful human communication."[26] Therefore, CPR should not be instituted when the patient's vital functions have already deteriorated despite maximal therapy (e.g., as in progressive septic or cardiogenic shock).

CPR should not be instituted when the patient's vital functions have already deteriorated despite maximal therapy (e.g., as in progressive septic or cardiogenic shock).

In neonates, withholding resuscitation attempts in the delivery room is appropriate when gestation, birth weight, or congenital anomalies are associated with almost certain early death and when unacceptably high morbidity is likely among the rare survivors.[6] This includes not initiating or discontinuing resuscitation in the delivery room of preterm newborns of <24 weeks' gestation or weighing <500 g, infants whose Apgar score remains zero at 10 minutes,[43] and newborns with confirmed or overt lethal malformations and/or chromosomal abnormalities.[44]

In the Hospital: Withdrawal of Ongoing Life Support

The decision to withdraw life support may be made minutes or even decades after the initial resuscitation. Usually it is the result of obtaining additional information from the patient, the discovery of advance directives, or a decision by the surrogate. Often the patient or surrogate requests that interventions be stopped because he or she believes that the "successful" resuscitation has not met the goal of an acceptable result or that the burden to the patient of continued treatment would exceed any benefits. Other reasons to withdraw support include the clinicians' determination that the interventions cannot ultimately be successful or that the patient is dead by brain criteria, in which case it is no longer technically "life support."

Goals of Therapy   While withdrawing life-support treatment may be an emotionally difficult decision for family and staff, it is ethically permissible under the circumstances described above. The goal is to avoid prolonging the dying process without degrading the quality of the patient's remaining life. This practice has widespread ethical and legal support.[45] Nevertheless, decisions about the withdrawal of artificially provided nutrition and hydration and, less commonly, about other modalities continue to be suffused with religiocultural polemics. If disagreement exists about the course of action, the institution's bioethics committee or consultant should be called in and, when necessary, asked to mediate between physicians, family, and staff.[46] In some circumstances, chaplains can effectively intervene, especially when families refuse to allow discontinuation of machines in "brain dead" patients because "a miracle" may occur.

In determining how to limit or withdraw treatments, clinicians and surrogates should carefully consider the patient's goals for therapy. For example, if a goal is to maintain the patient until loved ones arrive, it may be appropriate to continue mechanical ventilation. In general, interventions that do not contribute to achieving the patient's goals should be discontinued. Throughout this process, care must continue; comfort measures, including needed analgesics, must never be withdrawn.

Since the initial recommendations for discontinuing ventilator support were published in 1983, withdrawal of ventilators, dialysis, vasopressors, and other life-sustaining treatments has become more common.[47–49] The frequency with which treatments are withdrawn from intensive care unit (ICU) patients before death varies among institutions, with some never withdrawing treatments and others doing so in nearly all eligible patients.[51] It is unclear whether these differences reflect physician or institutional values regarding respecting patient preferences.[52]

Methods of Withdrawing Treatments   Critically ill patients often have multiple types of life-sustaining treatments. Withdrawing or foregoing these treatments may be done sequentially or simultaneously. The normal sequence in critical care units is to first withdraw dialysis, then to forego further diagnostic workups and discontinue vasopressors. Next, clinicians generally stop intravenous fluids, hemodynamic and electrocardiographic monitoring, and antibiotic treatment. The last interventions to be withdrawn usually are artificial nutrition and mechanical ventilation.[52]

The rationale for this "stepwise retreat" may not reflect optimal patient care. Rather, the order of withdrawal may relate to the intervention's symbolic importance, such as artificial feeding, or to how immediately its withdrawal will lead to death, as with a ventilator. Physicians appear reluctant to withdraw interventions that treat iatrogenic problems and are more comfortable withdrawing therapies related to their own subspecialty.[53,54] Surrogates are often more willing to eschew new interventions, such as antibiotics or dialysis, because the link between these decisions and death is not as obvious.[51]

After a decision to withdraw treatment is made, staff should continue to maintain the patient's comfort and dignity. Varying symptoms accompany the withdrawal of each life-support intervention. Appropriate therapies should be provided to minimize suffering associated with pain, dyspnea, delirium, convulsions, and other terminal complications. To accomplish this, it is ethically acceptable to gradually increase the dosage of narcotics and sedatives to relieve pain and other symptoms, even to levels that might concomitantly shorten the patient's life.[7]

For example, methods of withdrawing mechanical ventilation vary considerably among physicians and specialties. With any method, the goal is to keep the patient comfortable using appropriate medications, usually titrated opioids and benzodiazepines. Neuromuscular blocking agents should not be used and, if already in use, should be reversed. To achieve comfort, opioid-tolerant patients may need doses one order of magnitude higher than normal (e.g., 500–1,000 mg/hr). Documentation in the patient chart must specify that this medication is being used for comfort.[51]

If a patient has an implanted pacemaker or defibrillator ICD, this should normally be inactivated; although the residual rhythm that will persist is unpredictable, this may prevent automatic and uncomfortable defibrillations from the device at the end of life.[55] Most modern devices can be made ineffective by noninvasive reprogramming.[56] Before removing or inactivating such a device, the clinician should inform the patient or surrogate that such action could result in sudden death.[57]

Occasionally, in the process of withdrawing life support, clinicians may need to use terminal sedation (i.e., high doses of sedatives to relieve extremes of physical distress). This is a last-resort clinical response to extreme, unrelieved physical suffering. The purpose of the medications is to relieve suffering, not to intentionally end the patient's life. While it is an extraordinary measure, withholding such treatment in certain circumstances has been deemed "inhumane."[58] Terminal sedation is commonly used in critical care units to treat symptoms of suffocation when mechanical ventilation is withdrawn in dying patients.[59,60]

Decision-Making Capacity, Advance Directives, and Surrogate Decision Makers

Advance directives—such as living wills, durable powers of attorney for health care, and prehospital advance directives—are used to guide a patient's health care decisions *only* when they are unable to do so themselves (i.e., when they lack decision-making capacity). When a patient lacking decision-making capacity does not have an advance directive, a surrogate list may be used. The first step for clinicians, however, is to determine a patient's decision-making capacity at the bedside.

Decision-Making Capacity

In much of western culture, patient autonomy, also called self-determination, is a bedrock principle of modern biomedical ethics as well as law. Justice Benjamin Cardozo codified the principle in 1914 when he wrote that "Every human being of adult years and sound mind has a right to determine what shall be done with his own body...."[3] This means that adult patients with decision-making capacity may autonomously make their own health care decisions, including choosing between treatment options, refusing treatment, and designating someone else to make their health care decisions even if they are able to do so themselves. Exercising one's autonomy is the way to implement one's own values. In clinical practice, the word "competence" is often used to mean capacity. "Competence" is a legal term and can be determined only by the court.

The capacity to make one's own health care decisions may vary with the complexity of the decision, such as deciding between invasive or pharmacologic treatment of an arrhythmia or the seriousness of a decision's outcome, as with a heart transplant. Decision-making capacity can also vary over time. Elderly patients who "sundown" and patients partially incapacitated by drugs or physiologic events such as post–cardiac arrest or transient ischemic attack may not immediately be able to make their own health care decisions, although they may regain this capacity.

Clinicians must often decide whether patients currently have the capacity to make specific health care decisions. It is the treating physician's responsibility to determine the patient's decision-making capacity. The process of making this determination should be standardized and the results documented in the patient's medical record. Simply refusing a physician's recommendation for a commonly accepted treatment option such as thrombolytics or coronary angiography during an acute myocardial infarction does not, in itself, indicate that the person lacks decision-making capacity.

To have adequate decision-making capacity in any particular circumstance, an individual must understand the options, the consequences of acting on the various options, and the costs and benefits of these consequences, by relating them to a relatively stable framework of personal values and priorities.[61] One simple method, outlined below, for determining decision-making capacity at the bedside is to assess the patient's responses to three questions.[62] If any of them cannot adequately be answered, the capacity to make that decision is lacking.

Determining Decision-Making Capacity at the Bedside

After providing a patient with sufficient information to make an informed choice, information about the given condition and prognosis, the nature of the proposed intervention, alternatives, and risks and benefits, the patient is asked:

1. What options did the clinician present? (e.g., to be hospitalized or not.)

2. What are the risks and benefits to you for each option?
3. *Why* did you select the option you did?

To have decision-making capacity, the patient must provide coherent, appropriate answers to all three questions.

Assessing the last response requires weighing the patient's answer against what is known about his or her value system. The choice should be accepted if it seems to conform to the patient's values, even if it is not the choice most people would select (e.g., "I don't want any more medical treatment" or "I'm not sick enough to go into the hospital"). However, the answer may be bizarre and not consistent with reality (e.g., "They'll poison me like they do everyone else" or "The voices are telling me not to do it"). Such answers indicate a lack of decision-making capacity. Often, those accompanying the patient may be able to help determine how close the answer is to the patient's normal value system.[2,61]

It may be especially difficult to evaluate decision-making capacity for patients in the prehospital system via telephone or radio. In these cases, medics can ask the questions and transmit the answers, or the patient can be put on the telephone or radio while the physician asks the questions.

Unconscious patients, such as those in cardiopulmonary arrest, clearly lack decision-making capacity. Unless contradictory information is immediately available, such as a standard prehospital advance directive, consent for resuscitation procedures is presumed.[2]

Patients who retain decision-making capacity may still prefer to have a health care decision made by someone else. Many cultures, including some within western countries, rely on traditional decision-making models other than patient autonomy; usually this is family- or community-based decision making.[63] In those cases, the surrogates must be identified and given the same information the patient would need to make a decision.

When a patient lacks decision-making capacity, an advance directive or surrogate decision maker must be used. A significant number of patients in the hospital and in the acute setting have neither a directive nor an identifiable surrogate. In those cases, the clinician acts as surrogate.[64]

Advance Directives

The term "advance directives" includes several types of legal and quasi-legal documents. Advance directives indicate what medical interventions should be done for a patient in extremis who is no longer able to give or withhold permission for treatment. These forms, signed by the patient or surrogate, are usually written to avoid prolonging an inevitable, often painful or nonsentient dying process. Advance directives are usually variations of a living will, durable power of attorney for health care, or prehospital advance directive. Forms are specific to individual states; forms from other states have legal weight only if state statutes specifically permit it (e.g., Arizona). However, even if they carry no legal weight, these documents can provide caregivers and surrogates with valuable information about the person's wishes. State-specific statutes and forms can be obtained from the American Hospital Association, American Medical Association, American Bar Association, and American Association of Retired Persons or their state affiliates, and state governments. Most can be downloaded at no cost from the Internet.

Unfortunately, <50% of all patients needing others to make their health care decisions have advance directives.[65–72] People from some cultures may be less willing to discuss resuscitation status or to forego life-sustaining treatment and so may be less likely to complete advance directives.[73,74] Whites and individuals who are better educated are more likely to have advance directives.[75,76] The federal Patient Self-Determination Act of 1991 was designed to increase the use of advance directives.[77] It requires health care institutions and managed care organizations to ask newly admitted patients if they have advance directives and to facilitate the completion of these forms if they do not. Copies of any directives must be put in a patient chart if the patient desires it. However, there is little evidence that the act has increased the use of advance directives. In general, ignoring advance directives has no clear legal repercussions.

Advance directives are patient- or surrogate-initiated. These differ from physicians' orders regarding end-of-life treatment, which are discussed below.

Living Will

The living will is a relatively standardized form adopted in most states and the District of Columbia. Michigan and Massachusetts do not have statutes. This document usually requests that health care workers not perform resuscitative measures, but on occasion it requests the opposite—that all measures be taken to keep the patient alive. It goes into effect only if the individual lacks decision-making capacity; until that point, the patient continues to determine the medical course, despite anything said in the living will. Living wills normally require both that a physician certify an individual as terminally ill and that the patient has the mental capacity to understand its provisions at the time it is signed. Arizona, in a break with tradition, does not use "terminally ill," since all extant definitions are unclear. No ill effects have resulted.[78] States allow varying levels of specificity in the document, including, in some cases, the ability to refuse artificial nutrition and hydration.

Most living wills specify that the patient's physician must have seen and accepted the document's provisions in advance. This requirement establishes a physician who will act on the patient's behalf. For physicians, it protects those whose value systems will not allow them to abide by the documents' provisions. It also encourages families and physicians to discuss the circumstances surrounding the time of death and the actions they can take.[2]

The limitation of living wills is that they list specific actions—either to take or to eschew—in a limited set of circumstances. This reduces their usefulness and has led to a more flexible and powerful advance directive that names a trusted surrogate decision maker: the durable power of attorney for health care.

Durable Power of Attorney for Health Care (DPAH)

A more commonly used advance directive that specifies a surrogate decision maker is the durable power of attorney for health care. It goes by many names, including "durable power of attorney with medical provisions" and "medical directive." All states and the District of Columbia have statutes authorizing such directives. In its usual form, a durable power of attorney other than for health care takes effect immediately. However, a DPAH takes effect only when the individual no longer has the capacity to make his or her own medical decisions.

Typically, a relative or close friend is named as a surrogate, since he or she should know something about the individual's values related to medical treatment. More than one surrogate may be named; they are generally listed in preferential order, with the first one who is able to be contacted and is willing and able to act as surrogate making the decisions.[2]

The DPAH allows more flexibility than the living will because the surrogate is able to make any health care decisions that the patient would ordinarily make, including gathering new information and choosing among multiple treatment options as the medical situation changes. Optimally, the surrogate's decisions are guided by other written or oral directions the patient has left, including those in a living will. In reality, surrogates often consider many factors when making decisions.[79]

Prehospital Directives

Ambulances are often inappropriately called for patients in cardiopulmonary arrest who had previously expressed the desire not to be resuscitated. Many of these patients are chronically ill or have a terminal illness.[80–82] To avoid unwanted resuscitative efforts, prehospital directives were developed—first as local EMS protocols and then through legislation.[83]

As of 2003, 43 U.S. jurisdictions had enacted methods whereby patients outside of health care facilities could avoid unwanted resuscitation attempts. These usually take the form of either a prehospital DNAR order or a prehospital advance directive.[83] Often confused, the two forms differ greatly in their philosophies. The prehospital DNAR order is a physician-originated document.[84] The prehospital advance directive is generated by a patient or legal surrogate, with little or no involvement by health care personnel. Both instruct EMS personnel who have been inappropriately called at the time of death not to attempt to resuscitate the patient or to stop resuscitation efforts if they have already begun when such a form is found. Both types of form have proved effective.[83–86] The most common reason for having physician-initiated forms is the fear that murders and suicides could be aided by patient-initiated documents. In practice, this has not occurred. In EMS systems, prehospital DNAR policies provide direction and guidance for these situations. ACEP has provided general guidelines addressing the integration of public, EMS, and physician directives on a community-wide basis.

See Web site for ACEP policy statement on DNAR orders in the out-of-hospital setting.

Of the existing protocols, 34 were specifically authorized by statute, usually supplemented by regulation or guidelines. Eight states implemented protocols solely through regulations or guidelines, without a change in their legal code. Eight states have no statewide protocol in place. In an affront to patient autonomy, 39 are physician orders requiring a physician's signature; 7 states require only a physician's signature; and 33 states require signatures of both a physician and the patient.[84] Three protocols are patient-initiated advance directives that are valid with a witnessed patient signature, with no physician involvement required.[87] These instruments are of varying complexity; some include liability protection for EMS personnel and base-station providers and some may be usable for pediatric patients.[78,83] Table 37-2 contains a list of the elements ideally included in a prehospital advance directive/DNAR policy.

There is evidence that out-of-hospital health care providers can interpret and are willing to implement DNAR orders and other documents limiting treatment. Studies indicate that while emergency medical technicians (EMTs) and paramedics are willing to honor patient preferences, they need written, uniform directives or physician orders to do so.[17,88–90]

Prehospital DNAR orders or directives must be understandable to all involved (e.g., EMS personnel, physicians, patients, family members, and police, who may also respond to 911 calls). These documents can take many forms (e.g., uniform system or state forms, physician orders, standard wallet identification cards or identification bracelets, and other mechanisms approved by the local EMS system). As noted below (Table 37-2), the ideal prehospital directive should continue to be effective, at least in the emergency department, if the patient is transferred to a health care institution.[83]

Nonstandard Advance Directives

Clinicians occasionally encounter medallions, tattoos, or other information that purport to be advance directives. These may cause consternation, since they fall outside society's bounds for indicating life-determining decisions. What should clinicians do if these indicators are found during resuscitations?

To be useful, advance directives must be available to the treating clinicians when they are needed, be a product of the patient's or sometimes the surrogate's deliberations, be understandable, and be applicable in the patient's current medical situation. Nonstandard directives are usually abbreviated or abstract, such as a tattooed symbol for "do not defibrillate;" thus they fail to meet these requirements. One problem is that the nature of such indicators may make it unclear whether the patient or surrogate either understood how their "directive" might be interpreted or whether it was still what was desired. In general, emergency physicians should not rely on these indicators to make critical decisions.[12,13]

Surrogate Decision Makers

When patients do not have the capacity to make medical decisions for themselves and lack advance directives containing specific instructions or naming a surrogate, someone must make the decision for them. This works far better in the United States than it does in Europe, where physicians are reluctant to accept surrogate decision makers.[91]

Surrogates ideally make decisions based on two distinct standards: substituted judgment and best interests. Substituted judgment is used by surrogates who believe they know enough about the patient's values to make a decision similar to that which the patient would make. It is not clear that anyone can know that much about a person.[92]

Surrogates use the best interest standard when they do not know what the patient would want done in a particular situation but, as in the case of Karen Ann Quinlan, the patient once had the capacity to make such decisions.[93] In that case, a 22-year-old woman, after two apneic episodes a year previously, lay in a persistent vegetative state. Her parents requested that life support be removed. The court allowed her parents to use the patient's prior statements and behavior to attempt to extrapolate her values, making a decision as close as possible to what the she would have wanted. Some states may require explicit written directives for surrogates to follow.[94,95] The best-interest standard also applies, as in the Saikewicz case, when the patient has never had adequate decision-making capacity.[96] In that case, a 67-year-old profoundly retarded man with an IQ of 10 was diagnosed with leukemia. Painful and disabling chemotherapy offered only a 30% to 50% probability of producing a short remission. The court ruled that most people would not want such treatment and that decision could be made not to institute treatment. Refusal of such treatment, they said, should not be denied simply because the patient lacked decision-making capacity.

Although ethicists and clinicians expect surrogates to use substituted judgment or patients' best interests when making decisions, studies show that many surrogates rely on other factors, such as their own best interests or mutual interests of themselves and the patient.[79] In many cases, surrogates opt for far more medical treatment than the patient would have wanted, perhaps owing to a lack of understanding about end-of-life issues and options.[97–99]

There are five major classes of decision makers: family, statutory surrogates, bioethics committees, physicians, and the courts.[2]

Family Traditionally and usually in practice, a family member—especially a spouse—acts as the surrogate decision maker for a patient who lacks the capacity to make his or her own medical decisions. It should be understood, however, that even when there is a strong family tie, emotional or fiscal costs may sway the surrogate decision maker from certain courses of action the patient would wish taken.

| TABLE 37-2 • Guidelines for Developing a Policy for Out-of-Hospital Advance Directives

To ensure maximum coherence and compliance, a comprehensive out-of-hospital DNAR policy should be endorsed by the widest possible jurisdiction (i.e., local, regional, state, and the medical community, including the EMS governing body). Whenever feasible, legislative support for such a policy should be sought. The out-of-hospital DNAR policy should:

1. Note the established fact that current basic and advanced life support interventions may not be appropriate or beneficial in certain clinical settings.

    • Develop a means to educate the public about the appropriate use of 911 after expected deaths.

    • Establish the fact that comfort care and palliative care are affirmative actions for patients with DNAR orders. These appropriate interventions (e.g., hospice or respite care) do not require EMS activation and can often be arranged by calling the patient's physician in anticipation of death.

    • Develop a means to educate health care workers on topics of advance directives, including information on local out-of-hospital DNARs, community hospice alternatives, and bereavement services.

2. Establish consensus on the ideal identification device for DNAR directives to assure continuity of care across settings.

3. Reiterate that initial resuscitative attempts are usually indicated when the patient's wishes are not known.

4. Define the conditions under which an out-of-hospital DNAR order can be considered, including its use in long-term-care settings and in the emergency department.

5. Define which patients have the decisional capacity to agree to a DNAR order and whether surrogates can sign such orders.

6. Establish a mechanism for determining the precedence of various directives [e.g., living will, durable power of attorney for health care, prehospital advance directive (DNAR)].

7. Develop a statutory prioritized list of surrogates to use when there are no advance directives and the patient's decisional capacity is impaired.

8. Consider language acknowledging the growing home hospice movement as it concerns children and incorporate provisions for document use in minors.

9. Establish that the decision not to attempt resuscitation must be an informed decision made by the patient or surrogate.

10. Identify the information that should be contained in the DNAR order and the authority that will be responsible for developing such a mechanism.

11. Identify the clinical procedures that are to be provided and those withheld in the adherence with the DNAR order, or specify which authority will verify adherence.

12. Define the exact manner in which the DNAR order is to be followed, including the role of online medical direction. Each system should ensure that a communication path to access online medical direction is immediately available when necessary.

13. Establish legal immunity provisions for those who implement DNAR orders in good faith.

14. Establish data collection and protocol evaluation to perform periodic operational assessments.

15. Identify permissible exceptions to compliance with DNAR out-of-hospital directives. For example:

    • The patient is able to revoke a written directive at any time.

    • The EMS personnel can cancel the out-of-hospital DNAR order if there are doubts about the document's validity.

Source: From Schears RM, Marco CA, Iserson KV. "Do-not-attempt-resuscitation" (DNAR) policy in the out-of-hospital setting. *Ann Emerg Med* 2004;44(1):68–70, with permission.

Children represent a special situation. Individuals younger than the age of majority or who are unemancipated are usually deemed incapable of making their own medical decisions. Nevertheless, in most cases the same rules that apply to adult capacity apply to children. As the seriousness of the consequences increases, the child must have more understanding of the options, consequences, and values involved in order to make a decision. Even if a parent is pres-ent, it is not always clear that the adult is acting in the best interest of the child. In such cases, child protective services may become involved. Disagreements between parents are also possible. In some cases, this results in the involvement of bioethics committees or the courts.[100]

Statutory Surrogate Lists   If an adult patient lacks decision-making capacity and has no advance directive, many states allow individuals to automatically become the person's surrogate. In practice, this almost always means that the patient's spouse may act in that capacity. Some states have a statutory surrogate list, which simplifies the process. The most extensive list specifies, in order, spouse not divorced or legally separated, a majority of adult children who can be reasonably contacted, parents of an adult, domestic partner, sibling, close friend, and the attending physician in consultation with a bioethics committee.[78] For children, the parents are nearly always their health care decision makers.

Bioethics Committees and Consultants   Multidisciplinary bioethics committees now exist in most large hospitals to help solve bioethical dilemmas. These cases often involve surrogate decision making or patients who lack both advance directives and an identifiable surrogate. Bioethics committees also reconfirm prognoses and mediate between dissenting parties. Some smaller hospitals have bioethics consultants, rather than committees, to perform many of the same functions. These committees, composed of medical and nonmedical members, presumably help make decisions based on the best-interest standard.

Physicians   In the past, physicians often made unilateral decisions for their patients, whether or not the patients had the capacity to decide for themselves. This still occurs of course—especially in stressful situations, such as with acute and unexpected illnesses and injuries or in the relatively large patient population lacking both decision-making capacity and surrogates.[101] It may fall to the clinician both to determine decision-making capacity and, if it is absent, to make a medical treatment decision for the patient. These decisions are often made without judicial or institutional review.[64] Although physicians often try to discern their patients' best interests, patients' preferences are hard to predict. Assumptions based on quality of life, age, or functional status may be inaccurate, and physicians' choices may reflect their own preferences more than those of their patients.[102] In identical situations, different physicians may choose widely varying levels of care.[103] Rarely considered is that physicians should consider their conflicts of interest when making these decisions.[104]

When making unilateral decisions, physicians should recognize that they are not omniscient. Prognoses are often incorrect and medical knowledge is finite. In these situations, "buying time" with a bioethics consultation may be worthwhile.

Courts   The courts often act as the final adjudicators of disagreements over medical care. They appoint legal guardians and, in a select few cases, set precedent that is followed as health law. The courts, though, are usually neither expeditious nor necessarily cognizant of bioethical principles. They can only follow the societal values that are codified in the law. Many courts have suggested that, whenever possible, health care decisions should remain at the bedside rather than in legal chambers.[93-95]

Do-Not-Attempt Resuscitation (DNAR), Limitation-of-Treatment, and Do-Not-Hospitalize (DNH) Orders

Often lumped with advance directives, these documents are physician orders that dictate what is to be done for patients in the case of a cardiopulmonary arrest or other deterioration in the patient's condition. Physicians must write specific orders so that staff will not perform unwanted or nonbeneficial CPR and other resuscitation activities or to avoid inappropriately sending patients to the hospital from nursing homes. These orders can take several forms, including DNAR, DNH, Prehospital DNAR (PHDNAR), and limitation-of-treatment orders. The orders are normally written in hospitals, nursing homes, and hospices and for home-hospice patients.

Do-Not-Attempt-Resuscitation (DNAR) Orders

Unlike other medical interventions, CPR is expected to be initiated without a physician's order, based on presumed consent for emergency treatment. Therefore, a physician's order is necessary to withhold CPR. A DNAR order, sometimes called do-not-initiate-resuscitation (DNIR) or, less realistically, a do-not-resuscitate (DNR) order, is a physician's order in the hospital chart informing other medical personnel that they should not institute CPR in the event of cardiopulmonary arrest and explaining the rationale for the order. Ideally, this order is put on charts only after consultation with the patient possessing decision-making capacity and the family and is usually written for chronically ill patients with a poor prognosis for long-term survival.

These orders usually work well within a specific institution. But if patients are transferred, as from a nursing facility or home to a hospital, the act of transfer or the activation of the EMS system negates the order. This can be directly contrary to a patient's wishes for terminal care. However, if a patient arriving at the hospital still has the capacity to make a decision concerning resuscitation, it is the admitting physician's duty to document such a decision in the patient's chart, including the specific actions to be limited, the circumstances of the discussion, and the individuals present during the discussion.[2,105,106]

When DNAR orders are written after consultation with the patient or, if the patient lacks decision-making capacity, the surrogate decision maker, physicians should document their discussions and follow institutional guidelines on how to document the order in the patient's medical record. Oral DNAR orders are not acceptable, although if the attending physician is not physically present, nursing staff may accept a DNAR order by telephone with the understanding that the physician will sign the order promptly.[6] Some institutions require telephonic orders to be done with at least two nurses on the line with the attending physician. DNAR orders should be reviewed periodically, particularly if the patient's condition changes. Rather than automatically canceling them before surgery, as is done in some institutions, DNAR orders should be reviewed by the anesthesiologist, attending surgeon, and patient or surrogate to determine their applicability in the operating room and postoperative recovery room.[107–109]

Physicians must also make certain that the proper steps are taken to notify the rest of the patient's care team, including anyone who may be in a position to "call a code" or respond on a code team. This includes the nurses, consultants, other attending physicians, and house staff.

A grievous error in modern health care has often been to equate a DNAR order with decreasing the level of care provided to the patient. Unfortunately, orders to not attempt resuscitation can lead to near abandonment of patients or to denial of appropriate and necessary medical and nursing care. DNAR orders should never convey a sense of "giving up" to the patient, family, or health care providers at the patient's bedside.[26] Basic nursing and comfort care (i.e., oral hygiene, skin care, patient positioning, and measures to relieve pain and symptoms) must always be continued. DNAR orders withhold only resuscitative efforts and do not imply that other forms of treatment should be diminished.[6] When the intent is for specific other medical treatments to be withheld, these orders should be written separate from the DNAR order, preferably on a "limitation of medical treatment" form, after discussions with the patient or surrogate. See discussion below.

A DNAR order should not prohibit a patient from receiving appropriate diagnostic procedures or treatment interventions, including admission to intensive care or critical care units. If admitted to an intensive or critical care unit, routine orders for resuscitation should be modified on an individual basis.

Limitation-of-Treatment Orders

Many institutions have now recognized that simple DNAR forms may be inadequate to describe the limitations of medical treatment requested for some patients. A DNAR order does not automatically preclude interventions other than CPR. For clarity, some institutions have adopted limitation-of-treatment orders to specify exactly what treatments are to be withheld in addition to CPR. These may include cardioversion, intubation, mechanical ventilation, the administration of parenteral fluids or nutrition, oxygen, antibiotics, blood products, sedation, antiarrhythmics, or vasopressors. As an ethical matter, appropriate analgesia should never be withheld.

Problems can arise when these orders become inconsistent with rational medical treatment. Some patients, for example, may choose to accept defibrillation and chest compressions but not intubation and artificial ventilations. Such conflicts arise when patients or surrogates have not been fully briefed on the nature of the proposed medical treatments. It is the responsibility of the attending physician to ascertain that the order set is rational and that the patient or surrogate understands why it is being written as it is.

Do-Not-Hospitalize (DNH) Orders

One type of physician order that has been used successfully in many locales is the "do not hospitalize" order. Normally written for hospice and nursing home patients, it prevents many unwanted in-hospital resuscitation attempts and procedure-laden hospitalizations. Do-not-hospitalize physician orders instruct nurses not to send patients to the hospital when further medical interventions are not desired by either the patient or their surrogate decision maker. This allows people to die peacefully, rather than having the "last rites of CPR" performed when they are futile or unwanted. The only caveat to applying DNH orders is that staff must know that patients should still be sent to the hospital if they need palliative care not available in the nursing facility.[110]

Barriers to using DNH orders include unrealistic family expectations, fear of litigation, and staff discomfort with managing patients experiencing clinical decline.[111] Large variations in the use of DNH orders occur throughout the United States. Nursing home residents most likely to have a DNH order are those in independent facilities, in an urban location, who are white, with total functional dependence (usually advanced dementia), and having a living will or durable power of attorney for health care.[112,113]

EMS and extended or terminal care facilities should establish protocols that allow patients who decline resuscitative efforts, including transport and hospitalization, to still receive the full range of comfort care, emergency medical treatment, and ambulance transport.[26]

Issues Related to Out-of-Hospital Resuscitation

In situations in which the EMS personnel cannot obtain clear information about the patient's wishes, resuscitative measures should be initiated.

About 325,000 cardiac disease–related deaths occur in the prehospital setting and emergency departments in the United States annually.[114] About 60% of unexpected cardiac deaths are treated by EMS personnel.[115]

A basic principle for prehospital providers is that when in doubt, attempt to resuscitate. The key is knowing when not to start resuscitation: when patients have rigor mortis, livor mortis, injuries incompatible with life, or are burned beyond recognition. Bystanders doing CPR should call 911, and if EMS personnel have questions about whether to continue resuscitation, they can contact their base station for medical direction.

Many patients for whom 911 is called because of cardiac arrest have been chronically ill, have a terminal illness, or have a written advance directive. States and other jurisdictions have varying laws about prehospital DNAR orders and advance directives.[116] In some cases in which a DNAR order exists, especially where there are differing opinions among family members, it may be difficult to determine whether resuscitation should be initiated. In situations in which the EMS personnel cannot obtain clear information about the patient's wishes, resuscitative measures should be initiated.

INITIATION OF CPR IN PRESENCE OF DNAR ORDER OR DIRECTIVE

EMS professionals should initiate CPR and ACLS if they believe that:

1. There is reasonable doubt about the validity of a DNAR order or advance directive.

2. The patient may have changed his or her mind.

3. The best interests of the patient are in question.

CPR decisions are often made in seconds by rescuers who may not know the patient or if an advance directive exists. As a result, administration of CPR may sometimes conflict with a patient's desires or best interests. Neither bystanders nor EMS personnel should attempt to interpret unique, lawyer or personally written, or other non-standard advance directives. They should adhere only to standard, EMS system-approved forms.[2,83,117]

After starting a resuscitation attempt, relatives or other medical personnel may arrive and confirm that the patient had clearly expressed a wish that resuscitation not be attempted. If these instructions appear to be clear, CPR or other life-support measures may be discontinued. If possible, EMS should also confirm this with their base hospital.[6]

Issues Related to In-Hospital Resuscitation

CPR is the only medical intervention that requires an order to *not* do it. Given that, some unique issues arise.

Since many patients have DNAR orders, it is incumbent on those discovering a patient in cardiac arrest or responding with a "code team" to quickly obtain accurate information about the patient's DNAR status. It is tragic to prolong a patient's dying by providing inappropriate resuscitative measures. Even so, if there is any doubt about whether a patient should be resuscitated, begin CPR. Life support can always be

withdrawn if more information surfaces. Not initiating resuscitative procedures and discontinuing life-sustaining treatment are ethically equivalent. In situations in which the prognosis is uncertain, a trial of treatment should be considered while further information is gathered to help determine the likelihood of survival and the expected clinical course.[6]

Iatrogenic Cardiac Arrest

Should patients be resuscitated if the cardiopulmonary arrest or instability was directly due to a health care worker's actions or inactions (i.e., an iatrogenic cardiopulmonary arrest)? Many physicians seem to believe that DNAR orders do not apply in cases involving their error or another iatrogenic cause. Even when they believe the DNAR orders remain valid, health care personnel may still attempt resuscitation to assuage their feelings of guilt or responsibility for the event.[118] This abnegates patient self-determination. It also perpetuates the common misconception that errors are avoidable evils of medicine rather than expected results in modern practice.[119] There is now general agreement that these patients' DNAR orders should be respected.

DNAR Orders and the Operating Room

Should DNAR orders automatically be suspended during surgery? This may also apply to patients with prehospital advance directives undergoing outpatient surgery. Some anesthetic procedures—such as intubation, ventilation, and the use of vasopressors—are identical to those used during resuscitation. This has led many institutions to automatically discontinue DNAR orders for patients going to the operating room and during the perioperative period.

There is now widespread agreement that, while some modifications may need to be made in the DNAR orders, these should be discussed and clarified with the patient or surrogate and the surgeon and anesthesiologist. Automatically discontinuing a DNAR order preoperatively or reinstituting it postoperatively deprives patients of their right to self-determination.[107-109]

As the American College of Surgeons stated some years ago,

The best approach is a policy of 'required reconsideration' of previous advance directives. The patient and the physicians who will be responsible for the patient's care should discuss the new risks and the approach to potential life-threatening problems during the perioperative period. The results of such discussions should be documented in the record. The operative and anesthetic permit should indicate that the patient or the duly authorized patient's representative has had the opportunity to discuss and reconsider any advance directive.

The American Society of Anesthesiologists has suggested that the operative permit specify one of three options based on discussions with the patient or surrogate:

(1) full attempt at resuscitation, with revocation of the DNAR order during the perioperative period; (2) limited attempt at resuscitation defined with regard to specific procedures after the patient or surrogate is informed about which procedures (a) are essential to the success of the anesthesia and the proposed procedure, and (b) are not essential and may be refused; or (3) limited attempt at resuscitation defined with regard to the patient's goals and values, allowing the surgical team to determine whether the burden and outcome of resuscitation meets the patient's goals of therapy.[121]

Family Attendance at "Codes"

While prehospital resuscitation attempts often occur in the home with family present and the EMS team communicating with them during the process, family members and other survivors are often barred from witnessing these procedures in health care institutions. This may be owing to institutional tradition, to fear that family members may become disruptive or interfere with resuscitation procedures, to concern that they may faint and injure themselves, or to fears that their naive interpretation of events may increase the clinicians' exposure to legal liability. Health care providers' opinions vary widely about whether family should be present during resuscitation attempts. In general, nurses, EMS providers, pediatricians, and, most recently, emergency physicians have been more amenable to family presence during resuscitations than have other health care professionals.[122–130]

Many studies have shown that family members want to be offered the opportunity to be present for critical care procedures and during resuscitation, especially for a child.[131–137] Parents' presence during pediatric resuscitations has become relatively common and has been endorsed by the American Academy of Pediatrics and the Ambulatory Pediatric Association.[6,26]

The American Heart Association endorses giving family members the opportunity to be present as long as the patient has not previously raised objections. This position stems from the benefit families can derive from their presence during resuscitation attempts, the lack of harmful effects on them from viewing these resuscitations, and their quasi-right to be there based on the nature of their relationship to the patient.[6,26] ACEP endorses end-of-life measures directed at the patient and family.

 See Web site for ACEP policy statement on end-of-life issues in the emergency department.

Benefits

Both the survivors and the health care team benefit from family presence during the resuscitation process.

Most of those viewing resuscitations indicate that they would not be hesitant to do so again, saying that they felt that they had both helped their loved one and had eased their own grieving.[133,140–143] This has been confirmed by standard psychological questionnaires showing that family members present during resuscitative efforts demonstrate less anxiety and depression and more constructive grief behavior than family members absent from the resuscitation attempt.[135] Most spouses and family members who have not witnessed a resuscitation effort say they would want to be present.

Family members who witness resuscitation attempts recognize the enormous effort that goes into resuscitation and the skill and compassion that the health care team exhibits. Rather than being cloistered in a back room, awaiting news, they see for themselves the struggle to save their loved one's life. Afterward they rarely ask the question that so often accompanies an unsuccessful resuscitation attempt: Was everything done? They may also thank the resuscitation team for their efforts, something that rarely occurs otherwise.[133]

Procedure

EMS agencies and health care institutions should develop protocols to guide family member presence during resuscitations. These protocols will, by necessity, vary with the setting.

In the prehospital setting, EMS providers must be aware of stresses on family members who may not have wished to view the resuscitation. When possible, such family members should be removed to another area using the help of other bystanders. This may be especially important for children. When it will not compromise the resuscitative effort, it is vital that EMS personnel describe their activities in lay terms and communicate additional information to those survivors who remain to watch.[133]

Family members seldom ask if they can be present for resuscitations unless encouraged to do so by health care providers. But if encouraged, a surprisingly large number will speak up. Health care providers should extend the opportunity to family members whenever possible.[144] Resuscitation team members should be made aware that family members are present and be sensitive to their feelings. This, however, should never compromise the resuscitative effort. A calm, experienced, and knowledgeable staff member not involved in the resuscitation (e.g., chaplain, social worker, or charge nurse) should be assigned to the family members and remain with them during the resuscitation to see to their needs and to answer any questions they may have.[133,143–145] Being present during the resuscitation attempt demonstrates to the survivor that everything possible is being done—a question that is often asked if they are not present—and provides them with a sense of closure that they otherwise cannot achieve.[133,145]

If the resuscitation attempts fail, survivors witnessing the process should never be asked if the team should stop; that is a medical decision based on the clinical situation. Rather, they should be informed that the team will stop.[133,145]

An increasing number of institutions are developing these types of protocols.[133,146–154]

Providing Emotional Support to the Family: Death Notification

Despite our best efforts, most resuscitations fail. Notifying family members of a loved one's death is an important aspect of a resuscitation attempt. It should be done compassionately and in a manner that accommodates the family's cultural and religious beliefs and practices.[141,145]

Facing someone whose loved one has just died is one of the most difficult and stressful tasks health care professionals must do. Notifiers primarily fear the survivors' loss of control once they tell them that their loved one has died. Reactions are unpredictable and professionals must be prepared to respond appropriately. Notifiers also fear their own reactions, their interactions with survivors, their ability to communicate this news, and the questions survivors may ask. Additional fears involve being blamed by survivors for the death as well as fear of their own death or disabilities.[133,145]

Notifications[133,145]

The physician usually delivers the news, often accompanied by a chaplain, nurse, or social worker. If the physician is involved with another critical task, most survivors have no objection if a nurse, chaplain, or social worker gives them the news immediately as long as they have subsequent contact with the physician.[156] Notification, however, should never be relegated to the unit assistant, medical or nursing student, or other untrained or partially trained person unless that individual is in the process of being educated and is accompanied by an experienced, supervising mentor.

Directness, truth, consistency, and clarity are the key factors when delivering information about a sudden, unexpected death. Perceptive survivors can easily tell which notifiers care and which are only "going through the motions." A key psychological response that often diminishes notifiers' effectiveness is identifying too closely with survivors, producing a sense of awkwardness or inadequacy and causing notifiers to rush through the process to hide their own emotions. Consequently, their presentation may seem callous or insensitive and the exact opposite of what they desired.

Using a "D" word is one of the hardest parts of the process. "D" words are "Died," "Death," or "Dead," including "Dead by brain criteria." Notifiers often find euphemisms such as "passed away," "left us," "didn't make

it," "lost him," "gone," or "expired" easier to say, even though they should not be used, because these do not register with some people at this stressful time. If survivors don't seem to understand, another 'D' word should be used in a different context.[133,145]

Notifiers should also use "helpful," rather than the all too common "harmful," phrases to interact with survivors (Table 37-3). Helpful phrases allow the individual to emote and to begin to deal with their loss in a constructive manner. Harmful phrases often provoke anger, imply blame, and may raise unnecessary issues.[133,145]

TABLE 37-3 • Helpful and Harmful Phrases in Speaking With Survivors

Helpful Phrases
• I can't imagine how difficult this is for you.
• I know this is very painful for you.
• I'm so sorry for your loss (Inclusive rather than pitying).
• It's harder than most people think.
• It's okay to be angry with God.
• It must be hard to accept.
• Tell me how you're feeling.
• I know you are feeling totally overwhelmed right now.
• Tell me about (decedent's name) and your life together.
• May I just sit here with you?
• Is there anyone I can call for you?

Harmful Phrases
• It was actually a blessing because....(God cliché)
• Only the good die young. (God cliché)
• God never gives us more than we can handle. (God cliché)
• Aren't you lucky that at least....(Unhealthy expectation)
• You must be strong for your (other) children, spouse, etc. (Unhealthy expectation)
• You'll get over this. (Unhealthy expectation)
• You're young...you'll find someone else. (Unhealthy expectation)
• It must have been his or her time to go. (Ignorance)
• Everything is going to be okay. (Basic insensitivity)
• Did he or she make peace with God before the end? (Basic insensitivity)

Source: From Iserson KV: *Grave Words: Notifying Survivors About Sudden, Unexpected Deaths.* Tucson, AZ: Galen Press, 1999:49–51, with permission.

Notification After an Unsuccessful Resuscitation Attempt[133,145]

Death notifications after attempted resuscitations are common occurrences in emergency departments and ICUs. If a family arrives at the hospital while resuscitation attempts are ongoing, a chaplain, social worker, or nurse may be delegated to inform the family of the patient's status. Families may be grateful that these individuals may be more inclined to use nonmedical words to explain what is occurring than would a physician. To avoid miscommunication, health care workers who act as notifiers should use "heart attack" rather than "MI," "breathing machine" rather than "ventilator," and "heart stopped" rather than "cardiac arrest." These notifiers—the same person or at least one person from the group who initially spoke with the family—should continually update the family. Progressive notification that things are not looking good alerts survivors to the grave situation and gives them at least a little time to prepare for bad news. When the family speaks another language, either use a non–family member interpreter or a telephone interpreting service.

If the resuscitation attempts fail, any survivors who have not observed the resuscitation attempt should be asked if they want to view the body. Parents may be encouraged to hold their child and, in some cases, even get into the bed with the body.

Most hospitals find it useful to have information packets about transportation of the body from a home or hospital, death certification, and autopsy and medical examiner requirements. Information on body, organ, and tissue donation should be included.

Education

It is essential that those who deal with resuscitations and death notification on a regular basis pass their knowledge of how to care for survivors, the newest patients, on to the next generation of health care professionals. Professionals whose job includes delivering news about sudden unexpected deaths need to learn how to perform this difficult task before doing it. Unfortunately, most medical "short courses" dealing with resuscitation have not incorporated death notification into their training programs or manuals.[133]

Occasionally, physicians give the job of death notification to residents, medical students, or nurses. Although all three groups should be present to learn the techniques involved, they should not be left to deliver death notifications on their own. That is a form of professional abandonment and, in a teaching hospital, the worst form of student abuse.[2,133]

References

1. McCormick RA. Theology and bioethics. *Hastings Cent Rep* 1989;19(2):5–10.
2. Iserson KV. Bioethics. In Marx JA, Hockberger RS, Walls RM, et al, eds. *Rosen's Emergency Medicine: Concepts and Clinical Practice*, 6th ed. Philadelphia: Mosby, 2006:3127–3139.
3. *Schloendorff v Society of New York Hospital*, 105 NE 92, 93, 1914.
4. Curlin FA, Lawrence RE, Chin MH, et al. Religion, conscience, and controversial clinical practices. *N Engl J Med* 2007;356(6):593–600.
5. Iserson KV. Ethical principles—emergency medicine. In Schears RM, Marco CA, eds. Ethical issues in emergency medicine. *Emerg Clin North Am* 2006;24(3):513–545.
6. Ethical aspects of CPR and ECC. Part 2. European Resuscitation Council. *Resuscitation* 2000;46:17–27.
7. Landesman BM. Physician attitudes toward patients. In Iserson KV, Sanders AB, Mathieu D, eds. *Ethics in Emergency Medicine*, 2nd ed. Tucson, AZ: Galen Press, 1995:350–357.
8. Meisel A, Snyder L, Quill T. Seven legal barriers to end-of-life care: myths, realities and grains of truth. *JAMA* 2000;284:2495-2501.
9. Moskop J, Iserson KV. Emergency physicians and physician-assisted suicide: Part I. A review of the physician-assisted suicide debate. *Ann Emerg Med* 2001;38(5):570–575.
10. Moskop J, Iserson KV. Emergency physicians and physician-assisted suicide: Part II. Emergency care for patients who have attempted physician-assisted suicide. *Ann Emerg Med* 2001;38(5):576–582.
11. Iserson KV, Gregory DR, Christensen K, et al. Willful death and painful decisions: a failed assisted suicide. *Camb Q Healthcare Ethics* 1992;1(2):147–158.
12. Iserson KV. Nonstandard advance directives: a pseudoethical dilemma. *J Trauma* 1998;44:139–142.
13. Iserson KV. The "no code" tattoo: an ethical dilemma. *West J Med* 1992;156:309–312.
14. Iserson KV. Resuscitation termination. In Rosen P, Barkin RM, Haden SR, et al, eds. *5-Minute Emergency Medicine Consult*. Philadelphia: Lippincott Williams & Wilkins, 1999:974–975.
15. Reisinger J, Hollinger K, Lang W, et al. Prediction of neurological outcome after cardiopulmonary resuscitation by serial determination of serum neuron-specific enolase. *Eur Heart J* 2007;28(1):52–58.
16. Iserson KV, Stocking C. Standards and limits: emergency physicians' attitude toward prehospital resuscitation. *Am J Emerg Med* 1993;11:592–594.
17. Marco CA, Schears RM. Prehospital resuscitation practices: a survey of prehospital providers. *J Emerg Med* 2003;24:101–106.
18. Wijdicks EFM, Hijdra A, Young GB, et al. Practice parameter: prediction of outcome in comatose survivors after cardiopulmonary resuscitation (an evidence-based review): report of the Quality Standards Subcommittee of the American Academy of Neurology. *Neurology* 2006; 67(2):203–210.
19. Bleck TP. Prognostication and management of patients who are comatose after cardiac arrest. *Neurology* 2006;67(4):556–557.
20. Kaye P. Early prediction of individual outcome following cardiopulmonary resuscitation: systematic review. *Emerg Med J* 2005;22:700–705.
21. Sanders AB, Kern KB, Berg RA. Searching for a predictive rule for terminating cardiopulmonary resuscitation. *Acad Emerg Med* 2001;8(6):654–657.
22. Morrison LJ, Visentin LM, Kiss A, et al. Validation of a rule for termination of resuscitation in out-of-hospital cardiac arrest. *N Engl J Med* 2006;355(5):478–487.
23. Dueker CW. A predictive model for survival after in-hospital cardiopulmonary arrest. *Resuscitation* 2005;66(2):246.
24. Ewy GA. Cardiac resuscitation—when is enough enough? *N Engl J Med* 2006;355(5):510–512.
25. Brindley PG, Markland DM, Mayers I, et al. Predictors of survival following in-hospital adult cardiopulmonary resuscitation. *CMAJ* 2002;167(4):343–348.
26. Cummins RO, ed. Patients, families, and providers: ethical aspects of CPR and ECC. In *ACLS: Principles and Practice*. Dallas: American Heart Association, 2003:17–41.
27. Eisenberg MS, Cummins RO. Termination of CPR in the prehospital arena. *Ann Emerg Med* 1985;14:1106–1107.
28. Jones T, Woollard M. Paramedic accuracy in using a decision support algorithm when recognising adult death: a prospective cohort study. *Emerg Med J* 2003; 20:473–475.
29. Verbeek PR, Marian J, Vermeulen MJ, et al. Derivation of a termination-of-resuscitation guideline for emergency medical technicians using automated external defibrillators. *Acad Emerg Med* 2002;9(7):671–678.

30. Eckstein M, Stratton SJ, Chan LS. Termination of resuscitative efforts for out-of-hospital cardiac arrests. *Acad. Emerg. Med* 2005;12(1):65–70.

31. Bailey ED, Wydro GC, Cone DC, et al. Termination of resuscitation in the prehospital setting for adult patients suffering nontraumatic cardiac arrest: a position statement from the NAEMSP. *Prehosp Emerg Care* 2000;4:190–195.

32. Hall WL, Myers JH, Pepe PE, et al. The perspective of paramedics about on-scene termination of resuscitation efforts for pediatric patients. *Resuscitation* 2004;60(2):175–187.

33. Iserson KV. Withholding and withdrawing medical treatment: an emergency medicine perspective. *Ann Emerg Med* 1996;28:51.

34. Barzilay Z, Somekh M, Sagy M, et al. Pediatric cardiopulmonary resuscitation outcome. *J Med* 1998;19:229–241.

35. Weisfeldt ML, Becker LB. Resuscitation after cardiac arrest: a 3-phase time-sensitive model. *JAMA* 2002;288:3035–3038.

36. Schults SC, Cullinane DC, Pasquale MD, et al. Predicting in-hospital mortality during cardiopulmonary resuscitation. *Resuscitation* 1996;33:13–17.

37. Reis AG, Nadkarni V, Perondi MB, et al. A prospective investigation into the epidemiology of in-hospital pediatric cardiopulmonary resuscitation using the international utstein reporting style. *Pediatrics* 2002;109(2):200–209.

38. Graber J, Ummenhofer W, Herion H. Lightning accident with eight victims: case report and brief review of the literature. *J Trauma* 1996;40:288–290.

38a. Fontanarosa PB. Electrical shock and lightning strike. *Ann Emerg Med* 1993;22:378–385.

39. Lopez-Herce J, Garcia C, Rodriguez-Nunez A, et al. Long-term outcome of paediatric cardiorespiratory arrest in Spain. *Resuscitation* 2005;64:79–85.

40. Parra DA, Totapally BR, Zahn E, et al. Outcome of cardiopulmonary resuscitation in a pediatric cardiac intensive care unit. *Crit Care Med* 2000;28:3296–3300.

41. Peberdy MA, Kaye W, Ornato JP, et al. Cardiopulmonary resuscitation of adults in the hospital: a report of 14720 cardiac arrests from the National Registry of Cardiopulmonary Resuscitation. *Resuscitation* 2003;58:297–308.

42. Eckstein M. Termination of resuscitative efforts: medical futility for the trauma patient. *Curr Opin Crit Care* 2001;7(6):450–454.

43. Harrington DJ, Redman CW, Moulden M, et al. The long-term outcome in surviving infants with Apgar zero at 10 minutes: a systematic review of the literature and hospital-based cohort. *Am J Obstet Gynecol* 2007;196(5):422–423.

44. Goldsmith JP, Niermeyer S, Byme S. AHA worksheet on guideline on the use of specific clinical indicators for non-initiation or discontinuation of resuscitation in the delivery room. Dallas: American Heart Association, 2004.

45. Quill TE. The ambiguity of clinical intentions. *N Engl J Med* 1993;329:1039–1040.

46. Swetz KM, Crowley ME, Hook C, et al. Report of 255 clinical ethics consultations and review of the literature. *Mayo Clin Proc* 2007;82(6):686–691.

47. Grenvik A. Terminal weaning: discontinuance of life-support therapy in the terminally ill patient. *Crit Care Med* 1983;11:394–395.

48. Prendergast TJ, Luce JM. Increasing incidence of withholding and withdrawal of life support from the critically ill. *Am J Respir Crit Care Med* 1997;155:15–20.

49. Koch KA, Rodeffer HD, Wears RL. Changing patterns of terminal care management in an intensive care unit. *Crit Care Med* 1994;22:233–243.

50. Prendergast TJ, Claessens MT, Luce JM. A national survey of end-of-life care for critically ill patients. *Am J Respir Crit Care Med* 1998;158:1163–1167.

51. Faber-Langendoen K Lanken PN, ACP-ASIM end-of-life care consensus panel. Dying patients in the intensive care unit: forgoing treatment, maintaining care. *Ann Intern Med* 2000;133:886–893.

52. Faber-Langendoen K, Spomer A, Ingbar D. A prospective study of withdrawing mechanical ventilation from dying patients. *Am J Respir Crit Care Med* 1996;153:4S.

53. Christakis NA, Asch DA. Medical specialists prefer to withdraw familiar technologies when discontinuing life support. *J Gen Intern Med* 1995;10:491–494.

54. Christakis NA, Asch DA. Biases in how physicians choose to withdraw life support. *Lancet* 1993;342:642–646.

55. Quill TE, Barold SS, Sussman BL. Discontinuing an implantable cardioverter defibrillator as a life-sustaining treatment. *Am J Cardiol* 1994;74:205–207.

56. Braun TC, Hagen NA, Hatfield RE, et al. Cardiac pacemakers and implantable defibrillators in terminal care. *J Pain Symptom Manage* 1999;18:126–131.

57. Mueller PS, Hook CC, Hayes DL. Ethical analysis of withdrawal of pacemaker or implantable cardioverter-defibrillator support at the end of life. *Mayo Clin Proc* 2003;78:959–963.

58. Quill TE, Dresser R, Brock DW. The rule of double effect: a critique of its role in end-of-life decision making. *N Engl J Med* 1997;337:1768–1771.

59. Brody H, Campbell ML, Faber-Langendoen K, et al. Withdrawing intensive life-sustaining treatment-recommendations for compassionate clinical management. *N Engl J Med* 1997;336:652–657.

60. Quill TE, Byock IR. Responding to intractable terminal suffering: the role of terminal sedation and voluntary refusal of food and fluids. *Ann Intern Med* 2000;132:408–414.

61. Buchanan AE. The question of competence. In Iserson KV et al, eds. *Ethics in Emergency Medicine*, 2nd ed. Tucson, AZ: Galen Press, 1995.

62. Iserson KV, Sanders AB, Mathieu DR, eds. *Ethics in Emergency Medicine*, 2nd ed. Tucson, AZ: Galen Press, 1995.

63. Martinez JM, López JS, Martín A, et al. Organ donation and family decision-making within the Spanish donation system. *Soc Sci Med* 2001;53(4):405–421.

64. White DB, Curtis JR, Lo B, et al. Decisions to limit life-sustaining treatment for critically ill patients who lack both decision-making capacity and surrogate decision-makers. *Crit Care Med* 2006; 34:2053–2059.

65. Wenger NS, Oye RK, Desbiens NA, et al. The stability of DNR orders on hospital readmission. The SUPPORT Investigators. Study to Understand Prognoses and Preferences for Outcomes and Risks of Treatments. *J Clin Ethics* 1996;7:48–54.

66. Teno JM, Murphy D, Lynn J, et al. Prognosis-based futility guidelines: does anyone win? SUPPORT Investigators. Study to Understand Prognoses and Preferences for Outcomes and Risks of Treatment. *J Am Geriatr Soc* 1994;42:1202–1207.

67. Teno JM, Licks S, Lynn J, et al. Do advance directives provide instructions that direct care? SUPPORT Investigators. Study to Understand Prognoses and Preferences for Outcomes and Risks of Treatment. *J Am Geriatr Soc* 1997;45:508–512.

68. Teno JM, Hakim RB, Knaus WA, et al. Preferences for cardiopulmonary resuscitation: physician-patient agreement and hospital resource use. The SUPPORT Investigators. *J Gen Intern Med* 1995;10:179–186.

69. Phillips RS, Wenger NS, Teno J, et al. Choices of seriously ill patients about cardiopulmonary resuscitation: correlates and outcomes. SUPPORT Investigators. Study to Understand Prognoses and Preferences for Outcomes and Risks of Treatments. *Am J Med* 1996;100:128–137.

70. Hofmann JC, Wenger NS, Davis RB, et al. Patient preferences for communication with physicians about end-of-life decisions. SUPPORT Investigators. Study to Understand Prognoses and Preference for Outcomes and Risks of Treatment. *Ann Intern Med* 1997;127:1–12.

71. Lynn J, Teno JM, Phillips RS, et al. Perceptions by family members of the dying experience of older and seriously ill patients. SUPPORT Investigators. Study to Understand Prognoses and Preferences for Outcomes and Risks of Treatment. *Ann Intern Med* 1997;126:97–106.

72. The SUPPORT Principal Investigators. A controlled trial to improve care for seriously ill hospitalized patients: the Study to Understand Prognoses and Preferences for Outcomes and Risks of Treatments (SUPPORT). *JAMA* 1995;274:1591–1598.

73. Blackhall LJ, Murphy ST, Frank G, et al. Ethnicity and attitudes toward patient autonomy. *JAMA* 1995;274:820–825.

74. Garrett JM, Harris RP, Norburn JK, et al. Life-sustaining treatments during terminal illness: who wants what? *J Gen Intern Med* 1993;8:361–368.

75. Kiely DK, Mitchell S, Marlow A, et al. Racial and state differences in the designation of advance directives in nursing home residents. *J Am Geriatr Soc* 2001;49(10):1346–1352.

76. Lahn M, Friedman B, Bijur P, et al. Advance directives in skilled nursing facility residents transferred to emergency departments. *Acad Emerg Med* 2001;8(12):1158–1162.

77. Federal Patient Self Determination Act 1990. 42 U.S.C. 1395 cc (a).

78. Arizona Living Wills and Health Care Directives Act, *Ariz Rev Stat Ann* ss36-3201 to 36-3287, 2000.

79. Vig EK, Taylor JS, Starks H, et al. Beyond substituted judgment: how surrogates navigate end-of-life decision-making. *J Am Geriatr Soc* 2006;54:1688–1693.

80. Becker LJ, Yeargin K, Rea TD, et al. Resuscitation of residents with do-not-resuscitate orders in long-term care facilities. *Prehosp Emerg Care* 2003;7:303–306.

81. Dull SM, Graves J, Larsen MP, et al. Expected death and unwanted resuscitation in the prehospital setting. *Ann Emerg Med* 1994;23(5):997–1002.

82. Guru V, Veerbeck VP, Morrison LJ. Response of paramedics to terminally ill patients with cardiac arrest: an ethical dilemma. *CMAJ* 1999;161(10):1251–1254.

83. Iserson KV. A simplified prehospital advance directive law: Arizona's approach. *Ann Emerg Med* 1993;22:11:1703–1710.

84. Iserson KV. If we don't learn from history . . . ethical failings in a new prehospital directive. *Am J Emerg Med* 1995;13:241.

85. Crimmins TJ. Prehospital do-not-resuscitate orders. In Iserson KV et al, eds. *Ethics in Emergency Medicine*, 2nd ed. Tucson, AZ: Galen Press, 1995.

86. Iserson KV. Foregoing prehospital care: should ambulance staff always resuscitate? *J Med Ethics* 1991;17:19.

87. Schears RM, Marco CA, Iserson KV. Do not attempt resuscitation" (DNAR) in the out-of-hospital setting. *Ann Emerg Med* 2004;44(1):68–70.

88. Schmidt TA, Hickman S, Tolle SW, et al. The Physician Orders for Life-Sustaining Treatment (POLST) program: Oregon emergency medical technicians' practical experiences and attitudes. *J Am Geriatr Soc* 2004;52:1–7.

89. Naess AC, Steen E, Steen PA. Ethics in treatment decisions during out-of-hospital resuscitation. *Resuscitation* 1997; 35:245–256.

90. American College of Emergency Physicians. *Ethical Issues for Resuscitation*. Policy #400133; approved 1992; reaffirmed 1997 and 2001.

91. Moselli NM, Debernardi F, Piovano F. Forgoing life sustaining treatments: differences and similarities between North America and Europe. *Acta Anaesthesiol Scand* 2006;50:1177–1186.

92. Sonnenblick M, Friedlander Y, Steinberg A. Dissociation between the wishes of terminally ill patients and decisions by their offspring, *J Am Geriatr Soc* 1993;41:599–604.

93. *In re Quinlan*, 70 NJ 10, 355 A2d 647, 1976, *cert denied*, 429 US 922, 1976.

94. *Cruzan v Director, Missouri Department of Health*, US 58 LW 4916, 1990.

95. *Rasmussen v Fleming*, 154 Ariz 207, 741 P2d 674, 1987.

96. *Superintendent of Belchertown v Saikewicz*, 373 Mass 728, 370 NE 2d 417, 1977.

97. Li LLM, Cheong KYP, Yaw LK, et al. The accuracy of surrogate decisions in intensive care scenarios. *Anaesth Intens Care* 2007;35:46–51.

98. Silveira MJ, DiPiero A, Gerrity MS, et al. Patients' knowledge of options at the end of life—ignorance in the face of death. *JAMA* 2000;284:2483–2488.

99. Doig C, Murray H, Bellomo R, et al. Ethics roundtable debate: patients and surrogates want "everything done"—what does "everything" mean? *Crit Care* 2006;10:231–238.

100. Meisel A. Rights of minors. In Iserson KV, Sanders AB, Mathieu D, eds. *Ethics in Emergency Medicine*, 2nd ed. Tucson, AZ: Galen Press, 1995:72–76.

101. Siegel M. Alone at life's end: trying to protect the autonomy of patients without surrogates or decision-making capacity. *Crit Care Med* 2006;34(8):2238–2239.

102. Danis M, Patrick DL, Southerland LI, et al. Patients' and families' preferences for medical intensive care. *JAMA* 1988;260:797–802.

103. Cook DJ, Guyatt GH, Jaeschke R, et al. Determinants in Canadian health care workers of the decision to withdraw life support from the critically ill. *JAMA* 1995;273:703–708.

104. Veatch RM. Assault or homicide: treating and letting die without consent. *Crit Care Med* 2002;30:937–938.

105. Iserson KV. Getting advance directives to the public: a role for emergency medicine. *Ann Emerg Med* 1991;20:692.

106. Iserson KV. Federal advance directives legislation: potential effects on emergency medicine. *J Emerg Med* 1991;9:67.

107. Lo B. DNR in the OR and afterwards. *AHRQ WebM&M*. September 2006. Available at: http://www.webmm .ahrq.gov/case.aspx?caseID=135. Accessed July 7, 2007.

108. Veterans Health Administration. May do-not-resuscitate (DNR) orders be suspended for surgery? *EthicsRX*. January 2005. Available at: www.ethics.va.gov/ETHICS/docs/rx/EthicsRx_20050101_Suspending_DNR_Orders_For_Surgery.pdf. Accessed July 7, 2007.

109. Craig DB. Do-not-resuscitate orders in the operating room. *Can J Anaesth* 1996;43:(8):840–851.

110. Iserson KV. Ethical considerations in emergency care. *Israeli J Emerg Med* 2004;4(2):8–15.

111. Culberson J, Levy C, Lawhorne L. Do-not-hospitalize orders in nursing homes: a pilot study. *J Am Med Dir Assoc* 2005;6(1):22–26.

112. Mitchell SL, Teno JM, Intrator O, et al. Decisions to forgo hospitalization in advanced dementia: a nationwide study. *J Am Geriatr Soc* 2007;55:432–438.

113. Levy CR, Fish R, Kramer A. Do-not-resuscitate and do-not-hospitalize directives of persons admitted to skilled nursing facilities under the Medicare benefit. *J Am Geriatr Soc* 2005;53(12):2060–2068.

114. *Vital Statistics of the U.S., Data Warehouse, NCHS*. http://www.cdc.gov/nchs/datawh.htm Accessed July 7, 2007.

115. Chugh SS, Jui J, Gunson K, Stecker EC, et al. Current burden of sudden cardiac death: multiple source surveillance versus retrospective death certificate–based review in a large U.S. community. *J Am Coll Cardiol* 2004;44:1268–1275.

116. Tolle SW, Tilden VP, Nelson CA, et al. A prospective study of the efficacy of the physician order form for life-sustaining treatment. *J Am Geriatr Soc* 1998;46:1097–1102.

117. Bossaert L. European Resuscitation Council guidelines for resuscitation. In *The Ethics of Resuscitation in Clinical Practice*. Amsterdam: Elsevier; 1998:206–217.

118. Casarett DJ, Stocking CB, Siegler M. Would physicians override a do-not-resuscitate order when a cardiac arrest is iatrogenic? *J Gen Intern Med* 1999;14:35–38.

119. Casarett DJ, Ross LF. Overriding a patient's refusal of treatment after an iatrogenic complication. *N Engl J Med* 1997;336(26):1908–1909.

120. American College of Surgeons. [ST-19] Statement on advance directives by patients: "do-not-resuscitate" in the operating room. *Bul Am Coll Surg* 1994;79(9):29.

121. American Society of Anesthesiologists. *Ethical Guidelines for the Anesthesia Care of Patients with Do-Not-Resuscitate Orders*. Available at: http://www.asahq.org/publicationsAndServices/standards/09.html. Accessed July 7, 2007.

122. Engel KG, Desmond JS, Brandt M, et al. Provider experience and attitudes towards family presence during resuscitation procedures. *Acad Emerg Med* 2005;12(5 Suppl. 2):81.

123. Emergency Nurses Association. Position statement. *Family Presence at the Bedside During Invasive Procedures and Resuscitation*. 2001. Available at: http://ena.org/about/position/PDFs/4E6C256B26994E319F66C65748BFBDBF.pdf Accessed July 7, 2007.

124. Ellison S. Nurses' attitudes toward family presence during resuscitative efforts and invasive procedures. *J Emerg Nurs* 2003;29:515–521.

125. Sacchetti A, Paston C, Carraccio C. Family members do not disrupt care when present during invasive procedures. *Acad Emerg Med* 2005;12:477–479.

126. Heckendorn JT, Chakel SS, Ubel PA, et al. Family presence during critical resuscitation in the emergency department: do patients and family members agree? *Acad Emerg Med* 2005;12(5 Suppl 2):81.

127. Eichhorn DJ, Meyers TA, Guzzett CE, et al. Family presence during invasive procedures and resuscitation: hearing the voice of the patient. *Am J Nurs* 2001;101(5):48–55.

128. Fein JA, Ganesh J, Alpern ER. Medical staff attitudes toward family presence during pediatric procedures. *Pediatr Emerg Care* 2004;20(4):224–227.

129. Marrone L, Fogg C. Family presence during resuscitation: are policies allowing family into the trauma room humane and necessary—or just asking for trouble? *Nursing* 2005;35(8 ED Insider Suppl):21–22.

130. Merlevede E, Spooren D, Henderick H, et al. Perceptions, needs and mourning reactions of bereaved relatives confronted with a sudden unexpected death. *Resuscitation* 2004;61:341–348.

131. Boie ET, Moore GO, Brummett C, et al. Do parents want to be present during invasive procedures performed on their children in the emergency department? A survey of 400 parents. *Ann Emerg Med* 1999;34:70–74.

132. Boyd R. Witnessed resuscitation by relatives. *Resuscitation* 2000;43:171–176.

133. Iserson KV. *Grave Words: Notifying Survivors About Sudden, Unexpected Deaths.* Tucson, AZ: Galen Press, 1999.

134. Beckman AW, Sloan BK, Moore GP, et al. Should parents be present during emergency department procedures on children, and who should make that decision? A survey of emergency physician and nurse attitudes. *Acad Emerg Med* 2002;9:154–158.

135. Robinson SM, Mackenzie Ross S, et al. Psychological effect of witnessed resuscitation on bereaved relatives. *Lancet* 1998;352:614–617.

136. Barratt F, Wallis DN. Relatives in the resuscitation room: their point of view. *J Accid Emerg Med* 1998;15:109–111.

137. Piira T, Sugiura T, Champion GD, et al. The role of parental presence in the context of children's medical procedures: A systematic review. *Child Care Health Dev* 2005;31:233–243.

138. Gold KJ, Gorenflo DW, Schwenk TL, et al. Physician experience with family presence during cardiopulmonary resuscitation in children. *Pediatr Crit Care Med* 2006;7(5): 428–433.

139. Henderson DP, Knapp JF. Report of the national consensus conference on family presence during pediatric cardiopulmonary resuscitation and procedures. *J Emerg Nurs* 2006;32(1):23–29.

140. Doyle CJ, Post H, Burney RE, et al. Family participation during resuscitation: an option. *Ann Emerg Med* 1987;16:673–675.

141. UK Resuscitation Council. Bereavement. In: *Resuscitation Council UK Advanced Life Support Course Manual.* 1998:London: Resuscitation Council.

142. Adams S, Whitlock M, Higgs R, et al. Should relatives be allowed to watch resuscitation? *BMJ* 1994;308:1687–1692.

143. Eichhorn DJ, Meyers TA, Mitchell TG, et al. Opening the doors: family presence during resuscitation. *J Cardiovasc Nurs* 1996; 10:59–70.

144. Cobb LA, Eliastam M, Kerber RE, et al. Report of the American Heart Association Task Force on the Future of Cardiopulmonary Resuscitation. *Circulation* 1992;85:2346–2355.

145. Iserson KV. Gravest words: notifying survivors about sudden, unexpected deaths. *Res Staff Physician* 2001;47(7):66–68;71–72.

146. MacLean SL, Guzzetta CE, White C, et al. Family presence during cardiopulmonary resuscitation and invasive procedures: practices of critical care and emergency nurses. *Am J Crit Care* 2003;12:246–257.

147. Meyers TA, Eichhorn DJ, Guzzetta CE, et al. Family presence during invasive procedures and resuscitation: the experiences of family members, nurses, and physicians. *Am J Nurs* 2000;100:32–42.

148. McClenathan BM, Torrington KG, Uyehara CF. Family member presence during cardiopulmonary resuscitation: a survey of US and international critical care professionals. *Chest* 2002;122:2204–2211.

149. Emergency Nurses Association. *Presenting the Option for Family Presence.* 2nd ed. Des Plaines, Ill: Emergency Nurses Association; 2001.

150. Eichhorn DJ, Meyers TA, Guzzetta CE, et al. Family presence during invasive procedures and CPR: when pigs fly. In Mason DJ, Leavitt JK, Chaffee MW, eds. *Policy and Politics in Nursing and Health Care,* 4th ed. Philadelphia: Saunders, 2002:345–361.

151. Mason DJ. Family presence: evidence versus tradition. *Am J Crit Care* 2003;12:190–192.

152. McGahey PR. Family presence during pediatric resuscitation: a focus on staff. *Crit Care Nurse* 2002;22(6):29–34.

153. Sacchetti A, Carraccio C, Leva E, et al. Acceptance of family member presence during pediatric resuscitation in the emergency department: effects of personal experience. *Pediatr Emerg Care* 2000;16:85–87.

154. Helmer SD, Smith RS, Dort JM, et al. Family presence during trauma resuscitation: a survey of AAST and ENA members. American Association for the Surgery of Trauma. Emergency Nurses Association. *J Trauma* 2000;48:1015–1024.

155. Iserson KV. Notifying survivors about sudden, unexpected deaths. *West J Med* 2000;173:261–265.

156. Silverman PR. Services to the widowed: first steps in a program of preventive intervention. *Comm Mental Health J* 1967;3: 38–44.

Part

Eleven

Education and Research

Chapter 38
Careers in Resuscitation Medicine

Benjamin S. Abella and Lance B. Becker

A wide variety of individuals are interested in saving lives following sudden cardiac death and cardiac arrest. There are exciting options for career paths, funding, and collaborative models that make resuscitation science a rich and intriguing arena in which to contribute. Translational medical research provides a bridge to more directly connect basic research and patient care. Resuscitation science centers have been established, empowering translational science to provide models for collaborative interdisciplinary teams. Rich and rewarding careers are possible.

- Translational and resuscitation science provide an interdisciplinary foundation for basic and clinical investigation.
- Bench-to-bedside training is available for those interested in careers in resuscitation science. A wide range of interdisciplinary portals and funding is available and emerging.
- Collaboration between academic investigators and industry partners has proven to be fruitful in advancing resuscitation science.

Introduction

The daunting challenge of improving survival from cardiac arrest will require the collective energies of a wide variety of clinical investigators, basic scientists, public health experts, educators, paramedics, nurses, and physicians. In addition, given the importance of mechanical and electronic devices in emergency cardiovascular care (defibrillators, mechanical chest compression devices, biosensors, etc.), there is an enormous opportunity for contribution from the bioengineering industry as well. Collaboration between academic investigators and industry partners has proven to be particularly fruitful in advancing resuscitation science, and such interaction will provide wide opportunities in coming years.

Translational Science and Resuscitation Care

Resuscitation science, with its wide-ranging areas of inquiry and involvement from the laboratory to the community, is in many ways the ideal model for translational investigation. As the National Institutes of Health (NIH) and other funding organizations focus their interest on projects with a translational scope, resuscitation scientists, emergency cardiovascular care (ECC) community educators, bioengineers, and others have an opportunity to collaborate in teams that can truly move science into the clinical arena and bring clinical phenomena back to the laboratory. A recent body of work exemplifies this notion: the investigation of chest compression only cardiopulmonary resuscitation (CPR). Work by a variety of research teams has studied CPR physiology in the animal laboratory and others have furthered this work in clinical observational trials.[1-4] This will require further translation into educational, training, and community assessment work in coming years. Further iterations will require a return to the laboratory to better understand the role of respiration and oxygenation in more specific cardiac arrest models.

A number of resuscitation science centers have been established with translational science breadth and may serve as models for others as they form collaborative teams. The Safar Center for Resuscitation Research in Pittsburgh, the Center for Resuscitation Science in Philadelphia, and the Emergency Resuscitation Center in Chicago serve as examples of such organizations. Each of these centers comprises resuscitation-focused scientists and clinicians that carry out investigations and programs in cellular laboratories, animal facilities, and clinical trials. Having such collaborations within the same organization will allow for more rapid progress and innovation and neatly fits the NIH vision of translational science.

Opportunities for New Directions: Translational Science

There has been a recent appreciation for the importance of translational research in the biosciences, and this will likely have an important influence on careers and funding as it relates to ECC. As described on the NIH "roadmap" Web site:

As a field of study, resuscitation science could serve as a prime example for translational research, with its broad focus from basic science to the bedside, and for resuscitation beyond the bedside into the community. The NIH has specifically created special funding for translational research via Clinical and Translational Science Awards (CTSAs) and additional funding mechanisms. But there are those who criticize translational research, citing a lack of mechanistic

To improve human health, scientific discoveries must be translated into practical applications. Such discoveries typically begin at "the bench" with basic research—in which scientists study disease at the molecular or cellular level—then they progress to the clinical level, or the patient's "bedside." Scientists are increasingly aware that the bench-to-bedside approach to translational research is really a two-way street. Basic scientists provide clinicians with new tools for use in patients and for assessment of their impact, and clinical researchers make novel observations about the nature and progression of disease that often stimulate basic investigation. (http://nihroadmap.nih.gov/clinicalresearch/overview-translational.asp Dec2007)

focus, questioning the quality of the science, and noting that most researchers are not even sure what defines the boundaries of translational research. A consideration of what translational research is, why it may represent a particularly important opportunity for resuscitation science, and describing some models for how translational research can be organized is presented in the following section.

What really is translational research? There is general agreement that translational research is still somewhat poorly defined. Wikipedia defines translational research as "a branch of medical research that attempts to more directly connect basic research to patient care" but goes on to say "and is a term whose precise definition is in flux."[5]

The importance of translational research is growing in the health care industry and the most common notion is that it deals with the advancement of basic science into actual therapies for patients. This is the "bench-to-bedside" definition and is most often used in referring to drug or device development. However, others use "translational research" to mean something quite different. They refer to the broader dissemination of a therapy into the population or community. This definition often encompasses notions about education and training of providers, knowledge translation to various audiences, dissemination of knowledge, patient-oriented research, and putting known therapies into more common practice in a broad community. The American Heart Association's program "Get With the Guidelines" is termed a translational project under this definition.[6]

Career Opportunities

There are a wide variety of careers that directly impact emergency cardiac care and contribute toward saving lives from cardiac arrest. These career options span a large range of both educational backgrounds as well as areas of focus, including both research and nonresearch endeavors.

Clinical Investigator

A daunting number of clinical questions exist in our scientific knowledge of resuscitation and emergency cardiac care. Such questions will require a cadre of clinical scholars who practice medicine as well as conduct clinical trials and other human subject investigations. Questions that require further elaboration include the development and testing of novel drugs for ACLS and postarrest care, many of which have already been evaluated with promising results in the animal laboratory[7,8]; the further investigation of postarrest care and development of postarrest care pathways[9,10]; the implementation of different methods of CPR and defibrillation[4,11,12]; the evaluation of new CPR teaching and measurement techniques[3–15]; and the epidemiologic study of cardiac care processes and disease burden.[16–18] A number of other broad questions exist for aspiring clinical investigators, in such clinical fields as both adult and pediatric emergency medicine, cardiology, critical care, anesthesiology, epidemiology, general internal medicine, and cardiac surgery. Clinical investigators with medical and/or nursing backgrounds will both be required in these endeavors. In addition, EMS physicians, paramedics, and other field responders will be invaluable participants in clinical research processes and should be encouraged to consider study of ECC.

Basic Science Investigator

The realm of basic science investigation of cardiac arrest, ischemia–reperfusion, and the modeling of emergency cardiac conditions is in great need of further scholarship in numerous specific areas, including understanding the mechanisms of ischemia–reperfusion injury at the levels of the cell and subcellular organelles[19–23]; the modeling and understanding of ventricular fibrillation in isolated heart and heart tissues as well as computer models[24,25]; the evaluation of stem cell technology to improve repair and recovery from organ injury after ischemia–reperfusion[26,27]; the study of hormonal and neurologic influence on cardiac arrest and tissue response[28,29]; the physiology of CPR/CPR quality; and the impact of potential new therapeutic agents.[30,31] This list is by no means exhaustive, and investigators with both clinical and laboratory research background will be required to further develop these fields of inquiry. Expertise will be required from such domains as molecular biology, cellular physiology, bioengineering, veterinary critical care, computational biology, and neuroscience, to name just a few.

Public Health Education and Advocacy

At the level of policy development and public education, there is an enormous contribution to be made by those with a diverse set of educational and training backgrounds, including those with master's degrees in public policy or public health, advanced training in communications, public relations, government, and economics, to name just a few. Involvement in the legislative and public educational spheres will be critical to improve and broaden CPR education,[32] strengthen public access defibrillation programs,[33,34] and engender governmental support for such lifesaving programs. A formidable amount of work also exists to improve public education and legislative support to reduce risk factors for cardiac emergencies in the community, such as smoking cessation, hypertension screening and treatment,

and diabetes management. Positions for such careers exist not just in academia and government bodies, but also in the nonprofit organization sphere, including organizations such as the American Heart Association, the American Red Cross, and other public health–minded groups. Such organizations require individuals with research backgrounds as well as training in communications, marketing, and government affairs.

Bioengineering and Industry Careers

There are a wide array of careers available in ECC that reside within industry, and thus afford opportunities for those individuals trained in electrical, mechanical, or computer engineering, or marketing and business administration. ECC is dependent on high-quality industrial partners, and a number of corporate entities maintain important involvement in resuscitation device design, including monitors, defibrillators, and mechanical chest compression tools, drug development, as well as computer algorithms for data evaluation and processing for research and educational purposes. Exciting new frontiers in resuscitation care will include the development of better monitoring and sensors for assessment of physiology during and after arrest as well as optimization of treatment technology such as hypothermia equipment and telemedicine communication systems.

Funding Opportunities

Investigators in resuscitation science have historically received funding from a variety of sources, including federal and nonprofit agencies. The qualities of these funding entities and the nature of their funding programs are detailed below. This list is by no means exhaustive but reflects the collective experience of ECC professionals with regards to recent successful funding for research or other resuscitation-related projects.

Governmental Organizations

National Institutes of Health

The NIH has served as a major source of funding for biomedical research in the United States. Decisions regarding funds allocation are made by the 27 institutes and centers that make up the NIH (e.g., National Institute for Mental Health [NIMH], National Institute for Allergy and Infectious Diseases [NIAID], etc.). While the review process for NIH grants has some complexities and exceptions in unusual circumstances, grants are typically reviewed by a group of "peer" scientists through the Center for Scientific Review (CSR—termed a "study section"), which is an independent agency that serves primarily to rate each grant for scientific merit. This review process generates a "priority score" for each application as well as a narrative scientific critique. Following review of a grant by CSR, each individual agency will fund the highest-scored applications that are appropriate to the agencies' areas of interest and research. Funding applications for resuscitation science have historically been directed toward the National Heart Lung and Blood Institute (NHLBI), although other institutes might be considered, depending on specific research proposals. For example, a proposal that seeks to evaluate cardiac arrest treatment in the elderly could theoretically be directed to the National Institute of Aging (NIA). The success of a funding application depends in part on the "fit" between the described project and the goals and priorities of any given specific institute. Program officers within each institute can be consulted regarding the suitability of any given proposal. In general, to be successfully funded, most grants to the NIH must be clearly "hypothesis-driven," with a testable research question. Unless specifically described in a particular grant offering, the NIH generally does not fund educational or advocacy projects that do not have such hypotheses.

Agency for Health Research and Quality

This agency resides within the Department of Health and Human Services but is separate from the NIH structures described above. Certain resuscitation science proposals might be suitable for application to AHRQ, such as studies of health-care disparities or processes of care on a population level. AHRQ also provides competitive funding for small conferences and educational initiatives. Generally speaking, AHRQ does not fund laboratory-based projects, nor is it the optimal source for clinical trial funding.

Military Funding

Resuscitation science, involving the clinical goal of rapid care of acutely ill patients, has a number of clearly important links to the interests of military funding groups such as the Defense Advanced Research Projects Agency (DARPA), and military branch funding sources such as the Office of Naval Research (ONR) or the Army Research Office (ARO). Resuscitation from traumatic arrest and physiologic monitoring of the acutely ill serve as important starting points of interest for these agencies, and a number of resuscitation scientists have been successfully funded through their mechanisms for projects that span both clinical and laboratory investigations.

Nongovernmental Organizations

American Heart Association (AHA)

The sponsor of the U.S. version of international resuscitation guidelines for basic life support, advanced cardiac life support, and other emergency care protocols, the AHA has historically been a strong supporter of research into ECC and resuscitation science. AHA sponsors a number of funding opportunities through both the national organization and via regional chapters known as "affiliates." AHA also provides a large variety of opportunities for investigators (both young and senior) to become involved in education and policy surrounding resuscitation science through the Council for Cardiopulmonary Perioperative and Critical Care (CPCC) and the Emergency Cardiovascular Care (ECC) Committee. The AHA is also a sponsor of the annual Resuscitation Science Symposium (ReSS), held in conjunction with the American Heart Association Scientific Sessions.

Society for Academic Emergency Medicine

This society, composed of emergency medicine (EM) physicians, supports several young investigator, medical student, and resident grant opportunities in partnership with the affiliated Emergency Research Foundation (EMF). While generally preferring to support EM physicians, collaborations with non-EM personnel have been successfully funded as well.

American Thoracic Society

As the professional society of pulmonary/critical care physicians, this group supports a small grants portfolio that has historically focused on focused aspects of pulmonary/critical care medicine, earmarked for such topics as asthma, cystic fibrosis, etc. Unrestricted grants are also available and potentially might be considered for ECC-related projects championed by a pulmonary/critical care physician.

American Association of Critical Care Nurses (AACN)

This organization represents critical care nurses and nursing educators in a wide variety of disciplines, including cardiology, pulmonary medicine, medical and surgical critical care, and palliative care. AACN offers a variety of small grants annually, and ECC topics are specifically encouraged for several of these offerings. In addition, the grants portfolio encourages applications in quality of care and technology application to critical care nursing, which could certainly apply to resuscitation science.

Society for Critical Care Medicine

With a membership comprising medical intensivists, anesthesiologists, and surgical critical care specialists, this organization sponsors several grant opportunities annually that are available to the wide range of specialties represented.

Robert Wood Johnson (RWJ) Foundation

With a focus on health services and clinical research, RWJ sponsors a number of fellowship training programs nationally as well as hosting a variety of grant offerings. While fellowships and some grants are funding solely through the select institutions with established RWJ programs, other grant opportunities exist for applicants at other centers. Resuscitation topics that address health care costs, disparities, and systems of care may be appropriate for RWJ consideration.

Summary

For the wide variety of individuals who are interested in saving lives from cardiac arrest, there are exciting options for career paths, funding, and collaborative models that make resuscitation science a rich and intriguing arena in which to contribute. Given the enormous challenge to increase survival from such a deadly disease process, the ECC community will require the collective strengths of many to harness scientific advances and make them a reality for patients and the communities in which they live.

References

1. Dorph E, Wik L, Stromme TA, Eriksen M, et al. Oxygen delivery and return of spontaneous circulation with ventilation:compression ratio 2:30 versus chest compressions only CPR in pigs. *Resuscitation* 2004;60(3):309–318.

2. Berg RA, Kern KB, Sanders AB, et al. Bystander cardiopulmonary resuscitation. Is ventilation necessary? *Circulation* 1993;88(4 Pt 1): 1907–1915.

3. Berg RA, Sanders AB, Kern KB, et al. Adverse hemodynamic effects of interrupting chest compressions for rescue breathing during cardiopulmonary resuscitation for ventricular fibrillation cardiac arrest. *Circulation* 2001;104(20):2465–2470.

4. Cardiopulmonary resuscitation by bystanders with chest compression only (SOS-KANTO): an observational study. *Lancet* 2007;369 (9565):920–926.

5. *http://en.wikipedia.org/wiki/Translational_research*, accessed Dec 2, 2007.

6. Smaha LA. The American Heart Association Get With The Guidelines program. *Am Heart J* 2004;148(5 Suppl):S46–S48.

7. Gazmuri RJ, Ayoub IM, Hoffner E, et al. Successful ventricular defibrillation by the selective sodium–hydrogen exchanger isoform-1 inhibitor cariporide. *Circulation* 2001;104(2):234–239.

8. Huang L, Weil MH, Sun S, et al. Levosimendan improves postresuscitation outcomes in a rat model of CPR. *J Lab Clin Med* 2005;146(5):256–261.

9. Sunde K, Pytte M, Jacobsen D, et al. Implementation of a standardised treatment protocol for post resuscitation care after out-of-hospital cardiac arrest. *Resuscitation* 2007;73(1):29–39.

10. Oddo M, Schaller MD, Feihl F, et al. From evidence to clinical practice: effective implementation of therapeutic hypothermia to improve patient outcome after cardiac arrest. *Crit Care Med* 2006; 34(7):1865–1873.

11. Ong ME, Ornato JP, Edwards DP, et al. Use of an automated, load-distributing band chest compression device for out-of-hospital cardiac arrest resuscitation. *JAMA* 2006;295(22):2629–2637.

12. Kudenchuk PJ, Cobb LA, Copass MK, et al. Transthoracic incremental monophasic versus biphasic defibrillation by emergency responders (TIMBER): a randomized comparison of monophasic with biphasic ascending energy defibrillation for the resuscitation of out-of-hospital cardiac arrest due to ventricular fibrillation. *Circulation* 2006;114(19):2010–2018.

13. Wayne DB, Butter J, Siddall VJ, et al. Mastery learning of advanced cardiac life support skills by internal medicine residents using simulation technology and deliberate practice. *J Gen Intern Med* 2006;21(3):251–256.

14. Abella BS, Edelson DP, Kim S, et al. CPR quality improvement during in-hospital cardiac arrest using a real-time audiovisual feedback system. *Resuscitation* 2007;73(1):54–61.

15. Kramer-Johansen J, Edelson DP, Losert H, et al. Uniform reporting of measured quality of cardiopulmonary resuscitation (CPR). *Resuscitation* 2007;74(3):406–417.

16. Herlitz J, Svensson L, Engdahl J, et al. Characteristics of cardiac arrest and resuscitation by age group: an analysis from the Swedish Cardiac Arrest Registry. *Am J Emerg Med* 2007;25(9): 1025–1031.

17. Herlitz J, Engdahl J, Svensson L, et al. Is female sex associated with increased survival after out-of-hospital cardiac arrest? *Resuscitation* 2004;60(2):197–203.

18. Nichol G, Valenzuela T, Roe D, et al. Cost effectiveness of defibrillation by targeted responders in public settings. *Circulation* 2003;108(6):697–703.

19. Vanden Hoek TL, Li C, Shao Z, et al. Significant levels of oxidants are generated by isolated cardiomyocytes during ischemia prior to reperfusion. *J Mol Cell Cardiol* 1997;29:2571–2583.

20. Böttiger B, Teschendorf P, Krumnikl J, et al. Global cerebral ischemia due to cardiocirculatory arrest in mice causes neuronal degeneration and early induction of transcription factor genes in the hippocampus. *Mol Brain Res* 1999;65:135–142.

21. An J, Bosnjak ZJ, Jiang MT. Myocardial protection by isoflurane preconditioning preserves Ca^{2+} cycling proteins independent of sarcolemmal and mitochondrial KATP channels. *Anesth Analg* 2007;105(5):1207–1213, table of contents.

22. Giacomo CG, Antonio M. Melatonin in cardiac ischemia/reperfusion-induced mitochondrial adaptive changes. *Cardiovasc Hematol Disord Drug Targets* 2007;7(3):163–169.

23. Miyamoto S, Murphy AN, Brown JH. Akt mediates mitochondrial protection in cardiomyocytes through phosphorylation of mitochondrial hexokinase-II. *Cell Death Differ* 2008;15(3):521–529.

24. Abildskov JA. Additions to the wavelet hypothesis of cardiac fibrillation. *J Cardiovasc Electrophysiol* 1994;5(6):553–559.

25. Bernus O, Van Eyck B, Verschelde H, et al. Transition from ventricular fibrillation to ventricular tachycardia: a simulation study on the role of $Ca(2+)$-channel blockers in human ventricular tissue. *Phys Med Biol* 2002;47(23):4167–4179.

26. Kocher AA, Schlechta B, Gasparovicova A, Wolner E, Bonaros N, Laufer G. Stem cells and cardiac regeneration. *Transpl Int* 2007;20(9):731–746.

27. Gu Y, Yu J, Lum LG, Lee RJ. Tissue engineering and stem cell therapy for myocardial repair. *Front Biosci* 2007;12:5157–5165.

28. Little RA, Frayn KN, Randall PE, et al. Plasma catecholamines in the acute phase of the response to myocardial infarction. *Arch Emerg Med* 1986;3(1):20–27.

29. Kuhar P, Lunder M, Drevensek G. The role of gender and sex hormones in ischemic-reperfusion injury in isolated rat hearts. *Eur J Pharmacol* 2007;561(1–3):151–159.

30. Trevino RP, Bisera J, Weil MH, et al. End-tidal CO_2 as a guide to successful cardiopulmonary resuscitation: a preliminary report. *Crit Care Med* 1985;13(11):910–911.

31. Garnett AR, Ornato JP, Gonzalez ER, Johnson EB. End-tidal carbon dioxide monitoring during cardiopulmonary resuscitation. *JAMA.* 1987;257(4):512–515.

32. Lynch B, Einspruch EL, Nichol G, et al. Effectiveness of a 30-min CPR self-instruction program for lay responders: a controlled randomized study. *Resuscitation* 2005;67(1):31–43.

33. Ornato JP, Hankins DG. Public-access defibrillation. *Prehosp Emerg Care* 1999;3(4):297–302.

34. Riegel B, Mosesso VN, Birnbaum A, et al. Stress reactions and perceived difficulties of lay responders to a medical emergency. *Resuscitation* 2006;70(1):98–106.

Index

Page numbers followed by *f* indicate figures; those followed by *t* indicate tables.